Canine and Feline Anesthesia and Co-Existing Disease

Canine and Feline Anesthesia and Co-Existing Disease

Second Edition

Edited by

Rebecca A. Johnson, DVM, MS, PhD, DACVAA
Department of Surgical Sciences
School of Veterinary Medicine
University of Wisconsin–Madison
Madison, WI, USA

Lindsey B. C. Snyder, DVM, MS, DACVAA, CVA
Department of Surgical Sciences
School of Veterinary Medicine
University of Wisconsin–Madison
Madison, WI, USA

Carrie A. Schroeder, DVM, DACVAA
Department of Surgical Sciences
School of Veterinary Medicine
University of Wisconsin–Madison
Madison, WI, USA

WILEY Blackwell

This second edition first published 2022

Edition History
John Wiley & Sons, Inc. (1e, 2015)

Registered Offices
John Wiley & Sons, Inc., 111 River Street, Hoboken, NJ 07030, USA
John Wiley & Sons Ltd, The Atrium, Southern Gate, Chichester, West Sussex, PO19 8SQ, UK

Editorial Office
111 River Street, Hoboken, NJ 07030, USA

For details of our global editorial offices, customer services, and more information about Wiley products visit us at www.wiley.com.

Wiley also publishes its books in a variety of electronic formats and by print-on-demand. Some content that appears in standard print versions of this book may not be available in other formats.

Library of Congress Cataloging-in-Publication Data

Names: Johnson, Rebecca A. (Professor of anesthesia and pain management) editor. | Snyder, Lindsey B. C., editor. | Schroeder, Carrie A., editor.
Title: Canine and feline anesthesia and co-existing disease / edited by Rebecca A. Johnson, Lindsey Beth Culp Snyder, Carrie A. Schroeder.
Description: Second edition. | Hoboken, NJ : Wiley-Blackwell, 2022. | Includes bibliographical references and index.
Identifiers: LCCN 2021024496 (print) | LCCN 2021024497 (ebook) | ISBN 9781119604044 (hardback) | ISBN 9781119604051 (adobe pdf) | ISBN 9781119604068 (epub)
Subjects: MESH: Anesthesia–veterinary | Dog Diseases–surgery | Cat Diseases–surgery | Comorbidity
Classification: LCC SF914 (print) | LCC SF914 (ebook) | NLM SF 914 | DDC 636.089/796--dc23
LC record available at https://lccn.loc.gov/2021024496
LC ebook record available at https://lccn.loc.gov/2021024497

Cover Design: Wiley
Cover Images: © Carrie A. Schroeder, Rebecca A. Johnson

Set in 9.5/12.5pt STIXTwoText by Straive, Pondicherry, India

Printed in Singapore

M WEP355083 040425

This book is dedicated to our four-legged and two-legged families that inspired us personally and professionally to be the best teachers, researchers, veterinarians, partners, and mothers that we can be.

Contents

Preface

Since 1983, textbooks concerning anesthetic techniques and protocols associated with specific disease states have been published for humans (*Stoelting's Anesthesia and Co-Existing Disease*, first edition—currently on its eighth edition). Our veterinary patients are living longer lives and, thus, are experiencing increasingly complex, co-existing disease as well. *Canine and Feline Anesthesia and Co-Existing Disease* was published to discuss the most current concepts in the fields of veterinary anesthesia and analgesia, especially with regard to patients with co-existing disease. The second edition updates and expands upon these concepts, discussing clinically applicable concepts used in private practices and teaching institutions alike. Further, chapters addressing important emerging information (i.e., urogenital, genetic, and nociceptive diseases) have been added, along with a section concerning cardiopulmonary resuscitation.

Knowledge concerning veterinary anesthesia and analgesia is greatly expanding and continually developing as the breadth and depth of our profession is evolving with the emergence of species- and disease-specific research; this textbook is expanding accordingly. It not only provides foundational information for veterinary professionals to build upon (along with their own individual experiences and knowledge), but also details the most current anesthesia concepts necessary to manage each veterinary case safely and successfully.

List of Contributors

Turi K. Aarnes, DVM, MSc, DACVAA
Department of Veterinary Clinical Sciences
College of Veterinary Medicine
The Ohio State University
Columbus, OH, 43210, USA

Daniel Almeida, MedVet, MS, DACVAA
Veterinary Clinical Sciences Department
College of Veterinary Medicine
University of Minnesota
St. Paul, MN, 55108, USA

Benjamin Brainard, VMD, DACVAA, DACVECC
Department of Small Animal Medicine
& Surgery
College of Veterinary Medicine
University of Georgia
Athens, GA, 30602, USA

David B. Brunson, DVM, MS, DACVAA
Department of Surgical Sciences
School of Veterinary Medicine
University of Wisconsin–Madison
Madison, WI, 53706, USA

Andrew Claude, DVM, DACVAA, cVMA
Department of Small Animal Clinical Sciences
College of Veterinary Medicine
Michigan State University
East Lansing, MI, 48824, USA

Jonathan M. Congdon, DVM, MS, DACVAA
Veterinary Health & Wellness Center
College of Veterinary Medicine
North Carolina State University
Raleigh, NC, 27607, USA

Anderson Fávaro da Cunha, DVM, MS, DACVAA
Department of Specialty Medicine
College of Veterinary Medicine
Midwestern University
Glendale, AZ, 85308, USA

Carrie A. Davis, DVM, DACVAA
Animal Imaging
Irving, TX, 75039, USA

Thomas K. Day, DVM, MS, DACVAA, DACVECC, CVA
VCA Veterinary Emergency Service and
Specialty Center
Middleton, WI, 53562, USA

Berit L. Fischer, DVM, DACVAA, CCRP
Crown Veterinary Specialists
Lebanon, NJ, 08833, USA

Rebecca A. Johnson, DVM, MS, PhD, DACVAA
Department of Surgical Sciences
School of Veterinary Medicine
University of Wisconsin–Madison
Madison, WI, 53706, USA

Carolyn L. Kerr, DVM, DVSc, PhD, DACVAA
Department of Clinical Studies
Ontario Veterinary College
Guelph, Ontario, N1H 2W1, Canada

Philip Lerche, BVSc, PhD, DACVAA
Department of Veterinary Clinical Sciences
College of Veterinary Medicine
The Ohio State University
Columbus, OH, 43210, USA

Melissa A. Murdock, BVM&S, MS, DACVAA
BluePearl Specialty and Emergency
Pet Hospital
Levittown, PA, 19056, USA

Juliana Peboni Figueiredo, MV, MS, DACVAA
VCA West Coast Specialty and Emergency
Animal Hospital
Fountain Valley, Orange County,
CA, 92708, USA

Tania Perez Jimenez, DVM, MS, PhD, DACVAA
Veterinary Clinical Sciences
College of Veterinary Medicine
Program in Individualized Medicine (PrIMe)
Washington State University
Pullman, WA, 99164, USA

Verónica Salazar, LV, MSc, PhD, DACVAA
School of Veterinary Medicine
Universidad Alfonso X El Sabio
Madrid, 28691, Spain

Jusmeen Sarkar, DVM, MS, DACVAA
Anesthesia and Pain Management Service
Veterinary Specialty Center
Buffalo Grove, IL, 60089, USA

Carrie A. Schroeder, DVM, DACVAA
Department of Surgical Sciences
School of Veterinary Medicine
University of Wisconsin–Madison
Madison, WI, 53706, USA

Molly Shepard, DVM, DACVAA, cVMA
MedVet Medical and Cancer Center for Pets
3305 N California Ave
Chicago, IL, 60618, USA

Andre Shih, DVM, DACVAA
Department of Large Animal Clinical
Sciences
University of Florida
Gainesville, FL, 32608, USA
Capital Veterinary Specialists
Jacksonville, FL, 32609, USA

Bradley T. Simon, DVM, MSc, DACVAA
Department of Small Animal
Clinical Sciences
College of Veterinary Medicine and
Biomedical Science
Texas A&M University
College Station, TX, 77843,
USA

Christopher J. Snyder, DVM, DAVDC
Department of Surgical Sciences
School of Veterinary Medicine
University of Wisconsin–Madison
Madison, WI, 53706,
USA

Lindsey B. C. Snyder, DVM, MS, DACVAA, CVA
Department of Surgical Sciences
School of Veterinary Medicine
University of Wisconsin–Madison
Madison, WI, 53706,
USA

Jason W. Soukup, DVM, DAVDC
Department of Surgical Sciences
School of Veterinary Medicine
University of Wisconsin–Madison
Madison, WI, 53706,
USA

Paulo V. M. Steagall, MV, MS, PhD, DACVAA
Faculté de Médecine Vétérinaire
Université de Montréal
Saint-Hyacinthe, Québec, J2S 2M2, Canada

Erin Wendt-Hornickle, DVM, DACVAA, CVA
Veterinary Clinical Sciences Department
College of Veterinary Medicine
University of Minnesota
St. Paul, MN, 55108, USA

About the Companion Website

The book is accompanied by a website:

www.wiley.com/go/johnson/canine

The website features:

- Videos

1

Cardiovascular Disease

Jonathan M. Congdon

Veterinary Health & Wellness Center, College of Veterinary Medicine, North Carolina State University, Raleigh, NC, 27607, USA

Introduction

The most critical function of the cardiovascular system is to circulate blood continuously, ensuring adequate oxygen delivery and survival of cells and tissues. The body can survive food and water deprivation far longer than it can survive oxygen deprivation and lack of perfusion; absence of oxygen delivery can trigger the complicated cascade that leads to temporary, permanent, or irreversible cell death [1]. As such, the simplest definition of cardiovascular disease is the decreased ability of this system to ensure adequate oxygen delivery for day-to-day survival.

Nearly all anesthetic drugs compromise cardiovascular function via a single or multiple mechanism(s) and can severely compromise oxygen delivery in patients with underlying cardiac disease [2]. Cardiovascular goals during anesthesia target maintenance of oxygen delivery and homeostasis when using drugs that knowingly disturb the system. However, this goal becomes complicated in patients with underlying cardiovascular disease and increasingly more difficult when severe pathology is present. In patients with significant cardiovascular disease, the optimization of oxygen delivery requires a complete understanding of the mechanisms underlying the pathology, as well as the anesthetic drugs, patient support, and monitoring tools available. The most difficult challenge when faced with these patients is how to balance the pathophysiology of disease against the effects of anesthetic drugs and to subsequently individualize an anesthetic plan that minimizes cardiovascular compromise.

It is difficult to predict all possible combinations of patient signalment and temperament, cardiovascular and comorbid conditions, clinicopathologic abnormalities, surgical procedures, and their effects on anesthetic drug choices. Thus, studies have tended to focus more on describing the specific cardiac disease or cardiac effects of specific anesthetics and less on their combinations. This approach leaves the difficult task of knowing how to choose the appropriate anesthetic plan for an individual patient. The goal of this chapter is to provide an overview of cardiovascular physiology and pathophysiology, anesthetic agents, and cardiovascular patient evaluation, monitoring, and support during anesthesia to help the clinician prepare anesthetic plans for patients with mild to significant cardiovascular disease.

Canine and Feline Anesthesia and Co-Existing Disease, Second Edition. Edited by Rebecca A. Johnson, Lindsey B. C. Snyder and Carrie A. Schroeder.

Companion website: www.wiley.com/go/johnson/canine

Cardiovascular Physiology

Tissue Perfusion and Oxygen Delivery

The mathematical definition of oxygen delivery (DO_2) is the product of oxygen content (CaO_2, ml O_2 dl^{-1} blood) and cardiac output (CO, l min^{-1}; Figure 1.1) [3]. Perfusion and the ability to deliver oxygen suffer either if the ability of the heart to eject blood (CO) is compromised or if the ability of the blood to carry oxygen (CaO_2) is reduced. Although decreases in CaO_2 significantly affect tissue oxygenation, the focus of this chapter is on treating reductions in CO associated with cardiac disease.

Blood Pressure and Cardiac Output

It is critical to monitor blood pressure (BP) during anesthesia as it is our best, yet indirect, indicator of perfusion in veterinary medicine [4]. BP helps determine how anesthesia affects the patients' ability to perfuse their tissues and, as such, is used as a tool to treat perfusion abnormalities. However, BP is not a component of the mathematical definition of oxygen delivery: $DO_2 = CO \times CaO_2$. It is useful to assess BP to indirectly estimate changes in CO, as CO is rarely measured clinically in nonresearch patients.

Systolic arterial pressure (SAP) is the peak pressure measured in the artery or arteriole during one cardiac cycle, and is determined by several variables, including stroke volume (SV, volume ejected during one ventricular contraction), velocity of left ventricular ejection, arterial resistance, and blood viscosity [5]. Diastolic arterial pressure (DAP) is the lowest arterial pressure measured during the cycle, and is affected by blood viscosity, arterial compliance, and cardiac cycle length [5]. Mean arterial pressure (MAP) is not the arithmetic mean pressure in the vessel and is always a calculated number. Various formulae exist to calculate MAP such as:

$$MAP = DAP + 1/3\,(SAP - DAP) \text{ or}$$
$$MAP = (SAP + [2 \times DAP])/3.$$

Regarding perfusion, the most important of these values is MAP, as the total amount of time during the cardiac cycle (or during any one individual pulse) spent at SAP is very short, whereas the time spent at MAP is much longer (Figure 1.2) [6].

Mean Arterial Pressure and Autoregulation

Autoregulation is the automatic adjustment of blood flow through a tissue regardless of the MAP driving blood through the tissue (Figure 1.3). In other words, autoregulation is the unconscious adjustment of arterial and arteriolar smooth muscle tone to maintain a constant blood flow through a tissue across a wide range of pressures. Classically, this is thought to occur between a MAP of approximately 60–160 mmHg, and is due to adaptive metabolic, myogenic, and neurogenic feedback mechanisms. Outside of this interval, tissue or organ blood flow is substantially altered, potentially resulting in reduced or nonuniform perfusion patterns [7, 8].

Hypotension

MAPs <60 mmHg (or SAPs <90 mmHg) have historically been considered the minimum recommended pressures in small animals associated with adequate tissue oxygen delivery [9].

Oxygen Delivery	=	**Cardiac Output**	×	**Oxygen Content**
DO_2, mL min^{-1}		CO, L min^{-1}		CaO_2, mL dL^{-1} blood

Figure 1.1 Determinants of oxygen delivery. Oxygen delivery (ml min^{-1}) is the mathematical product of cardiac output (l blood min^{-1}) and oxygen content (ml dl^{-1} blood).

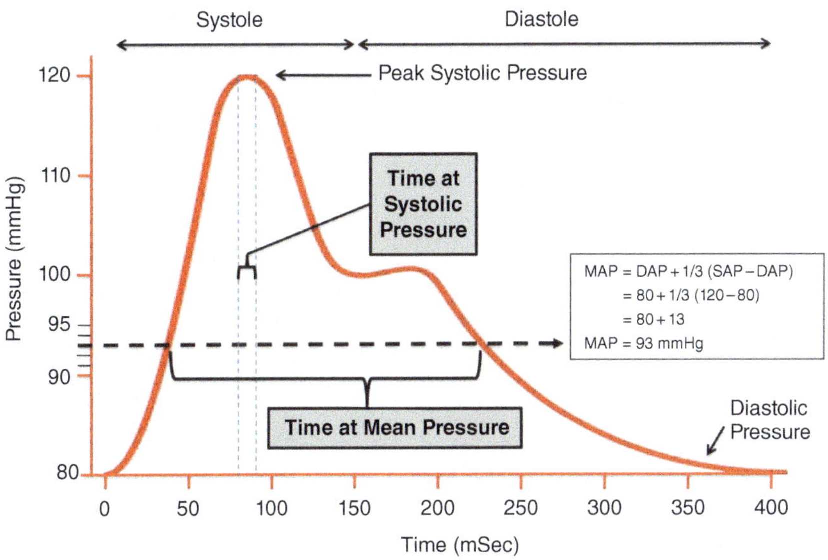

Figure 1.2 Arterial pulse pressure waveform. Mean arterial pressure (MAP) is 1/3 of the difference between systolic arterial pressure (SAP) added to the diastolic arterial pressure (DAP). MAP is considered the pressure of perfusion, as more time in the cardiac cycle is spent closer to MAP as compared to SAP. Total cycle length is 400 ms for illustration and is determined by the heart rate and other cardiovascular variables.

Figure 1.3 Between MAP of approximately 60 and 160 mmHg, blood flow through a tissue capillary bed is maintained at a relatively constant flow by autoregulatory mechanisms. At MAP lower than approximately 60 mmHg and greater than approximately 160 mmHg, autoregulation of blood pressure is lost and blood flow through capillary beds becomes pressure-dependent; tissues are either underperfused or overperfused, respectively.

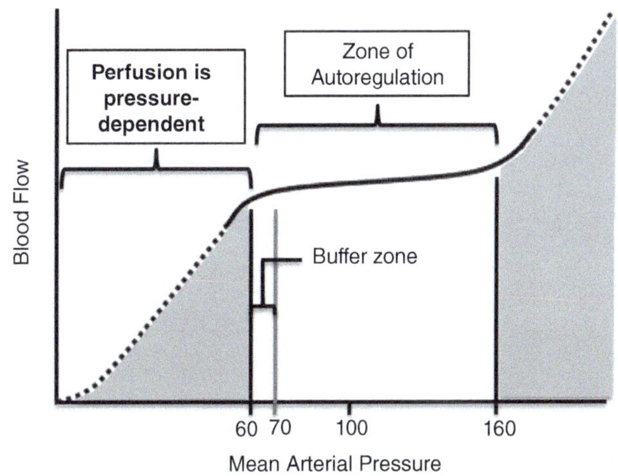

However, a MAP of approximately 60 mmHg may not actually reflect adequate perfusion for several reasons. First, studies investigating autoregulation are routinely performed in non-anesthetized patients [10]. Neurogenic mechanisms for autoregulation depend on sympathetic nervous system (SNS) input. Anesthetic agents depress both the conscious and unconscious (autonomic) nervous systems. Since SNS tone is substantially reduced during anesthesia, autoregulatory mechanisms are unavoidably depressed, either partially or completely, and autoregulation is impaired. Second, if a MAP of approximately 60 mmHg is considered the minimum acceptable BP but the patient is not yet considered to be truly hypotensive, then treatments may be delayed until the patient is in a state wherein oxygen delivery is pressure-dependent (i.e., to the left of the autoregulatory curve). As all hypotensive therapies are not instantaneously acting, there is concern that the patient may become increasingly hypotensive before treatments are efficacious. Thus, a MAP of approximately 70 mmHg (or SAP of approximately 90 mmHg) should be considered the minimum acceptable BP to build in a buffer zone so that treatments for hypotension can be applied and take effect before tissue perfusion is severely compromised, considering both altered autoregulatory mechanisms and the time-dependent treatment effects.

Relationship Between Mean Arterial Pressure and Cardiac Output

When considering the relationship of measured BP to the definition of oxygen delivery, one must understand the components that derive a measured BP [4]. MAP is the product of CO ($l\,min^{-1}$) and systemic vascular resistance (SVR) (dynes $s^{-1}\,cm^{-5}$). SVR is considered the degree of vasodilation (which reduces SVR) or vasoconstriction (which increases SVR) present in the systemic circulation. CO is the product of heart rate (HR, beats min^{-1}) and SV (ml ejected per heartbeat). SV is determined by preload (the venous return during diastole preloading the ventricle before contraction/ejection), afterload (the resistance that ventricular contraction must overcome in order to eject blood), and contractility (the force of contraction of ventricular muscle, independent of preload and afterload; Figure 1.4).

Increases in SVR, SV, preload, and contractility tend to increase BP, whereas increases in afterload tend to decrease SV, CO, and MAP. As MAP is a mathematical product, one cannot definitively determine if a decrease or increase in MAP is due to a decrease or increase in CO or SVR, as CO and SVR are not routinely measured in clinical patients. Choosing which mechanism for hypotension or hypertension is

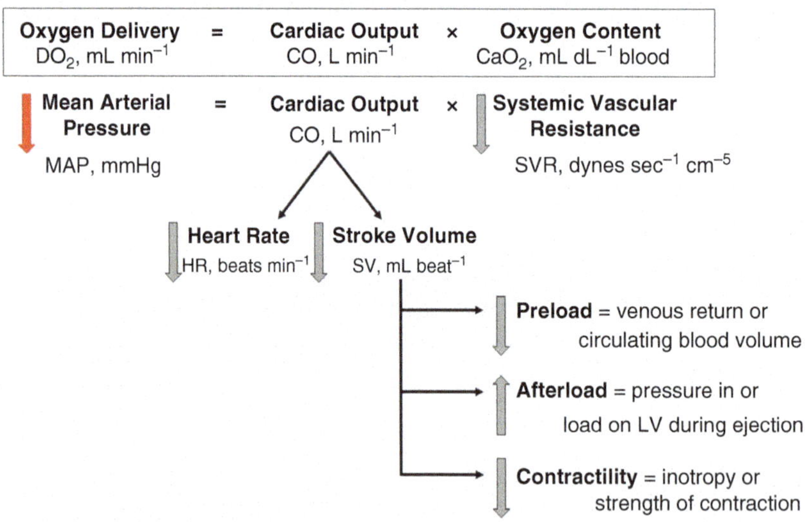

Figure 1.4 Mean arterial pressure (MAP) is the product of CO and systemic vascular resistance (SVR, the inherent tone or diameter of blood vessels). MAP is influenced by increased SVR (vasoconstriction) or decreased SVR (vasodilation). Note that MAP is not a direct component of oxygen delivery but is an indirect measurement of oxygen delivery. Cardiac output is the product of HR and SV (ml blood ejected by the heart per cardiac cycle). Stroke volume is determined by the volume of blood returning to the heart during diastole (preload), the resistance to ejection of blood during systole (afterload), and the strength of cardiac muscle contraction and relaxation (inotropy and lusitropy, respectively). Gray arrows indicate direction of change associated with hypotension (red arrow).

driving the change in pressure for a given patient requires understanding the effects of anesthetic drugs, autonomic physiology, and underlying pathophysiology, among many others.

The four mechanisms based on this algorithm are vasodilation, bradycardia, decreases in cardiac preload, and a decrease in myocardial contractility (Figure 1.4). These mechanisms of hypotension have a variety of causes (Figures 1.5–1.8) and treatments (Figure 1.9); lists within these figures are not meant to represent all causes and treatments but demonstrate common examples of those found in practice. For example, vasodilation can be treated either with (i) fluid boluses (crystalloids or colloids) to expand vascular volume to "fill" the vasodilated vasculature, or with (ii) administration of vasoconstricting agents to "offset" the vasodilation (phenylephrine, vasopressin, norepinephrine, etc.) or a positive inotrope that has vasoconstrictive properties (e.g., dopamine). Bradycardia can be treated with anticholinergics for sinus bradycardia or second-degree atrioventricular (AV) block, or with other antiarrhythmics directed at specific bradyarrhythmias. Decreases in cardiac filling can be treated with blood volume replacement (crystalloid or colloid boluses), or with reversal or removal of obstructions or compression of

Causes of Bradycardia

- Normal for breed/species
- Loss of SNS tone with anesthesia
- Arrhythmias
- Hypothermia
- Opioids
- Alpha-2-adrenergic agonists
- Beta-adrenergic antagonists
- Excessive anesthetic depth
- High vagal tone/stimulation
- Hypoxia (fetus, neonate)
- Low-dose anticholinergic
- Oculocardiac reflex
- Cushing's reflex
- Hyperkalemia

Figure 1.5 Example causes of decreased heart rate via disease, complications of a procedure (e.g., ocular or vagal stimulation), or drug side effects that can be used not only to treat a cause of bradycardia from patient comorbidities or procedures but also for management before or during anesthesia.

Causes of Vasodilation (Decreased SVR)

- Propofol
- Acepromazine
- Inhalant anesthetics
- Hypothermia
- Sepsis
- Anaphylaxis
- Hypercapnia
- Cardiac drugs
  - Nitroprusside
  - Nitroglycerine
  - Pimobendan
  - Hydralazine
  - ACE inhibitors
  - Amlodipine

Figure 1.6 Example causes of vasodilation (decreased SVR) via disease, complications of a procedure (e.g., septic shock or anaphylaxis), or drug side effects that can be used not only to treat a cause of vasodilation but also to predict potential vasodilation from patient comorbidities or diseases for management before or during anesthesia.

Causes of Decreased Preload

- Low total body water (geriatrics)
- Dehydration (vomiting, dehydration)
- 3rd spacing (effusions, ascites, GI fluid)
- Hemorrhage
- Hypovolemia
- Vascular occlusion/compression/obstruction
- Positive pressure ventilation
- Vasodilation

Figure 1.7 Example causes of decreased venous return (i.e., preload), either via disease or complications from drug side effects.

Causes of Decreased Contractility	
• Neonates/juveniles/pediatrics	• Propofol
• Dilated cardiomyopathy	• Hypocalcemia
• Secondary cardiomyopathies	• Acidosis
• Inhalant anesthetics	• Beta-adrenergic antagonists

Figure 1.8 Example causes of decreased contractility (or inotropy) via disease, complications of a disease, or drug side effects that can be used not only to treat a cause of decreased contractility but also to predict potential negative inotropy from patient comorbidities or anesthetics, or for management before or during anesthesia.

Mechanism of Hypotension	Treatments for Hypotension
1) Vasodilation	1a) Fluid boluses 1b) Vasopressors 1c) Reduce inhalant level
2) Bradycardia	2a) Anticholinergics 2b) Antiarrhythmics 2c) Treat underlying cause
3) Decreased preload	3a) Fluid boluses 3b) Decrease ventilation pressure 3c) Relieve obstruction/compression
4) Decreased contractility	4a) Positive inotropes 4b) Reduce inhalant level

Figure 1.9 Suggested treatment options for each underlying mechanism of hypotension are presented. Vasodilation can be treated with either volume resuscitation, vasoconstrictive agents, or reducing inhalant anesthetics. Bradycardia can be treated with anticholinergic or antiarrhythmic agents, or by treating the underlying cause of bradycardia (e.g., hyperkalemia). Decreased preload can be treated with volume boluses or correction of the inciting cause of loss of preload (e.g., obstruction to venous return or controlling hemorrhage). Decreased contractility can be treated with either minimizing the inciting cause (e.g., inhaled anesthetics) or with positive inotropic drugs (e.g., dopamine, dobutamine, etc.).

the cranial and caudal vena cava. Finally, decreases in myocardial contractility from any cause can be treated either by reducing or removing the cause or with positive inotropes that improve contractility. As inhalant anesthetics are moderately to severely depressant on myocardial contractility and vasodilation (depending on dose), reducing the inhaled anesthetic dose (or requirement) of a patient can dramatically improve contractility and hypotension.

It is critical to understand that these mechanism(s) and cause(s) exist not only in the anesthetized patient but also in the patient with preexisting disease or abnormal physiology (e.g., pregnancy, neonates, and geriatrics), and this approach can be used not only in the anesthetized patient but also in planning ahead for hypotension and other complications under anesthesia.

Preanesthetic Patient Assessment

Underlying cardiac disease necessitates a more extensive patient evaluation compared to non-cardiac patients [11, 12]. For example, patient history should include previous cardiovascular diagnoses, medications, and any recent changes in medication dosages. Historical radiographs, electrocardiography (ECG) or Holter monitor evaluation, BP, and echocardiogram findings should be available. Patients with severe disease should be evaluated within one to two weeks of a planned anesthetic procedure.

Although a complete physical examination (PE) should be performed before and on the day of anesthesia, attention must be paid to the cardiovascular and respiratory systems. The localization and characterization of heart murmurs, changes in lung sounds, increases in respiratory rate and effort, poor color and refill of mucous membranes, presence of jugular pulsations, and pulse irregularities or pulse deficits are obvious indicators of potential heart disease or changes in the patient's cardiovascular status.

A minimum database for cardiac disease should include assessments of organ function with a blood chemistry panel, electrolytes, and a complete blood count. Patients with cardiac disease should have some combination of preanesthetic ECG, BP, thoracic radiographs, and echocardiogram depending on the type of cardiac disease. Ideally, the entire workup should be completed for patients presenting with a cardiac murmur or arrhythmia and previously unrecognized cardiac disease.

Functional Classification of Cardiac Disease

Previous texts [12] have established a functional classification of cardiac disease based on clinical signs to help the clinician recognize which patients may have a higher risk of anesthetic complications and for whom anesthesia should be avoided until the patient has stabilized. If the presenting complaint necessitates anesthesia, this classification alerts the clinician to the high-risk nature of such patients for owner counseling, preanesthetic preparation, requirements for intensive patient monitoring, and patient support.

Classification I comprises all nonclinical patients with preexisting cardiac disease that can be anesthetized with no preanesthetic stabilization. Classification II includes patients who have preexisting cardiac disease with mild to moderate clinical signs of disease at rest or with exercise. These patients require significant stabilization with medications and/or hospitalization before anesthesia. If anesthesia is required for a life-saving procedure, immediate stabilization with parenteral medications before anesthesia is required. Aggressive and invasive monitoring is necessary due to their fragile nature. Classification III includes patients with ongoing, fulminant heart failure. Anesthesia is contraindicated until the patient can be stabilized. If anesthesia cannot be avoided due to a life-saving procedure, they carry the highest risk of anesthetic complications, including severe debilitation, morbidity, and mortality.

The American Society of Anesthesiologists (ASA) patient status classification scheme has been adapted by The American College of Veterinary Anesthesia and Analgesia (ACVAA; Table 1.1). The ASA patient status value is not intended to be a risk assessment; the assignment of patient status implies only the presence or absence of disease and that the clinician has evaluated the health status of the patient. The ASA physical status classification has limitations and is overly vague. However, the ASA does not (and presumably will not, as these definitions were accepted in 1963) expand on these limited definitions. Therefore, the clinician must individually determine the ASA status assignment of a patient with cardiac disease. Some authors have suggested classic types of patients who may be categorized into a physical status to help guide clinicians in the determination of ASA physical status [13].

Sedation Versus General Anesthesia

Sedation is defined as "a state characterized by central depression accompanied by drowsiness and some degree of centrally induced relaxation.

Table 1.1 American Society of Anesthesiologists (ASA) physical status classification.

Category	Physical status	Clinical examples
I	Normal, healthy patients	No detectable disease; patients presenting for ovariohysterectomy or castration
II	Patients with mild, systemic disease	Skin tumor, fracture without shock, uncomplicated hernia, cryptorchidectomy, localized infection, or compensated disease
III	Patients with severe, systemic disease fever, dehydration, anemia, cachexia, or moderate hypovolemia	
IV	Patients with severe, systemic disease that is a constant threat to life	Uremia, toxemia, severe dehydration and hypovolemia, cardiac decompensation, emaciation, or high fever
V	Moribund patients that are not expected to survive 24 h	Extreme shock, terminal malignancy or infection, severe trauma

Patient physical status adapted from the ASA physical status classification [13]. Clinical examples have been suggested by some authors; however, patient classification is highly variable and must be determined by the individual clinician.

The patient is generally unaware of its surroundings but can become aroused and is responsive to noxious stimulation" [13]. General anesthesia has been described as "insensibility"; it refers to the loss of sensation to any part of the body, or to its entirety. Anesthetic induction results from drugs that depress the nervous system locally, regionally, or centrally (central nervous system; CNS) [13]. Surgical anesthesia is "the state/plane of anesthesia that provides unconsciousness, amnesia, muscular relaxation, and hypoalgesia sufficient for painless surgery" [13]. The choice between whether to simply sedate a patient for a procedure or to use general anesthesia is important to consider. The degree of CNS depression that accompanies general anesthesia also depresses autonomic reflexes, the effects of which may be avoided if sedation is an acceptable alternative for the planned procedure. Systemic sedation that is appropriate for the patient's temperament and underlying disease in combination with locoregional analgesia may be sufficient for surgical analgesia in some cases [14–16].

Although sedation may appear to be a universally safer option due to the avoidance of CNS/autonomic depression, sedatives such as alpha-2-adrenergic receptor agonists and phenothiazines may be absolutely contraindicated with some types of cardiac disease [17, 18]. Moreover, the degree of cardiovascular depression may be difficult to treat (particularly in the case of the alpha-2-adrenergic agonists) without reversal of the sedative with an antagonist reversal agent. In some cases, sedation may be preferred; however, general anesthesia with cardiovascular-sparing protocols and appropriate patient monitoring and support may be the safer option. There is no single ideal anesthetic agent or anesthetic protocol for all cardiovascular disease; no one plan that will work for all patients and all procedures. All anesthetic plans should be individualized for the patient's cardiovascular status and coexisting disease. Optimizing the plan requires a complete understanding of anesthetic drug effects and side effects, as well as pathophysiology of disease, to combine the two for optimal outcome.

Anesthetic and Analgesic Agents

Premedicants

Premedication is an extremely important step in the process of anesthetizing patients because it provides sedation, analgesia, and a reduction in induction and maintenance drug doses [2].

As the induction and maintenance agents frequently are associated with severely depressant cardiovascular effects (albeit drug- and dose-dependent in most cases), a large step toward cardiovascular stability can be provided with mild to moderate sedation with appropriate premedication.

Opioids

Opioids are a mainstay of premedication, induction, and maintenance of anesthesia in patients with cardiac disease, as they have minimal cardiovascular effects [19–22]. Bradycardia is the major consequence of opioid use, as opioids have minimal to no effects on cardiac contractility or vascular tone [23–25]. Bradycardia can be controlled with treatment or concomitant premedication with an anticholinergic (such as atropine or glycopyrrolate). Differences among the large number of opioids can cause confusion in choosing the most appropriate drug in this class. Generally, opioids will produce better sedation in the very young, old, or compromised patient as compared to a normally healthy adult patient. This is especially important to consider in debilitated patients with cardiac disease. Opioids are traditionally described based on their receptor target (mu-, kappa-, delta-opioid receptors) and ability to exert desired clinical effects (e.g., efficacy) including sedation, analgesia, vomiting, etc.

Full Mu-Opioid Receptor Agonists

Morphine Morphine is considered the basis for comparison of all other opioids. Morphine is a full mu-opioid receptor agonist and provides very good sedation, often perceived as the best sedating choice in this class of drugs. It is also the most likely drug to induce vomiting [26]. It is absorbed rapidly when given intramuscularly (IM) [27], and its duration is 4–6 h. Intravenous (IV) bolus administration is not recommended due to the risk of histamine release [28]. Morphine can, however, be delivered by low dose constant rate infusion (CRI) and provides significant reductions in inhaled maintenance anesthetic requirements [29].

Hydromorphone/Oxymorphone Hydromorphone and oxymorphone have very similar profiles in small animals [30, 31]. Both are full mu-opioid receptor agonists and provide excellent analgesia. They are moderately sedating opioids and are slightly less likely to induce vomiting compared to morphine [26]. Hydromorphone (as well as morphine) may cause panting in clinical canine patients, which may be undesirable for sedated procedures. Hydromorphone has also been reported to cause postoperative hyperthermia in cats at standard clinical doses [32]; however, the clinical relevance of this is unclear [33].

Methadone Methadone is a synthetic full mu-opioid receptor agonist with dose-dependent [34], mild to moderate sedative effects [35], and minimal side effects. When given alone, panting and defecation are commonly reported [34, 36, 37], though vomiting is less common when compared to morphine [26]. Methadone delivered either intravenously or epidurally significantly reduces the requirement for isoflurane in dogs [38, 39], thus reducing the dose-dependent cardiovascular depression from isoflurane. Methadone is a superior analgesic in dogs when compared to butorphanol for postoperative analgesia following ovariohysterectomy [40]. Interestingly and different than other opioids, methadone also binds and is an antagonist at the N-methyl-D-aspartate (NMDA) receptor [41]. Methadone may also be a more effective analgesic for chronic pain based on this activity [42].

Fentanyl Fentanyl is a synthetic full mu-opioid receptor agonist that is 80–100 times more potent than morphine, implying that an equally effective dose is 80–100 times less than that of morphine [43]. Owing to its short duration of action (20–30 min after bolus administration), fentanyl is most useful for IV premedication, induction, or delivery by CRI [22]. Fentanyl is minimally sedating and is extremely unlikely to induce vomiting [44]. It is very well suited for use as a sole anesthetic induction agent at high doses or as part of a multidrug induction protocol.

Remifentanil, Sufentanil, and Alfentanil Remifentanil, sufentanil, and alfentanil are derivatives of fentanyl with similar beneficial effects regarding their analgesic efficacy and ability to profoundly decrease inhalant requirements. They all carry the same side effects of dose-dependent respiratory depression, bradycardia, and potential hypotension. Remifentanil is an ultrashort acting synthetic fentanyl derivative with a very short elimination time due to extrahepatic elimination by plasma esterase enzymes and thus must be delivered by constant infusion. Remifentanil decreases sevoflurane minimum alveolar concentration (MAC) in dogs by 30–60% in a dose-dependent fashion [45], and reduces isoflurane requirements in cats [46] and dogs [47].

Mixed Opioid Agonist–Antagonist Receptor Drugs

Butorphanol Butorphanol is a mixed opioid receptor agonist–antagonist; it is an agonist at the kappa-opioid receptor and an antagonist at the mu-opioid receptor [43]. Therefore, it is only indicated for mild to weakly moderate pain as it has analgesic effects only at the kappa-receptor; it is a very poor analgesic for moderate to severe pain [48]. Although it has a relatively short duration of analgesic action (45–90 min), it can be sedative in small animals and thus used for conscious procedures either as a sole IV sedative or in combination with other more potent sedatives, depending on the requirements. Bradycardia is less likely to occur after butorphanol administration than with full mu-opioid agonists. It is very unlikely to cause vomiting and demonstrates a “ceiling effect” in which no further sedation or analgesia is seen beyond 0.8 mg kg^{-1} [49, 50].

Nalbuphine Nalbuphine is a semi-synthetic mixed agonist–antagonist similar to butorphanol, historically used in human labor and delivery, but is less commonly used in veterinary medicine [51]. It is related chemically to oxymorphone and has a similar potency (though not efficacy) to morphine. As a kappa-agonist, it also appears to have a “ceiling effect” with fewer issues including respiratory depression, bradycardia, and others [52]. Epidural nalbuphine has been shown to reduce the isoflurane requirement by 26–38% in dogs [53]. Interestingly, despite reportedly similar opioid receptor effects, butorphanol may be a better sedative choice in dogs compared to nalbuphine when used alone [52], though this may not be observable when combined with dexmedetomidine/Telazol in cats [54].

Partial Mu-Opioid Receptor Agonists

Buprenorphine Buprenorphine is unique among the common opioids in that it is a partial mu-opioid receptor agonist. Buprenorphine has an extremely high affinity for the mu-opioid receptor, such that it outcompetes other opioids for receptor binding, but cannot evoke a full mu-opioid receptor response [55]. Therefore, it is not equally efficacious compared to full mu-opioid receptor agonists. It also demonstrates a “ceiling effect” in that doses above 0.04 mg kg^{-1} do not provide additional analgesia or sedation. Owing to receptor binding, buprenorphine is poorly reversible to irreversible with opioid antagonists [56]. It is very unlikely to cause bradycardia and vomiting and is a relatively poor sedative. In addition to its conventional formulation, buprenorphine is available in both sustained release [57] and high-concentration preparations [58].

Phenothiazines

Acepromazine is a common premedication and is an excellent tranquilizer in small animals. Sedation from phenothiazines is principally due to blockade of central G-protein-coupled, dopaminergic D2 receptors that lead to a decrease in cyclic AMP (cAMP), adenylate cyclase, and calcium conductance, and thus neuronal-firing activity [59]. However, it is an alpha-1-adrenergic receptor antagonist and administration may lead to peripheral vasodilation and hypotension [60] (along with potential negative inotropic effects). Although reductions in afterload may be beneficial in some patients with cardiac disease (such as mild aortic stenosis [AS]), and animals with stable, nonclinical disease may be able to compensate for the vasodilatory effects, it may be prudent to avoid acepromazine in patients with moderate to severe cardiac disease that cannot tolerate decreases in preload and/or afterload. In addition, hypotension may lead to a compensatory increase in HR, which can increase myocardial oxygen consumption. Acepromazine may protect the myocardium from epinephrine- and barbiturate-induced arrhythmias [61]; however, this benefit must be weighed against the hypotensive effects.

Benzodiazepines

Benzodiazepines (diazepam and midazolam) are good choices for sedation in patients with cardiac disease. They have minimal to no effects on HR, contractility, or vasomotor tone [62], and do not lead to hypotension across a wide range of doses ($0.5–2.5\,mg\,kg^{-1}$ IV). Although respiratory rate decreases, arterial blood gas values do not change appreciably [63]. The major disadvantage of benzodiazepines is that they are inconsistent sedatives in dogs [64, 65] and may be poor sedatives in cats. For example, IV premedication doses can lead to dysphoria, excitement, ataxia, arousal, and, potentially, violent aggression [64]; combinations of butorphanol and midazolam fail to provide sedation in healthy cats [65]. Although benzodiazepines decrease inhaled anesthetic requirements, this benefit can be achieved when they are combined with induction agents during the induction protocol as opposed to risking excitement when used as premedications [66, 67].

Alpha-2-Adrenergic Receptor Agonists

Alpha-2-adrenergic receptor agonists (dexmedetomidine, medetomidine, xylazine, etc.) may be relatively contraindicated in patients with cardiac disease. Alpha-2-adrenergic receptor agonists cause intense peripheral vasoconstriction and decrease sympathetic outflow from the CNS. The severe initial increase in SVR leads to a marked increase in BP, a significant increase in myocardial afterload, and a baroreceptor-mediated reflex bradycardia. Some patients may demonstrate a period of vasodilation and arterial hypotension after the initial hypertension. This is commonly seen with xylazine in horses, but appears to be less common with longer-acting agents such as dexmedetomidine [68]. The initial baroreceptor-mediated bradycardia is exacerbated by a decrease in centrally mediated descending sympathetic tone associated with reduced synaptic norepinephrine release. Alpha-2-adrenergic receptor agonists can also produce bradyarrhythmias such as AV blockade and ventricular escape cardiac rhythms. At sedative doses ($\geq 5\,\mu g\,kg^{-1}$ IV), dexmedetomidine will decrease CO by 50–60%, and medetomidine at $20\,\mu g\,kg^{-1}$ IV will decrease CO by at least 60% [69–71]. The increase in afterload from vasoconstriction, increase in left atrial pressure from centralization of blood volume, and decrease in CO are all mechanisms that can be detrimental to the function of a heart with underlying disease. Although alpha-2-adrenergic receptor agonists are extremely reliable sedatives, the cardiovascular side effects may be significant enough that the depth of sedation may be better sacrificed in the interest of cardiovascular safety. Some studies have shown promise for use of dexmedetomidine in cats with hypertrophic cardiomyopathy (HCM) [72], though further study is needed to clarify its cardiovascular effects in HCM.

Alfaxalone

Alfaxalone is a neuroactive steroid-like molecule that is capable of inducing general anesthesia through binding and interaction with the gamma aminobutyric acid (GABA) receptor [73]. Alfaxalone can be administered IV for anesthetic induction (discussed in the next section) or IM for sedation that has been reported in multiple species, including dogs, cats, and rabbits [74–78]. Typical IM dosing of alfaxalone for sedation ranges from 1 to $5\,mg\,kg^{-1}$ IM [74, 75]. It should be combined with other sedative/analgesics [79], as alfaxalone sedation alone has higher rates of side effects including paddling, twitching and ataxia [80]. Alfaxalone doses of up to 5–8 mg kg^{-1} IM have been reported but carry the risk of increased respiratory depression and/or inadvertent general anesthesia. Higher doses may require oxygen supplementation, pulse oximetry monitoring [70], or possibly endotracheal intubation and ventilatory support, as higher doses may precipitate general anesthesia rather than sedation [81].

Anticholinergics

Atropine and glycopyrrolate are parasympatholytic, anticholinergic agents used to increase HR amid vagally-mediated sinus bradycardia and AV block. Atropine has a faster onset time (1–2 min IV), shorter duration of action (20–30 min IV), and is more likely to incite tachyarrhythmias [82]. Glycopyrrolate has a longer onset time (2–4 min IV), longer duration of action (1 h IV), and may be less likely to cause tachyarrhythmias [82]. Low doses of atropine and glycopyrrolate can initially precipitate second-degree AV block (see the following sections), which may require additional doses of anticholinergic for treatment. Anticholinergics should not be indiscriminately combined with alpha-2-adrenergic agonist use, as while they will prevent or treat the bradycardia associated with alpha-2-agonist usage, the combination of a higher heart rate with increased systemic vascular resistance typical of alpha-2-receptor agonists places significant burden on the heart and might potentiate cardiac arrhythmias [70]. Routine premedication with anticholinergics has fallen out of favor, as the potential side effects including decreased gastrointestinal motility, thickened respiratory secretions, and potential for tachycardias are present. Anticholinergic use should be tailored to individual patient needs.

Induction Agents

Propofol

The main advantages of propofol are the rapid onset (15–20 s) and short duration of action (6–10 min of anesthesia) from an IV bolus that allow intubation and make it a suitable choice for a CRI [83]. The main mechanism of action [84] is stimulation of the GABA (the main inhibitory neurotransmitter in the CNS) receptor away from the binding site for other anesthetics such as thiopental [85]. Recoveries from propofol administration are generally smooth. However, propofol is a significant dose-dependent vasodilator [86] and can precipitate significant hypotension at moderate bolus doses. While patients with mild cardiac disease may tolerate hypotension associated with propofol, those with more severe disease or in whom a decrease in SVR will worsen cardiac function should be cautiously induced with propofol.

Alfaxalone

Alfaxalone was originally reported in 1971 as a new steroid hypnotic general anesthetic agent [87]. It is poorly water-soluble and so was formulated in a polyethoxylated castor oil vehicle which led to adverse reactions including hyperemia in cats [88] and anaphylactoid reactions in dogs [89]. A newer formulation [90] in a beta-cyclodextrin molecule allowed solubilization while avoiding previous side effects.

Alfaxalone provides rapid and smooth anesthetic induction of anesthesia when administered by bolus. Although it should always be administered "to effect," the manufacturer-recommended induction dose in dogs is 1.1–2.2 mg kg^{-1} IV (range: 0.2–4.5 mg kg^{-1} IV), and in cats it is 2.3–4.0 mg kg^{-1} IV (range: 1.1–10.8 mg kg^{-1} IV), with doses depending greatly on degree of sedation from premedication [91]. Similar to propofol, alfaxalone causes dose-dependent cardiorespiratory suppression (hypotension, apnea) in cats and dogs [92, 93]; however, clinically relevant doses show good cardiovascular stability. For example, IV alfaxalone administration increases heart rate, suggesting maintenance of the baroreceptor reflex post induction [77]. This property distinguishes alfaxalone from other induction agents and may contribute to its cardiovascular stability.

A comparison of propofol ($8\,mg\,kg^{-1}$ IV, to effect) and alfaxalone ($4\,mg\,kg^{-1}$ IV, to effect) for anesthetic induction found no significant differences in physiologic variables, quality of induction, duration of intubation, or quality of recovery [94]. Alfaxalone was associated with a higher likelihood of undesirable events (e.g., excitement, paddling, twitching, apnea), though these events were not thought to be clinically serious.

Dissociative Anesthetics

Dissociative anesthetics such as ketamine and tiletamine produce anesthesia by interrupting neuronal transmission, thus "dissociating" the centers responsible for consciousness and unconsciousness from the peripheral ascending inputs. The cardiovascular effects of dissociative anesthetics result from stimulation of the SNS, increasing HR, contractility, and MAP, with little change in SVR [95]. This leads to an increase in myocardial work and myocardial oxygen demand, which is compensated for by increased CO and coronary blood flow [96]. The increase in oxygen demand in patients with cardiac disease may worsen cardiac function or arrhythmias. Thus, ketamine, especially at high doses, should be used cautiously in patients where increases in myocardial contractility or work would be detrimental [97].

Etomidate

Etomidate is a nonopioid, nonbarbiturate sedative hypnotic drug that works similarly to propofol and barbiturates in that it enhances inhibitory GABA effects [98]. Etomidate has the distinct advantage of having minimal to no cardiovascular depression because it does not significantly change HR, contractility, afterload, or venous return [99, 100]. However, it has several drawbacks. Etomidate can cause adrenocortical suppression and has a very high osmolarity (approximately $4800\,mOsm\,l^{-1}$) that can lead to osmolar shifts, phlebitis, pain at the injection site, red blood cell crenation, and potential hemolysis [101]. Etomidate causes a reliable but relatively slow transition to unconsciousness when compared to propofol. Etomidate has poor muscle relaxation and can stimulate myoclonus, and so should be given with a benzodiazepine or opioid such as fentanyl to facilitate a smooth induction period [99].

High-Dose Opioids

High-dose, full mu-opioid receptor agonists such as fentanyl can be extremely effective in producing general anesthesia with uncomplicated placement of an endotracheal tube. High-dose opioids have the disadvantage of moderate to severe respiratory depression and bradycardia; however, both are easily controlled with intubation and anticholinergics, respectively. Unfortunately, transition to unconsciousness with fentanyl appears somewhat less reliable and slower compared to propofol [102]. Patients who are bright and energetic or are stimulated during the induction process by sound, touch, or pain may attempt to "override" the induction process, leading to poor induction quality. In these cases, a rescue induction agent (typically propofol for speed of onset or etomidate) can help push such a patient into unconsciousness. Quiet, dimly lit environments with little stimuli are ideal for fentanyl inductions, and fentanyl inductions usually work best in debilitated, older animals. Fentanyl should be given with a benzodiazepine for improved muscle relaxation.

Anesthetic Maintenance

Inhaled Anesthetics

Inhaled anesthetics are the most chosen drugs for maintenance of anesthesia. Although injectable maintenance protocols exist and are referred to as total intravenous anesthesia (TIVA) protocols (described in the following text; Table 1.2), inhaled anesthetics provide several unique advantages. Their pharmacokinetic properties allow for careful titration of and rapid changes in anesthetic depth. Inhaled anesthetic use requires an anesthetic vaporizer and a carrier gas flow (often 100% oxygen), which supports maximal arterial blood

Table 1.2 Selected propofol and alfaxalone infusion doses.

Propofol (dogs)	Induction dose IV	CRI dose
Bustamante et al. [103]	0.65–5 mg kg^{-1}	0.25 ± 4.7 mg kg^{-1} min^{-1}
Park et al. [104]		0.2–0.4 mg kg^{-1} min^{-1}
Kennedy and Smith [105]	4.0 ± 1.0 mg kg^{-1} (with ketamine 1:1)	0.3 ± 0.1 mg kg^{-1} min^{-1}
	5.3 ± 1.0 mg kg^{-1}	0.6 ± 0.1 mg kg^{-1} min^{-1}
Mohamadnia et al. [106]	8 mg kg^{-1}	0.3 mg kg^{-1} min^{-1}
Tsai et al. [107]	1.5–2.0 mg kg^{-1}	
Raisis et al. [108]	To effect	0.4 mg kg^{-1} min^{-1}
Murrell et al. [109]		0.33 mg kg^{-1} min^{-1}
Hughes and Nolan [110]	4 mg kg^{-1}	0.2–0.4 mg kg^{-1} min^{-1}
Smith et al. [111]	8.68 ± 0.57 mg kg^{-1}	0.68 ± 0.13 mg kg^{-1} min^{-1}
	6.13 ± 0.67 mg kg^{-1}	0.49 ± 0.16 mg kg^{-1} min^{-1}
	4.78 ± 0.39 mg kg^{-1}	0.26 ± 0.05 mg kg^{-1} min^{-1}
Alfaxalone (dogs)	Induction dose IV	CRI dose
Hunt et al. [112]	1.4 mg kg^{-1}	99 μg kg^{-1} min^{-1}
Bennell et al. [113]	1.5 mg kg^{-1}	
Dehuisser et al. [114]	2 mg kg^{-1}	150 μg kg^{-1} min^{-1}
Liao et al. [115]	1.5 mg kg^{-1}	268 μg kg^{-1} min^{-1}
	2.1 mg kg^{-1}	310 μg kg^{-1} min^{-1}
	0.62 mg kg^{-1}	83 μg kg^{-1} min^{-1}
	0.98 mg kg^{-1}	87 μg kg^{-1} min^{-1}
Conde Ruiz et al. [116]	3 mg kg^{-1}	200 μg kg^{-1} min^{-1}
Herbert et al. [117]	1.5 ± 0.57 mg kg^{-1}	0.11 (0.07–0.33) mg kg^{-1} min^{-1}
	1.2 (0–6.3) mg kg^{-1}	0.08 (0.06–0.19) mg kg^{-1} min^{-1}
Suarez et al. [118]	Propofol = 5.8 ± 0.30 mg kg^{-1}	Propofol = 0.37 ± 0.09 mg kg^{-1} min^{-1}
	Alfaxalone = 1.9 ± 0.07 mg kg^{-1}	Alfaxalone = 0.11 ± 0.01 mg kg^{-1} min^{-1}
Alfaxalone (cats)	Induction dose IV	CRI dose
Beths et al. [119]	1.7 (0.7–3.0) mg kg^{-1}	0.18 (0.06–0.25) mg kg^{-1} min^{-1}
Schwarz et al. [120]	2.57 ± 0.41 mg kg^{-1}	0.19–0.022 mg kg^{-1} min^{-1}

oxygenation. The use of an anesthesia machine with associated endotracheal intubation or laryngeal mask airway placement allows for more accurate monitoring of ventilation. In addition, ventilation can also be supplemented and/or supported more easily. The ability to monitor expired gases such as carbon dioxide or expired anesthetic concentrations allows for more robust patient monitoring and support. Unfortunately, inhaled anesthetics depress cardiovascular function, leading to dose-dependent CO and BP depression [121]. This is due to a moderate to severe dose-dependent reduction in myocardial contractility (i.e., negative inotropy) and subsequent decreases in SV and CO [121–124]. All modern inhalant anesthetics (isoflurane, sevoflurane, desflurane) also decrease SVR (i.e., vasodilation), which can incite or predispose to hypotension. Generally, these cardiovascular effects are managed either by minimizing the dose administered or by counteracting the side effects with interventions aimed at providing cardiovascular support. Many strategies are available to reduce the minimum alveolar concentration, or MAC, of inhaled anesthetic agents required to produce lack of response to a supramaximal noxious stimulus applied to a patient 50% of the time; means of reducing MAC and thereby reducing the inhaled anesthetic dose include use of premedicants, induction agents, bolus- or infusion-dose analgesics or sedatives, and local/regional anesthesia techniques. The ability to decrease the inhaled anesthetic requirements has been extensively studied (see Tables 1.3 and 1.4). The hypotensive effects of inhaled anesthetic agents can be treated by a variety of mechanisms, including optimizing HR and rhythm, judicious use of IV fluids (if not contraindicated by cardiovascular disease), increasing SVR with vasoactive medications, and directly increasing contractility with positive inotropic drugs (Figure 1.9).

Total Intravenous Anesthesia

TIVA is general anesthetic maintenance using titrated or computer-controlled infusions of anesthetic, sedative, and analgesic combinations, rather than anesthetic maintenance with inhaled anesthetics. Inhaled anesthetic use carries the disadvantages of dose-dependent patient cardiopulmonary depression, potential risk of waste-gas exposure to hospital staff, and the environmental impact of inhalants as greenhouse gases [134]. Inhaled anesthetics require a vaporizer for controlled dosing, an anesthesia machine for delivery, and waste anesthetic gas scavenging. Clinical circumstances may find inhalational anesthesia undesirable (e.g., head trauma, increased intracranial pressure) or

Table 1.3 Examples of MAC-reducing effects of common CRIs in cats.

Study	Loading dose ($mg\,kg^{-1}$)	CRI dose (μg $kg^{-1}min^{-1}$)	Inhalant	MAC (%)	MAC reduction	MAC reduction percentage
Remifentanil						
Brosnan et al. [125]	None	0.0625–16	Isoflurane	1.94 ± 0.8	None	None
Ferreira et al. [46]	None	0.25	Isoflurane	1.66 ± 0.08	1.27 ± 0.13	−23% ± 7.9%
	None	0.5	Isoflurane	1.66 ± 0.08	1.16 ± 0.17	−29.8% ± 8.3%
	None	1.0	Isoflurane	1.66 ± 0.08	1.22 ± 0.15	−26% ± 9.4%
Ketamine						
Pascoe et al. [126]	2.0	23	Isoflurane	1.51 ± 0.23	0.84 ± 0.33	−45% ± 17%
	2.0	46	Isoflurane	1.51 ± 0.23	0.57 ± 0.35	−63% ± 18%
	16.0	115	Isoflurane	1.51 ± 0.23	0.41 ± 0.35	−75% ± 17%

MAC is the minimum alveolar concentration of an inhaled anesthetic (the concentration of an inhalant at the pulmonary alveolar level) that prevents purposeful responses (i.e., not a reflex response) to noxious stimuli in 50% of patients. MAC reduction is typically defined as the percent reduction in MAC dose; the lower dose of inhalant that maintains 50% response to noxious stimuli with concurrent use of an example infusion during inhaled anesthesia. MAC reduction maintains a surgical plane of anesthesia at a lower inhalant level to reduce the side effects (e.g., vasodilation and decreased contractility).
μg = micrograms.

Table 1.4 Examples of MAC-reducing effects of common CRIs in dogs.

Study	Loading dose ($mg\,kg^{-1}$)	CRI dose ($\mu g\,kg^{-1}\,min^{-1}$)	Inhalant	MAC (%)	MAC reduction	MAC reduction percentage
Fentanyl						
Ueyama [127]	0.005	0.15	Isoflurane	1.42 ± 0.08	0.93 ± 0.04	−35%
Hellyer [128]	0.01	0.3	Isoflurane	1.8 ± 0.21	0.85 ± 0.14	−53%
Remifentanil						
Michelsen [129]	None	1.0	Enflurane	2.1 ± 0.2	NR	−63% ± 10.4%
Allweiler [130]	None	0.1	Isoflurane	1.28 ± 0.13	0.78 ± 0.17	−40%
	None	0.25	Isoflurane	1.28 ± 0.13	0.65 ± 0.16	−50%
Monteiro et al. [47]	None	0.15	Isoflurane	1.24 ± 0.18	NR	−43% ± 10%
	None	0.3	Isoflurane	1.24 ± 0.18	NR	−59% ± 10%
	None	0.6	Isoflurane	1.24 ± 0.18	NR	−66% ± 9%
	None	0.9	Isoflurane	1.24 ± 0.18	NR	−71% ± 9%
Ketamine						
Muir et al. [29]	None	10	Isoflurane	1.38 ± 0.08	1.3 ± 0.07	−25%
Queiroz-Castro [131]	1.0	25	Isoflurane	1.06 ± 0.02	0.73 ± 0.04	−28.7% ± 3.7%
Doherty [132]	1.5	50	Isoflurane	1.11 ± 0.05	0.56 ± 0.04	−49.6%
Love [133]	0.5	6.25	Sevoflurane	2.62 ± 0.21	2.61 ± 0.22	−0.4% ± 4%
	1.0	12.5	Sevoflurane	2.62 ± 0.21	2.06 ± 0.22	−22% ± 4%

MAC is the minimum alveolar concentration of an inhaled anesthetic (the concentration of an inhalant at the pulmonary alveolar level) that prevents purposeful responses (i.e., not a reflex response) to noxious stimuli in 50% of patients. MAC reduction is typically defined as the percent reduction in MAC dose; the lower dose of inhalant that maintains 50% response to noxious stimuli with concurrent use of an example infusion during inhaled anesthesia. MAC reduction maintains a surgical plane of anesthesia at a lower inhalant level to reduce the side effects (e.g., vasodilation and decreased contractility).
NR = not reported; μg = micrograms.

impossible (e.g., nonintubated procedures, long-term intensive care unit [ICU] ventilators without a vaporizer), and TIVA may be the best option. TIVA techniques require a delivery system such as a syringe pump, an intravenous catheter(s), and a dosing-control schedule. Despite avoiding inhaled anesthetics, endotracheal intubation and an anesthesia machine are strongly recommended with TIVA for delivery of oxygen, ability to monitor respiratory function and end-tidal gases (e.g., capnography), and to support or control ventilation.

TIVA dosing can be calculated to either a CRI where a consistent dose of drug is delivered, or with a target-controlled infusion (TCI) dose to target a consistent plasma concentration of drug. A complete description of TCI is beyond the scope of this text. However, in brief, TCI dosing requires previously determined pharmacokinetics for the drug of interest, including the species of interest and the effective plasma concentration; TCI infusions can be controlled manually or with computer programs, based on availability [135, 136]. To date, few publications are available for TCI use in clinical veterinary medicine. Thus, CRI dosing is currently the more common technique used clinically.

A wide variety of TIVA techniques have been employed and, though propofol has dominated the TIVA landscape [137], alfaxalone is a suitable alternative. Selected references for TIVA with alfaxalone and propofol are presented in Table 1.2 [103–120]. Dosing for CRI propofol infusions ranges 0.2–0.6 mg kg^{-1} min^{-1} (dog) and 0.2–1.0 mg kg^{-1} min^{-1} (cat). Dosing for alfaxalone infusions ranges 0.07–0.12 mg kg^{-1} min^{-1} (dog) and 0.18 mg kg^{-1} min^{-1} (cat).

Anesthetic Adjuncts

One major goal of adjunctive techniques or interventions is to increase cardiovascular stability and maximize CO and BP. In practice, this can be generally summarized as applying a technique that has fewer negative cardiovascular side effects as compared to patient management without that technique. As an example, fentanyl infusions have been shown to reduce the requirement for enflurane by as much as 65% [138] and of isoflurane by approximately 50% [128] at 0.8 and 0.3 μg kg^{-1} min^{-1}, respectively. As the primary cardiovascular effect of opioid infusions is bradycardia, which is easily corrected with anticholinergics, these infusions allow for decreased inspired inhalant concentrations, therefore reducing their cardiovascular compromise. This is presumed to be safer by providing improved cardiovascular stability than using higher doses of inhalants alone. Other anesthetic adjunctive techniques, including nonopioid analgesic CRIs (lidocaine and ketamine) and local and regional anesthesia (epidurals, peripheral nerve blocks, and local anesthetics), are aimed at reducing maintenance anesthetic requirements in the interest of cardiovascular stability.

Local and Regional Anesthesia and Analgesia

Local anesthetics have the distinct advantage of blocking peripheral nerve function as compared to other analgesic drug classes (opioids and nonsteroidal anti-inflammatory drugs [NSAIDs]) that modulate the ascending nociceptive stimuli. If nociceptive stimuli are completely prevented from reaching higher centers, then, theoretically, a patient would not require general anesthesia despite painful surgery or procedures. Although this may not be practical for most procedures, it reminds us that local anesthetics are a powerful tool in preventing pain perception or ascending nociceptive information. For patients under general anesthesia, local or regional anesthesia/analgesia can dramatically reduce systemic and inhaled anesthetic drug requirements. As local anesthetics have minimal cardiovascular compromise at appropriate doses, the reduction in systemic and inhaled anesthetic drug levels can minimize or prevent the cardiovascular depressant effects of these anesthetics, leading to a more stable patient. Numerous studies have shown a significant reduction in inhaled anesthetic requirements due to application of regional anesthesia techniques, including infraorbital nerve blocks [139] and opioid-based epidurals in dogs and cats [38, 140] as some examples. Thus, even though local anesthetics are associated with neurotoxicity and cardiotoxicity at high doses [141, 142], they are extremely valuable parts of multimodal anesthetic techniques. Newer texts focus on reviewing anatomy and approach for a large variety of locoregional anesthesia and analgesia techniques, both blindly and with ultrasound and/or or nerve stimulator guidance [143].

Systemic Analgesic Infusions

Much like local and regional techniques, systemically delivered analgesic infusions have the significant potential for reducing inhaled anesthetic drug doses and responsiveness to painful stimuli. If the cardiovascular side effects of the infusion(s) are not more detrimental than the inhaled anesthetic, the reduction in inhaled anesthetic dose can lead to a significant reduction in their negative consequences, such as negative inotropy, vasodilation, and respiratory depression, thus improving cardiovascular performance. As mentioned previously, IV opioid infusions are particularly beneficial in reducing inhaled anesthetic requirements (Tables 1.3 and 1.4) [46, 124–133] and are relatively safe infusions, as their primary side effect is bradycardia, easily treatable with anticholinergics. In horses anesthetized with sevoflurane, an IV lidocaine bolus of $1.3\,mg\,kg^{-1}$ followed by a CRI of $50\,\mu g\,kg^{-1}\,min^{-1}$ reduced sevoflurane MAC by 27% [144]. Intravenous lidocaine infusions have been studied in dogs repeatedly for their benefits in reducing both isoflurane- and sevoflurane-inhaled anesthetic concentrations. Lidocaine at $50\,\mu g\,kg^{-1}\,min^{-1}$ reduced isoflurane MAC by 29% [29] and sevoflurane MAC by 22.6% [145] in dogs. In another study at 50 and $200\,\mu g\,kg^{-1}\,min^{-1}$, no changes in cardiovascular parameters due to lidocaine infusion(s) were identified, and inhalant MAC was reduced by 15% and 37%, respectively [145].

Nonsteroidal Anti-Inflammatory Drugs

NSAIDs have been, and will remain, one of the most important analgesic options in veterinary medicine. A complete review of NSAID pharmacology, indications, guidelines, and adverse effects is beyond the scope of this text and is thoroughly discussed elsewhere [23, 146–150].

Cyclooxygenase-2 (COX-2) enzyme-selective inhibitors have been associated with increased risk of heart failure, myocardial infarction, strokes, and thromboembolic disease in humans due to their negative effects on platelet and vascular homeostasis via thromboxane A2 and prostacyclin [151–154]. Accordingly, rofecoxib (Vioxx™) and parecoxib (Celebrex™) were removed from the human market by the Food and Drug Administration (FDA) due to their increased risk of cardiovascular side effects in 2004 [155]. In veterinary medicine, emesis appears to be the most common adverse effect, with renal and hepatic adverse events found at low frequency with no cardiovascular effects reported [156, 157]. However, the use of NSAIDs is cautioned during periods of hemodynamic compromise (e.g., dehydration, hemorrhage, general anesthesia, heart failure, or renal/hepatic disease), as the kidney becomes more dependent on the vasodilatory effects of prostaglandins. Use of NSAIDs during these times could result in ischemic renal damage, and possible acute renal injury [150].

Sympathomimetic Drugs: Inotropes and Vasopressors

Inotropes and vasopressors are drugs aimed at improving BP and perfusion by taking advantage of SNS receptor targets. In effect, they mimic (mimesis in Greek, which means "to imitate") the SNS's effects on the cardiovascular system. In a normal sympathetic "fight or flight" response, epinephrine is released in response to a perceived or actual threat or injury and stimulates membrane-bound receptors. This response includes increases in heart rate (chronotropy), strength of myocardial contraction (inotropy), speed of cardiac conduction (dromotropy), increases in SVR, and bronchodilation. While the terms "inotropes" and "vasopressors" (or simply, "pressors") are often used interchangeably, in the strictest definition, an inotrope increases contractility, and a vasopressor increases SVR.

The receptor targets for epinephrine in the SNS are alpha-1 (α_1)-, alpha-2 (α_2)-, beta-1 (β_1)-, and beta-2 (β_2)-adrenergic receptors, and each receptor has a stereotypical response to stimulation (Table 1.5) [158]. Inotropes and vasopressors target these receptors, taking advantage of their cardiovascular effects, and each drug in these classes has one or more effects at these receptors. Choosing the appropriate drug to manage hypotension is a balance of the known receptor effects of the individual drug, the suspected mechanism for hypotension, potential risks of the drug, understanding of dosing and delivery techniques, and ability to deliver them safely. There are few absolute contraindications for any drug and gaining knowledge and comfort with them can often be a matter of training, clinical experience, and personal preference. It is important to note that, with few exceptions, the half-lives of these drugs are very short (approximately 1–3 min), and dosing of most sympathomimetic drugs is through CRI rather than by individual and/or intermittent bolus administration.

Dopamine

Dopamine is the immediate metabolic precursor to norepinephrine and, when delivered via CRI, has a dose-dependent positive inotropic effect. Dopamine has varied receptor effects based on the infusion dose. Between approximately 5 and 10 $\mu g\,kg^{-1}\,min^{-1}$, dopamine shows primarily β_1-adrenergic receptor-mediated increases in myocardial contractility, and occasionally β_1-mediated increases in HR. The recommended dose for improvement of CO is 7 $\mu g\,kg^{-1}\,min^{-1}$ [159], although the infusion rate should be tailored within the range to each patient's individual effect. Dopamine's actions are unique compared to other inotropes, as higher doses (above 10 $\mu g\,kg^{-1}\,min^{-1}$) activate α_1-adrenergic receptors and can increase SVR. Although this can also be beneficial for BP, an increase in SVR may in fact worsen cardiovascular performance and may be contraindicated in patients with specific cardiovascular diseases such as dilated cardiomyopathy (DCM), HCM, and regurgitant valvular disease. In addition, the higher dose of dopamine carries a higher potential for tachycardias, ventricular arrhythmias, and hypertension. It is also possible that higher doses of dopamine (or any vasoconstrictive agent), particularly when given by an inadvertent bolus (i.e., with a pump malfunction, medication-dosing error, or flushing an IV catheter in which a dopamine CRI has been delivered), may lead to acute vasoconstriction, hypertension, and reflex bradycardia.

Dobutamine

Dobutamine is a synthetic, nonspecific β-adrenergic agonist, activating both β_1- and β_2-receptors, and will increase both HR and contractility like the β_1-adrenergic receptor effects of dopamine. Higher doses (>10 $\mu g\,kg^{-1}\,min^{-1}$) have the potential to activate α_1-receptors, leading to increases in SVR [159]. The general recommended dose for dobutamine to achieve β_1-adrenergic effects is 1–5 $\mu g\,kg^{-1}\,min^{-1}$, though doses of 1–20 $\mu g\,kg^{-1}\,min^{-1}$ have been reported [160]. However, it is critically important to understand that dobutamine is also a β_2-adrenergic receptor agonist and will induce a decrease in SVR, leading to β_2-adrenergic-receptor-mediated vasodilation. The increase in HR and contractility may be offset by the vasodilation, and despite an increase in CO (and therefore perfusion), an increase in BP may not be

Table 1.5 Inotropes and vasopressors.

	Sympathetic nervous system receptor activation						
	Alpha-1	**Alpha-2**	**Beta-1**	**Beta-2**	**Dopamine (D1)**	**Vasopressin (V1)**	**Dose**
Effect	**Vasoconstriction bradycardia**	**Vasoconstriction**	**Inotropy chronotropy**	**Vasodilation bronchodilation**	**Vasodilation**	**Vasoconstriction**	
Drug							
Dopamine	+++ (High dose)	+	+++ (Low dose)	+ (Low dose)	+++	–	low: 5–10 μg kg^{-1} min^{-1} high: 10–20 μg kg^{-1} min^{-1}
Dobutamine	–	–	+++	++	–	–	1–10 μg kg^{-1} min^{-1}
Epinephrine	+++	+++	++	++	–	–	Bolus: 0.01–0.1 mg kg^{-1} CRI: 0.01–1.0 mg kg^{-1} min^{-1}
Isoproterenol	–	–	+++	+++	–	–	0.01–0.1 mg kg^{-1} min^{-1}
Norepinephrine	+++	–	++	+++	–	–	0.05–2.0 μg kg^{-1} min^{-1}
Phenylephrine	+++	–	–	–	–	–	Bolus: 1–5 μg kg^{-1} CRI: 0.5–3.0 μg kg^{-1} min^{-1}
Vasopressin	–	–	–	–	–	+++	Bolus: 0.1–0.6 mg kg^{-1} CRI: 1–4 mU kg^{-1} min^{-1}

Effects and doses of positive inotropic and vasoconstrictive infusions, with effects at various sympathetic and nonadrenergic receptors.

observed [159]. In general, dobutamine can be advantageous in patients with DCM.

Epinephrine

Epinephrine is a potent α- and β-adrenergic receptor agonist leading to intense peripheral vasoconstriction and increases in HR and contractility, respectively. It dramatically increases myocardial oxygen demand and is highly arrhythmogenic. It can be challenging to discriminate effects (i.e., β-adrenergic effects without α-adrenergic effects) with bolus-dose epinephrine, though dose recommendations exist to target β-adrenergic effects ($0.01\,\mathrm{mg\,kg^{-1}}$ IV) and avoid α-adrenergic effects ($0.1\,\mathrm{mg\,kg^{-1}}$ IV) [161]. In cats, dose-dependent effects of an epinephrine infusion occur between 0.125 and $2.0\,\mu\mathrm{g\,kg^{-1}\,min^{-1}}$ [162], though complete understanding of dose-dependent effects is lacking. With the availability of other, better-understood and lower-risk sympathomimetic drugs for management of hypotension, epinephrine may be a questionable choice for a routine inotropic agent, particularly due to the increase in oxygen demand and potential for arrhythmias. Ultimately and ideally, epinephrine should be limited to use for cardiopulmonary cerebral resuscitation (CPCR) or cardiopulmonary bypass.

Ephedrine

Ephedrine is a noncatecholamine sympathomimetic that acts both directly and indirectly (by causing norepinephrine release) at adrenergic receptors, though the effects are not as strong [163]. Ephedrine is one of the few inotropic/vasopressive agents that can be delivered by bolus injection, rather than by infusion, as the half-life for activity is longer than other sympathomimetic drugs. Typical bolus dose is $0.02–0.05\,\mathrm{mg\,kg^{-1}}$ IV [164] but higher doses ($0.2\,\mathrm{mg\,kg^{-1}}$ IV) have been used. Ephedrine bolus leads to increases in BP, cardiac index, and oxygen delivery in dogs anesthetized with isoflurane [165]. Onset time is rapid, and the duration of the increase in BP is shorter than that of the increase in CO. Unfortunately, repeated doses of ephedrine have diminishing returns, as norepinephrine stores are rapidly depleted [165]. As such, it is useful for short-term treatment of hypotension [166].

Vasopressin

Vasopressin (antidiuretic hormone, ADH) is an exception to the sympathomimetics, as it is a nonadrenergic hormone that participates in endogenous BP control and can be delivered exogenously for management of hypotension. Vasopressin acts via the vasopressin-1 (V1) endothelial receptor, increasing SVR and BP, but has no effect on HR, myocardial contractility, or CO [161]. Indirectly, the increase in SVR can lead to a decrease in CO and bradycardia at higher doses [7]. Actions at the vasopressin-2 (V2) receptor are responsible for the renal effects [163]. Since it is not a catecholamine, it is not arrhythmogenic, a significant advantage over other drugs in this group. Vasopressin has been shown to be comparable to phenylephrine for the treatment of hypotension in an endotoxic shock model [164]. Although intentionally titrated vasoconstriction can be an important strategy for treatment of refractory hypotension, high levels of SVR may potentially decrease CO and oxygen delivery, particularly in patients with heart disease (e.g., DCM) for which increases in afterload can be severely detrimental [167].

Norepinephrine

Norepinephrine is the major endogenous SNS neurotransmitter [168], and has both α- and β-adrenergic effects, although, in practice, the α_1-adrenergic receptor effect predominates, leading to its use primarily as a vasoconstrictor. At very low doses (approximately $0.025\,\mu\mathrm{g\,kg^{-1}\,min^{-1}}$), there is evidence that β_1 effects predominate, which can be beneficial in increasing HR and CO [169]. At higher doses in dogs ($0.1–0.8\,\mu\mathrm{g\,kg^{-1}\,min^{-1}}$), norepinephrine has shown dose-dependent increases in SAP, MAP, DAP, and resultant decreases in HR [170].

Phenylephrine

Phenylephrine is a pure α_1-adrenergic receptor agonist with no β_2-receptor activity, which leads to dose-dependent increases in SVR, and carries the benefits and drawbacks of pure vasoconstrictors as described previously [168]. Phenylephrine has been evaluated both in healthy cats [171] and for treatment of hypotension in cats with naturally existing hypertrophic obstructive cardiomyopathy (HOCM) [172]. Phenylephrine increases SVR and arterial BP, but does not increase HR, cardiac index, or calculated oxygen delivery; for treatment of isoflurane-induced hypotension via an increase in CO, dopamine would be a superior choice to phenylephrine, as dopamine increased CO and phenylephrine did not. However, if increases in SVR and BP are desired without increases in HR, phenylephrine remains a clinically useful option.

Patient Monitoring and Support

Fluid Therapy

As decreases in cardiovascular function and CO are inevitable effects of anesthetics, fluid therapy is recommended to maintain perfusion despite cardiovascular depression. Patients who present with compensated heart disease with no overt clinical signs may tolerate typical rates of IV fluids (balanced electrolyte solutions) during anesthesia, usually in the range of 3–5 $ml\,kg^{-1}\,h^{-1}$. Patients with evidence of noncompensated cardiovascular disease are often at risk for failure due to poor cardiac function or the cascade of neurohormonal mechanisms that leads to an increase in circulating blood volume such as activation of the renin–aldosterone–angiotensin system (RAAS) and increased secretion of ADH. Patients with a history of heart failure and/or chronic volume overload (mitral, tricuspid, and aortic valve insufficiency, left-to-right shunts including patent ductus arteriosus [PDA], and ventricular septal defects [VSDs]) may be less likely to tolerate high fluid rates during surgery; lower fluid rates should be used in these patients. Usually, 2–3 $ml\,kg^{-1}\,h^{-1}$ is sufficient to meet maintenance metabolic needs, but not increasing blood volume and risk precipitating heart failure. Furosemide may be used for its diuretic effects if the patient receives an excessive amount of IV crystalloid solution. The administration of synthetic colloids (i.e., hetastarch, pentastarch, dextran, and hemoglobin glutamer-200) is often avoided in patients with cardiac disease, as colloids can sustain plasma volume for significantly longer periods and are more difficult to treat/reverse with diuretics.

Patient Preoxygenation

Most anesthetic premedicants and induction agents are respiratory depressants; the most significant of which are the opioids, propofol, alfaxalone, and inhaled anesthetic agents. Ketamine is considered a minimal respiratory depressant as is etomidate [173]. The onset of respiratory depression can be very rapid, which can result in patient desaturation and cyanosis. The alveolar partial pressure of oxygen (PAO_2) is predicted by the alveolar gas equation (Table 1.6).

The following alveolar gas equations represent examples of differing $PaCO_2$ levels during normoxia (inspired oxygen = 21%):

$$PAO_2 = FiO_2\left(Patm - PH_2O\right) - PaCO_2 / 0.8 \tag{1.1}$$

$$PAO_2 = 0.21\left(760 - 47\right) - 40 / 0.8 = 99.7\ \text{mmHg} \tag{1.2}$$

$$PAO_2 = 0.21\left(760 - 47\right) - 60 / 0.8 = 74.7\ \text{mmHg} \tag{1.3}$$

and hyperoxemia (inspired oxygen = 40%):

$$PAO_2 = 0.40(760 - 47) - 40 / 0.8 = 235.2 \text{ mmHg} \quad (1.4)$$

$$PAO_2 = 0.40(760 - 47) - 60 / 0.8 = 210.2 \text{ mmHg} \quad (1.5)$$

where FIO_2 refers to the inspired fraction of oxygen, Patm is the atmospheric pressure (in mmHg), PH_2O is the partial pressure of water vapor (in mmHg), and $PaCO_2$ is the arterial partial pressure of carbon dioxide (in mmHg). In animals that are ventilating normally with a $PaCO_2$ of 40 mmHg (Table 1.6, Eq. (1.2)), the PAO_2 is nearly 100 mmHg. This pressure represents the alveolar pressure of oxygen able to diffuse down the oxygen concentration gradient into pulmonary arterial blood.

As patients hypoventilate, $PaCO_2$ increases (in this example, to 60 mmHg), which decreases the PAO_2 and results in clinical hypoxemia when PAO_2 is less than 80 mmHg (Table 1.6, Eq. (1.3)). When providing supplemental oxygen via a tight-fitting face mask (estimated to be a FIO_2 of approximately 40%), PAO_2 is subsequently increased (Table 1.6, Eq. (1.4)), which can blunt the effects of hypoxemia due to hypoventilation (Table 1.6, Eq. (1.5)). Thus, preoxygenation can be a critical component of maintaining a high PAO_2 and arterial partial pressure of oxygen (PaO_2) subsequent to anesthetic-related respiratory depression from premedication through the induction process. The general recommendation is to provide oxygen via a tight-fitting face mask for a minimum of 3 min before anesthetic induction [174]. This can be easily performed, as monitoring equipment (ECG, noninvasive blood pressure [NIBP], capnometry) is placed before induction of anesthesia.

Blood Pressure (BP)

Blood pressure is the most reliable clinical indicator of perfusion, despite the disadvantage that it is not a clear indicator of CO. BP is a standard monitoring tool for all anesthetized patients and has been the standard of care in humans for decades. The ACVAA guidelines on small animal patient monitoring recommend measurement of BP as part of basic patient care during anesthesia [175].

Methods of arterial BP monitoring include both invasive and noninvasive techniques.

Table 1.6 Alveolar and arterial oxygen partial pressure calculations, based on $PaCO_2$ and the alveolar gas equation.

$PaCO_2$ (mmHg)	**30**		**40**		**60**		**90**	
FiO_2 (%)	PAO_2	PaO_2	PAO_2	PaO_2	PAO_2	PaO_2	PAO_2	PaO_2
21	112.2	101.0	99.7	89.8	74.7	67.3	49.7	44.8
30	176.4	159.8	163.9	147.5	138.9	125.0	113.9	102.5
40	247.7	222.9	235.2	211.7	210.2	189.2	185.2	166.7
100	675.5	608.0	663.0	596.7	638.0	574.2	613.0	551.7

Alveolar partial pressure of oxygen is calculated using the alveolar gas equation: $PAO_2 = FiO_2 (P_{atm} - PH_2O) - PaCO_2/0.8$. PAO_2 is the alveolar partial pressure of oxygen. PaO_2 is the arterial partial pressure of oxygen, measured with arterial blood gas analysis. FiO_2 is the fraction of inspired oxygen (21–100%). P_{atm} is the atmospheric barometric pressure specific to the elevation at or above sea level, assumed in the example to be at sea level, where P_{atm} is 7-60 mmHg. PH_2O is the vapor pressure of water, which varies slightly by patient temperature generally assumed to be approximately 47 mmHg. $PaCO_2$ is the patient's current arterial pressure of carbon dioxide, measured on arterial blood gas analysis. $PaCO_2$ divided by 0.8 is respiratory quotient, which is the ratio of CO_2 molecules produced for O_2 molecules consumed in mitochondrial ATP synthesis. The normal alveolar to arterial gradient of oxygen is <10–15 mmHg in room air, and the PaO_2 values calculated in Table 1.5 assume a 105-mmHg difference between alveolar and arterial partial pressures. Refer to Eqs. (1.2)–(1.5) in the body of the text for values.

Noninvasive methods include automated oscillometric BP monitors and manual Doppler BP monitoring. Invasive (or direct) BP monitoring involves the placement of a catheter into a peripheral artery with connection to a fluid-filled pressure transducer system. All techniques have both advantages and disadvantages regarding the ease of placement, frequency and speed of measurement, invasive nature, and technical skill required for measurement and accuracy of measurement.

Invasive Blood Pressure

Invasive blood pressure (IBP) monitoring is the gold standard with which all other forms of BP measurement are compared [176–182]. Direct monitoring is the most accurate BP measurement and offers additional benefits of being a continuous, second-to-second monitor for SAP, DAP, and MAP. Acute changes in the patient's hemodynamic status can be appreciated rapidly, and alterations in the arterial pressure waveform can also provide information about patient status. The placement of an indwelling arterial catheter also allows for arterial blood gas sampling. IBP monitoring has significant drawbacks, including the skill required to place arterial catheters in potentially hypotensive, unstable patients, the requirement for a multiparameter patient monitor with the capability of connecting to a fluid-filled transducer system, the understanding of what causes error in the transducer system, and the need for an ability to troubleshooting of the system [183]. Despite these complexities, IBP monitoring is a mainstay of advanced cardiovascular monitoring.

Noninvasive Blood Pressure

NIBP monitoring includes both automated oscillometric monitoring devices and Doppler ultrasound BP monitoring [184]. Oscillometry uses an automated cuff that is inflated above SAP, occluding arterial blood flow. As cuff pressure is reduced, the arterial pulse begins to generate oscillations in the arterial wall that are transmitted to the cuff. These oscillations increase and then decrease in amplitude as cuff pressure is reduced, and eventually the oscillations are eliminated as blood flow becomes laminar. Although technology and calculation algorithms vary between oscillometric devices, generally, the onset of oscillations represents the SAP, the maximal oscillation amplitude represents MAP, and the cessation of oscillations is DAP. Oscillometry carries the advantage of automation and ease of use. However, oscillometric devices are fraught with error, including inappropriate cuff size. The cuff should be approximately 40% of limb circumference; oversized cuffs lead to inappropriately low readings, and inappropriately small cuffs lead to falsely elevated measurements [184]. Other issues with oscillometric devices include motion artifacts and interference from high HRs or cardiac arrhythmias [185]. Studies comparing the accuracy of oscillometric BP to direct BP found limited agreement with MAP and DAP in anesthetized dogs with 67% and 95% of readings within 10 and 20 mmHg of invasive pressure values, respectively [184]. Another study found poor correlation such that a 25-mmHg bias was identified between invasive and oscillometric pressure in anesthetized cats [177]. Oscillometric BP devices also carry the disadvantages of slow performance compared to continuous arterial catheters.

Doppler BP devices use a BP cuff that is manually inflated with a sphygmomanometer above SAP. A Doppler crystal is placed over a peripheral artery, and blood flow is audibly demonstrated with appropriate Doppler sound. When inflation of the cuff occludes flow, the Doppler signal is lost. As the cuff is manually deflated, blood flow begins to pass through the cuff and is again audible via the Doppler crystal. This is generally interpreted as the peak pressure or SAP. Blood pressure measured with the aid of a Doppler crystal can be checked manually more frequently than oscillometric devices and are simple to use. Furthermore, a Doppler crystal placed over a peripheral artery provides the anesthetist with an audible signal for blood flow, which can be a strong comfort for those moments in which the anesthetist's attention cannot be on the patient or patient monitor. Doppler crystal placement also allows for a second assessment of BP should an arterial catheter fail. Disadvantages of Doppler crystals include that they are somewhat fragile, require more skill for placement to obtain an audible signal, and may not accurately predict SAP. For example, multiple studies have evaluated the assessment of SAP with Doppler NIBP compared to IBP [182, 183, 186]. In cats, poor agreement was found between invasive SAP and Doppler BPs, such that the Doppler underestimated SAP by approximately 14 mmHg [168, 169, 175] to 25 mmHg [182, 183]. Doppler BP measurement was not recommended when accuracy is desired. However, in rabbits, direct SAP was found to have good agreement with Doppler BP [185]. Despite the potential inaccuracy of NIBP compared to IBP, NIBP can help identify relative changes, which may help the anesthetist choose intervention options.

Electrocardiography

ECG allows analysis of the cardiac rhythm. Understanding the components of the cardiac rhythm and how it relates to mechanical function of the heart helps the anesthetist to analyze the rhythm for changes that would indicate abnormalities. These abnormalities might imply that there is asynchrony in mechanical heart function and rhythm correction may improve mechanical function, CO, and perfusion. Although ECG monitoring does not "prove the patient is alive," as there can be dissociation between the electrical and mechanical activity (termed pulseless electrical activity, PEA), it is nevertheless a basic requirement of anesthetized patient monitoring.

Pulse Oximetry

Saturation of hemoglobin in arterial blood is an important component of the oxygen content (CaO_2) equation:

$$CaO_2 = \left(1.3 \times [Hb] \times \frac{SaO_2}{100}\right) + (0.003 \times PaO_2) \tag{1.6}$$

where the constant 1.3 is the amount of oxygen (ml at 1 atm) bound by 1 g of hemoglobin, [Hb] is the hemoglobin concentration, SaO_2 is the hemoglobin saturation with O_2, the constant 0.003 is the amount of O_2 dissolved in plasma, and PaO_2 is the arterial partial pressure of O_2. As most of the O_2 is carried in the hemoglobin molecule, the degree to which hemoglobin is saturated with oxygenated blood is a critical variable in oxygen delivery. The pulse oximeter is a simple tool that estimates the oxygen saturation of arterial blood ($SaO_2 \sim SpO_2$). Hemoglobin saturation of approximately 90% is correlated with a PaO_2 of approximately 60 mmHg, well into the hypoxic range. Therefore, a hemoglobin saturation of >93–94% is required to ensure normoxia. Many variables can interfere with the ability of the pulse oximeter to provide an accurate arterial saturation (Table 1.7) [187].

Core Body Temperature

Hypothermia has varying effects based on the amount of body temperature loss [2]. Essentially,

Table 1.7 Pulse oximetry (SpO_2): sources of error.

Motion artifact
Tissue thickness
Tissue hypoperfusion/hypotension
Vasoconstriction
Hypothermia
Tissue pigment
Methemoglobinemia (SpO_2 values approach 85% when MetHgb is approximately 30%)
Carboxyhemoglobinemia (SpO_2 values falsely elevated)
Intravenous dye injections (indocyanine green, methylene blue)
Ambient light at 660 and 920 nm wavelength(s)
Severe anemia (Hb < $5\,g\,dl^{-1}$)

all patients will become hypothermic to some degree because of premedication and induction of anesthesia, unless active heat support is provided. Causes of hypothermia include, but are not limited to, opioid-, phenothiazine-, and alpha-2-adrenergic-receptor agonist-mediated changes in thermoregulation, high surface area to body mass ratio, high cold-compressed O_2 flow rates, open body cavities, cold surfaces, room-temperature IV fluids, cold scrub solutions, and body cavity lavage (especially orogastric lavage with fluids below body temperature). Mechanisms for heat loss include evaporation, conduction, convection, and heat loss from respiration and radiant heat loss [186]. Anesthetized patients also have decreased heat production due to central depression and inability to shiver in response to hypothermia. It is far easier to prevent than it is to treat hypothermia, as the peripheral vasoconstrictive effects of hypothermia make external rewarming difficult and inefficient. Consideration of these variables for an individual patient or procedure will help the anesthetist generate a robust heat loss prevention or rewarming plan.

The physiologic effects of hypothermia vary with severity and include catecholamine release, decreased cerebral metabolic rate of O_2 consumption and intracranial pressure, and altered electroencephalogram and arterial blood gas results [188, 189]. At moderate levels, hypothermia decreases inhalant requirements, reduces concentrations of inhalant required to produce apnea, decreases CO and BP, and increases SVR. In addition, moderate hypothermia results in bradycardia, prolonged clotting times, decreased drug metabolism, prolonged nerve conduction and muscle contraction, and a left shift of the oxygen–hemoglobin dissociation curve (which favors hemoglobin loading) [190]. With these profound physiologic changes, it is clear that body temperature should be controlled in any anesthetized patient and especially in one who may have preexisting cardiovascular compromise, as they may lack the reserves to compensate.

Capnometry and Ventilation

Capnometry is the assessment of exhaled CO_2 as an indicator of ventilatory adequacy. Capnometry refers to the measurement of end-exhalation (end-tidal) CO_2; a capnograph provides a visual waveform display of the measurement of CO_2 over time. However, the term capnography is often used to imply all these components. Hypoventilation is defined by an increase in the $PaCO_2$ with a subsequent increase in end-tidal CO_2 levels. Hypoventilation leads to respiratory acidosis and should be avoided in patients with cardiac disease, as ideal cardiac function occurs at normal blood pH; acute respiratory acidosis has been shown to increase HR and CO but decrease myocardial contractility and SVR [191]. Hypercapnia increases catecholamine release [192, 193] and can result in tachyarrhythmias from the combination of acidosis, electrolyte changes due to acidosis, and CO_2-mediated increases in catecholamine release [194, 195]. It is possible to roughly estimate the change in pH on the basis of the increase in $PaCO_2$; for every approximately 10 mmHg acute increase in $PaCO_2$, arterial pH will decrease by approximately 0.1 pH unit [196].

Assisted or controlled ventilation can be helpful in maintaining normoventilation, to optimize oxygenation (SpO_2 or PaO_2) and improve inhaled anesthetic depth. Mechanical ventilation can be provided either with a controlled mechanical ventilator or with intermittent assisted manual ventilation ("bagging"). It is nearly impossible to provide the same consistency, tidal volume, respiratory rate, peak inspiratory pressure, and duration of inspiration with manual ventilation as compared to mechanical ventilation, and the use of mechanical ventilators is strongly recommended to maintain this consistency and allow the anesthetist to attend to other tasks.

However, mechanical ventilation can and very often will decrease BP by one of three mechanisms [197]. First, tidal volume via mechanical ventilation is very likely to be larger than that of a spontaneously taken breath. Therefore, mechanical ventilation represents an increase in anesthetic delivery via a larger number of volatile inhaled anesthetic molecules delivered within a larger tidal volume. Inhaled anesthetics subsequently cause dose-dependent decreases in BP, mediated by decreases in myocardial contractility and SVR. Second, increases in intrathoracic pressure during positive pressure ventilation decrease venous return (i.e., preload), leading to reduced SV, CO, and BP. The effects on CO are more pronounced with more frequent respiratory rates, longer inspiratory phase duration, and larger tidal volumes [198]. Finally, high $PaCO_2$ can increase sympathetic tone and improve BP, an effect that is reduced when patients are ventilated to a normal or even low end-tidal CO_2 [199, 200].

Arterial Blood Gases

Arterial blood gas analysis is a useful direct measurement of PaO_2 and $PaCO_2$ to evaluate pulmonary function and quality of ventilation. Serial monitoring of arterial blood gases helps the anesthetist to better direct ventilatory adjustments to maintain oxygenation and normal CO_2 levels. The availability of arterial catheterization allows for continuous IBP monitoring, as well as serial blood sampling for clinical pathology. Normal values for arterial blood gas values are presented in Table 1.6.

Central Venous Pressure (CVP)

Central venous pressure is the intraluminal pressure measured in the intrathoracic vena cava immediately outside the right atrium [201, 202]. Historically, it has been used as an indicator of right ventricular preload and overall patient intravascular volume status [203], as well as in assessment of right heart function and critical patient care monitoring [204]. However, right ventricular preload is truly defined by the difference between the intracardiac (i.e., right ventricular) and extracardiac transmural pressure gradient [195]. A variety of factors can reduce preload but lead to an increase in measured CVP, which may lead the clinician to erroneously interpret an increase in preload. These include changes in intrathoracic pressure (changes in stage of ventilation, pleural effusion, and abdominal hypertension) and blood volume or cardiac arrhythmias. Decreases in right ventricular compliance also can increase CVP, as end-diastolic filling pressures can be elevated with a "stiff" ventricle, pericardial disease, or pericardial tamponade. Ultimately, CVP represents the balance between volume return to the heart and cardiac function. There are many excellent, in-depth published reviews of CVP monitoring [201–204]. Although CVP monitoring requires a complete understanding of these variables and the ability to trend values over time, it can be a valuable tool in monitoring patients under anesthesia in select cases.

Arterial Pulse Pressure Variation (PPV)

Arterial PPV is a dynamic measurement and is defined as the difference between the maximum and minimum arterial pulse pressure during one mechanically ventilated breath [205]. While oscillometric techniques of measurement are under development, PPV typically requires arterial catheterization and specialized monitoring equipment. PPV was originally manually calculated, and expressed as percentage of the ratio of the difference between the maximal and minimal values of pulse pressure over the mean of these two values and expressed as a percentage [206]:

$$PPV\% = \left(PP_{max} - PP_{min}\right) / \left(\left[PP_{max} + PP_{min}\right] / 2\right) \tag{1.7}$$

PPV is an accurate predictor of fluid responsiveness in critically ill human patients [207–209] and in dogs [210], and is superior to CVP as a predictor of fluid responsiveness during open-abdomen surgical procedures in humans [211] and to pneumoperitoneum in dogs [212]. While PPV variation requires more study in veterinary medicine, it has potential to provide more continuous and dynamic monitoring of patient volume status. Readers are referred to additional texts for more complete information on equipment and tools to monitor fluid responsiveness as well as other cardiac parameters [2, 213].

Anesthetic and Pharmacologic Recommendations for Specific Cardiac Diseases

General Preanesthetic Evaluation

A common misconception is that most heart murmurs do not definitively require complete cardiac evaluation before anesthesia is planned, and that all patients with heart disease must be managed similarly when anesthetized. As with any anesthetic patient, patients with underlying cardiac disease should be evaluated with a complete history (detailing both the long- and short-term changes in underlying disease), PE, and minimum database of blood work/urinalysis relevant for their signalment. In addition, patients with cardiac disease should be evaluated with thoracic radiographs, ECG, BP, and echocardiogram, which are aimed at not only documenting presence of disease, but also assessing the severity of disease and possible response to previous treatments. As one of the main goals of perianesthetic management is maintenance of homeostasis, especially perfusion and oxygen delivery, preanesthetic cardiac evaluation should include assessments for cardiac pump function.

Valvular Heart Disease

Introduction

Valvular heart disease accounts for over 50% of congenital heart disease in dogs; chronic AV valvular disease is the most common cardiac disease in dogs, whereas mitral valve insufficiency is in the top three causes of cardiac disease in cats [214]. The prevalence of valvular disease in small animals necessitates a complete understanding of these comorbidities and how they affect and dictate the perianesthetic plan.

Degenerative Mitral Valve Disease (dMVD)

Incidence and Pathophysiology

Degenerative mitral valve disease is the most common cardiac disease in dogs, found in as much as 30% of the geriatric canine population [215]. dMVD is also referred to as myxomatous mitral valve degeneration, endocardiosis, degenerative valvular disease, and myxomatous degeneration; all terms describe the same constellation of pathophysiologic and clinical signs. In 2009, the American College of Veterinary Internal Medicine published a consensus for the diagnosis and treatment of myxomatous mitral valve disease in dogs, and the guidelines were updated in 2019 [216]. In this consensus, myxomatous mitral valve disease was categorized into stages A, B (B1, B2), C, and D:

Stage A

- Dogs at high risk of developing disease, but have no identifiable structural disease, and do not currently have a heart murmur.

Stage B

- Dogs with a heart murmur with structurally identifiable disease, but have never developed clinical signs of heart failure. This stage is divided into stages B1 and B2.
  - Stage B1: Dogs with no clinical signs, with no radiographic/echocardiographic evidence of disease, but have a heart murmur. Treatment is not warranted.
  - Stage B2: Asymptomatic dogs with more advanced disease that meet clinical criteria for starting treatment to delay progression of disease.

Stage C

- Dogs with current or past evidence of congestive heart failure (CHF), which requires hospitalization or outpatient treatment.

Stage D

- Dogs with ongoing, end-stage heart failure and are refractory to treatment. Advanced and specialized treatment is required, up to and including valve replacement.

dMVD is grossly seen as an idiopathic development of nodular irregularities on the free edge of mitral valve leaflets. These nodules consist of deposition of mucopolysaccharides in the layers of the valve leaflet, which can increase in size and number over time. Pathophysiology of dMVD may also include distortion of the chordae tendineae such that they lengthen and/or thicken [217]. When valve changes are severe, this leads to curling of the valve leaflet and subsequent AV valve incompetence. The valve may degenerate to the point at which valve leaflets can prolapse into the left atrium. When valvular changes are sufficient that leaflets do not oppose one another during ventricular systole, it results in regurgitant flow of blood into the left atrium. Mitral valve regurgitation may be trivial or severe, and volume of regurgitation is dictated by the size of the space between the valve leaflets, the pressure gradient between ventricle and atria, and the duration of systole [218]. Mitral regurgitation leads to a volume overload on the left atrium, as pulmonary venous return is complemented by regurgitant flow. CO suffers as regurgitant flow increases, and the body compensates with renal, neurohormonal, and cardiac remodeling (left ventricular eccentric hypertrophy). High atrial pressures due to volume overload lead to atrial dilation, as well as increases in pulmonary vein pressures and congestion of pulmonary venous flow, which will eventually lead to pulmonary edema. CHF is the result of chronic volume overload to the left atrium and pulmonary veins with eventual failure of adaptive mechanisms.

Physical Examination Findings

Dogs may present with lethargy, cough, exercise intolerance, weight loss, respiratory difficulty, or collapse [219]. Patients may also present with other complaints, and a murmur may be auscultated in a patient with no previous history of cardiac disease. It is these patients who often require a more cautious approach to evaluation and anesthesia planning; a lack of clinical signs may provide a false sense of security regarding potential anesthetic complications. The classic heart murmur for dMVD is a holosystolic murmur, loudest over the left apex of the heart. The intensity of the murmur tends to be consistent over the duration of systole, with no increase or decrease in the loudness of the murmur. Often, the second heart sound is inaudible. The murmur intensity is not correlated with the severity of regurgitant flow, but, in general, louder murmurs indicate worse regurgitation. Prolapse of the mitral valve may result in a mid-systolic click.

Anesthetic Management

Anesthetic management can cover the spectrum from patients with fully compensated, nonclinical disease to those at high risk for heart failure. No consensus exists regarding the management of either end of this spectrum. Patients with stable, compensated disease with no left atrial enlargement and no clinical signs of pulmonary edema or heart failure generally do not require intensive management. As a portion of left ventricular ejection regurgitates into the left atrium, CO is compromised, and the patient with dMVD is thought to compensate for this with increases in HR [215]. Normal to high-normal HRs are recommended for any signalment. Therefore, it is optimal to consider anticholinergics in the anesthesia plan, particularly if opioids are to be administered. Opioids are considered extremely safe for a patient with dMVD, as the cardiovascular effects are primarily limited to bradycardia, which is easily treated or prevented with the use of anticholinergics. Hypothermia should be avoided by using supplemental heat support to avoid hypothermia-related bradycardia. Stable patients should tolerate inductions with ketamine and diazepam/midazolam. Alternatively, they should tolerate the dose-dependent vasodilation with propofol or alfaxalone inductions; however, the induction agent dose should be minimized using preanesthetic sedatives and/or combining induction agents with benzodiazepines and/or opioids during induction. The severe negative inotropic effects and mild to moderate vasodilation associated with inhaled anesthetics can be minimized by additional use of local, regional, or systemic sedatives and analgesics. Opioids are well suited for this purpose. Alpha-2-adrenergic receptor agonists should be used with great caution due to the increase in afterload and the potential for increased regurgitant flow, as well as severe decreases in HR and CO.

Unstable patients, such as those at significant risk for onset of heart failure or with a previous history of heart failure, those with arrhythmias, or those with preexisting cardiovascular compromise, must be handled with extreme caution. Pre-induction stabilization of heart failure, hypotension, and arrhythmias must be attempted. Complete cardiac evaluation (PE, thoracic radiographs, ECG, BP, and echocardiogram) is optimal. Anesthetic management includes all efforts made to minimize or mitigate the cardiovascular compromise due to inhaled anesthetics and reliance on balanced anesthesia. As stated previously, alpha-2-adrenergic receptor agonists are not recommended in most cases. Sedation with opioids and benzodiazepines is useful, as they have minimal effects on cardiovascular function; opioid-mediated bradycardia can be minimized or prevented with anticholinergics. Although optimal sedation is ideal, oftentimes, good sedation must be sacrificed in the name of cardiovascular stability, as induction of anesthesia is approached. Midazolam followed quickly by etomidate is a good induction choice because both have minimal to no cardiovascular side effects. Fentanyl and midazolam may also be used for induction, provided opioid-associated bradycardias (and respiratory depression) are controlled and the patient is sufficiently sedated beforehand or is quite compromised. Alternatively, some patients may require induction with propofol despite the risk of dose-dependent vasodilation and hypotension. In these cases, alfaxalone may be a better choice for induction in unstable patients, as it has greater cardiovascular stability when compared to propofol [94, 115, 118]. In these situations, reducing the dose of propofol with pre-induction sedation and/or combining propofol with one (i.e., midazolam) or two (i.e., midazolam/fentanyl) additional induction drugs can minimize propofol dosage. Inhaled anesthetic concentration should similarly be minimized with additional local, regional, or systemic analgesics and sedatives. Monitoring in patients with severe mitral valve disease should include either Doppler NIBP or IBP monitoring.

Mitral Valve Stenosis (MVS)

Incidence and Pathophysiology

Mitral valve stenosis is a rare finding in dogs, with only 12 reported cases in a 10-year period [220] and 12 diagnosed cases in a cohort of 1779 patient records [221]. Stenotic lesions may involve the valve annulus, leaflets, chordae tendineae, or papillary muscles and present as a valvular or supravalvular lesion [222]. The heart murmur associated with MVS is a mid-diastolic low-frequency murmur and possibly a split-second heart sound (S2). The stenotic lesion creates a pressure gradient across the valve and leads to an increase in left atrial pressure, which is transmitted to the pulmonary vasculature and can lead to pulmonary edema with severe stenosis [214]. Diagnosis of MVS may be made only when a patient presents with left heart failure and the defect is identified with echocardiography. The treatment for MVS is frequently medical, as surgical options are extremely high risk and should only be considered when all alternatives have been exhausted. The goal of medical intervention is to manage signs of left-sided heart failure and to decrease left atrial pressure and signs of left heart failure with diuretics and angiotensin-converting enzyme (ACE) inhibitors. Sodium restriction is recommended.

Additional treatment may be required for supraventricular arrhythmias such as atrial fibrillation or supraventricular tachycardia (SVT).

Anesthetic Management

Anesthetic management largely depends on the severity of clinical presentation [223, 224]. The anesthetic goal is to prevent any situation in which CO is significantly impaired or the patient is put at risk for the development of pulmonary edema. With MVS, CO can be decreased by multiple mechanisms. For example, as MVS worsens in severity, ventricular filling depends increasingly on diastolic filling time and right atrial pressure. Tachycardia or tachyarrhythmias will decrease diastolic filling time and worsen ventricular filling and subsequently CO. Loss of association between atrial depolarization or the atrial kick boosting end-diastolic volume (10–30% of end-diastolic volume) and ventricular contraction/ejection will worsen CO. Therefore, arrhythmias affecting AV coordination should be treated rapidly in these cases. Atrial fibrillation and SVT can develop while anesthetized and the ECG should be evaluated before and through anesthetic induction. Acute vasodilation and decreases in atrial preload may worsen ventricular filling, as the normal response to acute hypotension is tachycardia. Finally, the pressure overload to the pulmonary vasculature from MVS can precipitate pulmonary edema [225]. Avoidance of increases in blood volume that can precipitate CHF is strongly recommended.

Patients with mild MVS can likely be managed with any anesthetic plan except for high dosages of ketamine and tiletamine. Both dissociative agents can increase catecholamine release, which increases sympathetic tone, potentially leading to tachycardia and increases in myocardial contractility. If diastolic filling time decreases significantly, CO can drop precipitously. Similarly, tachycardia from patient stress, anxiety, and pain can decrease CO. ACE inhibitors should be withheld for 24 h to reduce the potential for hypotension (see the section titled "Systemic Hypertension"). Moderate to profound preanesthetic sedation is optimal to prevent tachycardia. Opioids and benzodiazepines are attractive options, as they do not significantly decrease HR, contractility, or vascular tone. While some opioids are good sedatives, benzodiazepines are inconsistent sedatives in small animals and can precipitate mild dysphoria or excitement in dogs, and undesirable behavioral changes including potential aggression in cats [65, 67]. Anticholinergic agents are controversial in that they can precipitate tachycardia. However, anticholinergics can be indicated if there is a preexisting bradycardia or second-degree AV block. Patients with mild disease can likely tolerate the vasodilation associated with propofol for induction, but combination with an opioid (propofol–fentanyl) or benzodiazepine (propofol–midazolam) is recommended to reduce the total dosage of propofol. As mentioned in the earlier text, alfaxalone may provide increased cardiovascular stability compared to propofol. If patients have severe disease with significant cardiovascular compromise, anesthetic induction can be achieved with etomidate or fentanyl in combination with a benzodiazepine. Patient monitoring with MVS also depends on their degree of disease and anticipated complications. Patients with mild disease can be monitored as for any patient. Patients with advanced disease may require IBP monitoring, arterial blood gas assessment to evaluate pulmonary function, and CVP/PPV measurement. Patients with severe disease may warrant referral to specialty centers for consultations with veterinary cardiologists and anesthesiologists for management.

Tricuspid Valve Stenosis (TVS)

Incidence and Pathophysiology

Tricuspid valve stenosis as an independent finding is rare in small animals, and tricuspid valve incompetence is far more often due to tricuspid valve dysplasia or is the result of underlying cardiac disease. Like MVS, it may result from abnormalities of the annulus, valve leaflets, or papillary muscles. Labradors or breeds at risk for AV valve disease such as Newfoundlands and Bull Terriers may be at higher risk [167].

Anesthetic Management

Should TVS be identified as an isolated finding, recommendations for anesthetic management are the same as MVS. Given the rarity of isolated TVS, other causes for tricuspid valve incompetence must be investigated in patients who have suspicion of tricuspid valve disease.

Aortic Stenosis

Incidence and Pathophysiology

Aortic stenosis is the most common congenital cardiac disease of large breed dogs such as Boxers, Great Danes, Rottweilers, Golden Retrievers, German Shepherds, English Bulldogs, and Bouvier des Flandres, and has been described as heritable in Newfoundlands [214]. AS can be due to valvular, supravalvular, and subvalvular lesions (SAS); however, SAS is the most common finding in dogs representing more than 95% of lesions identified. The site of SAS is the left ventricular outflow tract (LVOT), which comprises the membranous and muscular portions of the basilar interventricular septum, the craniolateral left ventricular free wall, and the anterior mitral valve leaflet.

Aortic stenosis can be described as fixed or dynamic. Fixed SAS is due to an anatomic abnormality creating the stenotic lesion; the severity of the obstruction does not change with rate or velocity of flow through the area. Fixed SAS has been graded in cadavers depending on the anatomic findings. For example, Grade 1 has minor changes (endothelial nodules) in the subaortic endocardial surface, Grade 2 has a narrow fibrous band around part of the LVOT, and Grade 3 has a complete band of tissue surrounding the entire LVOT [226]. Dynamic SAS is an obstruction in the LVOT that changes based on the flow rate through the subaortic outflow tract. Increases in HR or cardiac contractility lead to a decrease in intraluminal pressure (based on the Bernoulli principle) and an increase in the degree of LVOT obstruction (LVOTO). Dynamic SAS is most identified in HCM and can be referred to as hypertrophic obstructive cardiomyopathy (HOCM).

The principal hemodynamic consequence of outflow tract obstruction is an increase in resistance to systolic ejection of blood from the ventricle, thereby decreasing flow through the outflow tract, increasing pressure across the stenosis, or both [227]. Left ventricular pressure is increased and results in compensatory concentric hypertrophy to maintain left ventricular output. Blood ejection through the stenotic area results in turbulence during systole and a resultant systolic murmur, typically described as an ejection murmur that increases and then decreases (crescendo–decrescendo) [228]. SAS and LVOTO along with the left ventricular hypertrophy typically do not lead to left-sided heart failure. However, left ventricular hypertrophy, a decrease in capillary density, and increased wall tension predispose to myocardial ischemia. Patients who develop this pathophysiology are at risk for syncope, ventricular arrhythmias, and sudden death, although it is unclear which of these is the definitive cause of death. Another possible explanation for sudden death is exercise-induced increases in left ventricular pressure (in addition to pathologically high resting left ventricular pressure) and activation of ventricular mechanoreceptors that lead to vasodilation and bradycardia; the Bezold–Jarisch reflex [224]. Aortic valve leaflet damage from high-velocity regurgitant jet flow can predispose the valves to bacterial endocarditis associated with bacterial shower from surgical or dental procedures or from concurrent noncardiac infection-causing bacteremia. Prophylactic antibiotics are recommended for all anesthetized procedures to minimize the risk of endocarditis.

Anesthetic Management

Anesthetic management in patients with SAS can become very complicated and requires intensive monitoring and antiarrhythmic treatments to maintain normal ventricular filling and optimal CO. Patients should remain in a normal sinus rhythm without sinus tachycardia or bradycardia, and one should be prepared to treat ventricular ectopy or atrial fibrillation. For example, left ventricular CO is dependent on the organization of atrial and ventricular contraction. Thus, AV blocks or atrial fibrillation will lead to loss of the atrial kick and reduction of left ventricular end-diastolic volume. Sinus tachycardia prevents diastolic filling time and should be avoided. Sinus bradycardia leads to poor CO and hypotension, subsequently leading to poor coronary and myocardial perfusion in a thickened left ventricle. Thus, HR should be kept in the normal range to prevent decreased tissue perfusion. Ventricular premature complexes (VPCs) cause contraction before complete ventricular filling and lead to a decrease in CO. Prompt treatment of ventricular ectopy is important, as the presence of ventricular rhythms can be a risk factor for sudden death [229].

Premedication in patients with moderate to severe AS should provide adequate sedation/analgesia to prevent anxiety, pain, or stress-related tachyarrhythmias. Anticholinergic agents are indicated to prevent bradycardia and AV blocks. The administration of acepromazine is controversial due to long-acting vasodilation but may be tolerated in the minimally affected patient if anxiety is present and tranquilization is required. Anesthetic drugs that should be used extremely cautiously (if at all) in AS include high-dose dissociative anesthetics (ketamine and tiletamine) and alpha-2-adrenergic receptor agonists (xylazine, medetomidine, and dexmedetomidine). High-dose anticholinergic agents are controversial in that it is difficult to predict the maximum HR a patient may develop in response to a typical dose of anticholinergic. It is worth considering titrating lower doses of anticholinergic agents for patients developing sinus bradycardia and assessing the response to low doses, rather than risk inducing tachyarrhythmias with standard or high doses of atropine or glycopyrrolate. Anesthetic induction can be accomplished with propofol, alfaxalone, etomidate, or opioid–benzodiazepine combinations.

Pulmonic Stenosis (PS)

Incidence and Pathophysiology

Pulmonic stenosis is rarely identified in cats but is the third most common cardiac defect identified in dogs [230]. Pulmonic valvular stenosis is the most common abnormality, with supravalvular and subvalvular stenosis being less common. Pulmonic stenosis is commonly identified as a sole lesion in dogs but can be identified in combination with other cardiac abnormalities such as tetralogy of Fallot (TOF). It is heritable in Beagles and Keeshonds, and a variety of breeds have increased risk for PS, including English Bulldogs, Cocker Spaniels, Mastiffs, Samoyeds, Miniature Schnauzers, Chihuahuas, and Chow Chows [230].

Pulmonic stenosis is due to variable congenital deformations and fusion of pulmonic valve leaflets. The degree of anatomical change and severity of pulmonary outflow tract obstruction are graded as either Grade 1 with minimal to mild fusion and trivial to mild outflow obstruction or Grade 2 that has moderate to severe valve deformation and fusion, with severe outflow obstruction [231]. Severe obstruction leads to poststenotic main pulmonary artery dilation in response to the turbulent blood flow downstream from the affected valve. The primary pathophysiologic hemodynamic effect of PS is an increase in resistance to right ventricular systolic ejection, leading to increased right ventricular pressure. This pressure overload leads to concentric hypertrophy of the right ventricle as a compensatory response, thereby returning right ventricular output to normal or near normal. The degree of pressure overload is related to the pressure gradient across the pulmonic valve and is correlated with disease severity. Right ventricular hypertrophy decreases right ventricular compliance, reduces ventricular filling, and leads to an increase in right atrial pressure. This mechanism also underlies the tricuspid regurgitation in patients with tricuspid dysplasia (whether preexisting or because of change in right ventricular size), which can result in right heart failure, jugular distension/pulsations, ascites, and pleural effusion.

Anesthetic Management

Definitive anesthetic recommendations for mild PS are lacking, but patients with clinically insignificant PS can likely be anesthetized with any technique. Intravenous crystalloid administration during anesthesia should be limited (2–5 ml kg^{-1} h^{-1}), and synthetic colloids should be avoided, as volume overload and right heart failure could be a concern, particularly in patients with concurrent tricuspid dysplasia. Patients with severe PS should be treated cautiously, and anesthetic management should be designed to minimize cardiovascular depression. Alpha-2-adrenergic receptor agonists are contraindicated due to the significant increase in right atrial pressure. Acepromazine is controversial due to the long lasting, irreversible vasodilation, hypotension, and reduced right atrial preload. However, opioids for patient analgesia and sedation as well as anticholinergics to prevent or treat opioid-associated bradycardia are recommended. Induction agents that preserve cardiac function and CO are preferred; combinations of etomidate or fentanyl with benzodiazepines have minimal cardiovascular depression, provided patients do not become bradycardic. Dissociative anesthetics are controversial and may be contraindicated in severe PS due to increases in SVR. Inhaled anesthetic doses should be minimized by opioid infusions to minimize vasodilation and significant decreases in contractility. Local and regional anesthetic techniques should be employed to reduce systemic and inhaled anesthetic requirements. Monitoring should consist of standard ECG, SpO_2, temperature, and capnography, as well as IBP management to allow observation in minute-to-minute changes in patient status.

Congenital Cardiac Disease

Congenital cardiac defects can be grouped according to their pathophysiologic mechanisms [232]. The most common examples include those with left-to-right shunting of blood and volume overload (PDA and VSD), pressure overload (PS and SAS), and those which present for cyanosis (TOF, PDA, and VSD with shunt reversal [right-to-left]).

Patent Ductus Arteriosus

Incidence and Pathophysiology

Patent ductus arteriosus is one of the most common congenital abnormalities identified in dogs but is rare in cats. Predisposed breeds include the Chihuahua, Bichon Frise, Collie, Cocker Spaniel, Keeshond, Maltese, Miniature Poodle, Pomeranian, and Yorkshire Terrier, among others [233]. The defect is genetic in the Miniature Poodle. The ductus arteriosus is a fetal structure that allows shunting of blood (80–90% of total flow) from the pulmonary artery to the aorta necessary to avoid blood flow through the high vascular resistance of the fetal lungs. Increases in oxygen tension in the ductus with neonatal ventilation should lead to constriction of the ductus and closure within the first week of life [234]. A PDA is the persistence of this fetal structure in the neonatal and juvenile patient. Morphology of a PDA can vary from a diverticular, funnel-shaped structure to a cylindrical tube between the descending aorta and main pulmonary artery [235]. Blood flow for a left-to-right shunt is determined by the diameter in the shunt and the pressure gradient between the aorta and pulmonary artery [236].

Left-to-right shunting of blood occurs continuously in patients with PDA throughout the cardiac cycle because of higher systemic BP as compared to pulmonary BP and is a function of relative resistances in the aorta as compared to pulmonary vascular resistance. This leads to constant volume overload of the left ventricle, as shunt flow is added to normal pulmonary venous return. The volume overload leads to atrial and ventricular dilation and ventricular hypertrophy. When pulmonary vascular resistance increases and exceeds SVR, shunt flow will reverse and become right-to-left, leading to clinical cyanosis, as shunt flow does not circulate through the lungs [234].

Anesthetic Management

Due to the risk of shunt reversal, cyanosis, development of heart failure, arrhythmias, and other complications, it is recommended that individuals intimately familiar with the pathophysiology of disease and the surgical/interventional procedures required to ligate/occlude PDA shunts anesthetize patients with PDA; evaluation and treatment by veterinary specialists trained to safely handle these patients are strongly recommended.

Anesthetic factors to consider are primarily directed at the patient's age and size. Neonatal or juvenile physiology leads to a variety of unique pharmacokinetic and pharmacodynamic alterations (see Chapter 19). For example, the cardiovascular system has lower myocardial contractile mass, low cardiac reserve, and high cardiac index; CO is HR-dependent primarily due to poor vasomotor control [237]. The ability to increase contractility or vasoconstrict may be reduced, and treatments aimed at increasing contractility or providing vasoconstriction may be reduced or ineffective. The respiratory system is very compliant with high elastic forces, leading to increased airway resistance. Respiratory rates and minute ventilation are greater than in the adult. The hepatic and renal systems are immature and drug effects may be pronounced or prolonged in these patients. Young patients have high body weight to surface area ratios and will lose body heat rapidly. Thus, heat support is critical in these patients. High body water content may lead to lower than adult packed cell volume (PCV) and albumin levels. Blood glucose regulation may be impaired; patient fasting should be shorter than adults, and supplemental dextrose may be warranted [237].

Patient size may present special challenges because patients are usually quite small at presentation for PDA ligation or coil placement, and patient size has been identified as a risk factor for anesthetic-related mortality. Placement of monitoring equipment may be difficult, and the ability to access the patient during surgery may be limited. Venous catheterization may be challenging, and access tubing should be confirmed and clearly labeled if the patient cannot be clearly visualized. Anticipated surgical or procedural complications can include hemorrhage, as well as complications from thoracotomy (pain, hypoventilation, hypoxia, ventilation/perfusion imbalance, etc.). Interventional catheterization carries the risk of hemorrhage, migration of the occlusive device into the pulmonary artery, and failure to occlude the PDA with conversion to thoracotomy.

Anesthetic drug selection is generally dictated by the unique neonatal/juvenile physiology; short-acting, reversible drugs are recommended. For example, a combination of opioids, benzodiazepines, and anticholinergics is frequently used for sedation, analgesia, and HR support. Examples for premedication may include hydromorphone, oxymorphone, methadone, or morphine with or without atropine. In very young patients, additional sedation may be achieved with midazolam or diazepam. Anticholinergics are recommended, as CO is HR-dependent, and bradycardia can lead to significant hypotension. Acepromazine is not recommended, as juvenile patients are relatively more vasodilated than adults, have difficulties in increasing cardiac contractility and SVR, and diastolic runoff through the PDA leads to very low DAPs. Induction agents including ketamine, etomidate, and fentanyl/benzodiazepine are recommended. Propofol is not recommended as a sole induction agent because of the dose-dependent vasodilation, though alfaxalone may provide improved cardiovascular stability and maintenance of baroreceptor reflexes [94]. Maintenance anesthetic requirements can be reduced by concurrent infusions of opioids and/or lidocaine. IBP monitoring is recommended, although Doppler BP measurement is a reasonable alternative, given the difficulty of arterial catheter placement in these patients. Regional anesthesia including intercostal or intrapleural nerve blocks can be considered as a part of a balanced analgesic plan for patients undergoing thoracotomy. Intercostal nerve blocks are performed by injection of local anesthetic along the caudal margin of the ribs, dorsal to the length of the incision. Injection of two to three intercostal spaces cranial and caudal to the incision location is recommended for lateral thoracotomy [238]. Total dose of lidocaine or bupivacaine is recommended to not exceed $2\,\text{mg}\,\text{kg}^{-1}$, as the highest plasma concentration of local anesthetics is seen after intercostal nerve blocks, suggesting significant drug uptake from intercostal injection [239]. Postoperative intrapleural analgesia can also be obtained by direct intrapleural infiltration of local anesthetic, again, not exceeding the $2\,\text{mg}\,\text{kg}^{-1}$ maximum dose. Typically, bupivacaine is chosen for these regional techniques due to the longer duration of action compared to lidocaine. Intraoperative glucose monitoring is recommended and supplemental dextrose at 1.25–2.5% in maintenance IV fluids can be considered as needed. Anesthetists should be aware and prepared for observing the Branham reflex, the decrease in heart rate, and increase in blood pressure immediately after PDA ligation [240]. Additional complications including hemorrhage, arrhythmias, hypothermia, and others are treated as needed.

Should an Amplatzer ductal occluder be the treatment option of choice, the anesthetist should be aware of the risk (3% of cases) of device migration from the PDA into the main pulmonary artery and lungs [241]. Thus, anesthetic recovery is a critical time for PDA occluder placement, as a poor or rough recovery may dislodge the device in the PDA. Reducing the risk for dysphoria from benzodiazepines or opioids may require carefully titrated reversal with flumazenil and/or naloxone, respectively. Butorphanol may also be used to reverse mu-opioid agonist effects while still providing some analgesia/sedation through kappa-opioid receptors. Similarly, titrating down inhalant doses toward the end of the anesthetic event may reduce the risk of emergence delirium. Vital signs including temperature, HR, and BP should continue. Postprocedural sedation with injectable acepromazine, benzodiazepines (dependent on patient temperament), or very low doses of alpha-2-adrenergic receptor agonists may be required. All care must be aimed at a smooth recovery to prevent device dislodgement.

Tetralogy of Fallot

Incidence and Pathophysiology

Tetralogy of Fallot is a common congenital anatomic malformation, which can cause cyanosis, polycythemia, stunted growth, exercise intolerance, collapse, and seizures [242]. Predisposed breeds include the English Bulldog, Keeshond, Miniature Poodle, and Schnauzer, as well as other dog breeds and cats. TOF is a combination of four anatomic derangements as follows: (i) VSD, (ii) dextrorotation with an overriding aorta, (iii) PS, and (iv) right ventricular hypertrophy due to obstruction in the right ventricular outflow tract (RVOT) [243].

Hemodynamic alterations are dependent on the degree of shunt through the VSD and the consequences of the PS. If PS is mild and resistance to RVOT flow is mild, then right ventricular pressures should be lower than left ventricular pressures and flow should be left-to-right [230, 243]. If PS is severe and represents significant outflow obstruction, then elevated right ventricular pressures can shunt blood right-to-left and lead to clinical cyanosis. Clinical cyanosis results in erythropoietin release and secondary polycythemia. Polycythemia (PCV>70–75%) can lead to increased blood viscosity and poor perfusion due to sludging of blood flow [244]; patients may seizure because of polycythemia.

Anesthetic Management

The primary consideration for anesthesia in a patient with TOF is maintenance of normal systemic BPs to prevent reduction in left ventricular pressure. Decreases in left ventricular pressure can lead to shunt reversal (i.e., right-to-left) if right ventricular pressures are higher than left ventricular pressures. Right ventricular desaturated blood can subsequently enter the systemic circulation, resulting in cyanosis and decreased oxygen delivery. Premedication, induction, and maintenance anesthetic agents should be selected to prevent systemic hypotension as much as possible. Due to their vasodilatory effects, avoiding or minimizing dosages of propofol and inhaled anesthetics is recommended. Alfaxalone can be considered in place of propofol for potential improved cardiovascular stability. Opioids are a mainstay of anesthetic management used to reduce inhaled anesthetic requirements. BP should be supported, and hypotension rapidly treated to prevent further right-to-left shunting; this may include positive inotropic agents such as dopamine or dobutamine, or vasopressors such as phenylephrine or norepinephrine. IBP monitoring is recommended for patients with significant cyanosis or right-to-left shunting for both gold-standard monitoring of systemic BP and arterial blood gas sampling in the event of desaturation. Preoxygenation and postoperative oxygen supplementation are strongly recommended.

Ventricular Septal Defect

Incidence and Pathophysiology

Ventricular septal defects represent the failure of complete development of the membranous or muscular interventricular septum. They are more likely seen in Keeshond and English Bulldogs but have been identified in many dog breeds [245]. The incidence in cats is unknown, but the prevalence in both dogs and cats is low. VSDs can vary in size and pathophysiology, and clinical presentation depends on the degree and direction of shunting. Simple VSDs show left-to-right shunting in both phases of the cardiac cycle, and volume of flow is dependent on the shunt diameter [245]. Small-to-medium size defects exhibit resistance to flow across the VSD, which typically minimizes the increase in right ventricular volume and does not result in increases in pulmonary circulation or pulmonary pressures. Large VSDs that do not cause resistance to flow across the VSD lead to pulmonary overcirculation and pulmonary hypertension (PHT). PHT can then increase right ventricular pressure and, if higher than left ventricular pressure, may lead to right-to-left shunting and clinical cyanosis. Increased pulmonary blood flow leading to increased left ventricular preload can lead to left ventricular hypertrophy and pulmonary edema because of the inability of the left ventricle to eject the increased pulmonary venous return.

Anesthetic Management

Similar to TOF, anesthetic management is directed at preventing right-to-left shunting by maintenance of systemic BP. Anesthetic plans should be designed to minimally impact BP, and rapid support for hypotension should be available with positive inotropic agents (dopamine and dobutamine) or vasopressors (phenylephrine and norepinephrine) if needed. Monitoring and interventions for patients are like those for TOF.

Abnormalities of Cardiac Conduction and Cardiac Rhythm

The importance of a normal cardiac rhythm cannot be overstated. The essential function of the cardiovascular system is to provide tissues with oxygen and nutrients while removing the waste products of metabolism. More than any other, the one essential micronutrient that the body cannot survive without is oxygen. As previously discussed, oxygen delivery is the product of CO ($l\,min^{-1}$) and CaO_2 ($ml\ O_2\,dl^{-1}$ blood). CaO_2 is the sum of oxygen bound by saturated hemoglobin and that found dissolved in blood (PaO_2). Cardiac output is the product of HR and SV (ml blood ejected per heartbeat). To maximize CO and optimize oxygen delivery, the contraction and relaxation of the heart must be sufficiently coordinated to allow diastolic ventricular filling and systolic ejection of blood. Cardiac arrhythmias, by definition, are disorganizations of the coordinated electrophysiologic and mechanical function of the heart and can rapidly lead to life-threatening reductions in CO and perfusion [246]. Identification and treatment of arrhythmias are critical components of patient management before and during anesthetic events, as well as into the recovery period.

The behavior of electrical impulses and of the cardiac rhythm is determined by the shape of the action potential. The ECG is the electrical representation of the summation of all cardiac vectors measured in standard Lead I, II, or III configurations at the limb electrodes placed on the patient, graphed in voltage versus time. Changes in the shape of the cardiac action potential or ECG are determined by shifts of ions, particularly sodium, potassium, and calcium across the cardiac myocyte cell membrane. The movement of ions is determined by cell surface receptors and the electrochemical gradients of these ions across the membrane, and is extensively reviewed elsewhere [246].

Electrophysiology of the Conduction System

The cardiac action potential is described in four phases, labeled as Phase 0 through 4, during the progression of the cardiac cycle (Figure 1.10) [246]. Phase 4 represents the resting phase and is described by the resting membrane potential (RMP), the voltage measured across the myocyte cell membrane during the unstimulated state. RMP varies by the type of myocyte; specialized myocytes such as the sinoatrial (SA) nodal cells (Figure 1.10) and AV nodal cells have a different RMP as compared to a nonspecialized working cardiac myocyte.

The transmembrane RMP measured in the generic cardiac myocyte is −90 mV but can vary from −50 to −90 mV depending on the type of cardiac myocyte. In Phase 4, the cell membrane is relatively permeable to potassium (inwardly rectifying potassium current, IK1) and impermeable to sodium and calcium; therefore, the RMP is determined mostly by potassium, as it moves out of the cell along the electrical and chemical gradients. The term "resting state" is somewhat misleading, as the RMP is also an active process due to the action of the basolateral Na^+-K^+-adenosine triphosphatase (ATPase) pump, which actively moves sodium out of the cell against the concentration gradient.

Phase 0 is characterized by myocyte cell membrane depolarization due to the rapid influx of sodium through rapidly opening voltage-gated sodium channels, down the electrochemical and concentration gradients such that the transmembrane potential reaches a positive value of approximately +30 mV [247]. The polarity reversal to positive in the cell membrane potential opens the L-type calcium channels, allowing the onset of inward calcium conductance that becomes important through Phase 2. The slope of Phase 0 represents the speed of depolarization of a single myocyte, and as conduction of the action potential through one myocyte dictates conduction to adjacent myocytes and spread of the action potential, the slope of Phase 0 determines conduction velocity through the heart. Pathologic states that slow sodium influx during Phase 0 reduce the speed of conduction of single myocytes through the heart and can be the origin of cardiac arrhythmias or reentry circuits.

Phase 1 results from the return of the RMP toward neutral due to the inactivation of Phase 0 voltage-gated sodium currents, the onset of inward calcium movement through L-type calcium channels, as well as transient inwardly rectifying potassium currents via voltage-gated potassium channels (I-to).

Phase 2 is the sustained depolarization of the cardiac myocyte termed "the plateau phase," which is a unique feature in electrically excitable tissues. The plateau is the balance of the inward calcium movement via L-type calcium channels and the outward potassium movement through a sodium/potassium exchanger current.

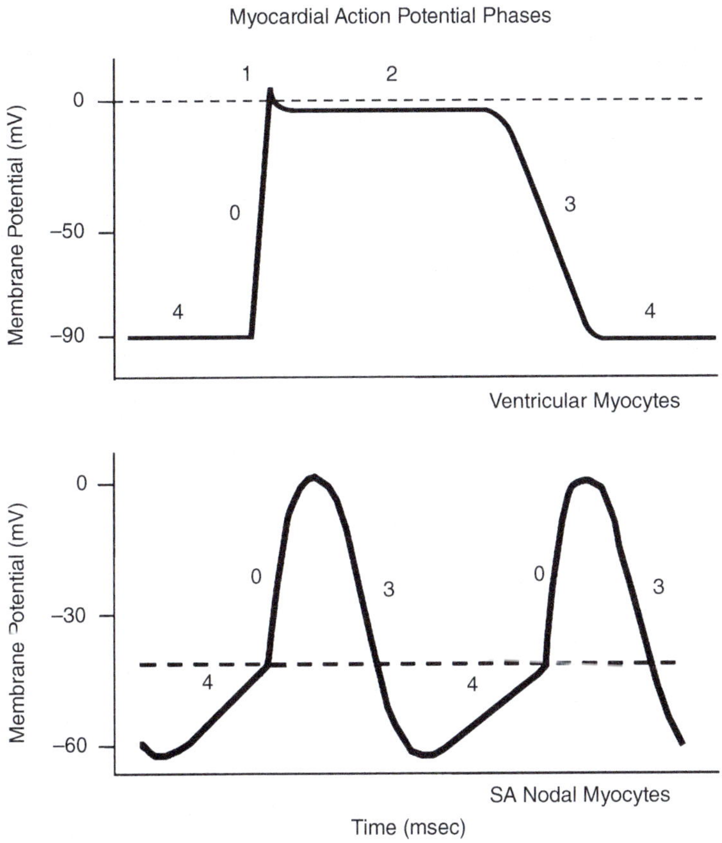

Figure 1.10 Representative myocardial action potential tracings of a ventricular myocyte (top) and SA nodal myocyte (bottom). Phase 4: resting membrane potential. Phase 0: rapid depolarization. Phase 1: initial repolarization. Phase 2: plateau phase. Phase 3: repolarization.

Phase 3 is the final repolarization of the cardiac myocyte and is primarily due to the increase in outward potassium conductance across the cell membrane via multiple slow, rapid, and delayed rectifier currents. At the same time, conductance of sodium and calcium decreases, allowing overall net movement of positive charge out of the cell and reestablishment of RMP at −50 to −90 mV. Another mechanism of arrhythmia generation is the reduction in overall potassium outward movement during Phase 3 in the failing heart, leading to events such as early afterdepolarizations.

After the end of Phase 3, the cardiac myocyte enters a refractory period, wherein further stimulation cannot result in the generation of an action potential. The refractory period allows the heart to relax during diastole and the ventricles to reach an appropriate end-diastolic volume such that when the refractory period ends, and the heart is again able to contract, a normal volume of blood is ejected, and SV/CO is maintained. The refractory period prevents cardiac tetany and depolarization of one myocyte from the adjacent one. This appropriately propagates the action potential in one direction, rather than allowing the passage of an action potential between two adjacent myocytes. The duration of the refractory period is roughly that of the action potential, such that the myocyte cannot be restimulated until the end of Phase 3. The refractory period can be divided into an (early) absolute refractory period, wherein no degree of stimulation can lead to depolarization, and a (later) relative refractory period, wherein a higher-than-normal stimulus has the potential to depolarize the myocyte.

Mechanisms Eliciting Cardiac Arrhythmias

Cardiac arrhythmias can be classified based on the electrophysiologic mechanism underlying the generation of the abnormal rhythm. These mechanisms include disorders of impulse generation, impulse conduction, and combined disorders. Specific arrhythmias of these classes are separated into sinus, supraventricular, and ventricular origin arrhythmias (Table 1.8) [243].

Table 1.8 Cardiac arrhythmia classification by mechanism.

Normal sinus impulse formation
- Normal sinus rhythm
- Sinus arrhythmia
- Wandering sinus pacemaker
- Disturbances of sinus impulse formation
- Sinus arrest
- Sinus bradycardia
- Sinus tachycardia

Disturbances of supraventricular impulse formation
- Atrial premature complexes
- Atrial tachycardia
- Atrial flutter
- Atrial fibrillation
- Atrioventricular junctional rhythm

Disturbances of ventricular impulse formation
- Ventricular premature complexes
- Ventricular tachycardia
- Ventricular asystole
- Ventricular fibrillation

Disturbances of impulse conduction
- Sinoatrial block
- Persistent atrial standstill ("silent" atrium)
- Atrial standstill (hyperkalemia)
- Ventricular pre-excitation
- Atrioventricular (AV) block

Normal Sinus Impulse Formation

The normal ECG waveform is generated from the coordinated conduction of the action potential from the SA node across the atria to the AV node, through the AV node to the bundle of His, and into the ventricular Purkinje system. The conduction is subsequently carried rapidly through the ventricles, leading to coordinated muscular ventricular contraction. Ventricular repolarization is the terminal event of a single ECG complex.

Atrial depolarization is seen as the P wave. P wave amplitude and duration can vary with changes in body position relative to electrode position, vagal tone, and with arrhythmias or cardiac disease. Action potential conduction through the AV node is represented by the P–R interval. Shortened P–R intervals can be due to accessory atrial pathways increasing rate of atrial conduction. P–R interval prolongation is the classic finding for first-degree AV block. Atrial repolarization occurs during ventricular depolarization and is not seen on the ECG waveform. The QRS complex is formed from ventricular depolarization (ventricular septum, left and right ventricular free walls; Figure 1.11). The S–T segment is the time between the end of ventricular depolarization and beginning of ventricular repolarization. Both S–T segment elevation and depression can be abnormal findings; elevation can be due to myocardial hypoxia, pericardial effusion, or digoxin toxicity (cats), and S–T segment depression can be due to hypoxia, hyperkalemia or hypokalemia, infarction, or digoxin toxicity [248]. Ventricular repolarization occurs after the QRS complex and is represented by the T wave.

Evaluation of the ECG Rhythm

Clinical evaluation of the ECG during anesthesia is typically performed in a Lead II arrangement. Each lead arrangement has a positive and a negative electrode, described by Einthoven's triangle (Figure 1.12). The principal cardiac

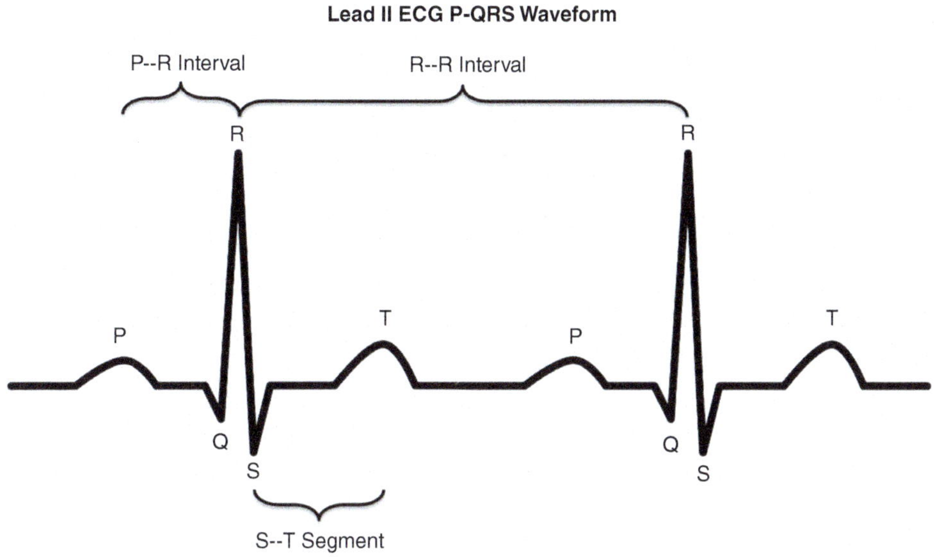

Figure 1.11 Representative Lead II ECG tracing to identify named peaks. The P wave represents atrial depolarization. The P–R interval represents AV nodal delay in conduction. The QRS complex represents ventricular depolarization. The T wave represents ventricular repolarization. The R–R interval determines overall heart rate and is evaluated for regularity during ECG assessment.

Figure 1.12 Einthoven's triangle illustrates electrical measurement vectors and polarity through the heart based on lead selection. A Lead II ECG shows the highest-amplitude ECG tracings as Lead II parallels electrical potentials from the SA node to the AV node and through the His–Purkinje system toward the ventricular myocardium. For this reason, Lead II is the most common ECG tracing used during general anesthesia.

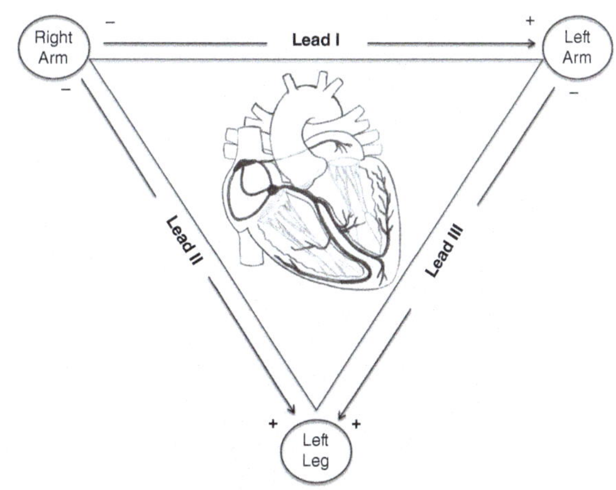

vector during normal sinus rhythm is from the SA node to the left ventricular free wall. Lead II ECG (negative right arm to positive left leg) measures parallel to this vector, typically resulting in the largest amplitude ECG waveform.

Evaluation of the ECG for arrhythmias requires a systematic approach to ensure arriving at an accurate diagnosis, and it is a common mistake to interpret the ECG and diagnose an arrhythmia with an "at-a-glance" approach. The following variables should be evaluated to identify ECG abnormalities.

Heart Rate

Heart rate will be averaged by the patient monitor over a specific duration of time, typically 6–10 s. Although this may be sufficient for some arrhythmias, manual calculation of the HR, whether an average over time or a calculated instantaneous rate (HR between two consecutive complexes), is recommended, as a patient monitor can incorrectly calculate HR with irregular rhythms or very tall/short complexes. Heart rate should never be taken from the ECG due to such inaccuracies. Heart rate analysis allows classification of tachyarrhythmias and bradyarrhythmias, which are species dependent.

P–Q-R-S Relationship

The anesthetist must ensure that there is a Q-R-S present for every P wave and a P wave for every Q-R-S complex. P waves not followed by a Q-R-S are typical of second- and third-degree AV block. In small animals, the P wave has a positive deflection. Rounded P waves indicate an abnormality in the SA node, and P waves of different or variable morphology may represent ectopic atrial contractions. An absence of P waves is seen with hyperkalemia, atrial standstill, atrial fibrillation, or P waves lost within a dissociated Q-R-S complex (third-degree AV block). Inverted P waves (negative in Lead II) indicate that the P wave origin is near the AV node and travel toward the Lead II negative electrode (right arm).

R-to-R Interval

Rhythm regularity is assessed by measuring the R-to-R interval between two successive Q-R-S complexes, most easily accomplished with calipers, though the edge of a piece of paper with markings or a ruler may suffice. A regular rhythm is one in which the R-to-R interval is consistent. Regular rhythms with a consistent R-to-R interval include normal sinus rhythm, sinus tachycardia, sinus bradycardia, SVT, and ventricular tachycardia. Irregularity can be described as "regularly irregular" where there is irregularity with a pattern (e.g., AV blocks, sinus arrhythmias, and wandering pacemakers), or as "irregularly irregular" where there is no pattern to the rhythm (e.g., atrial fibrillation). Usually, the faster the rhythm, the more difficult it is to detect regularity or irregularity. Printing ECG strips at faster paper speeds (e.g., $50\,\text{mm}\,\text{s}^{-1}$) can assist in unmasking irregularity if difficult to determine compared to slower paper speeds (e.g., 12.5 or $25\,\text{mm}\,\text{s}^{-1}$).

Q-R-S Morphology

Q-R-S complex morphology can aid in identification of supraventricular or ventricular origin waveforms. Ventricular origin ectopic complexes rarely conduct through the Purkinje system, and therefore the wave of depolarization must spread cell to cell. Cell-to-cell conduction is far slower (approximately $1\,\text{m}\,\text{s}^{-1}$) compared to conduction rates of the Purkinje system (approximately $100\,\text{m}\,\text{s}^{-1}$), and therefore the ECG trace of an ectopic ventricular complex is "wide and bizarre". Narrow-complex Q-R-S morphology is consistent with supraventricular origin complexes that pass through the AV node and spread via the Purkinje fibers and lead to extremely rapid (and therefore narrow) Q-R-S complexes.

Periodicity

Periodicity is the frequency of an arrhythmia and is described as either a sustained, incessant abnormality or nonsustained, paroxysmal rhythm. The term paroxysm is often reserved for an arrhythmia that converts from totally normal to totally abnormal between two Q-R-S complexes, for example, the sudden, acute paroxysm of SVT or ventricular tachycardia.

Specific Arrhythmias

Sinus Arrhythmia

Sinus arrhythmia is the most seen regularly irregular sinus rhythm during the respiratory cycle, wherein HR increases with inspiration and decreases with expiration [248]. This is due to changes in underlying vagal tone through the respiratory cycle and the effect of changing vagal tone on HR. It is common in the canine but is abnormal in the feline. If required, treatment is directed at increasing sympathetic tone or normalizing HR if bradycardic (usually with an anticholinergic agent). Owing to the effects of premedication and induction agents and subsequent effects on parasympathetic tone, sinus arrhythmia can be a normal finding while anesthetized.

Wandering Sinus Pacemaker

A wandering pacemaker is a sinus rhythm with variation in the origin of the P wave within the SA node and is likely due to variable vagal tone to the SA node [249]. It is seen as a cyclic variation in P wave configuration amid a normal sinus rhythm. The P wave may occasionally be isoelectric and therefore undetected on the ECG trace.

Sinus Arrest

Sinus arrest is the failure of the SA node to produce a depolarization and subsequent P–Q-R--S–T complex due to severely depressed automaticity of the SA node [250]. For a diagnosis of sinus arrest, the R-to-R interval of the period of arrest must be a minimum of twice the R-to-R interval of the underlying sinus rhythm. However, pauses of 5–12 s are not impossible and can be terminated by an escape ventricular complex, junctional escape complex, or sinus complex. Sinus arrest can result in clinical signs of weakness or syncope. Possible causes of sinus arrest include carotid sinus or ocular stimulation, SA nodal fibrosis, drug effects (digoxin, β-adrenergic blockers), or hyperexcitability of the vagus nerve ("vagotonia") with intrathoracic or cervical mass manipulation. Treatment of sinus arrest can include termination of the stimulating cause and attempts at anticholinergic therapy; however, if severe, mechanical pacemaker implantation may be required.

Sinus Bradycardia

Sinus bradycardia is a normal sinus rhythm of lower-than-normal expected rate. Assessment of normal HR varies with species and breeds. It may be a normal finding in a very calm, athletic, or sleeping patient, but can also be a consequence of drug therapy (e.g., opioids, alpha-2-adrenergic receptor agonists, propofol, β-adrenergic blockers, calcium channel blockers, and digoxin), pathophysiologic (e.g., hypothyroidism and hypothermia), or because of cardiac disease (e.g., sick sinus syndrome [SSS]) or elevations in vagal tone. Treatment for sinus bradycardia is recommended if there are signs of reduced perfusion, CO, or BP. If no contraindications exist, a bradycardic animal that is hypotensive should have the HR increased with anticholinergic therapy to improve CO and BP before other treatments to improve BP are attempted.

Sinus Tachycardia

Sinus tachycardia is a sinus rhythm more than the normal range, typically HR > 160 beats min^{-1} in dogs and >200–220 beats min^{-1} in cats [251]. It can be a normal physiologic response to pain, stress, or anxiety, due to drug overdoses of anticholinergics, catecholamines, or their derivatives (i.e., positive inotropes such as dopamine and dobutamine), or thyroid over-supplementation. Pathologic sinus tachycardia can be seen with pain, hyperthyroidism, fever, shock, CHF, and early stages of hypoxia (hypoxic, ischemic, hypemic, and/or histotoxic). Treatment of sinus tachycardia before or during anesthesia requires ruling out possible causes of tachycardia and treating as needed. Light anesthetic planes have been associated with sudden onsets of tachycardia and are due to increases in catecholamines as the patient mounts a physiologic response to noxious stimuli. Improvement of anesthetic depth or administration of analgesics typically resolves tachycardia due to this etiology. Rarely, β-adrenergic blockers may be required to treat a pathologic sinus tachycardia; however, identification and treatment of underlying causes should be the focus of treatment.

Atrial Premature Complexes (APCs)

Atrial premature complexes are ectopic foci of depolarization in the atria, which lead to premature atrial contractions [247]. Atrial contraction has been described as providing an atrial kick, increasing end-diastolic volume by 10–30% [252]. Loss of coordination and timing of the atrial contraction prevents this increase in end-diastolic volume and leads to a decrease in CO if sufficiently frequent. APCs are most frequently caused by cardiac disease, most commonly atrial enlargement secondary to AV valvular disease, valvular dysplasia, and PDA, but can also be seen with metabolic, neoplastic, and/or inflammatory diseases that affect the atria [253]. Any cause of atrial volume overload may lead to atrial enlargement and development of APCs. APCs may also precede worsening atrial arrhythmias such as atrial tachycardia, atrial flutter, or SVT.

The presence of APCs typically does not warrant specific treatment, provided overall perfusion is adequate, but when identified should alert the anesthetist to the possibility of occult cardiac disease and may suggest the need for further cardiac evaluation (thoracic radiographs, BP measurements, and/or echocardiogram) or the possibility that APCs could degrade into atrial tachycardia or atrial fibrillation.

Atrial Flutter

Atrial flutter is an atrial tachyarrhythmia (>300 beats min^{-1}) in which P waves are replaced by a "sawtooth pattern" of atrial depolarization, referred to as flutter or "f" waves [254]. Flutter wave conduction to the ventricles is variable, so that there may be a 4:1 ratio of atrial "f" waves to ventricular complexes or a 1:1 ratio that is difficult to differentiate from atrial tachycardia. Causes of atrial flutter are the same as those for other atrial tachyarrhythmias, particularly those causing atrial enlargement. Reentry rhythms can underlie atrial flutter, as can feline restrictive or hypertrophic cardiomyopathy, and ruptured chordae tendineae. Treatment of atrial flutter is not well described in veterinary medicine but is aimed at slowing ventricular rate. Options include diltiazem or digoxin administration, direct current cardioversion, or precordial thump in an emergency.

Atrial Fibrillation

Atrial fibrillation is a common rhythm in dogs and tends to be a sustained rhythm, although paroxysms have been described [255]. It is the classic "irregularly irregular" rhythm noted on auscultation, pulse palpation, or ECG analysis. There is complete loss of P waves, replaced by a chaotic isoelectric line of "f" waves and irregular R-to-R intervals. It is characterized mechanically by complete lack of coordinated atrial activity. Loss of all atrial coordination prevents the atrial kick in most if not all cardiac cycles and leads to significantly reduced CO when combined with the high ventricular rates. Atrial fibrillation is often the rhythm associated with DCM of large breed dogs, severe atrial enlargement of any cause, and cases with severe mitral regurgitation; "lone" atrial fibrillation is seen in giant breed dogs that have atrial fibrillation but no structural cardiac disease.

Treatment of atrial fibrillation focuses on medical therapy for rate control and includes digoxin, β-adrenergic blockers, and calcium channel blockers. Slowing of ventricular rate is important to prevent the development of heart failure and to extend diastolic filling time and improve CO. However, long-term conversion from atrial fibrillation to a sinus rhythm is often not possible with severe underlying cardiac disease. In cases with minimal underlying structural cardiac disease (typically those with lone atrial fibrillation and atrial enlargement only), cardioversion to a sinus rhythm may be considered. The decision to attempt cardioversion (medically or with electric cardioversion) is controversial, and there are no clear criteria for attempting cardioversion.

Atrioventricular Junctional Tachycardia

Atrioventricular junctional tachycardia is due to the presence of an ectopic focus of depolarization in the AV node. Intrinsic automaticity rate of the AV node is 40–60 beats min^{-1}. Therefore, an AV nodal tachycardia has only to be faster than this rate to be termed a tachycardia. The underlying mechanism is most commonly a reentry circuit. As the depolarization occurs in the AV node, the ventricular portion of the complex tends to be narrow. A noted variation in this rhythm is the presence of inverted P waves that can be seen before, during, or after the Q-R-S complex. It may not be possible to distinguish this rhythm from an atrial tachycardia at very high HRs, so the term SVT can be used to identify either rhythm. Treatment is aimed at breaking the reentry circuit with a calcium channel blocker (e.g., diltiazem) to reduce calcium entry into the myocyte and therefore reduce HR.

Ventricular Premature Complexes

Ventricular premature complexes (VPCs or PVCs) are due to ectopic depolarization foci located in the ventricular myocardium. They occur before the next expected Q-R-S complex based on the underlying R-to-R interval. Depolarization spreads cell to cell, resulting in a wide Q-R-S complex. Unifocal VPCs are individual wide Q-R-S complexes with the same morphology, indicating they come from the same focus of depolarization [256]. Multifocal VPCs have differing morphology and can be positive with different morphology, negative with different morphology, or both. Couplets (two consecutive wide complexes) and triplets are terms used to describe multiple VPCs occurring consecutively. A rhythm of alternating VPCs and sinus-origin beats is referred to as ventricular bigeminy. There is often a compensatory pause after the VPC, due to the refractory period of the VPC. When the VPC does not affect the R-to-R interval of the underlying sinus rhythm, it is referred to as an "interpolated VPC." R-on-T phenomenon occurs when the VPC occurs on the T wave of the previous sinus beat and can predispose to development of ventricular fibrillation (Vfib) [257].

The first line VPC treatment is a class 1b antiarrhythmic such as IV lidocaine or, less commonly, amiodarone. Recommended IV lidocaine doses range from 1 to 2 mg kg^{-1} in dogs or 0.25–1.0 mg kg^{-1} (up to 4 mg) for cats. Oral sotalol has also been recommended in cats but is not an option during anesthesia. Other therapies for ventricular arrhythmias have largely been unproven in the cat [252]. Mexiletine is an alternative for long-term management, as it is only available as an oral preparation. Class 1b antiarrhythmic drugs are believed to shorten the refractory period and terminate reentry rhythms by this mechanism. Triggers for treatment include multifocal VPCs (as more of the heart is presumed to be diseased/affected, and degradation to a worsening rhythm is likely), runs of couplets/triplets/ventricular tachycardia, R-on-T phenomenon, or any ventricular rhythm that has hemodynamic consequences. In cases of refractory life-threatening ventricular arrhythmias or shock-resistant ventricular fibrillation, amiodarone is recommended.

Causes of VPCs include hypoxia, cardiac disease (myocarditis, arrhythmogenic right ventricular cardiomyopathy [ARVC], neoplasia, trauma, and structural cardiac disease), splenic/hepatic neoplasia, gastric dilatation volvulus syndrome, acidosis, pain, and catecholamine or sympathomimetic therapy. Treatment of VPCs and ventricular rhythms must include evaluation, monitoring, and treatment of these mechanisms in addition to treatment for the arrhythmia itself.

Ventricular Tachycardia

Ventricular tachycardia is defined as a ventricular rhythm greater than 160–180 beats min^{-1} in dogs, whether paroxysmal or sustained [256]. Idioventricular rhythm is the ventricular escape rhythm seen with loss of supraventricular input such as in complete (third-degree) AV block, typically a pulse rate of 40–60 beats min^{-1} in dogs and 60–80 beats min^{-1} in cats. The most appropriate term for a complete ventricular rhythm with rates between 60 and 160 beats min^{-1} (in dogs) is an accelerated idioventricular rhythm; a ventricular rhythm that is not quite tachycardic. The major hemodynamic difference between accelerated idioventricular rhythm and ventricular tachycardia is the decrease in diastolic filling time as HR increases past 160–180 beats min^{-1}, as well as the decrease in CO that results. Causes of ventricular tachycardia are the same as for VPCs, and the same considerations apply for treatment.

Ventricular Fibrillation

Ventricular fibrillation is a chaotic organization of coarsely wandering electrical potentials of variable duration and amplitude with no P–Q-R-S–T organization. It is a nonperfusing rhythm, creating no mechanical activity in the heart, and CO is near zero. Ventricular fibrillation is a terminal rhythm and can result from severe ventricular tachycardia, severe systemic or cardiac disease, or cardiac surgery. The only treatment with a reasonable chance of converting Vfib to a perfusing rhythm is electrical defibrillation. However, the ability to convert to a sinus rhythm is often temporary, and fibrillation frequently recurs in minutes to hours.

Sinoatrial Block (SA Block)

Sinoatrial block is failure of a normally generated SA nodal-action potential to appropriately conduct to the atria and lead to atrial depolarization [253]. Sinoatrial block differs from sinus arrest in that SA block is a failure of conduction, while sinus arrest is failure of the SA node to depolarize (failure of impulse generation). It can be difficult to distinguish between them with routine Lead II ECG analysis in anesthetized patients. First-degree SA block is a prolonged period from SA nodal firing and atrial depolarization. This is undetectable on ECG, as SA nodal firing is not recorded. Second-degree SA block is identified by a pause after a sinus beat or beats, wherein the duration of the pause is an exact multiple of that of the underlying normal sinus rhythm P-to-P interval. SA block appears otherwise identical to sinus arrest. Sinus block can be the result of atrial disease (enlargement, fibrosis, cardiomyopathy, and neoplasia), drug toxicity (β-adrenergic and calcium channel blockers), or potentially SSS. SA nodal blocks typically do not require treatment. However, if severe bradycardia develops, treatment should be considered, as they may be responsive to atropine/glycopyrrolate. If the rhythm fails to respond to anticholinergics and the patient is clinical for the arrhythmia, transcutaneous or transvenous cardiac pacing may be required.

Persistent Atrial Standstill

Atrial standstill is failure of normally generated SA nodal potentials to depolarize the atria. The ECG appears as a flat line with no P waves. Atrial standstill can be due to diseased atrial myocardium that is unable to depolarize normally, or, more commonly, electrolyte disturbances such as hyperkalemia, where elevated serum potassium levels are sufficiently high to prevent atrial depolarization [251]. Common causes of hyperkalemia include urinary obstruction, renal failure, uroabdomen, and hypoadrenocorticism. At moderate to severe serum potassium levels, the SA node and ventricular myocardium maintain their ability to depolarize, albeit slowly, but no P waves are seen on the ECG; slowed and widened Q-R-S complexes can be seen. Elevations in serum potassium may not be correlated to the severity of arrhythmias; alterations in the ECG can be seen at severe hyperkalemia, and classic changes in the ECG waveform can be seen with low serum potassium levels. However, typically as potassium increases, the T waves become "tall and tented," P waves flatten, and the P-to-R interval increases in duration, progressing to atrial standstill followed by widening of the Q-R-S complex until the ECG appears as a sine wave. Ventricular arrhythmias may also present at any time.

Treatment for hyperkalemia is focused on identification and treatment of the underlying cause [258]. Immediate stabilization of the hyperkalemic patient involves decreasing serum potassium levels and treating underlying acid–base disturbances to move potassium intracellularly. These mechanisms are critically important in reducing serum potassium levels in a patient who requires general anesthesia to treat the underlying disease.

Calcium gluconate (50–100 mg kg^{-1} as a slow 5 min IV bolus) or calcium chloride (10 mg kg^{-1} as a similar bolus) can be given to counteract the electrochemical effects of hyperkalemia on resting membrane hyperpolarization and rapidly treat the ECG side effects of hyperkalemia. Improvements in ECG can be seen within minutes of administration and can last between 30 and 60 min, allowing time for other treatments to reduce the hyperkalemia. Calcium given too rapidly can cause bradycardia and worsen the rhythm, and so should be given slowly while monitoring the patient with an ECG placed.

Another strategy for decreasing serum potassium in the hyperkalemic patient is to cotransport potassium with glucose into cells under the influence of insulin. Recommendations for insulin/dextrose therapy are 0.25 units kg^{-1} of regular insulin IV given with 1–2 g of dextrose (diluted 3:1 with saline) for every full unit of insulin administered. Serial glucose monitoring is recommended, and patients may require a dextrose infusion (1.25–2.5%) to prevent hypoglycemia. In humans, onset time of insulin/dextrose therapy is 20 min, with a duration of 30–60 min [258].

Finally, sodium bicarbonate can be used to buffer an underlying acidosis and reverse the shift of transmembrane antiport of hydrogen ions and potassium, thus moving potassium back into cells. Once venous or arterial blood gas analysis is complete (pH, base excess, bicarbonate, and PCO_2), total bicarbonate deficit can be estimated with the formula: total deficit = 0.3 × base excess × body weight (in kilograms). If bicarbonate therapy is appropriate, it is recommended to replace no more than 1/3–1/2 of the deficit. Administration of a larger dose of bicarbonate risks overcorrection and development of an alkalosis. One of the more significant buffering mechanisms for bicarbonate therapy is the generation of CO_2 based on the carbonic anhydrase equation:

$$HCO_3^- + H^+ \leftrightarrow H_2CO_3 \leftrightarrow H_2O + CO_2 \quad (1.8)$$

where carbonic anhydrase catalyzes the reaction from carbonic acid to CO_2 and water. The patient must be capable of ventilating off the generated CO_2, an estimate of which is possible based on a normal or low partial pressure of CO_2 on blood gas analysis. If hypercapnic, further elevations in CO_2 associated with bicarbonate administration will generate a respiratory acidosis and can worsen blood pH. Slow bicarbonate administration is thus recommended. If the patient is anesthetized during bicarbonate administration, the anesthetist should be aware of the impending increase in CO_2 and adjust ventilation as necessary to maintain normal end-tidal CO_2. Finally, the administration of sodium bicarbonate will increase measured serum sodium and may potentially lead to increases in serum osmolarity, where calculated osmolarity = $2[Na^+ + K^+]$ + BUN/2.8 + Glucose/18 where BUN = blood urea nitrogen. Clinical signs of hyperosmolarity are not typically seen until osmolarity is >340 mOsm l^{-1}. Although it is unlikely that serum osmolarity will increase to this extent with sodium bicarbonate, if the patient is at risk for hyperosmolarity (unregulated diabetes, severe azotemia, etc.), bicarbonate must be carefully titrated and serum osmolarity monitored.

First-Degree AV Block

First-degree AV block is defined as the prolongation of the P-to-R interval due to slowed conduction of atrial depolarization action potentials through the AV node to >0.13 s in dogs and 0.09 s in cats [250]. Causes include AV nodal disease (fibrosis, ischemia, and cardiomyopathy), vagal stimulation, electrolyte imbalance (hyperkalemia and hypokalemia), and drug side effects (propranolol and digitalis toxicity). First-degree AV block is not usually clinically significant. However, it may be an indication of underlying disease or a predictor of worsening AV nodal function.

Second-Degree AV Block

Second-degree AV block is characterized by intermittent failure or delay in the association of the atrial depolarization through the AV node to the bundle of His and subsequent ventricular depolarization. This appears as one or more isolated P waves that are not followed by Q-R-S complexes.

Second-degree AV blocks are described either as Mobitz type I or II or as low- or high-grade. Mobitz type I is characterized by the increase in the duration of the P-to-R interval in successive sinus beats until a P wave is completely blocked and is not conducted through the AV node. Most Mobitz type I blocks are due to altered AV nodal physiology, AV nodal disease (as for first-degree AV block), or drug side effects (low-dose anticholinergics, digitalis toxicity, and alpha-2-adrenergic receptor agonists). Mobitz type I blocks may be normal in high vagal tone species such as the very athletic dog, juvenile animals, and horses [259].

Mobitz type II second-degree AV block is acute, intermittent failure of conduction of a P wave through the AV node, but the P-to-R intervals of successfully conducted P waves are of normal duration. If there are many P waves that are not conducted so that a P-to-R interval cannot be assessed, the term "high-grade" second-degree AV block is applied, especially when there are four or more nonconducted P waves for every conducted P wave and Q-R-S complex. High-grade second-degree AV block can be due to the same causes as less severe AV blocks, but may be a sign that AV nodal disease is severe and may degrade into complete AV dissociation (third-degree AV block). High-grade second-degree AV block may be more resistant to anticholinergic treatment and may require the placement of a permanent ventricular pacemaker.

Third-Degree AV Block

Third-degree AV block is complete failure of AV nodal conduction and subsequent dissociation [260]. While SA nodal function, atrial conduction pathways, and atrial depolarization are normal, the wave of depolarization is not conducted through to the ventricles. The cause of third-degree AV block is often idiopathic. The characteristic findings on ECG are normal P wave generation, with a regular P-to-P interval at a normal sinus rate. Owing to the lack of supraventricular input, the ventricles depolarize because of ventricular automaticity (30–50 beats min^{-1} in dogs and 60–80 beats min^{-1} in cats), and a superimposed ventricular rhythm develops (a wide Q-R-S ventricular escape rhythm) that has no association to the P waves, often with a regular R-to-R interval. It is critical that this escape rhythm not be interpreted and treated as VPCs, and the ECG be carefully evaluated for association between P waves and Q-R-S complexes. If no association exists, third-degree AV block must be strongly considered and ruled out before antiarrhythmics are considered. If the ventricular escape rhythm is treated with lidocaine, it may suppress the escape rhythm and lead to cardiac arrest.

Treatment for third-degree AV block most commonly requires placement of a permanent ventricular pacemaker. Temporary measures to support (ventricular) HR, CO, and perfusion include transcutaneous, transesophageal, or transvenous temporary cardiac pacing. Medical interventions are often unsuccessful and have included isoproterenol, epinephrine, atropine, dopamine, and dobutamine infusions [160].

Bundle Branch Blocks

The bundle branches are the first two divisions of the bundle of His as the conduction system travels from the AV node down the interventricular septum toward the ventricular myocardium. The left bundle branch divides into one anterior and one posterior fascicle. Bundle branch or fascicular blocks are the result of loss of rapid conduction through one or more of these bundles and result from combined rapid and slow conduction through the ventricular myocardium; the bundle branch that remains unblocked allows conduction through the bundle and into the Purkinje system, causing rapid depolarization of the ventricle and a narrow Q-R-S complex. The bundle block conduction from the AV node results in the cell-to-cell spread of depolarization and a resultant slow, wide Q-R-S complex. The combination of rapid and slow conduction leads to a Q-R-S complex that appears wide and bizarre but typically not as wide as a VPC.

Left bundle branch blocks can be due to significant underlying disease, including cardiomyopathy, degenerative conduction system disease, ischemia, AS, and drug toxicity (e.g., adriamycin), and can be secondary to left ventricular hypertrophy. Right bundle branch blocks can be normal in dogs and cats but can also develop because of right ventricular conduction abnormalities or because of right ventricular hypertrophy, in association with VSD, cardiomyopathy, and heartworm disease. Concurrent left and right bundle branch blocks have the same appearance and effects as third-degree AV block.

Bundle branch blocks will have a P wave present before the widened Q-R-S complex, as supraventricular and AV nodal function are normal. This is an important distinction from a VPC. Bundle branch blocks typically do not lead to impairment of cardiac performance, CO, and perfusion, but should alert the anesthetist to evaluate the patient for possible underlying causes of cardiac disease.

Cardiac Pacemakers and Pacing

The first report of a canine pacemaker implantation was published in 1968 [260] and the literature has many reports between 1999 and 2015 discussing indications and outcomes, many which demonstrate the fact that pacemaker implantation has become increasingly common [261–271]. In dogs, permanently placed cardiac pacemakers are indicated for third-degree AV block, advanced second-degree AV block, SSS, persistent atrial standstill (PAS), and vasovagal syncope [272]. In cats, the most common indication for pacemaker implantation is AV block (mainly third-degree AV block), or more rarely PAS [272].

While the first implanted pacemakers had very few components and short life span, current pacemakers have thousands of components and immense programmability. However, the basic components include a generator, pacing leads, and a battery. The generator contains components to sense intrinsic myocardial electrical potentials, a logic circuit to determine appropriate output (based on programming), and an output circuit that determines the voltage and duration of the output signal to the myocardium. Pacing leads are very thin wires of various materials that carry the signal from the generator to the myocardium. Given the frequency of stimulations to the myocardium and the movement under which the wires must flex while remaining implanted in the myocardium, the lead wires are the weakest link in the pacemaker chain, and the most likely to fail. Pacing leads can be actively or passively connected to the myocardium (e.g., sutured epicardial leads) or have a screw-like filament at the end of the lead that is anchored in the endocardium. Over decades, various battery materials (copper–zinc, nuclear, nickel–cadmium) have been tested and eventually rejected; current batteries are typically lithium–iodide and can have a life span of over 10 years. Most veterinary pacemakers have been collected from human patients and are repurposed, as new pacemakers are likely cost-prohibitive for dogs and cats. The structure and function of pacemakers have been reviewed elsewhere [273].

Anesthetic Management

The anesthetist will most likely encounter pacemakers in two clinical situations: either a patient presenting for permanent pacemaker implantation, or a patient with an existing pacemaker requiring an unrelated procedure under general anesthesia.

Permanent Pacemaker Implantation

As noted, dogs and cats presenting for pacemaker placement can present with a wide variety of bradyarrhythmias and most are placed in specialty or academic practices by veterinary cardiologists. Complete understanding of the arrhythmia by the anesthetist will guide choosing the anesthesia protocol, as well as any required advanced monitoring or patient support. Additionally, the cardiovascular depressant effects of anesthetics (bradycardia, decreased SVR, etc.) and the time required under general anesthesia for pacemaker placement rapidly destabilize a patient. Temporary cardiac pacing up until the point that the permanent pacemaker can be activated is commonly used.

Temporary pacing can be provided with either a temporary transvenous pacemaker or with transthoracic pacing via externally applied pads [274]. The temporary transvenous pacemaker can either be placed under sedation with a local anesthetic or with local anesthetic alone. Alternatively, but with higher risk, the temporary transvenous pacemaker can be introduced immediately after induction of general anesthesia. Equipment and experience with these techniques, either (or ideally both) from a veterinary cardiologist or veterinary anesthesiologist, are crucial to reduce patient morbidity, as transvenous pacing requires a high level of knowledge and technical skill [275].

Transthoracic temporary pacing is a noninvasive alternative method for temporary pacing that was introduced in the 1950s and has been a standard of care for decades in humans [276, 277]. It is safe and effective in dogs and is a simpler technique to apply. In short, two disposable transthoracic patch electrodes are placed directly over the heart on shaved skin and connected via lead wires to a defibrillator/cardioverter/pacemaker. Patch adhesion is supported with nonadhesive bandage material. The pacemaker lead and gain are adjusted until accurate sensing of the intrinsic cardiac rhythm could be detected. Once a sensing marker is seen on the pacemaker display, pacing rate and current are adjusted until ventricular capture is confirmed on the monitor and with palpation of an arterial pulse [278]. The major complications of transvenous pacing are excessive muscular movement (e.g., skeletal and intercostal muscles), the discomfort of external pacing, and failure of ventricular capture. Neuromuscular blockade with nondepolarizing agents (e.g., atracurium) is frequently employed to reduce skeletal muscle stimulation from transthoracic pacing [279], but may not be 100% effective due to direct electrical muscular depolarization. Other neuromuscular agents may be considered in place of atracurium, based on clinician preference. The pain and movement associated with transthoracic pacing require general anesthesia [274, 278].

Patient support should include standard monitoring including pulse oximetry, capnography, ECG, temperature, and BP monitoring. Additionally, for permanent pacemaker placement, the anesthetist should plan for IBP monitoring to evaluate moment-to-moment changes due to arrhythmias, changes in pulse rate due to pacing, hemorrhage, or other procedural complications. The ability to sample arterial blood for oxygenation/blood gas analysis may be of value in patients with signs of heart failure and potential ventilation/perfusion imbalances. Placement of a Doppler crystal on a peripheral artery brings most anesthetists great comfort as an audible indicator of arterial pulse as well as a backup BP monitor should an invasive catheter fail. The patient should have adequate padding to prevent myopathy/neuropathy, and temperature support that minimally interferes with the procedure should be provided. Fluid therapy should be guided by the state of the patient's underlying cardiac disease, and ongoing or potential heart failure.

A wide variety of drug protocols can be used to induce and maintain anesthesia for pacemaker implantation. The most important goals of drug selection are to minimally depress cardiovascular function, and to avoid precipitating changes in HR or significant arteriolar vasodilation that could lead to hypotension, tachyarrhythmias, bradyarrhythmias, and/or potential cardiac arrest. Once transthoracic or transvenous temporary pacing is achieved, the anesthetist or cardiologist can manipulate the settings to adjust HR as needed to support BP and perfusion.

Anticholinergics are controversial in that while there may be an increase in SA nodal firing and P wave rate, there may be no meaningful increase in the Q-R-S rate, pulse rate, and blood pressure [274]. Opioids remain a mainstay of anesthetic plans due to their benefits for analgesia, inhalant dose reduction, and reversibility. Patients on transthoracic pacing may require increased doses of opioids or an opioid infusion due to discomfort. Opioid doses should be chosen carefully to avoid inducing further significant bradycardia. In cases of severe bradyarrhythmias, it may be necessary to induce anesthesia and secure transthoracic pacing before administering opioids if the risk of exacerbating bradycardia with opioids is deemed too high. In this case, higher doses of induction agents may be required to maintain an appropriate anesthetic depth until opioids are administered. Benzodiazepines are excellent additions for cardiovascular cases, as they have minimal cardiovascular effects of their own [280], decrease isoflurane MAC requirements [128], and potentiate the effects of other anesthetics. Their major drawback can be paradoxical excitement or dysphoria, which is typically not seen when used as a co-induction agent. Both midazolam and diazepam can decrease myoclonus seen with etomidate [101] and are recommended as co-induction agents [279, 280]. While not absolutely contraindicated, acepromazine is likely best avoided due to its significant and irreversible decrease in SVR and potential to cause hypotension, as well as its inhibition of the alpha-1-adrenergic receptor and potential interference in using alpha-1-adrenergic receptor agonists for management of hypotension. Alpha-2-adrenergic receptor agonists such as medetomidine and dexmedetomidine are contraindicated due to their cardiovascular effects such as precipitously decreasing HR and CO while increasing BP and, potentially, the risk for hemorrhage.

Anesthetic induction can proceed with most induction agents. Propofol and alfaxalone are rapid, smooth induction agents which can be titrated to effect, reducing their dose-dependent decreases in blood pressure. Co-induction with a benzodiazepine is commonly recommended to further reduce induction drug doses. Dissociative induction agents such as ketamine or tiletamine can be beneficial in that they increase HR and BP indirectly by increasing sympathetic tone. They also have mild somatic analgesic effects. Etomidate is widely considered to be the most cardiovascular-sparing induction agent. A review of 57 dogs receiving pacemakers between 2002 and 2012 in one referral center showed dogs induced with etomidate were 10 times less likely to develop hypotension during the procedure, compared with propofol or alfaxalone for induction; the most common complications were hypothermia ($n = 19$), VPCs ($n = 7$), bradycardia ($n = 7$), hypotension ($n = 5$), and hypertension ($n = 2$) [279]. Transthoracic pacing was applied in 49/57 dogs [279].

Inhalant anesthetics remain the mainstay for maintenance of anesthesia for pacemaker placement. However, they cause dose-dependent decreases in BP via decreases in contractility and vasomotor tone. Reducing inhaled anesthetic doses with adjunctive sedatives and analgesics (opioid, lidocaine, and/or ketamine infusions, or with locoregional anesthesia) remains the best strategy to avoid or reduce cardiovascular compromise from inhalants. Currently, there are no reports of using TIVA in small animals for pacemaker placement. Further research is required to clarify if TIVA may be an effective alternative to inhalants for pacemaker placement, with less cardiovascular compromise.

As with PDA repair, anesthetic recovery is a crucial time, as a poor recovery with patient movement may dislodge the pacemaker lead wires from the myocardium. Reducing the risk of dysphoria from benzodiazepines or opioids may require carefully titrated reversal with flumazenil and/or naloxone, respectively. Butorphanol can also be administered to antagonize mu-opioid effects while still providing some analgesia/sedation through kappa-opioid effects. Decreasing inhalant doses slowly during recovery may reduce the risk of emergence delirium and paddling/patient movement. Vital sign monitoring should continue. Postprocedure sedation with injectable acepromazine, benzodiazepines (dependent on patient temperament), or very low doses of alpha-2-adrenergic receptor agonists may be required.

Existing Pacemaker for Noncardiac Procedures

Patients presenting with preexisting pacemakers for routine care requiring general anesthesia are becoming more common, and anesthesia for emergency procedures is always a possibility. Ideally, any elective anesthetic procedure should be performed at the center where the pacemaker was placed, as they will have the knowledge, experience, and equipment to adjust the pacemaker as needed. Often, pacemakers have a low limit setting for HR, and under anesthesia this may not be a sufficient rate to maintain BP and perfusion. In these cases, the pacemaker generator can be wirelessly interrogated and reprogrammed before and after the procedure to optimize the settings for anesthesia and return them to preanesthesia settings before discharge. Also, it is critical to evaluate the pacemaker for normal function before and after anesthesia, to ensure no loss of lead placement or overall function has occurred.

Provided the pacemaker can be adjusted and HR controlled as needed, the abovementioned comments on anesthesia plans and drug selection will essentially be the same for elective procedures. Dependent on patient status and comorbidities, intensive monitoring with IBP or arterial blood gases may not be required. Antibiotic prophylaxis is likely recommended for any procedure that may lead to bacteremia, to mitigate the risk of lead colonization and future complications.

Systemic and Pulmonary Arterial Hypertension

Systemic Hypertension

Incidence and Pathophysiology

Systemic hypertension is defined as a persistently elevated BP. Most authors agree that SAP >160–180 mmHg and DAP >90–100 mmHg define systemic hypertension [281, 282]. Systemic hypertension is often classified as either essential hypertension or secondary hypertension. Essential hypertension is defined as consistent, measurably repeatable high BP for which a cause cannot be identified despite a thorough diagnostic workup. Secondary hypertension is due to a known cause that changes either the components of CO or SVR.

Most patients with hypertension present during middle age. However, hypertension can also be caused by or is seen concurrent with many geriatric diseases. An important breed exception is Greyhounds, which have higher BP and CO due to cardiac hypertrophy unrelated to disease that does not lead to patient morbidity [283]. Essential hypertension has also been reported in a line of Siberian Huskies [284], which might be due to their selection for endurance.

Common causes for hypertension include chronic renal disease, hyperthyroidism, hyperadrenocorticism, and a variety of miscellaneous uncommon or rare causes, including pheochromocytoma, polycythemia, diabetes mellitus, increases in intracranial pressure (Cushing reflex), and hypercholesterolemia [285]. Drugs can also cause elevations in BP and include steroids, cyclosporine, phenylpropanolamine, and erythropoietin. Toxicities can also increase BP and include, but are not limited to, high salt, lead, nicotine, and Vitamin D intake, alpha-1- and beta-1-adrenergic receptor agonist administration, and steroid use [9].

As noted earlier, MAP is the product of CO and SVR. Cardiac output increases with increases in HR, vascular volume (preload), or myocardial contractility (Figure 1.4). Hypertension is caused by either increases in one variable contributing to CO or increases in SVR. Renal disease leads to neurohormonal activation, which increases sympathetic system activation and has direct effects on angiotensin II and RAAS, as well as changes in body fluid balance. Thyroid hormones increase HR (positive chronotropic effect) and result most commonly in a sinus tachycardia with hypertension [285, 286]. Thyrotoxicosis also leads to increases in contractility and peripheral vasodilation; yet, despite the decrease in SVR, the major cardiovascular side effect of hyperthyroidism is a significant increase in CO [285]. Increases in circulating glucocorticoids, whether endogenous due to hyperadrenocorticism or exogenously administered, lead to salt and water retention with subsequent increases in preload and CO and potential overproduction of renin with subsequent increases in SVR [284]. Pheochromocytoma is a malignant tumor of the catecholamine-producing chromaffin cells of the adrenal medulla. Epinephrine and norepinephrine secretion is intermittent and is thought to be unrelated to stressors; the increase in circulating catecholamines leads to hypertension and tachyarrhythmias among other clinical signs unrelated to hypertension [286]. Any medications that increase SVR (alpha-1-adrenergic receptor agonists or VP-1 receptor agonists) or HR and contractility (beta-1-adrenergic receptor agonists) have the potential to increase BP dramatically due to toxicity or inadvertent overdose.

Unfortunately, consequences of systemic hypertension can often go unrecognized for long periods, given the difficulty in recognizing and interpreting signs of hypertension by patient owners. Often, secondary hypertension is not recognized until signs of the primary disease are recognized [287]. Ophthalmic consequences of hypertension include acute blindness, retinal detachment, hyphema, retinal atrophy, or rare corneal ulcers. Renal hypertension can lead to potential pressure diuresis, glomerulonephritis, and renal failure. The cardiovascular system can exhibit gallop rhythms, heart murmurs, or other arrhythmias; patients can show exercise intolerance, dyspnea, and, rarely, CHF. The vascular system remodels the intimal and medial layers, resulting in atherosclerosis and vascular stiffening and can lead to hemorrhage exhibited as hyphema, epistaxis, or bleeding in other locations. Neurologic symptoms of hypertension can include stroke, infarction, or hemorrhage, and can lead to head tilt, seizures, paresis, or other neurologic signs.

Anesthetic Management

Treatment for hypertension should be aimed at identification and treatment of the underlying cause and consequences of hypertension and may subsequently be based on the severity of disease. Treatment of the underlying cause in itself may lead to resolution of the hypertension, and antihypertensive medication(s) may not be required. However, if hypertension is severe or if organ damage is identified (ophthalmic, cardiovascular, neurologic, renal, or vascular), treatment with antihypertensive agents may be necessary despite treatment of the underlying cause [287].

Antihypertensive agent options include vasodilators (arteriodilators or venodilators), beta-adrenergic receptor blockers, diuretics, ACE inhibitors, calcium channel blockers, and combinations of these. The choice of initial therapy has largely been extrapolated from human protocols and is a matter of species, identification of the underlying cause, and personal experience [281]. Generally, ACE inhibitors are recommended when hypertension is identified with chronic renal disease. ACE inhibitors will inhibit RAAS-mediated vasoconstriction and are indirect vasodilators. Alternatively, amlodipine is a calcium channel blocker, which also reduces SVR. Amlodipine has a slow onset of action and carries a lower risk for acute hypotension. Hydralazine is a direct arteriodilator and is generally not a first-line treatment for hypertension but is added to combination therapy for refractory hypertension.

Recommendations for anesthetic management of patients with systemic hypertension in veterinary patients are lacking. Human guidelines for anesthetic management are well accepted and can serve as guidelines for management of veterinary patients. Thus, recommendations for anesthetic management include evaluation for magnitude of preanesthetic hypertension, evaluation for end-organ damage due to hypertension, administration of prescribed antihypertensive agents according to treatment schedule before induction of anesthesia, and close monitoring of patient BP during anesthesia [288].

The ACE inhibitor enalapril given to healthy dogs without renal or cardiac disease on the day of an anesthetic event can result in clinically significant hypotension under isoflurane anesthesia, and more intra-anesthetic interventions for moderate to severe hypotension were necessary [289]. Similar results have been shown in cats receiving enalapril before isoflurane anesthesia [290]. Definitive recommendations for the time between stopping ACE inhibitor therapy and anesthesia are lacking; however, a 12-h interval between ACE inhibitor withdrawal and isoflurane anesthesia may still be insufficient to avoid hypotension [289], and a 12–24 h washout period with close BP monitoring before, during, and after anesthesia seems a prudent recommendation. Longer acting agents such as angiotensin receptor blockers (e.g., telmisartan) may require more prolonged washout periods.

Most anesthetics reduce BP by multiple mechanisms, including inducing bradycardia, peripheral vasodilation, and/or negative inotropy. It is generally accepted that the minimum acceptable MAP is >60–70 mmHg for healthy patients. However, it is unknown if higher minimum MAPs are required for veterinary patients with preexisting hypertension. The literature discussing anesthetic care for human patients with preexisting hypertension offers no consensus aside from recognizing that patients with preexisting hypertension are at higher risk for cardiovascular instability under anesthesia [291]. Minimum acceptable BP for veterinary patients remains an area for future research. However, anesthetic drugs that increase BP are generally avoided in patients with preexisting hypertension, including alpha-2-adrenergic receptor agonists and dissociative anesthetics. Excitement, stress, pain, and other causes of catecholamine release should be minimized, with sufficient sedation and analgesia throughout all phases of anesthesia. The choice of anesthetic agents for patients with systemic hypertension is equally reliant on the degree of hypertension, as well as any underlying disease(s).

Pulmonary Arterial Hypertension (PAH)

Incidence

PAH is defined as an abnormally high pressure in the blood vessels of the pulmonary circulation and can be due to either an increase in blood flow, an increase in blood viscosity, or an increase in pulmonary vascular resistance (i.e., pulmonary vasoconstriction). Pulmonary artery pressure >25–35 mmHg is considered abnormally high [292, 293]. Normal systolic pulmonary arterial pressure averages 15–25 mmHg, and normal diastolic pulmonary artery pressure averages 5–10 mmHg [202]. Classification of PAH can be divided by the mechanisms of disease and includes primary PAH, PAH due to left heart disease, to pulmonary hypoxia, or to thrombotic/embolic disease.

Typical breeds presenting with PAH are small to toy breed dogs and are typically middle age to older [293]. Primary PAH can be difficult to distinguish from those of underlying cardiac and pulmonary disease. Clinical features can include cough, dyspnea, lethargy, syncope or collapse, exercise intolerance, heart murmurs, and ascites [292, 293]. Signs of underlying disease may also be present and most commonly include those of right heart failure or heartworm disease, including cyanosis and tachypnea. Cardiopulmonary examination may reveal tricuspid or mitral murmurs, split heart sounds, increased bronchovesicular sounds or crackles, and abdominal fluid wave due to ascites.

Diagnosis of PAH is aimed at determining the magnitude of PAH and the underlying cause, and, most importantly, should include thoracic radiography and echocardiography. Thoracic radiography helps to identify underlying cardiorespiratory diseases that predispose to PAH. Right ventricular enlargement and dilated pulmonary arteries should increase suspicion of PAH. Characteristic echocardiographic findings include concentric right ventricular hypertrophy and dilation of the main pulmonary artery, although identification of underlying cardiac pathology can help assist in the identification of predisposing diseases [293]. Echocardiography also allows for grading of the severity of PAH from mild to severe by assessment of tricuspid valve regurgitation velocity, a number that estimates pulmonary artery systolic pressure. ECG can often be normal and may identify only arrhythmias because of underlying cardiac disease rather than be specific for PAH [293].

Treatment is aimed at reducing clinical signs, improving exercise tolerance, decreasing pulmonary arterial pressure, and identifying and treating underlying causes [294]. Unfortunately, treatment often fails unless the specific underlying cause can be identified and addressed before pulmonary vascular remodeling occurs and pulmonary vascular resistance becomes fixed. Vessel remodeling is characterized by vessel intimal proliferation, medial hypertrophy, and decreased compliance [293]. If the cause cannot be immediately identified, treatment is generally aimed at reducing pulmonary vascular resistance and controlling right ventricular pressure overload. The primary pulmonary vasodilator currently used in veterinary medicine is sildenafil, which appears to provide benefits by a number of pathways, of which direct pulmonary vasodilation is the most significant [295, 296]. Sildenafil improves survival and quality of life in dogs with PAH [295, 297, 298]. Recently, tadalafil, a newer phosphodiesterase (PDE)-5 inhibitor, has shown promise in treatment of canine PAH by offering a longer dosing window (every 24 h) compared to sildenafil (every 8 h), without decreases in treatment efficacy [299].

Anesthetic Management

The most important factor in planning anesthesia for patients with PAH is to be aware of the potential cardiopulmonary derangement associated with the disease. This assessment is based on PE, potential clinical signs consistent with PAH, and results of diagnostic tests. Treatment and stabilization of underlying diseases are optimal. Currently, no peer-reviewed publications exist regarding anesthetic management of PAH in veterinary patients; however, the topic has been extensively reviewed in human medicine [296, 300–303]. Therefore, symptomatic treatment is recommended based on the possible mechanisms of PAH. For example, providing oxygen by face mask before anesthetic induction will increase the FIO_2, PAO_2, and PaO_2, as described by the oxygen pathway (Figure 1.13).

Anesthetic maintenance with 100% oxygen is recommended, as oxygen is also a pulmonary vasodilator via stimulation of nitric oxide production [298]. Anesthetic goals are to maintain CO by optimizing preload and contractility and minimizing decreases in SVR. To that end, choosing anesthetic premedicants, induction, and maintenance agents should minimize cardiovascular depression, as outlined previously. It is crucial to avoid worsening or increasing pulmonary vascular resistance by preventing acidosis, hypoxia, hypercapnia, agitation, pain, and hypothermia [302]. Hypercapnia and hypoxia both worsen pulmonary arterial pressure and signs of PAH [304], and assurance of normocapnia while avoiding hypoxemia via mechanical or consistent manual ventilation is strongly recommended. IBP monitoring should be strongly considered, as it provides a continuous monitor of BP, as well as enables arterial blood gas sampling. Good sedation with premedicants is ideal to prevent stress and pain, which leads to increased catecholamine release and systemic and pulmonary vasoconstriction. Similarly, balanced anesthesia with a reliance on opioids (repeat boluses or infusions) is important to prevent catecholamine release due to nociception. Sildenafil is also recommended to be given 1–2 h before the induction of anesthesia.

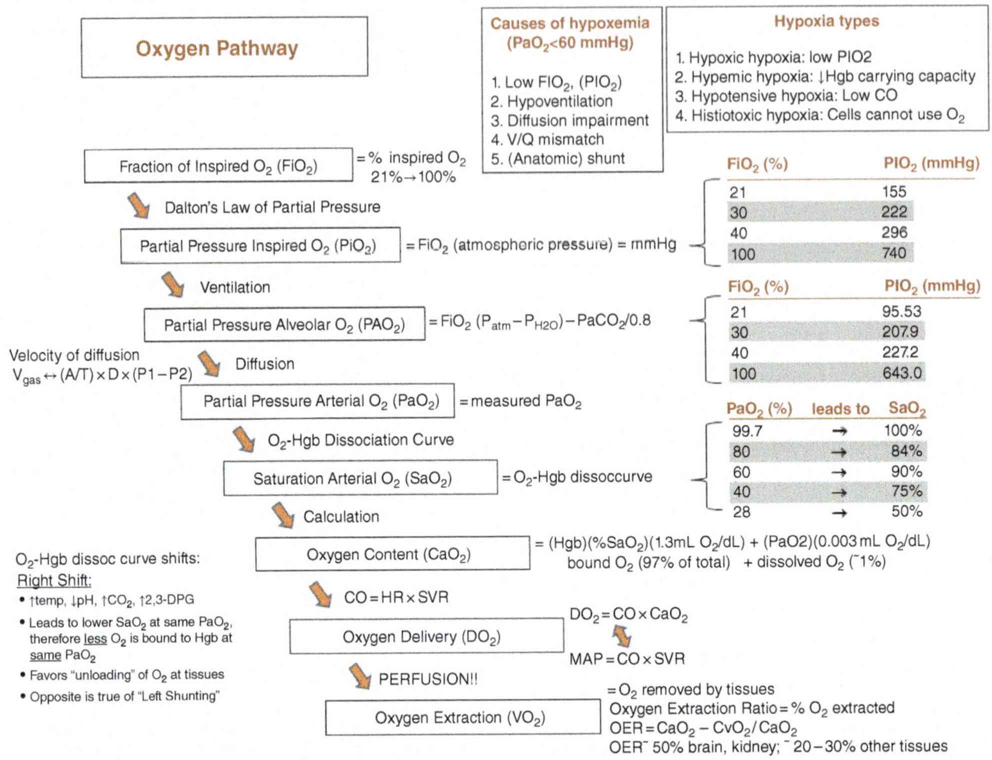

Figure 1.13 The physiologic pathways, principles, and equations that govern the movement of a molecule of oxygen in the environment to the tissue level. Causes and types of hypoxemia are included, with moderate hypoxemia at a P_aO_2 <60 mmHg. Calculated or measured variables are represented in the boxes along the pathway, with physiologic principles. Thus, all possible cases of hypoxemia should be represented at one point through this pathway, and this representation may aid the clinician in evaluating and pinpointing a cause or mechanism for hypoxemia.

Heart Failure

Introduction

Heart failure is defined as the inability of the heart to function as a pump and create forward flow (i.e., normal CO to meet tissue oxygen demands and systemic BP). It represents a final common pathway of several cardiac or pulmonary diseases and is associated with activation of neurohormonal and vascular mechanisms that compensate for the lack of forward flow. Initially, these mechanisms are beneficial in that they improve BP and perfusion, but eventually become detrimental as heart failure worsens. CHF is defined as the failure of the left or right ventricle and the subsequent mechanisms that lead to fluid accumulation in the lungs (pulmonary edema with left heart failure) or abdomen (ascites with right heart failure) [305].

Pathophysiology

The causes of heart failure or CHF are numerous and can be the result of a wide variety of cardiac diseases. The underlying mechanisms for heart failure can be classified into four categories as follows: (i) myocardial failure (primary or secondary), (ii) pressure overload, (iii) volume overload, and (iv) decreased ventricular filling due to poor venous return or abnormal ventricular compliance (Table 1.9).

Table 1.9 Mechanisms of heart failure [12].

Mechanisms of heart failure	Etiology category	Differentials
Myocardial failure		
Primary		Dilated cardiomyopathy
Secondary	Infectious	Bacterial, viral, protozoal, fungal
	Drug	Doxorubicin
	Trauma	Physical trauma, heat stroke, electrocution
	Infiltrative	Neoplasia
	Metabolic	Hypothyroidism, hyperthyroidism, uremia valvular insufficiency, shunt
	Other	
Pressure overload	Hypertension	Systemic or pulmonary hypertension
	Outflow obstruction (anatomic)	Aortic or pulmonic stenosis
	Outflow obstruction (dynamic)	Hypertrophic or obstructive cardiomyopathy
Volume overload	Valvular insufficiency	Mitral insufficiency
	Left-to-right shunt	PDA, VSD
	High-output state	Hyperthyroidism, anemia
Decreased ventricular filling	Pericardial disease	Pericardial effusion, restrictive pericarditis
	Diastolic dysfunction	Hypertrophic cardiomyopathy, restrictive pericarditis
	AV valve obstruction	Mitral or tricuspid stenosis
	Space-occupying lesion	Right atrial neoplasia, right ventricular outflow tract mass

Myocardial failure is characterized by loss of cardiac contractile strength, whether primary (e.g., DCM) or secondary to other etiologies. Myocardial failure leads to compensatory activation that increases circulating blood volume through sodium and water retention, thereby increasing end-diastolic volume leading to ventricular dilation. Stroke volume is initially maintained despite ventricular dilation, which can lead to AV valve insufficiency.

Pressure overload is due to an increase in myocardial wall stress after increases in ventricular systolic pressures. Most commonly, this results from valvular stenosis (PS and AS) or increases in systemic or pulmonary vascular resistance from either systemic hypertension or PAH, respectively. Pressure overload leads to concentric ventricular hypertrophy that can be identified on echocardiogram. Inner layers of hypertrophied muscle may be underperfused and become ischemic, which can lead to ventricular arrhythmias, fibrillation, and sudden death.

Volume overload is most seen with valvular insufficiency (usually AV valvular insufficiency) or anatomic shunts such as a PDA or VSD. It is defined as an increase in end-diastolic chamber size but normal end-systolic chamber size, an indicator that contractility is normal, and SV has increased. Volume overload leads to eccentric hypertrophy to manage the increase in ventricular volume and increase forward flow. Anatomic shunts also increase ventricular volume, as they allow an increase in ventricular filling. For example, a PDA allows aortic blood to backflow into the pulmonary artery, increasing left atrial and left ventricular blood volume. Eventually, myocardial failure can result.

Reduced ventricular filling occurs when there is a physical obstruction to blood flow, blood volume is reduced, or there is impaired relaxation (lusitropy) and filling of the ventricle. Physical obstruction to blood flow can occur because of enlarged abdominal organs (e.g., gastric dilatation volvulus, hepatic or splenic neoplasia, insufflation of hollow viscera, gravid uterus, etc.), surgical manipulation of vasculature responsible for venous return (i.e., cranial and caudal vena cava and tributaries), and positive pressure ventilation, among others. Reduced preload can be acute or chronic depending on the cause. For example, reduced blood volume can occur with dehydration, third spacing of fluids, or blood loss. Reductions in ventricular compliance occur with HCM and constrictive pericarditis, where stiffening due to muscular hypertrophy or a thickened pericardium prevents diastolic relaxation. Compliance is the pressure–volume relationship in the ventricle; poor compliance leads to abnormally high filling pressures with relatively normal filling volumes. Abnormally high ventricular pressures lead to blood backup to the atria and eventually organ congestion and/or edema.

Aside from the cardiac disease mechanisms and pathophysiology briefly described, compensatory mechanisms exist to maintain homeostasis in the face of poor heart function to maintain BP and tissue perfusion. While they have been extensively described elsewhere [306–308], a brief review is presented in this section. Compensatory mechanisms include the Frank–Starling mechanism and activation of the SNS, RAAS, and neuroendocrine pathways, which include endothelin and natriuretic peptides. In the acute phase of hypotension, decreased myocardial function activates baroreceptor responses to increase SNS tone, leading to vasoconstriction and increases in contractility and HR. The SNS also stimulates ADH and renin release. ADH causes fluid reabsorption in the kidneys, and renin stimulates the RAAS. The RAAS is further stimulated by reduced renal perfusion, SNS activation, and decreased sodium delivery to the macula densa. These mechanisms provide vasoconstriction and increase blood volume and venous return to restore normal perfusion. Although beneficial in the short term, chronic stimulation of these mechanisms is detrimental to homeostasis.

The New York Heart Association classifications [309] for heart failure have been adapted for veterinary use (Source: American Heart Association, Inc.) as follows: Class I: heart disease without clinical signs such as exercise intolerance, fatigue, shortness of breath or dyspnea; Class II: patients who present with mild exercise intolerance, but may not have radiographic evidence of disease, normal at rest; Class III: patients who have clinical signs of heart failure during normal activity and have multiple radiographic signs of heart failure, including cardiomegaly, pulmonary edema, distended vasculature, and left atrial enlargement; Class IV: patients are in obvious distress with signs of heart failure at rest. Radiographs have the aforementioned signs along with severe pulmonary infiltrates and potentially pleural or abdominal effusion [302]. Treatment strategies vary on the basis of the degree of heart disease and clinical signs along the spectrum of patients who present from mild to severe disease.

Anesthetic Management

Planning for and responding to complications during an anesthetic event in a patient at risk for heart failure, one who has recently been treated for heart failure, or one who has evidence of heart failure, test the knowledge and skill of the anesthetist. Patients can present anywhere along the spectrum of classification for heart failure from minimal to severe risks for anesthesia.

Preoperative assessment of patient status is a critical step in assessing risks and planning for potential complications, as well as choosing appropriate premedication/induction agents and preparing appropriate monitoring tools. It should include a complete history and PE, focusing on clinical signs of dyspnea, exercise intolerance, collapse, coughing, weakness, and other signs relevant to cardiopulmonary function. Of most importance are any recent changes in patient behavior. All medications for heart disease as well as the most recent dosing regimen should be noted. Although it is controversial to feed a patient anything before anesthesia, ensuring that the patient received morning doses of medications is prudent, except for ACE inhibitors or angiotensin receptor blockers, as they can precipitate significant hypotension under isoflurane anesthesia [289]. Physical exam should focus on parameters indicative of cardiopulmonary function such as mucous membrane color and capillary refill time, thoracic and cardiac auscultation, pulse rhythm and intensity, presence of jugular pulsations, and palpation/ballottement for organomegaly and/or fluid waves. Diagnostic procedures may consist of preanesthetic ECG, BP, thoracic radiography, abdominal ultrasonography, and echocardiography. Any abnormalities should prompt further investigation, as patient status may have changed since last examined. If the patient presenting with anesthesia is under the care of a veterinary cardiologist, patient reevaluation may be suggested and/or pursued.

The veterinary adaptation of the New York Heart Association classes of heart failure can be very useful in placing patients into an ASA status (Table 1.1). Although no classification system is optimal, and ASA status is not formally an assessment of risk of complications, it is reasonable to expect that as heart failure classification becomes more serious, ASA status will increase. The general strategies listed in the following section are intended to be specific to a patient presenting with heart failure. Obviously, if the nature of the procedure or the presence of comorbidities presents higher risk to the patient independent of the nature of their heart disease, ASA status would be higher than for the heart disease alone.

Patients who are Class I will likely be ASA status I or II and can likely be anesthetized with any combination of premedicants (opioids, anticholinergics, benzodiazepines, ketamine, and acepromazine) and induction agents (ketamine/benzodiazepine, propofol, alfaxalone, ±benzodiazepines), with the possible caveat that alpha-2-adrenergic receptor agonists would be best avoided. Standard monitoring of ECG, BP, SpO_2, and temperature is likely to be sufficient. Standard IV fluids administered at 3–5 $ml\,kg^{-1}\,min^{-1}$ are likely to be tolerated well.

Patients who are Class II present a higher potential for complications and are likely to be an ASA status III and should be treated accordingly. Depending on the pathophysiology of the cardiovascular disease, acepromazine and alpha-2-adrenergic receptor agonists should likely be avoided; reliance on opioids for sedation and dose reduction is recommended. Older, less stable patients may sedate well with a combination of an opioid and benzodiazepine. Induction agent dose, whether propofol, alfaxalone, or ketamine is used, should be reduced with good sedation from premedication and combination with a benzodiazepine. Inhaled anesthetic agent dose requirements should be reduced as much as possible with the combination of premedicants, opioids, or possibly other analgesic infusions (lidocaine and ketamine), as well as local or regional anesthesia techniques. Maintenance fluid rates may be normal or reduced depending on patient status. Positive inotropic agents and vasopressors should be available in case of hypotension unresponsive to reducing inhalant dose and optimization of HR and rhythm. Standard anesthetic monitoring may be sufficient; however, advanced monitoring (IBP and CVP ± PPV) may be required for unstable patients or for the nature of the procedure.

Patients who are Class III and IV present serious potential for decompensation and severe complications under anesthesia and are likely to be ASA status IV or V. The need for an anesthetic event must be carefully weighed against the benefit of a procedure, as the potential for life-threatening complications can be very high. These patients are very critical and require the highest level of intensive monitoring and support, including IBP monitoring, evaluation of arterial blood gases for oxygenation and acid–base balance, CVP and/or PPV monitoring, and advanced ECG interpretation. Positive inotropic agents, vasopressors, and antiarrhythmic agents should be available, and the anesthetist should be comfortable with their use. CPCR status should be discussed and known to the anesthesia team. Mechanical ventilation is extremely beneficial in optimizing ventilation and oxygenation, as well as preventing respiratory acidosis and the pH-related changes in cardiac function and electrolyte shifting. Premedication, induction, and maintenance phases of anesthesia should be aimed at minimally impacting cardiovascular function. Agents with short durations of action and/or reversibility are recommended should the patient decompensate. For this reason, opioids are good choices as premedication and induction agents. Acepromazine, ketamine, and alpha-2-adrenergic receptor agonists may be avoided; the use of benzodiazepines, opioids, and possibly anticholinergics is generally recommended. Anesthetic induction can be accomplished with combinations of opioids and benzodiazepines such as fentanyl and/or etomidate and midazolam.

Chamber, mask, or "box" inductions with inhaled anesthetics are not recommended due to slow and poorly controlled anesthetic induction and transition through the excitement phase, difficulty in monitoring of vital parameters, slow and poor airway access, and the dose of inhaled anesthetic required for intubation is higher (deeper) than is required for surgical procedures. These inhaled anesthetic doses invariably lead to moderate to severe cardiovascular depression, no matter how short they may (or may not) be. These inductions are a last-choice option for patients with severe cardiovascular disease and should only be considered for severely fractious patients for whom handling and premedication may lead to detrimental stress, catecholamine release, and potential arrhythmogenic effects. If a chamber induction cannot be avoided, it is recommended that patients not be anesthetized to the point of intubation (owing to depth required and cardiovascular depression), but rather to the point of safe handling (immediately deep to the excitement phase) and then removed to place a face mask of inhalant only. At that point, the patient can be removed, monitoring equipment and an IV catheter can be placed, and the induction completed with an option that provides less cardiovascular depression such as carefully titrated propofol or etomidate combined with a benzodiazepine. This typically leads to a more satisfactory and efficient intubation as compared to inhalant only.

Inhaled anesthetic agent requirements should be reduced to the lowest possible levels with the application of CRIs (Tables 1.2–1.4) and local/regional anesthesia techniques. Fluid rates should be significantly reduced to minimize the risk of volume overload; meeting metabolic requirements at 2–5 $ml\,kg^{-1}\,h^{-1}$ is recommended. Fluid boluses and colloids should be avoided or administered cautiously to avoid precipitating or worsening heart failure and pulmonary edema/ascites.

Canine and Feline Cardiomyopathies

Cardiomyopathy is a general term applied to diseases of the cardiac muscle tissue leading to structural impairment and subsequent decrease in cardiac function. This separates cardiomyopathies from valvular, congenital, electrical, or conduction abnormalities, and traumatic or metabolic disturbances.

A primary cardiomyopathy is due to intrinsic disease of the muscle; a secondary cardiomyopathy is due to derangements in a different organ system with secondary effects in the heart.

Hypertrophic Cardiomyopathy

Pathophysiology

Hypertrophic cardiomyopathy is due to idiopathic concentric thickening of the cardiac muscle, leading to stiffening of the myocardium and a failure of relaxation (lusitropy), a form of diastolic dysfunction wherein the heart fails to relax normally [310]. It is known to be autosomal-dominant in Maine Coon cats and is hereditary in Persians and some American Shorthairs [291]. Disease onset is seen as early as six months of age. Cats may be nonclinical even with severe disease, and sudden death is possible at any time. In these situations, a quantitative N-terminal pro-b-type natriuretic peptide (NT pro-BNP) assay (serum or pleural fluid) can be used to distinguish cats with severe subclinical HCM from normal cats or cats with mild disease. However, pro-BNP test results are not indicated to separate normal cats from those with mild to moderate, clinically evident disease, as a negative test cannot exclude the presence of disease [311, 312].

HCM tends to affect the left ventricular free wall and interventricular septum/papillary muscles preferentially. The etiology in most cases is idiopathic; however, other possible causes include hyperthyroidism, hypergonadotropism, and secondary to hypertension. This thickening leads to a decrease in the internal volume of the ventricle when relaxed (end-diastolic volume), and the inability to accept venous return leads to an eventual increase in left atrial pressure, mitral regurgitation, pulmonary edema, and the cascade of events leading to left heart failure. HOCM is a variant in which muscular hypertrophy can pull the anterior mitral valve leaflet into the LVOT and leads to dynamic obstruction of ventricular outflow. It is believed that increases in HR and velocity of blood flow through the LVOT can also predispose to systolic anterior motion (SAM) of the mitral valve leaflet and worsening of left ventricular CO. SAM may also worsen mitral regurgitation. Poor blood flow due to poor ventricular diastolic compliance leads to blood stasis and thrombus formation typically in the left atrium, leading to the potential for pulmonary thromboembolism. Diagnosis of HCM is typically due to identification of septal or free wall thickening in a nondilated ventricle with echocardiography. Poor diastolic ventricular filling also leads to poor CO and BP.

Treatment

Treatment for HCM typically involves identification and treatment of the underlying cause. No definitive treatments have been shown to achieve reversal of hypertrophy, although many veterinary cardiologists recommend empirical beta-adrenergic receptor blocker or calcium channel blocker therapy. Therefore, management is typically directed at treating the sequelae of reduced ventricular compliance: preventing myocardial ischemia, treatment of congestion and secondary arrhythmias, and potentially improving diastolic dysfunction.

Anesthetic Management

Anesthetic management of HCM varies based on the severity of disease. Patients with occult disease may fail detection and are likely successfully anesthetized with all combinations of anesthetic drugs. Patients with mild disease and heart murmurs with minimal structural change can similarly be anesthetized with nearly any combinations of anesthetics. However, the use of dissociative anesthetics such as ketamine and tiletamine is more controversial in mild cardiac disease. Dissociatives are generally considered contraindicated in more severe HCM, particularly if elevated BP or increased afterload is detrimental to heart function [310]. High-dose dissociative anesthetics cause an increase in HR, myocardial contractility, and BP due to SNS stimulation and increased sympathetic discharge [313–315]. This stimulation leads to an increase in myocardial work and oxygen demand. HCM is characterized by thickening of the myocardium leading to diastolic dysfunction, potential SAM, and LVOTO [309, 310]. Increases in blood flow velocity through the LVOT may worsen SAM and lead to ventricular ejection obstruction. Therefore, the sympathomimetic effects of dissociative anesthetics may be quite detrimental to ventricular outflow, and ketamine and tiletamine may be better off avoided in these cases. In addition, the increase in cardiac oxygen demand may not be met by tissues that are underperfused because of the pathologic remodeling of myocardial tissue, increasing the risk for myocardial ischemia and possible arrhythmias. Patients with severe disease characterized by previous history of CHF, arrhythmias, or HOCM require intensive monitoring and a complete understanding of strategies for management [316].

Regardless of disease severity, the primary focus for management should be to optimize perfusion and minimize myocardial oxygen demand. Typical treatments for hypotension include the following: (i) optimizing HR and rhythm, (ii) decreasing inspired inhaled anesthetic concentrations, (iii) providing adequate fluid therapy and volume, and (iv) administering positive inotropic agents or vasopressors (Figure 1.4).

Optimizing HR and rhythm is a combination of recognizing and treating bradycardia and underlying arrhythmias (SVT, ventricular ectopy, or ventricular tachycardia) while weighing the risks of anticholinergic therapy. Hypotensive cats with a sinus rhythm may be considered for anticholinergic therapy to improve CO and BP, and doses should be titrated to avoid inducing tachycardia. Although tachycardia may be less risky in cats with mild disease, patients with moderate to severe thickening or HOCM/SAM may have severe increases in myocardial oxygen demand (in poorly perfused, thickened muscle) due to tachyarrhythmias. Careful titration of anticholinergic therapy to prevent tachyarrhythmias is critical in these patients. Treatment for ventricular arrhythmias with lidocaine boluses (0.25–1.0 mg kg^{-1} with a total per cat dose of <4 mg IV) [239] or SVT (diltiazem 25–50 μg kg^{-1} titrated to lowest effective dose) should be considered. IBP monitoring is recommended in moderately to severely affected cats.

Fluid therapy and boluses are intended to improve venous return and are controversial in patients with mild HCM, as diastolic compliance, if affected, may not be able to tolerate additional venous return. In patients with severe disease, particularly with a history of CHF, high fluid rates and boluses are contraindicated, as the increase in preload may precipitate congestion and pulmonary edema. Colloids are contraindicated, as fluid overload with colloids is more difficult to treat compared to volume overload due to crystalloids because colloids have a long duration of action and rely on liver metabolism for elimination [317, 318].

Reduction in inhaled anesthetic concentrations is a critical tool in preventing anesthetic-induced hypotension. The anesthetist should consider all strategies to reduce inhaled anesthetic requirement, including analgesic boluses or infusions, local and regional analgesia, and potential for avoidance of general anesthesia if possible. Positive inotrope administration is controversial in cats with HCM. While positive inotropes primarily improve contractility, HCM is mainly associated with diastolic dysfunction (lusitropy, not inotropy), and typically systolic function is not reduced. Interestingly, positive inotropes, by increasing beta-1-adrenergic activity, also improve indices of relaxation (left ventricular change in pressure over change in time [LV dp/dt], lusitropy, etc.) [319], in addition to positive inotropic effects [320]. Increasing contractility may be detrimental, as it increases cardiac work (and myocardial oxygen demand in thickened, poorly perfused myocardium) and can worsen SAM in HOCM by increasing the flow velocity through the LVOT. Positive inotropes can also be arrhythmogenic and can precipitate or worsen underlying cardiac arrhythmias. For these reasons, vasopressors used to increase SVR have been recommended. Although new research has questioned these conclusions, more investigation is required.

Premedication of cats with HCM typically includes opioids for mild sedation, facilitation of catheter placement, and reduction of anesthetic induction doses. Acepromazine is controversial because it leads to long-acting vasodilation that is not reversible and can precipitate hypotension. Alpha-2-adrenergic receptor agonists, while controversial with respect to their use in heart disease, may in fact reduce LVOT obstruction in cats with obstructive HCM such that they are not contraindicated [321]. Benzodiazepines are very safe choices for patients with cardiac disease due to minimal cardiovascular effects but can be variable sedatives in cats and may lead to excitement and aggression. Alfaxalone delivered IM at 1–2 $mg\,kg^{-1}$ in combination with an opioid or benzodiazepine can provide rapid onset, excellent sedation in cats with HCM while avoiding typical side effects of dissociatives and alpha-2-adrenergic agonists [322–324].

Anesthetic induction can be achieved with combinations of propofol or alfaxalone with a benzodiazepine to reduce total induction dose in patients with mild to moderate disease. Patients with more severe disease can be induced with combinations of etomidate with a benzodiazepine. Although combinations of fentanyl with a benzodiazepine are attractive in that they cause minimal cardiovascular depression, the slow transition to unconsciousness (and potential to be overridden with sufficient stimuli), as well as the potential for severe dysphoria in cats, makes this combination successful in only the most debilitated cats. However, in these patients, it may offer an advantage if etomidate is unavailable.

As discussed previously, for patients with moderate to severe cardiovascular disease, mask, chamber, or "box" inductions with inhaled anesthetics are not recommended. Anesthetic induction is prolonged, and transition through the excitement phase is slow, leading to increased patient stress. Intensive monitoring that these patients require is impossible; ability to intubate is brief, slow to achieve, and poor in quality, and the dose of inhaled anesthetic for intubation causes moderate to severe cardiovascular depression for the duration of the slow induction process. Chamber inductions should only be considered for severely fractious patients for whom handling and premedication may lead to detrimental stress, catecholamine release, and potential arrhythmogenic effects.

Opioid infusions can be used to provide analgesia, as well as reduce inhaled anesthetic requirements. Doses may need to be lowered toward the end of anesthesia to allow metabolism and prevent dysphoria in recovery. Local and/or regional anesthesia techniques are strongly encouraged to reduce systemic drug requirements. Hypotension can be treated as stated previously. Ventilation should be supplemented to prevent respiratory acidosis, and patients with arrhythmias should be monitored with continuous ECG waveform. Pulse oximetry should be used to monitor for oxygen saturation in all patients with cardiac disease. IBP and arterial blood gas analysis are the gold standard of monitoring and should be strongly considered in patients with a recent or current history of CHF. Patients with CHF should be medically stabilized before anesthesia, provided it is not an emergency. Referral to a cardiologist or anesthesiologist may be considered for severe cases.

Dilated Cardiomyopathy

Incidence and Pathophysiology

DCM is the most common cardiovascular disease diagnosed in dogs, followed by mitral valve and heartworm diseases. It is most found in large breed dogs, including the Doberman Pinscher, Great Dane, Irish Wolfhound, Boxer dogs, and less commonly in mixed-breed dogs, with male dogs appearing to be more affected than the female dogs [325]. Although not proven, it is likely that there is a heritable component to canine DCM.

DCM is characterized by an idiopathic primary loss of myocardial contractility. Secondary causes of DCM include several nutritional deficiencies (e.g., taurine-deficiency-associated DCM in Cocker Spaniels and potentially in Labradors and Golden Retrievers), tachycardia-induced DCM (secondary to SVT or atrial flutter), and adriamycin toxicity [326]. Importantly, between 2015 and 2020, there has been a new association between grain-free diets and DCM in breeds not typically associated with DCM, including German Shepherds, Cocker Spaniels, and up to 5 cases in 25 different breeds [327]. Diets based on peas, lentils, other legumes, and potatoes and other novel ingredients have been implicated, but no clear correlation has been established. Research into potential causes of DCM separate from the known hereditary and/or nutritional deficiencies is ongoing to discriminate if grain-free or novel protein diets have a causal relationship with DCM and comprehensive reviews have been published [327, 328].

Loss of contractility leads to systolic dysfunction associated with reduced ejection fraction, fractional shortening, and rate of ejection, as well as an increase in end-systolic volume. These changes lead to progressive dilation of the ventricle followed by left-sided or biventricular CHF. The term "occult" DCM is used before clinical signs are seen and is characterized by the loss of contractility and ventricular remodeling. Clinical signs may include irregular pulse rhythm, decreased intensity of cardiac sounds, weak pulses, or jugular distension. The overt phase of DCM presents with clinical signs relative to onset of CHF, including lethargy, syncope, pulse deficits, dyspnea, cough, and/or abdominal distension. Patients can easily present with heart failure or sudden death as the first sign of DCM. Diagnosis is via demonstration of loss of systolic function without an identifiable cause. Patients may present with SVT, ventricular ectopy, atrial flutter, or atrial fibrillation.

Anesthetic Management

The goal of DCM treatment is to prevent or reverse the remodeling associated with the loss of contractility. Unfortunately, as most cases are idiopathic, therapy is limited to treatment/prevention of heart failure, treatment of cardiac arrhythmias, and improving quality of life. Treatment of heart failure must be tailored to the individual, as no single treatment strategy is sufficient for all patients; however, common strategies include removal of the grain-free diet, diuretics, positive inotropes, phosphodiesterase inhibitors, pimobendan, and antiarrhythmics. Long-term management may include diuretics, beta-adrenergic receptor blockers, ACE inhibitors, pimobendan, and/or oral antiarrhythmics.

Anesthetic management of patients diagnosed with DCM is multifactorial and includes planning for and maintenance of systolic function, prevention of heart failure, management of arrhythmias, and inotropic support. Since even nonclinical patients may already have significant systolic dysfunction and remodeling, the following techniques can likely be applied to all patients with occult or overt DCM. Patients presenting with heart failure are at severe anesthetic risks, and anesthesia should be postponed until the patient is stabilized.

Patients with overt DCM with reduced systolic function and forward flow develop heart failure, as they cannot eject diastolic preload. Therefore, perianesthetic fluid therapy should be titrated to the lowest effective dose for hydration and ongoing losses. Balanced electrolyte crystalloid administration rates should be 3–5 $ml\,kg^{-1}\,h^{-1}$; higher fluid rates may precipitate volume overload and heart failure. Colloids are contraindicated as previously discussed.

Common arrhythmias associated with DCM include VPCs, couplets, triplets, or more complicated ventricular ectopy, atrial fibrillation, and, rarely, atrial flutter or SVT. ECG monitoring should begin before induction of anesthesia, and the cardiac rhythm should be stabilized before anesthesia if possible. Antiarrhythmic agents including, but not limited to, lidocaine and diltiazem should be available.

For inotropic support, dobutamine is the clear choice over dopamine to increase contractility, SV, CO, and BP. While dopamine activates beta-1-adrenergic receptors and is a positive inotrope when delivered between 5 and 10 $\mu g\ kg^{-1}\ min^{-1}$, dopamine will cross to the alpha-1-adrenergic receptors at higher doses, subsequently inducing vasoconstriction and increasing afterload, which may severely reduce fractional shortening and CO. Dobutamine is preferred in these patients, as it has limited alpha-1-adrenergic effects. Dobutamine increases HR and contractility because of nonspecific beta-adrenergic receptor (mainly β_1) agonist effects.

Common premedication techniques for patients with DCM often include opioids because of their cardiovascular safety. Opioid-induced bradycardia may be treated with anticholinergics if necessary. Benzodiazepines are inconsistent sedatives in dogs. However, sedation with benzodiazepines is improved when combined with an opioid. Acepromazine is not recommended, as it leads to long-acting, irreversible vasodilation and can easily precipitate hypotension with variable effects on contractility and HR. Alpha-2-adrenergic receptor agonists are absolutely contraindicated due to the severe increase in afterload, as well as the decrease in CO.

Nearly all anesthetic induction agents are negative inotropes to some degree and will reduce contractility dose-dependently. Although patients with very mild disease may be successfully induced with propofol or alfaxalone while maintaining cardiovascular function, those with mild, moderate, or severe disease can most safely be induced with either etomidate or fentanyl and a benzodiazepine (midazolam or diazepam) or fentanyl. Etomidate has a more reliable transition to unconsciousness compared to fentanyl, but has other effects, including adrenocortical suppression, higher cost, lower availability, and very high osmolarity (approximately 4800 $mOsm\ l^{-1}$) [101, 329, 330]. While the sympathomimetic effects of ketamine will increase HR, contractility, and BP by increasing circulating norepinephrine concentrations, ketamine has a direct negative inotropic effect that is typically overwhelmed by the sympathomimetic effects [313–316]. The potential for further reductions in myocardial contractility in a patient with DCM may be severely detrimental to fractional shortening and ventricular ejection. As safer alternative induction options exist, ketamine is not recommended for induction of anesthesia in patients with DCM.

Maintenance with inhaled anesthetics is often unavoidable. However, all inhaled anesthetics produce a moderate to severe dose-dependent reduction in contractility and subsequent decrease in SV and CO. All attempts to minimize (or avoid) inhaled anesthetic doses must be applied. These include opioid infusions as well as local and regional anesthesia/analgesia.

Arrhythmogenic Cardiomyopathy

Incidence and Pathophysiology

ARVC (arrythmogenic right ventricular cardiomyopathy) is a variant of canine cardiomyopathy seen in Boxer dogs [331]. Patients often present with syncope or exercise intolerance; however, pulse deficits and arrhythmias may be identified incidentally. Unfortunately, sudden death may be the only identifier of the disease. A small percentage of dogs may develop systolic dysfunction and heart failure. Short periods of ECG monitoring may fail to identify abnormal ECG rhythms, and Holter monitoring is recommended to evaluate for extent of arrhythmogenic disease. Criteria for advanced diagnosis of occult ARVC are lacking. Treatment for affected dogs may not reverse or delay the onset of more severe clinical signs but may decrease syncopal events and is generally recommended for >1000 VPCs in a 24-h Holter period, if R-on-T phenomenon is identified or there are paroxysms of ventricular tachycardia.

Anesthetic Management

Anesthetic management is similar to patients with DCM. Pre-induction monitoring of the

ECG and treatment of ventricular ectopy are recommended before induction. Increases in sympathetic tone due to pain, stress, or excitement are to be avoided to reduce the potential for arrhythmogenic effects of catecholamine release.

Heartworm Disease

Incidence and Pathophysiology

Heartworm disease is prevalent across the United States and can affect all dogs and cats, regardless of age, environment, or gender. It is most common within 150 mi of the Gulf and Atlantic Coasts and along the Mississippi River Valley, with high seroprevalence in the South [332]. Other areas of the United States can see infection rates in up to 5% of the unprotected population. All dogs must be viewed as susceptible, and heartworm preventative is a mainstay of prophylactic veterinary medicine.

Heartworm infection is due to the parasite *Dirofilaria immitis* and is transmitted between dogs by mosquitoes, which transmit a larval stage of the parasite. Newly infected dogs develop adult heartworms that reside in the heart and pulmonary vasculature within five to six months of infection. Adult heartworms induce endothelial and myointimal thickening of both small and large pulmonary arteries from antigenic stimulation. Inflammatory mediators reacting to exposed subendothelial collagen and to adult worms lead to endothelial proliferation and development of villi-like projections on the arterial luminal surface. Arteries dilate and become torturous, leading to the classic radiographic findings. Altogether, these changes along with flow obstruction due to physical presence of worms lead to an increase in pulmonary vascular resistance and are the underlying cause of PHT. The development of PHT, if severe, can then lead to a pressure overload of the right ventricle, although the degree of PHT can vary from mild to severe. Right heart failure is a result of fulminant heartworm disease, although it is unclear if this is a direct result of PHT or some other mechanism. The fragmentation of dying or dead heartworms can lead to pulmonary thromboembolism and severe ventilation/perfusion imbalances. Pulmonary parenchymal disease characterized by inflammatory-mediated interstitial edema and eventual pulmonary fibrosis from chronic inflammation may also be seen.

Clinical signs of heartworm disease are dependent on worm burden in the heart and lungs. Early and mild infections may not have recognizable clinical signs; however, dogs with moderate worm burdens typically present with exercise intolerance, cough, and abnormal lung sounds. Dogs with severe worm burden can present with signs because of cardiac, pulmonary, hepatic, or renal dysfunction, including cough, exercise intolerance, dyspnea, hepatomegaly, syncope, ascites, heart murmurs, signs of right-sided heart failure, and/or acute death. Severe cases may also have signs of hypoxemia. Heart murmurs can auscult as left basilar ejection murmurs, split S2 sounds, systolic clicks, or murmurs supportive of tricuspid insufficiency. Severe disease can also present with pulmonary thromboembolism, disseminated intravascular coagulation, hemoptysis, or signs of allergic reactions directed against adult worms. Abnormalities may include eosinophilia and basophilia in mildly affected dogs. Severely affected dogs may show thrombocytopenia and anemia due to caval syndrome (see the following section), signs of organ damage due to hypoxemia, or decreased organ perfusion. Heartworm screening includes antigen and antibody testing in dogs.

Feline Heartworm Disease

Feline heartworm disease is far less common, as cats are not a typical target for mosquitoes, and microfilariae dose for clinical infection and disease is higher than dogs [333]. Physical exams of cats with heartworm disease are often normal. However, they may present with mild cough and may infrequently have heart murmurs, arrhythmias, or abnormal lung sounds.

Cats may present with asthmatic signs owing to immune system response to adult worms. No single abnormality on serum chemistry and blood count is diagnostic for adult heartworm infection. Combined antigen and antibody testing is recommended in cats, and a positive antigen test confirms infection, although infected cats are often antigen-negative [327].

Caval Syndrome

Caval syndrome is a life-threatening presentation of advanced heartworm disease and is characterized by a severe burden of adult worms with associated severe tricuspid regurgitation, decreased CO, intravascular hemolysis, marked hemoglobinemia, and hemoglobinuria. Clinical signs are due to acute accumulation of heartworms in the right ventricle and across the tricuspid valve, leading to severe ventricular dysfunction and tricuspid valve incompetence. It is unknown why the mass of heartworms invades the right heart, but moderate to severe PHT and a large worm burden are precipitating factors. Heartworms typically do not invade the right ventricle, as they are quickly moved into the pulmonary arteries because of downstream blood flow. Severe decreases in forward flow due to experimental administration of beta-adrenergic receptor blockers or thiopental have the potential to allow adult worms to "fall into" the right ventricle and precipitate caval syndrome. This argues that any severe decrease in forward flow, particularly in patients with high worm burdens or signs of PHT, has the potential to acutely develop caval syndrome in response to sudden decreases in CO. The lack of forward flow is the reason heartworms can recede into the right ventricle postmortem.

Anesthetic Management

In mildly to moderately affected dogs, no single anesthesia protocol appears to have significant advantages over others, and no particular anesthetics are contraindicated with positive heartworm antigen tests. As with any anesthetized patient, appropriate monitoring, including BP, pulse oximetry, and ECG, is critically important to evaluating patient stability and changes over time. Cardiovascular support for hypotensive patients can likely be provided as in normal patients.

In severely affected patients with moderate to severe worm burdens, particularly in those at risk for caval syndrome due to sudden decreases in CO, optimizing anesthetic plans to maintain CO and minimize changes in cardiac function and perfusion is strongly recommended. For patients with signs of right heart failure, anesthetic management has been previously described in this chapter. In patients who present with either heart failure or caval syndrome, choosing anesthetic plans that have minimal effects on CO or effects that are readily treatable is safest. If possible, avoidance of general anesthesia with sedation and/or locoregional anesthesia/analgesia is preferred to avoid the risks associated with general anesthesia.

Whether for sedation alone or as premedication before general anesthesia, sedation with opioids and benzodiazepines is preferred in that they have minimal cardiovascular effects, provided the opioid-mediated bradycardia is minimal or prevented with concurrent administration of anticholinergics. Premedication with alpha-2-adrenergic receptor agonists is contraindicated in patients at risk for caval syndrome or with high worm burdens due to the severe reductions in CO at typical premedication doses equal to or higher than 5 μg kg^{-1}. Acepromazine is controversial, as the alpha-1-adrenergic-receptor-antagonist-mediated decrease in SVR can lead to decreases in BP that are long-acting and irreversible.

Etomidate and fentanyl combined with a benzodiazepine have minimal effects on cardiac contractility and SVR and are ideal induction agents to maintain CO. Induction doses of opioids have the potential to significantly depress HR and ventilation, and these side effects must be controlled.

In addition to basic monitoring tools, advanced monitoring for severely affected patients is strongly recommended. Invasive arterial BP monitoring provides accurate, continuous BP monitoring. Access to arterial blood and availability of arterial blood gas analyses are critical tools for the assessment of ventilation/perfusion imbalances and can assist in the diagnosis of pulmonary thromboembolism. Doppler crystal placement also allows for a second assessment of BP should an arterial catheter fail.

Summary

The large variety of cardiovascular diseases and the wide range of severity and clinical presentation of cardiac diseases present a significant challenge to the clinician in planning for an anesthetic event. Thus, one of the most important concepts to understand is that the wide range of diagnoses and underlying pathophysiology should prompt the clinician to investigate the nature of any sign of cardiovascular disease carefully and completely and use that information to design an appropriate anesthetic and analgesic plan to maximize the safety of the patient through the anesthetic process. This chapter presents appropriate information for the clinician to prepare an individually tailored anesthesia plan for each patient presenting with cardiac disease.

References

1 Clarkson, A.N., Sutherland, B.A., and Appleton, I. (2005). The biology and pathology of hypoxia-ischemia: an update. *Arch. Immunol. Ther. Exp. (Warsz)* 53: 213–225.

2 Muir, W.W. (2015). Cardiovascular physiology. In: *Veterinary Anesthesia and Analgesia. The fifth edition of Lumb and Jones* (eds. K.A. Grimm, L.A. Lamont, W.J. Tranquilli, et al.), 417–472. Ames: Wiley Blackwell Updated Edition.

3 Mazzaferro, E. and Wagner, A.E. (2001). Hypotension during anesthesia in dogs and cats: recognition, causes, and treatment. *Compend. Contin. Educ. Pract. Vet.* 23: 7.

4 McGhee, B.H. and Bridges, E.J. (2002). Monitoring arterial blood pressure: what you may not know. *Crit. Care Nurse* 22 60-44, 66–70, 73.

5 Hall, J.E. and Hall, M.E. (2021). Local and humoral control of blood flow by the tissues. In: *Textbook of Medical Physiology*, 14e (eds. A.C. Guyton and J.E. Hall), 1152. Philadelphia: Elsevier.

6 Cooper, E. (2015). Hypotension. In: *Small Animal Critical Care Medicine*, 2e (eds. D.C. Silverstein and K. Hopper), 46–50. Philadelphia: Elsevier.

7 Dagal, A. and Lam, A.M. (2009). Cerebral autoregulation and anesthesia. *Curr. Opin. Anaesthesiol.* 22: 547–552.

8 Lassen, N.A. (1959). Cerebral blood flow and oxygen consumption in man. *Physiol. Rev.* 39: 183–238.

9 Littman, M.P. and Fox, P.R. (1999). Systemic hypertension: recognition and treatment. In: *Textbook of Canine & Feline Cardiology: Principles of Clinical Practice*, 2e (eds. P.R. Fox, D.D. Sisson and N.S. Moise), 798–800. Philadelphia: WB Saunders.

10 Torres Filho, I.P., Spiess, B.D., Pittman, R.N. et al. (2005). Experimental analysis of critical oxygen delivery. *Am. J. Physiol. Heart Circ. Physiol.* 288: H1071–H1079.

11 Kirk, R.W. and Bonagura, J.D. (eds.) (1992). *Kirk's Current Veterinary Therapy XI: Small Animal Practice*, 11e. WB Saunders: Philadelphia.

12 Kittleson, M.D. and Kienle, R.D. (eds.) (1998). *Small Animal Cardiovascular Medicine*. St. Louis: Mosby.

13 Tranquilli, W.J. and Grimm, K.A. (2015). Introduction: use, definitions, history, concepts, classification, and considerations for anesthesia and analgesia. In: *Veterinary*

Anesthesia and Analgesia. The Fifth Edition of Lumb and Jones (eds. K.A. Grimm, L.A. Lamont, W.J. Tranquilli, et al.), 3–11. Ames: Wiley Blackwell.

14 O'Hearn, A.K. and Wright, B.D. (2011). Coccygeal epidural with local anesthetic for catheterization and pain management in the treatment of feline urethral obstruction. *J. Vet. Emerg. Crit. Care* 21: 50–52.

15 Portela, D.A., Otero, P.E., Tarragona, L. et al. (2010). Combined paravertebral plexus block and parasacral sciatic block in healthy dogs. *Vet. Anaesth. Analg.* 37: 531–541.

16 Lemke, K.A. and Dawson, S.D. (2000). Local and regional anesthesia. *Vet. Clin. North Am. Small Anim. Pract.* 30: 839–857.

17 Sinclair, M.D. (2003). A review of the physiological effects of alpha 2-agonists related to the clinical use of medetomidine in small animal practice. *Can. Vet. J.* 44: 885–897.

18 Saponaro, V., Crovace, A., De Marzo, L. et al. (2013). Echocardiographic evaluation of the cardiovascular effects of medetomidine, acepromazine and their combination in healthy dogs. *Res. Vet. Sci.* 95: 687–692.

19 Psatha, E., Alibhai, H.I., Jimenez-Lozano, A. et al. (2011). Clinical efficacy and cardiorespiratory effects of alfaxalone, or diazepam/fentanyl for induction of anaesthesia in dogs that are a poor anaesthetic risk. *Vet. Anaesth. Analg.* 38: 24–36.

20 Covey-Crump, G.L. and Murison, P.J. (2008). Fentanyl or midazolam for co-induction of anaesthesia with propofol in dogs. *Vet. Anaesth. Analg.* 35: 463–472.

21 Ilkiw, J.E., Pascoe, P.J., Haskins, S.C. et al. (1994). The cardiovascular sparing effect of fentanyl and atropine, administered to enflurane anesthetized dogs. *Can. J. Vet. Res.* 58: 248–253.

22 Andreoni, V. and Lynne Hughes, J.M.L. (2009). Propofol and fentanyl infusions in dogs of various breeds undergoing surgery. *Vet. Anaesth. Analg.* 36: 523–531.

23 Lamont, L.A. and Matthews, K.A. (2007). Opioids, non-steroidal anti-inflammatories and analgesic adjuvants. In: *Lumb and Jones Veterinary Anesthesia and Analgesia*, 4e (eds. W.J. Tranquilli, J.C. Thurmon and K.A. Grimm), 241–272. Ames: Blackwell Publishing.

24 Gürkan, A., Birgül, Y., and Ziya, K. (2005). Direct cardiac effects in isolated perfused rat hearts of fentanyl and remifentanil. *Ann. Card Anaesth.* 8: 140–144.

25 Messenger, K.M., Hopfensperger, M., Knych, H.K. et al. (2016). Pharmacokinetics of detomidine following intravenous or oral-transmucosal administration and sedative effects of the oral-transmucosal treatment in dogs. *Am. J. Vet. Res.* 77: 413–420.

26 Monteiro, E.R., Junior, A.R., Assis, H.M. et al. (2009). Comparative study on the sedative effects of morphine, methadone, butorphanol or tramadol, in combination with acepromazine, in dogs. *Vet. Anaesth. Analg.* 36: 25–33.

27 Barnhart, M.D., Hubbell, J.A., Muir, W.W. et al. (2000). Pharmacokinetics, pharmacodynamics, and analgesic effects of morphine after rectal, intramuscular, and intravenous administration in dogs. *Am. J. Vet. Res.* 61: 24–28.

28 Robinson, E.P., Faggella, A.M., Henry, D.P. et al. (1988). Comparison of histamine release induced by morphine and oxymorphone administration in dogs. *Am. J. Vet. Res.* 49: 1699–1701.

29 Muir, W.W., Wiese, A.J., and March, P.A. (2003). Effects of morphine, lidocaine, ketamine, and morphine-lidocaine-ketamine drug combination on minimum alveolar concentration in dogs anesthetized with isoflurane. *Am. J. Vet. Res.* 64: 1155–1160.

30 Bateman, S.W., Haldane, S., and Stephens, J.A. (2008). Comparison of the analgesic efficacy of hydromorphone and oxymorphone in dogs and cats: a randomized blinded study. *Vet. Anaesth. Analg.* 35: 341–347.

31 Smith, L.J., Yu, K.J., Bjorling, D.E. et al. (2001). Effects of hydromorphone or oxymorphone, with or without acepromazine, on preanesthetic sedation, physiologic values, and histamine release in dogs. *J. Am. Vet. Med. Assoc.* 218: 1101–1105.

32 Posner, L.P., Gleed, R.D., Erb, H.N. et al. (2007). Post-anesthetic hyperthermia in cats. *Vet. Anaesth. Analg.* 34: 40–47.

33 Posner, L.P., Pavuk, A.A., Rokshar, J.L. et al. (2010). Effects of opioids and anesthetic drugs on body temperature in cats. *Vet. Anaesth. Analg.* 37: 35–43.

34 Menegheti, T.M., Wagatsuma, J.T., Pacheco, A.D. et al. (2014). Electrocardiographic evaluation and degree of sedation with three doses of methadone in healthy dogs [corrected]. *Vet. Anaesth. Analg.* 41: 97–104.

35 Vieira, B.H.B., Nishimura, L.T., Carvalho, L.L. et al. (2017). Cardiopulmonary and sedative effects of intravenous or epidural methadone in conscious dogs. *J. Vet. Pharmacol. Ther.* 40: e65–e68.

36 KuKanich, B. and Borum, S.L. (2008). The disposition and behavioral effects of methadone in Greyhounds. *Vet. Anaesth. Analg.* 35: 242–248.

37 Simon, B.T., Scallan, E.M., Siracusa, C. et al. (2014). Effects of acepromazine or methadone on midazolam-induced behavioral reactions in dogs. *Can. Vet. J.* 55: 875–885.

38 Campagnol, D., Teixeira-Neto, F.J., Peccinini, R.G. et al. (2012). Comparison of the effects of epidural or intravenous methadone on the minimum alveolar concentration of isoflurane in dogs. *Vet. J.* 192: 311–315.

39 Credie, R.G., Teixeira Neto, F.J., Ferreira, T.H. et al. (2010). Effects of methadone on the minimum alveolar concentration of isoflurane in dogs. *Vet. Anaesth. Analg.* 37: 240–249.

40 Shah, M.D., Yates, D., Hunt, J. et al. (2018). A comparison between methadone and buprenorphine for perioperative analgesia in dogs undergoing ovariohysterectomy. *J. Small Anim. Pract.* 59: 539–546.

41 Gorman, A.L., Elliott, K.J., and Inturrisi, C.E. (1997). The d- and l-isomers of methadone bind to the non-competitive site on the N-methyl-D-aspartate (NMDA) receptor in rat forebrain and spinal cord. *Neurosci. Lett.* 223: 5–8.

42 KuKanich, B. and Wiese, A.J. (2015). Opioids. In: *Veterinary Anesthesia and Analgesia. The Fifth Edition of Lumb and Jones* (eds. K.A. Grimm, L.A. Lamont, W.J. Tranquilli, et al.), 207–226. Ames: Wiley Blackwell.

43 Trescot, A.M., Datta, S., Lee, M. et al. (2008). Opioid pharmacology. *Pain Physician* 11: S133–S153.

44 Kamata, M., Nagahama, S., Kakishima, K. et al. (2012). Comparison of behavioral effects of morphine and fentanyl in dogs and cats. *J. Vet. Med. Sci.* 74: 231–234.

45 Murahata, Y., Hikasa, Y., Hayashi, S. et al. (2018). The effect of remifentanil on the minimum alveolar concentration (MAC) and MAC derivatives of sevoflurane in dogs. *J. Vet. Med. Sci.* 80: 1086–1093.

46 Ferreira, T.H., Aguiar, A.J., Valverde, A. et al. (2009). Effect of remifentanil hydrochloride administered via constant rate infusion on the minimum alveolar concentration of isoflurane in cats. *Am. J. Vet. Res.* 70: 581–588.

47 Monteiro, E.R., Teixeira-Neto, F.J., Campagnol, D. et al. (2010). Effects of remifentanil on the minimum alveolar concentration of isoflurane in dogs. *Am. J. Vet. Res.* 71: 150–156.

48 Wagner, A.E. (1999). Is butorphanol analgesic in dogs and cats? *Vet. Med.* 94: 4.

49 KuKanich, B. and Papich, M.G. (2009). Opioid analgesic drugs. In: *Veterinary Pharmacology and Therapeutics*, 9e (eds. J.E. Riviere and M.G. Papich), 301–336. Ames: Wiley-Blackwell.

50 Sawyer, D.C., Rech, R.H., Durham, R.A. et al. (1991). Dose response to butorphanol administered subcutaneously to increase visceral nociceptive threshold in dogs. *Am. J. Vet. Res.* 52: 1826–1830.

51 Narver, H.L. (2015). Nalbuphine, a non-controlled opioid analgesic, and its potential use in research mice. *Lab. Anim. (NY)* 44: 106–110.

52 Gomes, V.H., Oliveira, R.L., Marques, J.L. et al. (2018). Comparison of the sedative effects of nalbuphine and butorphanol, alone or in combination with acepromazine in dogs. *Vet. Anaesth. Analg.* 45: 68–72.

53 de Oliveira, F.F., DeRossi, R., de Affonseca Jardim, P.H. et al. (2014). Effects of epidural nalbuphine on intraoperative isoflurane and postoperative analgesic requirements in dogs. *Acta Cir. Bras.* 29: 38–46.

54 Kreisler, R.E., Cornell, H.N., Smith, V.A. et al. (2020). Use of nalbuphine as a substitute for butorphanol in combination with dexmedetomidine and tiletamine/zolazepam: a randomized non-inferiority trial. *J. Feline Med. Surg.* 22: 100–107.

55 Heit, H.A. and Gourlay, D.L. (2008). Buprenorphine: new tricks with an old molecule for pain management. *Clin. J. Pain* 24: 93–97.

56 Dahan, A., Aarts, L., and Smith, T.W. (2010). Incidence, reversal, and prevention of opioid-induced respiratory depression. *Anesthesiology* 112: 226–238.

57 Nunamaker, E.A., Stolarik, D.F., Ma, J. et al. (2014). Clinical efficacy of sustained-release buprenorphine with meloxicam for postoperative analgesia in beagle dogs undergoing ovariohysterectomy. *J. Am. Assoc. Lab Anim. Sci.* 53: 494–501.

58 Taylor, P.M., Luangdilok, C.H., and Sear, J.W. (2016). Pharmacokinetic and pharmacodynamic evaluation of high doses of buprenorphine delivered via high-concentration formulations in cats. *J. Feline Med. Surg.* 18: 290–302.

59 Rankin, D.C. (2015). Sedatives and tranquilizers. In: *Veterinary Anesthesia and Analgesia. The Fifth Edition of Lumb and Jones* (eds. K.A. Grimm, L.A. Lamont, W.J. Tranquilli, et al.), 196–206. Ames: Wiley Blackwell.

60 Farver, T.B., Haskins, S.C., and Patz, J.D. (1986). Cardiopulmonary effects of acepromazine and of the subsequent administration of ketamine in the dog. *Am. J. Vet. Res.* 47: 631–635.

61 Dyson, D. and Pettifer, G. (1997). Evaluation of the arrhythmogenicity of a low dose of acepromazine: comparison with xylazine. *Can. J. Vet. Res.* 61: 241–245.

62 Haskins, S.C., Farver, T.B., and Patz, J.D. (1986). Cardiovascular changes in dogs given diazepam and diazepam-ketamine. *Am. J. Vet. Res.* 47: 795–798.

63 Sunzel, M., Paalzow, L., Berggren, L. et al. (1988). Respiratory and cardiovascular effects in relation to plasma levels of midazolam and diazepam. *Br. J. Clin. Pharmacol.* 25: 561–569.

64 Ilkiw, J.E., Suter, C.M., Farver, T.B. et al. (1996). The behaviour of healthy awake cats following intravenous and intramuscular administration of midazolam. *J. Vet. Pharmacol. Ther.* 19: 205–216.

65 Biermann, K., Hungerbühler, S., Mischke, R. et al. (2012). Sedative, cardiovascular, haematologic and biochemical effects of four different drug combinations administered intramuscularly in cats. *Vet. Anaesth. Analg.* 39: 137–150.

66 Robinson, R. and Borer-Weir, K. (2013). A dose titration study into the effects of diazepam or midazolam on the propofol dose requirements for induction of general anaesthesia in client owned dogs, premedicated with methadone and acepromazine. *Vet. Anaesth. Analg.* 40: 455–463.

67 Sánchez, A., Belda, E., Escobar, M. et al. (2013). Effects of altering the sequence of midazolam and propofol during co-induction of anaesthesia. *Vet. Anaesth. Analg.* 40: 359–366.

68 Ringer, S.K., Schwarzwald, C.C., Portier, K.G. et al. (2013). Effects on cardiopulmonary function and oxygen delivery of doses of romifidine and xylazine followed by constant rate infusions in standing horses. *Vet. J.* 195: 228–234.

69 Yamashita, K., Tsubakishits, S., Futaok, S. et al. (2000). Cardiovascular effects of medetomidine, detomidine and xylazine in horses. *J. Vet. Med. Sci.* 62: 1025–1032.

70 Congdon, J.M., Marquez, M., Niyom, S. et al. (2011). Evaluation of the sedative and cardiovascular effects of intramuscular administration of dexmedetomidine with and without concurrent atropine administration in dogs. *J. Am. Vet. Med. Assoc.* 239: 81–89.

71 Kuo, W.C. and Keegan, R.D. (2004). Comparative cardiovascular, analgesic, and sedative effects of medetomidine, medetomidine-hydromorphone, and medetomidine-butorphanol in dogs. *Am. J. Vet. Res.* 65: 931–937.

72 Johard, E., Tidholm, A., Ljungvall, I. et al. (2018). Effects of sedation with dexmedetomidine and buprenorphine on echocardiographic variables, blood pressure and heart rate in healthy cats. *J. Feline Med. Surg.* 20: 554–562.

73 Olsen, R.W. (2018). GABA. *Neuropharmacology* 136: 10–22.

74 Deutsch, J., Jolliffe, C., Archer, E. et al. (2017). Intramuscular injection of alfaxalone in combination with butorphanol for sedation in cats. *Vet. Anaesth. Analg.* 44: 794–802.

75 Ribas, T., Bublot, I., Junot, S. et al. (2015). Effects of intramuscular sedation with alfaxalone and butorphanol on echocardiographic measurements in healthy cats. *J. Feline Med. Surg.* 17: 530–536.

76 Huynh, M., Poumeyrol, S., Pignon, C. et al. (2015). Intramuscular administration of alfaxalone for sedation in rabbits. *Vet. Rec.* 176: 255.

77 Cruz-Benedetti, I.-C., Bublot, I., Ribas, T. et al. (2018). Pharmacokinetics of intramuscular alfaxalone and its echocardiographic, cardiopulmonary and sedative effects in healthy dogs. *PLoS One* 13: e0204553.

78 Rodrigo-Mocholí, D., Escudero, E., Belda, E. et al. (2018). Pharmacokinetics and effects of alfaxalone after intravenous and intramuscular administration to cats. *N. Z. Vet. J.* 66: 172–177.

79 Tamura, J., Hatakeyama, N., Ishizuka, T. et al. (2016). The pharmacological effects of intramuscular administration of alfaxalone combined with medetomidine and butorphanol in dogs. *J. Vet. Med. Sci.* 78: 929–936.

80 Maney, J.K. (2017). Sedative and physiologic effects of low-dose intramuscular alfaxalone in dogs. *Vet. Anaesth. Analg.* 44: 1184–1188.

81 Tamura, J., Ishizuka, T., Fukui, S. et al. (2015). The pharmacological effects of the anesthetic alfaxalone after intramuscular administration to dogs. *J. Vet. Med. Sci.* 77: 289–296.

82 Mostafa, S.M. and Vucevic, M. (1984). Comparison of atropine and glycopyrronium in patients with pre-existing cardiac disease. *Anaesthesia* 39: 1207–1213.

83 Short, C.E. and Bufalari, A. (1999). Propofol anesthesia. *Vet. Clin. North Am. Small Anim. Pract.* 29: 747–778.

84 Wakita, M., Kotani, N., Nonaka, K. et al. (2013). Effects of propofol on GABAergic and glutamatergic transmission in isolated hippocampal single nerve-synapse preparations. *Eur. J. Pharmacol.* 718: 63–73.

85 Naguib, M. and Sari-Kouzel, A. (1991). Thiopentone-propofol hypnotic synergism in patients. *Br. J. Anaesth.* 67: 4–6.

86 Doursout, M.F., Joseph, P.M., Liang, Y.Y. et al. (2002). Role of propofol and its solvent, intralipid, in nitric oxide-induced peripheral vasodilatation in dogs. *Br. J. Anaesth.* 89: 492–498.

87 Child, K.J., Currie, J.P., Davis, B. et al. (1971). The pharmacological properties in animals of CT1341 - a new steroid anesthetic agent. *Br. J. Anaesth.* 43: 2–13.

88 Dodman, N.H. (1980). Complications of saffan anaesthesia in cats. *Vet. Rec.* 107: 481–483.

89 Gaudy, J.H., Sicard, J.F., Lhoste, F. et al. (1987). The effects of cremophor EL in the anaesthetized dog. *Can. J. Anaesth.* 34: 122–129.

90 Goodchild, C.S., Serrao, J.M., Kolosov, A. et al. (2015). Alphaxalone reformulated: a water-soluble intravenous anesthetic preparation in sulfobutyl-ether-β-cyclodextrin. *Anesth. Analg.* 120: 1025–1031.

91 Jurox Animal Health (2019). Alfaxalone mulitidose induction dose guidelines for dogs and cats. www.jurox.com (accessed 7 August 2019)

92 Muir, W., Lerche, P., Wiese, A. et al. (2008). Cardiorespiratory and anesthetic effects of clinical and supraclinical doses of alfaxalone in dogs. *Vet. Anaesth. Analg.* 35: 451–462.

93 Muir, W., Lerche, P., Wiese, A. et al. (2009). The cardiorespiratory and anesthetic effects of clinical and supraclinical doses of alfaxalone in cats. *Vet. Anaesth. Analg.* 36: 42–54.

94 Maney, J.K., Shepard, M.K., Braun, C. et al. (2013). A comparison of cardiopulmonary and anesthetic effects of an induction dose of alfaxalone or propofol in dogs. *Vet. Anaesth. Analg.* 40: 237–244.

95 Sinner, B. and Graf, B.M. (2008). Ketamine. *Handb. Exp. Pharmacol.* 182: 313–333.

96 Aroni, F., Iacovidou, N., Dontas, I. et al. (2009). Pharmacological aspects and potential new clinical applications of ketamine: reevaluation of an old drug. *J. Clin. Pharmacol.* 49: 957–964.

97 Waxman, K., Shoemaker, W.C., and Lippmann, M. (1980). Cardiovascular effects of anesthetic induction with ketamine. *Anesth. Analg.* 59: 355–358.

98 Berry, S.H. (2015). Injectable anesthetics. In: *Veterinary Anesthesia and Analgesia. The Fifth Edition of Lumb and Jones* (eds. K.A. Grimm, L.A. Lamont, W.J. Tranquilli, et al.), 277–296. Ames: Wiley Blackwell.

99 Rodríguez, J.M. et al. (2012). Comparison of the cardiopulmonary parameters after induction of anaesthesia with alphaxalone or etomidate in dogs. *Vet. Anaesth. Analg.* 39: 357–365.

100 Sams, L., Braun, C., Allman, D. et al. (2008). A comparison of the effects of propofol and etomidate on the induction of anesthesia and on cardiopulmonary parameters in dogs. *Vet. Anaesth. Analg.* 35: 488–494.

101 Muir, W.W. and Mason, D.E. (1989). Side effects of etomidate in dogs. *J. Am. Vet. Med. Assoc.* 194: 1430–1434.

102 Poulos, J.E., Kalogerinis, P.T., and Caudle, J.N. (2013). Propofol compared with combination propofol or midazolam/fentanyl for endoscopy in a community setting. *AANA J.* 81: 31–36.

103 Bustamante, R., Aguado, D., Cediel, R. et al. (2018). Clinical comparison of the effects of isoflurane or propofol anaesthesia on mean arterial blood pressure and ventilation in dogs undergoing orthopaedic surgery receiving epidural anaesthesia. *Vet. J.* 233: 49–54.

104 Park, J., Lee, H.B., and Jeong, S.M. (2018). Comparison of the effects of isoflurane versus propofol-remifentanil anesthesia on oxygen delivery during thoracoscopic lung lobectomy with one-lung ventilation in dogs. *J. Vet. Sci.* 19: 426–433.

105 Kennedy, M.J. and Smith, L.J. (2015). A comparison of cardiopulmonary function, recovery quality, and total dosages required for induction and total intravenous anesthesia with propofol versus a propofol-ketamine combination in healthy Beagle dogs. *Vet. Anaesth. Analg.* 42: 350–359.

106 Mohamadnia, A.R., Shahbazkia, H., Akhlaghi, M. et al. (2008). Clinical evaluation of repeated propofol total intravenous anesthesia in dog. *Pak. J. Biol. Sci.* 11: 1820–1824.

107 Tsai, Y.C., Wang, L.Y., and Yeh, L.S. (2007). Clinical comparison of recovery from total intravenous anesthesia with propofol and inhalation anesthesia with isoflurane in dogs. *J. Vet. Med. Sci.* 69: 1179–1182.

108 Raisis, A.L., Leece, E.A., Platt, S.R. et al. (2007). Evaluation of an anaesthetic technique used in dogs undergoing craniectomy for tumour resection. *Vet. Anaesth. Analg.* 34: 171–180.

109 Murrell, J.C., van Notten, R.W., and Hellebrekers, L.J. (2005). Clinical investigation of remifentanil and propofol for the total intravenous anaesthesia of dogs. *Vet. Rec.* 156: 804–808.

110 Hughes, J.M. and Nolan, A.M. (1999). Total intravenous anesthesia in greyhounds: pharmacokinctics of propofol and fentanyl–a preliminary study. *Vet. Surg.* 28: 513–524.

111 Smith, C.K., Seddighi, R., Cox, S.K. et al. (2017). Effect of dexmedetomidine on the minimum infusion rate of propofol preventing movement in dogs. *Vet. Anaesth. Analg.* 44: 1287–1295.

112 Hunt, J.R., Goff, M., Jenkins, H. et al. (2019). Clinical measurements performed during alfaxalone total intravenous anaesthesia for radiography and neurophysiological investigations in dogs. *Vet. Anaesth. Analg.* 46: 483–487.

113 Bennell, P.M., Whittem, T., and Tudor, E. (2019). A controlled randomized clinical trial to assess postoperative analgesia after thiopental-isoflurane anaesthesia or total intravenous anaesthesia with alfaxalone in dogs. *J. Vet. Pharmacol. Ther.* 42: 268–277.

114 Dehuisser, V., Bosmans, T., Kitshoff, A. et al. (2017). Cardiovascular effects, induction and recovery characteristics and alfaxalone dose assessment in alfaxalone versus alfaxalone-fentanyl total intravenous anaesthesia in dogs. *Vet. Anaesth. Analg.* 44: 1276–1286.

115 Liao, P., Sinclair, M., Valverde, A. et al. (2017). Induction dose and recovery quality of propofol and alfaxalone with or without midazolam co-induction followed by total intravenous anesthesia in dogs. *Vet. Anaesth. Analg.* 44: 1016–1026.

116 Conde Ruiz, C., Del Carro, A.P., Rosset, E. et al. (2016). Alfaxalone for total intravenous anaesthesia in bitches undergoing elective caesarean section and its effects on puppies: a randomized clinical trial. *Vet. Anaesth. Analg.* 43: 281–290.

117 Herbert, G.L., Bowlt, K.L., Ford-Fennah, V. et al. (2013). Alfaxalone for total intravenous anaesthesia in dogs undergoing ovariohysterectomy: a comparison of premedication with acepromazine or dexmedetomidine. *Vet. Anaesth. Analg.* 40: 124–133.

118 Suarez, M.A., Dzikiti, B.T., Stegmann, F.G. et al. (2012). Comparison of alfaxalone and propofol administered as total intravenous anaesthesia for ovariohysterectomy in dogs. *Vet. Anaesth. Analg.* 39: 236–244.

119 Beths, T., Touzot-Jourde, G., Musk, G. et al. (2014). Clinical evaluation of alfaxalone to induce and maintain anaesthesia in cats undergoing neutering procedures. *J. Feline Med. Surg.* 16: 609–615.

120 Schwarz, A., Kalchofner, K., Palm, J. et al. (1982). Minimum infusion rate of alfaxalone for total intravenous anaesthesia after sedation with acepromazine or medetomidine in cats undergoing ovariohysterectomy. *Vet. Anaesth. Analg.* 41: 480–490.

121 Pagel, P.S., Kampine, J.P., Schmeling, W.T. et al. (1991). Influence of volatile anesthetics on myocardial contractility in vivo: desflurane versus isoflurane. *Anesthesiology* 74: 900–907.

122 Warltier, D.C. and Pagel, P.S. (1992). Cardiovascular and respiratory actions of desflurane: is desflurane different from isoflurane? *Anesth. Analg.* 75: S17–S29; discussion S29-31.

123 Pagel, P.S., Kampine, J.P., Schmeling, W.T. et al. (1993). Evaluation of myocardial contractility in the chronically instrumented dog with intact autonomic nervous system function: effects of desflurane and isoflurane. *Acta Anaesthesiol. Scand.* 37: 203–210.

124 Boban, M., Stowe, D.F., Buljubasic, N. et al. (1992). Direct comparative effects of isoflurane and desflurane in isolated guinea pig hearts. *Anesthesiology* 76: 775–780.

125 Brosnan, R.J., Pypendop, B.H., Siao, K.T. et al. (2009). Effects of remifentanil on measures of anesthetic immobility and analgesia in cats. *Am. J. Vet. Res.* 70: 1065–1071.

126 Pascoe, P.J., Ilkiw, J.E., Craig, C. et al. (2007). The effects of ketamine on the minimum alveolar concentration of isoflurane in cats. *Vet. Anaesth. Analg.* 34: 31–39.

127 Ueyama, Y. (2009). Effects of intravenous administration of perzinfotel, fentanyl, and a combination of both drugs on the minimum alveolar concentration of isoflurane in dogs. *Am. J. Vet. Res.* 70: 1459–1464.

128 Hellyer, P.W., Mama, K.R., Shafford, H.L. et al. (2001). Effects of diazepam and flumazenil on minimum alveolar concentrations for dogs anesthetized with isoflurane or a combination of isoflurane and fentanyl. *Am. J. Vet. Res.* 62: 555–560.

129 Michelsen, L.G. (1996). The pharmacokinetics of remifentanil. *J. Clin. Anesth.* 8: 679–682.

130 Allweiler, S. (2007). The isoflurane-sparing and clinical effects of a constant rate infusion of remifentanil in dogs. *Vet. Anaesth. Analg.* 6: 388–393.

131 Queiroz-Castro, P. (2006). Effects of ketamine and magnesium on the minimum alveolar concentration of isoflurane in goats. *Am. J. Vet. Res.* 67: 1962–1966.

132 Doherty, T. (2007). Effect of intravenous lidocaine and ketamine on the minimum alveolar concentration of isoflurane in goats. *Vet. Anaesth. Analg.* 34: 125–131.

133 Love, L. (2011). The effect of ketamine on the MACBAR of sevoflurane in dogs. *Vet. Anaesth. Analg.* 38: 292–300.

134 Alexander, R., Poznikoff, A., and Malherbe, S. (2018). Greenhouse gases: the choice of volatile anesthetic does matter. *Can. J. Anaesth.* 65: 221–222.

135 Whittem, T., Beths, T., and Bauquier, S.H. (2015). General pharmacology of anesthetic and analgesic drugs. In: *Veterinary Anesthesia and Analgesia. The Fifth Edition of Lumb and Jones* (eds. K.A. Grimm, L.A. Lamont, W.J. Tranquilli, et al.), 147–176. Ames: Wiley Blackwell.

136 Levionnois, O.L. (2016). Target-controlled infusion in small animals: improving anaesthetic safety. *Vet. Rec.* 178: 501–502.

137 Joubert, K.E. (2009). Computer simulations of propofol infusions for total intravenous anaesthesia in dogs. *J. S. Afr. Vet. Assoc.* 80: 2–9.

138 Murphy, M.R. and Hug, C.C. (1982). The anesthetic potency of fentanyl in terms of its reduction of enflurane MAC. *Anesthesiology* 57: 485–488.

139 Snyder, C.J. and Snyder, L.B. (2013). Effect of mepivacaine in an infraorbital nerve block on minimum alveolar concentration of isoflurane in clinically normal anesthetized dogs undergoing a modified form of dental dolorimetry. *J. Am. Vet. Med. Assoc.* 242: 199–204.

140 Pypendop, B.H., Pascoe, P.J., and Ilkiw, J.E. (2006). Effects of epidural administration of morphine and buprenorphine on the minimum alveolar concentration of isoflurane in cats. *Am. J. Vet. Res.* 67: 1471–1475.

141 Liu, P.L., Feldman, H.S., Giasi, R. et al. (1983). Comparative CNS toxicity of lidocaine, etidocaine, bupivacaine, and tetracaine in awake dogs following rapid intravenous administration. *Anesth. Analg.* 62: 375–379.

142 Feldman, H.S., Arthur, G.R., Pitkanen, M. et al. (1991). Treatment of acute systemic toxicity after the rapid intravenous injection of ropivacaine and bupivacaine in the conscious dog. *Anesth. Analg.* 73: 373–384.

143 Campoy, L. and Read, M.R. (eds.) (2013). *Small Animal Regional Anesthesia and Analgesia*, 1e. Ames: Wiley Blackwell.

144 Rezende, M.L., Wagner, A.E., Mama, K.R. et al. (2011). Effects of intravenous administration of lidocaine on the minimum alveolar concentration of sevoflurane in horses. *Am. J. Vet. Res.* 72: 446–451.

145 Matsubara, L.M., Oliva, V.N., Gabas, D.T. et al. (2009). Effect of lidocaine on the minimum alveolar concentration of sevoflurane in dogs. *Vet. Anaesth. Analg.* 36: 407–413.

146 Innes, J.F., Clayton, J., and Lascelles, B.D. (2010). Review of the safety and efficacy of long-term NSAID use in the treatment of canine osteoarthritis. *Vet. Rec.* 166: 226–230.

147 KuKanich, B., Bidgood, T., and Knesl, O. (2012). Clinical pharmacology of nonsteroidal anti-inflammatory drugs in dogs. *Vet. Anaesth. Analg.* 39: 69–90.

148 Lascelles, D., McFarland, J.M., and Swann, H. (2005). Guidelines for safe and effective use of NSAIDs in dogs. *Vet. Ther.* 6: 237–251.

149 Sparkes, A.H. (2011). A summary of the ISFM and AAFP consensus guidelines on the long-term use of NSAIDS in cats. *Tijdschr. Diergeneeskd.* 136: 804–806.

150 McLean, M.K. and Khan, S.A. (2018). Toxicology of frequently encountered nonsteroidal anti-inflammatory drugs in dogs and cats: an update. *Vet. Clin. North Am. Small Anim. Pract.* 48: 969–984.

151 Rotunno, R., Oppo, I., Saetta, G. et al. (2018). NSAIDs and heart failure: a dangerous relationship. *Monaldi Arch. Chest Dis.* 88: 950.

152 Naumov, A.V., Tkacheva, O.N., and Khovasova, N.O. (2019). Safety of nonsteroidal anti-inflammatory drugs in patients with cardiovascular risk. *Ter. Arkh.* 91: 108–113.

153 Fuggle, N., Curtis, E., Shaw, S. et al. (2019). Safety of opioids in osteoarthritis: outcomes of a systematic review and meta-analysis. *Drugs Aging* 36: 129–143.

154 Masclee, G.M.C., Straatman, H., Arfe, A. et al. (2018). Risk of acute myocardial infarction during use of individual NSAIDs: a nested case-control study from the SOS project. *PLoS One* 13: e0204746.

155 Topol, E.J. (2004). Failing the public health–rofecoxib, Merck, and the FDA. *N. Engl. J. Med.* 351: 1707–1709.

156 Belshaw, Z., Asher, L., and Dean, R.S. (2016). The attitudes of owners and veterinary professionals in the United Kingdom to the risk of adverse events associated with using non-steroidal anti-inflammatory drugs (NSAIDs) to treat dogs with osteoarthritis. *Prev. Vet. Med.* 131: 121–126.

157 Hunt, J.R., Dean, R.S., Davis, G.N. et al. (2015). An analysis of the relative frequencies of reported adverse events associated with NSAID administration in dogs and cats in the United Kingdom. *Vet. J.* 206: 183–190.

158 Murrell, J.C. (2015). Adrenergic agents. In: *Veterinary Anesthesia and Analgesia. The Fifth Edition of Lumb and Jones* (eds. K.A. Grimm, L.A. Lamont, W.J. Tranquilli, et al.), 183–195. Ames: Wiley Blackwell.

159 Rosati, M., Dyson, D.H., Sinclair, M.D. et al. (2007). Response of hypotensive dogs to dopamine hydrochloride and dobutamine hydrochloride during deep isoflurane anesthesia. *Am. J. Vet. Res.* 68: 483–494.

160 Winter, R.L., Congdon, J., and Boscan, P. (2011). Anesthesia case of the month. Treating atrioventricular block in a dog during anesthesia. *J. Am. Vet. Med. Assoc.* 238: 854–858.

161 Abboud, F.M., Floras, J.S., Aylward, P.E. et al. (1990). Role of vasopressin in cardiovascular and blood pressure regulation. *Blood Vessels* 27: 106–115.

162 Silverstein, D.C. and Beer, K.A. (2015). Controversies regarding choice of vasopressor therapy for management of septic shock in animals. *J. Vet. Emerg. Crit. Care.* 25: 48–54.

163 Hemmings, H.C. and Hopkins, P.M. (2006). *Foundations of Anesthesia: Basic and Clinical Sciences*, 2e, 413–414, p. 502. London: Mosby.

164 Duke-Novakovski, T. and Carr, A. (2015). Perioperative blood pressure control and management. *Vet. Clin. North Am. Small Anim. Pract.* 45: 965–981.

165 Chen, H.C., Sinclair, M.D., and Dyson, D.H. (2007). Use of ephedrine and dopamine in dogs for the management of hypotension in routine clinical cases under isoflurane anesthesia. *Vet. Anaesth. Analg.* 34: 301–311.

166 Sinclair, M.D. and Dyson, D.H. (2012). The impact of acepromazine on the efficacy of crystalloid, dextran or ephedrine treatment in hypotensive dogs under isoflurane anesthesia. *Vet. Anaesth. Analg.* 39: 563–573.

167 Liu, S. and Fox, P.R. (2012). Cardiovascular pathology. In: *Textbook of Canine and Feline Cardiology: Principles of Clinical Practice*, 2e (eds. P.R. Fox, D. Sisson and N.S. Moise), 823–824. Philadelphia: WB Saunders.

168 Overgaard, C.B. and Dzavík, V. (2008). Inotropes and vasopressors: review of physiology and clinical use in cardiovascular disease. *Circulation* 118: 1047–1056.

169 Laks, M., Callis, G., and Swan, H.J. (1971). Hemodynamic effects of low doses of norepinephrine in the conscious dog. *Am. J. Physiol.* 220: 171–173.

170 Martínez, N.I., Panciera, D.L., Abbott, J.A. et al. (2005). Evaluation of pressor sensitivity to norepinephrine infusion in dogs with iatrogenic hyperadrenocorticism. Pressor sensitivity in dogs with hyperadrenocorticism. *Res. Vet. Sci.* 78: 25–31.

171 Pascoe, P.J., Ilkiw, J.E., and Pypendop, B.H. (2006). Effects of increasing infusion rates of dopamine, dobutamine, epinephrine, and phenylephrine in healthy anesthetized cats. *Am. J. Vet. Res.* 67: 1491–1499.

172 Wiese, A.J., Barter, L.S., Ilkiw, J.E. et al. (2012). Cardiovascular and respiratory effects of incremental doses of dopamine and phenylephrine in the management of isoflurane-induced hypotension in cats with hypertrophic cardiomyopathy. *Am. J. Vet. Res.* 73: 908–916.

173 Fresno, L., Andaluz, A., Moll, X. et al. (2008). The effects on maternal and fetal cardiovascular and acid-base variables after the administration of etomidate in the pregnant ewe. *Vet. J.* 177: 94–103.

174 McNally, E.M., Robertson, S.A., and Pablo, L.S. (2009). Comparison of time to desaturation between preoxygenated and nonpreoxygenated dogs following sedation with acepromazine maleate and morphine and induction of anesthesia with propofol. *Am. J. Vet. Res.* 70: 1333–1338.

175 ACVA (2009). Recommendations for monitoring anesthetized veterinary patients. https://acvaa.org/wp-content/uploads/2019/05/Small-Animal-Monitoring-Guidlines.pdf (accessed 9 September 2020).

176 Grandy, J.L., Dunlop, C.I., Hodgson, D.S. et al. (1992). Evaluation of the Doppler ultrasonic method of measuring systolic arterial blood pressure in cats. *Am. J. Vet. Res.* 53: 1166–1169.

177 Caulkett, N.A., Cantwell, S.L., and Houston, D.M. (1998). A comparison of indirect blood pressure monitoring techniques in the anesthetized cat. *Vet. Surg.* 27: 370–377.

178 Bodey, A.R., Michell, A.R., Bovee, K.C. et al. (1996). Comparison of direct and indirect (oscillometric) measurements of arterial blood pressure in conscious dogs. *Res. Vet. Sci.* 61: 17–21.

179 Meurs, K.M., Miller, M.W., and Slater, M.R. (1996). Comparison of the indirect oscillometric and direct arterial methods for blood pressure measurements in anesthetized dogs. *J. Am. Anim. Hosp. Assoc.* 32: 471–475.

180 Branson, K.R., Wagner-Mann, C.C., and Mann, F.A. (1997). Evaluation of an oscillometric blood pressure monitor on anesthetized cats and the effect of cuff placement and fur on accuracy. *Vet. Surg.* 26: 347–353.

181 Bosiack, A.P., Mann, F.A., Dodam, J.R. et al. (2010). Comparison of ultrasonic Doppler flow monitor, oscillometric, and direct arterial blood pressure measurements in ill dogs. *J. Vet. Emerg. Crit. Care* 20: 207–215.

182 Aarnes, T.K., Hubbell, J.A., Lerche, P. et al. (2012). Comparison of invasive and oscillometric blood pressure measurement techniques in anesthetized camelids. *Can. Vet. J.* 53: 881–885.

183 Lodato, R.F. (1997). Arterial pressure monitoring. In: *Principles and Practice of Intensive Care Monitoring*, 1e (ed. M.J. Tobin), 733–749. New York: McGraw-Hill.

184 Seliškar, A., Zrimšek, P., Sredenšek, J. et al. (2013). Comparison of high definition oscillometric and Doppler ultrasound devices with invasive blood pressure in anaesthetized dogs. *Vet. Anaesth. Analg.* 40: 21–27.

185 Harvey, L., Knowles, T., and Murison, P.J. (2012). Comparison of direct and doppler arterial blood pressure measurements in rabbits during isoflurane anaesthesia. *Vet. Anaesth. Analg.* 39: 174–184.

186 Guyton, A.C. and Hall, J.E. (2006). Body temperature, temperature regulations and fever. In: *Textbook of Medical Physiology*, 11e (eds. A.C. Guyton and J.E. Hall), 889–900. Philadelphia: Elsevier Saunders.

187 O., O. (2018). Pulse oximetry. In: *Veterinary Anesthetic and Monitoring Equipment* (eds. K.G. Cooley and R.A. Johnson), 227–228. Hoboken: Wiley-Blackwell.

188 Branson, K.R. (2007). Injectable and alternative anesthetic techniques. In: *Lumb and Jones Veterinary Anesthesia and Analgesia*, 4e (eds. W.J. Tranquilli, J.C. Thurmon and K.A. Grimm), 273–300. Ames: Blackwell Publishing.

189 Oncken, A.K., Kirby, R., and Rudloff, E. (2001). Hypothermia in critically ill dogs. *Compend. Contin. Educ. Pract. Vet.* 23: 15.

190 Dash, R.K. and Bassingthwaighte, J.B. (2004). Blood HbO2 and HbCO2 dissociation curves at varied O2, CO2, pH, 2,3-DPG and temperature levels. *Ann. Biomed. Eng.* 32: 1676–1693.

191 Walley, K.R., Lewis, T.H., and Wood, L.D. (1990). Acute respiratory acidosis decreases left ventricular contractility but increases cardiac output in dogs. *Circ. Res.* 67: 628–635.

192 Low, J.M., Gin, T., Lee, T.W. et al. (1993). Effect of respiratory acidosis and alkalosis on plasma catecholamine concentrations in anaesthetized man. *Clin. Sci. (Lond.)* 84: 69–72.

193 Brofman, J.D., Leff, A.R., Munoz, N.M. et al. (1985). Sympathetic secretory response to hypercapnic acidosis in swine. *J. Appl. Phys.* 69: 710–717.

194 Kerber, R.E., Pandian, N.G., Hoyt, R. et al. (1983). Effect of ischemia, hypertrophy, hypoxia, acidosis, and alkalosis on canine defibrillation. *Am. J. Physiol.* 244: H825–H831.

195 Orchard, C.H. and Kentish, J.C. (1990). Effects of changes of pH on the contractile function of cardiac muscle. *Am. J. Physiol.* 258: C967–C981.

196 Johnson, R.A. (2006). Respiratory acid-base disorders. In: *Fluid, Electrolyte and Acid-Base Disorders*, 3e (ed. D.B. SP), 283–296. Philadelphia: Elsevier Saunders.

197 Hopper, K. (2009). Basic & advanced mechanical ventilation. In: *Small Animal Critical Care Medicine*, 1e (eds. D.C. Silverstein and K. Hopper), 904–909. Philadelphia: Saunders Elsevier.

198 Kubitz, J.C. et al. (2006). The influence of PEEP and tidal volume on central blood volume. *Eur. J. Anaesthesiol.* 23: 954–961.

199 Yokoyama, I., Inoue, Y., Kinoshita, T. et al. (2008). Heart and brain circulation and CO2 in healthy men. *Acta Physiol. (Oxf.)* 193: 303–308.

200 Moreira, T.S., Takakura, A.C., Colombari, E. et al. (2006). Central chemoreceptors and sympathetic vasomotor outflow. *J. Physiol.* 577: 369–386.

201 Reems, M.M. and Aumann, M. (2012). Central venous pressure: principles, measurement, and interpretation. *Compend. Contin. Educ. Vet.* 34: E1.

202 de Laforcade, A.M. and Rozanski, E.A. (2001). Central venous pressure and arterial blood pressure measurements. *Vet. Clin. North Am. Small Anim. Pract.* 31: 1163–1174.

203 Kumar, A., Anel, R., Bunnell, E. et al. (2004). Pulmonary artery occlusion pressure and central venous pressure fail to predict ventricular filling volume, cardiac performance, or the response to volume infusion in normal subjects. *Crit. Care Med.* 32: 691–699.

204 Magder, S. (2005). How to use central venous pressure measurements. *Curr. Opin. Crit. Care* 11: 264–270.

205 Endo, Y., Tamura, J., Ishizu, T. et al. (2017). Stroke volume variation (SVV) and pulse pressure variation (PPV) as indicators of fluid responsiveness in sevoflurane anesthetized mechanically ventilated euvolemic dogs. *J. Vet. Med. Sci.* 79: 1437–1445.

206 Teboul, J.L., Monnet, X., Chemla, D. et al. (2019). Arterial pulse pressure variation with mechanical ventilation. *Am. J. Respir. Crit. Care Med.* 199: 22–31.

207 Lopes, M.R., Oliveira, M.A., Pereira, V.O. et al. (2007). Goal-directed fluid management based on pulse pressure variation monitoring during high-risk surgery: a pilot randomized controlled trial. *Crit. Care* 11: R100.

208 Michard, F., Chemla, D., Richard, C. et al. (1999). Clinical use of respiratory changes in arterial pulse pressure to monitor the hemodynamic effects of PEEP. *Am. J. Respir. Crit. Care Med.* 159: 935–939.

209 Michard, F., Boussat, S., Chemla, D. et al. (2000). Relation between respiratory changes in arterial pulse pressure and fluid responsiveness in septic patients with acute circulatory failure. *Am. J. Respir. Crit. Care Med.* 162: 134–138.

210 Berkenstadt, H., Friedman, Z., Preisman, S. et al. (2005). Pulse pressure and stroke volume variations during severe haemorrhage in ventilated dogs. *Br. J. Anaesth.* 94: 721–726.

211 Hussein, M.M. and Mostafa, R.H. (2018). Arterial pulse pressure variation versus central venous pressure as a predictor of fluid responsiveness during open major abdominal operations. *Open J. Anesthesiol.* 8: 10.

212 Di Bella, C., Lacitignola, L., Fracassi, L. et al. (2019). Pulse pressure variation can predict the hemodynamic response to pneumoperitoneum in dogs: a retrospective study. *Vet. Sci.* 6: 17.

213 Cooley, K.G. and Johnson, R.A. (eds.) (2018). *Veterinary Anesthetic and Monitoring Equipment*. Hoboken: Wiley-Blackwell.

214 Kittleson, M.D. (1998). Congenital abnormalities of the atrioventricular valves: mitral stenosis. In: *Small Animal Cardiovascular Medicine*, 1e (eds. M.D. Kittleson and R.D. Kienle), 275–281. St. Louis: Mosby.

215 Fox, P.R. (2012). Pathology of myxomatous mitral valve disease in the dog. *J. Vet. Cardiol.* 14: 103–126.

216 Keene, B.W. et al. (2019). ACVIM consensus guidelines for the diagnosis and treatment of myxomatous mitral valve disease in dogs. *J. Vet. Intern. Med.* 33: 1127–1140.

217 Oyama, M.A. (2009). Neurohormonal activation in canine degenerative mitral valve disease: implications on pathophysiology and treatment. *J. Small Anim. Pract.* 50: 3–11.

218 Kittleson, M.D. (1998). Myxomatous atrioventricular valve degeneration. In: *Small Animal Cardiovascular Medicine*, 1e (eds. M.D. Kittleson and R.D. Kienle), 297–304. St. Louis: Mosby.

219 Borgarelli, M. and Haggstrom, J. (2010). Canine degenerative myxomatous mitral valve disease: natural history, clinical presentation and therapy. *Vet. Clin. North Am. Small Anim. Pract.* 40: 651–663.

220 Fox, P.R., Miller, M.W., and Liu, S.K. (1992). Clinical, echocardiographic, and Doppler imaging characteristics of mitral valve stenosis in two dogs. *J. Am. Vet. Med. Assoc.* 201: 1575–1579.

221 Brambilla, P.G., Polli, M., Pradelli, D. et al. (2020). Epidemiological study of congenital heart diseases in dogs: prevalence, popularity, and volatility throughout twenty years of clinical practice. *PLoS One* 15: e0230160.

222 Lehmkuhl, L.B., Ware, W.A., and Bonagura, J.D. (1994). Mitral stenosis in 15 dogs. *J. Vet. Intern. Med.* 8: 2–17.

223 Shanewise, J.S. and Hug, C.C. (2005). Anesthesia for adult cardiac surgery. In: *Miller's Anesthesia*, 6e (ed. R.D. Miller), 1753–1804. Philadelphia: Elsevier Churchill Livingstone.

224 Hererra, A. (2012). Valvular heart disease. In: *Stoelting's Anesthesia & Co-Existing Disease*, 6e (eds. R.L. Hines and K. Marschall), 34–47. Philadelphia: Elsevier Saunders.

225 Borenstein, N., Daniel, P., Behr, L. et al. (2004). Successful surgical treatment of mitral valve stenosis in a dog. *Vet. Surg.* 33: 138–145.

226 Pyle, R.L., Patterson, D.F., and Chacko, S. (1976). The genetics and pathology of discrete subaortic stenosis in the Newfoundland dog. *Am. Heart J.* 92: 324–334.

227 Kittleson, M.K. (1998). Aortic stenosis, pathophysiology. In: *Small Animal Cardiovascular Medicine*, 1e (eds. M.K. Kittleson and R.D. Kienle), 262–263. St. Louis: Mosby.

228 Stern, J.A., Meurs, K.M., Nelson, O.L. et al. (2012). Familial subvalvular aortic stenosis in golden retrievers: inheritance and echocardiographic findings. *J. Small Anim. Pract.* 53: 213–216.

229 Meurs, K.M. (2004). Boxer dog cardiomyopathy: an update. *Vet. Clin. North Am. Small Anim. Pract.* 34: 1235–1244.

230 Bussadori, C., Amberger, C., Le Bobinnec, G. et al. (2000). Guidelines for the echocardiographic studies of suspected subaortic and pulmonic stenosis. *J. Vet. Cardiol.* 2: 15–22.

231 Strickland, K.N. (2008). Congenital heart disease. In: *Manual of Canine and Feline Cardiology*, 4e (eds. E.P. Tilley, F.W.K. Smith, M.A. Oyama and M.M. Sleeper), 227–236. St. Louis: Saunders, Elsevier.

232 Ware, W.A. and Ward, J.L. (2019). Congenital cardiac disease. In: *Small Animal Internal Medicine*, 6e (eds. R.W. Nelson and G. Couto), 100–118. Philadelphia: Elsevier.

233 Broaddus, K. and Tillson, M. (2010). Patent ductus arteriosus in dogs. *Compend. Contin. Educ. Vet.* 32: E3.

234 Smith, G.C. (1998). The pharmacology of the ductus arteriosus. *Pharmacol. Rev.* 50: 35–58.

235 Miller, M.W., Gordon, S.G., Saunders, A.B. et al. (2006). Angiographic classification of patent ductus arteriosus morphology in the dog. *J. Vet. Cardiol.* 8: 109–114.

236 Tobias, A.H. and Stauthammer, C.D. (2010). Minimally invasive per-catheter occlusion and dilation procedures for congenital cardiovascular abnormalities in dogs. *Vet. Clin. North Am. Small Anim. Pract.* 40: 581–603.

237 Grubb, T.L., Perez Jimenez, T.E., and Pettifer, G.L. (2015). Neonatal and geriatric patients. In: *Veterinary Anesthesia and Analgesia. The Fifth Edition of Lumb and Jones* (eds. K.A. Grimm, L.A. Lamont, W.J. Tranquilli, et al.), 983–987. Ames: Wiley Blackwell.

238 Read, M.R. (2013). The trunk. In: *Small Animal Regional Anesthesia and Analgesia*, 1e (eds. L. Campoy and M.R. Read), 169–186. Hoboken: Wiley Blackwell.

239 Kopacz, D.J., Emanuelsson, B.M., Thompson, G.E. et al. (1994). Pharmacokinetics of ropivacaine and bupivacaine for bilateral intercostal blockade in healthy male volunteers. *Anesthesiology* 81: 1139–1148.

240 Wattanasirichaigoon, S. and Pomposelli, F.B. (1997). Branham's sign is an exaggerated Bezold-Jarisch reflex of arteriovenous fistula. *J. Vasc. Surg.* 26: 171–172.

241 White, P. (2009). Treatment of patent ductus arteriosus by the use of an Amplatz canine ductal occluder device. *Can. Vet. J.* 50: 401–404.

242 Orton, E.C., Mama, K., Hellyer, P. et al. (2001). Open surgical repair of tetralogy of Fallot in dogs. *J. Am. Vet. Med. Assoc.* 219: 1089–1093.

243 Tilley, L.P. and Smith, F.W.K. (2016). Electrocardiography. In: *Manual of Canine and Feline Cardiology*, 5e (eds. L.P. Tilley, F.W.K. Smith, M.A. Oyama and M.M. Sleeper), 49–76. St. Louis: Saunders Elsevier.

244 Ringwald, R.J. and Bonagura, J.D. (1988). Tetralogy of Fallot in the dog: clinical findings in 13 cases. *J. Am. Anim. Hosp. Assoc.* 45: 10.

245 Buchanan, J.W. (1999). Prevalence of cardiovascular disorders. In: *Textbook of Canine and Feline Cardiology*, 2e (eds. P.R. Fox, D. Sisson and N.S. Moise), 461. Philadelphia: WB Saunders.

246 Guyton, A.C. and Hall, J.E. (2006). Membrane potentials and action potentials. In: *Textbook of Medical Physiology*, 11e (eds. A.C. Guyton and J.E. Hall), 152–153. Philadelphia: Elsevier Saunders.

247 Pappano, A.J. and Wier, W.G. (2013). Excitation: the cardiac action potential. In: *Cardiovascular Physiology*, 10e (eds. A.J. Pappano and W.G. Wier), 11–30. Philadelphia: Elsevier Mosby.

248 Tilley, L.P. and Bertnick, N.L. (1999). *Electrocardiography for the Small Animal Practitioner*. Jackson: Teton New Media.

249 Ben-Tal, A. (2012). Computational models for the study of heart-lung interactions in mammals. *Wiley Interdiscip. Rev. Syst. Biol. Med.* 4: 163–170.

250 Monfredi, O., Dobrzynski, H., Mondal, T. et al. (2010). The anatomy and physiology of the sinoatrial node–a contemporary review. *Pacing Clin. Electrophysiol.* 33: 1392–1406.

251 Pariaut, R. and Reynolds, C. (2014). Bradyarrhythmias and conduction abnormalities. In: *Small Animal Critical Care Medicine*, 2e (eds. D.C. Silverstein and K. Hopper), 246–249. Philadelphia: Saunders Elsevier.

252 Côté, E. (2010). Feline arrhythmias: an update. *Vet. Clin. North Am. Small Anim. Pract.* 40: 643–650.

253 Guyton, A.C. and Hall, J.E. (2006). Heart muscle: the heart as a pump and function of heart valves. In: *Textbook of Medical Physiology*, 11e (eds. A.C. Guyton and J.E. Hall), 107–110. Philadelphia: Elsevier Saunders.

254 Miller, M.S., Tilley, L.P., and Smith, F.W.K. (1999). Electrocardiography. In: *Textbook of Canine and Feline Cardiology: Principles and Clinical Practice*, 2e (eds. P.R. Fox, D. Sisson and N.S. Moise), 67–105. Philadelphia: WB Saunders.

255 Armentano, R.A., Schmidt, M.K., and Maisenbacher, H.W. (2010). ECG of the month. Atrial flutter. *J. Am. Vet. Med. Assoc.* 236: 51–53.

256 Pairaut, R. (2014). Ventricular tachyarrhythmias. In: *Small Animal Critical Care Medicine*, 2e (eds. D.C. Silverstein and K. Hopper), 250–254. Philadelphia: Saunders Elsevier.

257 Chiladakis, J.A., Karapanos, G., Davlouros, P. et al. (2000). Significance of R-on-T phenomenon in early ventricular tachyarrhythmia susceptibility after acute myocardial infarction in the thrombolytic era. *Am. J. Cardiol.* 85: 289–293.

258 Kim, H.J. and Han, S.W. (2002). Therapeutic approach to hyperkalemia. *Nephron* 92: 33–40.

259 Ohmura, H., Boscan, P.L., Solano, A.M. et al. (2012). Changes in heart rate, heart rate variability, and atrioventricular block during withholding of food in thoroughbreds. *Am. J. Vet. Res.* 73: 508–514.

260 Buchanan, J.W., Dear, M.G., Pyle, R.L. et al. (1968). Medical and pacemaker therapy of complete heart block and congestive heart failure in a dog. *J. Am. Vet. Med. Assoc.* 152: 1099–1109.

261 Sisson, D., Thomas, W.P., Woodfield, J. et al. (1991). Permanent transvenous pacemaker implantation in forty dogs. *J. Vet. Intern. Med.* 5: 322–331.

262 Flanders, J.A., Moïse, N.S., Gelzer, A.R. et al. (1999). Introduction of an endocardial pacing lead through the costocervical vein in six dogs. *J. Am. Vet. Med. Assoc.* 215: 46–48.

263 Oyama, M.A., Sisson, D.D., and Lehmkuhl, L.B. (2001). Practices and outcome of artificial cardiac pacing in 154 dogs. *J. Vet. Intern. Med.* 15: 229–239.

264 Domenech, O., Santilli, R., Pradelli, D. et al. (2005). The implantation of a permanent transvenous endocardial pacemaker in 42 dogs: a retrospective study. *Med. Sci. Monit.* 11: BR168–BR175.

265 Schrope, D.P. and Kelch, W.J. (2006). Signalment, clinical signs, and prognostic indicators associated with high-grade second- or third-degree atrioventricular block in dogs: 124 cases (January 1, 1997-December 31, 1997). *J. Am. Vet. Med. Assoc.* 228: 1710–1717.

266 Wess, G., Thomas, W.P., Berger, D.M. et al. (2006). Applications, complications, and outcomes of transvenous pacemaker implantation in 105 dogs (1997-2002). *J. Vet. Intern. Med.* 20: 877–884.

267 Johnson, M.S., Martin, M.W., and Henley, W. (2007). Results of pacemaker implantation in 104 dogs. *J. Small Anim. Pract.* 48: 4–11.

268 Hildebrandt, N., Stertmann, W.A., Wehner, M. et al. (2009). Dual chamber pacemaker implantation in dogs with atrioventricular block. *J. Vet. Intern. Med.* 23: 31–38.

269 Visser, L.C., Keene, B.W., Mathews, K.G. et al. (2013). Outcomes and complications associated with epicardial pacemakers in 28 dogs and 5 cats. *Vet. Surg.* 42: 544–550.

270 Genovese, D.W., Estrada, A.H., Maisenbacher, H.W. et al. (2013). Procedure times, complication rates, and survival times associated with single-chamber versus dual-chamber pacemaker implantation in dogs with clinical signs of bradyarrhythmia: 54 cases (2004–2009). *J. Am. Vet. Med. Assoc.* 242: 230–236.

271 Lichtenberger, J., Scollan, K.F., Bulmer, B.J. et al. (2015). Long-term outcome of physiologic VDD pacing versus non-physiologic VVI pacing in dogs with high-grade atrioventricular block. *J. Vet. Cardiol.* 17: 42–53.

272 Santilli, R.A., Giacomazzi, F., Porteiro Vázquez, D.M. et al. (2019). Indications for permanent pacing in dogs and cats. *J. Vet. Cardiol.* 22: 20–39.

273 DeForge, W.F. (2019). Cardiac pacemakers: a basic review of the history and current technology. *J. Vet. Cardiol.* 22: 40–50.

274 Bulmer, B.J. (2015). Cardiac pacemakers and anesthesia. In: *Veterinary Anesthesia and Analgesia. The Fifth Edition of Lumb and Jones* (eds. K.A. Grimm, L.A. Lamont, W.J. Tranquilli, et al.), 490–495. Ames: Wiley Blackwell.

275 Estrada, A.H., Maisenbacher, H.W., Jones, A.E. et al. (2019). Transvenous pacing implantation: techniques, tips, and lessons learned along the way. *J. Vet. Cardiol.* 22: 51–64.

276 Gammage, M.D. (2000). Temporary cardiac pacing. *Heart* 83: 715–720.

277 Hatlestad, D. (2002). The benefits of electricity: transcutaneous pacing in EMS. *Emerg. Med. Serv.* 31 38–40, 42, 44–45.

278 DeFrancesco, T.C., Hansen, B.D., Atkins, C.E. et al. Noninvasive transthoracic temporary cardiac pacing in dogs. *J. Vet. Intern. Med.* 17: 663–667.

279 Sanchis-Mora, S., Viscasillas, J., Mathis, A. et al. (2014). Anaesthetic management and complications of pacemaker implantation in dogs. *Vet. Rec.* 175: 303.

280 Jones, D.J., Stehling, L.C., and Zauder, H.L. (1979). Cardiovascular responses to diazepam and midazolam maleate in the dog. *Anesthesiology* 51: 430–434.

281 Stepien, R.L. (2005). Blood pressure assessment. In: *Textbook of Veterinary*

Internal Medicine, 6e (eds. S.J. Ettinger and E.C. Feldman), 470–476. Philadelphia: Elsevier Saunders.

282 Waddel, L.S. (2005). Management of hypotension. In: *Textbook of Veterinary Internal Medicine*, 6e (eds. S.J. Ettinger and E.C. Feldman), 480–485. Philadelphia: Elsevier Saunders.

283 Detweiler, D.K., Cox, R.H., and Alonso, F.R. (1975). Characteristics of the greyhound cardiovascular system. *Fed. Proc.* 34: 399.

284 Tippett, F.E., Padgett, G.A., Eyster, G. et al. (1987). Primary hypertension in a colony of dogs. *Hypertension* 9: 49–58.

285 Reusch, C.E., Schellenberg, S., and Wenger, M. (2009). Endocrine hypertension in small animals. *Vet. Clin. North Am. Small Anim. Pract.* 40: 335–352.

286 Syme, H.M. (2007). Cardiovascular and renal manifestations of hyperthyroidism. *Vet. Clin. North Am. Small Anim. Pract.* 37: 723–743.

287 Henik, R.A. and Brown, S.A. (2015). Systemic hypertension. In: *Manual of Canine and Feline Cardiology*, 5e (eds. L.P. Tilley, F.W.K. Smith, M.A. Oyama and M.M. Sleeper), 275–286. St. Louis: Saunders Elsevier.

288 Roizen, M.F. (2014). Anesthetic complications of concurrent diseases. In: *Miller's Anesthesia*, 8e (ed. R.D. Miller), 871–885. Philadelphia: Elsevier Churchill Livingstone.

289 Coleman, A.E., Shepard, M.K., Schmiedt, C.W. et al. (2016). Effects of orally administered enalapril on blood pressure and hemodynamic response to vasopressors during isoflurane anesthesia in healthy dogs. *Vet. Anaesth. Analg.* 43: 482–494.

290 Ishikawa, Y., Uechi, M., Ishikawa, R. et al. (2007). Effect of isoflurane anesthesia on hemodynamics following the administration of an angiotensin-converting enzyme inhibitor in cats. *J. Vet. Med. Sci.* 69: 869–871.

291 Goldman, L. and Caldera, D.L. (1979). Risks of general anesthesia and elective operation in the hypertensive patient. *Anesthesiology* 50: 285–292.

292 MacDonald, K.A. and Johnson, L.R. (2005). Pulmonary hypertension and pulmonary thromboembolism. In: *Textbook of Veterinary Internal Medicine*, 6e (eds. S.J. Ettinger and E.C. Felman), 1284–1288. Philadelphia: Elsevier Saunders.

293 Kellihan, H.B. and Stepien, R.L. (2010). Pulmonary hypertension in dogs: diagnosis and therapy. *Vet. Clin. North Am. Small Anim. Pract.* 40: 623–641.

294 Reinero, C., Visser, L.C., Kellihan, H.B. et al. (2020). ACVIM consensus statement guidelines for the diagnosis, classification, treatment, and monitoring of pulmonary hypertension in dogs. *J. Vet. Intern. Med.* 34: 549–573.

295 Bach, J.F., Rozanski, E.A., MacGregor, J. et al. (2006). Retrospective evaluation of sildenafil citrate as a therapy for pulmonary hypertension in dogs. *J. Vet. Intern. Med.* 20: 1132–1135.

296 Kellum, H.B. and Stepien, R.L. (2007). Sildenafil citrate therapy in 22 dogs with pulmonary hypertension. *J. Vet. Intern. Med.* 21: 1258–1264.

297 Kellihan, H.B., Waller, K.R., Pinkos, A. et al. (2015). Acute resolution of pulmonary alveolar infiltrates in 10 dogs with pulmonary hypertension treated with sildenafil citrate: 2005-2014. *J. Vet. Cardiol.* 17: 182–191.

298 Ueda, Y., Johnson, L.R., Ontiveros, E.S. et al. (2019). Effect of a phosphodiesterase-5A (PDE5A) gene polymorphism on response to sildenafil therapy in canine pulmonary hypertension. *Sci. Rep.* 9: 6899.

299 Jaffey, A., Leach, S.B., Kong, L.R. et al. (2019). Clinical efficacy of tadalafil compared to sildenafil in treatment of moderate to severe canine pulmonary hypertension: a pilot study. *J. Vet. Cardiol.* 24: 7–19.

300 Pritts, C.D. and Pearl, R.G. (2010). Anesthesia for patients with pulmonary hypertension. *Curr. Opin. Anaesthesiol.* 23: 411–416.

301 Fox, C., Kalarickal, P.L., Yarborough, M.J. et al. (2008). Perioperative management including new pharmacological vistas for patients with pulmonary hypertension for noncardiac surgery. *Curr. Opin. Anaesthesiol.* 21: 467–472.

302 Gordon, C., Collard, C.D., and Pan, W. (2010). Intraoperative management of pulmonary hypertension and associated right heart failure. *Curr. Opin. Anaesthesiol.* 23: 49–56.

303 Friesen, R.H. and Williams, G.D. (2008). Anesthetic management of children with pulmonary arterial hypertension. *Paediatr. Anaesth.* 18: 208–216.

304 Chuang, I.-C., Yang, R.-C., Chou, S.-H. et al. (2011). Effect of carbon dioxide inhalation on pulmonary hypertension induced by increased blood flow and hypoxia. *Kaohsiung J. Med. Sci.* 27: 336–343.

305 Teo, Y.W. and Greenhalgh, D.L. (2010). Update on anaesthetic approach to pulmonary hypertension. *Eur. J. Anaesthesiol.* 27: 317–323.

306 Erling, P. and Mazzaferro, E.M. (2008). Left-sided congestive heart failure in dogs: pathophysiology and diagnosis. *Compend. Contin. Educ. Vet.* 30: 79–90.

307 Häggström, J., Duelund Pedersen, H., and Kvart, C. (2004). New insights into degenerative mitral valve disease in dogs. *Vet. Clin. North Am. Small Anim. Pract.* 34: 1209–1226.

308 Sisson, D. and Kittleson, M.D. (1999). Management of heart failure: principles of treatment, therapeutic strategies and pharmacology. In: *Textbook of Canine and Feline Cardiology: Principles and Clinical Practice*, 2e (eds. P.R. Fox, D. Sisson and N.S. Moise), 225–226. Philadelphia: WB Saunders.

309 New York Heart Association Criteria Committee, Inc. Classes of heart failure. https://www.heart.org/en/health-topics/heart-failure/what-is-heart-failure/classes-of-heart-failure (accessed 2 September 2020).

310 Trehiou-Sechi, E. et al. (2012). Comparative echocardiographic and clinical features of hypertrophic cardiomyopathy in 5 breeds of cats: a retrospective analysis of 344 cases (2001-2011). *J. Vet. Intern. Med.* 26: 532–541.

311 Luis Fuentes, V., Abbott, J., Chetboul, V. et al. (2020). ACVIM consensus statement guidelines for the classification, diagnosis, and management of cardiomyopathies in cats. *J. Vet. Intern. Med.* 34: 1062–1077.

312 de Lima, G.V. and Ferreira, F.D.S. (2017). N-terminal-pro brain natriuretic peptides in dogs and cats: a technical and clinical review. *Vet. World* 10: 1072–1082.

313 Seeler, D.C., Dodman, N.H., Norman, W. et al. (1988). Recommended techniques in small animal anaesthesia. IV. Anaesthesia and cardiac disease. *Br. Vet. J.* 144: 108–122.

314 Ivankovich, A.D., Miletich, D.J., Reimann, C. et al. (1974). Cardiovascular effects of centrally administered ketamine in goats. *Anesth. Analg.* 53: 924–933.

315 Tweed, W.A., Minuck, M., and Mymin, D. (1972). Circulatory responses to ketamine anesthesia. *Anesthesiology* 37: 613–619.

316 Abbott, J.A. (2010). Feline hypertrophic cardiomyopathy: an update. *Vet. Clin. North Am. Small Anim. Pract.* 40: 685–700.

317 Smiley, L.E. (1992). The use of hetastarch for plasma expansion. *Probl. Vet. Med.* 4: 652–667.

318 Mensack, S. (2008). Fluid therapy: options and rational administration. *Vet. Clin. North Am. Small Anim. Pract.* 38: 575–586.

319 Pugsley, M.K., Guth, B., Chiang, A.Y. et al. (2017). An evaluation of the utility of LV dP/dt, QA interval, LV dP/dt min and Tau as indicators of drug-induced changes in contractility and lusitropy in dogs. *J. Pharmacol. Toxicol. Methods* 85: 1–21.

320 DeWitt, E.S., Black, K.J., Thiagarajan, R.R. et al. (2016). Effects of commonly used inotropes on myocardial function and oxygen consumption under constant ventricular loading conditions. *J. Appl. Physiol. (1985)* 121: 7–14.

321 Lamont, L.A., Bulmer, B.J., Sisson, D.D. et al. (2002). Doppler echocardiographic effects of medetomidine on dynamic left ventricular outflow tract obstruction in cats. *J. Am. Vet. Med. Assoc.* 221: 1276–1281.

322 Tamura, J., Ishizuka, T., Fukui, S. et al. (2015). Sedative effects of intramuscular alfaxalone administered to cats. *J. Vet. Med. Sci.* 77: 897–904.

323 Cremer, J. and Riccó, C.H. (2018). Cardiovascular, respiratory and sedative effects of intramuscular alfaxalone, butorphanol and dexmedetomidine compared with ketamine, butorphanol and dexmedetomidine in healthy cats. *J. Feline Med. Surg.* 20: 973–979.

324 Reader, R.C., Barton, B.A., and Abelson, A.L. (2019). Comparison of two intramuscular sedation protocols on sedation, recovery and ease of venipuncture for cats undergoing blood donation. *J. Feline Med. Surg.* 21: 95–102.

325 Bellumori, T.P., Famula, T.R., Bannasch, D.L. et al. (2013). Prevalence of inherited disorders among mixed-breed and purebred dogs: 27,254 cases (1995-2010). *J. Am. Vet. Med. Assoc.* 242: 1549–1555.

326 Tidholm, A., Häggström, J., Borgarelli, M. et al. (2001). Canine idiopathic dilated cardiomyopathy. Part I: aetiology, clinical characteristics, epidemiology and pathology. *Vet. J.* 162: 92–107.

327 Freeman, L.M., Stern, J.A., Fries, R. et al. (2018). Diet-associated dilated cardiomyopathy in dogs: what do we know? *J. Am. Vet. Med. Assoc.* 253: 1390–1394.

328 McCauley, S.R., Clark, S.D., Quest, B.W. et al. (2020). Review of canine dilated cardiomyopathy in the wake of diet-associated concerns. *J. Anim. Sci.* 98: 6.

329 Kruse-Elliott, K.T., Swanson, C.R., and Aucoin, D.P. (1987). Effects of etomidate on adrenocortical function in canine surgical patients. *Am. J. Vet. Res.* 48: 1098–1100.

330 Doenicke, A., Roizen, M.F., Hoernecke, R. et al. (1997). Haemolysis after etomidate: comparison of propylene glycol and lipid formulations. *Br. J. Anaesth.* 79: 386–388.

331 Caro-Vadillo, A., García-Guasch, L., Carretón, E. et al. (2013). Arrhythmogenic right ventricular cardiomyopathy in boxer dogs: a retrospective study of survival. *Vet. Rec.* 172: 268.

332 Bowman, D., Little, S.E., Lorentzen, L. et al. (2009). Prevalence and geographic distribution of *Dirofilaria immitis*, *Borrelia burgdorferi*, *Ehrlichia canis*, and *Anaplasma phagocytophilum* in dogs in the United States: results of a national clinic-based serologic survey. *Vet. Parasitol.* 160: 138–148.

333 Lee, A.C. and Atkins, C.E. (2010). Understanding feline heartworm infection: disease, diagnosis, and treatment. *Top. Companion Anim. Med.* 25: 224–230.

2

Respiratory Disease

Rebecca A. Johnson and David B. Brunson

Department of Surgical Sciences, School of Veterinary Medicine, University of Wisconsin–Madison, Madison, WI, 53706, USA

Introduction

Adequate respiratory function and support are critical for safe anesthetic management, especially if inhalants are used. When patients present with coexisting respiratory disease, safe anesthetic practices can become challenging. It is therefore important to understand normal physiology, as well as the physiological changes and pathological progression of any coexisting disease, especially regarding the respiratory system [1–3]. Dogs and cats with respiratory disease may require sedation or anesthesia for diagnostic or surgical procedures that are either related or unrelated to the primary problem. Fortunately, pulmonary function support in these cases can frequently be accomplished with minimal specialized equipment. A brief overview of relevant ventilatory concepts and strategies, respiratory physiology, sedative/anesthetic agents, and specific case management is presented in the following text. Readers are referred elsewhere for a full review of basic respiratory physiology and pathophysiology [2, 3].

Ventilatory Control

Ventilatory "drive" originates within respiratory centers of the central nervous system (CNS) ventral medulla. This brainstem circuitry of neurons and pathways is responsible for respiratory rhythm generation and respiratory pattern formation [4]. Although not yet fully elucidated, several models for this complex network have been proposed, many using reduced medullary slice preparations as models [5]. Respiratory rhythm and pattern are continuously altered by homeostatic control mechanisms that allow the animal to "adapt" to physiologic respiratory challenges (i.e., exercise, pregnancy) or pathologic conditions (i.e., neurologic or respiratory disease). This respiratory plasticity involves alterations via sensory (i.e., central and peripheral chemoreceptors and airway mechanoreceptors) and modulatory projections (i.e., serotonergic neurons), as well as many other conscious and unconscious processes that affect breathing (i.e., cortical inputs, cardiovascular disease, etc.). Collectively, inputs merge to form the spatiotemporal neural output that projects to the respiratory muscles. The primary inspiratory muscles are the diaphragm and inspiratory (external) intercostals which move the ribs forward and outward. However, accessory inspiratory muscles also play a role in breathing, especially during respiratory stress or disease (i.e., upper airway muscles innervated by the hypoglossal nerve) [6]. Altogether, synchronized respiratory muscle contraction generates a

Canine and Feline Anesthesia and Co-Existing Disease, Second Edition. Edited by Rebecca A. Johnson, Lindsey B. C. Snyder and Carrie A. Schroeder.

Companion website: www.wiley.com/go/johnson/canine

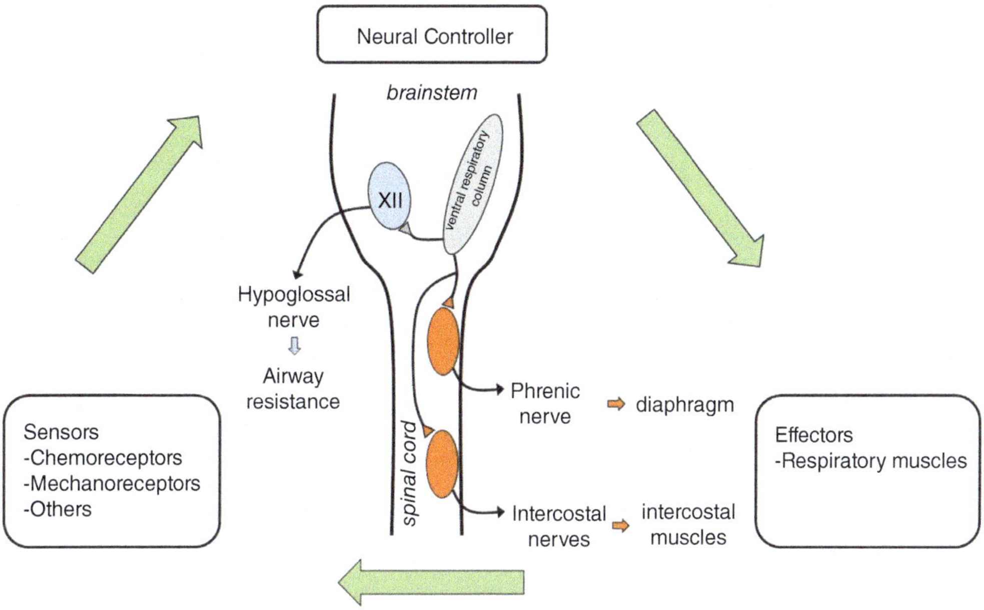

Figure 2.1 Graphic representation of the respiratory control system. The respiratory rhythm is generated within the brainstem and is modulated by multiple afferent inputs from various sensors such as mechanoreceptors and chemoreceptors. The detailed spatiotemporal output is projected to primary (diaphragm, inspiratory intercostal) and secondary (upper airway) respiratory muscles which contract to generate an adequate breath. During ventilation, respiratory mechanics and arterial oxygen and carbon dioxide levels change as conditions are altered, thus providing further sensory feedback to brainstem respiratory areas which imparts the respiratory continuum.

breath which ultimately drives alveolar ventilation and blood gas regulation (Figure 2.1) [7].

Respiratory Volumes and Ventilation

Normal respiratory volumes (Figure 2.2) can be affected in anesthetized/sedated patients or in patients with altered physiology (i.e., pregnancy, disease, etc.). Many respiratory volumes are not measured clinically. However, tidal volume (V_T) and functional residual capacity (FRC) can be measured in awake animals. Tidal volume refers to the air volume inspired or expired during a normal breath. The FRC is the amount of air remaining in the lungs after a normal expiration and can be affected by diaphragm position; although animal studies are sparse, this is especially important, as FRC likely decreases with pregnancy, bowel dilatation, abdominal masses, etc. [8]. The "inspiratory capacity" is the amount of air that can maximally inhaled beginning after a normal expiration. The "vital capacity" is the maximal amount of air that can be exhaled after filling them to their inspiratory capacity. The "residual volume" is the air left in the lungs following a maximal expiration. The "total lung capacity" is the lung volume following the greatest possible inspiratory effort (vital capacity and residual volume).

Alveolar ventilation ($\dot{V}_A$) is primarily driven by the arterial partial pressure of CO_2 ($PaCO_2$) sensed at central chemoreceptors such that, for a given metabolic state, $\dot{V}_A$ is directly and inversely related to $PaCO_2$ (see the section titled "Carbon Dioxide"). For example, if $\dot{V}_A$ increases by 50%, $PaCO_2$ is halved. It is defined as the rate that alveolar air is exchanged with atmospheric air. Although clinically it is frequently assumed to be minute ventilation ($\dot{V}_E$), these concepts are not the same due to anatomic (and potential mechanical) dead space (see in the following

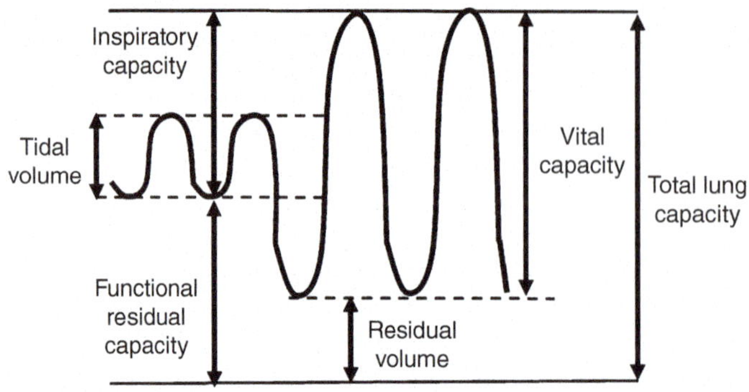

Figure 2.2 Graphical representation of lung volumes. Total lung capacity is the volume of air in the lungs following maximal inspiration; it is the inspiratory capacity plus the functional residual capacity or vital capacity plus the residual volume after peak expiration. A normal tidal volume represents only a small portion of the total lung capacity.

text). Minute ventilation is composed of the tidal volume (volume of each breath; V_T) and respiratory rate (f): $\dot{V}_E = V_T \times f$. For most species, the V_T is approximated at 8–20 ml kg^{-1}; however, breathing frequency is highly variable [9]. Although smaller animals usually breathe at higher frequencies than larger animals based on metabolic oxygen requirements, birds are an exception, as they have relatively slower respiratory rates than other mammals with similar body sizes due to large anatomical dead space in conducting airways [9, 10]. Typically, the respiratory rate of awake dogs and cats varies between 10 and 30 breaths min^{-1}. However, with sedation or general anesthesia, respiratory rates, as well as tidal volumes, are almost always reduced due to drug-induced respiratory muscle relaxation and respiratory center depression, hypothermia, body position, and other external factors such as bandages. For example, respiratory frequencies commonly range from 6 to 20 breaths min^{-1} in spontaneously breathing, anesthetized dogs and cats, and $\dot{V}_E$ is significantly reduced from normal values of approximately 150–250 ml kg^{-1} min^{-1} [9, 11]. Because of the high variability in respiratory frequency, and the influences of V_T on $\dot{V}_A$, respiratory rate alone is not an adequate indicator of ventilatory function.

An important concept in the assessment of small-animal ventilation is dead space (V_D). Mechanical dead-space ventilation occurs where two-way flow of gases is present with no gas exchange. This mainly occurs in the endotracheal tube extending from the mouth, any monitor adapters added to the circuit, and the end of the Y-piece before it splits into the inspiratory and expiratory tubing (Figure 2.3). Physiologic dead space is similar, except it occurs within the animal and is the arithmetic sum of both anatomic dead space and alveolar dead space. For example, no gas exchange occurs in the upper or conductive airways of the dog and cat (i.e., nares, larynx, pharynx, trachea, bronchi, nonrespiratory bronchioles). Thus, this portion of the V_T is referred to as anatomic dead-space ventilation. In addition, dead space also occurs in lung areas that are poorly perfused but adequately ventilated; little to no gas exchange occurs in these areas and this is referred to as alveolar dead-space ventilation. The ratio of physiological dead space to the tidal volume (V_D/V_T) has been clinically calculated by the Enghoff modification of the Bohr equation which uses arterial CO_2 ($PaCO_2$) in the place of alveolar CO_2 ($PACO_2$) [12, 13]:

$$V_D / V_T = \left(PaCO_2 - PECO_2\right) / PaCO_2 \quad (2.1)$$

$PECO_2$ is the expired CO_2 tension. V_D/V_T in awake dogs is approximately 35% but increases during inhalant anesthesia (to approximately 50% or more) [14]. Dead-space ventilation is

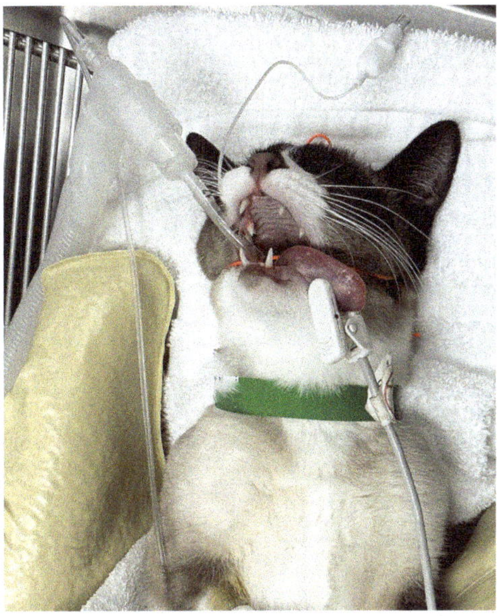

Figure 2.3 An anesthetized cat demonstrating considerable mechanical dead space containing two-way gas flow as the orotracheal tube extends at least 3–4 cm from the teeth to the capnometer adapter. In addition, the capnometer adapter adds to the mechanical dead space before attaching to the Y-piece which contains unidirectional gas flow due to the one-way valves of the rebreathing anesthetic system.

one reason that respiratory frequency should not be used to assess ventilation adequacy, since small, frequent breaths primarily ventilate only the anatomic dead space and alveolar ventilation may be inadequate. Rapid shallow ventilations may be effective for CO_2 removal that reaches the upper airways, but not effective for O_2 delivery to the alveoli. Slow deep ventilations are more likely to provide effective CO_2 removal and O_2 delivery, such as those seen in avian species. It is usually only the slow shallow ventilations that are easily recognized as ineffective by the anesthetist.

Respiratory Gases

The respiratory system is ultimately responsible for the effective transfer of O_2 and CO_2 between the atmosphere and the animal. Normally, the inspired air has only a trace percentage of CO_2, while the animal's arterial blood contains approximately 5% CO_2. This differential gradient promotes CO_2 movement out of the animal. By contrast, the normal atmospheric O_2 content is approximately 21%, which is higher than the O_2 in venous blood returning to the lungs, and O_2 diffuses from the alveoli into the blood. Respiratory gases such as O_2, CO_2, and nitrogen are measured as a part of the total gases in the animal. Since the animal lives normally at a pressure of 1 atm (approximately 760 mmHg at sea level), the units used to measure gases are also in mmHg. Evaluation of the pulmonary system requires an understanding of both O_2 and CO_2 transfer. Each gas is somewhat independent of the other (but not exclusively; see the section titled "Interactions Between CO_2 and O_2 Transport"), and assessment of pulmonary function requires measurement of both gases. Thus, the "gold standard" for measuring adequacy of ventilation and patient oxygenation is the use of arterial blood gas analysis in both dogs and cats (Table 2.1) [15, 16].

Carbon Dioxide (CO_2)

Although peripheral CO_2 receptors contribute to CO_2-induced ventilatory responses, the primary CO_2-/pH-sensitive chemoreceptors are located in the CNS throughout the brainstem (i.e., retrotrapezoid nuclei, serotonergic raphe neurons, noradrenergic neurons in the locus coeruleus, nucleus of the solitary tract, pre-Bötzinger complex, etc.) [7]. These chemoreceptors are extremely sensitive and even small deviations from a normal $PaCO_2$ level affect ventilation linearly and dramatically.

CO_2 diffuses rapidly from tissues into red blood cells where it forms bicarbonate according to the reaction: $CO_2 + H_2O \leftrightarrow H_2CO_3 \leftrightarrow H^+ + HCO_3^-$. The first reaction is slow in plasma, but rapid inside the red cell due to the presence of carbonic anhydrase. CO_2 is then transported mostly as bicarbonate (approximately 81%) with a small amount dissolved in plasma (approximately 8%) and combined with amino groups of blood proteins (approximately 11%) [4].

Table 2.1 Normal arterial blood gas values in the unanesthetized dog and cat while breathing room air (approximately 21% O_2).

	Dog	Cat
pH	7.41 (7.35–7.46)	7.39 (7.31–7.46)
PCO_2 (mmHg)	36.8 (30.8–42.8)	31.0 (25.2–36.8)
HCO_3^- (mEq/l)	22.2 (18.8–25.6)	18.0 (14.4–21.6)
PO_2 (mmHg)	92.1 (80.9–103.3)	106.8 (95.4–118.2)

Values are expressed as mean (range). When breathing 100% O_2 (as during anesthesia), PO_2 values are expected to approach 600 mmHg with ideal gas exchange [11, 12].

As previously mentioned, in the steady-state, $PaCO_2$ is inversely proportional to $\dot{V}_A$ based on the alveolar ventilation equation:

$$PaCO_2 = 0.863 \times \left(\dot{V}_{CO_2} / \dot{V}_A\right) \tag{2.2}$$

$\dot{V}_{CO_2}$ is the metabolic production of CO_2 and 0.863 is a constant that corrects for dissimilar units. CO_2 is approximately 20–24 times more diffusible than oxygen; as such, there is complete equilibration across the alveolar membrane under normal situations. Thus, the $PaCO_2$ is essentially the same as the $PACO_2$ (within a few mmHg, primarily due to a small amount of dead-space ventilation) in healthy animals. However, these values may significantly diverge in the presence of pulmonary disease states such as profound ventilation–perfusion inequalities or pulmonary shunting.

Overall ventilation is a measure of the animal's ability to regulate the level of CO_2 within the body; it is the only route for elimination. Adequate ventilation is present when CO_2 is maintained at an optimal partial pressure in arterial blood (Table 2.1) [11, 15, 17]. Accordingly, hyperventilation occurs when $\dot{V}_A$ is increased and the resultant $PaCO_2$ falls below normal values, while hypoventilation is defined as a reduction in $\dot{V}_A$, increasing $PaCO_2$ values from normal. Although blood gas analysis is the definitive way to assess the adequacy of ventilation, noninvasive technology such as the use of end-tidal CO_2 ($ETCO_2$) capnometers has become increasingly popular in small-animal (as well as exotic-animal) practice, since they closely approximate alveolar CO_2 levels under normal situations and can be easily used in most species (Figure 2.4). Since capnometry relies on adequate cardiac output to return CO_2 to the lungs, as well as pulmonary

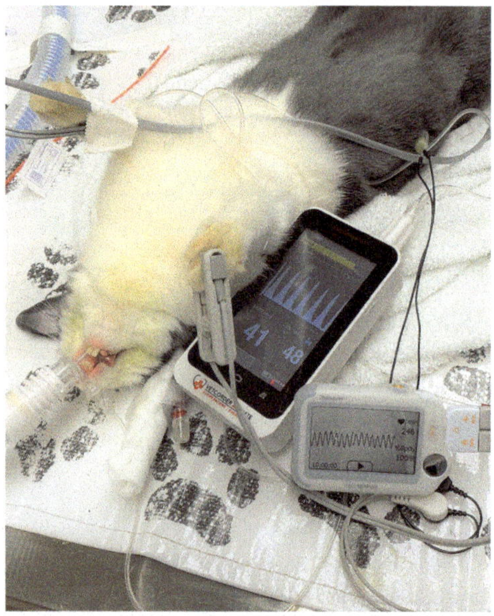

Figure 2.4 Capnometry (Vetcorder Airmate™ Capnograph, Sentier, Waukesha, WI) and pulse oximetry (Vetcorder™, Sentier, Waukesha, WI) used during isoflurane anesthesia on a domestic rabbit. Similar to the procedure in cats and dogs, the end-tidal sample is drawn directly from the oral end of the endotracheal tube via a low dead-space adapter. The capnometer produces a graphical waveform and is reading an end-tidal CO_2 level of 41 mmHg with a respiratory rate of 46 breaths min^{-1} in this rabbit (larger monitor). The pulse oximetry probe was placed on the foot and is reading a heart rate of 246 beats min^{-1} and hemoglobin saturation of 100% (smaller gray monitor). Inspired oxygen levels were approximately 100%.

function to eliminate CO_2 from the body, it is an essential piece of equipment in any case where respiratory impairment or dysfunction is a concern and should become a routine monitor for any veterinary practice [18].

Oxygen

Once oxygen is carried from the conducting airways to the respiratory exchange tissues (respiratory bronchioles and alveoli), it quickly diffuses into the blood where it is carried both dissolved in solution and bound to hemoglobin (Hb). Approximately 1.36–1.39 ml of O_2 can combine with 1 g of hemoglobin compared to only a small amount that is dissolved in blood (0.003 ml per 100 ml blood per mmHg PO_2) [4, 19]. The total oxygen content of blood (CaO_2) is therefore calculated as: $CaO_2 = (1.39 \times Hb \times SaO_2) + (0.003 \times PaO_2)$, where SaO_2 is the oxygen saturation of Hb. Thus, the amount combined with Hb impacts CaO_2 to a greater extent than does the dissolved amount, and altered Hb levels (i.e., anemia) will have a profound effect on not just CaO_2 but oxygen delivery (DO_2) to the tissues, since $DO_2 = CaO_2 \times$ cardiac output. However, in an anemic animal, the dissolved portion plays an increasing important role; increasing PaO_2 (through enriching inspired O_2 levels, for example) will be advantageous to these patients.

As determined by the oxygen–Hb dissociation curve, the amount of O_2 carried by Hb increases rapidly until PO_2 reaches approximately 60–70 mmHg where the curve flattens off (Figure 2.5). Many factors affect the curve placement including temperature, PCO_2, pH, and 2,3-diphosphoglycerate (2,3-DPG) levels, an enzyme which competes with O_2 for its binding site on Hb (Figure 2.5). Hemoglobin is normally nearly 100% saturated in healthy patients breathing room air (approximately 21% O_2) and should always be above 90–95% [20]. In most normal anesthetized patients, the PaO_2 is very high due to 100% O_2 used as a carrier gas for the inhalant (frequently >500 mmHg; Table 2.1). As per the oxygen–Hb dissociation curve, a very high percentage of Hb will therefore be bound with O_2. Since arterial blood gas analysis may not be available to every practitioner, pulse oximetry is a standard, yet indirect measure of oxygenation in anesthetized dogs

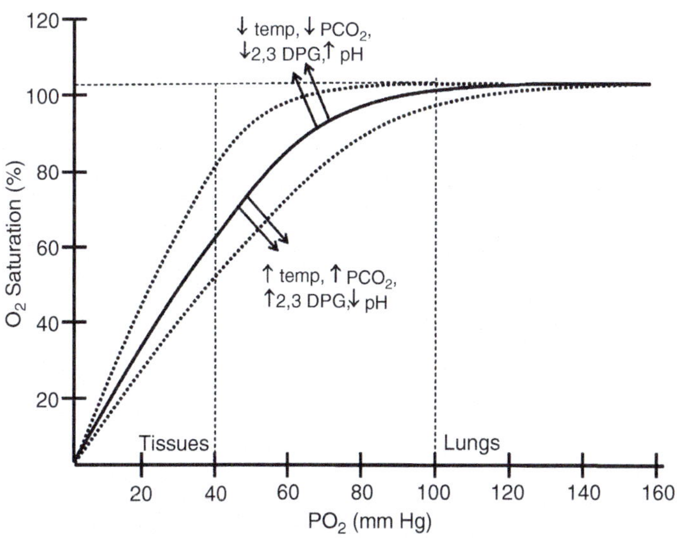

Figure 2.5 Example oxygen–hemoglobin dissociation curves. The amount of O_2 carried by hemoglobin increases rapidly until PO_2 reaches approximately 60–70 mmHg when the curve flattens off. High levels of PO_2 and hemoglobin saturation occur in the lung, whereas lower values occur in the tissues (near the bottom of the curve). The curve is shifted right by increases in temperature, PCO_2, and 2,3-DPG levels, and decreases in pH. Left shifts occur with opposite changes in temperature, PCO_2, pH, and 2,3-DPG levels.

and cats which measures pulse rate and estimates the Hb oxygen saturation (termed SpO_2; Figures 2.4 and 2.6) [21]. However, one must be cautious, since significant pathology must exist in the anesthetized patient administered 100% oxygen for the PaO_2 to drop to a level where the pulse oximeter will alert the anesthetist; a PaO_2 of approximately 60 mmHg corresponds to an SpO_2 of approximately 90%, and a PaO_2 of approximately 80 mmHg corresponds to an SpO_2 of approximately 95%. In addition, pulse oximetry does not indicate if adequate ventilation is present to remove CO_2, since the pulse oximeter only estimates the percentage of Hb saturation with O_2. Although this monitor has become one of the most widely used anesthetic monitors for a variety of species in veterinary medicine (Figures 2.4, 2.6, and 2.7), it provides little information concerning the animal's ventilatory status during anesthesia unless severe pathology is present and should be used with care.

Hypoxemia (low PaO_2) is commonly encountered in patients with respiratory impairment and is primarily due to one of the five reasons: low inspired O_2 fraction, hypoventilation, diffusion impairments, ventilation–perfusion mismatching, and right-to-left shunts (cardiac or pulmonary). Discerning between these causes is sometimes difficult. However, some information can be obtained from the alveolar gas equation which predicts that the arterial (a) or alveolar (A) O_2 tension will decrease with an increase in PCO_2: $PAO_2 = PIO_2 - (PACO_2/R)$, where PIO_2 is the inspired O_2 level and R is the respiratory

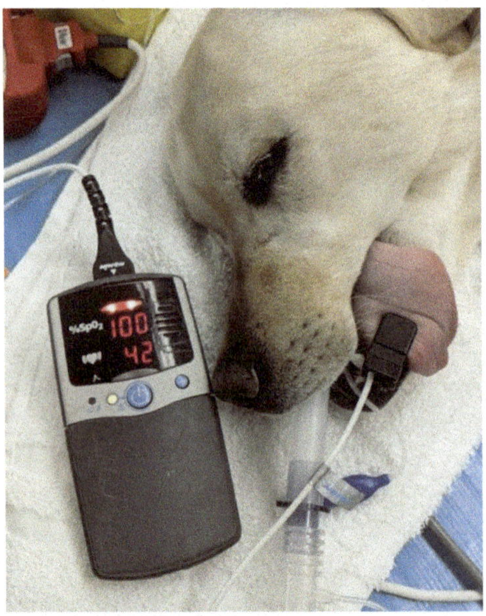

Figure 2.6 Pulse oximeter (Nonin Medical Incorporated, Plymouth, MN) used on an isoflurane-anesthetized dog. As measured with a lingual probe, the heart rate was 42 beats min^{-1} and SpO_2 read 100%. Isoflurane in 100% O_2 was delivered via the anesthesia machine and a large animal mechanical ventilator.

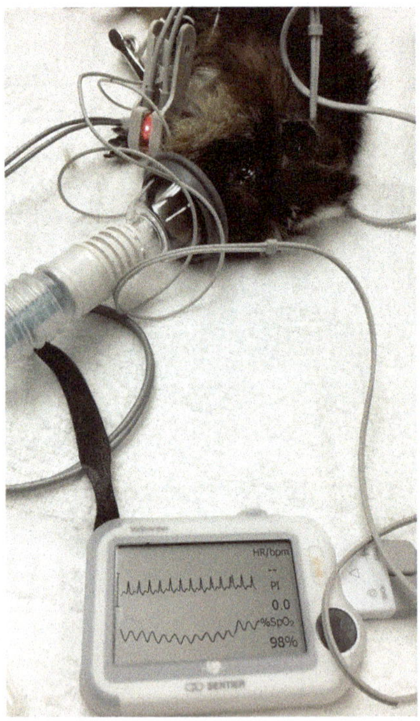

Figure 2.7 Pulse oximeter (Vetcorder™, Sentier, Waukesha, WI) used on an isoflurane-anesthetized domestic guinea pig (*Cavia porcellus*). This monitor can be a valuable tool to measure oxygenation in a variety of species (including cats and dogs). The probe is placed on the foot and displays a waveform (bottom trace) with an SpO_2 of 98%. In addition, this monitor is reading the electrocardiogram (top trace).

exchange ratio (approximately 0.8 in normal animals). The difference between alveolar and arterial oxygen levels is defined as the (A-a) gradient. Substituting $PaCO_2$ for $PACO_2$, the (A-a) oxygen gradient equation becomes: (A-a) gradient = $PAO_2 - PaO_2 = (PIO_2 - 1.25PaCO_2)$. Generally, values between 5 and 15 mmHg in animals breathing room air are considered normal [4].

Hypoxemia due to low inspired O_2 levels (i.e., low atmospheric pressure, use of nitrous oxide without appropriate O_2 flows) does not usually result in increased (A-a) O_2 gradients, since frequently there is a subsequent increase in $\dot{V}_A$ (thus, decreasing $PaCO_2$) secondary to hypoxemia. In addition, if hypoxemia is solely due to hypoventilation, the PAO_2 and PaO_2 decrease, while the $PaCO_2$ and $PACO_2$ must increase and the (A-a) difference should not change. However, in the case of ventilation–perfusion abnormalities or right-to-left shunting (both very common during anesthesia), the (A-a) gradients are significantly elevated. These two are differentiated from each other, as administration of 100% O_2 to patients with ventilation–perfusion abnormalities significantly increases the PaO_2, whereas PaO_2 levels fail to return to normal in patients with significant shunting, as blood traverses across the lungs or through the heart and does not pick up the oxygen [4].

Interactions Between CO_2 and O_2 Transport

Although management of CO_2 and O_2 within the body appears independent, they are not mutually exclusive of each other [9]. For example, acidity (lower pH) associated with carbonic acid produced from CO_2 in tissues promotes O_2 release from Hb with no change in dissolved oxygen levels, whereas CO_2 release from the lungs promotes oxygen uptake; this is known as the Bohr effect. In addition, the Haldane effect states that deoxygenation of Hb causes Hb to become a weaker acid, this increases its ability to carry hydrogen ions [9].

Ventilatory Cycle Phases and Ventilatory Support

Ventilatory Cycle

Normally, there are three ventilatory cycle phases: inspiration, expiration, and an expiratory pause (which are important to understand in evaluating breathing or during adjustments of ventilatory support). Inspiratory pauses are not normally present in conscious dogs and cats. Expiration, in most cases, is a passive process related to the elastic recoil of the chest. One exception is the horse in which expiration normally has an active phase even at rest [22]. The respiratory cycle is primarily changed by adjustments of the "pause" phase of the cycle. Ventilatory rates are usually increased by decreasing the pause time between each inhalation and exhalation. For mechanical ventilation, adjustment of the inspiratory to expiratory ratio (I:E) is possible and is important when changing the respiratory rate (Figure 2.8). As a guideline, the inspiratory time should be less than or equal to the expiratory time. Thus, the I:E ratio will be at least 1:1, but may vary to a ratio as high as 1:5. For example, if inspiratory time is kept at 1–2 s in duration and the respiratory rate is 10 breaths min^{-1}, then the I:E ratio will be between 1:5 and 1:2. Typically, the I:E ratio is usually not less than 1:1, which allows adequate time for lung filling and emptying.

Ventilatory Support with Intermittent Positive Pressure Ventilation (IPPV)

Mechanical ventilation differs significantly from spontaneous ventilation. Normally, air enters the respiratory system because of contraction of inspiratory intercostal muscles and the diaphragm. During normal inspiration, the change in alveolar pressure is only about 1 cm of water pressure [23]. However, IPPV is not a "normal" situation for the animal, as positive pressure is "forced" into the lungs; too much

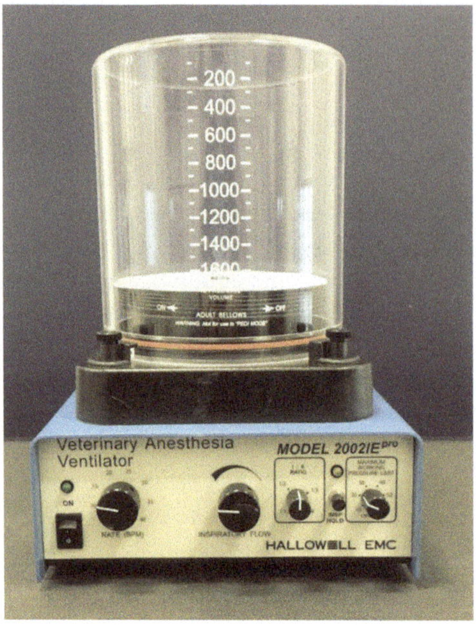

Figure 2.8 A mechanical ventilator used for small animals. Respiratory rate, inspiratory flow, maximum pressure, and I:E ratio can all be adjusted to reach the targeted end-tidal CO_2 level.

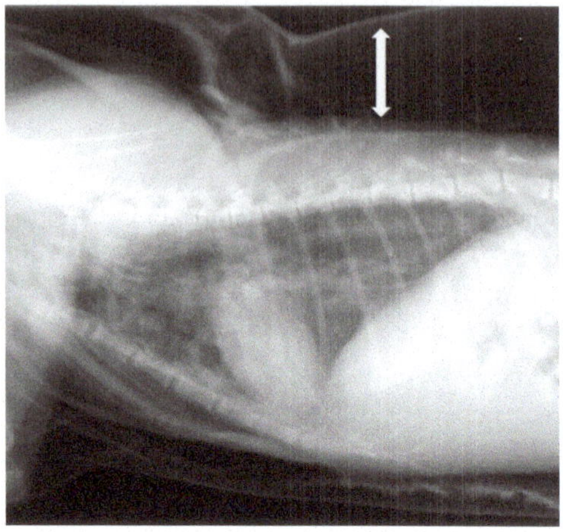

Figure 2.9 Thoracic radiograph depicting subcutaneous emphysema secondary to barotrauma following excessive intrathoracic pressure delivered to cat. The skin has been separated from the body wall by a large volume of radiolucent air (white arrow).

pressure can result in detrimental effects such as reducing cardiac output, volutrauma, barotrauma, etc. (Figure 2.9) [24].

Ultimately, the concern with IPPV is that intermittent high thoracic pressures can lead to tissue perfusion failure. For example, although during the positive pressure breath, pressurization of chest can augment cardiac ejection, increased intrathoracic pressure often exceeds central venous pressure, resulting in a decrease in venous return to the heart. The resulting decrease in ventricular filling may reduce cardiac output on the subsequent heartbeat and often decrease systolic arterial pressure [24]. To minimize the negative effects of IPPV, the inspiratory time should be kept short and should not exceed 2–3 s. Additionally, the lowest peak inspiratory pressure (PIP) capable of inflating the lungs should be used. In many animals, a PIP of less than 15 cmH_2O will be sufficient to fully inflate the lungs. In mammals, the guideline is to keep the PIP below 20 cmH_2O; for reptiles and birds the guideline is a maximum of 15 cmH_2O [25]. In animals with normal thoracic compliance, if PIP is set to approximately 10 cmH_2O, respiratory rate is approximately 10 breaths min^{-1}, and V_T is approximately 10–15 ml kg^{-1}, the $PaCO_2$ frequently approaches normal levels; minor adjustments can then be made to achieve the precise, desired $PaCO_2$ for the patient.

Because of the aforementioned concerns, mechanical ventilation may not be warranted in every patient. If the patient is healthy, having a short procedure (<1h), does not display airway obstruction, is not apneic, and is oxygenated, mild-to-moderate hypercapnia is usually well tolerated. However, ventilatory support should be available to all animals during general anesthesia and can include assisted "hand ventilation" by an anesthetist or the use of mechanical ventilation. This is because multiple factors contribute to an inability to adequately ventilate including drug-induced respiratory depression, age, body weight, and preexisting disease. Ventilation not only ensures that the patient is oxygenated and CO_2 is removed, but also ensures consistent delivery of anesthetic gases. Delivery, maintenance, and recovery from inhaled anesthetics uniquely depend on the movement of the agents through the lungs. Consistent and effective ventilation with controlled or assisted ventilation makes inhalant anesthesia both more precise and easier to perform. However, if the goal is to keep $PaCO_2$ or $ETCO_2$ at normal levels, consistent ventilation must occur, as CO_2 levels quickly rise when ventilation is stopped, even for a few minutes. Any patient can benefit from effective ventilatory support; however, in the patient with preexisting respiratory disease, it is essential.

Oxygen Supplementation

In many patients with respiratory insufficiency, O_2 supplementation can be beneficial. Criteria for preoxygenation include animals that are marginal or unable to maintain Hb O_2 saturation when breathing room air. Cyanosis is a sign of an oxygenation crisis that warrants immediate O_2 supplementation. The ability to see cyanosis indicates that approximately 5 g of Hb is in the reduced form or is not carrying O_2. However, it can be difficult to visually determine cyanosis in certain situations, such as in poor lighting conditions or if the animal is severely anemic. Oxygen can be administered via a face mask, an O_2 chamber, or via nasal O_2 cannulas (Figure 2.10). However, inspired O_2 levels may not reach 100% with these techniques. For example, low-flow nasal insufflation with 100% O_2 only resulted in approximately 32–61% inspired O_2 and was dependent on insufflation rate, respiratory rate, and tidal volume in cadaveric dog preparations [26]. However, high-flow nasal insufflation shows more promise [27]. In addition, mask oxygenation should not be forced on the patient if the process produces anxiety or stress due to increased patient O_2 demands associated with struggling. Unless the animal is cyanotic, the benefit of preoxygenation is that it provides a longer time before a patient becomes hypoxic during apneic periods; for example, following anesthetic induction [28, 29]. Specifically, 3 min of preoxygenation in dogs via tight-fitting face mask increased the time to Hb desaturation from approximately 70 s (room air) to 298 s (O_2 supplementation) following propofol induction [28].

Preoxygenation with 100% delivered O_2 theoretically fills the alveolus and FRC with a higher-than-normal O_2 concentration. If the animal becomes apneic or if tracheal intubation is delayed, additional O_2 is then available to the pulmonary blood. Effectively washing out gases normally found in the alveoli and replacing

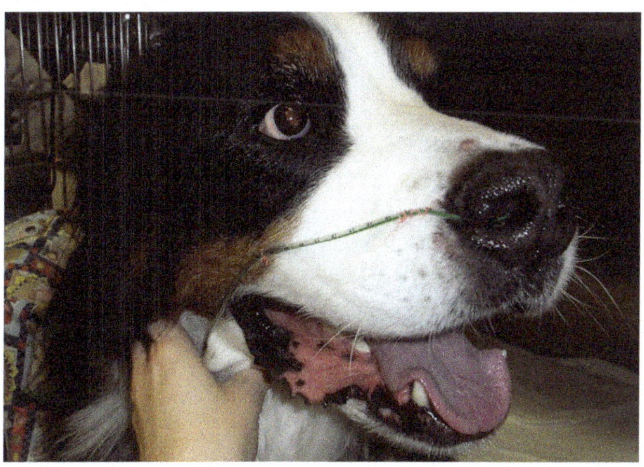

Figure 2.10 Bilateral nasal oxygen cannulas and supplementation in a dog. The tubing is secured to the lateral nasal area and upper lip to reduce the chances for dislodgment of the cannula. The tubing is further connected to an oxygen flowmeter to deliver gases enriched with oxygen.

them with a higher O_2 concentration take multiple minutes of preoxygenation [28], and any break in the breathing of the supplemental O_2 will require restarting of the oxygenation procedures. Thus, unless the animal is in respiratory distress and is hypoxic prior to anesthesia, preoxygenation may not benefit the animal and may actually precipitate additional failure through excitement or anxiety.

Ventilation in Conscious Patients

Adequate patient ventilation results from careful integration of all components of the respiratory system. For example, the (i) neural control system, (ii) upper and lower airways, (iii) pulmonary parenchyma, and (iv) thoracic bellows mechanism all need to function normally to maintain patient oxygenation and ventilatory capacity. If alterations occur in any or all these constituents, hypoxia or hypercapnia may occur; these untoward effects may be enhanced in anesthetized patients due to the inability to compensate for such changes. Thus, each part of the respiratory control system must be considered when creating an anesthetic plan for not just normal patients but also for patients with disorders of ventilation.

Pharmacologic Effects on Ventilation

Since respiratory function is frequently diminished simply by using respiratory-depressant agents such as inhalants [30, 31] and opioids (although variably) [32] in many species, respiratory complications from coexisting diseases can impair ventilation even further. Anesthetic management of these cases should focus on keeping the patient oxygenated, ventilated, and perfused. Frequently, the anesthetic agents themselves are not as important as the strict patient management associated with these high-risk cases.

Opioids

Many pure opioid analgesics depress minute ventilation via effects at mu-opioid receptors near and pathways projecting to brainstem respiratory centers. These dose-dependent effects can be seen as a reduction in respiratory frequency, tidal volume, or both [24], and are more pronounced with the pure mu-opioid receptor agonists when compared to the mixed agonist–antagonists or partial agonists [33, 34]. Mixed agonist–antagonists such as butorphanol may be used to reverse, at least in part, the respiratory depression seen with pure mu-opioid agonists [34, 35]. The ventilatory response to hypoxia is reduced and the CO_2 response is shifted to the right and the slope is decreased, resulting in a rightward shift of the apneic threshold (level of CO_2 where breathing no longer occurs and the animal becomes apneic; Figure 2.11) [24, 36]. Interestingly, ventilatory responsiveness may show maturational changes, as the newborn dog appears to have increased sensitivity to the respiratory-depressant effects of some opioids (e.g., morphine) [36]. In addition, these effects may be reversed with opioid receptor antagonists such as naloxone or naltrexone [24]. In any small-animal patient with significant respiratory disease, caution should be used when opioids are administered systemically; careful monitoring of ventilation ($PaCO_2$) and oxygenation (PaO_2) is highly recommended.

Other Sedatives and Tranquilizers

Similar to opioids, other tranquilizers and sedatives such as acepromazine [37] and alpha-2-adrenergic receptor agonists (e.g., medetomidine, dexmedetomidine) [38] may also have at least some respiratory-depressant effects in dogs and cats, although they appear to be minimal when the sedative agents are used alone and at clinical doses. For example, in dogs administered medetomidine, (the racemic mixture of levomedetomidine and dexmedetomidine (20 and $60 \mu g\, kg^{-1}$)), respiratory rate significantly decreased and $PaCO_2$

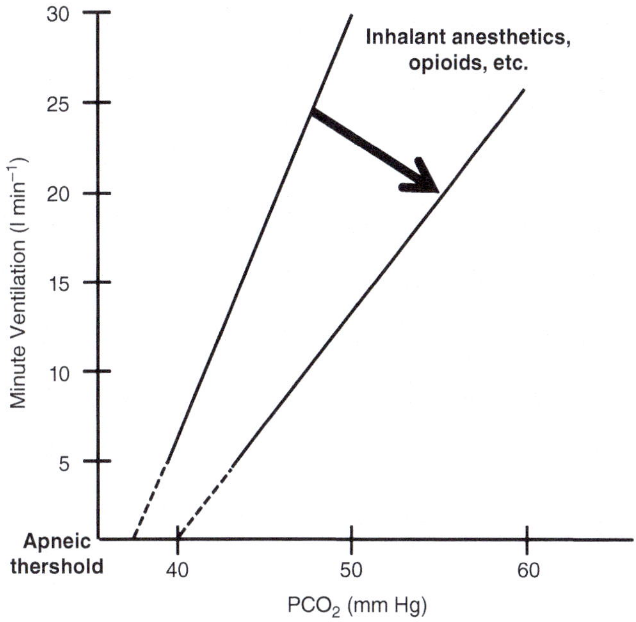

Figure 2.11 Example ventilatory response curves to inspired CO_2 levels. As CO_2 levels rise, ventilation increases rapidly as the central chemoreceptor system is tightly regulated. Pharmacologic agents such as inhalants and opioid analgesics may shift this curve to the right (decreasing sensitivity) and increase the apneic threshold (when ventilation ceases).

significantly increased, albeit with little effect on PaO_2 [33, 39–42]. By contrast, cats administered dexmedetomidine alone did not show decreased respiratory rates and medetomidine alone did not significantly alter arterial blood gas values significantly [43, 44]. It is important to recognize that the respiratory-depressant effects of the alpha-2-adrenergic receptor agonists are likely to be exaggerated when used in combination with other anesthetic/analgesic agents (i.e., propofol, opioids) [42].

Acepromazine has minimal effects on the respiratory control system in unanesthetized patients, at least at clinical doses. Studies in small animals show a reduction in respiratory rate following acepromazine administration with minimal changes in minute ventilation, PaO_2, $PaCO_2$, and arterial pH [34, 45, 46]. Similarly, benzodiazepines (diazepam, midazolam) are associated with minimal pulmonary effects in small animals [47]. However, as always, in animals with respiratory disease, care should be used when administration of the agents is required; proper respiratory monitoring should be performed.

Injectable and Inhalant Anesthetics

Similar to the pure mu-opioid agonists, most induction and inhalational agents depress minute ventilation significantly. $PaCO_2$ increases because of decreased respiratory rates and volumes; these changes are frequently dose-dependent. For example, propofol administered to small animals significantly reduces diaphragm contractility [48], arterial pH, and PaO_2 while significantly increasing $PaCO_2$; large doses can result in apnea [49]. Propofol also suppresses carotid body chemoreceptor activity involved in hypoxia-induced respiratory responses [50]. Alfaxalone dose-dependently decreases respiratory rate and minute volume similar to propofol in cats [51] and in dogs [52], although apnea appears to be more of an issue in dogs. By contrast, intravenous ketamine administration appears to have less respiratory-depressant effects than other agents, especially at low doses. Indeed, ketamine infusions improve respiratory (and cardiovascular) depressant effects associated with inhalant anesthetics in small animals when used as part of a balanced anesthesia technique [53].

All inhalant agents shift the CO_2–ventilatory response curve to the right and reduce the slope in a dose-dependent manner, and the CO_2 response curve is almost horizontal at high inhalant levels (2.0 × the minimum alveolar concentration) (Figure 2.11) [54, 55]. In addition, the ventilatory response to hypoxia is also diminished via significantly depressed carotid body chemoreflexes [56]. When inhalant anesthetics are used in animals with respiratory disease (as well as in normal patients), the anesthetist should be ready to assist or control ventilation, since the combination of anesthetic agents used (i.e., opioids along with sedatives and inhalants) is expected to result in significant respiratory depression in almost every anesthetized case.

Anesthetic Management of Specific Disorders

As previously stated, the choice of anesthetic/analgesic agents themselves is likely not as important as specific case management during respiratory disease (i.e., monitoring, ventilatory support, etc.). In normal anesthetized dogs and cats, as well as in patients with concurrent respiratory disease, general guidelines have been created by McDonell and Kerr (2015) when approaching ventilatory support: [9]

1) Endotracheal intubation is suggested for most canine and feline patients.
2) To reduce hypoxemia, enriched inspired oxygen levels of at least 30–35% should be used during general (injectable or inhalant) anesthesia, and in deeply sedated patients.
3) Although hypoxemia is infrequent in normal patients inspiring 100% oxygen, in patients with underlying disease, their status may become life-threatening during recovery when inspired oxygen levels are reduced to approximately 21%.
4) Application of "sighs" or delivery of intermittent large breaths (PIP ~ 20–30 cmH_2O) throughout anesthetic maintenance and into recovery may reduce the chance for continued atelectasis and associated ventilation–perfusion abnormalities.
5) Prolonged recumbency during surgery and large intravenous fluid volumes (i.e., approaching "shock" doses near 60–90 $ml\,kg^{-1}$) should be avoided during anesthesia when possible.

The following serve as examples of commonly occurring respiratory diseases in companion animal practice with some suggested approaches to case management [9]. They are separated into: (i) upper airway disease, (ii) lower airway or parenchymal disease, and (iii) extrapulmonary disease or disorders of the thoracic wall. Diseases may also be classified as obstructive (e.g., asthma, laryngeal paralysis [may also be restrictive], etc.) and restrictive respiratory disease (e.g., pneumonia, obesity, etc.). The main difference is that with obstructive disease, patients have difficultly exhaling a complete breath, whereas with restrictive disease, patients have difficulty in inhaling a complete lung volume. The clinical manifestation of restrictive disease is a decrease in the vital capacity of the lung (Figure 2.2); this contrasts with obstructive disease where inspiratory flow rates and volumes may be normal [1].

Upper Airway Disorders or Dysfunction

Disturbances in the upper airway include, but are not limited to, laryngeal paralysis, brachycephalic airway syndrome, collapsing trachea, intraluminal or extraluminal masses or abscesses, etc. Patients may present for anesthetic procedures unrelated to the airway disturbance or for surgical intervention to correct the primary airway problem. If an airway crisis is reached, patients frequently present anxious, dyspneic, and hypoxemic.

History, Signalment, and Diagnostics

Unless an emergent situation arises, a thorough history and physical exam should be performed, emphasizing respiratory system evaluation. Thoracic radiographs are almost always warranted in these patients to rule out concomitant pulmonary disease. Further diagnostics, including blood work, should be directed toward individual pathologic conditions. Arterial blood gas analysis and pulse oximetry measurements in the conscious patient should be performed as needed. In addition, these patients are more likely to overheat under conditions that would not make a normal dog hyperthermic and body temperature should be initially taken and monitored often during the perianesthetic period.

A thorough history and signalment can be highly suggestive for specific disorders. For example, brachycephalic airway syndrome is usually identified in younger to middle-aged animals and includes abnormalities such as stenotic nares, aberrant nasal conchae, elongated soft palate, everted laryngeal saccules, laryngeal collapse, hypoplastic trachea, and bronchial collapse, all of which may predispose to upper airway obstruction [57]. Brachycephalic dogs are at a higher risk for perianesthetic and postanesthetic complications compared with non-brachycephalic dogs, including aspiration pneumonia and regurgitation, among others [57]. However, corrective upper airway surgery in brachycephalic dogs reduced the odds of postanesthetic complications during subsequent anesthetic events in these same patients [58].

Laryngeal paralysis is recognized mostly in older dogs; however, it can also be found in cats [59]. It can slowly develop until it reaches a stage that causes significant dyspnea, as the larynx is unable to adduct properly to allow sufficient air flow into or out of the trachea (Figure 2.12). A sedated laryngeal exam may also be necessary to rule out laryngeal dysfunction in brachycephalic patients or patients with suspected laryngeal paralysis (see the sections titled "Sedation and Analgesia" and "Anesthetic Induction").

Tracheal collapse usually occurs in middle-aged, small-breed dogs that present with signs ranging from mild airway irritation to severe paradoxical cough and dyspnea [60]. Definitive diagnosis is made through dynamic radiographs, fluoroscopy, or bronchoscopy, and treatment consists of various medical and surgical corrective measures [60]. If the animal's disposition is anxious or easily stressed, and the situation is not emergent, Fear Free techniques, including the use of anti-anxiety drugs, should be used prior to entering the clinic [61]. For example, "Chill" protocols including agents such as gabapentin (10–30 $mg\,kg^{-1}$ PO), trazodone (2–10 $mg\,kg^{-1}$ PO), melatonin (0.5–3 $mg\,kg^{-1}$ PO), acepromazine (0.025–0.05 $mg\,kg^{-1}$ PO), dexmedetomidine solution (20–30 $\mu g\,kg^{-1}$ oromucosal; or Sileo (Zoetis, Kalamazoo, MI) 125 $\mu g\,m^{-2}$ oromucosal), and their combinations can be useful to reduce patient stress; however, debate about whether these drugs cause anxiolysis or simply sedation still exists [62].

Preanesthetic Considerations

Prior to anesthesia, systemic abnormalities should be treated, dehydration corrected, and the patient stabilized if possible. Preoxygenation as described in the preceding text is advised if tolerated by the patient. Food should be withheld as appropriate to reduce chances for aspiration, as this can be a complication associated with upper airway dysfunction (see "Sedation and Analgesia"). An IV catheter should always be placed in these patients as soon as possible either prior to or immediately following sedation.

Sedation and Analgesia

Sedatives should be chosen on an individual patient basis and doses adjusted toward

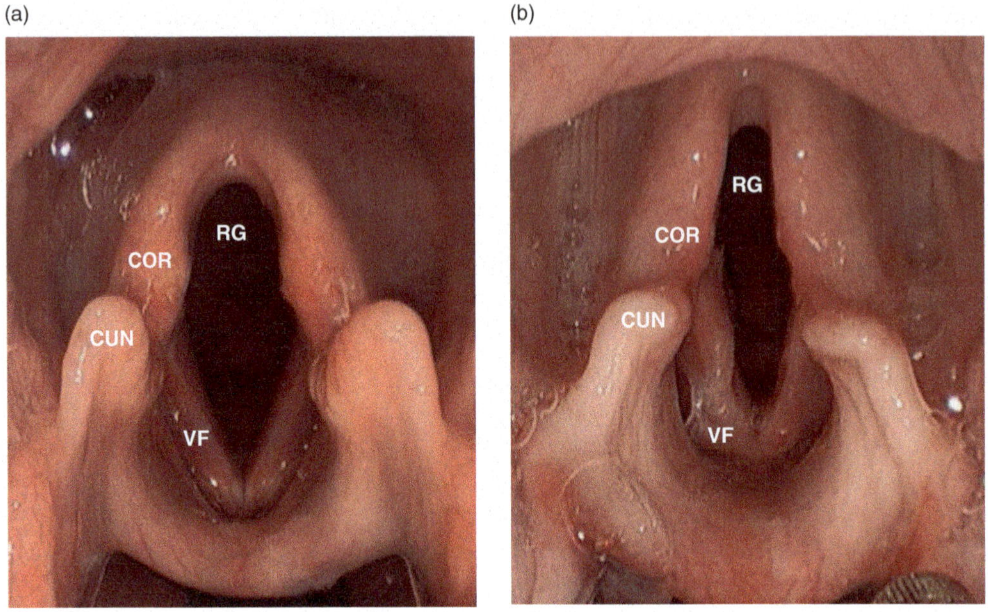

Figure 2.12 Laryngoscopic view of (a) the normal canine larynx and (b) a canine larynx with laryngeal paralysis showing the cuneiform (cun) and corniculate (cor) processes of the arytenoid cartilages. In the normal larynx, the arytenoid cartilages open, allowing sufficient air to move through the rima glottidis (rg) during a respiratory excursion (vf = vocal fold). With laryngeal paralysis, the arytenoid cartilages fail to adduct properly, resulting in a narrowed rima glottidis and increased resistance to breathing. *Source:* Photo courtesy of Dr. Robert Hardie, University of Wisconsin.

individual pathologies. However, sedation with low doses of tranquilizers (i.e., acepromazine 0.01–0.05 mg kg^{-1} IM, IV) or anxiolytics (i.e., dexmedetomidine at 0.001–0.010 mg kg^{-1} IM, IV) and nonstressful handling are important during the preanesthetic period. Although some upper airway disorders (i.e., laryngeal paralysis, tracheal collapse, brachycephalic airway syndrome, etc.) are not believed to be painful conditions in and of themselves, opioid analgesics are frequently administered (i.e., butorphanol at 0.02–0.05 mg kg^{-1} IM, IV; hydromorphone at 0.1–0.2 mg kg^{-1} IM, IV, etc.). If respiratory depression is a concern, and any anticipated pain is considered mild-to-moderate, buprenorphine (0.02–0.05 mg kg^{-1} IV, IM, TM in cats) can also be used. The synergism of sedatives with the opioid often reduces anxiety and stress and improves the animal's comfort and breathing without significant respiratory depression; if inhalant anesthetics are subsequently used, levels may be reduced.

One caveat associated with sedation in patients with upper airway disease is the potential for vomiting and subsequent aspiration. Thus, if possible, antiemetics such as maropitant (1 mg kg^{-1} IV, SC; 2–4 mg kg^{-1} PO) should be administered at least 1–2 h prior to sedation (depending on route) and/or general anesthesia [63]. In addition, mu-opioid agonists and alpha-2-adrenergic receptor agonists should be administered cautiously, especially when used in combination. The IV route should be considered over IM opioid administration, since IV use may somewhat reduce the chances for vomiting [64].

In any case, if the procedure is anticipated to be painful, opioid agonists should not be withheld; however, the analgesic plan should be tailored to the specific case. For example, a multimodal approach including the use of ketamine and nonsteroidal anti-inflammatory drugs (NSAIDs) may be warranted. However, if steroid administration is likely to occur during the procedure to reduce airway inflammation, NSAIDs should be avoided. If appropriate, local anesthetic techniques including nerve blocks, fascial plane blocks, and epidurals should be used if appropriate. Depending on required duration of action, lidocaine, bupivacaine, mepivacaine, or ropivacaine can be chosen. In addition, the intraincisional use of liposomal bupivacaine (Nocita®, Elanco Animal Health, Greenfield, IN) may be an excellent adjunct in the analgesic plan, as analgesia occurs locally with no systemic sedative effects. However, no studies exist concerning the use of liposomal bupivacaine in airway surgeries.

Ventilatory Support

Along with preoxygenation, securing an airway quickly is quite important in these patients. All equipment including orotracheal tubes, laryngoscopes, tics, and cuff inflators should be organized and accessible. Orotracheal intubation is the most common and efficient means to deliver 100% oxygen and inhalants. However, in an emergent situation, supraglottic airway devices (v-gel®, Jorgensen Laboratories, Loveland, CO) may be used in cats (and rabbits) (Figure 2.13).

An important factor associated with respiratory fatigue is airway resistance. Resistance to laminar flow is governed by the Hagen–Poiseuille law, and is estimated by:

$$\text{Resistance} = \left(8 \times \text{viscosity} \times \text{tube length}\right) / \text{radius}^4 \quad (2.3)$$

Based on this formula, resistance is directly proportional to the airway or tube length, an important factor when choosing anesthetic tubes. But, more importantly, the diameter (or radius) also significantly influences resistance, such that if diameter increases by 50%, resistance decreases 16-fold. Thus, if the upper airway is obstructed/narrowed with disease or dysfunction, or if a small orotracheal tube is used, airway resistance may become excessive, and ventilatory support may be required throughout the procedure to avoid respiratory fatigue; when choosing an orotracheal tube, the largest, yet safest tube possible should be used to minimize airway resistance.

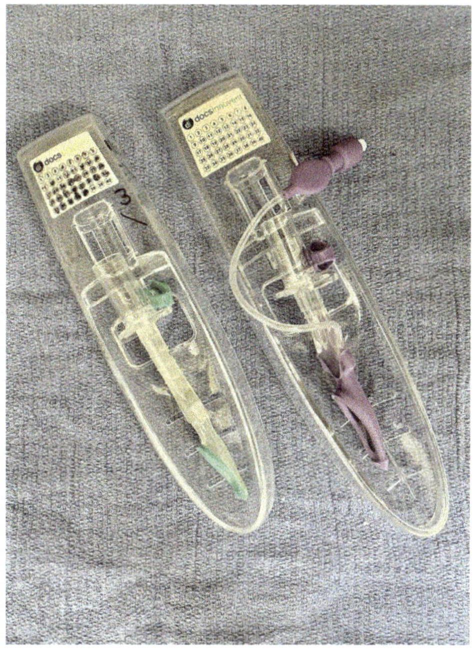

Figure 2.13 Example of a supraglottic airway device for use in cats (purple, right) and rabbits (green, left) (v-gel®, Jorgensen Laboratories, Loveland, CO). The device sits securely in the pharynx, producing a seal over the tracheal entrance.

Anesthetic Induction

Induction is frequently performed with short-acting intravenous anesthetics such as propofol (1–6 $mg\,kg^{-1}$ IV), alfaxalone (0.5–2 $mg\,kg^{-1}$ IV), or a dissociative/benzodiazepine combination (ketamine 2–4 $mg\,kg^{-1}$ with midazolam/diazepam 0.1–0.2 $mg\,kg^{-1}$ IV) to effect, avoiding apnea. Inhalant inductions are not recommended due to the inability to gain airway access quickly, chance for aspiration, and exposure to personnel. In the specific example of laryngeal paralysis, a laryngeal exam may require small doses of induction agent to allow for sufficient relaxation and to facilitate laryngeal examination at the lightest anesthetic plane possible. Since all induction inhalants may affect laryngeal motion to at least some degree, and premedications may affect the exam, there does not appear to be a clear choice for dogs and cats undergoing diagnostic airway exams [65–69]. In many patients, acepromazine (0.03 mg kg^{-1} IV) and butorphanol (0.2 mg kg^{-1} IV), followed by approximately 1–2 mg kg^{-1} IV of propofol, will be sufficient for effective examination of laryngeal movement [69]. In addition, administration of doxapram (1.1 mg kg^{-1} IV) may be useful for differentiating normal dogs from dogs with laryngeal paralysis in some situations [69, 70]. Once diagnosis of laryngeal paralysis is confirmed, the dog can be intubated and maintained on inhalant anesthetics for the surgical procedure.

Anesthetic Maintenance and Monitoring

Anesthetic maintenance is usually accomplished with inhalant agents in 100% oxygen such as isoflurane or sevoflurane. However, in special circumstances such as bronchoscopy, or intratracheal or laryngeal surgery where tracheal intubation is not possible, injectable agents may be advisable. Most commonly, propofol, delivered as a constant rate infusion, is used (0.1–0.6 mg kg^{-1} min^{-1} IV); however, alfaxalone can also be used as a constant rate infusion (4–9 mg kg^{-1} h^{-1}); exact doses depend on premedications chosen. Anesthetic monitoring should be accomplished as with any anesthetized patient, albeit focusing on the airway system. Capnometry and pulse oximetry are essential and blood gas analysis is recommended. Electrocardiography, blood pressure, and body temperatures should also be monitored.

Anesthetic Recovery

Patients should be monitored well into the recovery period, as airway obstruction, hypoxemia, and hypercapnia can still be significant issues during this period. The patient should be kept quiet and comfortable and should remain in sternal recumbency if possible. The goal is to have the patient regain full consciousness without pain or distress, so they can more readily protect their airway and ventilate adequately. Continuing pain management into the recovery period is important. However, administration of high-dose sedatives or pure mu-opioid agonists may result in overly sedate postanesthetic patients, which can further contribute to aspiration pneumonia, particularly associated with the "tie-back" surgery for laryngeal paralysis [71, 72]. Thus, buprenorphine administration or butorphanol constant rate infusions are commonly performed in the postoperative period (0.2–0.4 mg kg^{-1} h^{-1} IV) to provide mild analgesia with minimal sedation. If moderate or profound analgesia is required, patients should be monitored for excessive sedation and the analgesic plan altered accordingly. The anesthetist should stay with the animal until it is fully conscious and can maintain ventilation without assistance. The endotracheal tube should be left in place until they are able to swallow and any blood or mucous should be cleared from the upper airways before extubation. Oxygen should be supplemented as needed and equipment/drugs required to reintubate the animal should be kept nearby.

Lower Airway and Parenchymal Diseases

Patients with lower airway or pulmonary parenchymal disorders commonly present for anesthetic procedures required for concurrent problems unrelated to the respiratory disturbance, although some require anesthesia to correct the primary lung problem. Examples of lower respiratory disease include feline asthma, pneumonia, pulmonary neoplasia, pulmonary edema, etc. Anesthetic management of these patients is similar to those with upper airway disorders with some adjustments [9].

History, Signalment, Diagnostics, and Preanesthetic Considerations

A thorough history and signalment should be completed in these patients because clinical signs may again lead to a diagnosis. For example, an animal with fever, cough, and history of regurgitation may suggest pneumonia. More specifically, aspiration pneumonia is a common example of a restrictive, parenchymal lung disease. Aspiration pneumonia occurs when material enters the lung through the larynx resulting in an inflammatory airway reaction, which is frequently diagnosed with history and radiographs. Although mild aspiration usually results in minor gas exchange problems, deposition of caustic or severely damaging material into the lung can cause severe tissue destruction. Vomiting, regurgitation, and aspiration of intestinal contents can occur during sedation and anesthesia of any patient [73–77]. Thus, patient monitoring for signs of fluid and/or intestinal contents in the mouth or airway is critical. If signs of regurgitation or vomiting are observed, the opening of the oral cavity should be lowered to facilitate gravitational drainage and cleaning should be immediately performed. A stomach tube can then be passed to facilitate removal of additional gastric material. Lavage with clean water and instillation of bicarbonate to increase esophageal pH have been recommended [77]. Antibiotics are also recommended to decrease the likelihood of pneumonia.

In addition, feline bronchial asthma is one of the most diagnosed respiratory conditions of young to middle-aged cats and patients present with increased efforts to move air into (and especially out of) the lungs; coughing and open mouth breathing are commonly observed in severe cases [78].

Despite the disease process, radiographic evaluation of the lungs is essential and disease stabilization prior to anesthesia is recommended. Further, preoxygenation will aid in reducing hypoxemia associated with the disease itself in patients that will tolerate it. Fear Free techniques [61] and "Chill" protocols [62] should be used when necessary to reduce the chances of disease exacerbation as patients enter the clinic.

Anesthetic and Postanesthetic Management and Monitoring

Sedation, analgesic, and anesthetic management in these patients will be similar to those with upper airway disease. Patients will benefit from being kept calm and quiet if possible. Use of analgesics and sedatives is recommended to limit excitement during handling and IV catheterization if needed. If significant respiratory compromise is present, midazolam or diazepam ($0.1–0.2\,mg\,kg^{-1}$ IV) with or without an opioid as described in the preceding text may help reduce anxiety in these patients; however, patient excitement may also be associated with these drugs. Analgesia should always be provided using a multimodal approach with systemic and local techniques. Rapid induction techniques and airway intubation allow for delivery of light levels of isoflurane or sevoflurane which may cause bronchodilation [79]. In addition, ketamine premedication or induction (approximately $5–7\,mg\,kg^{-1}$ IM, SC, and $1–2\,mg\,kg^{-1}$ to effect IV, respectively) is often recommended, since it is associated with bronchodilation via central release of catecholamines, stimulating beta-2-adrenergic receptors, and inhibits vagal pathways resulting in an anticholinergic effect on airway smooth muscle [80, 81]. These drugs increase lower airway size and decrease the resistance to inflation of the alveoli.

Monitoring should be as with any patient and should always include capnometry, pulse oximetry, and blood gas analysis if possible (along with electrocardiography and blood pressure and temperature monitoring). Hypoventilation and hypoxemia associated with ventilation–perfusion abnormalities are common in these patients and should be treated with appropriate ventilation strategies while minimizing further disease progression. Low tidal volumes and positive end-expiratory pressures (PEEPs) to keep alveoli open may be warranted. Oxygen should be supplemented well into recovery, as hypoxemia is common when patients are returned to room air (approximately 21% O_2).

Extrapulmonary or Thoracic Wall Disease

These categories of respiratory dysfunction include diseases of the pleural space (i.e., pleural effusion, pneumothorax, hemothorax, pyothorax) (Figure 2.14), obesity, diaphragmatic hernia, penetrating chest wounds, large intraabdominal masses, and diseases associated with respiratory muscle weakness or rigidity (i.e., neuromuscular disorders, spinal cord injury, etc.). In all cases, one should be prepared to support ventilation during sedation and/or anesthesia, as the patients have increased work of breathing and respiratory muscle fatigue may ensue if not already present.

History, Signalment, Diagnostics, and Preanesthetic Considerations [9]

Diagnostic procedures vary with history and signalment, but thoracic and abdominal radiography is almost always indicated. In pleural space disease, extrapulmonary, yet intrathoracic fluid or air should be removed prior to anesthesia if possible; this may require sedation. Because these diseases may be acutely life-threatening, all supplies necessary for tracheal intubation and ventilatory support should be readily available.

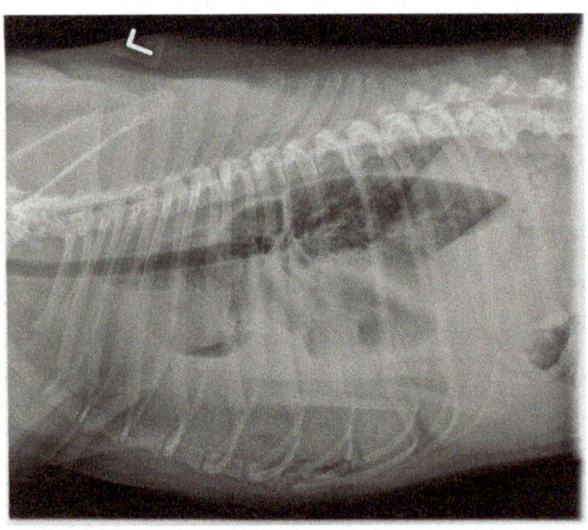

Figure 2.14 Thoracic radiograph depicting pulmonary effusion in a cat. The radiolucent lungs do not extend throughout the thorax, and fissure lines can be seen between lobes due to restriction by intrathoracic fluid. Prior to anesthesia, the fluid should be evacuated if possible, to reduce chances for hypoxemia. If chronic, the lungs should not be reexpanded quickly with positive pressure as reexpansion pulmonary edema may develop.

Anesthetic and Postanesthetic Management and Monitoring

Sedation, analgesic, and anesthetic management in these patients will be similar to that for patients with upper airway, lower airway, or pulmonary parenchymal disease. Sedatives should be used to reduce stress and facilitate fluid removal if necessary and multimodal analgesic techniques used as appropriate. Many of these patients have significant cardiovascular or respiratory compromise; use of a benzodiazepine ($0.1–0.2\,mg\,kg^{-1}$ IV) with or without an opioid may be recommended. Anesthetic induction should be quick and ventilatory support initiated as soon as possible. Since concurrent pulmonary parenchymal pathology is usually present in these patients as well, low tidal volume/airway pressure techniques should be used if possible.

Anesthetic monitoring should include electrocardiography, blood pressure, body temperature, capnometry, pulse oximetry, and blood gas analysis if possible. Because lungs cannot expand properly, hypoventilation and hypoxemia are common. In cases where the lungs have been chronically atelectatic, slow alveolar reexpansion is recommended to reduce development of pulmonary edema from changes in vascular permeability, abnormal shear forces, free-radical release, and cellular infiltration [82]. However, when reexpansion pulmonary edema does result, it is usually, but not always, self-limiting and treatment is supportive [82]. Thus, oxygen should be supplemented well into recovery, as hypoxemia is common when patients are returned to room air (approximately 21% O_2).

Summary

Anesthetic management of dogs and cats with respiratory diseases can usually be performed if care is provided to ensure adequate oxygenation and CO_2 elimination. Clinicians should review and be familiar with the normal function of the respiratory system and ensure that the patient is stabilized prior to anesthesia. A critical consideration is to minimize patient stress and anxiety during handling and induction; proper premedication with analgesics and sedatives including "Chill" protocols should be standard for dogs or cats with respiratory disease. Rapid airway control with a properly placed endotracheal tube and ventilatory support is essential for the anesthetic care of animal with respiratory disease. Capnometry, pulse oximetry, and potentially blood gas analysis should be routine monitoring methods for all animals during anesthesia and are especially essential for all animals with respiratory disease.

References

1 Hines, R.L. and Marschall, K.E. (2018). *Stoelting's Anesthesia and Co-Existing Disease*, 7e. Philadelphia: Elsevier Saunders.

2 West, J.B. and Luks, A.M. (2021). *West's Respiratory Physiology: The Essentials*, 11e. Philadelphia: Wolters Kluwer.

3 West, J.B. (2013). *West's Pulmonary Pathophysiology: The Essentials*, 8e. Philadelphia: Lippincott Williams & Wilkins.

4 Johnson, R.A. and deMorais, H.A. (2012). Respiratory acid-base disorders. In: *Fluid, Electrolyte, and Acid-Base Disorders*, 4e (ed. S.P. DiBartola), 287–301. St. Louis: Elsevier Saunders.

5 Funk, G.D. and Greer, J.J. (2013). The rhythmic, transverse medullary slice preparation in respiratory neurobiology: contributions and caveats. *Respir. Physiol. Neurobiol.* 186: 236–253.

6 Johnson, R.A. and Mitchell, G.S. (2013). Common mechanisms of compensatory respiratory plasticity in spinal neurological disorders. *Respir. Physiol. Neurobiol.* 189: 419–428.

7 Mitchell, G.S., Baker-Herman, T.L., McCrimmon, D.R. et al. (2009). Respiration. In: *Encyclopedia of Neuroscience* (ed. L.R. Squire), 121–130. Oxford: Academic Press.

8 McDonell, W.N. and Hall, L.W. (1974). Functional residual capacity in conscious and anaesthetized horses. *Br. J. Anaesth.* 46: 802–803.

9 McDonell, W.N. and Kerr, C.L. (2015). Physiology, pathophysiology, and anesthetic management of patients with respiratory disease. In: *Veterinary Anesthesia and Analgesia. The Fifth Edition of Lumb and Jones* (eds. K.A. Grimm, L.A. Lamont, W.J. Tranquilli, et al.), 513–555. Ames: Wiley.

10 McLelland, J. (1989). Larynx and trachea. In: *Form and Function in Birds*, vol. 4 (eds. A.S. King and J. McLelland), 69–103. London: Academic.

11 Robertson, S.A. (2002). Oxygenation and ventilation. In: *Veterinary Anesthesia and Pain Management Secrets*, 1e (ed. S.A. Greene), 15–20. Philadelphia: Hanley & Belfus.

12 Bohr, C. (1887). *Uber die Lungenathmung. Centralblatt fur Physiologie* 1: 236–268.

13 Enghoff, H. (1938). Volumen inefficax. Bemerkungen zur Frage des schadlichen Raumes. *Uppsala Lakareforen Forhandl* 44: 191–218.

14 McDonell WN. 1969. Ventilation and acid-base equilibrium with methoxyflurane anesthesia in dogs. MSc thesis. Guelph, Canada: University of Guelph.

15 Haskins, S.C. (1983). Blood gases and acid-base balance: clinical interpretation and therapeutic implications. In: *Current Veterinary Therapy VIII* (ed. R.W. Kirk), 201. Philadelphia: Saunders.

16 Murray, J.F. (1986). Gas exchange and oxygen transport. In: *The Normal Lung* (ed. J.F. Murray), 194. Philadelphia: WB Saunders.

17 Ilkiw, J.E., Rose, R.J., and Martin, I.C.A. (1991). A comparison of simultaneously collected arterial, mixed venous, jugular venous and cephalic venous blood samples in the assessment of blood gas and acid base status in dogs. *J. Vet. Intern. Med.* 5: 294–298.

18 O'Dwyer, L. (2018). Gas monitoring. In: *Veterinary Anesthetic and Monitoring Equipment* (eds. K.G. Cooley and R.A. Johnson), 199–211. Hoboken: Wiley.

19 Robinson, N.E. (2009). The respiratory system. In: *Equine Anesthesia*, 2e (eds. W.W. Muir and H. JAE), 11–36. Saunders St. Louis: Elsevier.

20 West, J.B. and Luks, A.M. (2021). Gas transport by the blood. How gases are moved to and from the peripheral tissues. In: *Respiratory Physiology: The Essentials*, 11e (eds. J.B. West and L. uks AM), 94–115. Philadelphia: Wolters Kluwer.

21 O O. (2018). Pulse oximetry. In: *Veterinary Anesthetic and Monitoring Equipment* (eds. K.G. Cooley and R.A. Johnson), 223–232. Hoboken: Wiley.

22 Koterba, A.M. (1988). Breathing strategy of the adult horse (*Equus caballus*) at rest. *J. Appl. Physiol.* 64: 337–346.

23 West, J.B. and Luks, A.M. (2021). Mechanics of breathing. How the lung is supported and moved. In: *Respiratory Physiology: The Essentials*, 11e (eds. J.B. West and A.M. Luks), 116–150. Philadelphia: Wolters Kluwer.

24 Kerr, C.L. and McDonell, W.N. (2009). Oxygen supplementation and ventilator support. In: *Equine Anesthesia*, 2e (eds. W.W. Muir and H. JAE), 332–352. Saunders St. Louis: Elsevier.

25 Hawkins, M.G., Zehnder, A.M., and Pascoe, P.J. (2014). Cagebirds. In: *Zoo Animal and Wildlife Immobilization and Anesthesia*, 2e (eds. G. West, D. Heard and N. Caulkett), 399–434. Ames: Wiley.

26 Zimmerman, M.E., Hodgson, D.S., and Bello, N.M. (2013). Effects of oxygen insufflation rate, respiratory rate, and tidal volume on fraction of inspired oxygen in cadaveric canine heads attached to a lung model. *Am. J. Vet. Res.* 74: 1247–1251.

27 Jagodich, T.A., Bersenas, A.M.E., Bateman, S.W. et al. (2020). High-flow nasal cannula oxygen therapy in acute hypoxemic respiratory failure in 22 dogs requiring oxygen support escalation. *J. Vet. Emerg. Crit. Care* 30: 364–375.

28 McNally, E.M., Robertson, S.A., and Pablo, L.S. (2009). Comparison of time to desaturation between preoxygenated and nonpreoxygenated dogs following sedation with acepromazine maleate and morphine and induction of anesthesia with propofol. *Am. J. Vet. Res.* 70: 1333–1338.

29 Sirian, R. and Wills, J. (2009). Physiology of apnoea and the benefits of preoxygenation. *Contin. Edu. Anaesth. Crit. Care Pain* 9: 105–108.

30 Steffey, E.P. and Howland, D. Jr. (1977). Isoflurane potency in the dog and cat. *Am. J. Vet. Res.* 38: 1833–1836.

31 Stuth, E.A., Tonkovic-Capin, M., Kampine, J.P. et al. (1992). Dose-dependent effects of isoflurane on the CO_2 responses of expiratory medullary neurons and the phrenic nerve activities in dogs. *Anesthesiology* 76: 763–774.

32 Ramirez, J.-M., Burgraff, N.J., Wei, A.D. et al. (2021). Neuronal mechanisms underlying opioid-induced respiratory depression: our current understanding. *J. Neurophysiol.* 125: 1899–1919.

33 Ko, J.C., Bailey, J.E., Pablo, L.S. et al. (1996). Comparison of sedative and cardiorespiratory effects of medetomidine and medetomidine-butorphanol combination in dogs. *Am. J. Vet. Res.* 57: 535–540.

34 Talavera, J., Kirschvink, N., Schuller, S. et al. (2006). Evaluation of respiratory function by barometric whole-body plethysmography in healthy dogs. *Vet. J.* 172: 67–77.

35 McCrackin, M.A., Harvey, R.C., Sackman, J.E. et al. (1994). Butorphanol tartrate for partial reversal of oxymorphone-induced postoperative respiratory depression in the dog. *Vet. Surg.* 23: 67–74.

36 Bragg, P., Zwass, M.S., Lau, M. et al. (1995). Opioid pharmacodynamics in neonatal dogs:

differences between morphine and fentanyl. *J. Appl. Physiol.* 79: 1519–1524.

37 Farver, T.B., Haskins, S.C., and Patz, J.D. (1986). Cardiopulmonary effects of acepromazine and of the subsequent administration of ketamine in the dog. *Am. J. Vet. Res.* 47: 631–635.

38 Sabbe, M.B., Penning, J.P., Ozaki, G.T. et al. (1994). Spinal and systemic action of the alpha 2 receptor agonist dexmedetomidine in dogs. Antinociception and carbon dioxide response. *Anesthesiology* 80: 1057–1072.

39 Vainio, O. and Palmu, L. (1989). Cardiovascular and respiratory effects of medetomidine in dogs and influence of anticholinergics. *Acta Vet. Scand.* 30: 401–408.

40 Pettifer, G.R. and Dyson, D.H. (1993). Comparison of medetomidine and fentanyl-droperidol in dogs: sedation, analgesia, arterial blood gases and lactate levels. *Can. J. Vet. Res.* 57: 99–105.

41 Pypendop, B. and Verstegen, J. (1999). Cardiorespiratory effects of a combination of medetomidine, midazolam, and butorphanol in dogs. *Am. J. Vet. Res.* 60: 1148–1154.

42 Sinclair, M.D. (2003). A review of the physiological effects of α2-agonists related to the clinical use of medetomidine in small animal practice. *Can. Vet. J.* 44: 885–897.

43 Lamont, L.A., Bulmer, B.J., Grimm, K.A. et al. (2001). Cardiopulmonary evaluation of the use of medetomidine hydrochloride in cats. *Am. J. Vet. Res.* 62: 1745–1749.

44 Selmi, A.L., Mendes, G.M., Lins, B.T. et al. (2003). Evaluation of the sedative and cardiorespiratory effects of dexmedetomidine, dexmedetomidine-butorphanol, and dexmedetomidine-ketamine in cats. *J. Am. Vet. Med. Assoc.* 222: 37–41.

45 Popovic, N.A., Mullane, J.F., and Yhap, E.O. (1972). Effects of acetylpromazine maleate on certain cardiorespiratory responses in dogs. *Am. J. Vet. Res.* 33: 1819–1824.

46 Colby, E.D. and Sanford, B.S. (1981). Blood pressure and heart and respiratory rates of cats under ketamine/xylazine, ketamine/acepromazine anesthesia. *Feline Pract.* 11: 19–24.

47 Haskins, S.C., Farver, T.B., and Patz, J.D. (1986). Cardiovascular changes in dogs given diazepam and diazepam-ketamine. *Am. J. Vet. Res.* 47: 795–798.

48 Pavlidou, K., Savvas, I., Moens, Y.P.S. et al. (2013). The effect of four anaesthetic protocols for maintenance of anaesthesia on trans-diaphragmatic pressure in dogs. *PLoS One* 8: e75341.

49 Maney, J.K., Shepard, M.K., Braun, C. et al. (2013). A comparison of cardiopulmonary and anesthetic effects of an induction dose of alfaxalone or propofol in dogs. *Vet. Anaesth. Anal.* 40: 237–244.

50 Ponte, J. and Sadler, C.L. (1989). Effect of thiopentone, etomidate and propofol on carotid body chemoreceptor activity in the rabbit and the cat. *Br. J. Anaesth.* 62: 41–45.

51 Taboada, F.M. and Murison, P.J. (2010). Induction of anaesthesia with alfaxalone or propofol before isoflurane maintenance in cats. *Vet. Record* 167: 85–89.

52 Muir, W., Lerche, P., Wiese, A. et al. (2008). Cardiorespiratory and anesthetic effects of clinical and supraclinical doses of alfaxalone in dogs. *Vet. Anesth. Anal.* 35: 451–462.

53 Boscan, P., Pypendop, B.H., Solano, A.M. et al. (2005). Cardiovascular and respiratory effects of ketamine infusions in isoflurane-anesthetized dogs before and during noxious stimulation. *Am. J. Vet. Res.* 12: 2122–2129.

54 Munson, E.S., Larson, C.P. Jr., Babad, A.A. et al. (1966). The effects of halothane, fluorxene, and cyclopropane on ventilation: a comparative study in man. *Anesthesiology* 27: 716–728.

55 Mutoh, T., Nishimura, R., Kim, H.Y. et al. (1997). Cardiopulmonary effects of sevoflurane, compared with halothane, enflurane, and isoflurane, in dogs. *Am. J. Vet. Res.* 58: 885–890.

56 Pandit, J.J., Winter, V., Bayliss, R. et al. (2010). Differential effects of halothane and isoflurane on carotid body glomus cell intracellular Ca^{2+} and background K^+ channel responses to hypoxia. *Adv. Exp. Med. Biol.* 669: 205–208.

57 Gruenheid, M., Aarnes, T.K., McLoughlin, M.A. et al. (2018). Risk of anesthesia-related complications in brachycephalic dogs. *J. Am. Vet. Med. Assoc.* 253: 301–306.

58 Doyle, C.R., Aarnes, T.K., Ballash, G.A. et al. (2020). Anesthetic risk during subsequent anesthetic events in brachycephalic dogs that have undergone corrective airway surgery: 45 cases (2007–2019). *J. Am. Vet. Med. Assoc.* 257: 744–749.

59 Hardie, R.J., Gunby, J., and Bjorling, D.E. (2009). Arytenoid lateralization for treatment of laryngeal paralysis in 10 cats. *Vet. Surg.* 38 (4): 445–451.

60 Tappin, S.W. (2016). Canine tracheal collapse. *J. Small Anim. Pract.* 57: 9–17.

61 Fear Free, LLC. Available at: www.fearfreepets.com (accessed February 26, 2021).

62 Love, L. (2019). Oral sedatives and anxiolytics for veterinary visits. Available at: http://www.mynavas.org/post/oral-sedatives-and-anxiolytics-for-veterinary-visits (accessed 26 February 2021).

63 Krause, B.L.H. (2013). Efficacy of maropitant in preventing vomiting in dogs premedicated with hydromorphone. *Vet. Anaesth. Anal.* 40: 28–34.

64 KuKanich, B., Hogan, B.K., Krugner-Higby, L.A. et al. (2008). Pharmacokinetics of hydromorphone in healthy dogs. *Vet. Anaesth. Anal.* 35: 256–264.

65 Muir, W.W. and Gadawski, L.E. (1998). Respiratory depression and apnea induced by propofol in dogs. *Am. J. Vet. Res.* 59: 157–161.

66 Gross, M.E., Dodam, J.R., Pope, E.R. et al. (2002). A comparison of thiopental, propofol, and diazepam-ketamine anesthesia for evaluation of laryngeal function in dogs premedicated with butorphanol-glycopyrrolate. *J. Am. Anim. Hosp. Assoc.* 38: 503–506.

67 Jackson, A.M., Tobias, K., Long, C. et al. (2004). Effects of various anesthetic agents on laryngeal motion during laryngoscopy in normal dogs. *Vet. Surg.* 33: 102–106.

68 Nelissen, P., Corletto, F., Aprea, F. et al. (2012). Effect of three anesthetic induction protocols on laryngeal motion during laryngoscopy in normal cats. *Vet. Surg.* 41: 876–883.

69 Radkey, D.I., Hardie, R.J., and Smith, L.J. (2018). Comparison of the effects of alfaxalone and propofol with acepromazine, butorphanol and/or doxapram on laryngeal motion and quality of examination in dogs. *Vet. Anaesth. Anal.* 45: 241–249.

70 Tobias, K.M., Jackson, A.M., and Harvey, R.C. (2004). Effects of doxapram HCl on laryngeal function of normal dogs and dogs with naturally occurring laryngeal paralysis. *Vet. Anaesth. Anal.* 31: 258–263.

71 Mercurio, A. (2011). Complications of upper airway surgery in companion animals. *Vet. Clin. North Am. Small Anim. Pract.* 41: 969–980.

72 Wilson, D. and Monnet, E. (2016). Risk factors for the development of aspiration pneumonia after unilateral arytenoid lateralization in dogs with laryngeal paralysis: 232 cases (1987–2012). *J. Am. Vet. Med. Assoc.* 248: 188–194.

73 Kraus, B.L.H. (2012). Efficacy of maropitant in preventing vomiting in dogs premedicated with hydromorphone. *Vet. Anaesth. Anal.* 40: 28–34.

74 Wilson, D.V., Evans, A.T., and Miller, R. (2005). Effects of preanesthetic administration of morphine on gastroesophageal reflux and regurgitation during anesthesia in dogs. *Am. J. Vet. Res.* 66: 386–390.

75 Wilson, D.V., Boruta, D.T., and Evans, A.T. (2006). Influence of halothane, isoflurane, and sevoflurane on gastroesophageal reflux during anesthesia in dogs. *Am. J. Vet. Res.* 67: 1821–1825.

76 Wilson, D.V., Evans, A.T., and Mauer, W.A. (2007). Pre-anesthetic meperidine: associated vomiting and gastroesophageal

reflux during the subsequent anesthetic in dogs. *Vet. Anaesth. Anal.* 34: 15–22.

77 Wilson, D.V. and Evans, A.T. (2007). The effect of topical treatment on esophageal pH during acid reflux in dogs. *Vet. Anaesth. Anal.* 34 (5): 339–343.

78 Venema, C.M. and Patterson, C.C. (2010). Feline asthma: what's new and where might clinical practice be heading? *J. Feline Med. Surg.* 12 (9): 681–692.

79 Rooke, G., Choi, J.-H., and Bishop, M.J. (1997). The effect of isoflurane, halothane, sevoflurane, and thiopental/nitrous oxide on respiratory system resistance after tracheal intubation. *Anesthesiology* 86: 1294–1299.

80 Lau, T.T. and Zed, P.J. (2001). Does ketamine have a role in managing severe exacerbation of asthma in adults? *Pharmacotherapy* 21: 110–116.

81 Craven, R. (2007). Ketamine. *Anesthesiology* 62 (Suppl 1): 48–53.

82 Verhagen, M., van Buijtenen, J.M., and Geeraedts, L.M.G. Jr. (2015). Reexpansion pulmonary edema after chest drainage for pneumothorax: a case report and literature overview. *Respir. Med. Case Rep.* 14: 10–12.

3

Neurologic Disease

Erin Wendt-Hornickle and Daniel Almeida

Veterinary Clinical Sciences Department, College of Veterinary Medicine, University of Minnesota, St. Paul, MN, 55108, USA

Introduction

Patients with diseases involving the nervous system often require anesthesia for diagnostic imaging, sample collection, or treatment of the disease pathology. Others will require anesthesia for procedures unrelated to the disease of the nervous system. Understanding the physiology and pathology of the nervous system is important when considering an anesthetic plan during which the goal should be optimization of cerebral blood flow (CBF) and perfusion and prevention of increases in intracranial pressure (ICP). Anesthesia of patients with some neurologic conditions may be technically challenging and clinically complex. The requirement of advanced knowledge and specialized equipment may make some of these cases better suited for a clinical setting with an anesthesiologist.

Nervous System Physiology

Cerebral Blood Flow

Cerebral blood flow is regulated by several factors, including the cerebral metabolic rate of oxygen ($CMRO_2$), arterial partial pressure of carbon dioxide ($PaCO_2$), and arterial partial pressure of oxygen (PaO_2). The $CMRO_2$ is proportional to cerebral (neuronal) activity; CBF needs to match metabolic requirements and it does so by the mechanism of flow–metabolism coupling. Acutely, $PaCO_2$ exerts a significant influence on CBF, where flow varies directly with $PaCO_2$ (each 1 mmHg change in $PaCO_2$ causes CBF to change 1–2 ml $100\,g^{-1}\,min^{-1}$). Those changes are due to rapid diffusion of CO_2 across the cerebrovascular endothelium and consequent pH changes in the extracellular fluid of the brain. Although PaO_2 exerts an influence in CBF, it is minimal until the PaO_2 falls below 50 mmHg at which point CBF increases [1]. Hemodynamically, it is also helpful to understand CBF in light of Ohm's law, where blood flow to the brain is a dependent variable and cerebral perfusion pressure (CPP) and cerebral vascular resistance (CVR) are the independent variables that control flow [2]. The brain receives a significant share of cardiac output considering the total tissue volume; in humans, the brain accounts for 2% of total body weight and receives 12–15% of total cardiac output [3]. In clinically normal canines, the CBF is approximately 67–90 ml min^{-1} $100\,g^{-1}$ tissue [4–6]. In clinically normal felines, the CBF is approximately 40 ml min^{-1} $100\,g^{-1}$ tissue [4, 5, 7].

Canine and Feline Anesthesia and Co-Existing Disease, Second Edition. Edited by Rebecca A. Johnson, Lindsey B. C. Snyder and Carrie A. Schroeder.

Companion website: www.wiley.com/go/johnson/canine

The brain is unique in that an intact, bony, noncompliant skull encases the intracranial structures. All intracranial structures (tissue, cerebrospinal fluid [CSF], and blood) must have a fixed volume to maintain normal intracranial volume. Any increases in the volume of tissue, CSF, or blood without a concomitant decrease in the volume of another constituent will lead to an increase in intracranial volume and therefore an increase in ICP. This is illustrated by the Monro–Kellie doctrine (Eq. (3.1)) [8, 9]. The total volume (*V*) of intracranial constituents is equal to brain volume, CSF volume, and blood volume combined:

$$V_{\text{intracranial}} = V_{\text{brain}} + V_{\text{CSF}} + V_{\text{blood}} \tag{3.1}$$

If ICP continues to increase, herniation of brain tissue from its normal position within the skull may occur. Signs of brain herniation may include increasing systolic and pulse pressures, bradycardia, and irregular breathing, collectively known as the Cushing reflex [6, 9]. Efforts at preventing and treating increased ICP should be aimed at decreasing the volume of the intracranial constituents. This can be achieved with therapeutic interventions such as hyperventilation, hyperosmotic therapy, or diuretics.

Though measurement of CBF is not commonly employed in veterinary medicine, there are both noninvasive and invasive methods described in human patients. Noninvasive techniques include ultrasonography of optic nerve sheath diameter, transcranial Doppler (TCD) ultrasonography, and near-infrared spectroscopy (NIRS). TCD ultrasonography measures linear CBF velocity and pulsatility index within the intracranial arteries. NIRS is based on the differences in absorption of near-infrared light by oxyhemoglobin and deoxyhemoglobin in cerebral tissue, reflecting the mixed venous–capillary–arterial oxygenation state of the brain tissue in the location of interest. Invasive methods of CBF include jugular venous oximetry, brain tissue oxygen monitoring, cerebral microdialysis, external ventricular drain, intracranial ventricular pressure measurement, and laser Doppler or diffusion flowmetry. A full review of CBF measurement modalities is beyond the scope of this chapter; however, there are many available resources reviewing the mechanisms of these measurement tools [10–12].

Autoregulation

Autoregulatory mechanisms are those that help maintain the internal environment of the central nervous system (CNS), which can include hemodynamic responses and flow–metabolism coupling. The mechanism described here is the hemodynamic response which helps maintain adequate CBF over a range of perfusion pressures.

It was long believed that under normal conditions CBF was strictly autoregulated, keeping it constant over a wide range of CPPs and mean arterial pressures (MAPs) between 60 and 140 mmHg (Figure 3.1). It is possible, however, that the lower limit of CBF autoregulation may vary between individual patients. Data in humans point to a higher limit for autoregulation, suggesting an MAP range of 70–150 mmHg; in patients undergoing cardiopulmonary bypass, the lower MAP limit of CBF autoregulation ranged from 40 to 90 mmHg [14].

Typically, during autoregulation when systemic pressure increases, cerebral capillary, arteriolar, and arterial constriction occurs, and when systemic pressure decreases, cerebral capillary, arteriolar, and arterial vasodilation occurs [4]. Once the ability to mount appropriate vasoactive responses is exhausted, CBF becomes completely dependent on changes in CPP [2].

Vascular responses are mediated by several cellular mechanisms, including nitric oxide, vasoactive peptides, potassium channels, and prostaglandins, as well as by markers of metabolic demands of neurovascular units (i.e., glutamate, adenosine, vasoactive intestinal peptide, and hydrogen and potassium ions). Several disease processes, including hypertension, intracranial space-occupying lesions, traumatic brain injury (TBI), and the dose-dependent

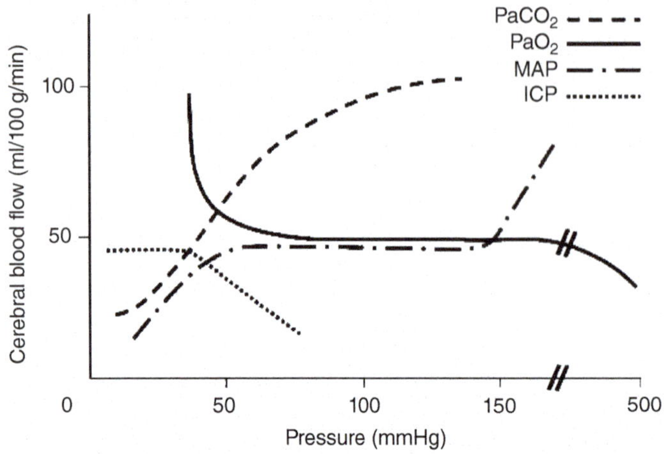

Figure 3.1 Impact of intracranial pressure (ICP), partial pressure of oxygen (PaO_2), partial pressure of carbon dioxide ($PaCO_2$), and mean arterial pressure (MAP) on cerebral blood flow in milliliters per 100 g of brain tissue per minute [4, 13]. *Source:* Canine and Feline Anesthesia and Co-Existing Disease, 2015, with permission.

presence of volatile anesthetics, affect autoregulation. Thus, blood flow patterns may be altered by the disease process itself in addition to general anesthetics.

Cerebral Perfusion Pressure and Mean Arterial Pressure

As previously mentioned, as an independent variable, CPP has a large effect on CBF. CPP is defined as the difference between MAP and the higher of either ICP or central venous pressure (CVP) (Eq. (3.2)):

$$CPP = MAP - ICP \tag{3.2}$$

In healthy dogs, ICP is 5–10 mmHg and CPPs are approximately 70–85 mmHg [15]. Although subtle species differences in these values may exist, the concept remains as follows: when ICP increases, MAP must also increase to maintain CPP. Since hypotension is common during anesthesia, low MAP must be monitored vigilantly and treated aggressively.

Cerebral Metabolic Rate

Typically, the CBF and $CMRO_2$ are directly related (i.e., under physiologic conditions, flow and metabolism are coupled). As regional $CMRO_2$ increases or decreases, CBF changes in the same direction to meet metabolic requirements. The $CMRO_2$ is influenced by several factors, including temperature and anesthetic drugs such as inhalants, sedatives, and analgesics [4]. Flow–metabolism coupling is critical in stressful physiologic conditions, such as hypothermia, hypotension, and hypoxia, which are not uncommon complications in small-animal anesthesia. In humans, intravenous anesthetic agents seem to preserve CBF–$CMRO_2$ coupling better than inhalant anesthetics [2].

Arterial Partial Pressure of Carbon Dioxide and Oxygen

The $PaCO_2$ rapidly affects CBF; therefore, CO_2 is often targeted in the treatment of increased ICP. Changes in $PaCO_2$ will result in directionally proportional changes in CBF (Figure 3.1); CBF increases or decreases by approximately $2\,ml\,min^{-1}\,100\,g^{-1}$ of brain tissue for every 1 mmHg increase or decrease in arterial carbon dioxide within the range of $PaCO_2$ from 20 to 80 mmHg [16]. This is mediated by the changes in the pH of the CSF surrounding the arterioles.

The pH decrease with hypercapnia results in cerebral vasodilation, increased CBF, and increased ICP. Thus, it is important to maintain normocapnia ($PaCO_2$ is approximately 35 mmHg, end-tidal CO_2 is approximately 30–35 mmHg) to prevent or treat cerebral vasodilation. Normocapnia is achieved through mechanical ventilation. Controlling $PaCO_2$ can be instrumental in controlling cerebral blood volume and ICP in the short term.

The PaO_2 has an effect on CBF as well, but not until levels are below 50 mmHg (Figure 3.1). At this level of hypoxemia, cerebral vasodilation will occur, increasing CBF and ICP. Although monitoring oxygenation with arterial blood gases is the definitive way to accurately determine PaO_2, it may not be available. As such, pulse oximetry can be used as a surrogate with the understanding that recognition of hypoxemia will be delayed while on 100% oxygen, according to the oxygen–hemoglobin dissociation curve [17].

Central Venous Pressure

Blood flows continuously out of the brain when ICP is higher than CVP. Under normal conditions, CVP has almost no effect on CBF. In situations wherein CVP is increased, however, CBF will also increase. Some conditions that may increase CVP include poor right ventricular contractility, increased venous return due to venoconstriction or hypervolemia, tension pneumothorax, heart failure, tamponade, pleural effusion, mechanical ventilation, positive end-expiratory pressure, pulmonary hypertension, and pulmonary embolism.

Spinal Cord Blood Flow

While much is published about CBF, there is comparatively much less known about the specifics of spinal cord blood flow. Similar to the cerebral circulation, the blood flow to the spinal cord is under autoregulation within a range of MAPs. Additionally, both hypercapnia and hypoxemia increase spinal cord blood flow. In general, when assessing anesthetic drug effects on spinal cord blood flow, attention is better spent on the hemodynamic effects of those drugs until more is known about their specific effects on spinal cord blood flow. In humans, the spinal cord has significant collateral blood flow, which can represent a "double-edged sword," as it may be protective against ischemia in normal conditions but may also lead to spinal cord hypoperfusion in conditions of systemic hypotension such as general anesthesia, as blood gets shunted away. It is reported that high spinal cord injuries can also lead to changes in CBF by affecting both the autoregulatory response and neurovascular coupling [2].

Anesthesia of Patients with Neurologic Conditions

Preanesthetic Considerations

For patients who are unstable before anesthesia, extracranial stabilization should be the priority. Optimizing hemodynamic parameters such as cardiac output and blood pressure by initiating adequate volume replacement is of utmost importance. Certain neurologic conditions may affect ventilatory centers; therefore, adequate oxygenation and ventilation must also be a priority. After the most life-threatening problems have been addressed, intracranial stabilization should follow shortly. This includes maintaining normal CBF, CPP, and ICP.

Glycemic Control

Hyperglycemia is a common sequela to head trauma and is significantly associated with the severity of injury in both dogs and cats [18]. Hyperglycemia in the face of head trauma leads to higher mortality rates and worsened neurologic outcomes [19–21]. Glucose levels above 180 $mg\,dl^{-1}$, specifically, are associated with poorer outcomes in patients with brain injuries [22]. However, because glucose is essential to cerebral metabolism and mental alertness, levels below 60 mg dl^{-1} should be treated with glucose supplementation [23].

Other Nursing Strategies

Measures should be taken to prevent iatrogenic increases in CVP and ICP. Harnesses, not neck leads, should be used for restraint during ambulation. Also, jugular phlebotomy and, therefore, occlusion should be avoided. During periods of jugular occlusion in healthy dogs, ICP elevated to an average of 30 mmHg with some dogs reaching ICPs above that [15].

Methods to Manage Increased Intracranial Pressure

It is currently not practical to measure ICP in veterinary patients; changes in clinical signs that suggest increases in ICP must be assessed before anesthesia and closely monitored during and after anesthesia. The measurement of intraocular pressure (IOP) has been investigated as a noninvasive surrogate for ICP. Several human studies suggest that IOP and ICP are positively correlated when measured simultaneously [24]. Given the ease of measurement and the implications that early diagnosis of elevated ICP can have, it seems a beneficial diagnostic tool to add to the overall clinical picture. Absent or abnormal pupillary reflexes, mentation, and ventilatory pattern changes may be appreciated on physical examination. The Cushing reflex is a result of increased sympathetic discharge to the peripheral vasculature and a reflex increase in parasympathetic discharge to the heart, respectively [9]. These events occur because of increasing ICP and happen to maintain cerebral perfusion. Physiologic changes seen during this response include an increase in systemic blood pressure followed by a decrease in heart rate.

Patient Positioning

Current recommendation in human post-craniotomy patients and those with a history of head injury is to place the head in an elevated position relative to the heart and body. A head elevation of 30°–45° decreased and helped prevent further increases in ICP, respectively, by encouraging venous outflow [25–29]. In awake, healthy dogs, a head-down position increased ICP by >100% compared to an elevated head position [15]. Veterinary patients with intracranial hypertension would also likely benefit from head elevation.

Controlled Ventilation

Hyperventilation, thus lowering $PaCO_2$, is the most effective method for rapidly reducing ICP by decreasing CBF [30–32]. This response is maintained during both inhaled and intravenous anesthesia [33]. A common recommendation is to maintain the $PaCO_2$ between 30 and 35 mmHg in patients with increased ICP [4]. Because this approach mechanistically requires changes in the pH of extracellular spaces and CSF, once buffering systems neutralize these, continued hypocapnia beyond several hours will result in alkalosis and will no longer be effective at decreasing CBF. Furthermore, continued hypocapnia can have deleterious effects on many other systems. It can cause cerebral ischemia, especially in areas of the CNS with a lower basal CBF [34]. It can worsen cerebral ischemia in cases of traumatic brain injuries [35]. Hypocapnia can also decrease perfusion to splanchnic organ and myocardial and musculoskeletal tissues. It affects coagulation by provoking an increase in adhesion and platelet aggregation. Hypocapnia can also cause acute lung injury and other less-severe pulmonary changes such as bronchoconstriction and attenuation of hypoxic pulmonary vasoconstriction [35]. It is not currently recommended in humans to hyperventilate patients prophylactically, as it will not prevent increases in ICP, nor is it recommended to abruptly discontinue hyperventilation, as rebound increases in CBF may develop [34]. For these reasons, maintaining a low-normal $PaCO_2$ (approximately 35 mmHg) is recommended for veterinary patients.

Hyperosmotic Therapy

The evidence that hyperosmotic therapy improves outcomes in patients with neurologic injury is limited. The most common hyperosmotic agents administered are mannitol and hypertonic saline.

Mannitol is an osmotic diuretic and may be used to reduce ICP in patients with elevated ICP [36]. Mannitol increases plasma osmolarity, theoretically causing a movement of water down an osmotic gradient from the intracellular and interstitial areas of neuronal tissue to the intravascular space within the brain and ultimately to the systemic circulation. Mannitol may also reduce ICP by increasing cerebral perfusion, causing cerebral vasoconstriction [37, 38], and by decreasing the production of CSF [39]. Mannitol's effects peak around 30–45 min after administration and last roughly 6 h [40]. Despite its many mechanisms of ICP reduction, mannitol may cause elevations in ICP through reversal of the initial plasma-to-blood osmotic gradient in patients without an intact blood–brain barrier [41], or through acute expansion of the intravascular fluid volume causing an elevation in CVP. In these cases, hypertonic saline may be a viable alternative.

Hypertonic saline works similarly to mannitol, causing a net loss of water from intracranial structures to the systemic circulation. It may be used in patients with intracranial pathology to reduce or prevent increases in ICP [42–44]. In cases of TBI, hypertonic saline is more effective than mannitol in treating elevated ICP [45–48]. In humans with traumatic brain injuries, administration of hypertonic saline correlated with reduced intracranial hypertension in addition to improving mortality and neurologic outcome [49]. Hypertonic saline's effect on decreasing intracranial volume, however, may be limited to <90 min [50], limiting its use for long-term control of elevated ICP. Recently, the COBI (*co*ntinuous hyperosmolar therapy for traumatic *b*rain-*i*njured patients) trial was being conducted, which may shed more light on the outcomes of patients receiving hyperosmotic therapy post TBI [51].

Anesthetic Management (Box 3.1)

Sedatives and Analgesics

Acepromazine has historically been implicated in decreasing the seizure threshold in patients with a history of seizure activity. A retrospective study has since indicated that acepromazine can be used without the risk of increasing the likelihood of seizure [52]. Since acepromazine exerts antagonist effects on alpha-1-adrenergic receptors leading to vasodilation and subsequent hypotension, this sedative should be used with caution in patients with intracranial or spinal pathology (Table 3.1). MAP should be closely monitored to maintain CPP (Eq. 3.1).

Dexmedetomidine is an excellent choice in patients with intracranial disease, provided systemic hypotension is avoided. Dexmedetomidine decreases CBF in dogs anesthetized with halothane or isoflurane [53, 54]. Animal and human studies indicate that there is likely a neuroprotective effect in part through reduction of neuroendocrine hormones and inflammatory mediators such as tumor necrosis factor-alpha (TNF-α) and IL-6 [55]. In addition, dexmedetomidine also significantly reduces postoperative cognitive dysfunction when compared to other sedatives [55].

Midazolam is a reasonable choice for sedation of neurologic patients. Midazolam reduces CBF by decreasing the $CMRO_2$ consumption; [56] additionally, midazolam is effective as an anticonvulsant. Caution should be exercised, as benzodiazepines may cause paradoxical excitement when used as a preanesthetic agent.

Opioids are an acceptable choice for premedication and analgesia in neurologic patients, as they have minimal direct effects on CBF and ICP [57]. Opioids, however, can indirectly increase ICP, as administration may cause emesis [58, 59], which can cause increases in ICP. They can also cause hypoventilation, leading to an increase in ICP secondary

Box 3.1 Summary of recommendations.

Preoperative
- General patient stabilization
- Hemodynamic status
- Biochemical abnormalities
- Management of comorbidities
- Management of stress and anxiety
- Avoid drugs that cause respiratory depression and/or hypotension if suspected ICP elevated
- Avoid iatrogenic causes of elevated ICP or CVP
- Avoid emesis
- Avoid jugular occlusion
- Preoxygenate with tight-fitting face mask for 3–5 min at 3–5 l min^{-1}

Induction
- Goals of anesthesia
- Assure proper level of CNS depression before attempting intubation as to avoid laryngeal stimulation that may lead to coughing or retching
- Maintain proper patient positioning (head elevated above heart)
- Choose drugs that do not cause increased CBF

Maintenance
- Mechanical ventilation readily available—goal $ETCO_2$ 30–35 mmHg
- Maintain SpO_2 >95%
- Maintain CPP
- Maintain MAP
- Avoid iatrogenic increases in ICP or CVP
- Avoid increases in $CMRO_2$ or CBF
- Choose drugs that decrease or do not change $CMRO_2$
- Treat any seizure activity promptly
- Choose drugs that do not directly increase CBF
- Monitor $ETCO_2$ or $PaCO_2$ and maintain normocapnia
- Monitor SpO_2 or PaO_2 and maintain oxygenation
- If using inhalants, keep expired levels below 1 MAC

Postoperative
- Provide a smooth recovery
- Avoid coughing, retching, and emesis
- Administer adequate analgesia
- Continue to monitor ventilation
- Delay neurologic examination until fully recovered

to hypercapnia; therefore, assisted, or mechanical ventilation during general anesthesia is recommended [60]. Because pain can also cause respiratory depression, avoiding the use of opioids as analgesics in these situations cannot be recommended. Further exploration into alternatives to opioid analgesia may allow for an eventual decrease in opioid use.

Injectable Anesthetics

Barbiturates, etomidate, propofol, and alfaxalone all decrease CBF and ICP and contribute to the decrease in $CMRO_2$ seen with CNS depression [61–65], and have all been used in patients with neurologic injury. Historically, thiopental blocks sodium, potassium, and calcium flux, scavenges free radicals, blocks seizures, and improves regional blood flow [66]. Because of the negative effects on cardiovascular physiology and immune function, barbiturates are typically reserved for patients with refractory increases in ICP. Though etomidate decreases $CMRO_2$, it has not been proven to provide neuroprotection or improve outcomes in cases with cerebral ischemia. In addition, etomidate can cause retching and myoclonic muscle activity, potentially increasing ICP. Propofol is the current standard for control of ICP in human intensive care units and is an appropriate choice for anesthesia in veterinary patients with intracranial pathology. At this time, the evidence for using the current formulation of alfaxalone in

Table 3.1 Effects of opioids, sedatives, and anesthetics on intracranial pressure (ICP).

Drug or drug class	Effect on ICP
Opioids	Decrease[a]
Benzodiazepines	No change or decrease
Acepromazine	Potential increase secondary to cerebral vasodilation and increase CBF
Alpha-2-adrenergic agonists	No change
Propofol	Decrease
Etomidate	Decrease[b]
Barbiturates	Decrease
Ketamine	Increase[c]
Isoflurane, sevoflurane, desflurane	In general, no change if <1 MAC Increase if >1 MAC or if hypercapnia occurs
Nitrous oxide	Profound increase

[a] Can indirectly increase through hypoventilation or emesis
[b] May cause increases secondary to retching
[c] May cause no change if used with other sedatives and controlled ventilation

human or veterinary patients under these circumstances is limited.

Ketamine use in patients with intracranial pathology is slowly becoming more favorable. Unlike other injectable anesthetics, ketamine does not reduce CBF, ICP, or $CMRO_2$ [13]. Early studies examining ketamine's effect on intracranial hemodynamics were performed in humans without concurrent sedation or mechanical ventilation. However, the use of ketamine in patients with controlled ventilation has demonstrated no increase in ICP [67]; the use of other sedative agents will also blunt increases in CBF caused by ketamine. Therefore, with the use of mechanical ventilation and its use combined with sedatives/muscle relaxants, ketamine may be a reasonable choice in veterinary patients with intracranial pathology. An analysis of human TBI literature [68] demonstrated that not only did ketamine administration not increase ICP but that there were no adverse events associated with its use. In a retrospective study of human trauma patients receiving sedative agents, those that received ketamine had lower mortality rates after controlling for type of injury [69]. The effects of ketamine on N-methyl-D-aspartate (NMDA) receptors and glutamate may impart a protective effect in patients with TBI.

Intravenous lidocaine has been shown to be neuroprotective in experimental studies of hypoxia and ischemia. This seems to be effective when given prior to and shortly after the injury, limiting its clinical use. The mechanism of action is not entirely known; however, it is likely a combination of its effects on sodium channels, preservation of cellular mitochondria and adenosine triphosphate (ATP), and the reduction of neuroinflammation [70].

Total intravenous anesthesia (TIVA) is the sole use of injectable anesthetic agents for the maintenance of anesthesia. TIVA has been recommended for patients with intracranial pathology to prevent further increases in CBF and thus ICP. In humans undergoing anesthesia for the surgical treatment of acute subdural hematomas, propofol-based TIVA provided better brain relaxation and maintained a lower ICP and better hemodynamics when compared to inhalational anesthesia [71]. Few disadvantages exist. They include cumulative drug effects, reliance on hepatic or other means of drug biotransformation, and the need for specialized equipment or proficiency in dosage and infusion calculations for adequate delivery.

Inhalant Anesthetics

In general, inhalant anesthetics increase CBF and decrease $CMRO_2$, causing an uncoupling of the two. The effect on CBF is a result of opposing actions on cerebral vasculature: vasodilation due to direct action on vascular smooth muscle versus decreases in blood flow due to a reduction in $CMRO_2$ [72]. Most volatile anesthetics minimally affect CBF when used at concentrations below 1 minimum alveolar concentration (MAC). Above the MAC, however, cerebral blood vessels will continue to dilate and cause increased CBF and possibly increased ICP. The changes in CBF are inhalant- and dose-dependent. Sixty percent nitrous oxide increases CBF and $CMRO_2$ by up to 203% in dogs [73]. Of the volatile anesthetics, halothane appears to have the most effect on CBF, whereas enflurane, isoflurane, sevoflurane, and desflurane are similar in their effect on CBF [74]. Halothane produces significant increases in CBF at 0.5–1.5 times the MAC in cats, whereas isoflurane does not [75]. Sevoflurane and isoflurane have minimal effects on CBF at concentrations of anesthetic up to 2.15 MAC in anesthetized dogs [76]. Similarly, desflurane concentrations from 0.5 to 1.5 MAC cause dose-dependent increases in the CBF of anesthetized dogs [77]. The magnitude of $CMRO_2$ reduction is least with halothane, but similar with isoflurane, sevoflurane, and desflurane [75–79]. In mechanically ventilated anesthetized dogs, both isoflurane and sevoflurane significantly decrease CPP at two times the MAC, with mean CPP lower during isoflurane anesthesia at all MAC tested [80]. The inhalant anesthetics increase ICP in parallel to the increases in CBF [78, 81]. These effects, however, can be minimized by hyperventilating to mild hypocapnia [82]. It important to use a balanced or multimodal approach to anesthesia, which will permit reduction in the inhalant levels required for a surgical anesthetic plane, but minimally affect the oxygen supply to the CNS.

Neurospecific Monitoring

In humans, several methods of monitoring neurophysiology during anesthesia exist; they include continuous electroencephalogram (EEG), brain tissue oxygen monitoring, ICP, CPP, and pressure reactivity index [83]. Unfortunately, none are currently readily available or practical in veterinary patients.

Anesthetic Management of Specific Disease Processes

Traumatic Brain Injury

TBI is divided into primary and secondary events. Primary injuries are the result of the initial traumatic event (Figure 3.2) and irreversible, whereas secondary injuries occur immediately after the event and can lead to global and local ischemia, the death of more neuronal tissue, and worsening survival if not prevented or promptly treated. The etiology of secondary brain injury includes hypoxemia, hypotension, decreased cerebral perfusion, increased ICP, and decreased CBF [84–86].

Diagnostic imaging or decompressive measures may be necessary in these patients after initial extracranial stabilization. Additional procedures requiring anesthesia may be performed, such as the management of intrathoracic and intra-abdominal injuries or fracture stabilization. The goals of anesthesia should be aimed at maintaining oxygenation, systemic blood pressure, and CPP, while preventing further increases in ICP, thus contributing to the prevention of secondary injury.

Premedication should focus on providing analgesia and decreasing induction doses of injectable drugs and maintenance doses of volatile anesthetics. Rarely is a sedative indicated. Anesthetic agents that increase CBF (halothane and nitrous oxide) should be avoided. Most injectable anesthetics (barbiturates, propofol, alfaxalone, and etomidate) reduce $CMRO_2$ and decrease CBF; therefore, these are reasonable induction choices for patients with TBI. Rapid intubation with minimal laryngeal stimulation, as to not provoke coughing, and a resultant increase in ICP, should be performed. If a difficult intubation is suspected, preoxygenation ($100\,ml\,kg^{-1}\,min^{-1}$) of the patient with a tight-fitting mask for 3 min will attenuate hemoglobin desaturation for approximately 5 min [87]. Assisted or mechanical ventilation should be instituted to avoid hypercapnia and cerebral vasodilation.

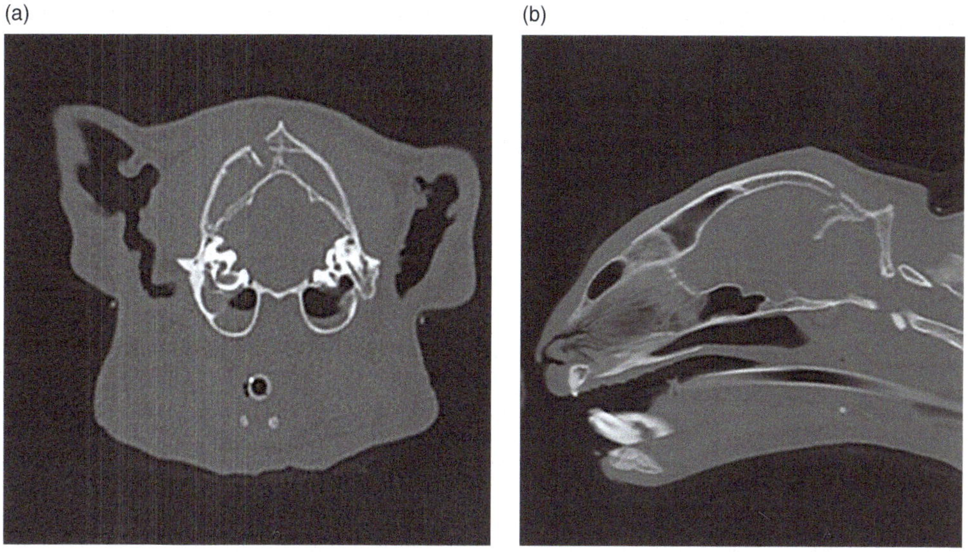

Figure 3.2 (a) Axial and (b) sagittal CT images of a feline skull fracture. The left caudal parietal bone has a depression fracture measuring approximately 3.5 mm diameter. A cortical fragment of the same diameter is ventrally depressed into the left caudal parietal lobe of the brain.

Hypocapnia should also be avoided, as it can worsen cerebral ischemia in TBI [35]. Maintenance of anesthesia may include continuous infusions of intravenous analgesics such as a combination of fentanyl and propofol or low-dose volatile anesthetics.

In the recovery period, continuous monitoring of neurologic status is prudent. The use of standardized scoring systems for neurologic injury and outcome, such as the Glasgow Coma Scale, has been validated and widely used in human patients. A modified Glasgow Coma Scale has been used in veterinary medicine with some success [88]. More typically, veterinary clinicians rely on serial neurologic assessments and response to treatment to predict the severity of injury and the overall prognosis. Care must be taken to ensure that the sedative effects of drugs given during anesthesia are not affecting patients' neurologic assessments.

Several pharmacologic agents and their effects on neurologic outcomes in TBI have been examined. Some examples include progesterone, erythropoietin, cyclosporine A, magnesium, and nitric oxide. None are currently considered standard of care or used in veterinary medicine.

Current research and recommendations for patients with TBI can be found at the Brain Trauma Foundation (www.braintrauma.org).

Intracranial Tumors

Tumors found within the brain may be primary or metastatic. Meningiomas are the most common primary intracranial tumor in dogs and cats followed closely by astrocytomas and oligodendrogliomas in dogs and lymphoma in cats [89–91]. The most common dog breeds affected are Golden Retrievers and Boxers [90, 92], whereas domestic shorthaired cats seem to be predisposed [89, 91]. Clinical signs can be extremely variable. Dogs present most frequently with seizures, changes in mentation, vestibular syndrome, blindness, and neck pain [90, 92], whereas cats present with altered consciousness, circling, and seizures [89, 91, 93].

Diagnosis of intracranial tumors requires the use of imaging techniques such as computed tomography (CT) or magnetic resonance imaging (MRI) (Figure 3.3), while treatment may require surgical intervention or radiation therapy. All the aforementioned require anesthesia for veterinary patients. If intramuscular premedication is necessary, drugs that have minimal effects on ICP should be administered. The intramuscular administration of pure mu-opioid receptor agonists, such as morphine and hydromorphone, may cause emesis which can increase ICP.

Anesthesia should be induced with drugs that cause unconsciousness rapidly and reliably without increasing the ICP. Laryngeal stimulation leading to coughing should be avoided by using intravenous lidocaine ($2\,mg\,kg^{-1}$) in dogs or topically administered lidocaine in cats, and the patient should be mechanically ventilated to avoid hypercapnia and cerebral vasodilation. Anesthetic maintenance should be aimed at providing a balanced approach. Fluid therapy should be instituted with either isotonic crystalloids or hyperosmolar solutions, being careful to avoid hypervolemia. Monitoring should include the placement of an arterial catheter for the measurement of invasive blood pressures, as well as pulse oximetry, capnography, and electrocardiography. In the recovery period, the assessment of neurologic status may be postponed to ensure that the sedative effects of drugs given during anesthesia do not exacerbate pre-existing neurologic conditions.

Seizure Disorders

Seizures are caused by transient, paroxysmal, and synchronous discharge of neurons in the brain [4]. Clinical presentations depend on the extent of brain involved and the specific area of the brain that is affected. Causes can be classified into two categories. Extracranial causes of seizures, such as metabolic disturbances, toxicosis, and systemic disease, necessitate treatment of the underlying cause, which is often curative. Intracranial causes of seizures include many disorders such as degenerative, anomalous, neoplastic, infectious, inflammatory, idiopathic, traumatic, and vascular conditions. Treatment typically involves maintaining normal temperatures, ensuring adequate perfusion, oxygenation and ventilation, and instituting therapies to decrease the development of cerebral edema and stop any continued seizure activity [94, 95].

Anesthetic management in patients with a history of seizures must include consideration of the effect of antiepileptic drugs on anesthesia. Anticonvulsants that result in sedation can

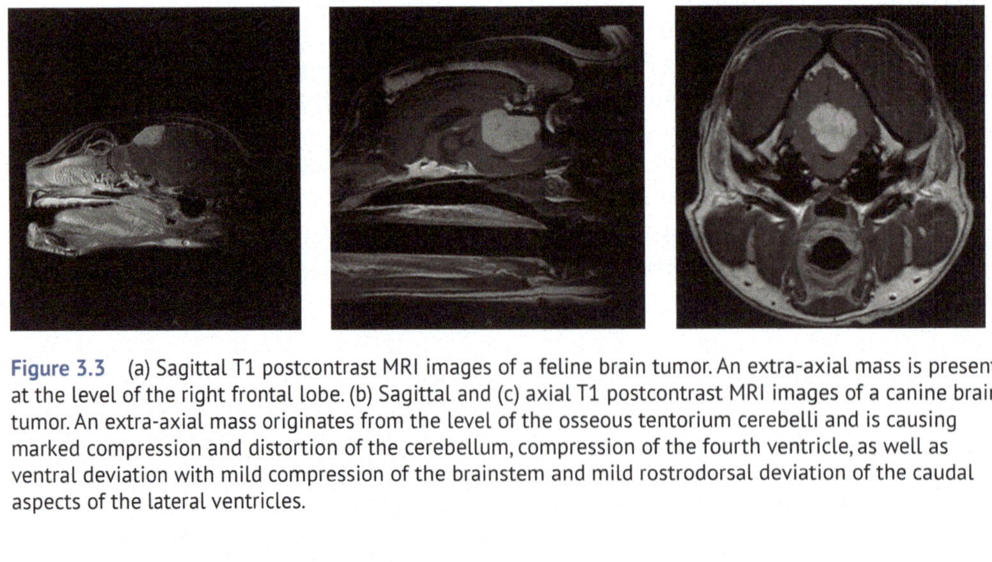

Figure 3.3 (a) Sagittal T1 postcontrast MRI images of a feline brain tumor. An extra-axial mass is present at the level of the right frontal lobe. (b) Sagittal and (c) axial T1 postcontrast MRI images of a canine brain tumor. An extra-axial mass originates from the level of the osseous tentorium cerebelli and is causing marked compression and distortion of the cerebellum, compression of the fourth ventricle, as well as ventral deviation with mild compression of the brainstem and mild rostrodorsal deviation of the caudal aspects of the lateral ventricles.

have additive effects, leading to decreased doses of other CNS depressants, whereas drugs that induce hepatic enzymes (barbiturates) could alter the pharmacokinetics and pharmacodynamics of anesthetic drugs such that increased doses are necessary [4]. Avoid the use of epileptogenic drugs such as methohexital; historically, acepromazine was avoided owing to the suspected increase in seizure activity associated with administration. However, a retrospective study has since indicated that acepromazine does not potentiate seizure activity [52]. Opioids, benzodiazepines, alfaxalone, propofol, and barbiturates are reasonable choices for the anesthetic period. During the recovery period, continued monitoring for seizure activity is important and treatment with anticonvulsants instituted if necessary.

Hydrocephalus

Hydrocephalus is the active distension of the ventricular system of the brain that results from the accumulation of an abnormal amount of CSF from the point of production within the ventricles to its point of absorption. CSF is produced by the choroid plexus in the lateral, third, and fourth ventricles, the ependymal lining, the external pial-glial membrane on the surface of the brain, and by the blood vessels in the pia-arachnoid. Most CSF absorption occurs in the arachnoid villi; some occurs via venous and lymphatic drainage around spinal and cranial nerves. Hydrocephalus can be congenital, with signs becoming apparent within the first year of life or acquired. Diagnosis of hydrocephalus is done with a combination of clinical signs and imaging modalities such as ultrasound, CT, and MRI (Figure 3.4). Treatment is directed at the underlying cause. For cases that cannot be treated medically, ventriculoperitoneal shunting may be performed.

Anesthetic management is similar to other intracranial disorders and should be aimed at preventing intracranial hypertension and maintaining CPP. Induction should be performed with drugs that induce unconsciousness rapidly and reliably without increasing the ICP. Laryngeal stimulation during intubation should be avoided to reduce the chances of coughing or gagging. The patient should be mechanically ventilated to avoid hypercapnia and resultant cerebral vasodila-

(a)

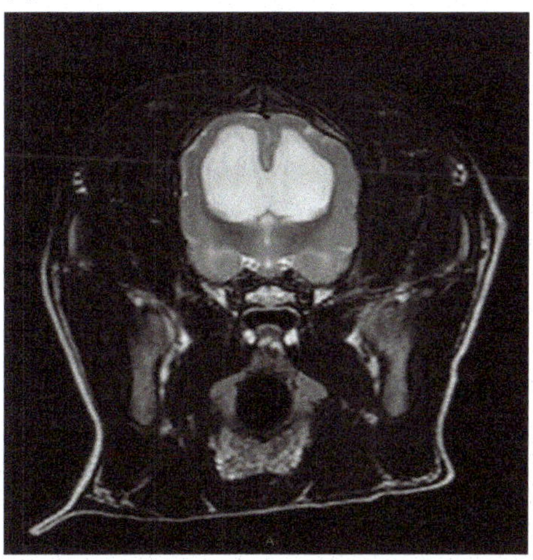

(b)

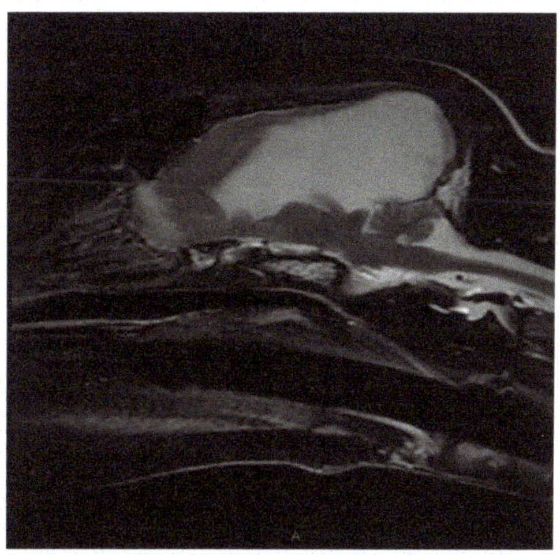

Figure 3.4 (a) Axial and (b) sagittal T1 postcontrast MRI images of a canine brain with hydrocephalus. Severe hydrocephalus involves the lateral ventricles and results in essentially complete atrophy of the occipital lobes and severe atrophy of the parietal and temporal lobe cortex.

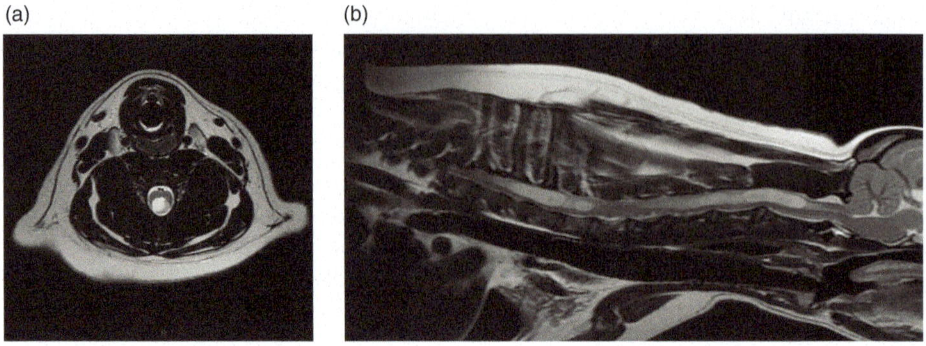

Figure 3.5 (a) Axial T2 MRI images of a canine spinal cord with syringomyelia. There is an extensive syrinx formation within the central to dorsal central aspect of the cervical spinal cord. (b) Sagittal T2 MRI images of a canine brain and spinal cord with Chiari-like malformation and cervical and thoracic syringomyelia. The syrinx begins over the level of the C2 vertebral body and extends caudally throughout the cervical spine ending in the mid-thoracic spine. The cerebellum is crowded in the caudal fossa against the occipital bone and there is indentation in the ventral aspect of the cerebellar vermis. The vermis is moderately herniated and contacts the dorsal aspect of the brainstem.

tion. Maintenance of anesthesia should be aimed at providing a balanced approach. Conservative fluid therapy should be instituted with isotonic crystalloids being careful to avoid hypervolemia. Hyperosmolar solution administration should be reserved for the treatment of elevated ICP unresponsive to other means. Invasive blood pressure should be monitored when possible. Pulse oximetry, capnography, and electrocardiography should also be continuously monitored. In the recovery period, continued assessment of neurologic status should be performed, but may be postponed to ensure that the sedative effects of drugs given during anesthesia are not exacerbating preexisting neurologic conditions.

Chiari-Like Malformation and Syringomyelia

Cavalier King Charles Spaniels have a 100% incidence of Chiari-like malformation and up to 70% have concurrent syringomyelia. Other small and toy breeds may also be afflicted with this condition. Some of the most common clinical signs in dogs with syringomyelia secondary to a Chiari-like malformation are cervical pain, allodynia, and dysesthesia [96–99], but it is also common for patients to be asymptomatic. Patients may present with a suspected Chiari-like malformation or syringomyelia diagnosed definitively with MRI (Figure 3.5). When planning the anesthetic management of these patients, one must consider using a balanced anesthetic technique by providing adequate analgesia. Focus should also be on preventing increases in ICP and providing analgesia for ongoing pain.

Intervertebral Disc Disease and Other Spinal Injuries

Intervertebral disc disease and vertebral trauma leading to spinal cord dysfunction are major causes of neurologic injury in small-animal patients. Traumatic injuries cause disruption of neural tissue leading to demyelination, axonal injury, and neuronal and axonal destruction [100]. Pain results either from instability of local tissues or from the compression of spinal structures.

Patients with suspected spinal cord injury may undergo some form of diagnostic imaging, either spinal radiography, myelography, CT, or MRI that necessitates the use of general anesthesia. They may also undergo surgical intervention.

Several goals should be addressed during this time. Sedation, induction, and maintenance techniques and drug choices should focus on providing necessary analgesia and using balanced anesthetic techniques. If a fracture or luxation is suspected, immobilization and stabilization of the spine before anesthesia are extremely important, as relaxation of paraspinal musculature can lead to instability and further damage. Maintaining physiologic parameters such as heart rate and blood pressure is imperative. Certain breeds of dogs, such as Dachshunds, are more susceptible to developing bradycardia during spinal imaging [101]. The treatment of bradycardia with an anticholinergic such as glycopyrrolate or atropine may help maintain normal heart rates during anesthesia. Hypothermia is a frequent anesthetic complication in veterinary patients [102, 103]. The maintenance of normothermia can be challenging; however, using intravenous fluid-warming devices [104] and forced air-warming devices [105] may attenuate drops in temperature. Patients receiving radiographic imaging studies or myelography may undergo frequent position changes under anesthesia predisposing patients to tracheal trauma [106, 107]. Paying particular attention to reducing endotracheal tube movement and briefly disconnecting from the anesthesia circuit, as needed, during patient movement positioning may decrease this risk. Patients with cervical lesions may experience respiratory compromise if innervation to the diaphragm or accessory muscles is affected.

Dogs anesthetized for the treatment of intervertebral disc disease are at risk for developing pneumonia postoperatively [108]. Efforts to shorten the duration of anesthesia and prevent postanesthetic vomiting and regurgitation may decrease this risk. Post-myelography seizures are reported in 3–14% of dogs [109, 110]. Acute anticonvulsant therapy should be instituted as described elsewhere [94, 95].

Patients with nervous system dysfunction or injury to nervous system tissues, similar to that which might occur in patients with intervertebral disc disease, are at risk for developing neuropathic pain. Mechanisms thought to be responsible for the reorganization of sensory transmission within the nervous system include central sensitization, central disinhibition, and phenotypic changes to A-beta fibers [96]. Because of this neurochemical transformation, perioperative analgesia regimes using opioids may not be sufficient for these patients. Adjunct analgesics, such as a ketamine constant rate infusion, are beneficial. The reader is referred elsewhere for an extensive review of the pathophysiology and treatment of neuropathic pain [96].

Spinal Shock

Spinal shock is a reversible phenomenon that can occur after an acute spinal cord injury. It is described as a profound physiologic depression in segmental spinal reflexes caudal to the injury, even though reflex arcs remain physically intact. In a retrospective evaluation, the prevalence of spinal shock in dogs presenting for thoracolumbar MRI was 6% [111]. Patients with cervical or high thoracolumbar injuries may experience neurogenic shock that results in autonomic dysfunction and hemodynamic instability. These patients will require cardiovascular stabilization with anticholinergics, inotropic agents, vasopressors, or a combination of these substances throughout the perianesthetic period.

Other Nervous System Disorders

Dysautonomia

Dysautonomia is a rare idiopathic condition characterized by degeneration of neurons in the autonomic nervous system ganglia. Clinical signs and physical examination findings reflect the severity of degeneration in both sympathetic and parasympathetic nervous systems. Dysuria with a distended urinary bladder, mydriasis with absent pupillary light reflexes, xerostomia, decreased tear production, decreased anal tone, and vomiting or regurgitation are common in dogs with dysautonomia [112, 113]. In cats, lethargy, inappetence, vomiting, dysphagia, stranguria, mydriasis with absent pupillary light reflexes, xerostomia, prolapse of the nictitans, and bradycardia are reported [114]. In general, dysautonomia has a grave prognosis with very high mortality rates in both dogs and cats [112, 114]. Patients needing anesthesia should be managed similarly to any critically ill patient, paying particular attention to heart rate and potential for regurgitation.

Myasthenia Gravis

Myasthenia gravis is a congenital or an acquired autoimmune disease that causes a decrease in functional acetylcholine receptors at the neuromuscular junction. Clinical signs include muscle weakness and megaesophagus, making pulmonary aspiration of gastric contents a risk. Treatment includes anticholinesterase drugs in combination with immunosuppressive therapies when indicated. Patients with myasthenia gravis may need anesthesia for procedures unrelated to the disease. Special attention should be paid to the increased risk of gastroesophageal reflux and aspiration of gastric contents. Preoperative treatment with antiemetics and prokinetics is often recommended and may be instituted. The combination of esomeprazole and cisapride therapy has been shown to decrease gastroesophageal reflux events in healthy dogs under general anesthesia [115]. Patients should be induced and intubated rapidly with frequent laryngeal and proximal esophageal suctioning. Extubation should be performed when a patient demonstrates the ability to adequately maintain respiration and to protect their airway via the return of the ability to swallow.

Because of the decrease in functional acetylcholine receptors, these patients may have an increased sensitivity to nondepolarizing muscle relaxants such as atracurium [116, 117]. If the use of nondepolarizing muscle relaxants is necessary, the dose should be reduced by one half to two thirds and the response monitored with a peripheral nerve stimulator [118, 119]. Interestingly, human patients with myasthenia gravis are somewhat resistant to the effects of depolarizing muscle relaxants [120]. However, this has not been described in veterinary patients.

Peripheral Neuropathies

Peripheral neuropathies can be associated with several other conditions, including cancer [121] and diabetes mellitus [122, 123]. Paraneoplastic peripheral neuropathies occur in patients with malignant disease and have been reported with several tumor types in the veterinary literature [124–135]. Patients with diabetes mellitus are more susceptible to peripheral nerve ischemia due to compression and stretching. During anesthesia, positioning and padding are extremely important to prevent further injury to nerves. In addition, peripheral neuropathies may increase the effects of nondepolarizing muscle relaxants because of neural damage and the possibility of denervation-induced upregulation [136].

Nerve Sheath Tumors

Nerve sheath tumors originate from nerve roots or peripheral nerves, most commonly the cervical nerve roots or brachial plexus [137]. Clinical signs are dependent on the tissues involved, but commonly include unilateral forelimb lameness with varying degrees of pain. Muscle atrophy and neurologic deficits may also be present. Diagnostic imaging such as radiographs, CT, or MRI may be necessary for surgical planning (Figure 3.6). The goals of anesthetic management should focus on using a balanced, multimodal approach while providing adequate analgesia. Because these patients may be experiencing neuropathic pain, opioids alone will not be sufficient [96].

Postoperative Cognitive Dysfunction

Postoperative cognitive dysfunction or decline (POCD) is a condition recognized clinically in humans and experimentally in animals. It is

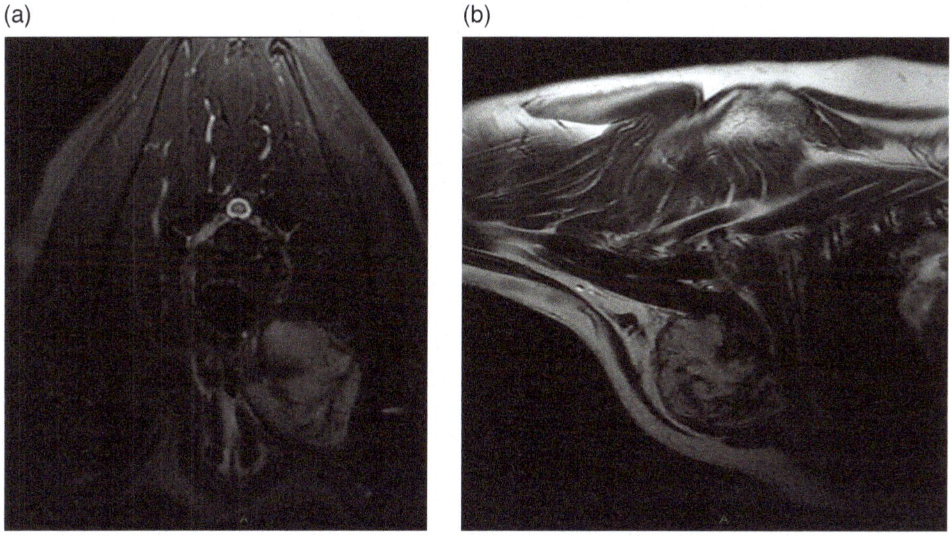

Figure 3.6 (a) Axial and (b) sagittal T2 MRI images of a canine peripheral nerve sheath tumor of the left brachial plexus. The mass arises from the C6–C7 nerve root 3–4 cm from the intervertebral foramen.

described as acute or persistent deficits in attention, concentration, learning, and memory following surgery and anesthesia that are not attributable to an overt complication or insult arising from the procedure [138, 139]. Aged patients are at greater risk for developing POCD. The pathophysiology is incompletely understood, but the presence of elevated inflammatory markers such as IL-6, IL-β, and TNF-α both peripherally and within the CNS seems instrumental to its development. Studies in aged rats and mice suggest that inhalant anesthesia alone (without surgery) induced cognitive dysfunction associated with microglial activation and CNS inflammation, as well as memory impairments and alterations in proteins associated with synaptic plasticity and neuronal signaling [140, 141]. There is evidence that the addition of some pharmacologic agents such as lidocaine and vitamin C may attenuate the loss in cognitive function after anesthesia [142, 143], but this is certainly an area of future interest and examination.

Though not likely to be of large clinical relevance in the anesthesia of most companion animals, there are few populations worth mentioning. Aged working animals (police, military, etc.) may be affected and less able to complete their tasks for some time after anesthesia. In addition, geriatric animals with preoperative cognitive decline may have further decreases in quality of life after anesthesia; therefore, necessitating clear communications and expectations with caregivers prior to anesthesia.

References

1 Lemkuil, B.P., Drummond, J.C., and Patel, P.M. (2013). Central nervous system physiology: cerebrovascular. In: *Pharmacology and Physiology for Anesthesia: Foundations and Clinical Applications*, 1e (eds. H.C. Hemmings Jr. and T.D. Egan), 123–136. Elsevier: Philadelphia.

2 Ellis, J.A., Yocum, G.T., Ornstein, E. et al. (2017). Cerebral and spinal cord blood flow.

In: *Neuroanestheisa*, 6e (eds. J.E. Cottrell and P. Patel), 19–58. Philadelphia: Elsevier.

3 Meng, L. and Flexman, A. (2018). Central nervous system disease. In: *Basics of Anesthesia*, 7e (eds. M.C. Pardo Jr. and R.D. Miller), 511–523. Elsevier: Philadelphia.

4 Pasternak, J.J. and Lanier, W.L. Jr. (2018). Diseases affecting the brain. In: *Stoelting's Anesthesia and Co-existing Disease*, 7e (eds. R.L. Hines and K.E. Marschall), 265–304. Elsevier: Philadelphia.

5 Busija, D.W., Heistad, D.D., and Marcus, M.L. (1981). Continuous measurement of cerebral blood flow in anesthetized cats and dogs. *Am. J. Physiol.* 241 (2): 228–234.

6 Peterson, K.L., MacLeod, A.G., Wisner, E.R. et al. (2008). Quantitative assessment of blood volume, blood flow, and permeability of the brain of clinically normal dogs by use of dynamic contrast-enhanced computed tomography. *Am. J. Vet. Res.* 69 (1): 45–50.

7 Ewing, J.R., Branch, C.A., Fagan, S.C. et al. (1990). Fluorocarbon-23 measure of cat cerebral blood flow by nuclear magnetic resonance. *Stroke* 21 (1): 100–106.

8 Walters, F.J. (1990). Neuro anaesthesia–a review of the basic principles and current practices. *Cent. Afr. J. Med.* 36 (2): 44–51.

9 Fodstad, H., Kelly, P.J., and Buchfelder, M. (2006). History of the Cushing reflex. *Neurosurgery* 59: 1132–1137.

10 Cyrous, A., O'Neal, B., and Freeman, W.D. (2012). New approaches to bedside monitoring in stroke. *Expert Rev. Neurother.* 12 (8): 915–928.

11 Kalanuria, A., Nyquist, P.A., Armonda, R.A. et al. (2013). Use of transcranial doppler (TCD) ultrasound in the neurocritical care unit. *Neurosurg. Clin. North Am.* 24 (3): 441–456, Philadelphia, Elsevier.

12 Thewissen, L., Caicedo, A., Lemmers, P. et al. (2018). Measuring near-infrared spectroscopy derived cerebral autoregulation in neonates: from research tool toward bedside multimodal monitoring. *Front. Pediatr.* 14 (6): 117.

13 Harvey, R., Greene, S., and Thomas, W. (2015). Physiology, pathophysiology, and anesthetic management of patients with neurologic disease. In: *Veterinary Anesthesia and Analgesia: The Fifth Edition of Lumb and Jones* (eds. K.A. Grimm, L.A. Lamont, W.J. Tranquilli, et al.), 559–583. Wiley Blackwell Publishing: Ames.

14 Joshi, B., Ono, M., Brown, C. et al. (2012). Predicting the limits of cerebral autoregulation during cardiopulmonary bypass. *Anesth. Analg.* 114 (3): 505–510.

15 Sturges, B.K., Dickinson, P.J., Tripp, L.D. et al. (2019). Intracranial pressure monitoring in normal dogs using subdural and intraparenchymal miniature strain-gauge transducers. *J. Vet. Intern. Med.* 33 (2): 708–716.

16 Grubb, R.L. Jr., Raichle, M.E., Eichling, J.O. et al. (1974). The effects of changes in $PaCO_2$ on cerebral blood volume, blood flow, and vascular mean transit time. *Stroke* 5 (5): 630–639.

17 Antonini, E. (1979). History and theory of the oxyhemoglobin dissociation curve. *Crit. Care Med.* 7: 360–367.

18. Syring, R.S., Otto, C.M., and Drobatz, K.J. (2001). Hyperglycemia in dogs and cats with head trauma: 122 cases (1997–1999). *J. Am. Vet. Med. Assoc.* 218 (7): 1124–1129.

19 Tude Melo, J.R., Di Rocco, F., Blanot, S. et al. (2010). Mortality in children with severe head trauma: predictive factors and proposal for a new predictive scale. *Neurosurgery* 67 (6): 1542–1547.

20 Prisco, L., Iscra, F., Ganau, M. et al. (2012). Early predictive factors on mortality in head injured patients: a retrospective analysis of 112 traumatic brain injured patients. *J. Neurosurg. Sci.* 56 (2): 131–136.

21 Seyed Saadat, S.M., Bidabadi, E., Seyed Saadat, S.N. et al. (2012). Association of persistent hyperglycemia with outcome of severe traumatic brain injury in pediatric population. *Childs Nerv. Syst.* 28 (10): 1773–1777.

22 Claassen, J., Vu, A., Kreiter, K.T. et al. (2004). Effect of acute physiologic derangements on outcome after subarachnoid hemorrhage. *Crit. Care Med.* 32: 32–38.

23 Grubb, T.L., Perez-Jimenez, T.E., and Pettifer, G.R. (2015). Neonatal and pediatric patients. In: *Veterinary Anesthesia and Analgesia: The Fifth Edition of Lumb and Jones* (eds. K.A. Grimm, L.A. Lamont, W.J. Tranquilli, et al.), 983–987. Ames: Wiley Blackwell Publishing.

24 Yavin, D., Luu, J., James, M.T. et al. (2014). Diagnostic accuracy of intraocular pressure measurement for the detection of raised intracranial pressure: meta-analysis: a systematic review. *J. Neurosurg.* 121 (3): 680–687.

25 Rosner, M.J. and Coley, I.B. (1986). Cerebral perfusion pressure, intracranial pressure, and head elevation. *J. Neurosurg.* 65 (5): 636–641.

26 Schneider, G.H., von Helden, G.H., Franke, R. et al. (1993). Influence of body position on jugular venous oxygen saturation, intracranial pressure and cerebral perfusion pressure. *Acta Neurochir. Suppl. (Wien)* 59: 107–112.

27 Ng, I., Lim, J., and Wong, H.B. (2004). Effects of head posture on cerebral hemodynamics: its influences on intracranial pressure, cerebral perfusion pressure, and cerebral oxygenation. *Neurosurgery* 54 (3): 593–597.

28 Agbeko, R.S., Pearson, S., Peters, M.J. et al. (2012). Intracranial pressure and cerebral perfusion pressure responses to head elevation changes in pediatric traumatic brain injury. *Pediatr. Crit. Care Med.* 13 (1):39–47.

29 Jiang, Y., Ye, Z., You, C. et al. (2015). Systematic review of decreased intracranial pressure with optimal head elevation in postcraniotomy patients: a meta-analysis. *J. Adv. Nurs.* 71 (10): 2237–2246.

30 Jackson, R.T., Clairmont, A.A., and Pollock, R.A. (1974). The effect of carbon dioxide inhalation on cerebral blood flow: a two-hour duration study in dogs with microspheres. *Stroke J.* 5 (3): 344–349.

31 Detre, J.A., Subramanian, V.H., Mitchell, M.D. et al. (1990). Measurement of regional cerebral blood flow in cat brain using intracarotid $2H_2O$ and 2H NMR imaging. *Magn. Reson. Med.* 14 (2): 389–395.

32 Oertel, M., Kelly, D.F., Lee, J.H. et al. (2002). Efficacy of hyperventilation, blood pressure elevation, and metabolic suppression therapy in controlling intracranial pressure after head injury. *J. Neurosurg.* 97 (5): 1045–1053.

33 Flood, P. and Shafer, S. (2015). Neurophysiology. In: *Stoelting's Pharmacology & Physiology in Anesthetic Practice*, 5e (eds. P. Flood, J. Rathmell, S. Shafer and R.K. Stoelting), 45–97. Philadelphia: Wolters Kluwer Health.

34 Godoy, D.A., Seifi, A., Garza, D. et al. (2017). Hyperventilation therapy for control of posttraumatic intracranial hypertension. *Front. Neurol.* 17 (8): 250.

35. Curley, G., Kavanagh, B.P., and Laffey, J.G. (2010). Hypocapnia and the injured brain: more harm than benefit. *Crit. Care Med.* 38 (5): 1348–1359.

36 Bagley, R.S., Keegan, R.D., Greene, S.A. et al. (1995). Intraoperative monitoring of intracranial pressure in five dogs with space-occupying intracranial lesions. *J. Am. Vet. Med. Assoc.* 207 (5): 588–591.

37 Rosner, M.J. and Coley, I. (1987). Cerebral perfusion pressure: a hemodynamic mechanism of mannitol and the post-mannitol hemogram. *Neurosurgery* 21: 147–156.

38 Hartwell, R.C. and Sutton, L.N. (1993). Mannitol, intracranial pressure, and vasogenic edema. *Neurosurgery* 32: 444–450.

39 Donato, T., Shapira, Y., Artru, A. et al. (1994). Effect of mannitol on cerebrospinal fluid dynamics and brain tissue edema. *Anesth. Analg.* 78 (1): 58–66.

40 Hastie, M. and Shanewise, J. (2015). Diuretics. In: *Stoelting's Pharmacology & Physiology in Anesthetic Practice*, 5e (eds. P. Flood, J. Rathmell and S. Shafer), 533–541. Philadelphia: Wolters Kluwer Health.

41 Palma, L., Bruni, G., Fiaschi, A.I. et al. (2006). Passage of mannitol into the brain around gliomas: a potential cause of rebound phenomenon. A study on 21 patients. *J. Neurosurg. Sci.* 50 (3): 63–66.

42 Prough, D.S., Johnson, J.C., Poole, G.V. Jr. et al. (1985). Effects on intracranial pressure

of resuscitation from hemorrhagic shock with hypertonic saline versus lactated Ringer's solution. *Crit. Care Med.* 13 (5): 407–411.

43 Gunnar, W., Jonasson, O., Merlotti, G. et al. (1988). Head injury and hemorrhagic shock: studies of the blood brain barrier and intracranial pressure after resuscitation with normal saline solution, 3% saline solution, and dextran-40. *Surgery* 103 (4): 398–407.

44 Qureshi, A.I., Wilson, D.A., and Traystman, R.J. (2002). Treatment of transtentorial herniation unresponsive to hyperventilation using hypertonic saline in dogs: effect on cerebral blood flow and metabolism. *J. Neurosurg. Anesthesiol.* 14 (1): 22–30.

45 Vialet, R., Albanese, J., Thomachot, L. et al. (2003). Isovolume hypertonic solutes (sodium chloride or mannitol) in the treatment of refractory post traumatic intracranial hypertension: 2 ml/kg 7.5% saline is more effective than 2 ml/kg 20% mannitol. *Crit. Care Med.* 31: 1683–1687.

46 Battison, C., Andrews, P.J., Graham, C. et al. (2005). Randomized, controlled trial on the effect of a 20% mannitol solution and a 7.5% saline/6% dextran solution on increased intracranial pressure after brain injury. *Crit. Care Med.* 33: 196–202.

47 Cottenceau, V., Masson, F., Mahamid, E. et al. (2011). Comparison of effects of equiosmolar doses of mannitol and hypertonic saline on cerebral blood flow and metabolism in traumatic brain injury. *J. Neurotrauma* 28: 2003–2012.

48 Alnemari, A.M., Krafcik, B.M., Mansour, T.R. et al. (2017). A comparison of pharmacologic therapeutic agents used for the reduction of intracranial pressure after traumatic brain injury. *World Neurosurg.* 106: 509–528.

49 Mangat, H.S. (2018). Hypertonic saline infusion for treating intracranial hypertension after severe traumatic brain injury. *Crit. Care* 22 (1): 37.

50 Ito, N., Suzuki, K., Koie, H. et al. (2006). The effect of 7.2% hypertonic saline solution on the duration of sodium gradient between the cerebrospinal fluid and the venous circulation in the dog. *J. Vet. Med. Sci.* 68 (2): 183–185.

51 Roquilly, A., Lasocki, S., Moyer, J.D. et al. (2017). COBI group COBI (COntinuous hyperosmolar therapy for traumatic Brain-Injured patients) trial protocol: a multicentre randomised open-label trial with blinded adjudication of primary outcome. *BMJ Open* 7 (9): e018035.

52 Tobias, K.M., Marioni-Henry, K., and Wagner, R. (2006). A retrospective study on the use of acepromazine maleate in dogs with seizures. *J. Am. Anim. Hosp. Assoc.* 42 (4): 283–289.

53 Zornow, M.H., Fleischer, J.E., Scheller, M.S. et al. (1990). Dexmedetomidine, an alpha 2-adrenergic agonist, decreases cerebral blood flow in the isoflurane-anesthetized dog. *Anesth. Analg.* 70 (6): 624–630.

54 Karlsson, B.R., Forsman, M., Roald, O.K. et al. (1990). Effect of dexmedetomidine, a selective and potent alpha 2-agonist, on cerebral blood flow and oxygen consumption during halothane anesthesia in dogs. *Anesth. Analg.* 71 (2): 125–129.

55 Yang, W., Kong, L.S., Zhu, X.X. et al. (2019). Effect of dexmedetomidine on postoperative cognitive dysfunction and inflammation in patients after general anaesthesia: a PRISMA-compliant systematic review and meta-analysis. *Medicine (Baltimore)* 98 (18): e15383.

56 Nugent, M., Artru, A.A., and Michenfelder, J.D. (1982). Cerebral metabolic, vascular and protective effects of midazolam maleate. *Anesthesiology* 56: 172–176.

57 KuKanich, B. and Wiese, A. Opioids. In: *Veterinary Anesthesia and Analgesia: The Fifth Edition of Lumb and Jones* (eds. K.A. Grimm, L.A. Lamont, W.J. Tranquilli, et al.), 207–226. Ames: Wiley Blackwell Publishing.

58 Valverde, A., Cantwell, S., Hernández, J. et al. (2004). Effects of acepromazine on the incidence of vomiting associated with opioid administration in dogs. *Vet. Anaesth. Analg.* 31 (1): 40–45.

59 Self, I.A., Hughes, J.M., Kenny, D.A. et al. (2009). Effect of muscle injection site on preanaesthetic sedation in dogs. *Vet. Rec.* 164 (11): 323–326.

60 Marsh, M.L., Marshall, L.F., and Shapiro, H.M. (1977). Neurosurgical intensive care. *Anesthesiology* 47 (2): 149–163.

61 Pierce, E.C. Jr., Lambertsen, C.J., Deutsch, S. et al. (1962). Cerebral circulation and metabolism during thiopental anesthesia and hyper-ventilation in man. *J. Clin. Invest.* 41: 1664–1671.

62 Prior, J.G., Hinds, C.J., Williams, J. et al. (1983). The use of etomidate in the management of severe head injury. *Intensive Care Med.* 9: 313–320.

63 Vandesteene, A., Trempont, V., Engelman, E. et al. (1988). Effect of propofol on cerebral blood flow and metabolism in man. *Anaesthesia* 43 (Suppl): 42–43.

64 Artru, A.A., Shapira, Y., and Bowdle, T.A. (1992). Electroencephalogram, cerebral metabolic, and vascular responses to propofol anesthesia in dogs. *J. Neurosurg. Anesthesiol.* 4 (2): 99–109.

65 Branson, K. (2007). Injectable and alternative anesthetic techniques. In: *Lumb and Jones' Veterinary Anesthesia and Analgesia*, 4e (eds. W.J. Tranquilli, J.C. Thurman and K.A. Grimm), 273–299. Ames: Blackwell Publishing.

66 Drummond, J.C. and Patel, P.M. (2010). Neurosurgical anesthesia. In: *Miller's Anesthesia*, 7e (eds. R.D. Miller, L.I. Eriksson, L.A. Fleischer, et al.), 2045–2087. Philadelphia: Elsevier.

67 Chang, L.C., Raty, S.R., Ortiz, J. et al. (2013). The emerging use of ketamine for anesthesia and sedation in traumatic brain injuries. *CNS Neurosci. Ther.* 19 (6): 390–395.

68 Zeiler, F.A., Sader, N., Gillman, L.M. et al. (2016). The cerebrovascular response to ketamine: a systematic review of the animal and human literature. *J. Neurosurg. Anesthesiol.* 28 (2): 123–140.

69 Cornelius, B.G., Webb, E., Cornelius, A. et al. (2018). Effect of sedative agent selection on morbidity, mortality and length of stay in patients with increase in intracranial pressure. *World J. Emerg. Med.* 9 (4): 256–261. https://doi.org/10.5847/wjem.j.1920-8642.2018.04.003.

70 Leng, T., Gao, X., Dilger, J.P., and Lin, J. (2016). Neuroprotective effect of lidocaine: is there clinical potential? *Int. J. Physiol. Pathophysiol. Pharmacol.* 8 (1): 9–13.

71 Preethi, J., Bidkar, P.U., Cherian, A. et al. (2019). Comparison of total intravenous anesthesia vs. inhalational anesthesia on brain relaxation, intracranial pressure, and hemodynamics in patients with acute subdural hematoma undergoing emergency craniotomy: a randomized control trial. *Eur. J. Trauma Emerg. Surg.* 47 (3): 831–837.

72 Drummond, J.C., Todd, M.M., Scheller, M.S. et al. (1986). A comparison of the direct cerebral vasodilating potencies of halothane and isoflurane in the New Zealand white rabbit. *Anesthesiology* 65: 462–468.

73 Sakabe, T., Kuramoto, T., Inoue, S. et al. (1978). Cerebral effects of nitrous oxide in the dog. *Anesthesiology* 48 (3): 195–200.

74 Patel, P.M., Drummond, J.C., and Lemkuil, B.P. (2020). Cerebral physiology and the effects of anesthetics and techniques. In: *Miller's Anesthesia*, 9e (eds. M.A. Gropper, N.H. Cohen, L.I. Eriksson, et al.), 294–332. Philadelphia: Elsevier.

75 Todd, M.M. and Drummond, J.C. (1984). A comparison of the cerebrovascular and metabolic effects of halothane and isoflurane in the cat. *Anesthesiology* 60: 276–282.

76 Scheller, M.S., Nakamura, K., Fleischer, J.E. et al. (1990). Cerebral effects of sevoflurane in the dog: comparison with isoflurane and enflurane. *Br. J. Anaesth.* 65 (3): 388–392.

77 Lutz, L.J., Milde, J.H., and Milde, L.N. (1990). The cerebral functional, metabolic, and hemodynamic effects of desflurane in dogs. *Anesthesiology* 73 (1): 125–131.

78 Scheller, M.S., Tateishi, A., Drummond, J.C. et al. (1988). The effects of sevoflurane on cerebral blood flow, cerebral metabolic rate for oxygen, intracranial pressure, and the electroencephalogram are similar to those of isoflurane in the rabbit. *Anesthesiology* 68: 548–552.

79 Cucchiara, R.F., Theye, R.A., and Michenfelder, J.D. (1974). The effects of isoflurane and canine cerebral metabolism and blood flow. *Anesthesiology* 40: 571–574.

80 Chohan, A.S., Greene, S.A., Keegan, R.D. et al. (2013). Intracranial pressure and cardiopulmonary variables during isoflurane or sevoflurane anesthesia at various minimum alveolar concentration multiples in normocapnic dogs. *Am. J. Vet. Res.* 74 (3): 369–374.

81 Artru, A.A. (1983). Relationship between cerebral blood volume and CSF pressure during anesthesia with halothane or enflurane in dogs. *Anesthesiology* 58 (5): 33–39.

82 Drummond, J.C. and Todd, M.M. (1985). The response of the feline cerebral circulation to $PaCO_2$ during anesthesia with isoflurane and halothane and during sedation with nitrous oxide. *Anesthesiology* 62: 268–273.

83 Makarenko, S., Griesdale, D.E., Gooderham, P. et al. (2016). Multimodal neuromonitoring for traumatic brain injury: a shift towards individualized therapy. *J. Clin. Neurosci.* 26: 8–13.

84 Shackford, S.R., Mackersie, R.C., Davis, J.W. et al. (1989). Epidemiology and pathology of traumatic deaths occurring at a level I trauma center in a regionalized system: the importance of secondary brain injury. *J. Trauma* 29: 1392–1397.

85 Pietropaoli, J.A., Rogers, F.M., Shackford, S.R. et al. (1992). The deleterious effects of intraoperative hypotension on outcome in patients with severe head injuries. *J. Trauma* 33: 403–407.

86 Jones, P.A., Andrews, P.J., Midgley, S. et al. (1994). Measuring the burden of secondary insults in head-injured patients during intensive care. *J. Neurosurg. Anesthesiol.* 6: 4–14.

87 McNally, E.M., Robertson, S.A., and Pablo, L.S. (2009). Comparison of time to desaturation between preoxygenated and non-preoxygenated dogs following sedation with acepromazine maleate and morphine and induction of anesthesia with propofol. *Am. J. Vet. Res.* 70 (11): 1333–1338.

88 Platt, S.R., Radaelli, S.T., and McDonnell, J.J. (2001). The prognostic value of the modified Glasgow Coma Scale in head trauma in dogs. *J. Vet. Intern. Med.* 15 (6): 581–584.

89 Troxel, M.T., Vite, C.H., Van Winkle, T.J. et al. (2003). Feline intracranial neoplasia: retrospective review of 160 cases (1985–2001). *J. Vet. Intern. Med.* 17 (6): 850–859.

90 Snyder, J.M., Shofer, F.S., Van Winkle, T.J. et al. (2006). Canine intracranial primary neoplasia: 173 cases (1986–2003). *J. Vet. Intern. Med.* 20 (3): 669–675.

91 Tomek, A., Cizinauskas, S., Doherr, M. et al. (2006). Intracranial neoplasia in 61 cats: localisation, tumour types and seizure patterns. *J. Feline Med. Surg.* 8 (4): 243–253.

92 Greco, J.J., Aiken, S.A., Berg, J.M. et al. (2006). Evaluation of intracranial meningioma resection with a surgical aspirator in dogs: 17 cases (1996–2004). *J. Am. Vet. Med. Assoc.* 229 (3): 394–400.

93 Negrin, A., Cherubini, G.B., Lamb, C. et al. (2010). Clinical signs, magnetic resonance imaging findings and outcome in 77 cats with vestibular disease: a retrospective study. *J. Feline Med. Surg.* 12 (4): 291–299.

94 Dewey, C.W. (2006). Anticonvulsant therapy in dogs and cats. *Vet. Clin. North Am. Small Anim. Pract.* 36 (5): 1107–1127.

95 Fletcher, D. (2010). Seizures and anticonvulsant therapy. In: *16th International Veterinary Emergency and Critical Care Society Proceedings*, 325–328. San Antonio: The international Veterinary Emergency and Critical Care Society.

96 Mathews, K.A. (2008). Neuropathic pain in dogs and cats: if only they could tell us if they hurt. *Vet. Clin. North Am. Small Anim. Pract.* 38 (6): 1365–1414.

97 Lu, D., Lamb, C.R., Pfeiffer, D.U. et al. (2003). Neurological signs and results of magnetic resonance imaging in 40 Cavalier King Charles spaniels with Chiari type 1-like malformations. *Vet. Rec.* 153 (9): 260–263.

98 Rusbridge, C., MacSweeney, E. Jr., Davies, J.V. et al. (2000). Syringohydromyelia in Cavalier King Charles spaniels. *J. Am. Anim. Hosp. Assoc.* 36: 64–65.

99 Rusbridge, C. (2007). Chiari-like malformation with syringomyelia in the Cavalier King Charles spaniel: long-term outcome after surgical management. *Vet. Surg.* 36: 396–405.

100 Jeffery, N.D. (2010). Vertebral fracture and luxation in small animals. *Vet. Clin. North Am. Small Anim. Pract.* 40 (5): 809–828.

101 Harrison, R.L., Clark, L., and Corletto, F. (2012). Comparison of mean heart rate in anaesthetized dachshunds and other breeds of dog undergoing spinal magnetic resonance imaging. *Vet. Anaesth. Analg.* 39 (3): 230–235.

102 Redondo, J.I., Suesta, P., Serra, I. et al. (2012). Retrospective study of the prevalence of postanaesthetic hypothermia in cats. *Vet. Rec.* 170 (8): 206.

103. Redondo, J.I., Suesta, P., Serra, I. et al. (2012). Retrospective study of the prevalence of postanaesthetic hypothermia in dogs. *Vet. Rec.* 171 (15): 374.

104 Steinbacher, R., Mosing, M., Eberspächer, E. et al. (2010). Perioperative use of fluid warmers reduces hypothermia in cats. *Tierarztl. Prax. Ausg. K Kleintiere Heimtiere* 38 (1): 15–22.

105 Kibanda, J.O. and Gurney, M. (2012). Comparison of two methods for the management of intraoperative hypothermia in dogs. *Vet. Rec.* 170 (15): 392.

106 Mitchell, S.L., McCarthy, R., Rudloff, E. et al. (2000). Tracheal rupture associated with intubation in cats: 20 cases (1996–1998). *J. Am. Vet. Med. Assoc.* 216 (10): 1592–1595.

107 Alderson, B., Senior, J.M., and Dugdale, A.H. (2006). Tracheal necrosis following tracheal intubation in a dog. *J. Small Anim. Pract.* 47 (12): 754–756.

108 Java, M.A., Drobatz, K.J., Gilley, R.S. et al. (2009). Incidence of and risk factors for postoperative pneumonia in dogs anesthetized for diagnosis or treatment of intervertebral disk disease. *J. Am. Vet. Med. Assoc.* 235 (3): 281–287.

109 Lexmaulova, L., Zatloukal, J., Proks, P. et al. (2009). Incidence of seizures associated with iopamidol or iomeprol myelography in dogs with intervertebral disk disease: 161 cases (2000–2002). *J. Vet. Emerg. Crit. Care. (San Antonio)* 19 (6): 611–616.

110 da Costa, R.C., Parent, J.M., and Dobson, H. (2011). Incidence of and risk factors for seizures after myelography performed with iohexol in dogs: 503 cases (2002–2004). *J. Am. Vet. Med. Assoc.* 238 (10): 1296–1300.

111 Full, A.M., Heller, H.L., and Mercier, M. (2016). Prevalence, clinical presentation, prognosis, and outcome of 17 dogs with spinal shock and acute thoracolumbar spinal cord disease. *J. Vet. Emerg. Crit. Care (San Antonio)* 26 (3): 412–418.

112 Longshore, R.C., O'Brien, D.P., Johnson, G.C. et al. (1996). Dysautonomia in dogs: a retrospective study. *J. Vet. Intern. Med.* 10: 103–109.

113 Harkin, K.R., Andrews, G.A., and Nietfeld, J.C. (2002). Dysautonomia in dogs: 65 cases (1993–2000). *J. Am. Vet. Med. Assoc.* 220 (5): 633–639.

114 Kidder, A.C., Johannes, C., O'Brien, D.P. et al. (2008). Feline dysautonomia in the Midwestern United States: a retrospective study of nine cases. *J. Feline Med. Surg.* 10 (2): 130–136.

115 Zacuto, A.C., Marks, S.L., Osborn, J. et al. (2012). The influence of esomeprazole and cisapride on gastroesophageal reflux during anesthesia in dogs. *J. Vet. Intern. Med.* 26 (3): 518–525.

116 Smith, C.E., Donati, F., and Bevan, D.R. (1989). Cumulative dose-response curves for atracurium in patients with myasthenia gravis. *Can. J. Anaesth.* 36 (4): 402–406.

117 Nilsson, E. and Meretoja, O.A. (1990). Vecuronium dose-response and maintenance requirements in patients with myasthenia gravis. *Anesthesiology* 73: 28–32.

118 Jones, R.S., Brown, A., and Watkins, P.E. (1988). Use of muscle relaxant atracurium in a myasthenic dog. *Vet. Rec.* 122: 611.

119 Marschall, K.E. (2018). Skin and musculoskeletal diseases. In: *Stoelting's Anesthesia and Co-existing Disease*, 7e (eds. R. Hines and K. Marschall), 507–538. Philadelphia: Elsevier.

120 Eisenkraft, J.B., Book, W.J., Mann, S.M. et al. (1988). Resistance to succinylcholine in myasthenia gravis. *Anesthesiology* 69: 760–763.

121 Cavana, P., Sammartano, F., Capucchio, M.T. et al. (2009). Peripheral neuropathy in a cat with renal lymphoma. *J. Feline Med. Surg.* 11 (10): 869–872.

122 Kramek, B.A., Moise, N.S., Cooper, B. et al. (1984). Neuropathy associated with diabetes mellitus in the cat. *J. Am. Vet. Med. Assoc.* 184 (1): 42–45.

123 Morgan, M.J., Vite, C.H., Radhakrishnan, A. et al. (2008). Clinical peripheral neuropathy associated with diabetes mellitus in 3 dogs. *Can. Vet. J.* 49 (6): 583–586.

124 Griffiths, I.R., Duncan, I.D., and Swallow, J.S. (1977). Peripheral polyneuropathies in dogs: a study of five cases. *J. Small Anim. Pract.* 18: 101–116.

125 Cardinet, G.H. and Holliday, T.A. (1979). Neuromuscular diseases of domestic animals: a summary of muscle biopsies from 159 cases. *Ann. N.Y. Acad. Sci.* 317: 290–313.

126 Chrisman, C.L. (1980). Postoperative results and complications of insulinomas in dogs. *J. Am. Anim. Hosp. Assoc.* 16: 677–684.

127 Sorjonen, D.C., Braund, K.G., and Hoff, E.J. (1982). Paraplegia and subclinical neuromyopathy associated with a primary lung tumor in a dog. *J. Am. Vet. Med. Assoc.* 180: 1209–1211.

128 Shahar, R., Rousseaux, C., and Steiss, J. (1985). Peripheralpolyneuropathy in a dog with functional islet B-cell tumor and widespread metastasis. *J. Am. Vet. Med. Assoc.* 187: 175–177.

129 Dyer, K.R., Duncan, I.D., Hammang, J.P. et al. (1986). Peripheral neuropathy in two dogs: correlation between clinical, electrophysiological and pathological findings. *J. Small Anim. Pract.* 27: 133–146.

130 Presthus, J. and Teige, J. (1986). Peripheral neuropathy associated with lymphosarcoma in a dog. *J. Small Anim. Pract.* 27: 463–469.

131 Braund, K.G., McGuire, J.A., Amling, K.A. et al. (1987). Peripheral neuropathy associated with malignant neoplasms in dogs. *Vet. Pathol.* 24 (1): 16–21.

132 Braund, K.G., Steiss, J.E., Amling, K.A. et al. (1987). Insulinoma and subclinical peripheral neuropathy in two dogs. *J. Vet. Int. Med.* 1: 86–90.

133 Braund, K.G. (1990). Remote effects of cancer on the nervous system. *Semin. Vet. Med. Surg. (Small Anim.)* 5 (4): 262–270.

134 Villiers, E. and Dobson, J. (1998). Multiple myeloma with associated polyneuropathy in a German shepherd dog. *J. Small Anim. Pract.* 39 (5): 249–251.

135 Mariani, C.L., Shelton, S.B., and Alsup, J.C. (1999). Paraneoplastic polyneuropathy and subsequent recovery following tumor removal in a dog. *J. Am. Anim. Hosp. Assoc.* 35 (4): 302–305.

136 Fikes, L.L., Dodman, N.H., and Court, M.H. (1990). Anaesthesia for small animal patients with neuromuscular disease. *Br. Vet. J.* 146: 487–499.

137 Bradley, R.L., Withrow, S.J., and Snyder, S.P. (1982). Nerve sheath tumors in the dog. *J. Am. Anim. Hosp. Assoc.* 18: 915–921.

138 Terrando, N., Brzezinski, M., Degos, V. et al. (2011). Perioperative cognitive decline in the aging population. *Mayo Clin. Proc.* 86 (9): 885–893.

139 Tsai, T.L., Sands, L.P., and Leung, J.M. (2010). An update on postoperative cognitive dysfunction. *Adv. Anesth.* 28 (1): 269–284.

140 Wang, H.L., Ma, R.H., Fang, H. et al. (2015). Impaired spatial learning memory after isoflurane anesthesia or appendectomy in aged mice is associated with microglia activation. *J. Cell Death* 8: 9–19.

141 Kawano, T., Yamanaka, D., Aoyama, B. et al. (2018). Involvement of acute neuroinflammation in postoperative delirium-like cognitive deficits in rats. *J. Anesth.* 32 (4): 506–517.

142 Li, J., Zhu, X., Yang, S. et al. (2019). Lidocaine attenuates cognitive impairment after isoflurane anesthesia by reducing mitochondrial damage. *Neurochem. Res.* 44 (7): 1703–1714.

143 Cheng, B., Zhang, Y., Wang, A. et al. (2015). Vitamin C attenuates isoflurane-induced caspase-3 activation and cognitive impairment. *Mol. Neurobiol.* 52 (3): 1580–1589.

4

Hepatobiliary Disease

Carrie A. Schroeder

Department of Surgical Sciences, School of Veterinary Medicine, University of Wisconsin, Madison, WI, 53706, USA

Introduction

The liver is a highly complex organ that is vital to several functions. Derangements in hepatic function can present many challenges to the anesthetist. Liver dysfunction can range from an elevation in liver enzymes with no clinical disease to fulminant liver failure. Fortunately, veterinary patients rarely present for anesthesia with severe liver disorders leading to hepatic failure such as cirrhosis or hepatitis. However, many liver conditions require surgical interventions such as liver biopsy or portosystemic venous shunt attenuation, and thus require sedation or general anesthesia. The anesthetist must understand the disease extent, the abnormalities associated with the disease, and their repercussions on drug metabolism and patient homeostasis before formulating an anesthetic plan.

Anatomy and Physiology

Blood flow to the liver comprises 25–30% of total cardiac output and is provided via dual blood supplies: the hepatic artery and portal vein. The portal vein accounts for 75% of the blood flow, but, owing to the relatively low oxygen saturation of portal venous blood, provides only 50–55% of hepatic oxygen requirements. However, the hepatic artery provides only 25% of blood flow, but 45–50% of oxygen requirements. Owing to the constitutively high hepatic blood flow, increases in hepatic oxygen demand are met with increased oxygen extraction from the blood rather than further increases in blood flow to the organ itself [1].

Under normal circumstances, decreases in cardiac output or systemic blood pressure with accompanying decreases in portal venous flow are usually compensated for by increases in hepatic arterial flow. The hepatic vasculature is richly innervated with alpha-1-adrenergic receptors; sympathetic nervous system activation results in hepatic artery vasoconstriction and, therefore, reduced hepatic blood flow [2]. Hepatic blood flow is also decreased in the face of increased portal pressure and is directly related to central venous pressure (CVP); such increases in CVP may be associated with congestive heart failure or positive pressure ventilation. Circumstances such as these will impair outflow of blood from the liver, increasing portal venous pressure and decreasing hepatic blood flow.

In healthy animals, the liver provides multiple essential functions, which include bile for-

Canine and Feline Anesthesia and Co-Existing Disease, Second Edition. Edited by Rebecca A. Johnson, Lindsey B. C. Snyder and Carrie A. Schroeder.

Companion website: www.wiley.com/go/johnson/canine

mation and excretion, metabolic functions, plasma protein synthesis, and glycogen storage. Although the liver serves a wide array of functions, it has substantial reserve, and significant disease may be present before clinical abnormalities are evident. Bile salts and acids are synthesized in hepatocytes, and bile is carried from hepatic lobules by bile ducts, with the gallbladder serving as a reservoir in most species. The common bile duct releases bile into the duodenum on relaxation of the sphincter of Oddi. Morphine administration may cause spasm of the sphincter of Oddi in several species and was once contraindicated in the face of acute pancreatitis [3]. However, human research suggests that morphine is safe for analgesic use in acute pancreatitis and there is no clinical evidence to avoid the use of morphine in patients with hepatobiliary disease for this reason (see the section titled "Opioids") [4].

Multiple enzymatic pathways are present in the liver, thereby metabolizing carbohydrates, proteins, fats, and pharmacological agents. Carbohydrate metabolism results in glucose synthesis and its storage in the form of glycogen. Abnormalities in glucogenesis can lead to hypoglycemia, a common presenting complaint in patients with severe hepatic dysfunction. Protein metabolism through deamination provides further vital energy substrates to the organism but produces ammonia as a byproduct. Under normal circumstances, ammonia is cleared from the body, but can be elevated in certain hepatic disease states and is a key contributor in the clinical presentation of hepatic encephalopathy (HE) [5]. Anesthetic and analgesic agent metabolism may also be impaired in the patient with hepatic disease, leading to prolonged drug effects. With few exceptions, most anesthetic agents undergo hepatic biotransformation to active or inactive compounds. Many of these reactions rely on the hepatic cytochrome P450 enzymes (CYP). The hepatic CYP enzymes can be induced by drugs such as barbiturates and inhibited by multiple drugs such as chloramphenicol, ketoconazole, and cimetidine (Table 4.1) [6–10]. Enzyme induction can cause a degree of drug tolerance and cross-tolerance, thus requiring an increase in patient drug dosages, especially with chronic administration of enzyme inducers such as phenobarbital. Conversely, drug dosages should be decreased when enzyme inhibitors have been chronically administered, as enzyme inhibition may lead to a decrease in hepatic drug metabolism. Greyhounds appear to have decreased CYP activity, accounting in part for the increased anesthetic drug duration observed in this breed [8, 10–12]. This has been extrapolated to all members of the sighthound family; drugs that rely heavily on the CYP system for biotransformation, such as methadone, should be titrated carefully in these breeds to avoid an exaggerated response [10].

Table 4.1 Enzyme inhibitors and inducers commonly encountered in veterinary medicine.

Enzyme inhibitors	Enzyme inducers
Ciprofloxacin	Rifampicin
Erythromycin	Phenytoin
Chloramphenicol	Phenobarbital
Ketoconazole	Omeprazole
Itraconazole	St. John's wort
Fluconazole	Insulin
Fluoxetine	Dexamethasone
Omeprazole	Tramadol
Cimetidine	
Ranitidine	
Quinidine	
Amiodarone	
Chlorpromazine	
Methadone	
Propofol	
Synthetic cannabinoids	

Note that some pharmacological agents may act as both an enzyme inhibitor and an inducer, depending on the CYP enzyme form [6].

One of the most vital roles of the liver is protein synthesis. Nearly all proteins are formed in the liver. This includes albumin, coagulation factors, and cholinesterase [2]. Albumin is critical in providing plasma oncotic pressure and transport of multiple substances including anesthetic drugs. Hypoalbuminemia, azotemia, and acidosis reduce drug binding to albumin. This subsequently increases the free, unbound drug portion and potentially increases the drug effect. Albumin has a half-life of approximately 21 days; due to this prolonged half-life, acute liver disease typically will not manifest with hypoalbuminemia [1]. By contrast, all coagulation factors except III, IV, and VIII (thromboplastin, calcium, and von Willebrand factor) are synthesized by hepatocytes and, unlike albumin, have relatively short half-lives; coagulation factors may be affected by acute liver disease [2, 6]. While liver dysfunction is often associated with prolonged coagulation times, various liver disease states may trigger a hypercoagulable state [13]. Patients with acute liver dysfunction should have coagulation testing performed before anesthesia and surgery. In addition to coagulations times such as prothrombin time (PT) and partial thromboplastin time (PTT), assays that evaluate the dynamic process of coagulation, such as thromboelastography (TEG), may be indicated if coagulopathy is suspected (see Chapter 14).

Table 4.2 Biochemical markers and commonly encountered abnormalities associated with hepatic dysfunction.

Biochemical markers	Clinical signs and abnormalities
↑ Ammonia	Hepatic encephalopathy
↑ Bile acids	Ascites
↓ BUN	Hypotension
↓ Cholesterol	Impaired drug biotransformation
↓ Blood glucose	Coagulopathy
↓ Serum albumin	
↑ Coagulation times (PT/PTT)	
↓ K	
↑ AST, ALT, ALP, GGT (nonspecific and often do not reflect true liver function)	

Markers of Hepatic Dysfunction

Unfortunately, biochemical markers of hepatic dysfunction can be both nonspecific and insensitive (Table 4.2). Liver function tests include serum albumin, ammonia, bile acids, blood glucose, blood urea nitrogen (BUN), and cholesterol measurements [14]. Owing to variability in serum half-lives, deviations in these markers of hepatic function may not be present immediately. Due to the relatively long half-life of albumin (approximately 21 days), hypoalbuminemia may not be seen until hypoglycemia, hypocholesterolemia, and decreased BUN become evident. Coagulation factors have a relatively short half-life, and as previously mentioned, abnormal coagulation may appear with acute disease. As abnormalities associated with liver disease may induce a hypocoagulable or hypercoagulable state, the patient's overall coagulation status is best performed by TEG; however, many clinically relevant coagulopathies may be detected by evaluation of PT/PTT, platelet count, and fibrinogen measurement [15, 16].

Hepatic enzyme elevations suggest hepatocellular damage rather than true dysfunction. The laboratory abnormalities associated with hepatocellular injury and evaluation of serum biomarkers of hepatocellular damage have been reviewed elsewhere [14]. In short, serum aminotransferases such as aspartate aminotransferase (AST) and alanine aminotransferase (ALT) are released with hepatocellular injury and are of some diagnostic use. AST is present in the liver as well as multiple extrahepatic sites, such as skeletal muscle and erythrocytes. ALT is found in large concentrations within hepatocytes and, as such, is more specific for hepatocellular damage that AST [14]. The absolute values of these enzymes can be related to the extent of hepatocellular injury but not the reversibility of injury; in general, injury that is less extensive is associated with a more minor increase in measured value as compared to the more significant enzyme elevations associated with widespread hepatocellular injury [14]. Serum alkaline phosphatase (ALP) is produced by the liver, bone, small intestine, and kidney. Mild elevations in this enzyme are consistent with hepatocellular injury, but elevations may also be present in pediatric patients, patients with bone disease, or patients chronically administered drugs such as phenobarbital, phenytoin, and corticosteroids [14]. Increased γ-glutamyl transferase (GGT) is generally associated with cholestasis or biliary hyperplasia and is a more sensitive biomarker for hepatobiliary disease than ALP in cats [14].

A more sensitive and specific test for hepatobiliary dysfunction is preprandial and postprandial measurement of bile acids. Elevations in preprandial and postprandial bile acids can be present in portal venous shunts, cirrhosis, hepatic necrosis, and inflammation, steroid hepatopathy, cholestasis, and intestinal obstruction [17].

Ultimately, it is difficult to definitively diagnose hepatobiliary disease solely based on blood work. Diagnosis should be made by careful physical examination and clinical presentation in addition to biochemical evaluation. Diagnostic imaging, such as abdominal ultrasound or computed tomography (CT), and hepatic biopsy may be necessary to provide a definitive diagnosis.

Perioperative Effects on Hepatic Function

General Anesthetic Effects

Of the modern anesthetics, there is limited direct adverse impact on hepatic function. However, it is important to note that nearly all injectable anesthetics and analgesics rely on varying degrees of hepatic biotransformation for drug elimination. While hepatic injury may not adversely impact the enzymatic processes of the liver, disease states that impact hepatic function such as portosystemic shunt (PSS) may result in altered drug pharmacokinetics and exaggerated or prolonged anesthetic effects. More common than true alterations in hepatic function are alterations in hepatic blood flow associated with general anesthesia. Decreases in cardiac output and mean arterial pressure by volatile anesthetics subsequently decrease portal blood flow in a dose-dependent manner [2, 18]. Modern volatile anesthetics better preserve hepatic arterial blood flow, largely preserving total hepatic blood flow [18]; however, the overall impact of general anesthesia may result in altered drug pharmacokinetics administered in the perioperative period. Drugs with a low intrinsic clearance, with little reliance on the liver for metabolism, are minimally affected by changes in hepatic blood flow; drugs with a high intrinsic clearance are directly impacted by changes in hepatic blood flow [19]. Drugs with low intrinsic clearance relative to total hepatic blood flow, such as theophylline, will likely not have alterations in pharmacokinetics, while drugs with high intrinsic clearance relative to hepatic blood flow, such as morphine and ketamine, may have exaggerated or prolonged effects in the perioperative period. A number of other factors, including extrahepatic clearance of drugs, protein binding, and autoregulation of local blood flow, can profoundly affect anesthetic agent biotransformation and it may be difficult to predict the true clinical effects that may result from anesthetic-induced alterations in hepatic blood flow. As is the case in when approaching an anesthetic plan in nearly all patients with coexisting diseases; an individualized plan, the use of agents with drug antagonists, and careful anesthetic titration are key to successful management in the perioperative period.

Mechanical or assisted ventilation using high peak inspiratory pressures, mean pressures, and/or positive end-expiratory pressures (PEEP) reduce hepatic blood flow because of venous congestion and decreases in both cardiac output and portal blood flow [20, 21]. On the other hand, hypercarbia, which can be associated with spontaneous ventilation under general anesthesia, can also decrease hepatic blood flow [22]. Since the liver and diaphragm/thoracic cavity are in close proximity, surgical manipulation may impinge on lung and thoracic wall excursions, resulting in hypoventilation. Care must be taken to reduce the mechanical restriction of breathing, especially in small patients. Mechanical ventilation may therefore be indicated in these cases. However, close peak airway pressure monitoring is necessary to avoid barotrauma and to avoid unnecessarily high airway pressures.

Surgical Effects

Not only can perfusion of the liver and other organs be compromised by factors associated with general anesthesia, but the stress associated with surgery as well as mechanical factors can greatly impact hepatic blood flow. The hepatic vasculature is richly innervated with alpha-1-adrenergic receptors; activation of the sympathetic nervous system associated with surgical stress and pain may lead to catecholamine release resulting in an initial vasoconstriction, thereby reducing hepatic arterial flow [2]. Intra-abdominal surgery can result in decreased hepatic blood flow due to the direct compression of hepatic vasculature by surgical manipulation; direct compression of vasculature leading to the liver either by manipulation of large tumors or by surgical instruments or hands may temporarily decrease arterial supply, portal blood flow, or venous return. Abdominal insufflation, utilized with laparoscopic techniques, may induce temporary increases in intra-abdominal pressure (IAP) that may compromise splanchnic and abdominal organ blood flow. Intra-abdominal hypertension (IAH) is defined as a sustained elevation in IAP above 12 mmHg, while pressures greater than 20 mmHg define abdominal compartment syndrome [23]. Most laparoscopic surgeries do not result in sustained pressures that may compromise blood flow, but other perioperative conditions such as fluid or blood accumulation, bowel distension, or abdominal wall rigidity may result in sustained IAH. Unfortunately, noninvasive means of measuring IAP are not readily available, but it is important to note that consequences of surgical interventions on hepatic blood flow may reach into the postoperative period and result in increased morbidity [23, 24].

Hepatic Dysfunction and Pharmacological Agents

Sedative Agents

Phenothiazines

Acepromazine is commonly used in veterinary medicine for its sedative properties. Acepromazine is a phenothiazine derivative that causes dopaminergic and alpha-1-adrenergic receptor blockade, leading to vasodilation [25]. Drug metabolism is via hepatic biotransformation, and no antagonist is available. As such, caution should be exercised when administering this agent to patients with hepatobiliary disease. The direct effects of acepromazine on hepatic blood flow and hepatic function have not been well characterized in veterinary medicine. The combined administration of ketamine, xylazine, and acepromazine does not appear to have adverse effects on liver function, graft liver regeneration, inflammatory response, or hepatic pathologic changes in rodent hepatic transplantation studies [26]. However, acepromazine should be used with caution in patients with hepatic disease; the vasodilation associated with acepromazine administration may lead to systemic hypotension [25]. Patients with hypoalbuminemia and/or patients presenting with PSS may have preexisting hypotension due to a decrease in colloidal osmotic pressure; acepromazine administration may further decrease systemic blood pressure. Furthermore, the coadministration of acepromazine and atropine induces abnormalities in platelet aggregation [27]. However, subsequent research evaluating the platelet function following acepromazine administration by TEG failed to detect platelet function inhibition in normal dogs [28]. Since patients with hepatic dysfunction may present with coagulopathies, caution should be exercised with acepromazine administration in the face of coagulation disorders or before procedures such as ultrasound-guided liver biopsy. Caution should also be exercised in acepromazine administration prior to laparoscopic procedures, as systemic vasodilation may lead to splenic engorgement, decreasing visibility, or limiting available access points in the abdomen.

Alpha-2-Adrenergic Receptor Agonists

Alpha-2-adrenergic receptor agonists such as dexmedetomidine offer excellent sedative properties at the cost of significant cardiovascular depression. Alpha-2-adrenergic receptor agonists significantly decrease heart rate and cardiac output while increasing systemic vascular resistance [29–31]. Dogs administered dexmedetomidine under experimental conditions demonstrated a delay in contrast delivery to the liver, suggesting decreased blood flow that was not antagonized by MK-467, a peripheral alpha-2-adrenergic antagonist [32]. However, most studies suggest that hepatic blood flow may be well-preserved. For example, dogs undergoing thoracotomy did not show significant decreases in hepatic blood flow after dexmedetomidine administration, and hepatic blood flow was preserved in human patients in early stages of septic shock when a dexmedetomidine infusion was administered. [33]. In fact, there are liver-protective and other organ-protective effects associated with dexmedetomidine administration [34].

Dexmedetomidine metabolism relies on hepatic biotransformation, but alpha-2-adrenergic receptor antagonists such as atipamezole are available in the event of increased effect or duration of effects. Overall, dexmedetomidine does not appear to have negative effects on the liver and is not contraindicated in patients with liver disease. However, caution should be used, as this agent can induce extreme sedation and cardiovascular depression and has not been extensively evaluated in veterinary clinical patients with preexisting liver disease. Careful dosage titration to the desired clinical effect and close monitoring of sedated patients are advised.

Benzodiazepines

The benzodiazepines, such as midazolam and diazepam, exert their sedative effect via enhancement of endogenous inhibitory neurotransmitter enhancement, namely, gamma-aminobutyric acid (GABA) [35]. These agents have minimal cardiovascular effects and are generally well tolerated in patients with many disease states [36]. However, fulminant liver failure has been associated with oral administration of diazepam in cats [37]. This adverse event has not been reported after oral administration of alprazolam or parenteral administration of diazepam or midazolam, and both are considered safe for administration in the perioperative period. Metabolism occurs through hepatic biotransformation and a GABA receptor antagonist, flumazenil, is available if sedation is prolonged or excessive.

Benzodiazepine administration for preoperative sedation of most patients with liver dysfunction is an excellent choice. However, care must be exercised in patients with HE. Neurons from animals with HE have increased sensitivity to benzodiazepines and increased "GABAergic tone" due to the presence of endogenous benzodiazepines, and the administration of exogenous benzodiazepines can aggravate HE [38]. The benzodiazepine antagonist flumazenil temporarily alleviates the HE symptoms, although there is no evidence for its use in providing long-term management [39, 40]. Owing to the effect of HE on the benzodiazepine sensitivity, diazepam and midazolam dosages should be closely considered and may need to be greatly decreased or avoided in animals demonstrating hepatic encephalopathic signs.

Opioids

Opioids are classified based on their effects on opioid receptors [41]. Mu-opioid agonists exert a pharmacological effect via activation of the mu-opioid receptor; these agents include, but are not limited to, morphine, hydromorphone, fentanyl, and methadone. Butorphanol, classified as an opioid agonist–antagonist, acts as an antagonist at the mu-opioid receptor and as an agonist at the kappa-opioid receptor. Buprenorphine is a partial agonist at the mu-opioid receptor and, as such, exhibits a submaximal clinical response.

In general, opioids are safe for use in patients with liver disease. Most opioids rely on hepatic biotransformation, and the duration of effect may be prolonged in cases of liver dysfunction [42]. Similar to benzodiazepines, patients with HE may demonstrate an increased sensitivity to opioids, owing to increased opioid receptor density in the brain [43]. In patients with significant liver function compromise, drug dosages may need to be decreased and carefully titrated to effect. Naloxone, a nonselective opioid receptor antagonist, may be given if drug duration is prolonged or opioid agonist effects are profound. However, one must consider that most analgesic effects may also be reversed with the administration of naloxone. Locoregional anesthesia can supplement analgesic needs without inducing protracted sedation or systemic effects; for instance, the epidural administration of morphine successfully provides postoperative analgesic needs for patients undergoing surgical PSS attenuation [44].

As discussed previously, morphine contracts the sphincter of Oddi in several species, increasing biliary pressure [3]. Although previously considered unsafe for use in patients with acute pancreatitis, human research suggests that morphine is indeed safe for analgesic use in these cases [4]. At this time, there is no clinical evidence to suggest that morphine should be avoided in patients with hepatobiliary disease.

Most opioids primarily undergo hepatic biotransformation followed by renal excretion. Remifentanil is a notable exception: metabolism is entirely extrahepatic, via ester hydrolysis [45]. It has an ultrashort duration of approximately 5 min and should be administered as a constant rate infusion to provide analgesia of any appreciable duration [46]. Remifentanil is advantageous in animals with liver disease, as duration of effect should be unchanged in the presence of liver dysfunction. In humans, duration and drug clearance were unchanged in severe, chronic liver disease and during the anhepatic phase of liver transplantation [47, 48]. Remifentanil has an isoflurane-sparing effect in both dogs and cats and has been used in combination with isoflurane to provide anesthesia for liver biopsy in dogs [49–52]. As significant respiratory depression and bradycardia can result with bolus administration, close cardiovascular and ventilatory status monitoring is imperative, as anticholinergic administration and positive pressure ventilation may be required.

Nonsteroidal Anti-Inflammatory Agents

Nonsteroidal anti-inflammatory drugs (NSAIDs) are a critical component of most perioperative analgesic regimens and are administered chronically in many patients presenting for surgery and anesthesia. Using clinically relevant dosages, all NSAIDs have the potential to cause idiosyncratic hepatotoxicity with clinical signs of hepatic dysfunction and liver enzyme elevation, largely due to oxidative stress [53, 54]. Dogs treated with carprofen for postoperative pain exhibited acute ALT elevations without any clinical indicators of hepatobiliary dysfunction, while dogs chronically treated with carprofen did not demonstrate elevations in liver enzymes [55, 56]. In another study of long-term administration of NSAIDs, meloxicam and etodolac were associated with increased GGT levels [57]. Overall, although not contraindicated, caution should be used when administering NSAIDs to animals with liver disease owing to the potential for this hepatotoxicity or oxidative stress. Furthermore, NSAIDs may adversely affect platelet aggregation. Platelet dysfunction occurred in dogs after administration of deracoxib and coagulation; coagulation times were increased in dogs receiving long-term carprofen, meloxicam, ketoprofen, and flunixin [57–59]. As liver disease may be accompanied by impaired coagulation and multiple NSAIDs have been implicated in causing platelet dysfunction, it is prudent to avoid NSAIDs in cases of hepatic dysfunction with coagulopathy.

Induction Agents

Alfaxalone

Alfaxalone is a synthetic neurosteroid that rapidly induces anesthesia through interactions with $GABA_A$ receptor in the central nervous system [60]. It is rapidly biotransformed by the liver, although less significant extrahepatic metabolism may also be involved [60, 61]. Cardiovascular and respiratory effects include dose-dependent and generally well-tolerated decreases in cardiac output, systemic vascular resistance, and mean arterial pressure, as well as respiratory depression [60]. No studies have evaluated the direct effect on hepatic blood flow in veterinary species, but there is no evidence that hepatic blood flow decreases out of proportion to cardiac output and there is no evidence for contraindications in patients with hepatobiliary disease. As is recommended for most anesthetic induction agents, careful titration to effect in hemodynamically stabilized and preoxygenated patients is the key to successful administration with minimal adverse effects.

Propofol

Propofol similarly provides hypnosis and rapid induction through $GABA_A$ interactions [62]. It is rapidly metabolized in the liver to inactive metabolites; extrahepatic metabolism occurs as well, most notably in the lungs and kidneys [62]. Bolus propofol dosing is known to cause systemic hypotension via decreases in cardiac output and systemic vascular resistance; hepatic blood flow may be reduced due to this cardiovascular depression [62]. However, hepatic arterial flow increased in dogs while portal blood flow was unchanged [63]. Propofol is an excellent choice for anesthetic induction in patients with liver dysfunction. It does not exacerbate HE and is safe for postoperative use in canine PSS patients and human patients with cirrhosis [64–66].

Etomidate

Etomidate offers the advantage of greater cardiovascular stability as compared to other injectable agents [62]. Bolus dosing provides rapid anesthetic induction and recovery through precipitous redistribution out of the central nervous system. Metabolism is via ester hydrolysis, and drug clearance is not significantly altered in the presence of severe liver dysfunction [67]. Despite the cardiovascular stability offered by etomidate, hepatic blood flow and oxygen delivery are decreased after administration [68]. However, etomidate is considered safe for use in patients with liver dysfunction due to its minimal cardiovascular effects and rapid recovery profile.

Dissociatives

The dissociative agents ketamine and tiletamine rely on hepatic biotransformation for metabolism in most species; ketamine is metabolized to its less-active metabolite, norketamine, by CYP hepatic enzymes [69]. Cats, however, rely more extensively on renal excretion of dissociatives than other species [70]. After experimental ketamine administration to dogs, hepatic arterial and portal venous flows were not significantly altered from baseline, although hepatic oxygen delivery was decreased [71]. Overall, dissociative agents are considered safe induction agents for use in patients with hepatic dysfunction. However, recovery relies more significantly on hepatic metabolism as compared to other induction agents, so alternative induction agents may be considered in the face of severe disease. Dosages consistent with analgesia rather than anesthesia (0.25–1 $mg\,kg^{-1}$ bolus, 2–10 $\mu g\,kg^{-1}\,min^{-1}$ IV constant rate infusion) may be considered without significant concern, although accumulation could occur after long-term administration; it is important to observe patients closely for increased sedation or increased locomotor activity consistent with dissociative administration and titrate drug infusion rates to effect. Interestingly, long-term use and abuse of ketamine in human subjects may lead to sclerosing cholangitis; this has not been reported in veterinary species [72, 73].

Inhalational Agents

Historically, halothane was associated with hepatotoxicity in several animal species [74–78]. Modern anesthetics are not directly associated with hepatotoxicity, but several adverse physiologic effects can occur. In general, all halogenated anesthetics decrease overall hepatic blood flow to varying degrees in a dose-dependent manner, while some studies report an increase in hepatic arterial flow [79–82]. Reduced hepatic blood flow, largely a result of dose-dependent hypotension, results in decreased drug clearance and, in extreme cases, hepatocellular damage. As hypercarbia also decreases hepatic blood flow, the dose-dependent respiratory depression associated with volatile anesthetics must additionally be considered [22]. Ventilatory status should be monitored, and positive pressure ventilation instituted as necessary to maintain arterial CO_2 levels. All modern volatile anesthetics are minimally metabolized via CYP hepatic enzymes [83]; however, anesthetic recovery is nearly entirely via expiration of inhaled anesthetics rather than metabolism and is, therefore, generally unaltered directly by hepatic dysfunction. These agents are considered safe, although ALT, AST, and GGT levels can be elevated after anesthesia with isoflurane and sevoflurane [84, 85]. Collectively, isoflurane, sevoflurane, and desflurane are all acceptable for use in patients with liver dysfunction and choice should be based on availability and familiarity with the agent of choice.

Nitrous oxide administration causes dose-dependent decreases in hepatic arterial and portal venous blood flow [86]. Centrilobular necrosis occurs in the hypoxic rat model; no such hepatotoxicity has been reported in clinical patients under normoxic conditions [87] and nitrous oxide is largely considered safe for patients with hepatic dysfunction. Nitrous oxide can be advantageous to decrease the amount of halogenated anesthetic needed, thus attenuating the adverse cardiorespiratory effects of these agents.

Anesthetic Management of Patients with Hepatic Dysfunction

As previously mentioned, there can be a broad spectrum of hepatic dysfunction, ranging from nonclinical liver enzyme elevation detected on preoperative serum biochemistry profile to fulminant liver failure. Several underlying disease processes can cause these abnormalities, and the case presentation can be quite variable. Table 4.2 lists the commonly encountered physiological abnormalities in patients with hepatic dysfunction. It is important to consider that most anesthetic agents that rely heavily on hepatic biotransformation for metabolism and duration of effect may be prolonged if liver function is impaired. Fortunately, in veterinary medicine, patients presenting with fulminant liver failure for general anesthesia are rare. It is far more likely that patients may present for surgery or procedures that require anesthesia with unrelated hepatopathy or nonspecific hepatic enzyme elevations. Some of the most common case presentations seen in veterinary medicine are surgical or ultrasound-guided liver biopsy, PSS diagnosis and/or surgical ligation, hepatic neoplasia resection, and biliary surgery. General considerations for anesthesia are presented in Table 4.3.

Table 4.3 General recommendations for anesthesia in patients with hepatobiliary disease.

Preoperative evaluation of albumin or total solids, blood glucose, coagulation status
Prepare for management of hypotension (i.e., positive inotropes, vasopressors)
Choose reversible drugs for premedication/sedation
Add anesthetic adjuncts to decrease inhalant requirements
Invasive blood pressure measurement should be utilized for surgical procedures
Positive pressure ventilation when surgery is performed on the liver
Manage coagulopathy with plasma, vitamin K_1, blood transfusion, as necessary

General Considerations

Patient Monitoring with Hepatic Dysfunction

Patients with hepatobiliary dysfunction should be carefully outfitted with anesthetic monitors before draping, especially those of small stature that may become poorly accessible after surgical draping. Temperature, pulse oximetry, electrocardiography, blood pressure, and end-tidal carbon dioxide should be closely monitored. Intraoperative fluid boluses to increase stroke volume may be required and visible pulse waveforms to assess dynamic indicators of fluid status, such as pulse pressure variation (PPV; see Chapter 8) or pulse oximeters with technology to evaluate plethysmography variability index (PVI) may be used to guide fluid therapy. Invasive arterial blood pressure measurement should be used in patients with baseline hypotension, severe hypoalbuminemia, or when intraoperative hemorrhage is anticipated. If arterial cannulation is not possible, a noninvasive blood pressure measurement should be noted every 5 min, either by a reliable oscillometric monitor or by Doppler ultrasonic device accompanied by a sphygmomanometer. Management of hypotension should follow assessments of heart rate, stroke volume, and systemic vascular resistance with interventions as needed.

Postoperatively, it is important to carefully monitor and evaluate the patient with hepatic dysfunction. Blood pressure, temperature, hematocrit, albumin, and blood glucose should be measured to provide an immediate postoperative baseline measurement and to gauge further therapy in the postoperative period. Delayed anesthetic recovery can result from residual or prolonged drug effects, hypothermia, and hypoglycemia. Drug antagonism, temperature support, and supplementation of dextrose should be provided as necessary.

Anesthetic and Analgesic Choices

Drug choice should be tailored to patient temperament, degree of hepatic dysfunction, and procedure type. Preference should be given to drugs that may be antagonized in the event of untoward or prolonged effects. In general, it is safe to use a benzodiazepine/opioid combination either intramuscularly (IM) or intravenously (IV) prior to anesthetic induction, but other agents may be more suitable (see the section titled "Sedative Agents"). The IV route is preferable for drug administration, as drugs can be titrated to effect and the minimum effective doses can be given.

As intraoperative hypotension may be encountered during many procedures involving the liver, it is important to choose anesthetic adjuncts that may decrease the inhalant amount required to maintain a surgical anesthetic plane. Constant rate infusions of fentanyl or remifentanil, ketamine, and lidocaine may be considered to provide intraoperative analgesia as well as decrease inhalant concentrations. It is important to consider the dosages and long-term use of constant rate infusions with agents that rely on hepatic biotransformation in patients with compromised liver function. If the hepatic metabolic capacity is in question, dosages should be significantly decreased or agents that utilize extrahepatic metabolism (e.g., remifentanil) should be used. Regional anesthetic blocks, including epidurals and fascial plane blocks, should be utilized as much as possible to decrease sympathetic stimulation, decrease the need for systemically administered agents, and provide analgesia. The use and techniques of these blocks have been described extensively elsewhere [88]. Perioperative antiemetics, such as maropitant, should be considered in all cases with hepatobiliary disease, as these patients may present with anorexia or vomiting.

Liver Biopsy

Animals presenting for workup of liver enzyme elevation often have sufficient functional hepatic reserve and do not present many unexpected anesthetic challenges apart from what has been discussed previously. Note that elevations in hepatic enzymes may be nonspecific (see the section titled "Markers of Hepatic Dysfunction"), but often do not indicate abnormalities in hepatic function. Indicators of hepatic dysfunction (Table 4.2) should trigger concern for delayed or abnormal anesthetic agent metabolism and signal the need for perioperative management of derangements such as hypoglycemia, hypoalbuminemia, and coagulopathy. Before an anesthetic plan is formulated, it is important to have a complete physical exam, serum chemistry, electrolyte panel, and coagulation times (platelet count, PT/PTT, or TEG) to evaluate fitness for anesthesia as well as biopsy. Applicable preanesthetic stabilization should be performed if concerns are raised by this evaluation.

In general, sedation with agents that have available antagonist agents such as alpha-2-adrenergic receptor agonists or benzodiazepines combined with an opioid are excellent choices. Choice of sedative agent and opioid should be guided by the patient's underlying cardiovascular status, comorbidities, and anticipated analgesic requirements. Depending on the patient's cardiovascular status, propofol, alfaxalone, or etomidate will allow sufficient relaxation for endotracheal intubation. All these agents may be excellent choices, as they allow rapid anesthetic induction and rely on redistribution followed by hepatic and extrahepatic metabolism for recovery (see the section titled "Induction Agents"). Patients should be closely monitored following liver biopsy for evidence of pain or hemorrhage.

In the case of ultrasound-guided biopsy, preanesthetic sedation may be unnecessary. If the patient requires sedation or general anesthesia, an intravenous dose of butorphanol (0.1–0.3 $mg\,kg^{-1}$), a kappa-opioid agonist with mild sedative and analgesic properties, followed by propofol titrated to effect to allow sufficient relaxation may be adequate.

Laparoscopic liver biopsy requires special consideration regarding patient positioning and insufflation of the peritoneal cavity. Nonphysiologic positions, such as reverse Trendelenburg (head up, rear down) positioning, may be required to facilitate exposure; these positions may decrease venous return and subsequently decrease blood pressure. Pneumoperitoneum from insufflation may hinder diaphragmatic excursions and lead to hypercapnia; positive pressure ventilation should be initiated to prevent atelectasis and hypoventilation with subsequent hypercapnia and respiratory acidosis. Intraabdominal hypertension, discussed previously, is a potential transient effect that may decrease hepatic blood flow [23, 24]. Caution should be exercised to avoid excessively high pressures with abdominal insufflation. Vasodilation associated with anesthetic administration may lead to splenic engorgement; surgeons should use caution to avoid inadvertent splenic puncture with port incision sites.

Portosystemic Shunts

Patients presenting with portosystemic venous shunts are typically the most severe cases of hepatic dysfunction encountered by the veterinary anesthetist. PSSs may be intrahepatic or extrahepatic and allow portal blood to enter the systemic circulation, bypassing the liver [89]. Patients with congenital PSS are typically pediatric patients that are abnormally small and present with clinical signs that may be consistent with hepatic failure and/or HE. Laboratory abnormalities consistent with hepatic failure include low BUN, low cholesterol, prolonged coagulation times, hypoglycemia, and hypoalbuminemia. It is important to manage these abnormalities throughout the entire perioperative period, not just while on the operating table. Hypoglycemia is often present in these patients due to impaired hepatic glucose metabolism and should be closely monitored throughout the perioperative period. Fasting should be kept to a minimum; for instance, a small amount of baby food or moistened canned food may be offered approximately 2 h prior to surgery. Blood glucose should be checked prior to sedation, at anesthetic induction, every 30–60 min while under anesthesia (if possible), and on recovery. Intravenous dextrose should be administered (0.5–1.0 ml kg^{-1} of 50% dextrose diluted 1:4) or IV fluids supplemented with 2.5–5% dextrose as needed to maintain blood glucose above 70 mg dl^{-1} [90]. Hypoglycemia should be suspected and ruled out in the event of delayed anesthetic recovery. Hypoalbuminemia, due to multiple factors including impaired protein synthesis, can cause several anesthetic challenges. Drug protein binding will be altered, and highly protein-bound drugs such as diazepam will exert a greater effect due to a greater proportion of unbound, active drug [90]. As many anesthetic agents have a high degree of protein binding, anesthetic drug dosages should be decreased in the face of significant hypoalbuminemia. Albumin plays a critical role in providing oncotic support to plasma; decreases in this oncotic support can lead to hypotension and edema. For example, severe hypoalbuminemia (albumin concentration <1.5 g dl^{-1}) can lead to pulmonary and/or peripheral edema with perioperative crystalloid administration [91]. The perioperative administration of plasma should be considered in cases of severe hypoalbuminemia as IV fluid support; volumes sufficient to significantly increase albumin concentration would likely lead to volume overload.

HE is the result of several factors, key of which is hyperammonemia, and presentation may vary anywhere from behavioral abnormalities to seizures to coma [92]. Chronic management of HE has been described elsewhere [92] and medical stabilization measures should be performed prior to anesthesia. PSS patients that present with HE are more likely to experience seizures; nearly 5% of dogs experience seizures in the postoperative period and approximately 11% of patients experience other neurological signs [93, 94]. It is critically important to closely monitor PSS patients in the postoperative period for seizure activity and neurologic abnormalities. Seizures may be treated with antiepileptic medications as needed. Studies evaluating the prophylactic treatment of dogs with levetiracetam (Keppra, UCB Pharmaceuticals, Brussels, Belgium) to reduce the incidence of postattenuation seizures have shown mixed results [95, 96]. Owing to a high concentration of endogenous benzodiazepine receptor agonists in HE patients, these patients are uniquely sensitive to drugs that exert action through the GABA receptor such as benzodiazepines [38, 97]. While benzodiazepines may be used in both the premedication of patients and control of postattenuation seizures, profound sedation can result if drug dosages are not appropriately decreased or titrated carefully to effect.

Hypotension due to hypovolemia, hypoalbuminemia, and/or hypothermia is often encountered. Surgical manipulation in the abdomen of small patients may worsen hypotension by impeding venous return, resulting in sudden blood pressure swings. Invasive blood pressure measurement via arterial catheterization should be used in patients with severe liver disease, although the small size of many portal venous shunt patients can make this difficult. In the absence of invasive blood pressure measurement, a noninvasive blood pressure measurement should be noted every 5 min, either by a reliable oscillometric monitor or by Doppler ultrasonic device accompanied by a sphygmomanometer. Hypotension management should follow assessments of heart rate, stroke volume, and systemic vascular resistance with interventions as needed. Crystalloid boluses (3–5 ml kg^{-1}) to increase stroke volume should be limited to prevent fluid overload in hypoalbuminemic patients, and dynamic indicators of fluid status such as PPV (see Chapter 8) should guide fluid therapy. Hypotension should first be addressed by assessing anesthetic depth and decreasing inhalational agents as needed; anesthetic requirements may be reduced by the administration of anesthetic adjuncts such as ketamine. Vasopressors (e.g., norepinephrine [0.05–0.3 μg kg^{-1} min^{-1} IV]) may be considered to increase systemic vascular resistance, increase mean arterial pressure, and improve venous return from peripheral blood pooling.

Due to the small stature of these patients, vascular cannulation may be difficult; the application of a eutectic local anesthetic cream with lidocaine and prilocaine (e.g., EMLA®, Astra Pharmaceuticals, Wayne, PA) before IV catheterization can aid in patient comfort. Intramuscular sedation may be required prior to attempting catheterization. Sedative choice should be based on patient presentation and considerations for the presence of laboratory abnormalities, HE, and any comorbidities. Preference should be given to anesthetic agents that can be reversed with drug antagonists and/or agents with extrahepatic metabolism. Furthermore, small patients are highly prone to hypothermia, which may further delay drug biotransformation and contribute to prolonged anesthetic recovery or adverse effects. Heat support should be provided upon sedation and throughout the entire anesthetic period and patient temperature closely monitored.

Hepatic Neoplasia Resection

Like many hepatobiliary diseases, the presence of space-occupying lesions associated with the liver can be associated with any number of abnormalities, ranging from minor liver enzyme elevations to fulminant liver failure. Anesthetic plans should be formulated with considerations that have been described within this chapter and book and tailored to the specific patient's disease process, presentation, and comorbidities. Many anesthetic concerns unique to hepatic neoplasia relate more to the mechanical effects of a space-occupying lesion and the risk of severe hemorrhage with their resection. General considerations are presented in Table 4.3.

Ascites, while not specific to liver disease, may be present in animals with significant portal hypertension and/or severe hypoalbuminemia [98]. A large volume of ascitic fluid will impair lung expansion on recumbency. In these cases, fluid should be removed before anesthesia, with care to not remove large volumes of fluid rapidly. Ascitic fluid that is removed too rapidly can cause a shift in intravascular volume to the abdominal cavity, resulting in profound hypovolemia and potential cardiovascular collapse. Animals with considerable ascitic fluid should be preoxygenated with 100% oxygen delivered by face mask before anesthetic induction, as time to desaturation with apnea may occur more rapidly in these patients.

In any patient with liver dysfunction presenting for anesthesia and invasive procedures, it is important to check the coagulation status to rule out coagulopathy. At a minimum, platelet count and PT/PTT should be checked before anesthesia. However, further coagulation testing may be warranted, such as TEG. Coagulopathy can be treated with fresh frozen plasma and administration of vitamin K_1 [99]. Even in the event of normal coagulation times, the anesthetist should be prepared for hemorrhage with all invasive procedures, as the liver is highly vascular. Blood products should be available, and the animal cross-matched as needed to blood donors. A central line or a second IV catheter should be placed preoperatively if rapid fluid or blood product administration may be needed due to hemorrhage or the administration of vasoactive agents is anticipated. Fluid boluses may be required in the event of hemorrhage to replace losses. Generally, crystalloids should be administered as replacement of hemorrhage less than 15–20% of blood volume, while blood products may be considered if blood loss exceeds 15–20% or if hemoglobin loss is sufficient to compromise oxygen-carrying capacity.

While multiple electrolyte abnormalities may be present, hypokalemia may be the most critical in the perianesthetic period. Potassium levels <3.5 $mEq\,l^{-1}$ should be treated before anesthesia. This can be accomplished through IV fluid supplementation with potassium at a rate not to exceed 0.5 $mEq\,kg^{-1}\,h^{-1}$ of supplementation (see Chapter 8).

Venous return may be compromised due to surgical manipulation around the liver and great vessels or the mass itself. Continuous, invasive blood pressure monitoring should be utilized and, if arterial cannulation is not possible or not successful, noninvasive blood pressure should be evaluated every 3–5 min. Hypotension should be managed as needed, with heart rate, stroke volume, and systemic vascular resistance evaluation guiding management strategies. Vasodilation associated with inhalational anesthetic administration should be minimized using anesthetic adjuncts to decrease the amount of inhalant needed. Different strategies such as using fentanyl, ketamine, lidocaine, and the regional anesthetic blocks such as epidural or fascial plane blocks may decrease the need for inhalational anesthetics. Vasopressors (e.g., norepinephrine), positive inotropic agents (e.g., dopamine, dobutamine), and anticholinergics should be utilized as needed (Table 4.3).

Cholecystectomy

Patients presenting with cholecystitis also represent a wide range of comorbidities, instability, and acuity. General anesthesia may be required for diagnostic evaluation, a procedure unrelated to the patient's cholestatic disease, or cholecystectomy due to biliary obstruction. Blood work typically reveals that increases in ALT, AST, ALP, and GGT with increases in total bilirubin and electrolyte abnormalities may be consistent with vomiting [100, 101]. Patients may present with cranial abdominal pain (Figure 4.1), lethargy, anorexia, vomiting, and fever, or, in cases of gallbladder rupture, present with bile peritonitis and/or clinical signs consistent with sepsis. As the clinical presentation is variable, it is important to evaluate all abnormalities, triage, and stabilize as needed. Surgical procedures of the biliary system may be quite prolonged, and it is critically

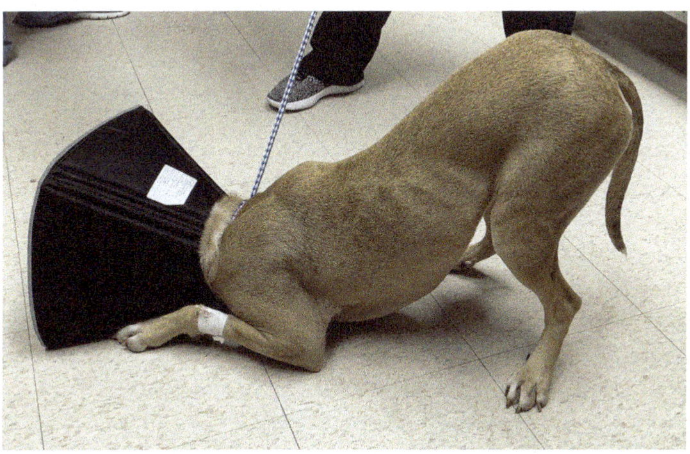

Figure 4.1 Dog presenting with cranial abdominal pain associated with cholecystitis.

important to optimize fluid deficits and electrolyte abnormalities prior to surgery if possible.

Intraoperative hypotension is extremely common in dogs undergoing cholecystectomy, with rates reported anywhere form 54–74% of cases [102, 103]. It is important to anticipate this common occurrence and prepare. Consideration should be given to the preplacement of a second IV catheter or central line for vasoactive substances administration. Continuous, invasive blood pressure monitoring should be utilized and, if arterial cannulation is not possible or not successful, noninvasive blood pressure should be evaluated every 3–5 min. Hypotension should be managed as needed, with evaluation of heart rate, stroke volume, and systemic vascular resistance guiding management strategies. Vasodilation associated with inhalational anesthetic administration should be minimized using anesthetic adjuncts to decrease required inhalant. Different strategies using fentanyl, ketamine, lidocaine, and the regional anesthetic blocks may decrease the need for inhalational anesthetics. Vasopressors (e.g., norepinephrine [0.05–0.3 $\mu g\,kg^{-1}\,min^{-1}$ IV]) may be used to increase systemic vascular resistance as needed; if cardiac contractility is suspected to be a cause of hypotension, positive inotropes (e.g., dobutamine [5–10 $\mu g\,kg^{-1}\,min^{-1}$ IV] or dopamine [5–10 $\mu g\,kg^{-1}\,min^{-1}$ IV]) may be used.

Patients should be closely and continuously monitored following surgery. Monitoring of blood pressure should continue into the postoperative period. Postoperative hypotension is a negative prognostic indicator; a retrospective evaluation of cholecystectomy patients found a 20-fold increase in mortality associated with the presence of hypotension in the postoperative period [104].

Summary

Patients with liver disease can have highly variable case presentations; close attention to clinical abnormalities with a plan for careful management of each is advised. The anesthetist must have a thorough understanding of the repercussions of liver dysfunction, as well as any possible confounding issues of the procedure requiring anesthesia. Although true of all patients, it is especially important for patients with liver dysfunction to be carefully monitored not only intraoperatively, but also postoperatively. With careful attention, monitoring, and management, these patients can be successfully managed through the entire perioperative course.

References

1 Murray, M.J. (2014). Gastrointestinal physiology. In: *Stoelting's Pharmacology & Physiology in Anesthetic Practice*, 5e (eds. P. Flood, J. Rathmell, S. Shafer and R.K. Stoelting), 45–97. Philadelphia: Wolters Kluwer Health.

2 Njoku, D.B., Chitilian, H.V., and Kronish, K. (2020). Hepatic physiology, pathophysiology, and anesthetic considerations. In: *Miller's Anesthesia*, 9e (eds. M.A. Gropper, N.H. Cohen, L.I. Eriksson, et al.), 420–443. Philadelphia: Elsevier.

3 Coelho, J.C., Senninger, N., Runkel, N. et al. (1986). Effect of analgesic drugs on the electromyographic activity of the gastrointestinal tract and sphincter of Oddi on biliary pressure. *Ann. Surg.* 204: 53–58.

4 Thompson, D.R. (2001). Narcotic analgesic effects on the sphincter of Oddi: a review of the data and therapeutic implications in treating pancreatitis. *Am. J. Gastroenterol.* 96: 1266–1272.

5 Perazzo, J.C., Tallis, S., Delfante, A. et al. (2012). Hepatic encephalopathy: an approach

to its multiple pathophysiological features. *World J. Hepatol.* 43 (3): 50–65.

6 Sweeney, B.P. and Bromilow, J. (2006). Liver enzyme induction and inhibition: implications for anesthesia. *Anesthesia* 61: 159–177.

7 Myre, S.A., Schroeder, T.J., Grund, V.R. et al. (1991). Critical ketoconazole dosage range for ciclosporin(sic) clearance inhibition in the dog. *Pharmacology* 43: 233–241.

8 Sams, R. and Muir, W. (1993). Effects of phenobarbital on thiopental pharmacokinetics in greyhounds. *Am. J. Vet. Res.* 49: 245–249.

9 Aidasani, D., Zaya, M.J., Malpas, P.B. et al. (2008). in vitro drug-drug interaction screens for canine veterinary medicines: evaluation of cytochrome P450 reversible inhibition. *Drug Metab. Dispos.* 36: 1512–1518.

10 Kukanich, B., Kukanich, K.S., and Rodriguez, J.R. (2011). The effects of concurrent administration of cytochrome P450 inhibitors on the pharmacokinetics of oral methadone in healthy dogs. *Vet. Anaesth. Analg.* 35: 224–230.

11 Kukanich, B., Coetzee, J.F., Gehring, R. et al. (2007). Comparative disposition of pharmacologic markers for cytochrome P-450 mediated metabolism, glomerular filtration rate, and extracellular and total body fluid volume of greyhound and beagle dogs. *J. Vet. Pharmacol. Ther.* 30: 314–319.

12 Martinez, S.E., Andresen, M.C., Zhu, Z. et al. (2020). Pharmacogenomics of poor drug metabolism in greyhounds: cytochrome P450 (CYP) 2B11 genetic variation, breed distribution, and functional characterization. *Sci. Rep.* 10 (1): 69.

13 Fry, W., Lester, C., Etedali, N.M. et al. (2017). Thromboelastography in dogs with chronic hepatopathies. *J. Vet. Intern. Med.* 31 (2): 419–426.

14 Lawrence, Y.A. and Steiner, J. (2017). Laboratory evaluation of the liver. *Vet. Clin. Small Anim. Pract.* 47 (3): 539–553.

15 Webster, C.R.L. (2017). Hemostatic disorders associated with hepatobiliary disease. *Vet. Clin. Small Anim. Pract.* 47 (3): 601–615.

16 Thawley, V. (2017). Acute liver insufficiency and failure. *Vet. Clin. Small Anim. Pract.* 47 (3): 617–630.

17 McCord, K.W. and Webb, C.B. (2011). Hepatic dysfunction. *Vet. Clin. Small Anim. Pract.* 41: 745–758.

18 Frink, E.K., Morgan, S.E., Coetzee, A. et al. (1992). The effects of sevoflurane, halothane, enflurane, and isoflurane on hepatic blood flow and oxygenation in chronically instrumented greyhound dogs. *Anesthesiology* 76: 85–90.

19 Nies, A.S., Shand, D.G., and Wilkinson, G.R. (1976). Altered hepatic blood flow and drug distribution. *Clin. Pharmacokinet.* 1: 135–155.

20 Putensen, C., Wrigge, H., and Hering, R. (2006). The effects of mechanical ventilation on the gut and abdomen. *Curr. Opin. Crit. Care* 12: 160–165.

21 Soni, N. and Williams, P. (2008). Positive pressure ventilation: what is the real cost? *Br. J. Anaesth.* 101: 446–457.

22 Fujita, Y., Sakai, T., Ohsumi, A. et al. (1989). Effects of hypocapnia and hypercapnia on splanchnic circulation and hepatic function in the beagle. *Anesth. Analg.* 69: 152–157.

23 Inal, M.T., Memis, D., Sezar, Y.A. et al. (2011). Effects of intra-abdominal pressure on liver function assessed with the LiMON in critically ill patients. *Can. J. Surg.* 54: 161–166.

24 Malbrain, M.L., Viaene, D., Kortgen, A. et al. (2012). Relationship between intra-abdominal pressure and indocyanine green plasma disappearance rate: hepatic perfusion may be impaired in critically ill patients with intra-abdominal hypertension. *Ann. Intensive Care* 2 (Suppl. 1): S19.

25 Ludders, J.W., Reitan, J.A., Martucci, R. et al. (1983). Blood pressure response to phenylephrine infusion in halothane-anesthetized dogs given acetylpromazine maleate. *Am. J. Vet. Res.* 44: 969–999.

26 Songqing, H., Atkinson, C., Qiao, F. et al. (2010). Ketamine-xylazine-acepromazine compared with isoflurane for anesthesia

during liver transplantation in rodents. *J. Am. Assoc. Lab. Anim. Sci.* 49: 45–51.

27 Barr, S.C., Ludders, J.W., Looney, A.L. et al. (1992). Platelet aggregation in dogs after sedation with acepromazine and atropine and during subsequent general anesthesia and surgery. *Am. J. Vet. Res.* 53: 2067–2070.

28 Conner, B.J., Hanel, R.M., and Hansen, B.D. (2012). Effects of acepromazine maleate on platelet function assessed by use of adenosine diphosphate activated- and arachidonic acid-activated modified thromboelastography in healthy dogs. *Am. J. Vet. Res.* 73: 595–601.

29 Selmi, A.L., Mendes, G.M., Lins, B.T. et al. (2003). Evaluation of the sedative and cardiorespiratory effects of dexmedetomidine, dexmedetomidine-butorphanol, and dexmedetomidine-ketamine in cats. *J. Am. Vet. Med. Assoc.* 222: 37–41.

30 Murrell, J.C. and Hellebrekers, L.J. (2005). Medetomidine and dexmedetomidine: a review of cardiovascular effects and antinociceptive properties in the dog. *Vet. Anaesth. Analg.* 32: 117–127.

31 Congdon, J.M., Marquez, M., Niyom, S. et al. (2011). Evaluation of the sedative and cardiovascular effects of intramuscular administration of dexmedetomidine with and without concurrent atropine administration in dogs. *J. Am. Vet. Med. Assoc.* 239: 81–89.

32 Restitutti, F., Laiitinen, M.R., Raekallio, M.R. et al. (2013). Effect of MK-467 on organ blood flow parameters detected by contrast-enhanced ultrasound in dogs treated with dexmedetomidine. *Vet. Anaesth. Analg.* 40: e48–e56.

33 Memis, D., Kargi, M., and Sut, N. (2009). Effects of propofol and dexmedetomidine on indocyanine green elimination assessed with LiMON to patients with early septic shock: a pilot study. *J. Crit. Care* 24: 603–608.

34 Bao, N. and Tang, B. (2020). Organ-protective effects and the underlying mechanism of dexmedetomidine. *Mediat. Inflamm.* May: 6136105.

35 Rathmell, J.P. and Rosow, C.E. (2015). Intravenous sedatives and hypnotics. In: *Stoelting's Pharmacology & Physiology in Anesthetic Practice*, 5e (eds. P. Flood, J. Rathmell, S. Shafer and R.K. Stoelting), 160–203. Philadelphia: Wolters Kluwer Health.

36 Jones, D.J., Stehling, L.C., and Zauder, H.L. (1979). Cardiovascular responses to diazepam and midazolam maleate in the dog. *Anesthesiology* 51: 430–434.

37 Center, S.A., Elston, T.H., Rowland, P.H. et al. (1996). Fulminant hepatic failure associated with oral administration of diazepam in 11 cats. *J. Am. Vet. Med. Assoc.* 209: 618–625.

38 Jones, E.A., Yurdaydin, C., and Basile, A.S. (1993). The role of endogenous benzodiazepines in hepatic encephalopathy: animal studies. *Alcohol Suppl.* 2: 175–180.

39 Goulenok, C., Bernard, B., Cadrenel, J.F. et al. (2002). Flumazenil vs placebo in hepatic encephalopathy in patients with cirrhosis: a meta-analysis. *Aliment. Pharmacol. Ther.* 16: 361–372.

40 Goh, E.T., Andersen, M.L., Morgan, M.Y. et al. (2017). Flumazenil versus placebo or no intervention for people with cirrhosis and hepatic encephalopathy. *Cochrane Database Syst. Rev.* 7: CD002798.

41 Kukanich, B. and Wiese, A. (2015). Opioids. In: *Veterinary Anesthesia and Analgesia: The Fifth Edition of Lumb and Jones* (eds. K.A. Grimm, L.A. Lamont, W.J. Tranquilli, et al.), 207–226. Ames: Wiley Blackwell Publishing.

42 Tegeder, I., Lotsch, J., and Geisslinger, G. (1999). Pharmacokinetics of opioids in liver disease. *Clin. Pharmacokinet.* 37: 17–40.

43 Zeneroli, M.L., Ventura, E., and Pinelli, G. (1985). Opiate receptors and beta-endorphin levels in brain areas of dogs with portal-systemic encephalopathy. *J. Hepatol.* 1: 619–627.

44 Dancker, C., MacFarlane, P.D., and Love, E.J. (2020). The effect of neuraxial morphine on postoperative pain in dogs after extrahepatic portosystemic shunt attenuation. *Vet. Anaesth. Analg.* 47 (1): P111–P118.

45 Chism, J.P. and Rickert, D.E. (1996). The pharmacokinetics and extra-hepatic clearance of remifentanil, a short acting opioid agonist, in male beagle dogs during constant rate infusions. *Drug Metab. Dispos.* 24: 34–40.

46 Michelsen, L.G., Salmenpera, M., and Hug, C.C. (1996). Anesthetic potency of remifentanil in dogs. *Anesthesiology* 84: 865–872.

47 Dershwitz, M., Hoke, J.F., Rosow, C.E. et al. (1996). Pharmacokinetics and pharmacodynamics of remifentanil in volunteer subjects with severe liver disease. *Anesthesiology* 84: 812–820.

48 Navapurkar, V.U., Archer, S., Gupta, S.K. et al. (1998). Metabolism of remifentanil during liver transplantation. *Br. J. Anaesth.* 81: 881–886.

49 Allweiler, S., Brodbelt, D.C., Borer, K. et al. (2007). The isoflurane-sparing and clinical effects of a constant rate infusion of remifentanil in dogs. *Vet. Anaesth. Analg.* 34: 388–393.

50 Anagnostou, T.L., Kazakos, G.M., Savvas, I. et al. (2011). Remifentanil/isoflurane anesthesia in five dogs with liver disease undergoing liver biopsy. *J. Am. Anim. Hosp. Assoc.* 47: e103–e109.

51 Ferreira, T.H., Aguiar, A.J., Valverde, A. et al. (2009). Effect of remifentanil hydrochloride administered *via* constant rate infusion on the minimum alveolar concentration of isoflurane in cats. *Am. J. Vet. Res.* 70: 581–588.

52 Akashi, N., Murahata, Y., Kishida, H. et al. (2020). Effects of constant rate infusions of dexmedetomidine, remifentanil and their combination on minimum alveolar concentration of sevoflurane in dogs. *Vet. Anaesth. Analg.* 47: 490–498.

53 MacPhail, C.M., Lappin, M.R., Meyer, D.J. et al. (1998). Hepatocellular toxicosis associated with administration of carprofen in 21 dogs. *J. Am. Vet. Med. Assoc.* 212: 1895–1901.

54 Galati, G., Tafazoli, S., Sabzevari, O. et al. (2002). Idiosyncratic NSAID drug induced oxidative stress. *Chem. Biol. Interact.* 142: 25–41.

55 Raekallio, M.R., Hielm-Bjorkman, A.K., and Kejonen, J. (2006). Evaluation of adverse effects of long-term orally administered carprofen in dogs. *J. Am. Vet. Med. Assoc.* 228: 876–880.

56 Hernandez-Avalos, I., Valverde, A., and Ibancovichi-Camarillo, J.A. (2020). Clinical evaluation of postoperative analgesia, cardiorespiratory parameters and changes in liver and renal function tests of paracetamol compared to meloxicam and carprofen in dogs undergoing ovariohysterectomy. *PLoS One* 15 (2): e0223697.

57 Luna, S.P.L., Basilio, A.C., Steagall, P.V. et al. (2007). Evaluation of adverse effects of long-term oral administration of carprofen, etodolac, flunixin meglumine, ketoprofen, and meloxicam in dogs. *Am. J. Vet. Res.* 68: 258–264.

58 Blois, S.L., Allen, D.G., Wood, R.D. et al. (2010). Effects of aspirin, carprofen, deracoxib, and meloxicam on platelet function and systemic prostaglandin concentrations in healthy dogs. *J. Vet. Res.* 71: 349–358.

59 Brainard, B.M., Meredith, C.P., Callan, M.B. et al. (2007). Changes in platelet function, hemostasis, and prostaglandin expression after treatment with nonsteroidal anti-inflammatory drugs with various cyclooxygenase selectivities in dogs. *Am. J. Vet. Res.* 68: 251–257.

60 Whittem, T., Pasloske, K.S., Heit, M.C. et al. (2008). The pharmacokinetics and pharmacodynamics of alfaxalone in cats after single and multiple intravenous administration of Alfaxan at clinical and supraclinical doses. *J. Vet. Pharm.* 31: 571–579.

61 Warne, L.N., Beths, T., Whittem, T. et al. (2015). A review of the pharmacology and clinical application of alfaxalone in cats. *Vet. J.* 203: 141–148.

62 Vuyk, J., Sitsen, E., and Reekers, M. (2020). Intravenous anesthetics. In: *Miller's*

Anesthesia, 9e (eds. M.A. Gropper, N.H. Cohen, L.I. Eriksson, et al.), 638–679. Philadelphia: Elsevier.

63 Wouters, P.F., Van de Velde, M.A., Marcus, M.A.E. et al. (1995). Hemodynamic changes during induction of anesthesia with eltanolone and propofol in dogs. *Anesth. Analg.* 81: 125–131.

64 Gommeren, K., Claeys, S., and de Rooster, H. (2010). Outcome from status epilepticus after portosystemic shunt attenuation in 3 dogs treated with propofol and phenobarbital. *J. Vet. Emerg. Crit. Care* 20: 346–351.

65 Khamaysi, I., William, N., Olga, A. et al. (2011). Sub-clinical hepatic encephalopathy in cirrhotic patients is not aggravated by sedation with propofol compared to midazolam: a randomized controlled study. *J. Hepatol.* 54: 72–77.

66 Sharma, P., Singh, S., Sharma, B.C. et al. (2011). Propofol sedation during endoscopy in patients with cirrhosis, and utility of psychometric tests and critical flicker frequency in assessment of recovery from sedation. *Endoscopy* 43: 400–405.

67 Van Beem, H., Manger, F.W., Van Boxtel, C. et al. (1983). Etomidate anaesthesia in patients with cirrhosis of the liver: pharmacokinetic data. *Anaesthesia* 38 (Suppl): 61–62.

68 Thomson, I.A., Fitch, W., Hughes, R.L. et al. (1986). Effects of certain I.V. anaesthetics on liver blood flow and hepatic oxygen consumption in the greyhound. *Br. J. Anaesth.* 58: 69–80.

69 Capponi, L., Schmitz, A., Thormann, W. et al. (2009). in vitro evaluation of differences in phase 1 metabolism of ketamine and other analgesics among humans, horses, and dogs. *Am. J. Vet. Res.* 70: 77–86.

70 Hanna, R.M., Borchard, R.E., and Schmidt, S.L. (1988). Pharmacokinetics of ketamine HCl and metabolite I in the cat: a comparison of IV, IM, and rectal administration. *J. Vet. Pharmacol. Ther.* 11: 84–93.

71 Thomson, I.A., Fitch, W., Campbell, D. et al. (1988). Effects of ketamine on liver blood flow and hepatic oxygen consumption. Studies in the anaesthetized greyhound. *Acta Anaesthesiol. Scand.* 32: 10–14.

72 Turkish, A., Luo, J.J., and Lefkowitch, J.H. (2013). Ketamine abuse, biliary tract disease, and secondary sclerosing cholangitis. *Hepatology* 58: 825–827.

73 Knooihuizen, S.A.I., Aday, A., and Lee, W.M. (2020). Ketamine-induced sclerosing cholangitis (KISC) in a critically ill patient with COVID-19. *Hepatology* 23: e10.1002.

74 O'Brien, T.D., Raffe, M.R., Cox, V.S. et al. (1986). Hepatic necrosis following halothane anesthesia in goats. *J. Am. Vet. Med. Assoc.* 189: 1591–1595.

75 Peters, R.L., Edmondson, H.A., Reynolds, T.B. et al. (1969). Hepatic necrosis associated with halothane anesthesia. *Am. J. Med.* 47: 748–764.

76 Van Dyke, R.A. (1982). Hepatic centrilobular necrosis in rats after exposure to halothane, enflurane, or isoflurane. *Anesth. Analg.* 61: 812–819.

77 Gaunt, P.S., Meuten, D.J., and Pecquet-Goad, M.E. (1984). Hepatic necrosis associated with use of halothane in a dog. *J. Am. Vet. Med. Assoc.* 184: 478–480.

78 Gopinath, C., Jones, R.S., and Ford, E.J.H. (1970). The effect of repeated administration of halothane on the liver of the horse. *J. Pathol.* 102: 107–114.

79 Manohar, M. and Parks, C.M. (1984). Porcine systemic and regional organ blood flow during 1.0 and 1.5 minimum alveolar concentrations of sevoflurane anesthesia with and without 50% nitrous oxide. *J. Pharmacol. Exp. Ther.* 231: 640–648.

80 Gelman, S.I., Fowler, K.C., and Smith, L.R. (1984). Liver circulation and function during isoflurane and halothane anesthesia. *Anesthesiology* 61: 726–730.

81 Conzen, P.F., Vollmar, B., Habazetti, H. et al. (1992). Systemic and regional hemodynamics of isoflurane and sevoflurane in rats. *Anesth. Analg.* 74: 79–88.

82 Frink, E.J., Morgan, S., Coetzee, A. et al. (1992). The effect of sevoflurane, halothane, enflurane, and isoflurane on hepatic blood flow and oxygenation in chronically instrumented greyhound dogs. *Anesthesiology* 76: 85–92.

83 Forman, S.A. and Ishizawa, Y. (2020). Inhaled anesthetic uptake, distribution, metabolism, and toxicity. In: *Miller's Anesthesia*, 9e (eds. M.A. Gropper, N.H. Cohen, L.I. Eriksson, et al.), 509–539. Philadelphia: Elsevier.

84 McEwen, M., Gleed, R.D., and Ludders, J.W. (2000). Hepatic effects of halothane and isoflurane anesthesia in goats. *J. Am. Vet. Med. Assoc.* 217: 1697–1700.

85 Topal, A., Gul, N., and Ilcol, Y. (2003). Hepatic effects of halothane, isoflurane or sevoflurane anaesthesia in dogs. *J. Vet. Med. A Physiol. Pathol. Clin. Med.* 50: 530–533.

86 Thomson, I.A., Hughes, R.L., Fitch, W. et al. (1982). Effects of nitrous oxide on liver haemodynamics and oxygen consumption in the greyhound. *Anesthesia* 37: 548–553.

87 Fassoulaki, A., Eger, E., Johnson, B. et al. (1984). Nitrous oxide, too, is hepatotoxic to rats. *Anesth. Analg.* 63: 1076–1080.

88 Read, M.R. and Schroeder, C.A. (2013). Truncal Blocks. *Small Animal Regional Anesthesia and Analgesia*, 1e (eds. L. Campoy and M. Read), 167–198. Ames: Wiley Blackwell Publishing.

89 Thieman Mankin, K.M. (2015). Current concepts in congenital portosystemic shunts. *Vet. Clin.Small Anim.* 45: 477–487.

90 de Brito Galvao, J.F. and Center, S.A. (2012). Fluid, electrolyte, and acid-base disturbances in liver disease. In: *Fluid, Electrolyte, and Acid-Base Disorders in Small Animal Practice*, 4e (ed. S.P. DiBartola), 456–499. St Louis: Elsevier.

91 DiBartola, S.P. and Bateman, S. (2012). Introduction to fluid therapy. In: *Fluid, Electrolyte, and Acid-Base Disorders in Small Animal Practice*, 4e (ed. S.P. DiBartola), 331–350. St Louis: Elsevier.

92 Gow, A.G. (2017). Hepatic encephalopathy. *Vet. Clin.Small Anim.* 47: 585–599.

93 Strickland, R., Tivers, M.S., and Adamantos, S.E. (2018). Incidence and risk factors for neurological signs after attenuation of single congenital portosystemic shunts in 253 dogs. *Vet. Surg.* 47: 745–755.

94 Mullins, R.A., Sanchez Villamil, C., Selmic, L.E. et al. (2020). Prognostic factors for short-term survival of dogs that experience postattenuation seizures after surgical correction of single congenital extrahepatic portosystemic shunts: 93 cases (2005–2018). *Vet. Surg.* 49: 958–970.

95 Fryer, K.J., Levine, J.M., Peycke, L.E. et al. (2011). Incidence of postoperative seizures with and without levetiracetam pretreatment in dogs undergoing portosystemic shunt attenuation. *J. Vet. Intern. Med.* 25: 1379–1384.

96 Mullins, R.A., Sanchez Villamil, C., and de Rooster, H. (2019). Effect of prophylactic treatment with levetiracetam on the incidence of postattenuation seizures in dogs undergoing surgical management of single congenital extrahepatic portosystemic shunts. *Vet. Surg.* 48: 164–172.

97 Basile, A.S., Pannell, L., Jaouni, T. et al. (1990). Brain concentrations of benzodiazepines are elevated in an animal model of hepatic encephalopathy. *Proc. Natl Acad. Sci. USA* 87: 5263–5267.

98 O'Neill, E. (2020). Approach to the patient with liver disease. In: *Clinical Small Animal Internal Medicine*, vol. 1 (eds. D.S. Bruyette, N. Bexfield, J.D. Chretin, et al.), 639–658. Hoboken: Wiley Blackwell Publishing.

99 Berent, A. (2015). Hepatic Failure. In: *Small Animal Critical Care Medicine*, 2e (eds. D.C. Silverstein and K. Hopper), 615–621. St Louis: Elsevier.

100 Rondeau, M.P. (2015). Acute cholecystitis. In: *Small Animal Critical Care Medicine*, 2e (eds. D.C. Silverstein and K. Hopper), 606–609. St Louis: Elsevier.

101 Harris, B. (2020). Diseases of the gallbladder and extrahepatic biliary ducts. In: *Clinical Small Animal Internal Medicine*, vol. 1 (eds. D.S. Bruyette, N. Bexfield, J.D. Chretin, et al.), 721–726. Hoboken: Wiley Blackwell.

102 Burns, B.R., Hofmeister, E.H., and Brainard, B.M. (2014). Anesthetic complications in dogs undergoing hepatic surgery: cholecystectomy versus non-cholecystectomy. *Vet. Anaesth. Analg.* 41: 186–190.

103 Hattersley, R., Downing, F., Gibson, S. et al. (2020). Impact of intra-operative hypotension on mortality rates and post-operative complications in dogs undergoing cholecystectomy. *J. Small Anim. Pract.* 61: 624–629.

104 Malek, S., Sinclair, E., Hosgood, G. et al. (2013). Clinical findings and prognostic factors for dogs undergoing cholecystectomy for gall bladder mucocele. *Vet. Surg.* 42: 418–426.

5

Gastrointestinal Disease

Juliana Peboni Figueiredo

VCA West Coast Specialty and Emergency Animal Hospital, Fountain Valley, Orange County, CA, 92708, USA

Gastrointestinal (GI) Tract Function

The digestive system provides the body with a continual supply of water, electrolytes, and nutrients. To achieve these larger global functions, several physiological functions need to be occurring normally. Food must be appropriately taken, ingested, and moved through the gastrointestinal (GI) tract: the stomach must secrete digestive enzymes, and, at the same time, the homeostatic function of the stomach must be maintained. Nutrients, water, and electrolytes must be absorbed by the small intestines; circulation of the GI organs must be adequate to carry away the absorbed substances, and motility of the GI tract must be maintained [1].

Any alteration in function or structure in the segments of the GI tract can disturb these physiological processes, resulting in anorexia, dehydration, hypovolemia, acid–base and electrolyte disturbances, protein loss, abdominal pain, and patient emaciation. All these derangements can have significant implications in the anesthetic management of dogs and cats undergoing diagnostic procedures (e.g., endoscopy), feeding tube placement, or surgery.

Oropharyngeal Diseases

Anatomically, the oral cavity is generally composed of the lips, cheeks, hard and soft palates, lower and upper dental arcades and associated bones (i.e., incisive, maxillary, palatine, mandible), tongue, and oropharynx [2]. In dogs and cats, endotracheal (ET) intubation is commonly achieved orally, and injury or disease of the oral cavity can present unique challenges to accomplish this task, in addition to other complications during the perianesthetic period (Table 5.1). Oral cavity diseases in dogs and cats that require surgical intervention include congenital and traumatic abnormalities, infectious disorders, foreign bodies, neoplasia, and salivary gland and dental diseases.

Clinical Signs

Patients with oral disease may present with ptyalism, abnormal food prehension, dysphagia, inappetence, weight loss, and halitosis. Attempts to ingest food can cause trauma to the oropharyngeal mucosa, resulting in oral pain and bleeding [2, 3]. Patients with pharyngeal dysphagia may be more prone to regurgitation and aspiration, particularly in cases where a large space-occupying mass is compressing

Canine and Feline Anesthesia and Co-Existing Disease, Second Edition. Edited by Rebecca A. Johnson, Lindsey B. C. Snyder and Carrie A. Schroeder.

Companion website: www.wiley.com/go/johnson/canine

Table 5.1 Potential perianesthetic considerations in patients with oral cavity and oropharyngeal disorders undergoing anesthesia for surgical procedures.

Common oral surgical diseases		Anesthetic considerations
Dogs		
Congenital	Primary cleft palate	Pediatric patient Dysphagia—potential for preoperative aspiration pneumonia Low body condition score (BCS)
Infectious	Lingual abscesses	Large ventral cervical swelling—potential for pain and airway obstruction
Trauma	Lip avulsion, jaw fracture, tooth fracture	Pain
	Foreign body (tongue, palate, oropharynx)	Difficult intubation (e.g., wood stick in oral cavity) Surgical ventral midline approach of oropharynx—potential for laryngeal paralysis in recovery if laryngeal recurrent nerve is damaged
	Chemical burns	Careful handling of tongue with ET intubation
Neoplasia	Oral melanomas, nontonsillar squamous cell carcinoma (SCC), fibrosarcoma, osteosarcoma, canine acanthomatous ameloblastoma (CAA)	Potential for preoperative aspiration pneumonia when dysphagia is present[a] Difficult ET intubation[a] Hemorrhage, pain[b] Postoperative aspiration of fluid and blood Postoperative airway obstruction if gauze sponges are left in oropharynx
	Tonsillar SCC	Potential for preoperative aspiration pneumonia when dysphagia is present[a] Preoperative stridor, airway obstruction, dyspnea[a] Difficult ET intubation[a] Hemorrhage, pain, postoperative aspiration of fluid and blood[c] Postoperative airway obstruction if gauze sponges are left in oropharynx Postoperative airway obstruction or dyspnea due to pharyngeal swelling secondary to tissue trauma
Sialocele	Pharyngeal sialoceles	Potential for preoperative aspiration pneumonia when dysphagia and regurgitation are present[a] Preoperative stridor, airway obstruction, dyspnea[a] Difficult ET intubation[a] Postoperative airway obstruction if gauze sponges are left in oropharynx
Cats		
Feline orofacial pain syndrome (FOPS)		Pain
Neoplasia	Oral SCC, mast cell tumor, fibrosarcoma, osteosarcoma, peripheral odontogenic fibroma (POF)	Hemorrhage, pain[d] Postoperative aspiration of fluid and blood Postoperative airway obstruction if gauze sponges are left in oropharynx

[a] Large space-occupying pharyngeal mass.
[b] In dogs, mandibulectomy or maxillectomy is recommended for the treatment of malignant oral neoplasms involving bones.
[c] Tonsillectomy.
[d] In cats, rostral mandibulectomy is recommended for the treatment of malignant oral neoplasms involving the rostral mandible.

cranial nerves IX and X. These nerves are responsible for a series of involuntary movements that transport food through the pharynx and cricopharyngeal sphincter into the esophagus and protect the airway during swallowing [4]. Patients with pharyngeal-stage dysphagia have repeated unsuccessful attempts at swallowing and food may stay in the pharynx. Because the epiglottis relaxes at the termination of swallowing and leaves the airway unprotected, affected animals are at risk for aspiration pneumonia. Difficulty associated with eating and swallowing can lead to weight loss and poor body condition score, which can compromise redistribution of lipid-soluble drugs such as propofol [2, 3, 5]. In addition, animals with large oropharyngeal neoplasia may be at risk of partial or complete airway obstruction, and anesthesia may have to be induced in an emergency in order to intubate the trachea and relieve the obstruction [3].

Laboratory Data

Before anesthesia is performed, a thorough physical examination, complete blood count (CBC), serum biochemistry profile, and urinalysis should be performed. The prothrombin time, partial thromboplastin time, and buccal mucosal bleeding time tests should be considered when a coagulopathy is suspected, or a large, vascularized mass is to be resected. Blood typing should be performed before surgery in dogs and cats undergoing mandibulectomy or maxillectomy to ensure safety, in case blood product transfusion is necessary, and blood cross-matching should always be performed in dogs and cats that have previously been transfused [3]. CBC and serum biochemical profile results can be nonspecific for these patients; however, low hematocrit values owing to continuous small bleeding from trauma of the oropharyngeal mucosa may be noted (Figure 5.1) [2, 3].

Anesthetic Management

Perianesthetic Considerations

Anemic patients with packed cell volume (PCV) lower than 20% should receive a packed red blood cell (pRBC) transfusion before surgery because the oxygen-carrying capacity of blood and the oxygen delivery to tissues are significantly impaired below this point. pRBC transfusion must also occur in patients with severe anemia undergoing mandibulectomy and maxillectomy owing to the increased risk of hemorrhage during these procedures [2]. The inferior alveolar artery, a branch of the maxillary artery, runs through the horizontal ramus of the mandible and is almost always ligated and transected during mandibulectomy (Figure 5.1). Blood supply to the maxillary region is provided by two major arteries, the major palatine, and the infraorbital arteries, both branches from the maxillary artery.

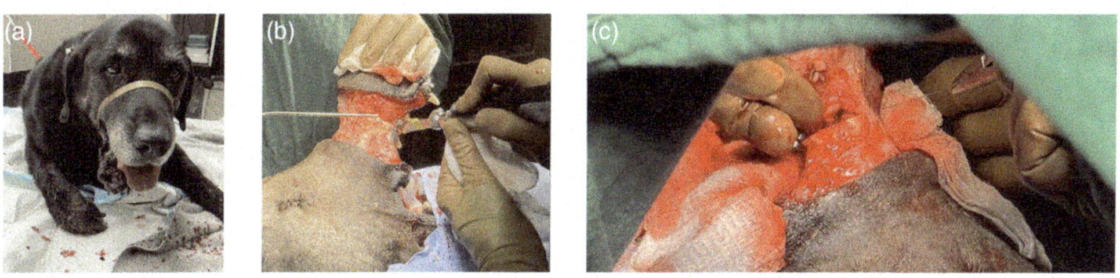

Figure 5.1 (a) Twelve-year-old male neutered Labrador Retriever presented for an actively hemorrhagic and necrotic rostral mandibular mass, previously diagnosed as osteosarcoma. On presentation, PCV was 30% and TP was 6.0 g dl^{-1}. Surgery was scheduled on the following day. Preoperative PCV was 17% and TP 4.8 g dl^{-1}. Patient received pRBCs prior and during surgery. (b) Rostral mandibulectomy. (c) Inferior alveolar artery ligation prior mandibular horizontal ramus resection.

Depending on the location of the tumor, one or both arteries may be ligated before maxillectomy. Rostral maxillectomy can be accompanied by diffuse bleeding from the highly vascularized nasal turbinates [6]. In this regard, the placement of two intravenous (IV) catheters may be prudent, as this allows simultaneous administration of blood, fluids, and inotropic support, if necessary.

Preoperative thoracic radiographs or computed tomography (CT) for the detection of pulmonary metastases is indicated for dogs and cats with oral neoplasia; the presence of visible pulmonary metastases may indicate an extremely poor prognosis and surgery may not be indicated [6]. Careful lung auscultation and thoracic radiographs are advised for evaluation of aspiration pneumonia in patients with clinical signs of dysphagia and diagnosed with large oropharyngeal masses or swelling [3].

Laryngeal visualization is often challenging in dogs and cats with large oral cavity masses (Figure 5.2) or masses located in the temporomandibular joint, which can complicate ET intubation and maintenance of a patent airway. General anesthesia without a secure airway may result in aspiration of gastric contents and blood, which can lead to pneumonia and small airway obstruction, respectively. In cases where ET intubation is expected to be difficult (i.e., patients with large pharyngeal masses, difficulty of opening the mouth, or for those already presenting dyspnea), preoxygenation with 100% oxygen via a tight-fitting mask should be considered before anesthetic induction. In addition, diverse diameters of ET tubes, stylets, a laryngoscope with adequate lighting, and several laryngoscope blade sizes should be readily available. A flexible endoscope can also be valuable in visualizing the airway for ET intubation, if available. Alternatively, retrograde ET intubation can be performed in patients with restricted mouth opening. In this case, the anesthetist punctures the cricothyroid membrane with a needle or an IV catheter, a guide wire is inserted through the needle or catheter and advanced retrograde to the mouth opening. The guide wire is grasped with forceps once it is observed in the oral cavity and a cuffed ET tube is passed caudally over the wire into the larynx. The guide wire is removed, and the ET tube is advanced further caudally into the trachea [7]. Regardless of the selected ET intubation technique, a surgical tracheostomy pack should always be available, as tracheostomy may be necessary if several attempts at ET intubation fail.

(a) (b) (c)

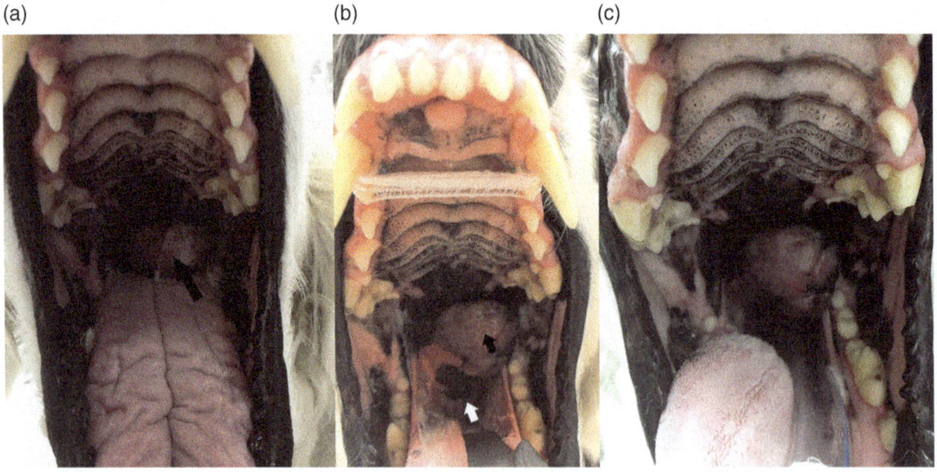

Figure 5.2 (a) Oropharyngeal mass (black arrow) hindering laryngeal visualization. (b) Possible laryngeal visualization (white arrow) with the aid of a tie gauze around the muzzle to widely open the oral cavity and a long-blade laryngoscope. (c) Successful ET intubation.

An orally placed ET tube can sometimes hinder oral cavity and oropharyngeal surgery. In these cases, the portion of the ET tube that remains in the oral cavity can be deviated through a pharyngotomy or tracheotomy incision (see Chapter 13; Figure 5.3). For all methods of intubation, it is important that the ET tube and its cuff are properly inflated and lubricated to prevent blood and fluid from entering the lower airways. Gauze sponges are frequently placed in the oropharynx around the ET tube to help absorb fluids. However, these gauze sponges must be removed before the end of anesthesia and removal of the ET tube to prevent airway obstruction [2, 3]. Tying umbilical tape around the gauze to stack them together in the oropharynx and leaving the other end of the umbilical tape long enough to exit the mouth is a common way to prevent leaving packing material in the pharynx (Figure 5.4) [3].

Proper patient and anesthetic equipment positioning maximize the surgeon's ability to visualize the surgical field. In some situations, the anesthetist and anesthetic equipment will be away from the patient head, which can make it difficult for the anesthetist to monitor the signs associated with anesthetic depth, and therefore changes associated with heart rate, arterial blood pressure, and respiratory rate and pattern should be used to help predict anesthetic depth.

A mouth gag is often needed to facilitate exposure of the oral cavity. However, in cats, spring-loaded mouth gags have been associated with neurological deficits, including post-operative blindness. Blood flow to the feline brain is primarily supplied via the maxillary artery. The high and constant forces between the maxilla and the mandible applied by spring-loaded mouth gags can compromise cerebral blood flow by stretching the maxillary

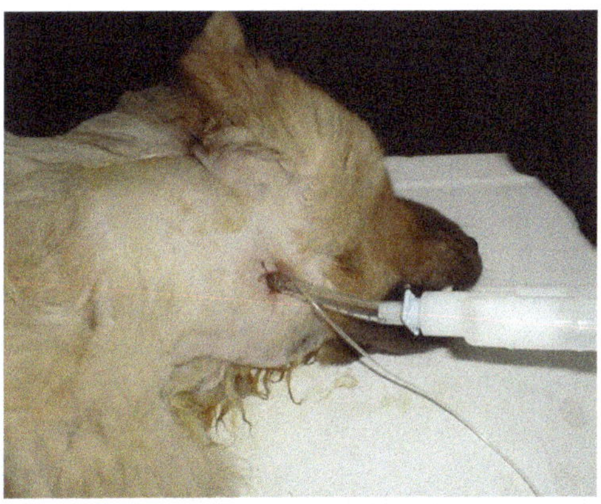

Figure 5.3 Introduction of the proximal end of the ET tube through a pharyngotomy. After the ET tube is orally placed and connected to the breathing system, inhalational anesthesia is started. A pharyngotomy is performed, and the adaptor of the ET tube is removed. A hemostat is inserted through the skin at the entry site of the pharyngotomy. The proximal end of the ET tube (without the adaptor) is grasped with the hemostat and pulled through the pharyngotomy. The adaptor is reattached to the ET tube, and the latter is reattached to the breathing system. Inhalational anesthesia can be continued at this time. *Source:* Photo courtesy of Dr. M. Martinez, Dr. V. Cairoli, and Dr. R. Bruhl Day.

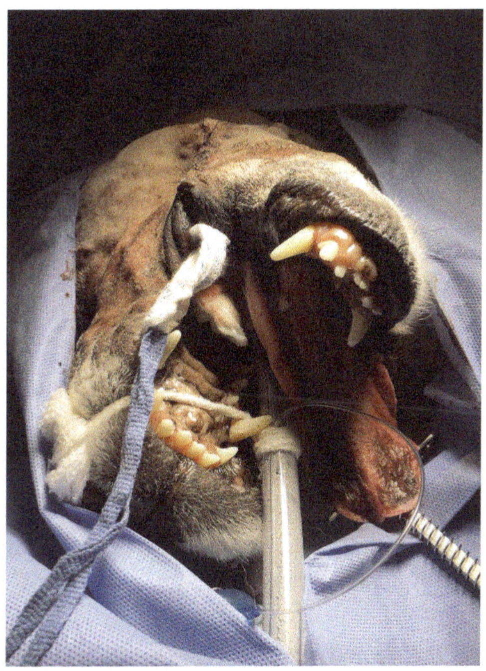

Figure 5.4 Laparotomy sponge used to pack oropharynx and prevent fluid from entering airway. The tie of the laparotomy sponge is left exiting the oral cavity to remind the anesthetist to remove it before anesthetic recovery.

artery. If a mouth gag is necessary, the use of a smaller and plastic mouth gag (e.g., a plastic needle cap or a 20 mm, cut 1 ml syringe barrel, depending on the size of the cat) between the upper and lower arcades is advised [8, 9]. Decreased duration of open-mouth procedures should also be exercised during feline oral cavity surgery to minimize reduced maxillary artery blood flow.

Preanesthetic Medication

Sedative drug selection will depend on multiple factors, including patients' signalment, temperament, physical status, and disease localization (Table 5.2). In patients with partial airway obstruction and those in whom preoxygenation is included before induction of anesthesia, sedative drugs that decrease anxiety may be desired.

The potential for severe pain exists in patients undergoing mandibulectomy and maxillectomy, as bone and nerves will be resected during these procedures. Therefore, these cases warrant a multimodal analgesic approach [10]. Full mu-opioid agonist drugs should be included in the premedication with the goal of providing preemptive analgesia (Table 5.2).

Vomiting after premedication should be avoided in patients with an inability to open the oral cavity and with partial airway obstruction. Therefore, drugs such as alpha-2-adrenergic agonists [11] and full mu-agonist opioids [12, 13] should be used with caution or via appropriate routes (e.g., IV versus IM). Meperidine and methadone are notable exceptions, as they are less likely to cause vomiting in small-animal patients [14, 15]. The advantage of using full mu-opioid agonists (i.e., intense analgesia) must be weighed against several factors, including options of opioids available, procedural pain level, and the risks associated with emesis. Therefore, in patients in whom vomiting is undesirable, but analgesia is required, methadone may be a better premedication drug to administer if the chosen route is IM [14].

Anesthetic Induction

In patients with airway obstruction or an inability to open the oral cavity, anesthetic induction should be rapidly achieved without excitement (Table 5.2). For this reason, IV anesthetic induction techniques with propofol (2.0–8.0 $mg\,kg^{-1}$ IV), alfaxalone (0.5–4.0 $mg\,kg^{-1}$ IV), or ketamine–diazepam or ketamine–midazolam (5.0 $mg\,kg^{-1}$, 0.25 $mg\,kg^{-1}$ IV) are overwhelmingly preferred to mask induction with inhalation anesthetics.

Anesthetic Maintenance

Anesthetic maintenance in patients undergoing oral cavity surgery should be achieved using inhalation anesthetics (e.g., isoflurane, sevoflurane, or desflurane) or injectable techniques (total or partial IV anesthesia; TIVA or PIVA). Intraoperative analgesia can be accomplished by combining nitrous oxide with the inhalation anesthetic or by using a multimodal approach. Local or regional blocks can be very effective for providing analgesia for mandibulectomy and maxillectomy. Depending on the resected area, regional blocks of the infraorbital, maxillary, mental, or mandibular nerves can be performed with the administration of 0.5–1.0 $ml\,kg^{-1}$ of lidocaine, bupivacaine, or ropivacaine (Table 5.3) [16]. Ultrasound-guided techniques can be used to allow local anesthetic visualization and distribution in the region of the maxillary nerve [17], and a nerve stimulator can aid in the localization of the proximal mandibular nerve [18]. Specific descriptions of these techniques can be found elsewhere [17, 18]. Intraoperatively, analgesia can also be achieved by a continuous rate infusion (CRI) of an opioid (e.g., fentanyl, morphine, hydromorphone, or methadone) or combined with multimodal CRIs such as IV lidocaine and/or ketamine (Table 5.2). This approach provides the additional benefit of reducing the amount of inhalation anesthetic required, which will improve hemodynamic stability for the patient and may also prevent central sensitization of pain [10, 19].

Table 5.2 Preanesthetic, induction, and adjunct agents used in the anesthetic management of patients with gastrointestinal diseases.

	Dogs		Cats
	Dose (mg kg^{-1}) and route	LD (mg kg^{-1}); CRI (mg kg^{-1} h^{-1}) (IV route)	Dose (mg kg^{-1}) and route
Premedication			
Phenothiazines			
Acepromazine	0.02–0.05 IV, IM		0.05–0.1 IV, IM
Alpha-2-adrenergic agonists			
Dexmedetomidine	0.002–0.01 IV, IM		0.003–0.02 IV, IM
Opioids			
Morphine	0.3–1.0 IM		0.1–0.3 IM
Meperidine	1.0–5.0 IM		0.5–1.0 IM
Methadone	0.1–1.0 IV, IM		0.1–0.3 IV, IM
Hydromorphone	0.05–0.2 IV, IM		0.05–0.1 IV, IM
Oxymorphone	0.05–0.2 IV, IM		0.05–0.1 IV, IM
Buprenorphine	0.01–0.03 IV, IM		0.01–0.02 IV, IM
Butorphanol	0.1–0.4 IV, IM		0.1–0.4 IV, IM
Benzodiazepines			
Diazepam	0.2–0.4 IV		0.2–0.4 IV
Midazolam	0.2–0.4 IV, IM		0.2–0.4 IV, IM
Induction			
Propofol	2.0–8.0 IV[a]		2.0–8.0 IV[a]
Alfaxalone	0.5–4.0 IV[a]		0.5–4.0 IV[a]
Ketamine + diazepam OR midazolam	K: 5.0 IV + D/M: 0.25 IV		K: 5.0 IV + D/M: 0.25 IV
Fentanyl + diazepam OR midazolam	F: 0.005–0.01 IV + D/M: 0.2–0.5 IV		
Adjuncts and analgesics			
Opioids			
Morphine		CRI: 0.1–0.3	
Hydromorphone		CRI: 0.01–0.05	
Methadone		CRI: 0.12–0.036	
Fentanyl		LD: 0.002–0.005 CRI: 0.002–0.04	
Remifentanil		LD: 0.002–0.005 CRI: 0.002–0.04	
NSAIDs			
Carprofen	2.0–4.0 SC		2.0–4.0 SC[b]
Meloxicam	0.2 SC		0.1–0.2 SC[b]

(continued)

Table 5.2 (Continued)

	Dogs		Cats
	Dose (mg kg^{-1}) and route	LD (mg kg^{-1}); CRI (mg kg^{-1} h^{-1}) (IV route)	Dose (mg kg^{-1}) and route
Robenacoxib	2.0 SC		2.0 SC
NMBAs			
Atracurium	0.1 IV		0.1 IV
Vecuronium	0.1 IV		0.1 IV
Local anesthetics			
Lidocaine		LD: 1.0–2.0 IV CRI: 3.0 IV	
N-methyl-D-aspartate receptor (NMDA) antagonist			
Ketamine		LD: 0.5 CRI: 0.6 IV	
Opioid antagonist or partial reversal			
Naloxone	0.001–0.002 IV		0.001–0.002 IV
Butorphanol	0.1 IV		0.1 IV

LD: loading dose; CRI: continuous rate infusion; IV: intravenously; IM: intramuscularly; SC: subcutaneously.
[a] Administered to effect.
[b] Single dose in cats.

Table 5.3 Perineural anesthesia of the head according to the location of mandibulectomy and maxillectomy.

Surgery location	Type of perineural block
Rostral hemimandibulectomy	Ipsilateral mental nerve block
Rostral mandibulectomy	Left and right mental nerve blocks
Central, caudal, or total hemimandibulectomy	Ipsilateral mandibular nerve block
Rostral hemimaxillectomy	Ipsilateral infraorbital nerve block
Rostral maxillectomy	Left and right infraorbital nerve blocks
Central, caudal, or total hemimaxillectomy	Ipsilateral maxillary nerve block

Although rarely reported in veterinary medicine, maxillofacial surgery can trigger the trigeminovagal reflex, which produces increases in vagal tone and bradycardia when a branch of the trigeminal nerve is stimulated [20, 21]. Therefore, anesthetic monitoring should include an electrocardiogram (ECG), a means to detect heart rate or pulse rate (e.g., Doppler oscillometry, pulse oximetry, esophageal stethoscope), and blood pressure measuring to accurately and rapidly diagnose severe hypotension that may be associated with bradycardia or asystole. Upon recognition of the trigeminovagal reflex, rapid communication between anesthetist and surgeon should occur in an attempt to discontinue the stimulation of the surgical region followed by IV treatment with anticholinergics (e.g., atropine or

Table 5.4 Fluids and therapeutic agents used to treat cardiovascular derangements during anesthesia in patients with gastrointestinal diseases.

Fluids and therapeutic agents	Dose regimen
Maintenance fluid rate during anesthesia	
Balanced crystalloid (e.g., LRS)	5–10 ml kg^{-1} h^{-1} IV
Fluids for hypovolemia	
6% HES	20 ml kg^{-1} d^{-1} IV[a]
6% HES	1–2 ml kg^{-1-1} IV[a]
6% HES bolus	3–5 ml kg^{-1} IV[a]
7% hypertonic saline	4–6 ml kg^{-1} IV
Isotonic crystalloid shock dose	60–90 ml kg^{-1} IV
Isotonic crystalloid bolus	10–20 ml kg^{-1}
Treatment for intraoperative bradycardia	
Glycopyrrolate	0.005–0.02 mg kg^{-1} IV
Atropine	0.02–0.04 mg kg^{-1} IV
Treatment for intraoperative hypotension	
Dopamine	5–20 μg kg^{-1} min^{-1} IV
Dobutamine	1–10 μg kg^{-1} min^{-1} IV
Norepinephrine	0.01–2.0 mcg kg^{-1} min^{-1} IV
Phenylephrine	0.5–3.0 mcg kg^{-1} min^{-1} IV
Vasopressin	0.5–2.0 mU kg^{-1} min^{-1}
Treatment for ventricular tachycardia	
Lidocaine	Bolus: 2–4 mg kg^{-1} IV Infusion: 3.0–4.5 mg kg^{-1} h^{-1} IV
Procainamide	Bolus: 2–8 mg kg^{-1} slow IV Infusion: 1.5–2.4 mg kg^{-1} h^{-1}

[a] Use is controversial; see text for details.

glycopyrrolate) or beta-1-adrenergic receptor agonists (e.g., dopamine, dobutamine) in case of a refractory response to anticholinergics (Table 5.4) [21].

Intraoperatively, a balanced isotonic crystalloid solution (e.g., lactated Ringer's solution [LRS]) should be administered IV at a rate of up to 5–10 ml kg h^{-1} (Table 5.4). The surgery magnitude and the likelihood of hemorrhage, due to the extensive vascular supply of the oral and nasal cavity, should be considered when selecting modalities of arterial blood pressure monitoring. Intra-arterial catheter placement with invasive arterial blood pressure measurements is preferred when large, vascularized masses are excised. Hypertonic saline (7.0–7.5%), hydroxyethyl starches (HESs; 6% hetastarch 600/0.75 [Hespan®] or 6% tetrastarch 130/0.4 [VetStarch™]), a combination of 23.4% saline with HES, whole blood or pRBC, and fresh frozen plasma (FFP) should be available in the event of severe hemorrhage (Table 5.4) [2]. In situations of significant blood loss, an approach combining several types of fluids is desirable, since large volumes of crystalloids are required to replace intravascular volume. HES solutions are commonly used for the treatment of hemorrhagic shock in dogs and cats. In the recent years, controversies related to their use have been raised in both human and veterinary medicine, particularly in critically ill patients or patients with sepsis [22–27]. Negative outcomes, such as acute kidney injury, need for renal replacement therapy, and mortality, have been associated with the administration of HES in critically ill human patients, but are likely related to HES solutions with higher concentrations, molecular weights (MWs), and molar substitutions (MSs), as well as administration of large cumulative doses over several days of hospitalization [28]. These conclusions have been extrapolated to veterinary medicine and prospective controlled studies are still lacking in critically ill dogs and cats. However, 6% tetrastarch (HES 130/0.4) in noncritically ill dogs and cats at recommended doses for intraoperative volume replacement (dogs: 5–20 $ml\,kg^{-1}$, cats: 3–15 $ml\,kg^{-1}$) has been shown to effectively expand plasma volume during anesthesia or in hemorrhagic shock states without evidence of acute kidney injury or long-lasting effects on coagulation function [29–35].

Anesthetic Recovery

On termination of inhalation anesthetics, gauze sponges should be removed from the caudal pharynx and the oral cavity [2]. Fluid evacuation with a suction tube before termination of anesthesia may also prevent fluid aspiration. Postoperative swelling of the oral mucous membranes may cause airway obstruction. This can be minimized by the administration of corticosteroids (e.g., dexamethasone 0.1–0.2 $mg\,kg^{-1}$ IV).

Tracheal extubation should be delayed until a well-developed swallowing reflex is present. When the patient is ready for extubation, the ET tube should be removed with the cuff at least partially inflated to help ensure that any blood clots and fluid left in the pharynx are expelled through the mouth rather than being aspirated or swallowed [36]. During recovery, these patients should be monitored for signs of airway obstruction or pain.

Analgesics such as opioids (e.g., fentanyl, hydromorphone, methadone) and nonsteroidal anti-inflammatory drugs (NSAIDs) (e.g., carprofen [2.0–4.0 $mg\,kg^{-1}$ in dogs; 2.0–4.0 $mg\,kg^{-1}$ single dose in cats], meloxicam [0.2 $mg\,kg^{-1}$ in dogs; 0.1–0.2 $mg\,kg^{-1}$ single dose in cats], robenacoxib [2.0 $mg\,kg^{-1}$ for up to 3 days in dogs and cats]) should be provided as needed. However, if corticosteroids have been previously administered to the patient, caution should be taken when deciding if NSAIDs are an appropriate analgesic to administer.

Esophageal Diseases

The esophagus carries food, water, and saliva from the pharynx to the stomach. Impairment of these functions can lead to gastroesophageal reflux (GER), esophagitis, regurgitation of the ingesta back to the oral cavity, and aspiration of this content, resulting in pneumonia [2].

Esophageal diseases in dogs and cats are related to obstructive, motility (e.g., megaesophagus), or inflammatory (e.g., esophagitis from chronic vomiting or GER) disorders [37]. In certain situations, these patients require anesthesia for feeding tube placement (e.g., percutaneous endoscopic gastrostomy [PEG] tube and gastrostomy tube), further diagnostics (e.g., esophagoscopy and biopsy), or treatment of the primary problem (e.g., esophagoscopy for foreign body removal, esophageal balloon dilation, and vascular ring anomaly correction).

Esophageal Anatomy

The esophagus connects the pharynx to the stomach and is responsible to transport ingesta and fluid. It is the only visceral organ that contains striated muscle. In the dog, the muscular layers of the esophagus are made entirely of striated muscle, whereas in the cat, only the proximal two- thirds contain striated muscle. The esophagus is divided into cervical and thoracic portions. The upper esophageal sphincter (composed of cricopharyngeus and thyropharyngeus muscles) is located at the proximal end of the esophagus. The lower esophageal sphincter (LES) is located at the distal end, at the gastroesophageal junction. In this area, dogs have a thick muscle layer created by a circular arrangement of striated muscle. Combined with the diaphragm crura and the angle at which the esophagus and stomach meet, a zone of higher intraluminal pressure at the gastroesophageal junction is created [38–40].

Esophageal Obstruction

Esophageal obstruction usually occurs in dogs and cats because of foreign bodies, benign strictures, neoplasia, hiatal hernias, gastroesophageal intussusceptions, and vascular ring anomalies [2]. Depending on the degree of obstruction, food and secretions accumulate cranially to the obstruction leading to segmental distention of the esophagus, disruption of normal neuromuscular function, and decreased esophageal peristalsis [40].

Esophageal foreign bodies are relatively common in small-animal patients. Foreign material usually lodges where the esophagus narrows. These locations include the thoracic inlet, the base of the heart, and the esophageal hiatus in the diaphragm. Dogs, particularly small breed and younger than 3 years old [41], are the most frequently diagnosed with esophageal foreign bodies. Esophageal injuries secondary to the foreign body can occur, and the extent of these injuries depends on the type of object, its size and shape, and the duration in contact with the mucosa [37]. Previous unsuccessful attempts at endoscopic foreign material removal can also lead to a significant increase in secondary esophageal injury. Esophageal perforation prior to or during foreign body removal can lead to significant morbidity and mortality due to pneumothorax, pleuritis, pyothorax, and respiratory distress [42].

Esophagitis is caused by esophageal mucosal inflammation and, in more severe cases, these lesions can extend into the submucosa and muscularis layers, leading to esophageal stricture formation. Causes associated with esophagitis include persistent vomiting, gastroesophageal emptying, hiatal hernia, ingestion of corrosive substances, thermal burns, and esophageal foreign bodies. However, esophagitis with resulting esophageal stricture related to GER during general anesthesia is the most common cause of benign esophageal stricture in dogs and cats (46–83%) [43–47] and may occur when protective mechanisms are diminished (i.e., reduced LES pressure, absence of swallowing saliva, reduced esophagus clearance) by general anesthesia itself and anesthetic/analgesic drugs (Box 5.1). During anesthesia, the acidic gastric contents, particularly with pH ≤4.0, that contact the esophageal mucosa can severely damage the esophagus if they are not neutralized by saliva or removed by peristalsis within a few minutes. The most common signs of esophagitis/esophageal stricture include hypersalivation, dysphagia, esophageal pain, anorexia, weight loss, and regurgitation. These signs may take as little as a few days or up to 3 weeks after the general anesthetic event to present [44, 45, 47]. Despite the most common cause of esophageal stricture being associated with anesthesia, the overall incidence of esophageal stricture following anesthesia appears to be low (0.07–0.1%). However, when it occurs, the cost associated with diagnosis and treatment of this disorder is extremely large, with a subsequent high mortality rate (12–30%) [44, 45, 47]. These patients usually return for several subsequent anesthetic events in which esophageal bougienage or dilation with balloon catheters is performed to treat the strictures.

Brachycephalic dogs presented with signs of brachycephalic obstructive airway syndrome are known to have a higher incidence of gastroesophageal abnormalities due to the generation of high negative intrathoracic pressures during increased inspiratory effort [70]. Although they are at increased risk of GER, regurgitation, and vomiting preoperatively and postoperatively [70, 71], one study failed to show that they are at increased risk of GER

Box 5.1 Factors that increase GER or decrease LES pressure in dogs and cats during anesthesia.

Factors
Age: older animals [48]
Age: younger animals [49]
Dogs weighing >40 kg (regurgitation) [50]
Large-sized, deep-chested dogs and sternal recumbency [51, 52]
Prolonged fasting time (>10 h) [53–56]
Shorter fasting time (3 h) [49]
Dorsal recumbency [49, 57]
Change in body position during anesthesia [58]
Intraabdominal surgery (including laparoscopic procedures) [48, 58]
Anesthesia in the second half of pregnancy [59]
Anesthetic duration (>105 min) [58, 60]
Atropine [53, 61–63]
Acepromazine [53, 62, 64]
Xylazine [62]
Opioids [15, 60]
Diazepam [64]
Injectable anesthetics (thiopental, alphaxalone-alphadolone, propofol, ketamine–xylazine, and ketamine[a]) [65–67]
Inhalant anesthetic (halothane, isoflurane, sevoflurane, and nitrous oxide) [68, 69]

[a] Least decrease in LES compared to other injectable agents.

and regurgitation during anesthesia [72]. However, this study was underpowered and brachycephalic dogs presented in respiratory distress were excluded from the data if they had received corticosteroids prior to anesthesia. Therefore, when anesthetizing brachycephalic breeds, the anesthetist should still closely monitor for intraoperative regurgitation and signs of esophagitis and aspiration pneumonia in the immediate postoperative period.

Megaesophagus

Megaesophagus may occur with esophageal motility disorders. The causes of esophageal hypomotility are extensive, varying from a primarily idiopathic origin in dogs (most common) or secondary to neuromuscular, muscular, infectious, or autoimmune disorders. Patients with megaesophagus may require anesthesia for esophagoscopy or other diagnostic tests and procedures for the suspected primary disease. These may include electromyography and nerve conduction velocity, muscle biopsy, cerebrospinal fluid collection, or thymoma removal [2, 37].

Clinical Signs

Clinical signs of esophageal diseases include abnormalities of prehension and swallowing, regurgitation, and ptyalism. Vomiting can occur if both the esophagus and stomach have significant disease such as with hiatal hernia, gastroesophageal intussusception, or GER [37].

It is important to differentiate regurgitation from vomiting because regurgitation is more likely to occur in patients with primary pharyngeal or esophageal disorders. In addition, the clinical consequences of vomiting and regurgitation may be different and, as such, can influence the clinician's anesthetic plan. Regurgitation is a passive flow of food, water, or saliva from the esophagus to the oral cavity [73]. The primary complication of regurgitation is aspiration pneumonia. Alternatively, vomiting is a forceful expulsion of gastroduodenal contents mediated by the central nervous system. The presence of vomiting usually indicates the presence of GI or systemic disease [73, 74].

Chronic regurgitation can lead to anorexia, weight loss, stunted growth compared to littermates (e.g., vascular ring anomalies, congenital megaesophagus), depression, and emaciation [2]. Esophageal pain may be suspected when patients are observed having signs of neck stretching while swallowing and repeated swallowing [45, 47].

Respiratory distress, coughing, pulmonary crackles, and fever may suggest aspiration pneumonia secondary to regurgitation. In the case of foreign bodies, respiratory distress can also be associated with pneumothorax or compression of the upper airway by the foreign material. Therefore, it is recommended to closely examine thoracic radiographs, not only for the diagnosis of a foreign body but also to evaluate for signs of aspiration pneumonia, pleural effusion, pneumothorax, pneumomediastinum, or tracheal compression [40].

Patients with esophageal motility disorders (e.g., megaesophagus) can also present with generalized muscle weakness or atrophy, neurologic deficits, and/or oropharyngeal dysphagia when generalized myasthenia gravis is present [2, 37].

Laboratory Data

A minimum database of tests, including a CBC and serum biochemical profile, should be performed in patients with esophageal disease. PCV, total protein (TP), blood urea nitrogen (BUN), and creatinine may be elevated because of dehydration. A neutrophilia with left shift may be consistent with aspiration pneumonia. Metabolic acidosis with lactatemia can occur in dehydrated patients and metabolic alkalosis can be seen with gastroesophageal disorders (e.g., hiatal hernia) [37]. Patients with megaesophagus secondary to hypoadrenocorticism may have electrolyte disturbances such as hyperkalemia and hyponatremia [73, 75].

Anesthetic Management

Perianesthetic Considerations

The purpose of preoperative fasting is to withhold liquids and solids for a specified period before surgery to reduce gastric volume and acidity. These goals are particularly important for patients with gastroesophageal diseases that are prone to regurgitation. When considering preoperative fasting, one needs to balance the risk of dehydration, administration of preoperative oral medications, and hypoglycemia versus the risk of GER, regurgitation, esophageal injury, and aspiration pneumonia. Traditionally, in small-animal medicine, preoperative fasting times have been 8–12 h for scheduled procedures with the rationale that the stomach would be empty prior to anesthetic induction, since complete gastric emptying in dogs and cats ranges from 7–15 h [76]. More recently, the American Society of Anesthesiologists (ASA) has modified their guidelines for preoperative fasting in healthy humans undergoing elective procedures; these guidelines may additionally need to be adjusted for people with coexisting diseases or conditions that can affect gastric emptying or fluid volume. With that in mind, the ASA Practice Guidelines for Preoperative Fasting recommend: (i) clear liquids may be ingested for up to 2 h before anesthetic procedures; (ii) a light meal may be ingested for up to 6 h before elective procedures; and (iii) fasting time of 8 h or more may be needed in cases of patient intake of fatty foods and/or meat. These conclusions were based on randomized clinical trials that showed no differences in findings regarding gastric volume and pH when people could have a light meal 4–6h before a procedure compared to overnight fasting [77].

In veterinary medicine, the incidence of GER in healthy dogs after shorter fasting time has been reported (Box 5.1). When fed a light meal (one-half of their daily ration in canned food) approximately 3h before elective procedures, 3/60 dogs experienced GER during anesthesia compared to 12/60 dogs that were fed the same amount and type of food but 10h prior to anesthetic induction [56]. These results were confirmed as dogs did not have significantly increased gastric volume when fed canned food at one-half of their daily ration 3h before anesthesia; in addition, the gastric acidity was reduced [54]. However, in a more recent report, dogs that were fed a light meal 3h prior to anesthesia were associated with significantly greater odds of both GER and regurgitation compared to dogs fasted for 18h [49]. The differences can be due to diet composition which may have different gastric emptying time or the preanesthetic administration of opioids (or other drugs) that could have also influenced gastric motor function and affected residual gastric volume content. While shorter preoperative fasting may be desirable in veterinary medicine and has been the new standard of practice in people, there have been no randomized controlled trials assessing the impact of preoperative fasting for dogs and cats with GI disorders, and veterinarians have followed recommendations based on small clinical studies and experience. Based on that, the American Animal Hospital Association (AAHA) has recommended shorter preoperative fasting times for water and food for healthy dogs and cats [78]. For patients with a history of, or at risk for, regurgitation, fasting times for food and water should be kept between 6 and 12h. In addition, the clinician should consider feeding 10–25% of the normal amount of food in the form of a wet ration 4–6h prior to induction. Regardless of fasting duration, the anesthetist should recognize that esophageal diseases can increase the likelihood of GER, regurgitation, and related morbidities, and that additional strategies may be appropriate, such as rapid induction and ET intubation, as well as readiness to suction the pharynx and airway. GI foreign bodies are considered medical emergencies, and fasting is usually not possible. If patients are not fasted, preoperative and intraoperative regurgitation may occur with potential of aspiration.

Preoperative fasting for young animals (i.e., 8–16 weeks of age) undergoing surgery, such as ligation and transection of the ligamentum arteriosum in puppies and kittens with persistent right aortic arch (Figure 5.5), should be kept to a minimum and limited to no greater than 4–6h. In cases of malnourished animals,

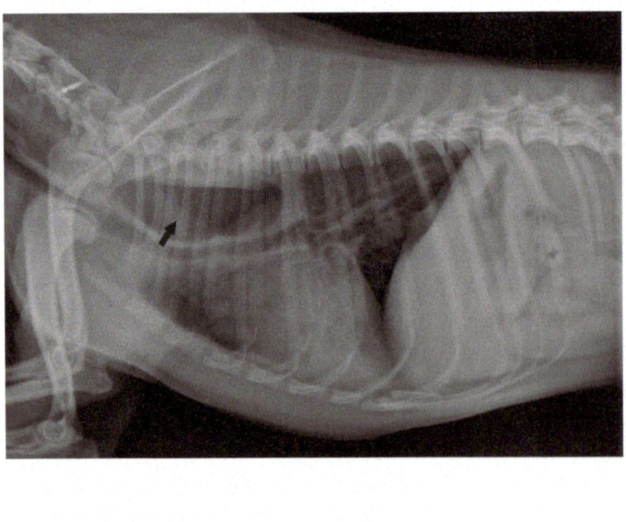

Figure 5.5 Right lateral thoracic radiograph showing esophageal dilation cranial to the base of the heart (black arrow) secondary to a vascular ring anomaly (persistent right aortic arch in this case). *Source:* Photo courtesy Dr. G. Sepulveda.

preoperative fasting should be decreased to 1–2 h [2, 39]. In these young animals, other anesthetic considerations regarding size and nourishment must also be considered. For example, blood glucose should be monitored during the procedure, maintenance fluids may have to be supplemented with dextrose, and hypothermia should be aggressively prevented [2, 42].

GER may still happen during anesthesia regardless the duration of food withholding. The incidence at which patients with esophageal diseases have GER during anesthesia is unknown, but one can assume that this occurs at higher rate than in patients without GI disease, especially in patients with clinical signs of esophagitis. In dogs and cats without history of esophageal or GI disorders, GER during anesthesia occurs frequently with an incidence rate varying from 12% to 67% [15, 48, 49, 52–56, 58–60, 66, 67, 69, 72, 79–81]. However, clinically, GER is usually not diagnosed during anesthesia because it requires the use of an esophageal pH meter or a pH impedance catheter to be detected. Only a minority of patients that experience GER regurgitate (0–15%) during anesthesia [15, 48, 50, 53, 58–60, 66, 67, 69, 80, 81], making it an insensitive clinical sign for recognizing GER. For this reason, medications to prevent GER and reflux events, to increase the pH of gastric secretions, or to improve GI motility preoperatively have been advocated by some clinicians. It should be noted that the efficacy of these drugs, when administered preoperatively, in reducing the frequency of reflux events in healthy dogs and cats that experienced GER during anesthesia is equivocal. In part, the lack of drug efficacy in reducing reflux may be due to differences in methodology of measuring pH. In some cases, administration of these drugs preoperatively, particularly proton-pump inhibitors (PPIs), may still be beneficial in reducing gastric acidity, helping to reduce esophageal mucosal and lung damage after aspiration if reflux or regurgitation does occur [2, 81, 82]. In humans, the ASA guideline for preoperative fasting and the use of pharmacologic agents found inconclusive evidence to routinely recommend administration of metoclopramide, histamine-2 antagonists (H2As), PPIs, or antiemetics prior to anesthesia to reduce the incidence of GER, emesis, or pulmonary aspiration. As such, these drugs are only recommended in people at increased risk of aspiration pneumonia [77]. Similarly, the AAHA Anesthesia and Monitoring Guidelines for Dogs and Cats recommend antiemetic, antiacid, and promotility drugs prior to anesthesia for patients with history of, or at risk for, regurgitation [78]. Clinically, H2As and PPIs are commonly administered prior to anesthesia with the goal to decrease gastric acidity. Ranitidine ($2\,\text{mg}\,\text{kg}^{-1}$ IV) administered 6 h prior to anesthesia did not prevent or decrease the frequency of GER in dogs [83]. Although famotidine administered every 12 h is superior to famotidine every 24 h or ranitidine to decrease gastric acid secretion and increase gastric pH, H2As are overall less efficacious than PPIs in dogs and cats to treat gastroduodenal ulceration or reflux esophagitis [84]. In addition, H2A tachyphylaxis may occur within 3–13 days [85], which could give a false sense of security if patients with esophageal diseases receiving this therapeutic regimen for that period would reflux or regurgitate during anesthesia. Currently, there are no studies in dogs and cats that determine if the preanesthetic administration of H2As and, potentially, a short period of increasing esophageal pH present any benefit in the anesthetized patient [86]. Therefore, additional studies of H2As prior to anesthesia to reduce esophageal pH are warranted before they are routinely recommended. In clinically healthy dogs and cats, PPIs such as omeprazole and pantoprazole are the most effective in increasing gastric pH compared to H2As [86]. In addition, omeprazole administered orally to dogs as a single dose 4 h before anesthesia and to cats twice, 18–24 h and 4 h before anesthesia, decreased the incidence of GER with pH <4. However, reflux event frequency was not decreased in both dogs and cats that had GER [81, 82]. In addition, esomeprazole administration IV 12–18 h and 1.0–1.5 h before anesthetic induction in dogs undergoing orthopedic surgery significantly increased the gastric and esophageal pH. Like the studies with omeprazole, the preanesthetic administration of esomeprazole did not decrease reflux event frequency. By contrast, esomeprazole administration IV combined with cisapride, a prokinetic drug, before anesthesia significantly decreased GER events [87], likely due to increase in LES pressure [88]. Therapy with PPIs (omeprazole 0.5–1.0 mg kg^{-1} PO or pantoprazole 1.0 mg kg^{-1} IV) should be started at least 2 days before anesthesia in order to be most effective [82, 84]. Recently the American College of Veterinary Internal Medicine published a Consensus Statement on the administration of gastroprotectants to dogs and cats and has made several recommendations to the practice of acid suppressants for the management of GI diseases, including the prevention of reflux esophagitis. The consensus opinions on the use of acid suppressants for management and prevention of reflux esophagitis, which pertains to the scope of this chapter, including: (i) there is lack of benefit for administration of H2As on a once-daily basis in dogs and cats to treat reflux esophagitis; (ii) monotherapy with an H2A given twice daily is inferior to PPIs given twice daily to dogs and cats; (iii) acid-suppressing agents may be beneficial for prevention of esophagitis secondary to GER, particularly in animals when these are associated with an anesthetic procedure; and (iv) administration of PPIs does not decrease GER, but may prevent injury by increasing the pH of the refluxate [86].

Metoclopramide is a dopaminergic receptor antagonist with antiemetic properties. In addition, it is thought to increase the LES resting tone and promote gastroduodenal motility. However, metoclopramide at 0.5 mg kg^{-1} PO did not increase LES pressure measured by high-resolution manometry in unpremedicated awake healthy Beagles [88]. Clinically, metoclopramide is recommended as a prokinetic in the treatment of esophagitis because esophageal inflammation may cause esophageal hypomotility. Also, it is routinely administered to patients who are at risk of GER and regurgitation during anesthesia; however, clinical studies are conflicting in this regard and there is no consensus if metoclopramide administration perioperatively decreases the risk of GER, esophagitis, and aspiration pneumonia. For example, high-dosage IV administration (1.0 mg kg^{-1}) followed by a high-dosage CRI (1.0 mg kg^{-1} h^{-1}) in healthy dogs undergoing orthopedic surgery decreased the risk of GER by 54% [79]. By contrast, the same high-dosage CRI (1.0 mg kg^{-1} h^{-1}) did not influence the incidence of GER in dogs undergoing ovariohysterectomy, which could have been a result of a small number of dogs experiencing GER in the studied groups [83]. Lower dosages similar to that required to attain an antiemetic and gastric prokinetic effect (0.4 mg kg^{-1} IV followed by a 0.3 mg kg^{-1} h^{-1} CRI) also did not decrease the incidence of GER compared to a negative control group [79]. Interestingly, preoperative metoclopramide at a lower dosage CRI (2.0 mg kg^{-1} d^{-1}) combined with maropitant (1 mg kg^{-1} IV) did not decrease the incidence of postoperative clinical GER, defined in the study as passive gastric reflux observed in the oral cavity (i.e., regurgitation) combined with signs of nausea. The authors speculated that metoclopramide could also have increased gastro-oral reflux due to anxiety from metoclopramide-induced extrapyramidal effects [89]. When metoclopramide (0.5 mg kg^{-1}) was administrated in combination with famotidine or omeprazole in brachycephalic dogs undergoing airway surgery, there was a lower incidence of postoperative regurgitation, and preoperative administration of these drugs is recommended for brachycephalic breeds. However, brachycephalic dogs with history of regurgitation are still more likely to regurgitate intraoperatively regardless of treatment with GI-protectant drugs [71]. Therefore, it can be concluded that the risk of GER and regurgitation during anesthesia still exists when metoclopramide is administered regardless of the CRI dose in healthy patients, and observation of clinical signs for esophagitis is warranted postoperatively. Care must be taken when extrapolating these data from healthy patients to patients with esophageal disorders who already have a predisposition to GER and regurgitation (e.g., brachycephalic breeds), and, therefore, these patients, when receiving metoclopramide perioperatively, should be closely monitored for signs of regurgitation and aspiration pneumonia.

Maropitant (1.0 mg kg^{-1}), an antiemetic drug that acts as a neurokinin-1 receptor (NK1) antagonist, administered IV 45–60 min prior to anesthetic premedication with acepromazine and hydromorphone did not significantly decrease the incidence of GER in dogs undergoing elective surgical procedures when compared to dogs treated with saline [90]. Similarly, preoperative administration of maropitant (1.0 mg kg^{-1} IV) did not prevent postoperative GER/regurgitation in dogs [89]. Currently, there is not sufficient evidence that maropitant decreases the incidence of GER or regurgitation, and therefore maropitant should not be recommended with the intent to prevent anesthesia-induced GER.

However, both metoclopramide (0.2 mg kg^{-1} IM) [91, 92] and maropitant (1.0 mg kg^{-1} SC or IV) [90, 91, 93–99] are effective antiemetics administered prior to opioids combined with dexmedetomidine or acepromazine in healthy dogs and cats. Their administration in dogs and cats with esophageal disease preoperatively may be desirable with the goal of preventing vomiting, thus decreasing further damage to the esophagus and the risk of aspiration pneumonia. Metoclopramide should be administered 30–45 min in dogs and maropitant 30–60 min in dogs and 20 h in cats before the administration of an opioid or an alpha-2-adrenergic agonist premedication to be most effective.

In cases where the patient is emaciated, anesthesia should be postponed until the animal has an improvement in body condition score. However, in certain situations, treatment for nutritional debilitation requires the placement of a gastrostomy or PEG tube, both of which require general anesthesia. In these situations, the anesthesia period should be kept as short as possible with perianesthetic considerations aimed at the individual patients' physical status and comorbidities.

Since regurgitation is commonly associated with esophageal disease, thoracic radiographs should be taken preoperatively to evaluate for the presence of aspiration pneumonia. Patients with aspiration pneumonia should be treated aggressively before being anesthetized for esophagoscopy, surgery, or feeding tube placement. If anesthesia cannot be delayed until aspiration pneumonia resolves, preoxygenation with 100% oxygen before anesthetic induction is recommended [2]. In addition, the trachea should be immediately intubated after induction, and positive pressure ventilation should be instituted to maintain oxygen saturation above 90%.

Dogs presenting with esophageal diseases that appear to be dehydrated or hypovolemic based on physical examination, CBC, and serum biochemical variables should receive fluid resuscitation before anesthesia. Tachycardia, pale mucous membranes, prolonged capillary refill time, and cold extremities are signs of hypovolemic shock and should be treated with isotonic crystalloids (60–90 ml kg^{-1} in one-quarter dose increments) and/or HES solutions (5–20 ml kg^{-1}, when indicated) and reassessed before anesthetic induction (Table 5.4). It should be noted that cats in shock might present with bradycardia and hypothermia [100]. Treatment of acid–base and electrolyte disturbances should be initiated before anesthesia if possible (see the subsection titled "Laboratory Data" under the section titled "Gastric and Small Intestinal Diseases").

In general, the anesthetic protocol is not aimed at avoiding drugs that decrease LES pressure because many of the drugs administered with the purpose of producing anesthesia or analgesia will interfere with protective mechanisms against GER (Box 5.1). Most drug selection is based on the physical status of the patient, mentation, pain level, and surgical procedure (Table 5.2). Whenever possible, drugs that produce emesis should be avoided to prevent further damage to esophagus and aspiration pneumonia.

Preanesthetic Medication

The GI effects of anticholinergic drugs have been well described. Atropine and glycopyrrolate decrease LES tone at doses commonly used for prevention or treatment of bradycardia [53, 61–63]. At high doses, they inhibit hydrogen-ion secretion by gastric parietal cells, and at the standard recommended doses for preanesthetic medication, they have minimal effect on the pH of gastric secretions in dogs [101]. Therefore, the argument for including anticholinergic drugs in the preanesthetic medication is not justifiable due to their effect on the LES, likelihood of GER, and lack of effect to reduce gastric acidity at clinical doses.

The administration of drugs that may induce vomiting or GER (e.g., alpha-2-adrenergic agonists and full mu-opioids) in the preanesthetic period of patients with an esophageal foreign body is questionable. Sharp foreign body objects may abrade or lacerate the esophageal mucosa, causing esophagitis. Sharp objects may also perforate the esophagus and, occasionally, the great vessels. If emesis is induced by preanesthetic drugs in these patients, further damage may occur [2, 102]. Acidic gastric-fluid reflux can induce further damage to the esophagus. Even so, opioids are usually included in the preanesthetic medication of these patients to provide analgesia even if foreign body removal is performed with noninvasive techniques (e.g., esophagoscopy) wherein pain is less intense. However, opioids that do not cause vomiting such as butorphanol (0.1–0.4 $mg\,kg^{-1}$), buprenorphine (0.01–0.03 $mg\,kg^{-1}$), methadone (0.1–1.0 $mg\,kg^{-1}$), and fentanyl (0.002–0.005 $mg\,kg^{-1}$) have been recommended for this type of procedure [42]. The administration of morphine, hydromorphone, and oxymorphone has been shown to increase the risk of regurgitation, GER, or vomiting significantly [13–15, 50, 60]. Therefore, methadone or fentanyl is preferred in the case of esophageal surgery where pain is more likely to be more intense. In addition, IV administration may result in less vomiting altogether, as drugs may bypass the chemoreceptor trigger zone (which induces vomiting) and act to suppress vomiting at the vomiting center [103]. Maropitant may be administered 30–60 min prior to opioid administration to prevent emesis [90, 91, 93–99].

Acepromazine (0.02–0.05 $mg\,kg^{-1}$) can be administered to provide sedation in patients with esophageal foreign bodies that are hemodynamically stable. When administered before opioids, acepromazine decreases the incidence of vomiting [13], although it increases the chances of GER [53]. Diazepam or midazolam (0.2 $mg\,kg^{-1}$) may be preferred in depressed and hypovolemic patients. Furthermore, diazepam has been associated with a significant reduction in GER episodes [53].

Intense sedation or muscle relaxation should be avoided in patients with megaesophagus. Muscle relaxation of the striated muscle layer of the esophagus can increase the likelihood of regurgitation before anesthetic induction. Intense sedation may impair the patients' ability to protect their airway, increasing the chances of aspiration pneumonia. Acepromazine, alpha-2-adrenergic agonists, and benzodiazepines should be used with caution in these patients.

Anesthetic Induction

Dogs and cats with esophageal disease are at high risk of regurgitation and aspiration pneumonia. For this reason, it is advised to have a suctioning system set up during the induction period. Anesthetic induction should be rapid with immediate ET intubation. Therefore, mask induction with inhalation anesthetic should be avoided, and IV anesthetic techniques are preferred. Propofol (2.0–8.0 $mg\,kg^{-1}$ IV) or alfaxalone (0.5–4.0 $mg\,kg^{-1}$ IV) are rapid-acting, and the airway can be immediately secured, particularly in patients with megaesophagus. Alternatively, other drugs with fast onset, such as ketamine–diazepam/midazolam, can be used in patients with esophageal disorders [42].

Endotracheal intubation should be performed with the patient in sternal recumbency with the head elevated. Application of pressure to the cricoid region has been documented in humans to reduce regurgitation [104]; however, this has not been advocated for dogs and cats. If regurgitation is observed during induction, the airway of the patient should be secured with a properly sized and lubricated cuffed ET tube and its cuff immediately inflated. Afterward, the patient's head should be dropped below the thoracic inlet, and the airway and oropharynx should be suctioned. The ET tube should be connected to a breathing system and 100% oxygen supplemented. Oxygenation and ventilation with the aid of a pulse oximeter and capnograph should be monitored at this time. If the procedure can be delayed, it is advised to allow the patient to recover from anesthesia and be observed for signs of aspiration pneumonia.

Anesthetic Maintenance

Anesthetic maintenance in patients with esophageal obstruction or megaesophagus is achieved with inhalation anesthetics (e.g., isoflurane, sevoflurane, or desflurane) diluted in 100% oxygen. Nitrous oxide should be avoided in patients with esophageal obstruction, as it can accumulate in viscous organs and dilate the esophageal portion distal to the obstruction [2].

Owing to the striated muscle layer in the esophagus, especially in dogs, central muscle relaxant administration (e.g., diazepam and midazolam) or short-acting neuromuscular blocking agents (e.g., atracurium 0.1–0.4 $mg\,kg^{-1}$ IV) may be indicated for patients with esophageal foreign bodies. These drugs may help to relax the striated muscular layer of the esophagus, reduce esophageal tone, and facilitate endoscopic manipulations and foreign body removal [2, 42]. Positive pressure ventilation is required in patients that receive neuromuscular blocking agents, and, ideally, neuromuscular function should be monitored by accelerometry. Deep anesthetic planes required with inhalation anesthetics to achieve muscle relaxation are not recommended in patients who are hemodynamically unstable.

Intraoperatively, a balanced isotonic crystalloid solution (e.g., LRS) should be administered up to a rate of 5–10 $ml\,kg^{-1}\,h^{-1}$. Supplemental fluid boluses of isotonic crystalloids may be indicated depending on the patient's hydration and hemodynamic status. In most cases, blood pressure can be monitored noninvasively, and pulse oximetry and capnography can provide valuable information in the event of esophageal perforation or aspiration [42].

Most general anesthetics can increase the chances of GER or regurgitation because of their effects on the LES tone in dogs and cats [65–69]. Although the incidence of regurgitation is low in healthy anesthetized patients [15, 48, 50, 53, 58–60, 66, 67, 69, 80, 81], it is more likely to occur in patients with esophageal disorders. Continuous monitoring for regurgitation during anesthetic maintenance, and immediate treatment if regurgitation occurs, can help prevent complications from occurring.

If regurgitation is observed during anesthesia, suctioning the refluxate from the oropharyngeal cavity and esophagus can minimize the chances of the patient aspirating and avoids damage to the esophageal mucosa, respectively. However, only suctioning of the refluxate from the esophagus has minimal impact in increasing the pH within the lumen of the esophagus. If regurgitation is observed, suctioning should be followed by esophageal lavage and sodium bicarbonate instillation [105]. Esophageal lavage with tap water can increase esophageal pH above 4.0, and infusion of a small volume of sodium bicarbonate can increase the pH above 6.0–7.0 for up to 3 h [105, 106]. However, esophageal lavage with tap water after esophageal suctioning may not be necessary if sodium bicarbonate is instilled, especially when all or most of the regurgitant volume is suctioned from the esophagus. Although esophageal lavage with tap water increases the esophageal pH, instillation of sodium bicarbonate after suctioning the esophagus readily buffers the pH of the esophageal lining, rendering any dilutional effect of the lavage inconsequential. The esophagus can be suctioned using a smooth tipped 8–12 Fr catheter. To ensure correct placement of the catheter and avoid suctioning from the stomach, the distance from the mandibular incisors to the 10th rib should be measured. Caution should be taken when inserting the catheter into the oropharynx to not enter the trachea. Therefore, it is critical that the airway is protected, and the ET tube cuff appropriately inflated. Esophageal suctioning should only be applied, as the catheter is withdrawn to avoid trauma to the esophagus. If the esophagus is lavaged with tap water, the lavage should be continued until clear fluid is retrieved. Sodium bicarbonate solution can be prepared using a 1:1 ratio of 8.4% sodium bicarbonate and water for injection; a volume of $0.6\,ml\,kg^{-1}$ of this solution has been recommended for instillation into the esophagus [105, 106]. Pantoprazole ($1.0\,mg\,kg^{-1}$ IV) may be administered to dogs and cats following regurgitation.

If reflux aspiration is observed while the animal is anesthetized, the airway should be suctioned to remove irritants, and oxygen saturation and breathing patterns should be monitored. If oxygen saturation starts to drop, positive pressure ventilation should be instituted. Peak inspiratory pressure generated by a normal tidal volume ($10–20\,ml\,kg^{-1}$) should be observed. Generation of high peak inspiratory pressure (>20 cm H_2O) with a normal tidal volume can indicate bronchospasm. Blood gas analysis can help assess the degree of oxygen exchange impairment.

Esophageal perforation with life-threatening tension pneumothorax should be suspected with sudden changes in breathing patterns, subsequent drops in oxygen saturation, decreased breath sounds on thoracic auscultation, and increased resistance to manual ventilation [42]. If these occur, immediate thoracocentesis should be performed and positive pressure ventilation instituted. A decision of exploratory thoracotomy should then be made to remove the esophageal foreign body and repair the esophagus [2, 40]. In cases of thoracotomy for esophageal surgery, positive pressure ventilation must be continued, and appropriate pain management should be administered intraoperatively and postoperatively. Air and fluid must be evacuated via a thoracostomy tube or thoracocentesis after the procedure.

Anesthetic Recovery

Observing for regurgitation and airway protection during recovery is still crucial. Premature extubation can lead to aspiration if regurgitation occurs. Patients should be maintained in sternal recumbency, with the head elevated until the animal regains full consciousness and laryngeal reflexes. The ET tube cuff should be kept inflated (at least in part) during extubation to remove any fluid or content proximal to the ET tube cuff, which will minimize the chances of aspiration [36]. If the patient regurgitates on extubation, its head should be dropped below the thoracic inlet, and suctioning of the airway should be provided. Oxygenation with the aid of a pulse oximeter must be monitored during recovery from anesthesia.

Postoperative analgesia should be provided accordingly to the intensity of pain produced by the procedure and damage to the esophageal mucosa in the case of foreign bodies. NSAIDs have been identified as a factor associated with intraoperative regurgitation [50]; therefore, these drugs should be avoided in patients with esophageal disorders.

Gastric and Small Intestinal Disease

Gastric surgery is commonly performed to remove foreign bodies and to correct gastric dilatation–volvulus (GDV). Gastric foreign bodies usually cause vomiting and regurgitation because of mechanical irritation to the mucosa, outflow tract obstruction, or gastric distention. Vomiting often is intermittent, occurring when the object is forced into the pyloric antrum [2, 74].

Gastric ulceration, hemorrhage, and neoplasia are less common indications for surgery. However, patients with these disorders may require endoscopic diagnostic procedures or feeding tube placement. Gastric mucosal bleeding should be considered in patients with gastroduodenal ulceration or esophagitis due to chronic vomiting and, less often, due to malignancy [107].

Gastroscopy or gastrotomy is often indicated for the removal of large, sharp, or potentially toxic foreign bodies, whereas partial gastrectomy is performed for the removal of ulcers and neoplasms or necrosis from GDV. Pylorectomy with gastroduodenal anastomosis is indicated for the removal of the pylorus due to neoplasia, outflow tract obstruction caused by hypertrophic pyloric gastropathy, or gastric outflow tract ulceration [2, 74, 108].

Small intestinal surgery (enterotomy, intestinal resection, and anastomosis) is most often indicated for GI obstruction (i.e., foreign bodies). Foreign body material can result in partial or complete intestinal luminal obstruction, tissue necrosis, intestinal perforation, or a combination of these. With intraluminal GI obstructions, the intestine rostral to the lesion distends with gas and fluid. Fluid accumulation is caused both by fluid retention in the intestinal lumen and by fluid secretion by intestinal glands. During obstruction, secretion increases, and absorption diminishes; gas also accumulates. Eventually, fluid shifts not only into the lumen, but also from the serosa into the peritoneal cavity. Circulation in the mucosa and submucosa becomes impaired, and the mucosa becomes ischemic. Full thickness wall necrosis may occur at the obstruction site. Small intestinal stasis leads to luminal bacterial overgrowth. If the normal mucosal barrier is impaired by distention and ischemia, permeability may increase, with subsequent bacterial translocation, absorption of toxins into the systemic circulation or peritoneal cavity, or both [2].

Other indications for small intestine surgery include trauma (e.g., perforation, ischemia), malpositioning (e.g., volvulus, intussusception), neoplasia, and diagnostic procedures (e.g., full thickness biopsy). In addition, patients with suspected protein-losing enteropathy require stomach and intestinal biopsies in order to confirm the diagnosis. These patients may undergo gastroduodenoscopy or exploratory laparotomy with gastrotomy and enterotomy [109].

Clinical Signs

Visual examination provides the following information about dogs and cats with GI disease: the animal's mental state, temperament, nutritional state, and comfort. Most animals with gastric diseases have vomiting, regurgitation, anorexia, or depression, and, occasionally, abdominal pain and weight loss. Patients with primary small intestinal disorders usually present for signs of vomiting, diarrhea, anorexia, depression, and/or weight loss [2]. Fever and abdominal pain may result from severe GI disease such as complete GI obstruction or perforation [2, 74]. These patients usually become severely dehydrated due to fluid loss and a reduced fluid intake, resulting in acute volume depletion and signs of shock [2, 42, 73]. Abdominal distention may be evident if pyloric outflow obstruction or intestinal perforation is present.

Upper GI hemorrhage is an important cause of blood loss and anemia and is potentially life-threatening in dogs [107]. Hematemesis or melena may indicate gastroduodenal ulceration or coagulopathy [2]. If blood loss exceeds 25% of total blood volume, these patients may experience hypotension and tachycardia and may be poor anesthetic candidates.

Coughing, dyspnea, and cyanosis can indicate that aspiration pneumonia has occurred in vomiting animals. However, aspiration pneumonia is a less common complication of vomiting than it is of regurgitation because reflex closure of the glottis occurs during emesis. Regurgitation may also occur because of esophagitis in animals that experience chronic vomiting [2, 73].

Laboratory Data

A full CBC, serum biochemistry profile, and venous blood gas (if possible) should be performed in any patient presenting with vomiting and/or diarrhea, as GI disease can lead to electrolyte and acid–base disturbances [42, 73, 109].

Laboratory parameters may be normal or may show only changes caused by dehydration (e.g., high PCV, TP, BUN, and creatinine), especially in animals with acute GI foreign bodies [2]. The metabolic consequences of vomiting due to foreign bodies are variable, but can be severe [74, 110]. The most common electrolyte and acid-base abnormalities, regardless of the site (stomach or small intestine) or type of foreign body, are hypochloremia, metabolic alkalosis, hypokalemia due to loss of acid-rich gastric secretions, and hyponatremia. Paradoxical aciduria occurs in consequence of hypovolemia and hypokalemia [73, 74, 110]. This also suggests that foreign bodies distal to the duodenum can produce metabolic alkalosis by increased secretion of chloride and potassium into the intestinal lumen. This combined with vomiting of acid-rich gastric secretions and volume contraction act to perpetuate any initial metabolic alkalosis [110]. However, metabolic acidosis might occur depending on the composition and volume of expelled GI contents and the degree of dehydration [73, 74]. In patients with more chronic vomiting, hyperlactatemia with subsequent metabolic acidosis may occur because of GI ischemia or systemic hypoperfusion [2, 73].

Hematocrit in patients with acute and severe gastric bleeding may be normal early during acute gastroduodenal hemorrhage due to insufficient time for plasma volume equilibration. Once plasma volume is equilibrated and fluid resuscitation is administered, anemia becomes more overt [74]. Acute upper GI bleeding is associated with a normocytic normochromic regenerative anemia, whereas chronic blood loss is characterized by iron deficiency and microcytic hypochromic anemia. In addition, a mild to moderate thrombocytosis may also be noted with chronic GI blood loss. With active bleeding, anemia is accompanied by hypoproteinemia [74]. BUN levels are typically increased in these cases because of the absorbed nitrogen load from the blood in the small intestine. A high BUN-to-creatinine ratio has been reported with upper GI hemorrhage [107].

Gastrointestinal loss accounts for approximately 40% of the normal daily turnover of plasma proteins, and, for this reason, protein-losing enteropathy (e.g., inflammatory bowel disease) can lead to hypoproteinemia [111]. The mechanism of protein loss may be related to GI barrier inflammation or damage. Albumin is one of the proteins lost into the GI tract and, as it contributes significantly to oncotic pressure, intravascular fluid loss can occur second to hypoalbuminemia [73]. As albumin decreases ($<1.5\,\mathrm{g\,dl^{-1}}$), effusions (e.g., pleural and peritoneal effusions) and edema can occur [111].

Anesthetic Management

Perianesthetic Considerations

The degree of dehydration should be evaluated based on physical examination and laboratory findings. Ideally, fluid deficit and electrolyte and acid–base abnormality correction should take place before anesthesia to improve the patient's hemodynamic stability throughout the anesthetic procedure [42]. Isotonic (0.9%) saline is the fluid of choice for metabolic alkalosis. Since hypokalemia can lead to skeletal muscle weakness, decreased GI motility/ileus, and cardiac arrhythmias, it should be corrected with potassium chloride supplementation before anesthesia. When administered IV, potassium chloride generally should not be infused at rates >0.5 mEq kg^{-1} h^{-1} to avoid potential adverse cardiac effects [112]. Hypokalemia can also predispose the myocardium to the refractory effects of class I antiarrhythmic drugs such as lidocaine and procainamide. These drugs are commonly used during anesthesia in patients with diseases that can cause ventricular arrhythmias such as GDV. Hypokalemic patients in shock should be resuscitated with an isotonic crystalloid solution (e.g., 0.9% saline or LRS) before adding potassium chloride to the fluids. If a patient is severely hypokalemic (serum potassium <2 mEq), it is prudent to start potassium as a separate infusion and not with the resuscitation fluid bag to not exceed the recommended potassium infusion rate (0.5 mEq kg^{-1} h^{-1}) [73]. Dehydration from vomiting in patients with metabolic acidosis should be corrected with a balanced isotonic crystalloid solution containing lactate or acetate as a buffer. The administration of sodium bicarbonate is necessary only in the treatment of patients with severe metabolic acidosis who have not responded to fluid therapy (pH <7.15) [113]. In these patients, bicarbonate deficit should be corrected with sodium bicarbonate according to the following equation:

$$\text{Bicarbonate deficit}\left(\text{mEq}\right) = 0.3 \times \text{base excess}\left(\text{mEq l}^{-1}\right) \times \text{body weight}\left(\text{kg}\right) \tag{5.1}$$

Initially one-third to one-half of the calculated sodium bicarbonate should be administered slowly [42]. The administration of sodium bicarbonate should be withheld in hypokalemic patients [73].

Patients with GI foreign bodies or GDV should have surgery performed as soon as possible after the animal's condition has been stabilized. They should be assumed to have a full stomach when they come for surgery [2].

Patients with signs of profuse GI bleeding (i.e., hematemesis or melena) should be hemodynamically stabilized with fluid resuscitation [2, 74, 107]. If PCV is <20%, these patients should be blood-typed or cross-matched (if they have previously received a blood transfusion), and pRBC or whole blood transfusions should be administered or at least started before gastroduodenoscopy or surgery [2, 74]. These patients should also be evaluated for coagulation defects by measuring prothrombin time, activated partial thromboplastin time, platelet count, fibrinogen, and fibrin degradation products [74]. FFP transfusions should be considered if clotting times are prolonged or if albumin is <1.5 g dl^{-1} [2]. Medications known to cause ulcers (e.g., NSAIDs and steroids) should be discontinued [107]. Since gastroduodenal ulceration is the most common cause of GI bleeding and GER may occur during general anesthesia, the administration of drugs that increase gastric secretion pH is advised [84]. Administration of PPIs should be considered as standard of care with gastroduodenal ulceration, since they are superior to H2As and other gastric acid suppressants (see the section titled "Esophageal Diseases") [86].

Preanesthetic Medications

Sedative drug selection should be based on the patient's attitude and disease severity (Table 5.2). Debilitated animals do not require drugs that produce intense sedation (e.g., alpha-2-adrenergic agonists). Alternatively, benzodiazepines combined with opioids should be considered because they produce adequate sedation in depressed dogs and cats. Opioids are usually part of the premedication protocol for patients undergoing exploratory laparotomy because they produce analgesia and spare inhalational anesthetics [42]. Acepromazine has central antiemetic effects and can be included in the preanesthetic medication. However, caution should be taken when administering acepromazine to dehydrated or hypovolemic patients due to vasodilation [74].

In animals with gastric foreign bodies (Figure 5.6), vomiting can be induced with preanesthetic medication in dogs and cats, but only if the object is small and has rounded

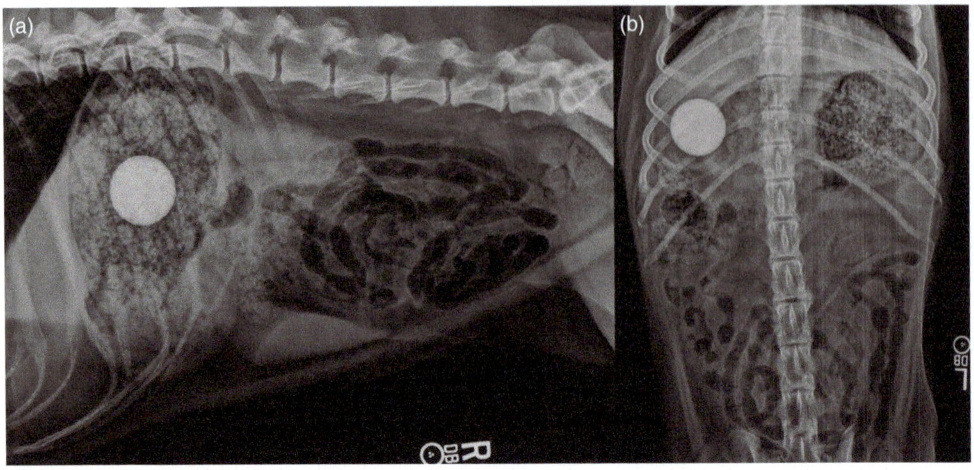

Figure 5.6 (a) Lateral abdominal radiograph showing a round radiopaque foreign body in the stomach of a dog. (b) Ventrodorsal radiograph showing the same round radiopaque foreign body in the stomach of a dog. Gastroscopic study of the dog revealed that the round radiopaque foreign body was a golf ball.

edges so that no harm will occur to the esophagus during expulsion. Trauma to the esophagus could be potentially life-threatening or could lead to future esophageal stricture [2]. In dogs, xylazine is more likely to induce vomiting than medetomidine [11]. In cats, xylazine, medetomidine, and dexmedetomidine have a high incidence of inducing emesis [11, 98]. Alpha-2-adrenergic agonists can be used as emetic agents, if patients are hemodynamically stable. On the other hand, if vomiting is undesirable due to concerns of potential gastric perforation, opioids that are less likely to cause vomiting [14] can be included in the preanesthetic medication. Butorphanol or buprenorphine can be administered to dogs and cats undergoing gastric foreign body removal via endoscopy; however, if retrieval of the foreign material is unsuccessful, analgesia provided by these drugs may not be sufficient for laparotomy/gastrotomy. In this case, methadone or fentanyl administration would be more appropriate. In addition, maropitant or metoclopramide can be administered 30–60 min prior to premedication with an opioid or alpha-2-adrenergic agonist–opioid combination [90–99].

Anticholinergic and opioid agents may increase pyloric sphincter tone in dogs and cats. The drug effects on the difficulty and time required to pass an endoscope into the proximal duodenum have been evaluated in dogs and cats. In dogs, atropine, morphine, and methadone administration prior to gastroscopy resulted in significant difficulty in passing an endoscope into the duodenum [114, 115]. While in cats, hydromorphone alone, hydromorphone and glycopyrrolate, medetomidine alone, or butorphanol alone in the premedication did not affect the duration or difficulty of endoscope passage through the pylorus [116]. Experience of the endoscopist can also play an important role in achieving duodenal intubation in a timely fashion independently of preanesthetic medication administered to dogs and cats. In addition, overdistention of the stomach with air during gastroscopic examination may increase pyloric tone and impede duodenal intubation.

Anesthetic Induction

Induction agent selection depends on the cardiovascular and nutritional status of the patient. If patients are hemodynamically stable, virtually any IV anesthetic technique can be used. In hemodynamically compromised patients, ketamine (5.0 mg kg^{-1}) and diazepam or midazolam (0.25 mg kg^{-1}) should be considered. Neuroleptanalgesia techniques with an opioid (e.g., fentanyl 0.005–0.01 mg kg^{-1}, oxymorphone 0.05–0.1 mg kg^{-1}, hydromorphone 0.05–0.2 mg kg^{-1}, or methadone 0.1–0.6 mg kg^{-1}) and benzodiazepines (diazepam 0.2 mg kg^{-1} or midazolam 0.2 mg kg^{-1}) can also be administered IV in very debilitated animals. Rapid induction and immediate intubation are essential if vomiting is a concern, and mask induction should be avoided.

Anesthetic Maintenance

Any halogenated inhalational anesthetic can be administered for GI procedures commonly performed in small animals. However, the concentration of these gases should be as low as possible in hypovolemic patients by using drug infusions that produce minimal cardiovascular depression and have inhalation-anesthetic-sparing effects. Nitrous oxide increases the volume of air trapped in body viscera and therefore should be avoided in patients with intestinal obstruction [2]. Constant rate infusions of opioids (e.g., fentanyl or remifentanil 0.005–0.04 mg kg^{-1} h^{-1}) and lidocaine (3 mg kg^{-1} h^{-1}) can achieve this goal in dogs in addition to providing analgesia. Although lidocaine CRIs decrease isoflurane requirement in cats, they are not recommended because of greater cardiovascular depression than an equipotent dose of isoflurane alone [117]. Abdominal wall regional anesthetic techniques such as fascial plane blocks are quite anesthetic sparing. One such block can be accomplished by infiltration of bupivacaine or ropivacaine 0.125–0.25% (0.25–0.5 ml kg^{-1} $site^{-1}$) into the interfascial plane formed by the transversus abdominis and the internal oblique muscles, also known as the transversus abdominis plane (TAP) block [118, 119]. In humans, the TAP block with liposomal bupivacaine has proven to be efficacious in providing long-lasting analgesia and decreasing postoperative use of IV and oral opioids [120]. To date, the benefit of liposomal bupivacaine has not been determined in dogs and cats for abdominal procedures, and future studies on the efficacy and duration of TAP block with liposomal bupivacaine are warranted.

Body heat is lost from exposed viscera during abdominal surgery. This may lead to hypothermia, which may reduce the need for anesthesia. Care should be taken during surgery to try to maintain the patient's body temperature above 95°F (35°C), especially in nutritionally debilitated animals with poor body condition scores [2].

Routine anesthetic monitoring is recommended in these patients. Patients with hypovolemia undergoing GI surgery of long duration will benefit from invasive blood pressure monitoring. Serial arterial blood gas analysis allows evaluation of oxygenation and ventilation status of patients with severe abdominal distention, as well as the metabolic status, lactate concentration, and electrolyte levels. During gastroscopy, gastric inflation and distention can impair ventilation, oxygenation, and circulation [42]. Therefore, monitoring with capnography, pulse oximetry, noninvasive blood pressure, and heart rate can help the anesthetist judge the degree of stomach inflation and associated complications. Excessive air in the stomach can be removed with the use of suction through the endoscope. Prolonged gastric distention can result in decreased venous return to the heart and vasovagal stimulation, leading to bradycardia [102]. A decrease in heart rate and blood pressure should be treated with anticholinergic agents.

A balanced isotonic crystalloid solution should be administered throughout surgery or the endoscopic procedure at a maintenance rate of 5–10 ml kg^{-1} h^{-1}. Fluids supplemented with potassium that are used in hospitalized patients should be used with caution during anesthesia, as they may increase the risk of potassium chloride overdose if fluid boluses are administered. If potassium supplementation is required, use a secondary IV line or fluid pump containing a potassium-supplemented fluid and a primary IV line containing nonsupplemented fluids for the purpose of fluid maintenance and boluses.

Patients with protein-losing enteropathy who present with hypoalbuminemia are more likely to become hypotensive because of decreased oncotic pressure and leakage of intravascular fluid to the interstitium. Although somewhat controversial, HES solutions ($1–2\,ml\,kg^{-1}\,h^{-1}$) can also be administered perioperatively in hypoalbuminemic patients to improve oncotic pressure, and balanced isotonic crystalloid therapy should be decreased.

Intraoperative hypotension in patients with gastric and small intestine diseases can be treated with balanced isotonic crystalloid boluses (e.g., LRS $10–20\,ml\,kg^{-1}$) if hypoalbuminemia is not present, HES ($3–5\,ml\,kg^{-1}$), or sympathomimetic drugs such as dopamine, dobutamine (starting at approximately $5.0\,\mu g\,kg^{-1}\,min^{-1}$), or norepinephrine (starting at approximately $0.05\,\mu g\,kg^{-1}\,min^{-1}$) (Table 5.4).

Anesthetic Recovery

Pain should be estimated and treated accordingly in patients recovering from laparotomy for gastrotomy, enterotomy, and intestinal resection and anastomosis. Fentanyl and lidocaine infusions can still be administered postoperatively. If these medications are discontinued, analgesia should be supplemented with methadone, hydromorphone, or oxymorphone as needed.

Nonsteroidal anti-inflammatory drugs may cause gastric ulceration by inhibiting prostaglandin synthesis, which decreases mucosal blood flow and alters gastric mucus production [121]. In addition, prostaglandin synthesis inhibition may impair renal blood flow in the event of hypovolemia and hypotension, potentially leading to renal ischemia and acute renal insufficiency. Therefore, NSAIDs should be used with caution in patients with GI diseases, hypovolemia, or hypotension.

Gastric Dilatation–Volvulus

GDV is an acute, life-threatening disorder that affects 40 000 to 60 000 dogs (with an increased risk in large breeds) per year in the United States [74, 122, 123]. The disease refers to acute stomach distention associated with rotation on its mesenteric axis, resulting in complete gastric outflow obstruction. Concurrent gastroesophageal junction obstruction precludes relief of fluid and gas accumulation by vomiting [2, 74, 124]. The GDV syndrome has a mortality rate of approximately 10–45% in treated animals [123, 125–129]. One study showed an overall mortality rate of 35.9%; however, when the preoperatively euthanized dogs were excluded from the study, mortality among treated dogs decreased to 16.5% [130], similar to other reports [131]. Increased mortality is usually associated with septic shock or peritonitis secondary to gastric necrosis or perforation, gastrectomy and splenectomy, and preoperative cardiac arrhythmias [2, 127, 129, 132]. Reperfusion injury, associated with correction of the mispositioned stomach, has also been implicated as a factor associated with high mortality [2].

The initiating cause for gastric distention is not entirely clear; however, once the stomach dilates, normal physiological means of removing air (i.e., eructation, vomiting, and pyloric emptying) are hindered because the esophagus and pylorus become obstructed. The stomach becomes enlarged, as gas and fluid accumulate in the lumen. Normal gastric secretion and fluid transudation into the gastric lumen because of venous congestion contribute to fluid accumulation. The stomach rotates and the duodenum, pylorus, and spleen are displaced (Figure 5.7). Splenomegaly can occur secondary to displacement [2]. Impairment of venous return to the heart occurs, as the caudal vena cava, portal vein, and splanchnic vasculature are compressed by massive gastric distention and an increase in intraabdominal pressure, ultimately decreasing cardiac output, tissue perfusion, and systemic arterial pressures, causing myocardial ischemia [74, 124, 133, 134]. As a result, dogs with GDV can develop multiple types of shock, including obstructive, hypovolemic, and distributive shocks affecting multiple organs, including the kidneys, heart, pancreas, stomach, and small intestines [2]. In addition, multiple factors can lead to gastric mucosal ulceration, hemorrhage, and necrosis. These factors include an increase in intragastric pressure, decreases in gastric mucosal perfusion, and increased gastric secretion. Necrosis and perforation can lead to peritonitis [124].

Gastric distention also prevents caudal displacement of the diaphragm, decreasing pulmonary compliance and impeding normal thoracic expansion (Figure 5.7). Respiratory rate and effort are increased as a compensatory mechanism. If these efforts are inadequate, then minute volume ventilation is decreased, and respiratory acidosis and hypoxemia occur [124].

Cardiac arrhythmias such as sinus tachycardia, atrial fibrillation, idioventricular tachycardia, paroxysmal ventricular tachycardia, and ventricular tachycardia (Figure 5.8) are frequently observed in dogs with GDV, particularly those with gastric necrosis [125, 126, 135]. Arrhythmias may contribute to mortality and require appropriate monitoring and treatment [125]. The cause of ventricular arrhythmias is unknown, but reduced cardiac output, myocardial ischemia, epinephrine release, and the release of myocardial depressant factor may be the contributing factors [124, 134–136].

Clinical Signs

Dogs with GDV present with acute abdominal distention and may appear to have signs of abdominal pain (e.g., arched back). Nonproductive retching, hypersalivation, distended abdomen, restlessness, and respiratory

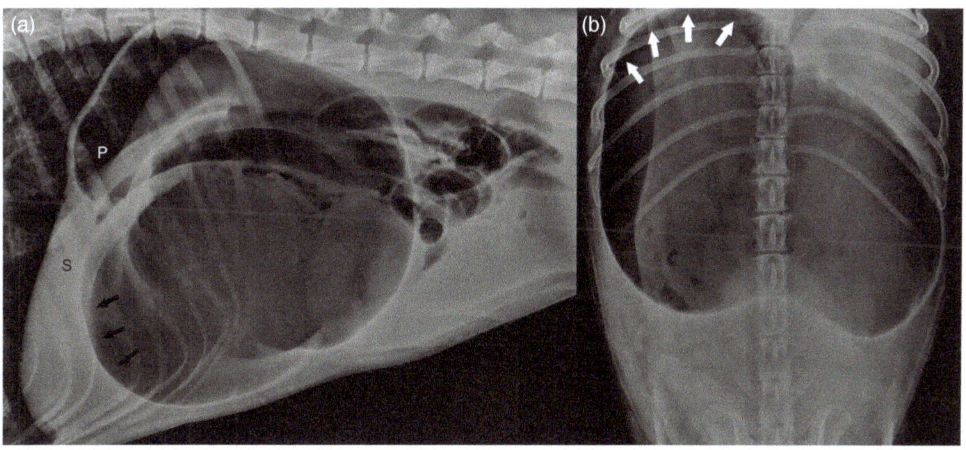

Figure 5.7 (a) Right lateral radiographic view of a dog with gastric dilatation–volvulus (GDV). The pylorus (P) and spleen (S) are displaced cranially. The major radiographic feature observed is accumulation of gas and distention of the stomach (black arrows). All these abnormalities lead to decreased venous return from compression of the caudal vena cava, portal vein, and splanchnic vasculature, as well as cranial displacement of the diaphragm (shown in [b], white arrows) and respiratory compromise. *Source:* Photo courtesy Dr. G. Sepulveda.

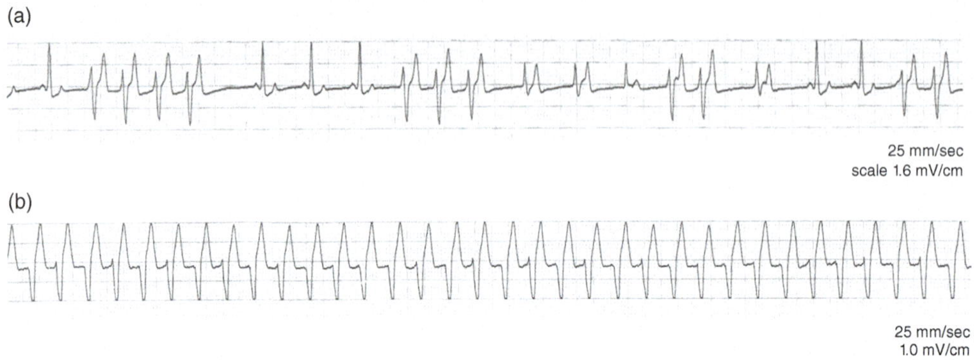

Figure 5.8 (a) Paroxysmal ventricular tachycardia in a dog. (b) Ventricular tachycardia in a dog.

distress are common. Clinical signs of shock may be present, including depressed mentation, weak peripheral pulses, tachycardia, prolonged capillary refill time, injected or pale mucous membranes, dyspnea, and hypothermia. Arrhythmias (commonly ventricular) can often be auscultated along with palpable pulse deficits [2, 74, 124, 135].

Laboratory Data

GDV can be associated with several metabolic and electrolyte derangements which are not always consistently present [137, 138]. Hypokalemia is present in approximately 33% of dogs with GDV; however, potassium may also be elevated or normal. Hypochloremic metabolic alkalosis may develop from gastric sequestration of hydrogen and chloride ions [138]. Later in the disease progression, metabolic acidosis may occur from decreased effective circulating blood volume, resulting in tissue hypoxia and lactate production. Plasma lactate concentrations can help to predict gastric necrosis and therefore guide disease prognosis. Survival rates for dogs without gastric necrosis may be as high as approximately 98–100%. In most situations, low lactate levels (below 4–6 mmol l^{-1}) at preresuscitation or more than a 50% decrease in lactate levels within 12 h from initial presenting concentration suggest that gastric necrosis is not present, and therefore a fair prognosis is warranted [139–141]. However, there are exceptions in both cases where lactate values of expected survivors and expected nonsurvivors overlap, and care must be taken when applying specific cutoff values to individual patients. Monitoring serial lactate levels throughout resuscitation and intraoperatively may help guide therapy and determine outcome [142].

Respiratory acidosis is likely to occur secondary to gastric impingement on the diaphragm and diminished ventilatory compliance. Once anesthesia is induced, respiratory acidosis may become severe because of the respiratory depressant effects of anesthetics. Hypoventilation combined with ventilation perfusion mismatch can lead to hypoxemia.

Blood glucose levels may also decrease in the later stages of shock, as energy demands cannot be met by the inefficient production of adenosine triphosphate (ATP) through anaerobic metabolism [124]. PCV and TP may reveal evidence of hemoconcentration. Platelets may be consumed leading to thrombocytopenia. These patients may have increased BUN and creatinine owing to prerenal azotemia due to decreased renal perfusion [124]. Increased alanine aminotransferase (ALT) and total bilirubin are associated with hepatocellular damage due to biliary stasis.

Anesthetic Management

Perianesthetic Considerations

Gastric distention and abdominal vasculature compression lead to cardiopulmonary and GI compromise that can severely affect the stability of these dogs during anesthesia. Therefore, stabilizing the patient's condition is the initial goal before induction. At least two large-bore (14–18 gauge) IV catheters should be placed in either a jugular and a cephalic vein or both cephalic veins (Figure 5.9). More than one catheter allows rapid fluid resuscitation and multiple drug administration simultaneously, some of which may be incompatible in the same line. Blood samples for CBC, serum biochemistry profile, and blood gas analysis can be collected at the same time of catheter placement [2, 74, 143].

During the initial patient examination and up to anesthetic induction, oxygen should be supplemented via a tight-fitting mask if the patient is amenable. Restoration of circulating plasma volume should be initiated using high volumes of isotonic solutions. These solutions can be given alone or with hypertonic saline solution or HES solutions over 5–15 min [2, 124, 144, 145]. However, hypertonic saline should not be administered to patients with severe sodium derangements; HES solutions should be avoided or used with caution in patients that are potentially septic (see the section titled "Secondary Septic Peritonitis"), and severely hypernatremic/hyperchloremic. The shock dose for isotonic crystalloid fluids is equivalent to the patient's blood volume (approximately $90\,\mathrm{ml\,kg^{-1}}$) and should be calculated and administered in aliquots of one-third to one-quarter of the total dose. These aliquots can be administered in combination with 7% hypertonic saline (4–$6\,\mathrm{ml\,kg^{-1}}$) or aliquots of one-quarter of the daily HES ($5\,\mathrm{ml\,kg^{-1}}$). A small volume fluid resuscitation with a combination of hypertonic saline and synthetic colloid (e.g., HES solution) has been advocated as a more efficient method than high volume during resuscitation of dogs with GDV [141, 142]. In this case, a mixture of approximately 7% hypertonic saline and 6% HES can be prepared by calculating $1\,\mathrm{ml\,kg^{-1}}$ 23.4% saline and $2\,\mathrm{ml\,kg^{-1}}$ of 6% HES, mixing them in the same syringe, and administering the total volume ($3\,\mathrm{ml\,kg^{-1}}$) of the combination over 5 min. If 7% hypertonic saline and/or HES solutions are administered, the rate of subsequent crystalloid administration must be adjusted. After initial resuscitation, cardiovascular parameters (e.g., heart rate, arterial blood pressure, mucous membrane color) and

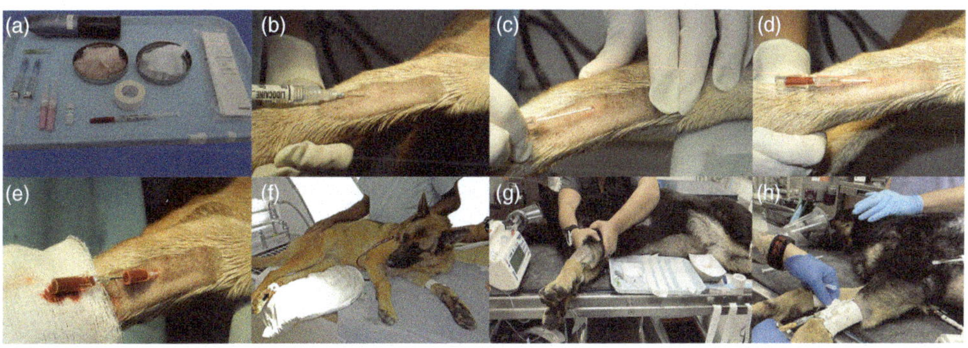

Figure 5.9 Desensitization of the dorsal skin of the hock and catheter placement in the dorsal pedal artery before anesthetic induction. (a) All material required for arterial catheterization. (b) The hair of the skin over the dorsal pedal artery is clipped and aseptically prepared. Lidocaine (2%) is injected subcutaneously over the dorsal pedal artery. To avoid the artery and subsequent hematoma formation, the artery should be palpated and the skin over the artery pulled to the side before injection. (c) The dorsal pedal artery should be palpated before catheter placement. (d) The catheter and stylet are introduced into the artery. (e) The catheter is fed into the artery. (f) Successful arterial catheter placement in a dog with GDV before anesthetic induction. (g) Placement of second IV cephalic vein catheter for volume resuscitation. (h) Anesthetic induction with neuroleptanalgesic drug combination (midazolam and fentanyl).

mentation should be reassessed before further administration of fluids. If hypotension persists after appropriate volume expansion, inotropic and/or vasopressor therapy should be considered. Significant electrolyte and acid–base abnormalities should be corrected along fluid resuscitation and blood gas analysis should be performed as needed [2, 124].

Debilitated moribund dogs usually will often allow catheterization of the dorsal pedal artery after the skin over the artery is desensitized with lidocaine (Figure 5.9). Arterial catheterization will allow monitoring of arterial blood pressures, pressure waveforms, and gas analysis, which can be used as a guide to fluid therapy before and during anesthesia [143]. If arterial catheterization is not possible before anesthesia, blood pressure should be monitored noninvasively with the aid of an oscillometric blood pressure device, or an ultrasonic Doppler device combined with a sphygmomanometer.

Continuous ECG monitoring will provide valuable information regarding the cardiac rhythm in these patients. Preoperative arrhythmia treatment should include correction of hypovolemia and electrolyte imbalances. This is especially important if hypokalemia is present because lidocaine is less effective in the presence of hypokalemia [146]. Ventricular arrhythmias should be treated if they interfere with cardiac output and should be primarily treated with IV lidocaine boluses of 2.0–4.0 mg kg^{-1}. Clinical findings that may suggest poor cardiac output due to ventricular arrhythmias may include poor blood pressure or lack of palpable pulse during tachycardia, multiform ventricular arrhythmias, the presence of subsequent premature beats inscribed on the T wave of the previous complex (R-on-T), or a sustained ventricular rate of >160 beats per min. After the initial bolus is given, lidocaine treatment can be continued with a CRI of 3.0–4.5 mg kg^{-1} h^{-1} (50–75 μg kg^{-1} min^{-1}) [135]. Signs of lidocaine toxicity should be monitored in the awake patient, including muscle tremors, vomiting, and seizures. If any of these occur, lidocaine administration should be decreased or discontinued. If seizures occur, they should be treated with IV diazepam or midazolam (0.5 mg kg^{-1}). Procainamide (2.0–8.0 mg kg^{-1} IV bolus and CRI at 1.5–2.4 mg kg^{-1} h^{-1}) may be administered if lidocaine fails to convert the rhythm back to a normal sinus rhythm, or if improvement in variables indicative of circulation (e.g., heart rate, peripheral pulse pressure quality, arterial blood pressure, mucous membrane colors, and capillary refill time) is not seen [2, 124, 135].

Gastric decompression should be performed to remove air and fluid from the stomach as soon as the dog is hemodynamically stabilized. This can be achieved preferably via orogastric intubation, or percutaneously via an over-the-needle catheter or a trocar into the distended stomach. Decompression of the stomach may improve the patient's cardiopulmonary status. When an orogastric tube is placed, the clinician should have an ET tube and laryngoscope available in case the dog refluxes around the orogastric tube or is too sedate to protect its airway [74, 124]. Drugs that increase the gastric pH such as PPIs should be considered preoperatively (see the section titled "Esophageal Diseases").

Preanesthetic Medication

Sedation may be necessary for gastric decompression via orogastric tube placement or percutaneous gastrocentesis. However, drugs that produce moderate to intense sedation are not necessary because dogs presented with GDV are usually depressed and have decreased cardiac output. Therefore, the use of alpha-2-adrenergic agonists should be avoided in these cases because of their depressant effects on cardiac output, despite the initial increase in blood pressure [11]. Acepromazine should be avoided because its vasodilatory effect can further decrease venous return to the heart and lead to hypotension [122].

Preanesthetic drugs that produce vomiting should be avoided because dogs may not be able to expel their gastric contents due to gastroesophageal obstruction. Increases in abdominal pressure may lead to stomach rupture and decreased venous return to the heart [133].

Intravenous drug administration is preferred because doses can be administered as needed; total drug doses are often reduced, and the effects are more predictable. The combination of diazepam or midazolam (0.1–0.2 $mg\,kg^{-1}$) with butorphanol (0.2–0.4 $mg\,kg^{-1}$) has been commonly recommended for GDV because of the antiemetic properties of butorphanol and minimal cardiovascular effects of both drugs [74, 143]. However, dogs with volvulus require surgery, and full mu-opioid agonists will produce more effective analgesia. Butorphanol is an agonist–antagonist with a 1–2 h duration of action and, if still present in therapeutic concentrations in the plasma at surgery, can decrease the effectiveness of a full mu-agonist. Full mu-agonist opioids are the drugs of choice to minimize the amount of inhalation anesthetics because of their anesthetic-sparing and minimal cardiovascular effects. As an alternative to butorphanol, methadone (0.1–0.5 $mg\,kg^{-1}$), hydromorphone (0.05–0.2 $mg\,kg^{-1}$), oxymorphone (0.05–0.1 $mg\,kg^{-1}$), or fentanyl (0.002–0.005 $mg\,kg^{-1}$) combined with diazepam or midazolam can be used [143]. As previously discussed, maropitant may be administered to prevent vomiting reflexes, preferably 30–60 min before sedation if time permits.

Anesthetic Induction

Induction agents should produce minimal cardiovascular depression. Drugs that produce significant vasodilation, myocardial depression, or are arrhythmogenic should be avoided [42, 122]. Neuroleptanalgesic combinations such as diazepam or midazolam (0.2–0.5 $mg\,kg^{-1}$ IV) and fentanyl (0.005–0.02 $mg\,kg^{-1}$ IV) administered to effect produce minimal cardiovascular changes and are appropriate for anesthetic induction in dogs with unstable cardiovascular function (Table 5.2). Propofol (2.0–8.0 $mg\,kg^{-1}$ IV) or alfaxalone (1.0–4.0 $mg\,kg^{-1}$ IV) titrated to effect and ketamine (5.0 $mg\,kg^{-1}$ IV) combined with diazepam or midazolam (0.25 $mg\,kg^{-1}$ IV) have been suggested as appropriate options for anesthetic induction [143]. Care must be taken when inducing severely sick patients with ketamine–benzodiazepine because ketamine may potentially cause negative inotropy when sympathetic depletion is present, which often occurs in the later stages of shock [42]. Once the ET tube is placed, the cuff should be inflated. An orogastric tube should be placed soon after induction to minimize the risk of regurgitation and aspiration.

Anesthetic Maintenance

Because inhalation anesthetics produce dose-dependent vasodilation and myocardial depression, their concentrations during maintenance of anesthesia in dogs with GDV should be decreased using balanced anesthetic techniques. Sevoflurane and desflurane can be considered in these cases because they are relatively insoluble agents and end-expiratory concentrations can be rapidly changed in the case of cardiovascular instability. However, it is also possible to achieve a reasonably rapid change of anesthetic depth with isoflurane as well [42]. Nitrous oxide is contraindicated before permanent gastric decompression is achieved because it rapidly diffuses into gas-filled compartments, causing additional organ distention and increasing the intragastric volume. This can crowd the operative field, limit diaphragmatic movement, and compromise respiration [2].

Fentanyl or remifentanil (loading dose: 0.002–0.005 $mg\,kg^{-1}$, CRI: 0.005–0.04 $mg\,kg^{-1}\,h^{-1}$) and lidocaine (loading dose: 1.0–2.0 $mg\,kg^{-1}$, CRI: 3.0 $mg\,kg^{-1}\,h^{-1}$) are usually administered for their anesthetic-sparing effects [147, 148]. In addition, fentanyl and remifentanil produce effective analgesia, whereas lidocaine has been shown to have analgesic, antiarrhythmic, anti-inflammatory, and possibly GI prokinetic effects [147–152]. Furthermore, lidocaine administration as a bolus followed by a CRI starting before surgery in dogs with GDV decreased the occurrence of cardiac arrhythmias and resulted in a shorter hospitalization stay [153]. Benzodiazepines (e.g., diazepam/midazolam 0.05–0.2 $mg\,kg^{-1}$ IV) or nondepolarizing neuromuscular blocking agents (NMBAs; e.g., atracurium 0.1–0.4 $mg\,kg^{-1}$ IV) can be supplemented as part of balanced anesthetic technique. If NMBAs are administered, ideally, neuromuscular function should be monitored with accelerometry [42].

Intraoperatively, a balanced isotonic solution (e.g., LRS) should be administered at a rate of up to 5–10 $ml\,kg^{-1}\,h^{-1}$. If an arterial catheter has not been placed before induction, an attempt should be made after induction for monitoring of invasive blood pressure because patients are often hypotensive [133]. Because a variety of acid–base abnormalities may occur during anesthetic maintenance, the monitoring of serial blood gas and electrolyte is advised. Sodium bicarbonate should only be administered if severe acidosis occurs (pH <7.15) [113]. As discussed previously, the administration of sodium bicarbonate should be withheld in hypokalemic patients [75].

Hypertonic saline, HES, and FFP should be available for hypotension with or without tachycardia. Fluid therapy during anesthesia should be continuously reassessed and based on central venous pressure, invasive arterial blood pressure and waveform analysis, arterial blood gas analysis, lactate concentration, PCV, TP, heart rate, capillary refill time, and mucous membrane color [122]. For example, changes of invasive systolic blood pressure values or the pulse oximeter pulse pressure wave immediately after a delivered breath by a mechanical ventilator, termed systolic pressure variation (SPV), pulse pressure variation (PPV), or plethysmographic waveform variation (plethysmographic variability index; PVI), can provide early information regarding volume depletion and guide response to fluid challenges (Figure 5.10). SPV, PPV, or PVI are noninvasive dynamic indices of stroke volume; in anesthetized humans, they have been shown to be the most accurate predictor of fluid responsiveness [154–161]. In veterinary patients, dogs must be mechanically ventilated with a constant tidal volume of at least 10 $ml\,kg^{-1}$, have no arrhythmias, and have minimal alterations in

(a) (b)

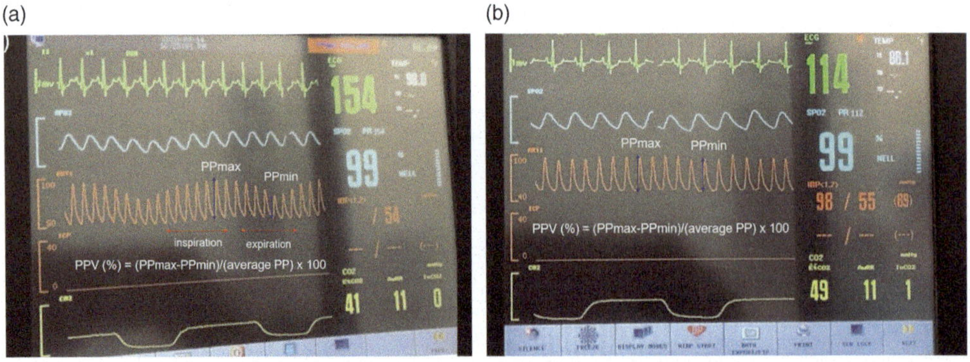

Figure 5.10 Pulse pressure variation (PPV) in a dog with GDV that underwent exploratory laparotomy. Heart and pulse rates were 154 beats min^{-1} (green ECG trace and blue plethysmograph, speed 25 mm s^{-1}). Arterial blood pressure was monitored invasively by the means of an arterial catheter (red plethysmograph, speed 12.5 mm s^{-1}) and the dog was mechanically ventilated with positive pressure ventilation without spontaneous effort and with a tidal volume of 12 ml kg^{-1}. (a) Before volume resuscitation, PP_{max} (mmHg) during inspiration = $P_{systolic}$ (mmHg) – $P_{diastolic}$ (mmHg) was 95–54 = 41 mmHg; and PP_{min} (mmHg) during expiration = $P_{systolic}$ (mmHg) – $P_{diastolic}$ (mmHg) was 86–52 = 34 mmHg. PPV (%) = 18.6%. (b) After volume resuscitation, heart and pulse rates were markedly decreased (114 beats min^{-1}); PP_{max} and PP_{min} were minimally changed during mechanical ventilation without spontaneous effort and with a tidal volume of 12 ml kg^{-1}.

chest compliance (e.g., open chest) in order to correctly interpret this variation. PPV and PVI are determined by multiparameter monitors based on the following equations [161]:

$$PPV(\%) = (PP_{max} - PP_{min}) / (\text{average PP}) \times 100 \quad (5.2)$$

$$PVI(\%) = (PI_{max} - PI_{min}) / (PI_{max}) \times 100 \quad (5.3)$$

where PP = pulse pressure and PI = pulse index. In humans, PPV >12–13% is predictive of fluid responsiveness [156, 157]; and in dogs, PPV and PVI >7–15% seems to distinguish dogs that would benefit from volume expansion [159–161]. In addition, urine output can also be used as an assessment of renal perfusion, cardiac output, and fluid therapy efficacy. Therefore, it should be considered in hemodynamically compromised patients.

Inotrope administration using dobutamine or dopamine (starting at approximately 5.0 μg kg^{-1} min^{-1} [2–20 μg kg^{-1} min^{-1}]) can help maintain mean arterial pressure above approximately 60 mmHg [143]. In septic patients or in patients with refractory response to fluids and inotropic support, administration of vasopressor drugs such as norepinephrine (0.01–2.0 μg kg^{-1} min^{-1}), phenylephrine (0.1–3.0 μg kg^{-1} min^{-1}), or vasopressin (0.5–2.0 mU kg^{-1} min^{-1}) may be warranted. High dosages of sympathomimetic agents may result in tachycardia and arrhythmias. Continuous ECG monitoring will allow detection of arrhythmias and help to evaluate the efficacy of antiarrhythmic drugs when administered.

Positive pressure ventilation should be instituted to correct respiratory acidosis, as well as to recruit collapsed alveoli and improve blood oxygenation. However, as mentioned before, intrathoracic positive pressure caused by mechanical ventilation may decrease venous return, thus worsening hypotension, especially in dogs with ineffective circulatory volume. In this case, a fluid challenge may be warranted, as well as decreases in tidal volume until intravascular volume is replaced in the hemodynamically unstable patient.

Anesthetic Recovery

Mucous membrane color, capillary refill time, ECG, heart rate, blood pressure, and oxygen saturation should still be monitored in recovery. PCV and TP measurements can be helpful in determining if hemodilution produced by fluid therapy has occurred. These measurements can also be used to determine if blood products will be needed postoperatively. Lactate and urine output are useful indicators of tissue perfusion and can guide the postoperative administration of fluids, inotropic drugs, and vasopressors [124]. Acid–base and electrolyte abnormalities should still be monitored, as prevention or correction of hypokalemia may decrease the incidence of muscle weakness in recovery from anesthesia. NSAIDs should likely be avoided due to mucosal damage and potential GI and renal hypoperfusion. Analgesia can be achieved by fentanyl and lidocaine CRIs. In cases of prolonged recovery where dogs received high doses of opioid agonist drugs, partial reversal may be required with incremental doses of naloxone (0.001–0.002 mg kg^{-1} IV) or butorphanol (0.1 mg kg^{-1} IV); however, analgesia may also be reversed, and the level of pain should be closely assessed. Temperature should still be monitored during recovery and treated accordingly, especially if the dog is experiencing a prolonged recovery.

Colonic, Rectal, Anal, and Perineal Surgery

Colonic surgery is indicated for lesions associated with perforation, obstruction, neoplasia, colonic inertia, trauma, or chronic intussusception (Box 5.2). Colotomy/colectomy is often avoided for foreign bodies, since there is great concern regarding colonic healing and leakage of intestinal content, which can lead to life-threatening complications. Any prolonged large intestine (e.g., foreign body, neoplasia, intraluminal strictures) or pelvic area (e.g., pelvic fractures or masses, prostatomegaly) obstruction leading to chronic constipation

Box 5.2 Most common surgical diseases of the colon, rectum, anus, and perineum in dogs and cats.

- Linear foreign body
- Intestinal intussusception
- Colonic and rectal perforation
- Intestinal neoplasms
- Colonic or cecocolic volvulus
- Idiopathic megacolon in cats
- Secondary megacolon
- Rectal prolapse
- Rectal neoplasms
- Perianal (circumanal) gland adenoma or adenocarcinoma
- Apocrine gland anal sac adenocarcinoma
- Non-neoplastic anal sac diseases: impaction, sacculitis, and abscessation
- Atresia ani
- Perineal hernias

can result in megacolon in cats and dogs. Cats with idiopathic megacolon may require general anesthesia for enemas, but ultimately most cats will have to undergo anesthesia for total or subtotal colectomy, which is the current treatment for idiopathic megacolon (Figure 5.11) [162, 163]. Rectal surgery is usually performed to resect neoplasia and to repair rectal prolapses or perforations. Perianal surgeries are often indicated for anal, perianal, and anal sac neoplasia removal, non-neoplastic anal sac diseases, and, less often, for congenital defects such as atresia ani (Figure 5.12), the most common congenital anorectal anomaly in dogs. Perineal surgery is most often performed to treat perineal hernias and to remove neoplasia (Box 5.2). Perineal hernia occurs because of weakness and separation of the components of the pelvic diaphragm. Loss of support from the pelvic diaphragm allows deviation of the rectum and caudal protrusion of various abdominal organs (prostate gland, bladder, and intestine) into the perineum. Older and intact males are most likely to acquire perineal hernias, as they rarely occur in female dogs and cats [2, 164].

Clinical Signs

In general, patients with large intestine or perianal/perineal region diseases will present with tenesmus, dyschezia, and constipation due to either some degree of obstruction or lesions that cause pain during defecation. Patients with large intestinal strangulation or perforation and those with incarcerated small intestines within

(a) (b)

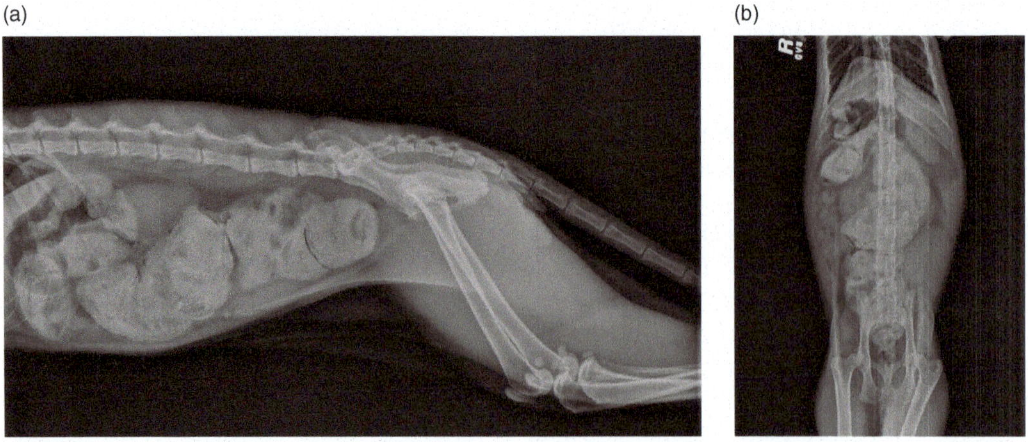

Figure 5.11 (a) Right lateral abdominal radiographic view of a cat with megacolon. (b) Ventrodorsal abdominal radiographic view of a cat with megacolon. *Source:* Photo courtesy Dr. G. Sepulveda.

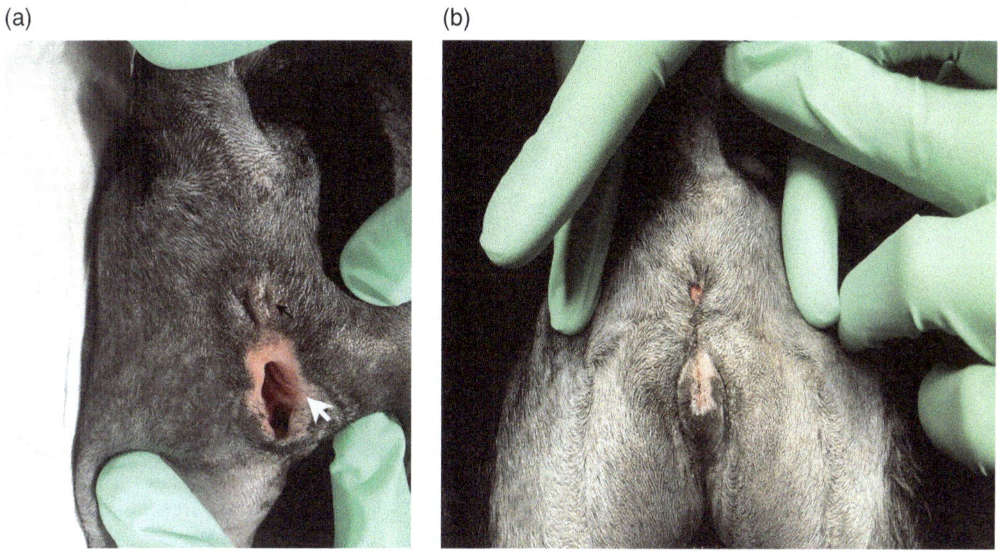

Figure 5.12 Four-month-old, female, Miniature Schnauzer puppy diagnosed with atresia ani. (a) Before surgery - black arrow: closed anus visualized as "dimple" instead of an anal opening; white arrow: vulva and vaginal canal with rectovaginal fistula. (b) Anal reconstruction and vaginal fistula correction.

a perineal hernia may present with signs of shock and require emergency exploratory laparotomy once stabilized [2, 122, 163, 164].

Patients with colonic diseases may also have diarrhea, vomiting, anorexia, or abdominal enlargement. In more chronic diseases, significant weight loss may occur. Hematochezia may also be present in colonic and rectal neoplastic diseases [163, 164]. Presence of a mass or swelling in the anal or perianal region is an indication of perianal gland or anal sac neoplasia but can also be associated with non-neoplastic anal sac abnormalities. Other clinical signs associated with perianal neoplasia or swelling include lesion ulceration and draining tracts, pain, or irritation of the region. Patients may also scoot, lick, or bite the perianal area, and are uncomfortable when sitting. Metastatic disease from malignant perianal gland adenocarcinoma and apocrine gland anal sac adenocarcinoma can be evidenced by sublumbar lymph node enlargement, which can, in some cases, contribute to constipation and dyschezia. In addition, dogs with apocrine gland anal sac adenocarcinoma can present with polyuria, polydipsia, anorexia, muscular weakness, vomiting, and constipation due to paraneoplastic pseudohyperparathyroidism producing hypercalcemia [164].

Large unilateral or bilateral perineal swellings in the perineal area highly suggest the presence of perineal hernias, and a firm painful swelling usually is associated with incarcerated or strangulated organs. Clinical signs include those of obstruction, incarceration, or strangulation of herniated organs such as tenesmus and constipation (when intestines and rectum are present in the hernia); dysuria and stranguria may occur in patients with prostatic disease or bladder retroflexion. Patients with urinary tract obstruction and electrolyte abnormalities should be treated with urinary catheterization or bladder decompression and fluids until they are stable [160].

Puppies with atresia ani often develop clinical signs beginning at the time of or after weaning (approximately 4 weeks of age). These signs vary from constipation and tenesmus to unthriftiness, anorexia, enlarged abdomen, absence of defecation, and perianal bulging. Vomiting and dehydration may also develop [164].

Laboratory Data

Most patients with neoplastic intestinal diseases and perineal hernias are geriatric and laboratory data should include CBC, biochemical profile, and urinalysis. Conversely, puppies with atresia ani may be malnourished and, depending on their age, hypoglycemia should be considered. Patients with obstructive or strangulating intestinal disease showing systemic clinical signs should also have complete blood work and a urinalysis performed. Laboratory data may reveal dehydration, prerenal azotemia, and electrolyte or acid–base abnormalities. If the patient is not rapidly deteriorating, hydration and acid–base and electrolyte deficits should be corrected before anesthetic induction. Postrenal azotemia and hyperkalemia may occur in cases of perineal hernia with bladder retroflexion and obstruction. Hypoglycemia and hypercalcemia/hypophosphatemia may occur as a result of paraneoplastic syndrome in the case of intestinal leiomyosarcoma and apocrine gland anal sac adenocarcinoma, respectively. Therefore, patients with suspected neoplasia in the GI system should be screened for these abnormalities.

Anesthetic Considerations

Anesthetic complications may arise from uncorrected dehydration and electrolyte or acid–base abnormalities. Therefore, correction should be addressed before anesthesia whenever possible. Severe hyperkalemia in patients with perineal hernia owing to bladder retroflexion should be corrected with the administration of 0.9% saline solution, dextrose and insulin, or sodium bicarbonate (see Chapter 8). Balanced crystalloids can also be used in mild hyperkalemia. Calcium gluconate or chloride administration should be considered to normalize the difference between resting and threshold potential of the myocardium, thus helping to restore membrane excitability [112]. Fluid therapy should also be initiated to treat azotemia. The urinary bladder can be decompressed by cystocentesis, paracentesis via the perineal skin, or urethral catheterization [2]. Fluid obtained by bladder decompression should be confirmed as urine by comparing its creatinine or potassium concentration to that of peripheral blood. Mildly to moderately hypercalcemic animals, based on ionized calcium measurements, should be rehydrated and diuresed with a 0.9% saline solution [2]. Fasting of pediatric patients with atresia ani and patients with intestinal neoplasia with documented hypoglycemia should be limited to 1–2 h, and maintenance fluids may have to be supplemented with dextrose [2, 42]. Serial blood glucose measurements should be taken during the anesthetic period.

Anesthetic protocols should be based on patient signalment, attitude, blood work abnormalities, and severity of systemic clinical signs as previously discussed. In colorectal junction and cranial rectal surgeries, pelvic canal exposure may be necessary by performing pelvic symphysiotomy, or pubic and/or ischial osteotomies. In these cases, analgesia can be provided by administration of a full mu-opioid agonist CRI (fentanyl, morphine, hydromorphone, or methadone) or combined with multimodal CRIs such as IV lidocaine in dogs and/or ketamine in dogs and cats. Fascial plane blocks such as the TAP block with bupivacaine or ropivacaine 0.125–0.25% (0.25–0.5 $ml\,kg^{-1}$ $site^{-1}$) may provide abdominal wall analgesia and muscle relaxation for laparotomy surgery [119]. If there are no contraindications (e.g., sepsis, bleeding disorders, and hypovolemia), epidural administration (lumbosacral or sacrococcygeal) of bupivacaine or ropivacaine alone (0.1 $ml\,kg^{-1}$) or combined with preservative-free morphine (0.1 $mg\,kg^{-1}$) should be considered to provide balanced anesthesia and multimodal analgesia for all rectal, perianal, or perineal surgeries [42].

All dogs and cats undergoing perineal/perianal or intestinal surgeries require basic monitoring (e.g., noninvasive or invasive blood pressure, ECG, and body temperature). Patients requiring surgery for perineal hernia repair, anal gland sacculectomy, or perineal mass removal are positioned in ventral recumbency placed on a rectal stand or with their hind-end elevated and their head down (Trendelenburg position). This results in diaphragmatic compression and impaired ventilation. Positive pressure ventilation and devices to monitor ventilation (e.g., capnograph) and oxygenation (e.g., pulse oximeter) are required in these patients [42]. A rolled towel can be placed under the thoracic limbs and cranial thorax to position the dog more horizontally and decrease pressure on the diaphragm. Patients positioned in this manner must also be carefully positioned to avoid pressure points, myopathy, or neuropathy.

Secondary Septic Peritonitis

Recognizing peritonitis secondary to GI perforation caused by necrosis or ulceration is critical and must be treated promptly and aggressively. In dogs undergoing GI tract surgery, low preoperative serum albumin and intraoperative hypotension were associated with increased risk to develop secondary septic peritonitis postoperatively [165]. Secondary peritonitis is the predominant form of peritonitis in dogs and usually is caused by bacteria (i.e., septic peritonitis). It is particularly common in young animals that have perforating foreign bodies and in those with abdominal trauma (e.g., hit by a car or bite wounds) [166, 167]. In addition, older animals on chronic NSAID or glucocorticoid therapy can have perforation of the GI tract with consequent peritonitis [165]. Once diagnosed, treatment of septic peritonitis is directed toward the correction of electrolyte and fluid abnormalities, and exploratory laparotomy to determine and surgically correct the underlying cause of the peritonitis. Mortality rates with septic peritonitis secondary to leaking intestinal anastomosis may be as high as approximately 70–85% [162, 168]. With septic peritonitis, most present for treatment of lethargy, anorexia, vomiting, diarrhea, fever, and/or abdominal pain. Some may be hypothermic, particularly cats. Abdominal distention may be noted if sufficient fluid has accumulated, which may interfere with ventilation. Prolonged capillary refill times, pale mucous membranes, and tachycardia may indicate shock, although some animals may show hyperdynamic shock with injected mucous membranes, rapid capillary refill times, and bounding pulses. Dehydration and arrhythmias may also occur [166]. Massive fluid and protein movement to the peritoneal cavity results in a fluid shift away from the intravascular space, causing hemoconcentration, azotemia, and eventual hypovolemic shock. Free bacteria and endotoxin release cause massive neutrophil shifts to the abdomen, visceral vasculature vasodilation, high hepatic energy demand (hypoglycemia), metabolic acidosis (hyperlactatemia), and often fatal septic shock [162]. Glucose and lactate analyses from abdominal effusion and comparison of the values to blood may help with the diagnosis of septic peritonitis. Abdominal effusion with a glucose concentration below 5 mg dl^{-1} was 100% specific for bacterial peritonitis [169]. When blood glucose measured by a blood chemistry analyzer was compared to peritoneal effusion, a difference greater of 20 mg dl^{-1} in blood was 100% sensitive and 100% specific in dogs and 86% sensitive and 100% specific in cats [170]. A cutoff difference of 38 mg dl^{-1} for blood to peritoneal fluid is more accurate if a veterinary point-of-care glucometer is used [171]. Lactate in both blood and peritoneal effusion can be measured and compared to support a septic peritonitis diagnosis. Blood-to-peritoneal effusion lactate difference below −2.0 to 2.5 mmol l^{-1} combined with clinical findings and other fluid analysis is supportive of septic peritonitis in dogs [170, 172].

Anesthetic Considerations

Animals with septic peritonitis often are endotoxic and hypotensive. IV fluid resuscitation should be initiated as soon as possible, particularly if the animal is dehydrated or in shock. Aggressive fluid therapy combined with vasopressor drug support is usually necessary to maintain arterial blood pressure in patients with septic peritonitis. Synthetic colloids such as 6% HES may be beneficial, particularly if vasculitis is present and TP is under $4\,g\,dl^{-1}$ or albumin levels are under $1.5\,g\,dl^{-1}$ [165]. However, synthetic colloid use has been controversial in patients with sepsis. In veterinary critically ill patients, studies are conflicting regarding increased creatinine concentrations, acute kidney injury, and mortality following HES administration [24, 25, 29]. It is important to point it out that in many studies, dogs received HES for several days, and a cumulative dose seemed to play a role in risk of side effects [29]. Six percent HES (130/0.4) at doses administered for fluid resuscitation (up to $20\,ml\,kg^{-1}$) has not been associated with increased renal injury and may be appropriate for improving hemodynamic variables in the perioperative period [28]. Anesthetic management, monitoring, preanesthetic and anesthetic drug selection, and inotropic and vasopressor support in patients with septic peritonitis are similar to patients with GDV, as both syndromes produce acid–base and electrolyte abnormalities combined with hypovolemic and distributive shock.

Summary

Canine and feline patients with GI disease commonly require sedation and/or anesthesia for diagnostic and surgical procedures. They frequently have alterations in function and/or structure of the GI tract resulting in anorexia, dehydration, hypovolemia, acid–base and electrolyte disturbances, protein loss, abdominal pain, and emaciation. Since these changes can alter the anesthetic management of these patients, attempts should be made, if possible, to treat these derangements before general anesthesia.

References

1 Hall, J.E. (2016). General principles of gastrointestinal function – motility, nervous control, and blood circulation. In: *Guyton and Hall Textbook of Medical Physiology*, 13e. E-book (ed. J.E. Hall). Philadelphia, PA: Elsevier Health Sciences.

2 Radlinsky, M. and Fossum, T.W. (2019). Surgery of the digestive tract. In: *Small Animal Surgery*, 5e (ed. T.W. Fossum), 331–511. Philadelphia, PA: Elsevier.

3 Anderson, G.M. (2018). Soft tissue of the oral cavity. In: *Veterinary Surgery: Small Animal*, 2e (eds. S.A. Johnston and K.M. Tobias), 1637–1652. St. Louis, MO: Elsevier.

4 Watrous, B.J. and Suter, P.F. (1979). Normal swallowing in the dog: a cineradiographic study. *Vet Radiol. Ultrasound* 20: 99–109.

5 Reiter, A.M. and Saltero-Rivera, M.M. (2017). Oral and salivary gland disorders. In: *Textbook of Veterinary Internal Medicine*, 8e (eds. S.J. Ettinger and E.C. Feldman), 1469–1475. St. Louis, MO: Elsevier.

6 Berg, J. (2018). Mandibulectomy and maxillectomy. In: *Veterinary Surgery: Small Animal*, 2e, 1663–1677. St. Louis, MO: Elsevier.

7 Vieitez, V., Ezquerra, L.J., Rámis, V.L. et al. (2018). Retrograde intubation in a dog with severe temporomandibular joint ankylosis: case report. *BMC Vet. Res.* 14: 118–123.

8 Stiles, J., Weil, A.B., Packer, R.A. et al. (2012). Post-anesthetic cortical blindness in cats: twenty cases. *Vet. J.* 193: 367–373.

9 Martin-Flores, M., Scrivani, P.V., Loew, E. et al. (2014). Maximal and submaximal mouth opening with mouth gags in cats: implications for maxillary artery blood flow. *Vet. J.* 200: 60–64.

10 Gaynor, J.S. and Muir, W.W. (2015). Acute pain management: a case-based approach. In: *Handbook of Veterinary Pain Management*, 3e (eds. J.S. Gaynor and W.W. Muir), 444–471. St. Louis, MO: Mosby Elsevier.

11 Sinclair, M.D. (2003). Review of the physiological effects of α_2-agonists related to the clinical used of medetomidine in small animal practice. *Can. Vet. J.* 44: 885–897.

12 Takahashi, T., Tsuchida, D., and Pappas, T.N. (2007). Central effects of morphine on GI motility in conscious dogs. *Brain Res.* 1166: 29–34.

13 Valverde, A., Cantwell, S., Hernández, J. et al. (2004). Effects of acepromazine on the incidence of vomiting associated with opioid administration in dogs. *Vet. Anaesth. Analg.* 31: 40–45.

14 Monteiro, E.R., Junior, A.R., Assis, H.M. et al. (2009). Comparative study on the sedative effects of morphine, methadone, butorphanol or tramadol, in combination with acepromazine, in dogs. *Vet. Anaesth. Analg.* 36: 25–33.

15 Wilson, D.V., Evans, T.A., and Mauer, W.A. (2007). Pre-anesthetic meperidine: associated vomiting and gastroesophageal reflux during the subsequent anesthetic in dogs. *Vet. Anaesth. Analg.* 34: 15–22.

16 Campoy, L. and Read, M. (2015). Local and regional anesthetic techniques. In: *Handbook of Veterinary Pain Management*, 3e (eds. J.S. Gaynor and W.W. Muir), 224–265. St. Louis, MO: Mosby Elsevier.

17 Klaumann, P.R., Menzies, R.A., Briganti, A. et al. (2019). Nerve blocks of the upper jaw. In: *Manual of Small Animal Regional Anesthesia. Illustrated Anatomy for Nerve Stimulation and Ultrasound-Guided Nerve Blocks*, 2e (eds. P.E. Otero and D.A. Portela), 319–325. República Argentina: Editorial Inter-médica.

18 Carotenuto, A.M., Ravasio, G., Fonda, D. et al. (2011). Proximal mandibular nerve block, using electrolocation, for rostral mandibulectomy in a geriatric dog. *Can. Vet. J.* 52: 515–518.

19 Muir, W.W., Wiese, A.J., and March, P.A. (2003). Effects of morphine, lidocaine, ketamine, and morphine-lidocaine-ketamine drug combination on minimum alveolar concentration in dogs anesthetized with isoflurane. *Am. J. Vet. Res.* 64: 1155–1160.

20 Vezina-Audette, R., Benedicenti, L., Castejon-Gonzalez, A. et al. (2017). Anesthesia case of the month. *J. Am. Vet. Med. Assoc.* 250: 1104–1106.

21 Bellini, L., Perazzi, A., Carobbi, B. et al. (2018). Maxillomandibulocardiac reflex in a dog. *Acta Vet. Scand.* 60: 64–68.

22 Dart, A.B., Mutter, T.C., Ruth, C.A. et al. (2010). Hydroxyethyl starch (HES) versus other fluid therapies: effects on kidney function. *Cochrane Database Syst. Rev.* (20): CD007594.

23 Gattas, D.J., Dan, A., Myburgh, J. et al. CHEST Management Committee (2012). Fluid resuscitation with 6% hydroxyethyl starch (130/0.4) in acutely ill patients: an updated systematic review and meta-analysis. *Anesth. Analg.* 114: 159–169.

24 Hayes, G., Benedicenti, L., and Mathews, K. (2016). Retrospective cohort study on the incidence of acute kidney injury and death following hydroxyethyl starch (HES 10% 250/0.5:5:1) administration in dogs (2007–2010). *J. Vet. Emergency Crit. Care* 26: 35–40.

25 Yozova, I.D., Howard, J., and Adamik, K.N. (2016). Retrospective evaluation of the effects of administration of tetrastarch (hydroxyethyl starch 130/0.4) on plasma creatinine concentration in dogs (2010–2013): 201 dogs. *J. Vet. Emergency Crit. Care* 26: 568–577.

26 Sigrist, N.E., Kälin, N., and Dreyfus, A. (2017). Changes in serum creatinine concentration and acute kidney injury (AKI) grade in dogs treated with hydroxyethyl starch 130/00.4 from 2013 to 2015. *J. Vet. Intern. Med.* 31: 434–441.

27 Boyd, C.J., Claus, M.A., Raisis, A.L. et al. (2018). Hypocoagulability and platelet dysfunction are exacerbated by synthetic colloids in a canine hemorrhagic shock model. *Front. Vet. Sci.* 13: 279.

28 Weiss, R., Wenk, M., Aken, H.V. et al. (2018). HES or how to end science. *Anesth. Analg.* 127: 1440–1444.

29 Glover, P.A., Rudloff, E.R., and Kirby, R. (2014). Hydroxyethyl starch: a review of pharmacokinetics, pharmacodynamics, current products, and potential clinical risks, benefits, and use. *J. Vet. Emergency Crit. Care* 24: 642–661.

30 McBride, D., Hosgood, G., Raisis, A. et al. (2016). Platelet closure time in anesthetized greyhounds with hemorrhagic shock treated with hydroxyethyl starch 130/0.4 or 0.9% sodium chloride infusions. *J. Vet. Emergency Crit. Care* 26: 509–515.

31 McBride, D., Raisis, A., Hosgood, G. et al. (2017). Hydroxyethyl starch 130/0.4 compared with 0.9% NaCl administered to greyhounds with haemorrhagic shock. *Vet. Anaesth. Analg.* 44: 444–451.

32 Diniz, M.S., Teixeira-Neto, F.J., Celeita-Rodríguez, N. et al. (2018). Effects of 6% tetrastarch and lactated Ringer's solution on extravascular lung water and markers of acute renal injury in hemorrhaged, isoflurane-anesthetized healthy dogs. *J. Vet. Intern. Med.* 32: 712–721.

33 Diniz, M.S., Teixeira-Neto, F.J., Gonçalves, D.S. et al. (2018). Effects of 6% tetrastarch or lactated Ringer's solution on blood coagulation in hemorrhaged dogs. *J. Vet. Intern. Med.* 32: 1927–1933.

34 Boyd, C.J., Claus, M.A., Raisis, A.L. et al. (2019). Evaluation of biomarkers of kidney injury following 4% succinylated gelatin and 6% hydroxyethyl starch 130/0.4 administration in a canine hemorrhagic shock model. *J. Vet. Emergency Crit. Care* 29: 132–142.

35 Zersen, K.M., Mana, K., and Mathis, J.C. (2019). Retrospective evaluation of paired plasma creatinine and chloride concentrations following hetastarch administration in anesthetized dogs (2002–2015): 244 cases. *J. Vet. Emergency Crit. Care* 29: 309–313.

36 Vance, A., Hofmeister, E.H., Laas, C. et al. (2011). The effects of extubation with an inflated versus deflated endotracheal tube cuff on endotracheal fluid volume in the dog. *Vet. Anaesth. Analg.* 38: 203–207.

37 Johnson, S.E. and Sherding, R.G. (2006). Diseases of the esophagus and disorders of swallowing. In: *Saunders Manual of Small Animal Practice*, 3e (eds. S.J. Birchard and R.G. Sherding), 636–654. St. Louis, MO: Saunders Elsevier.

38 Nickel, R., Schummer, A., Seiferle, E., and Sack, W.O. (1973). *The Viscera of the Domestic Animals*, 2e, 21–202. New York: Springer-Verlag.

39 Bright, R.M. (2006). Surgery of the esophagus. In: *Saunders Manual of Small Animal Practice*, 3e (eds. S.J. Birchard and R.G. Sherding), 655–663. St. Louis, MO: Saunders Elsevier.

40 Kyles, A.E. and Huck, J.L. (2018). Esophagus. In: *Veterinary Surgery: Small Animal*, 2e (eds. S.A. Johnston and K.M. Tobias), 1678–1700. St. Louis, MO: Elsevier.

41 Ryan, W.W. and Greene, R.W. (1975). The conservative management of esophageal foreign bodies and their complications: a review of 66 cases in dogs and cats. *J. Am. Anim. Hosp. Assoc.* 11: 243–249.

42 Bennett, R. (2007). Gastrointestinal and hepatic disease. In: *BSAVA Manual of Canine and Feline Anaesthesia and Analgesia*, 2e (eds. C. Seymour and T. Duke-Novakovski), 244–256. Gloucester: British Small Animal Veterinary Association.

43 Galatos, A.D., Rallis, T., and Raptopoulos, D. (1994). Post anaesthetic oesophageal stricture formation in three cats. *J. Small Anim. Pract.* 35: 638–642.

44 Leib, M.S., Dinnel, H., Ward, D.L. et al. (2001). Endoscopic balloon dilation of benign esophageal strictures in dogs and cats. *J. Vet. Intern. Med.* 15: 547–552.

45 Adamama-Moraitou, K., Rallis, T.S., Prassinos, N.N. et al. (2002). Benign esophageal stricture in the dog and cat: a retrospective study of 20 cases. *Can. J. Vet. Res.* 66: 55–59.

46 Kushner, L.I. and Shofer, F.S. (2004). Incidence of esophageal strictures and esophagitis after general anesthesia. In: *Proceeding of the 8th World Congress of*

Veterinary Anesthesia, 184. Knoxville, TN: World Congress of Veterinary Anesthesia.

47 Wilson, D.V. and Walshaw, R. (2004). Postanesthetic esophageal dysfunction in 13 dogs. *J. Am. Anim. Hosp. Assoc.* 40: 455–460.

48 Galatos, A.D. and Raptopoulos, D. (1995). Gastro-oesophageal reflux during anaesthesia in the dog: the effect of age, positioning and type of surgical procedure. *Vet. Rec.* 137: 513–516.

49 Viskjer, S. and Sjöström, L. (2017). Effect of the duration of food withholding prior to anesthesia on gastroesophageal reflux and regurgitation in healthy dogs undergoing elective orthopedic surgery. *Am. J. Vet. Res.* 78: 144–150.

50 Lamata, C., Loughton, V., Jones, M. et al. (2012). The risk of passive regurgitation during general anaesthesia in a population of referred dogs in the UK. *Vet. Anaesth. Analg.* 39: 266–274.

51 Pratschke, K.M., Bellenger, C.R., Mcallister, H. et al. (2001). Barrier pressure at the gastroesophageal junction in anesthetized dogs. *Am. J. Vet. Res.* 62: 1068–1072.

52 Anagnostou, T., Kazakos, G.M., Savvas, I. et al. (2017). Gastro-oesophageal reflux in large-sized, deep-chested versus small-sized, barrel-chested dogs undergoing spinal surgery in sternal recumbency. *Vet. Anaesth. Analg.* 44: 35–41.

53 Galatos, A.D. and Raptopoulos, D. (1995). Gastro-oesophageal reflux during anaesthesia in the dog: the effect of preoperative fasting and premedication. *Vet. Rec.* 137: 479–483.

54 Savas, I. and Raptopoulos, D. (2000). Incidence of gastro-esophageal reflux during anaesthesia, following two different fasting times in dogs. *Vet. Anaesth. Analg.* 27: 59–60.

55 Savvas, I., Rallis, T., and Paptopoulos, D. (2009). The effect of pre-anaesthetic fasting time and type of food on gastric content volume and acidity in dogs. *Vet. Anesth. Analg.* 36: 539–546.

56 Savvas, I., Raptapoulos, D., and Rallis, T. (2016). A "light meal" three hours preoperatively decreases the incidence of gastro-esophageal reflux in dogs. *J. Am. Anim. Hosp. Assoc.* 52: 357–363.

57 Waterman, A.E., Hashim, M.A., and Pearson, H. (1995). Effect of body position on oesophageal and gastric pressures in the anaesthetised dog. *J. Small Anim. Pract.* 36: 196–200.

58 Torrente, C., Vigueras, I., Manzanilla, E.G. et al. (2017). Prevalence of and risk factors for intraoperative gastroesophageal reflux and postanesthetic vomiting and diarrhea in dogs undergoing general anesthesia. *J. Vet. Emergency Crit. Care* 27: 397–408.

59 Anagnostou, T.L., Savvas, I., Kazakos, G.M. et al. (2015). The effect of the stage of the ovarian cycle (anoestrous or dioestrus) and of pregnancy on the incidence of gastro-oesophageal reflux in dogs undergoing ovarioshysterectomy. *Vet. Anaesth. Analg.* 42: 502–511.

60 Wilson, D.V., Evans, A.T., and Miller, R. (2005). Effects of preanesthetic administration of morphine on gastroesophageal reflux and regurgitation during anesthesia in dogs. *Am. J. Vet. Res.* 66: 386–390.

61 Laitinen, S., Mokka, R.E., Valanne, J.V. et al. (1978). Anaesthesia induction and lower oesophageal sphincter pressure. *Acta Anaesthesiol. Scand.* 22: 16–20.

62 Strombeck, D.R. and Harrold, D. (1985). Effect of atropine, acepromazine, meperidine, and xylazine on gastroesophageal sphincter pressure in the dog. *Am. J. Vet. Res.* 46: 963–965.

63 Hashim, M.A. and Waterman, A.E. (1993). Effects of acepromazine, pethidine and atropine premedication on lower oesophageal sphincter pressure and barrier pressure in anaesthetised cats. *Vet. Rec.* 133: 158–160.

64 Hall, J.A., Magne, M.L., and Twedt, D.C. (1987). Effect of acepromazine, diazepam, fentanyl-droperidol, and oxymorphone on gastroesophageal sphincter pressure in healthy dogs. *Am. J. Vet. Res.* 48: 556–567.

65 Hashim, M.A. and Waterman, A.E. (1991). Effects of thiopentone, propofol, alphaxalone-alphadolone, ketamine and xylazine-ketamine on lower oesophageal sphincter pressure and barrier pressure in cats. *Vet. Rec.* 129: 137–139.

66 Raptopoulos, D. and Galatos, A.D. (1997). Gastro-esophageal reflux during anaesthesia induced with either thiopentone or propofol in the dog. *J. Vet. Anaesth.* 24: 20–22.

67 Galatos, A.D., Savas, I., Prassinos, N.N. et al. (2001). Gastro-oesophageal reflux during thiopentone or propofol anaesthesia in the cat. *J. Vet. Med. Assoc.* 48: 287–294.

68 Hashim, M.A., Waterman, A.E., and Pearson, H. (1995). A comparison of the effects of halothane and isoflurane in combination with nitrous oxide on lower oesophageal sphincter pressure and barrier pressure in anaesthetised dogs. *Vet. Rec.* 137: 658–661.

69 Wilson, D.V., Boruta, D.T., and Evans, A.T. (2006). Influence of halothane, isoflurane, and sevoflurane on gastroesophageal reflux during anesthesia in dogs. *Am. J. Vet. Res.* 67: 1821–1825.

70 Poncet, C.M., Dupre, G.P., Freiche, V.G. et al. (2005). Prevalence of gastrointestinal tract lesions in 73 brachycephalic dogs with upper respiratory syndrome. *J. Small Anim. Pract.* 46: 273–279.

71 Costa, R.S., Abelson, A.L., Lindsey, J.C. et al. (2020). Postoperative regurgitation and respiratory complications in brachycephalic dogs undergoing airway surgery before and after implementation of a standardized perianesthetic protocol. *J. Am. Vet. Med. Assoc.* 256: 899–905.

72 Shaver, S.L., Barbu, L.A., Jimenez, D.A. et al. (2017). Evaluation of gastroesophageal reflux in anesthetized dogs with brachycephalic syndrome. *J. Am. Anim. Hosp. Assoc.* 53: 24–31.

73 Chapman, S.R. (2015). Regurgitation and vomiting. In: *Small Animal Critical Care Medicine*, 2e (eds. D.C. Silverstein and K. Hopper), 634–638. St. Louis, MO: Saunders Elsevier.

74 Johnson, S.E., Sherding, R.G., and Bright, R.M. (2006). Diseases of the stomach. In: *Saunders Manual of Small Animal Practice*, 3e (eds. S.J. Birchard and R.G. Sherding), 664–690. St. Louis, MO: Saunders Elsevier.

75 Dowling, P.M. (2015). Motility disorders. In: *Small Animal Critical Care Medicine*, 2e (eds. D.C. Silverstein and K. Hopper), 626–630. St. Louis, MO: Saunders Elsevier.

76 Wyse, C.A., McLellan, J., Dickie, A.M. et al. (2003). A review of methods for assessment of the rate of gastric emptying in the dog and cat: 1989-2002. *J. Vet. Intern. Med.* 17: 609–621.

77 ASA (2017). Practice guidelines for preoperative fasting and the use of pharmacologic agents to reduce the risk of pulmonary aspiration: application to healthy patients undergoing elective procedure: an updated report by the American Society of Anesthesiologists task force of preoperative fasting and the use of pharmacologic agents to reduce the risk of pulmonary aspiration. *Anesthesiology* 126: 376–393.

78 Grubb, T., Sager, J., Gaynor, J.S. et al. (2020). 2020 AAHA anesthesia and monitoring guidelines for dogs and cats. *J. Am. Anim. Assoc.* 56: 59–82.

79 Wilson, D.V., Evans, A.T., and Mauer, W.A. (2006). Influence of metoclopramide on gastroesophageal reflux in anesthetized dogs. *Am. J. Vet. Res.* 67: 26–31.

80 Sideri, A.I., Galatos, A.D., Kazakos, G.M. et al. (2009). Gastro-oesophageal reflux during anaesthesia in the kitten: comparison between use of a laryngeal mask airway or an endotracheal tube. *Vet. Anaesth. Analg.* 36: 547–554.

81 Garcia, R.S., Belafsky, P.C., Maggiore, A.D. et al. (2017). Prevalence of gastroesophageal reflux in cats during anesthesia and effect of omeprazole on gastric pH. *J. Vet. Intern. Med.* 31: 734–742.

82 Panti, A., Bennett, R.C., Corletto, F. et al. (2009). The effect of omeprazole on oesophageal pH in dogs during anaesthesia. *J. Small Anim. Pract.* 50: 540–544.

83 Favarato, E.S., Souza, M.V., Costa, P.R. et al. (2012). Evaluation of metoclopramide and ranitidine on the prevention of gastroesophageal reflux episodes in anesthetized dogs. *Res. Vet. Sci.* 93: 466–467.

84 Bersenas, A.M., Mathews, K.A., Allen, D.G. et al. (2005). Effects of ranitidine, famotidine, pantoprazole, and omeprazole on intragastric pH in dogs. *Am. J. Vet. Res.* 66: 425–431.

85 Tolbert, M.K., Graham, A., Odunayo, A. et al. (2017). Repeated famotidine administration results in a diminished effect on intragastric pH in dogs. *J. Vet. Intern. Med.* 31: 117–123.

86 Marks, S.L., Kook, P.H., Papich, M.G. et al. (2018). ACVIM consensus statement: support for rational administration of gastrointestinal protectants to dogs and cats. *J. Vet. Intern Med.* 32: 1823–1840.

87 Zacuto, A.C., Marks, S.L., Osborn, J. et al. (2012). The influence of esomeprazole and cisapride on gastroesophageal reflux during anesthesia in dogs. *J. Vet. Intern. Med.* 26: 518–525.

88 Kempf, J., Lewis, F., Reusch, C.E. et al. (2014). High-resolution manometric evaluation of the effects of cisapride and metoclopramide hydrochloride administration orally on lower esophageal sphincter pressure in awake dogs. *Am. J. Vet. Res.* 75: 361–366.

89 Jones, C.T. and Fransson, B.A. (2019). Evaluation of the effectiveness of preoperative administration of maropitant citrate and metoclopramide hydrochloride in preventing postoperative clinical gastroesophageal reflux in dogs. *J. Vet. Med. Assoc.* 255: 437–445.

90 Johnson, R.A. (2014). Maropitant prevented vomiting but not gastroesophageal reflux in anesthetized dogs premedicated with acepromazine-hydromorphone. *Vet. Anaesth. Analg.* 41: 406–410.

91 Lorenzutti, A.M., Martin-Flores, M., Litterio, N. et al. (2017). A comparison between maropitant and metoclopramide for the prevention of morphine-induced nausea and vomiting in dogs. *Can. Vet. J.* 58: 35–38.

92 Brioschi, F.A., Gioeni, D., Jacchetti, A. et al. (2018). Effect of metoclopramide on nausea and emesis in dogs premedicated with morphine and dexmedetomidine. *Vet. Anaesth. Analg.* 45: 190–194.

93 Kraus, B.L.H. (2013). Efficacy of maropitant in preventing vomiting in dogs premedicated with hydromorphone. *Vet. Anaesth. Analg.* 40: 28–34.

94 Koh, R.B., Isaza, N., Xie, H. et al. (2014). Effects of maropitant, acepromazine, and electroacupuncture on vomiting associated with administration of morphine in dogs. *J. Am. Vet. Med. Assoc.* 244: 820–829.

95 Claude, A.K., Dedeaux, A., Chiavaccini, L. et al. (2014). Effects of maropitant citrate or acepromazine on the incidence of adverse events associated with hydromorphone premedication in dogs. *J. Vet. Intern. Med.* 28: 1414–1417.

96 Kraus, B.L.H. (2014). Effect of dosing interval on efficacy of maropitant for prevention of hydromorphone-induced vomiting and signs of nausea in dogs. *J. Am. Vet. Med. Assoc.* 245: 1015–1020.

97 Lorenzutti, A.M., Martin-Flores, M., Litterio, N.J. et al. (2016). Evaluation of the antiemetic efficacy of maropitant in dogs medicated with morphine and acepromazine. *Vet. Anaesth. Analg.* 43: 195–198.

98 Martin-Flores, M., Sakai, D.M., Learn, M.M. et al. (2016). Effects of maropitant in cats receiving dexmedetomidine and morphine. *J. Am. Vet. Med. Assoc.* 248: 1257–1261.

99 Kraus, B.L.H. (2017). Spotlight on the perioperative use of maropitant citrate. *Vet. Med.* 8: 41–51.

100 De Laforcade, A.M. and Silverstein, D.C. (2009). Shock. In: *Small Animal Critical Care Medicine* (eds. D.C. Silverstein and K. Hopper), 41–45. St. Louis, MO: Elsevier Saunders.

101 Roush, J.K., Keene, B.W., Eicker, S.W. et al. (1990). Effects of atropine and glycopyrrolate on esophageal, gastric, and tracheal pH in anesthetized dogs. *Vet. Surg.* 19: 88–92.

102 Tams, T.R. (2011). Gastroscopy. In: *Small Animal Endoscopy*, 3e (eds. T.R. Tams and C.A. Rawlings), 97–172. St. Louis, MO: Mosby Elsevier.

103 Blancquaert, J.P., Lefebvre, R.A., and Willems, J.L. (1986). Emetic and antiemetic effects of opioids in the dogs. *Eur. J. Pharmacol.* 128: 143–150.

104 Tantawy, H. and Myslajek, T. (2018). Diseases of the gastrointestinal system. In: *Stoelting's Anesthesia and Co-Existing Disease*, 7e (eds. R.L. Hines and K.E. Marschall), 359–375. Philadelphia, PA: Elsevier.

105 Wilson, D.V. and Evans, A.T. (2007). The effect of topical treatment on esophageal pH during acid reflux in dogs. *Vet. Anaesth. Analg.* 34: 339–343.

106 Allison, A., Italiano, M., and Robinson, R. (2020). Comparison of two topical treatments of gastro-oesophageal regurgitation in dogs during general anaesthesia. *Vet. Anaesth. Analg.* 47: 672–675.

107 Boysen, S.R. (2015). Gastrointestinal hemorrhage. In: *Small Animal Critical Care Medicine*, 2e (eds. D.C. Silverstein and K. Hopper), 630–634. St. Louis, MO: Saunders Elsevier.

108 Cornell, K. (2018). Stomach. In: *Veterinary Surgery: Small Animal*, 2e (eds. S.A. Johnston and K.M. Tobias), 1700–1731. St. Louis, MO: Elsevier.

109 Hume, D.Z. (2015). Diarrhea. In: *Small Animal Critical Care Medicine*, 2e (eds. D.C. Silverstein and K. Hopper), 639–642. St. Louis, MO: Saunders Elsevier.

110 Boag, A.K., Coe, R.J., Martinez, T.A. et al. (2005). Acid-base and electrolyte abnormalities in dogs with gastrointestinal foreign bodies. *J. Vet. Intern. Med.* 19: 816–821.

111 Sherding, R.G. and Johnson, S.E. (2006). Diseases of the jejunum. In: *Saunders Manual of Small Animal Practice*, 3e (eds. S.J. Birchard and R.G. Sherding), 702–738. St. Louis, MO: Saunders Elsevier.

112 DiBartola, S.P. and DeMorais, H.A. (2012). Disorders of potassium: hypokalemia and hyperkalemia. In: *Fluid, Electrolyte, and Acid-Base Disorders in Small Animal Practice*, 4e (ed. S.P. DiBartola), 92–119. St. Louis, MO: Saunders Elsevier.

113 Hopper, K. (2017). Is bicarbonate therapy useful? *Vet. Clin. N. Am. Small Anim. Pract.* 47: 343–349.

114 Donaldson, L.L., Leib, M.S., Boyd, C. et al. (1993). Effect of preanesthetic medication on ease of endoscopic intubation of the duodenum in anesthetized dogs. *Am. J. Vet. Res.* 54: 1489–1495.

115 McFadzean, W.J., Hall, E.J., and Van Oostrom, H. (2017). Effect of premedication with butorphanol or methadone on ease of endoscopic duodenal intubation in dogs. *Vet. Anaesth. Analg.* 44: 1296–1302.

116 Smith, A.A., Posner, L.P., Goldstein, R.E. et al. (2004). Evaluation of the effects of premedication on gastroduodenoscopy in cats. *J. Am. Vet. Med. Assoc.* 225: 540–544.

117 Pypendop, B.H. and Ilkiw, J.E. (2005). Assessment of the hemodynamic effects of lidocaine administered IV in isoflurane-anesthetized cats. *Am. J. Vet. Res.* 100: 97–101.

118 Bruggink, S.M., Schroeder, K.M., Baker-Herman, T.L. et al. (2012). Weight-based volume of injection influences cranial to caudal spread of local anesthetic solution in ultrasound-guided transversus abdominis plane block in canine cadavers. *Vet. Surg.* 41: 455–457.

119 Portela, D.A., Fuensalida, S.E., Viscasillas, J. et al. (2019). Transversus abdominis plane block. In: *Manual of Small Animal Regional Anesthesia. Illustrated Anatomy for Nerve Stimulation and Ultrasound-Guided Nerve Blocks*, 2e (eds. P.E. Otero and D.A. Portela), 254–261.

120 Moon, R.C., Lastrapes, L., Wier, J. et al. (2019). Preoperative transversus abdominis plane (TAP) block with liposomal bupivacaine for bariatric patients to reduce the use of opioid analgesics. *Obesity Surg.* 29: 1099–1104.

121 Khan, S.A. and McLean, M.K. (2012). Toxicology of frequently encountered nonsteroidal anti-inflammatory drugs in dogs and cats. *Vet. Clin. N. Am. Small Anim. Pract.* 41: 289–306.

122 Aronson, L.R., Brockman, D.J., and Brown, D.C. (2000). Gastrointestinal emergencies. *Vet. Clin. N. Am. Small Anim. Pract.* 30: 555–579.

123 Glickman, L.T., Glickman, N.W., Schellenberg, D.B. et al. (2000). Incidence of and breed-related risk factors for gastric dilatation-volvulus in dogs. *J. Am. Vet. Med. Assoc.* 216: 40–45.

124 Sharp, C.R. (2015). Gastric dilatation-volvulus. In: *Small Animal Critical Care Medicine*, 2e (eds. D.C. Silverstein and K. Hopper), 649–653. St. Louis, MO: Saunders Elsevier.

125 Muir, W.W. (1982). Gastric dilatation-volvulus in the dog, with emphasis on cardiac arrhythmias. *J. Am. Vet. Med. Assoc.* 180: 739–742.

126 Brockman, D.J., Washabau, R.J., and Drobatz, K.J. (1995). Canine gastric dilatation/volvulus syndrome in a veterinary critical care unit: 295 cases (1986–1992). *J. Am. Vet. Med. Assoc.* 207: 460–464.

127 Beck, J.J., Staatz, A.J., Pelsue, D.H. et al. (2006). Risk factors associated with short-term outcome and development of perioperative complications in dogs undergoing surgery because of gastric dilatation-volvulus: 166 cases (1992–2003). *J. Am. Vet. Med. Assoc.* 229: 1934–1939.

128 Buber, T., Saragusty, J., Ranen, E. et al. (2007). Evaluation of lidocaine treatment and risk factors for death associated with gastric dilatation and volvulus in dogs: 112 cases (1997–2005). *J. Am. Vet. Med. Assoc.* 230: 1334–1339.

129 Mackenzie, G., Barnhart, M., Kennedy, S. et al. (2010). A retrospective study of factors influencing survival following surgery for gastric dilatation-volvulus syndrome in 306 dogs. *J. Am. Anim. Hosp. Assoc.* 46: 97–102.

130 Sharp, C.R., Rozanski, E.A., Finn, E. et al. (2020). The pattern of mortality in dogs with gastric dilatation and volvulus. *J. Vet. Emergency Crit. Care* 30: 232–238.

131 O'Neill, D.G., Case, J., Boag, A.K. et al. (2017). Gastric dilation-volvulus in dogs attending UK emergency-care veterinary practices: prevalence, risk factors and survival. *J. Small Anim. Pract.* 58: 629–638.

132 Brourman, J.D., Schertel, E.R., Allen, D.A. et al. (1996). Factors associated with perioperative mortality in dogs with surgically managed gastric dilatation-volvulus: 137 cases (1988–1993). *J. Am. Vet. Med. Assoc.* 208: 1855–1858.

133 Orton, E.C. and Muir, W.W. (1983). Hemodynamics during experimental gastric dilatation-volvulus in dogs. *Am. J. Vet. Res.* 44: 1512–1515.

134 Muir, W.W. and Weisbrode, S.E. (1982). Myocardial ischemia in dogs with gastric dilatation-volvulus. *J. Am. Vet. Med. Assoc.* 181: 363–366.

135 Muir, W.W. and Lipowitz, A.J. (1978). Cardiac dysrhythmias associated with gastric dilatation-volvulus in the dog. *J. Am. Vet. Med. Assoc.* 172: 683–689.

136 Schober, K.E., Cornand, C., Kirbach, B. et al. (2002). Serum cardiac troponin I and cardiac troponin T concentrations in dogs with gastric dilatation-volvulus. *J. Am. Vet. Med. Assoc.* 221: 381–388.

137 Wingfield, W.E., Twedt, D.C., Moore, R.W. et al. (1982). Acid-base and electrolyte values in dogs with acute gastric dilatation-volvulus. *J. Am. Vet. Med. Assoc.* 180: 1070–1072.

138 Muir, W.W. (1982). Acid-base and electrolyte disturbances in dogs with gastric dilatation-volvulus. *J. Am. Vet. Med. Assoc.* 181: 229–231.

139 De Papp, E., Drobatz, K.J., and Hughes, D. (1999). Plasma lactate concentration as a predictor of gastric necrosis and survival among dogs with gastric dilatation-volvulus: 102 cases (1995–1998). *J. Am. Vet. Med. Assoc.* 215: 49–52.

140 Zacher, L.A., Berg, J., Shaw, S.P. et al. (2010). Association between outcome and changes in plasma lactate concentration during presurgical treatment in dogs with gastric dilatation-volvulus: 64 cases (2002–2008). *J. Am. Vet. Med. Assoc.* 236: 892–897.

141 Green, T.I., Tonozzi, C.C., Kirby, R. et al. (2011). Evaluation of initial plasma lactate values as a predictor of gastric necrosis and initial and subsequent plasma lactate values as a predictor of survival in dogs with gastric dilatation-volvulus: 84 dogs (2003–2007). *J. Vet. Emergency Crit. Care* 21: 36–44.

142 Mooney, E., Raw, C., and Hughes, D. (2014). Plasma lactate concentration as a prognostic biomarker in dogs with gastric dilation and volvulus. *Top. Comp. Anim. Med.* 29: 71–76.

143 Wong, P.L. (1992). Anesthesia for gastric dilatation/volvulus. *Vet. Clin. N. Am. Small Anim. Pract.* 22: 471–474.

144 Allen, D.A., Schertel, E.R., Muir, W.W. et al. (1991). Hypertonic saline/dextran resuscitation of dogs with experimentally induced gastric dilatation-volvulus shock. *Am. J. Vet. Res.* 52: 92–96.

145 Schertel, E.R., Allen, D.A., Muir, W.W. et al. (1997). Evaluation of a hypertonic saline-dextran solution for treatment of dogs with shock induced by gastric dilatation-volvulus. *J. Am. Vet. Med. Assoc.* 210: 226–230.

146 Pariaut, R. (2015). Ventricular Tachyarrhythmias. In: *Small Animal Critical Care Medicine*, 2e (eds. D.C. Silverstein and K. Hopper), 255–259. St. Louis, MO: Saunders Elsevier.

147 Matsubata, L.M., Oliva, V.N.L.S., Gabas, D.T. et al. (2009). Effect of lidocaine on the minimum alveolar concentration of sevoflurane in dogs. *Vet. Anesth. Analg.* 36: 407–413.

148 Valverde, A., Doherty, T.J., Hernandez, J. et al. (2004). Effect of lidocaine on the minimum alveolar concentration of isoflurane in dogs. *Vet. Anaesth. Analg.* 31: 264–271.

149 Lahav, M., Levite, M., Bassani, L. et al. (2002). Lidocaine inhibits secretion of IL-8 and IL-1beta and stimulates secretion of IL-1 receptor antagonist by epithelial cells. *Clin. Exp. Immunol.* 127: 226–233.

150 Yardeni, I.Z., Beilin, B., Mayburd, E. et al. (2009). The effect of perioperative intravenous lidocaine on postoperative pain and immune function. *Anesth. Analg.* 109: 1464–1469.

151 McCarthy, G.C., Megalla, S.A., and Habib, A.S. (2010). Impact of intravenous lidocaine infusion on postoperative analgesia and recovery from surgery: a systematic review of randomized controlled trials. *Drugs* 70: 1149–1163.

152 Rimback, G., Cassuto, J., and Tollesson, P.O. (1990). Treatment of postoperative paralytic ileus by intravenous lidocaine infusion. *Anesth. Analg.* 70: 414–419.

153 Bruchim, Y., Itay, S., Shira, B.H. et al. (2012). Evaluation of lidocaine treatment on frequency of cardiac arrhythmias, acute kidney injury, and hospitalization time in dogs with gastric dilatation volvulus. *J. Vet. Emergency Crit. Care* 22: 419–427.

154 Preisman, S., Pfeiffer, U., Lieberman, N. et al. (1997). New monitors of intravascular volume: a comparison of arterial pressure waveform analysis and the intrathoracic blood volume. *Intensive Care Med.* 23: 651–657.

155 Westphal, G.A., Silva, E., Gonçalvez, A.R. et al. (2009). Pulse oximetry wave variation as a noninvasive tool to assess volume status in cardiac surgery. *Clinics* 64: 337–343.

156 Marik, P.E., Cavallazi, R., Vasu, T. et al. (2009). Dynamic changes in arterial waveform derived variables and fluid responsiveness in mechanically ventilated patients: a systematic review of literature. *Crit. Care Med.* 37: 2642–2647.

157 Michard, F. (2005). Changes in arterial pressure during mechanical ventilation. *Anesthesiology* 103: 419–428.

158 Klein, A.V., Teixeira-Neto, F.J., Garofalo, N.A. et al. (2016). Change in pulse pressure variation and plethysmographic variability index caused by hypotension-inducing hemorrhage followed by volume replacement in isoflurane-anesthetized dogs. *Am. J. Vet. Res.* 77: 280–287.

159 Endo, Y., Tamura, J., Ishizuka, T. et al. (2017). Stroke volume variation (SVF) and pulse pressure variation (PPV) as indicators of fluid responsiveness in sevoflurane anesthetized mechanically ventilated euvolemic dogs. *J. Vet. Med. Sci.* 79: 1437–1445.

160 Fantoni, D.T., Ida, K.K., Gimenes, A.M. et al. (2017). Pulse pressure variation as a guide for volume expansion in dogs undergoing orthopedic surgery. *Vet. Anaesth. Analg.* 44: 710–718.

161 Sano, H., Seo, J., Wightman, P. et al. (2018). Evaluation of pulse pressure variation and pleth variability index to predict fluid responsiveness in mechanically ventilated isoflurane-anesthetized dogs. *J. Vet. Emergency Crit. Care* 28: 301–309.

162 Ellison, G.W. (2011). Complications of gastrointestinal surgery in companion animals. *Vet. Clin. N. Am. Small Anim. Pract.* 41: 915–934.

163 Williams, J.M. (2018). Colon. In: *Veterinary Surgery: Small Animal*, 2e (eds. S.A. Johnston and K.M. Tobias), 1761–1782. St. Louis, MO: Elsevier.

164 Baines, S.J. and Aronson, L.R. (2018). Rectum, anus, and perineum. In: *Veterinary Surgery: Small Animal*, 2e (eds. S.A. Johnston and K.M. Tobias), 1783–1828. St. Louis, MO: Elsevier.

165 Grimes, J.A., Schmiedt, C.W., Cornell, K.K. et al. (2011). Identification of risk factors for septic peritonitis and failure to survive following gastrointestinal surgery in dogs. *J. Am. Vet. Med. Assoc.* 238: 486–494.

166 Fossum, T.W. (2019). Surgery of the abdominal cavity. In: *Small Animal Surgery*, 5e (ed. T.W. Fossum), 512–539. Philadelphia, PA: Elsevier.

167 Hosgood, G. and Salisbury, S.K. (1988). Generalized peritonitis in dogs: 50 cases (1975-1986). *J. Am. Vet. Med. Assoc.* 193: 1448–1450.

168 Ralphs, S.C., Jessen, C.R., and Lipowitz, A.J. (2003). Risk factors for leakage following intestinal anastomosis in dogs and cats: 115 cases (1991-2000). *J. Am. Vet. Med. Assoc.* 223: 73–77.

169 Hughes, D. and Swann, H. (2000). Diagnosis and management of peritonitis. *Vet. Clin. N. Am. Small Anim. Pract.* 30: 603–615.

170 Bonczynski, J.J., Ludwig, L., Barton, L.J. et al. (2003). Comparison of peritoneal fluid and peripheral blood pH, bicarbonate, glucose, and lactate concentration as a diagnostic tool for septic peritonitis in dogs and cats. *Vet. Surg.* 32: 161–166.

171 Koenig, A. and Verlander, L.L. (2015). Usefulness of whole blood, plasma, peritoneal fluid, and peritoneal fluid supernatant glucose concentrations obtained by a veterinary point-of-care glucometer to identify septic peritonitis in dogs with peritoneal effusion. *J. Am. Vet. Med. Assoc.* 247: 1027–1032.

172 Levin, G.M., Bonczynski, J.J., Ludwig, L.L. et al. (2004). Lactate as a diagnostic test for septic peritoneal effusions in dogs and cats. *J. Am. Anim. Hosp. Assoc.* 40: 364–371.

6

Renal Disease

Carrie A. Schroeder

Department of Surgical Sciences, School of Veterinary Medicine, University of Wisconsin–Madison, Madison, WI, 53706, USA

Introduction

General anesthesia has profound effects on the body, greatly affecting cardiac output, blood pressure, and perfusion of vital organs. The anesthetist's task is to minimize these detrimental effects, with the goal of maximizing the resemblance to patient homeostasis. This is no simple task in the healthy patient and can be a daunting task in the face of disease. Renal disease is a common pathology faced when providing anesthesia to today's pet population. The estimated prevalence of chronic kidney disease (CKD) is 0.5–1.0% in dogs and 1.0–3.0% in cats, increasing to 80% among older cats [1].

Before anesthetizing a patient with either acute kidney injury (AKI) or CKD, it is paramount to understand the effects of renal dysfunction on the patient, and the anesthetic and surgical effects on the kidneys; only then can an anesthetic plan be tailored to the patient and the disease process. Although anesthetic procedures and drug choices may have profound renal effects, the maintenance of normotension, euvolemia, and adequate cardiac output sufficient to maintain renal perfusion has the greatest effect on the prevention of initial or ongoing renal insult.

Anatomy and Physiology

The kidneys serve several functions, including metabolic waste products and toxin excretion, blood volume, extracellular fluid volume, osmolality regulation, and electrolyte balance. The kidneys also serve important roles in acid–base regulation, erythrocyte production, and hormone secretion.

Each kidney is divided into cortical and medullary portions and is made up of thousands of nephrons, the functional kidney units [2]. The nephron comprises the glomerulus and the renal tubule (Figure 6.1a). The glomerulus is a unique ball of capillaries interposed between two sets of arterioles with a high hydrostatic pressure, favoring fluid filtration. Fluid filtered from the glomerulus enters the renal tubule, where, depending on several factors, reabsorption and secretion occur, resulting in the end product of urine (Figure 6.1b).

Despite their relatively small size, the kidneys receive an impressively high proportion of cardiac output, roughly 20–25% [2, 3]. The vast majority (90–95%) of blood flow is directed to the renal cortex, with the remainder perfusing the renal medulla [3]. High blood flow serves to match the extremely high oxygen

Canine and Feline Anesthesia and Co-Existing Disease, Second Edition. Edited by Rebecca A. Johnson, Lindsey B. C. Snyder and Carrie A. Schroeder.

Companion website: www.wiley.com/go/johnson/canine

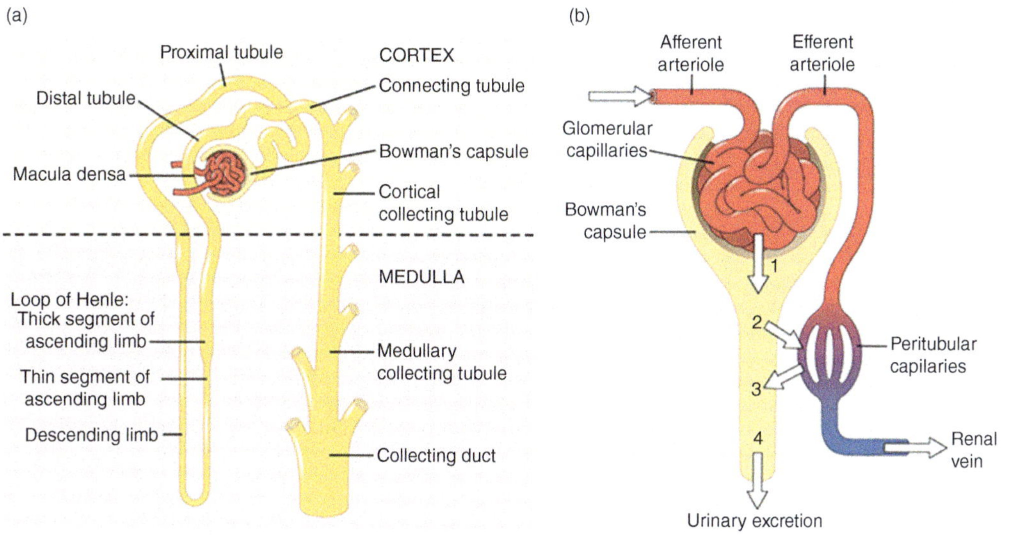

Figure 6.1 (a) Schematic representation of the nephron and glomerulus. (b) Schematic representation of urine formation. [1] Filtration of blood at the level of the glomerulus. [2] Reabsorption of substances from renal tubules by peritubular capillaries. [3] Secretion of substances from peritubular capillaries into renal tubules. [4] Excretion of the urine. Urinary excretion is the net result of filtration minus reabsorption plus secretion (excretion = filtration − reabsorption + secretion). Source: Adapted from Guyton and Hall Textbook of Medical Physiology, 2021, with permission.

consumption of the kidneys. On a per-gram basis, the kidneys have roughly twice the oxygen consumption of the brain, but nearly seven times the blood flow [4]. As oxygen delivery to the kidneys exceeds the consumption under normal circumstances, the arteriovenous difference in the kidneys is relatively low.

In general, renal blood flow (RBF) is directly related to glomerular filtration rate (GFR). However, renal autoregulation serves to stabilize GFR, despite large swings in blood pressure (Figure 6.2). This occurs via several extrinsic and intrinsic [4] mechanisms at mean arterial blood pressures from approximately 70–180 mmHg [4]. Although GFR is preserved within this autoregulatory range, several factors can alter this process and lead to renal ischemia, despite apparent normotension. For example, sympathetic activation, as occurs in the presence of pain or surgical stimulation, can lead to renal vasoconstriction and hypoperfusion of the kidney [3]. Although autoregulation is preserved with most anesthetics, anesthetic drugs may cause a redistribution of blood flow away from the renal cortex [3]. Autoregulation may also be altered in the presence of chronic hypertension, acute renal failure, and sepsis [3]. In the face of these disease processes, mean arterial pressure must be maintained at a higher range to preserve autoregulation of RBF.

Pathophysiology

Renal disease is broadly classified as AKI or CKD. AKI can occur over a period of hours to days and is due to several processes, including toxicities, infection, and inflammatory conditions. Broadly, perioperative injury can be due to prerenal AKI (e.g., hypovolemia or severe dehydration), direct renal injury, or postrenal AKI (e.g., urinary obstruction) [5]. Perioperative acute tubular necrosis may be due to ischemia–reperfusion injury or nephrotoxicity (sources may include antibiotic therapy or myoglobin) [5]. Some of the more common perioperative causes of AKI include urethral obstruction, sepsis, and infectious disease.

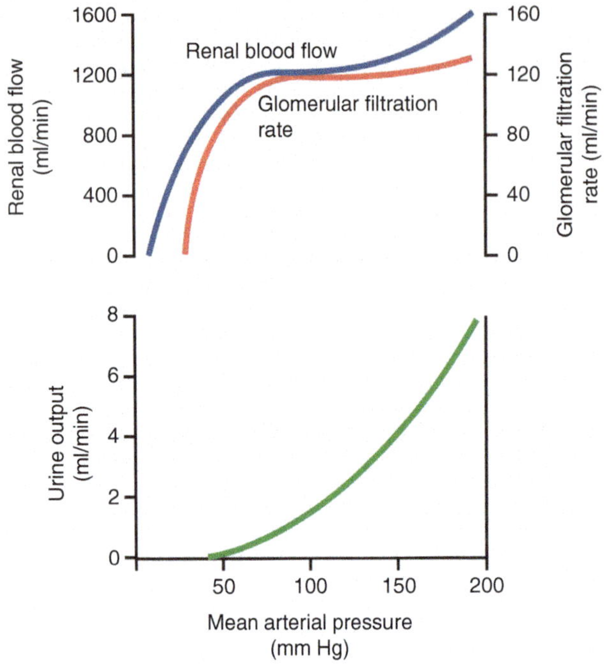

Figure 6.2 Autoregulation of renal blood flow (RBF) and glomerular filtration rate (GFR). Renal autoregulation stabilized GFR within a range of mean arterial pressures of approximately 70–180 mmHg, while urine output is directly related to changes in blood pressure. Source: Guyton and Hall Textbook of Medical Physiology, 2021, with permission.

Indeed, AKI has been reported to occur in 12% of dogs with abdominal sepsis [6]. In bitches presenting with pyometra, 20 out of 20 dogs presented with some degree of renal tissue injury including tubular degeneration or necrosis and/or glomerulonephritis, meeting the criteria for AKI [7]. Despite this presence of damage, only 40% of those patients met the criteria for sepsis via the sequential organ failure assessment score. It is important to be aware that kidney injury may be present or impending in any animal presenting with an acute abdomen-type condition that may lead to sepsis or renal damage.

Animals with AKI may present for any number of procedures, from brief urethral catheter placement to major exploratory laparotomy. AKI can also result from anesthesia and surgery. In humans, this is often due to a combination of prerenal azotemia and acute tubular necrosis [8]. While idiosyncratic cases can occur with no apparent intraoperative insults, tubular necrosis can occur perioperatively resulting from a prolonged decrease in renal perfusion due to decreased cardiac output, severe hypotension, or inflammatory processes [8–10]. Fortunately, the healthy kidney is relatively tolerant of perioperative insults, and multiple and/or severe insults are generally required to produce injury enough to cause a significant decrease in renal function [8]. Judicious fluid use and blood pressure maintenance, in addition to avoiding nephrotoxic agents and ischemia, are often sufficient to prevent perioperative AKI. Patients with AKI can present with coexisting abnormalities in acid–base status, electrolytes, and the biochemical profile that may affect patient anesthetic management (Table 6.1). Thus, before attempting general anesthesia, it is important to perform a thorough patient evaluation, including assessment of hydration, hemodynamics, electrolyte and acid–base status, blood pressure, and biochemical profile.

Table 6.1 Physiological abnormalities commonly associated with acute kidney injury (AKI).

Abnormalities commonly associated with acute renal injury
↑ BUN
↑ Creatinine
↑, ↓, or – Na^+
↑ K^+
↑ P
↑, ↓, or – urine output
Metabolic acidosis
↑ Respiratory rate
Hypertension or hypotension
Cardiac dysrhythmias
Nausea and vomiting

↑ and ↓ indicate an increase and decrease, respectfully, in a parameter, – indicates no change.

AKI describes a wide range of severity and prognoses. Many classification schemes have been described in humans, including the RIFLE (risk, injury, failure, loss of kidney function, and end-stage kidney disease) and AKIN (acute kidney injury network) systems [11]. In veterinary medicine, the International Renal Interest Society (IRIS) has developed recommendations for AKI grading in dogs and cats on a scale of I to V (Table 6.2) [12]. Prognosis is based on grading; animals with IRIS AKI Grades I and II that are appropriately managed may regain renal function within 2–5 days, while animals that fall in Grades IV to V may die within 5–10 days [12]. Overall, patient prognosis with AKI can be quite poor, with an overall mortality rate of 45–53% in small animals [13]. The risks versus benefits of performing general anesthesia on patients with AKI need to be assessed, and, if necessary, anesthesia should be delayed until appropriate patient stabilization has been achieved. However, the reality is that many patients with AKI, such as patients presenting with urethral obstruction (see Chapter 7), may require general anesthesia to attain appropriate stabilization, especially if sedation or regional anesthesia is not an option.

CKD is the structural or functional disease of one or both kidneys that has been present for a longer duration, generally 3 months and longer [14]. CKD is due to a myriad of underlying problems and, unlike AKI, is considered progressive and irreversible. The diagnosis can be made based on several hallmark abnormalities, and a single test is generally insufficient to diagnose CKD. Like AKI, The IRIS has developed guidelines to stage renal disease on a scale of 1–4 based on renal function tests (Table 6.3). Patients are then substaged based on the presence or absence of proteinuria and hypertension. Complete guidelines for renal disease staging, as well as current algorithms for staging in small animals, can be found on the IRIS website (http://www.iris-kidney.com). Based on the animal's IRIS stage, appropriate prognosis and treatment can be pursued by the managing clinician. Animals presenting for general anesthesia with a history of CKD, especially those that have had a diagnostic workup and have been assigned an IRIS stage, generally are accompanied by a history of diagnostic tests and have been chronically managed medically. Newly diagnosed patients should be staged and stabilized with medical treatment before undergoing general anesthesia. Unfortunately, this is not always the case. All patients presenting with CKD should have baseline diagnostic tests performed before formulating an anesthetic plan, including a thorough evaluation of hydration, cardiovascular status, blood pressure, complete blood count, biochemical profile, and evaluation of electrolytes and acid–base status. In addition to standard biochemical screening that includes blood urea nitrogen (BUN) and creatinine, a fasting symmetric dimethylarginine (SDMA) immunoassay should be performed. SDMA is a biomarker that reflects GFR and is a more sensitive indicator of renal function [15]. Generally, SDMA levels below 14 $\mu g\ dl^{-1}$ are considered acceptable and are within the reference interval.

It is important to realize that these patients can present with several abnormalities

Table 6.2 International Renal Interest Society (IRIS) staging of acute kidney injury (AKI) [12].

AKI grade	Creatinine (mg dl^{-1})	Clinical description
I	<1.6	Nonazotemic AKI Documented AKI (historical or clinical) Progressive increases in creatinine (≥0.3 mg dl^{-1} within 48 h) Oliguria or anuria over 6 h
II	1.7–2.5	Mild AKI Documented AKI Static or progressive increases in creatinine (≥0.3 mg dl^{-1} within 48 h) Oliguria or anuria over 6 h
III	2.6–5.0	Moderate to severe AKI
IV	5.1–10.0	Documented AKI
V	>10.0	Increasing severity of azotemia Functional renal failure

(Table 6.4). Age-related comorbidities such as diabetes mellitus and cardiovascular disease are also frequently encountered [7]. Stabilization and management of sequelae of the primary disease, as well as any comorbidities, are keys to successful management of CKD.

Renal Disease and Surgery

Stress and pain associated with surgery can have significant effects on the kidney. Catecholamine, renin, arginine vasopressin (AVP), and aldosterone release associated with surgical stimulation often lead to an increase in renal vascular resistance and decrease in RBF and GFR [5, 16]. Systemic analgesic drugs or regional anesthetic techniques may attenuate this response, but even patients without preexisting renal disease can experience perioperative kidney dysfunction because of anesthesia and/or surgery. The perioperative period is a time of extreme physiologic stress and it is important to anticipate possible negative consequences of anesthesia and surgical procedures. Patients that present with preexisting AKI or CKD should be optimized prior to surgery to minimize the detrimental effects of the perioperative period (see the section titled "Pre-anesthetic Stabilization").

Table 6.3 International Renal Interest Society (IRIS) staging of chronic kidney disease (CKD).

IRIS stage	Creatinine (mg dl^{-1})		SDMA (μg dl^{-1})	
	Dog	Cat	Dog	Cat
1	<1.4	<1.6	<18	<18
2	1.4–2.8	1.6–2.8	18–35	18–35
3	2.9–5.0	2.9–5.0	36–54	26–38
4	>5.0	>5.0	>54	>38

Source: Complete details and substaging may be found at www.iris-kidney.com.

Surgical manipulation may compromise RBF either through direct compression of vasculature associated with the kidneys or through increases in intra-abdominal pressure. Renal hypoperfusion and venous congestion can occur through abdominal organ manipulation and elevations of central venous pressure [16]. Pneumoperitoneum associated with the insufflation in laparoscopic surgery can increase intra-abdominal

Table 6.4 Physiological abnormalities commonly associated with chronic renal disease.

Abnormalities commonly associated with chronic renal disease
↑ BUN
↑ Creatinine
↑ SDMA
↑ or ↓ K^+
↑ Mg
Ca^{2+}
↑ P
Metabolic acidosis
↑ Respiratory rate
Hypertension
Anemia
Uremic coagulopathy
Hypoalbuminemia
Dehydration
Nausea, vomiting

↑ and ↓ indicate an increase and a decrease, respectfully, in a parameter.

pressures significantly; abdominal compartment syndrome, defined as sustained increases in intra-abdominal pressure >20 mmHg, may lead to organ dysfunction [5]. However, more modest increases in intra-abdominal pressure (>12 mmHg) have been associated with a higher risk of renal damage [17]. AKI and oliguria may be consequences of intraoperative and postoperative intra-abdominal hypertension and abdominal compartment syndrome [17, 18].

In addition, any intervention that decreases cardiac output can similarly affect RBF and GFR. This includes the cardiac depression that may be associated with general anesthesia, positive pressure ventilation (PPV), and positive end-expiratory pressure (PEEP). It is important to closely monitor blood pressure and cardiorespiratory parameters as surrogate measures of cardiac output and address concerns accordingly to maintain adequate RBF. Optimizing hydration status and achieving euvolemia should attenuate the hemodynamic responses associated with positive pressure ventilation such as decreased venous return and pulse pressure variation, but increased airway and pleural pressures associated with PPV and PEEP can lead to renal vasoconstriction, antidiuresis, and anti-natriuresis [15]. Increasing levels of PEEP can lead to increases in renin and aldosterone and depression of cardiac output, RBF, GFR, and urine volume [15]. When utilizing PPV and/or PEEP, more conservative ventilator settings are recommended.

Renal Disease and Pharmacologic Agents

Pre-anesthetic Agents

Phenothiazines

Acepromazine is a relatively common sedative utilized in modern veterinary practice. It belongs to the phenothiazine class of neuroleptics and produces mild to moderate sedation lasting anywhere from 1–6 h, depending on dosage, and no direct-acting drug antagonist is available [19, 20]. Acepromazine causes blockade of dopaminergic and alpha-1-adrenergic receptors, inducing vasodilation that may lead to hypotension below the range of renal autoregulation [21, 22]. The concurrent use of volatile anesthetics and their accompanying vasodilation and hypotension may worsen phenothiazine-induced hypotension. However, incremental dosages of acepromazine administered intravenously under isoflurane anesthesia increase cardiac index and oxygen delivery and preserve systemic blood pressures [23]. Renal function as measured by GFR, RBF, and blood analytes was preserved in dogs administered acepromazine prior to anesthetic induction, despite systemic hypotension [21]. Since no drug antagonist is available, one must use caution in choosing this agent in patients that may not tolerate prolonged sedation or the possible accompanying systemic hypotension associated with its use. Careful blood pressure monitoring is advised following administration of acepromazine, especially to patients with preexisting renal disease.

Alpha-2-Adrenergic Receptor Agonists

This drug class includes agents such as xylazine, detomidine, romifidine, medetomidine, and dexmedetomidine. In small-animal patients, the most relevant alpha-2-adrenergic agent is dexmedetomidine. Each of these agents significantly decreases heart rate and cardiac output while increasing systemic vascular resistance [24–27]. Medetomidine administration, the racemic mixture of levomedetomidine and dexmedetomidine, along with propofol induction decreased cardiac output by approximately 60% and decreased RBF by approximately 50% in dogs [28]. However, GFR was increased despite these changes. Another study evaluating the renal effects of medetomidine in dogs revealed variable effects dependent on the method of drug administration. For example, intramuscular administration of medetomidine induced decreases in RBF and GFR, whereas intravascular administration induced opposite effects, increasing RBF and GFR [29]. These contradictory effects may be attributed to the immediate systemic hypertension following intravenous administration, an effect less drastically observed with intramuscular administration [29]. Slow administration may attenuate the hemodynamic responses associated with rapid or bolus administration. Constant rate infusion (CRI) of dexmedetomidine in dogs anesthetized with sevoflurane decreased cardiac index but had no effect on GFR or RBF [27].

A diuretic effect is often observed with these agents owing to several possible mechanisms, including inhibition of AVP, natriuresis, and osmotic diuresis due to insulin inhibition and resulting hyperglycemia [27, 29]. Therefore, the use of alpha-2-adrenergic agonists in patients with unresolved urinary obstruction should be avoided.

Owing to the hemodynamic instability and possible associated decreases in RBF as well as wide blood pressure variations, alpha-2-adrenergic agonists should be used judiciously. When administered intravenously, agents should be administered slowly and titrated to effect. Doses administered intramuscularly should be carefully calculated and kept to a minimum. This can be achieved by the coadministration with other agents with minimal cardiac effects, such as opioids or benzodiazepines. Blood pressure and heart rate should be monitored, at minimum, when these agents are administered.

Benzodiazepines

The benzodiazepines, most commonly midazolam and diazepam, exert a sedative effect via enhancement of the endogenous inhibitory neurotransmitter, gamma-aminobutyric acid (GABA) [30]. Their cardiovascular effects are mild, and they are well-tolerated in patients with many disease states, including renal disease [31]. Although benzodiazepine use is generally recommended and considered safe, caution must be exercised in using these agents in animals that may demonstrate paradoxical excitement on administration, most notoriously juvenile patients, and young cats [32]. Sole administration of benzodiazepines to most veterinary patients is generally not suggested for this reason, and, to improve sedation, coadministration with an opioid or other sedative is advised. When used appropriately, benzodiazepines are an excellent choice for patients either with preexisting renal disease or in disease states that may predispose them to renal damage (e.g., sepsis, hypovolemic shock).

Opioids

The opioids can be broadly classified into agonists, agonist–antagonists, and partial agonists based on their effects on opioid receptors [33]. Opioid agonists include, among others, morphine, hydromorphone, fentanyl, and methadone; these exert a pharmacologic effect via interaction with the mu-opioid receptor. Butorphanol is a commonly used agent in veterinary medicine and is classified as an opioid agonist–antagonist, acting as an antagonist at the mu-opioid receptor and an agonist at the kappa-opioid receptor. Buprenorphine, a partial agonist, acts as an agonist at the mu-opioid receptor but exhibits a submaximal response as compared to opioid agonists [34]. This submaximal response does not necessarily reflect analgesia, as buprenorphine has proven moderate, although variable, analgesic efficacy in several species, especially as part of a multimodal analgesic plan [35, 36]. Direct adverse renal effects of the opioids are generally mild and of little consequence for patients with renal disease [37, 38]. However, bradycardia associated with high opioid dosages may lead to decreases in the cardiac index, potentially impacting RBF [39]. Significant bradycardia should be treated as necessary to restore hemodynamic stability.

The profound analgesic effects of this pharmacologic class may attenuate the sympathetic response associated with surgical pain, thus minimizing renal vasoconstriction. Furthermore, minimal alveolar concentration (MAC) of volatile anesthetics is reduced with concurrent opioid use. For example, oxymorphone and hydromorphone administration decreased the MAC of isoflurane in dogs by approximately 45%, while fentanyl decreases isoflurane MAC in a similar, dose-dependent manner [40, 41]. Decreases in MAC associated with opioid use, which have minimal direct effects on blood pressure, may attenuate the systemic hypotension associated with volatile anesthetics.

Multiple opioids are metabolized by extrarenal pathways, and duration and effect are largely unaffected by renal failure [42, 43]. However, active morphine and meperidine metabolites rely on renal excretion; significant renal disease may result in untoward effects such as prolonged sedation, respiratory depression, or neuroexcitation [42, 44–48]. For example, morphine is metabolized in most species to morphine-3-glucuronide and morphine-6-glucuronide, both eliminated by glomerular filtration. Morphine-6-glucuronide has similar activity to the parent drug, and significant renal impairment resulting in compromised excretion of this metabolite has been shown to lead to prolonged clinical effects in human patients [44–46]. Similarly, the metabolite of meperidine, normeperidine, has been reported to cause seizures in humans with renal impairment [47, 48].

Nonsteroidal Anti-Inflammatory Drugs (NSAIDs)

Nonsteroidal anti-inflammatory drugs exert their effects via inhibition of the cyclooxygenase (COX) and lipoxygenase (LOX) enzymes that oxidize arachidonic acid to various prostaglandins and leukotrienes. The result is inhibition of important mediators of pain and inflammation, such as prostaglandin E_2 and prostacyclin [49–51].

COX enzyme isoforms, including COX-1 and COX-2, are constitutively expressed in multiple species, including dogs and cats [52]. Protective prostaglandins are derived largely from the COX-1 isoform; such prostaglandins are thought to induce renal protection under conditions of renal ischemia. Under stressful conditions such as that induced by general anesthesia and surgery, RBF can become prostaglandin-dependent. Furthermore, animals with CKD may have altered COX expression [52]. COX-1-sparing NSAIDs such as meloxicam and carprofen and selective COX-2 inhibitors such as robenacoxib are considered more kidney-sparing than nonpreferential NSAIDs such as aspirin [53, 54]. Multiple studies evaluating these agents in healthy canine and feline patients have failed to reveal detrimental renal effects, even under conditions of moderate hypotension [28, 54–62]. However, adverse effects have been reported, including renal insufficiency in cats following use of meloxicam, and the safety of these drugs in small animals with preexisting renal disease in the perioperative period is still questionable [63]. Evidence of renal dysfunction following periods of experimentally induced dehydration has been documented [64]. Subclinical renal damage in patients receiving perioperative NSAIDs that experience periods of hypotension or hypoperfusion cannot be fully ruled out, and the perioperative safety of these agents under conditions of true clinical hypovolemia, hypotension, and hypoperfusion has not been definitively proven. In the acute perioperative period, judicious use of these agents is recommended. Administration should only occur in patients that have not experienced hypotensive episodes, and extreme caution should be exercised in patients with preexisting renal dysfunction or patients at risk for AKI (e.g., sepsis). For long-term analgesia in animals with chronic pain and concurrent CKD, the documented benefit may far outweigh any possible risk, and safety of these agents for long-term administration has been documented [65, 66].

Relatively new NSAIDs that inhibit the prostaglandin E_2 EP_4 receptor (EP_4 prostaglandin receptor antagonist, or PRA), such as grapiprant, are effective analgesics used primarily for osteoarthritis [67]. At this time, no significant adverse effects have been reported in long-term, oral use [68]. However, efficacy for acute, perioperative pain has not been evaluated. Until clinical studies demonstrate the utility of these EP_4 antagonists for acute pain, agents of this class cannot be recommended for surgical analgesia.

Induction Agents

Alfaxalone

Alfaxalone is a synthetic neurosteroid that, like many other anesthetic agents, potentiates the inhibitory action of GABA with the $GABA_A$ receptor [69]. This agent is unique among anesthetic induction agents in that it can produce this effect and induce varying levels of sedation and anesthetic induction through administration by either intramuscular or intravenous routes. Following administration of alfaxalone, cardiovascular function is reasonably well-maintained and significant decreases in cardiac output are not to be expected [70–73]. Biotransformation is primarily via the liver, although extrahepatic metabolism may be involved [69]. Adequate renal function is required for elimination of metabolites, although there are no documented studies at this time that have evaluated change in recovery characteristics in patients with renal disease. Alfaxalone, along with sedatives such as benzodiazepines, is an excellent choice for pre-anesthetic sedation and induction in patients with renal disease.

Propofol

Propofol is a rapidly acting induction agent that potentiates GABA-induced chloride currents, thus creating a hypnotic effect [30]. Although data are not available for all species, propofol does not induce significant changes in RBF or GFR in dogs and is an excellent choice in patients with renal disease [74, 75]. Furthermore, the pharmacokinetic profile of propofol is not significantly altered in the face of chronic renal disease in human patients and some studies have suggested a renoprotective effect of propofol in renal transplantation [76, 77]. These effects have not been evaluated in veterinary species. It is important to note, however, that hypotension can occur following bolus administration of propofol, potentially leading to decreases in RBF; this is a transient effect and can be attenuated by volume loading and preadministration of sedative agents and/or opioids [78].

Etomidate

Etomidate is widely considered the safest induction agent in patients with cardiovascular disease, exerting minimal cardiovascular effects following administration. Similar to propofol, etomidate exerts its anesthetic effect via an interaction with the GABA receptor [30]. Etomidate does not induce significant decreases in RBF or GFR and is generally considered safe for use in patients with renal disease [74]. Drug dosage should be tailored to the severity of the underlying disease, as plasma protein binding of etomidate is markedly decreased in human patients with renal failure, potentially leading to an unexpected increase in drug effect; the lower end of the etomidate dosage range (1–2 mg kg^{-1}) should be used in patients with significant renal disease [79].

Ketamine

Ketamine is unique among anesthetic induction agents in its mode of action, causing immobilization via antagonism of the *N*-methyl-D-aspartate (NMDA) receptor [80]. Ketamine administration induces catecholamine release, increasing blood pressure and renal vascular resistance [81]. Ketamine preserves GFR, increases RBF, and, under experimental conditions, preserves RBF during hemorrhage [47, 81–83]. Ketamine is metabolized by the liver in most species; renal disease should have little effect on the metabolism of moderate doses of ketamine. However, elimination of ketamine relies more extensively on renal excretion in cats, and, therefore, dosages required for anesthetic induction (5 mg kg^{-1} IV) should be avoided or used with caution in cats with renal impairment to avoid impaired drug elimination [84].

Inhalational Agents

All inhalational anesthetics cause a dose-dependent and significant decrease in RBF and GFR; these effects are directly related to the depressant effects of the inhalants on cardiac output [85–88]. Methods to reduce the MAC of inhaled anesthetics, such as anesthetic adjuncts, and pre-anesthetic fluid optimization may attenuate these responses.

Historically, methoxyflurane was associated with nephrotoxicity due to metabolic breakdown to free fluoride ions [89]. Of the modern agents, sevoflurane is the most metabolized, approximately 5% as compared to approximately 0.2% and 0.02% for isoflurane and desflurane, respectively, leading to the release of inorganic fluoride ions [87]. These ions have the potential to induce nephrotoxicity, but there appears to be no relationship between serum inorganic fluoride concentration and renal toxicity following anesthesia with inhalational agents [90–93]. Sevoflurane also produces Compound A, a potentially nephrotoxic agent that is formed by the reaction with potassium or sodium hydroxide found in soda lime or Baralyme® (withdrawn from the market) carbon dioxide absorbents [94, 95]. However, modern carbon dioxide absorbents contain considerably lower levels of these chemicals, nearly eliminating degradation to Compound A. Although healthy human volunteers administered sevoflurane for multiple hours did reveal some biochemical evidence of glomerular injury, multiple studies have failed to provide sufficient evidence to preclude the use of sevoflurane in patients with renal dysfunction [91–93, 96, 97]. The avoidance of low-flow anesthesia, carbon dioxide absorbents containing potassium and/or sodium hydroxide, and carbon dioxide absorbent desiccation will greatly decrease the formation of potential nephrotoxic degradation products [98]. Isoflurane and desflurane are minimally metabolized to inorganic fluoride and do not create Compound A. Therefore, some practitioners choose these agents over sevoflurane. However, all of the modern volatile anesthetics are appropriate choices for anesthetic maintenance of patients with renal disease, and choice of agent should be based primarily on availability, practitioner familiarity and comfort level, and considerations based on blood:gas solubility, if applicable.

Nitrous oxide exerts mild decreases on RBF, but to a lesser extent than the other inhalants, and can be used safely in patients with renal disease [99]. However, in patients with CKD and severe anemia, the use of nitrous oxide must be weighed against the need to provide supplemental oxygen, as these patients may present with reduced oxygen-carrying capacity. Nitrous oxide should be avoided if the patient cannot tolerate a fraction of inspired oxygen <0.7.

Adjunctive Drugs

Historically, the administration of a low-dose infusion of dopamine (1–3 μg kg^{-1} min^{-1}) was commonly used in the management of patients with both AKI and CKD. Dopamine infused at these rates acts via the dopamine-1 (D1) and dopamine-2 (D2) receptors in multiple species to produce vasodilation of renal arteries, leading to increased RBF and natriuresis via inhibition of Na^+-K^+-adenosine triphosphatase (ATPase) activity [100–102]. Despite these effects, this regimen appears to be ineffective, and the use of low-dose dopamine in the management of animals with renal disease is no longer recommended [103–108]. In fact, low-dose dopamine might induce negative renal effects. For example, dopamine infusion inhibits renal tubuloglomerular feedback, a protective mechanism induced within the kidney under conditions of ischemia [109]. Furthermore, dopamine increases renal medullary blood flow, while the intrarenal partial pressure of oxygen remains unchanged, suggesting that dopamine increases tubular work and negatively impacts renal function [110]. Overall, there is insufficient evidence to suggest a positive effect of low-dose dopamine in patients with renal disease, and the effects of low-dose dopamine infusions may prove detrimental.

However, more moderate doses of dopamine (5–10 μg kg^{-1} min^{-1}) or dobutamine (5–10 μg kg^{-1} min^{-1}) acting through beta-adrenergic receptors may be indicated for inotropic support in hypotensive patients. Blood pressure maintenance via these agents may support RBF through enhancement of cardiac output rather than direct renal effects. Blood pressure support via beta-1-adrenergic agonists such as dopamine or dobutamine is highly recommended in hypotensive patients that require inotropic support. Dopamine has been used in several species, although some believe that dopamine is ineffective in cats due to a lack of intrarenal dopamine receptors. However, cats do possess a unique putative D1 receptor, and dopamine infusions for inotropic support are indeed effective [111–114].

Mannitol has been used to support renal function; this agent induces natriuresis and causes renal arteriole dilation, decreased vascular resistance, increased urine output, and scavenging of oxygen-free radicals [115]. Mannitol also improves GFR, RBF, and urine output in small animals as a bolus dose (0.5–0.8 g kg^{-1} over 15 min), although the effect may be short-lived in animals under experimental conditions [115–117]. Mannitol-induced acute renal failure, however, has been reported in humans and animals from osmotic nephrosis, histologically appearing as vacuolization of the renal tubular epithelium [118–122]. A meta-analysis reviewing mannitol administration for AKI prevention in human patients concluded that there is no benefit in patients at risk of AKI [123]. Due to the potential for renal damage, caution should be exercised in the administration of mannitol to patients with preexisting renal disease or along with other potential nephrotoxic agents.

Furosemide is a loop diuretic used to differentiate between oliguria of hypovolemia versus that from redistribution of RBF. Furosemide administration increases urine output without increasing GFR. However, animal studies that provide definitive evidence for the benefit of furosemide in renal disease are lacking, and meta-analyses evaluating furosemide use for renal disease management in human patients revealed conflicting but encouraging evidence for improved outcome in patients with renal disease administered with furosemide [124–126]. Furosemide use may have a role in the management of AKI, but likely not in the perioperative period; perioperative management should focus on management of cardiac output (CO), RBF, GFR, and euvolemia. Initial diagnosis of perioperative oliguria should also focus on evaluation of cardiovascular parameters and fluid status.

Anesthetic Management of Patients with Renal Disease

There is no single anesthetic plan when it comes to management of patients with renal disease. Although all anesthetic agents have effects on RBF and GFR, some more than others, there is no combination of drugs that is far more effective in the management of these cases than other drugs. Rather than focusing on the perfect combination of anesthetic agents, it is instead more important to focus on management of the individual sequelae of the renal disease and any coexisting disease while striving to avoid significant depression of cardiac function or RBF while maintaining normotension and euvolemia.

Pre-anesthetic Stabilization

With both AKI and CKD, it is extremely important to medically stabilize the patient as much as possible before sedation and general anesthesia. If stabilization cannot be achieved, the value of the procedure requiring anesthesia must be questioned when weighed against the risks of sedation and anesthesia. The case should be delayed or rescheduled until the patient has been sufficiently managed medically and presents less of an anesthetic risk. Unfortunately, this is often not a possibility, and general anesthesia must be induced in patients who are highly unstable, which increases the risk of significant morbidity and, in extreme cases, mortality. Therefore, stabilization of the patient must be attempted quickly with prioritization of clinical signs and their threat to life.

Preanesthetic stabilization should be geared toward each individual problem; however, attaining adequate hydration status is often the most valuable step taken before anesthetic induction. This optimizes cardiac output and RBF while helping to attenuate variations in blood pressure that may accompany anesthetic induction and maintenance. Ideally, a patient with CKD presenting for an elective procedure should be admitted to the hospital and maintained on intravenous fluids for 12–24 h before anesthesia. This assumes that the patient has a baseline level of dehydration or, in extreme cases, hypovolemia. Fluid rate should be calculated based on maintenance fluids (40–60 ml kg^{-1} d^{-1}) plus replacement of any fluid deficit, in addition to fluids to account for ongoing losses such as vomiting, if present. Patients presenting for emergent conditions with either AKI or CKD should be administered fluids to, at minimum, replace fluid deficits. This can be estimated by assessing the patient's level of dehydration and replacing the deficit over 6 h or longer, if time allows. For example, a 10-kg patient presenting with 7% dehydration should be administered 700 ml of intravenous fluids (10 000 g × 7% = 700 ml) spread over at least 6 h, in addition to maintenance fluids [127]. Fluid choice should be made based on the patient's electrolyte status; typically, a polyionic balanced crystalloid, such as lactated Ringer's solution, is an excellent choice. Saline (0.9%) may be chosen if the patient is hyperkalemic, but care should be taken to avoid worsening any preexisting metabolic acidosis with a large chloride load. Fluid administration should be carefully monitored to achieve adequate hydration while avoiding overhydration, especially in patients with concurrent cardiovascular disease (see Chapter 8).

Tables 6.1 and 6.4 list problems often associated with AKI and CKD. Anesthetic case management is highly dependent on the patient presentation, comorbidities, and current medical management. Although multiple abnormalities can be present, those that are most relevant to anesthetic management are azotemia, acidosis, hyperkalemia, and anemia.

Azotemia is often encountered with both AKI and CKD but may not reflect the severity of the disease process. Azotemia may be due to dehydration (i.e., prerenal), intrinsic kidney damage or disease (i.e., renal), or due to urinary blockage (i.e., postrenal). BUN level is a non-specific test that may be altered by several non-renal processes. Elevated levels of BUN should not be used as a definitive diagnostic for renal disease; rather, elevated BUN should warrant a further diagnostic workup. Azostix® reagent strips (Santa Cruz Biotechnology, Dallas, Texas) may be used as a preoperative screening tool if a chemistry panel is impractical due to time or financial constraints. Creatinine is a biomarker that is more specific to renal disease but may be falsely decreased in animals with cachexia or muscle wasting [128]. The reference ranges often provided for serum creatinine are quite wide and mild elevations that fall within the reference range may be falsely interpreted as normal renal function. Kidney function often needs substantial decline before elevations are detected. Furthermore, there is high individual, age, and even breed variability; trending of serum creatinine in individual patients may be of more value [128]. SDMA is a biomarker that is a more kidney-specific diagnostic test and is a direct reflection of GFR, elevating earlier in CKD than creatinine [15, 128]. Serum creatinine and SDMA are tools that are used to stage CKD by IRIS guidelines (Table 6.3). Patients may then be substaged based on systemic blood pressure and urine protein to creatinine ratio (UP/C).

Not only is azotemia suggestive of prerenal or renal disease, it can also alter blood–brain barrier permeability [129]. This becomes clinically relevant in that anesthetic agents which rely on passage across the blood–brain barrier into the central nervous system and can have more profound effects in the presence of azotemia. Furthermore, azotemia, in addition to acidemia and hypoalbuminemia may cause a decrease in drug–protein binding [130]. Highly protein-bound drugs such as midazolam will, theoretically, exert more profound effects, as there will be more unbound, active drug in circulation. However, it is difficult to say what the clinical significance of this would be in all patients. Taking these factors into account, sedative and induction agent dosages may need to be decreased in the azotemic patient, as well as those demonstrating acidosis and hypoalbuminemia. It is important to tailor the anesthetic plan to each individual patient and titrate agents to effect.

Patients with AKI or CKD should have an electrolyte panel analyzed prior to anesthesia, ideally just prior to sedation or the anesthetic event. Acute and chronic management of electrolyte disorders has been discussed elsewhere, but it is important to be able to acutely recognize and respond to abnormalities that accompany AKI and CKD in the perioperative period [127, 131]. Although multiple electrolyte abnormalities can accompany both AKI and CKD, hyperkalemia is the most life-threatening and may require immediate correction. In the absence of serum potassium measurement, an electrocardiogram (ECG) can aid in the diagnosis, as characteristic waveform changes are often associated with increased serum potassium. These changes are often progressive, with mild elevations in potassium (5.5–7.5 mEq l^{-1}), resulting in increased amplitude and narrowing of the T wave, or "tenting," as well as shortening of the Q-T interval. Prolongation of the P-R interval, widening of the Q-R-S complex, and a decrease in amplitude and widening of the P wave are consistent with moderate hyperkalemia (7.0–8.0 mEq l^{-1}). In cases of severe hyperkalemia (8.0–9.0 mEq l^{-1}), P waves are absent, and bradycardia occurs (Figure 6.3). Finally, in extreme cases (>10.0 mEq l^{-1}), a sine wave appearance on the ECG, ventricular fibrillation, or asystole may occur [132, 133]. These electrical disturbances are due to an increase in the resting membrane potential of the cardiac myocyte from hyperkalemia, decreasing automaticity, conductivity, contractility, and excitability [133]. It is paramount to treat hyperkalemia immediately and closely monitor the ECG for characteristic changes and dysrhythmias. Induction of anesthesia should not be attempted in patients with serum potassium

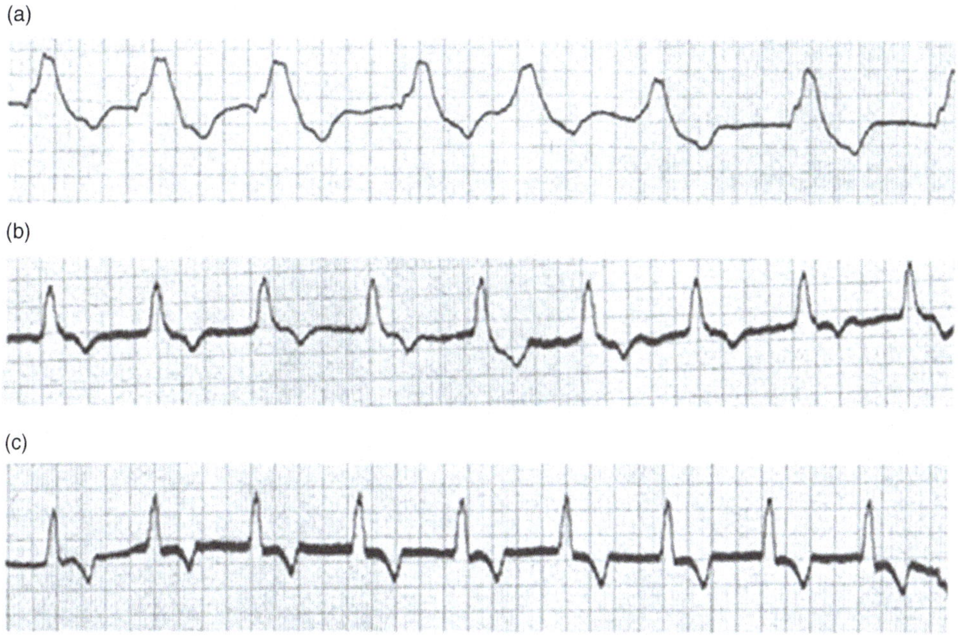

Figure 6.3 (a) Electrocardiogram from a hyperkalemic cat ($[K^+]$ = 10 mEq l^{-1}) presenting with urinary obstruction and heart rate approximately 58 beats per min^{-1}. Note the bradycardia, absence of P waves, and widened Q-R-S complexes. (b) Electrocardiogram from the same patient after administration of calcium gluconate (0.5 mg kg^{-1} IV; heart rate approximately 69 beats per min^{-1}). (c) Electrocardiogram after completion of calcium therapy (1.0 mg kg^{-1} IV, heart rate approximately 73 beats per min^{-1}). Calcium was administered as initial therapy for its membrane stabilization effects; definitive treatment was administered after cardiovascular stabilization. Source: Canine and Feline Anesthesia and Coexisting Disease, 2015, with permission.

concentrations exceeding 6.0 mEq l^{-1}. Although, ultimately, hyperkalemia may resolve with resolution of the underlying renal insult, treatment is geared toward shifting potassium intracellularly where it is not free to exert effects on cardiac action potentials. This can be accomplished through intravenous administration of regular insulin (0.5–1.0 U kg^{-1}) and dextrose (1–2 g per unit of administered insulin, diluted at least 1:3 due to hyperosmolarity) [131, 132]. Acidosis worsens hyperkalemia by shifting potassium extracellularly, increasing serum potassium. In patients under anesthesia, mechanical hyperventilation should be initiated to avoid the addition of respiratory acidosis through respiratory depression-induced hypercarbia, or a slight compensatory respiratory alkalosis can be induced through mild hyperventilation. Extreme cases may be treated with intravenous administration of sodium bicarbonate (1–2 mEq kg^{-1} IV) [131]. Sodium bicarbonate administration is not frequently recommended or performed; it is important to note that exogenous administration of bicarbonate will result in carbon dioxide production, potentially creating a respiratory acidosis if the patient is unable to ventilate appropriately. If bicarbonate is administered under anesthesia, only 1/3 of the calculated dose should be administered initially, and mechanical ventilation should be instituted. Although calcium administration does not directly affect serum potassium concentration, the presence of hypocalcemia can potentiate the cardiovascular effects of hyperkalemia, such as bradycardia or ECG changes; if cardiovascular effects are present, this should be the first line of therapy. To counteract adverse cardiac effects, 10% calcium gluconate can be slowly administered (0.5–1.5 ml kg^{-1} IV over 20–30 min; Figure 6.3b,c) [131].

Patients with both AKI and CKD often present with metabolic acidosis because of dehydration and hypoperfusion, leading to lactic acidosis, decreased urinary H^+ excretion, and decreased urinary HCO_3^- reabsorption [131]. Acid–base disorders and dehydration should be corrected before general anesthesia is induced. Once anesthesia is induced, it is important to control ventilation to prevent worsening acidemia with a concurrent respiratory acidosis. End-tidal carbon dioxide should be monitored and maintained at approximately 30–35 mmHg, and in cases of moderate to severe metabolic acidosis, arterial blood gas measurements should be taken.

Patients with CKD may have moderate to severe anemia owing to increased red blood cell fragility and decreased production of erythropoietin [14]. Anemia is often chronic and is fairly well-tolerated or may be due to therapeutic measures such as hemodialysis [134]. However, with severe anemia (Hgb <7.0 g dl^{-1}), oxygen-carrying capacity can be critically impaired, and the animal may have a greater reliance on the dissolved fraction of oxygen. Therefore, it is imperative that oxygen be supplemented throughout the entire case: before induction through recovery. Furthermore, hemoglobin levels <7.0 g dl^{-1} are consistent with critical decreases in oxygen-carrying capacity and may require transfusion of red blood cells to maintain adequate oxygen-carrying capacity. Anesthesia should be delayed until the hemoglobin is >7.0 g dl^{-1}. Note that pulse oximetry measurements will not be directly affected by anemia. Anemic animals may have normal SpO_2 values, yet the delivery of oxygen will be adversely impacted due to a decreased carrying capacity of oxygen.

Hypertension can be present in patients with CKD and will cause shifts in individual organ autoregulatory ranges [3, 135]. For instance, while RBF is autoregulated at blood pressures of approximately 80–180 mmHg in normal patients (Figure 6.2), the patient with chronic hypertension may have autoregulatory ranges shifted to a higher range from chronic compensation. These patients may not tolerate hypotension to the degree of a healthy patient and may require earlier intervention in the event of hypotension. Attempts should be made to maintain mean arterial blood pressure within approximately 20% less than baseline (ideally at least 70–80 mmHg). Many patients with underlying renal disease are treated with angiotensin-converting enzyme inhibitors (ACEIs), such as enalapril or benazepril, or an angiotensin receptor blocker such as telmisartan [135]. Refractory hypotension may occur under general anesthesia if these agents are not withheld for 12–24 h prior to anesthesia [136, 137]. Even with appropriate withdrawal of these agents, significant hypotension can occur, and vigilant monitoring of blood pressure is required.

Intraoperative Management

There is no single protocol for all patients, and patient temperament must be considered. However, it is generally safe to use a benzodiazepine/opioid combination as a pre-anesthetic sedative. For instance, midazolam (0.05–0.2 mg kg^{-1} IM) and hydromorphone (0.1–0.2 mg kg^{-1} IM) may be administered to dogs or cats. Lower ends of the dosage range should be used when administering drugs intravenously or in patients with moderate to severe disease. Following sedation and intravenous catheter placement, 100% oxygen should be supplemented by face mask for 5 min at a flow of 1–5 l min^{-1}, especially in anemic animals, wherein oxygen-carrying capacity is compromised. Anesthetic induction can be achieved with intravenous propofol (2–6 mg kg^{-1} IV) or alfaxalone (0.5–2 mg kg^{-1}) to facilitate intubation and transition to gas anesthetic. Intravenous fluids should be supplemented at a rate of 10 ml kg^{-1} h^{-1} for the first hour and then decreased to 5 ml kg^{-1} h^{-1} for the remainder of the case if prior fluid overload is not present. Note that comorbidities such as cardiovascular disease will alter the fluid rates and dynamic fluid status indicators, such as pulse pressure variation, should be monitored throughout the perianesthetic period. It is especially important in these patients to allow a slow transition to euvolemia through pre-anesthetic hospitalization and maintenance fluid therapy over 12–24 h, described earlier. The degree of anesthetic monitoring depends on the severity of the patient's condition and any coexisting disease. At a minimum, capnometry, pulse oximetry, and noninvasive blood pressure monitors should be placed. With a history of or existing hyperkalemia, an ECG should be closely monitored for dysrhythmias. If there is anticipated difficulty in obtaining accurate noninvasive blood pressure measurements or if variations in blood pressure are anticipated, an arterial catheter should be placed to monitor beat-to-beat invasive blood pressure accurately, as well as to measure arterial blood gas tensions.

Summary

Although patients with renal disease can have highly variable underlying conditions and presentation, pre-anesthetic stabilization with careful tailoring of the anesthetic plan to the patient problem list, and close monitoring of the patient to maintain normotension and euvolemia will maximize patient management success in the perioperative period.

References

1 Roura X. 2019. Risk factors in dogs and cats for development of chronic kidney disease. Available at: http://www.Iris-Kidney.com/education (accessed 28 February 2021).

2 Hall, J.E. and Hall, M.E. (2021). The urinary system: functional anatomy and urine formation by the kidneys. In: *Guyton and Hall Textbook of Medical Physiology*, 14e (eds. J.E. Hall and M.E. Hall), 321–330. Philadelphia: Elsevier.

3 Hastie, J. and Shanewise, J.S. Renal physiology. In: *Stoelting's Pharmacology & Physiology in Anesthetic Practice*, 5e (eds. P. Flood, J. Rathmell, S. Shafer and R.K. Stoelting), 45–97. Philadelphia: Wolters Kluwer Health.

4 Hall, J.E. and Hall, M.E. (2021). Glomerular filtration, renal blood flow, and their control. In: *Guyton and Hall Textbook of Medical Physiology*, 14e (eds. J.E. Hall and M.E. Hall), 331–342. Philadelphia: Elsevier.

5 Liu, K.D., Burkhardt, D.H., and Pearse, R.M. (2020). Renal pathophysiology and treatment for perioperative ischemia and nephrotoxic injury. In: *Miller's Anesthesia*, 9e (eds. M.A. Gropper, N.H. Cohen, L.I. Eriksson, et al.), 1340–1353. Philadelphia: Elsevier.

6 Kenney, E.M., Rozanski, E.A., Rush, J.E. et al. (2010). Association between outcome and organ system dysfunction in dogs with sepsis: 114 cases. *J. Am. Vet. Med. Assoc.* 236: 83–87.

7 Gasser, B., Uscategui, R.A.R., Maronezi, M.C. et al. (2020). Clinical and ultrasound variables for early diagnosis of septic acute kidney injury in bitches with pyometra. *Sci. Rep.* 10: 88–94.

8 Wagener, G. and Brentjens, T.E. (2010). Anesthetic concerns in patients presenting with renal failure. *Anesthesiol. Clin.* 28: 39–54.

9 Gu, W.J., Hou, B.L., Kwong, J.S. et al. (2018). Association between intraoperative hypotension and 30-day mortality, major adverse cardiac events, and acute kidney injury after non-cardiac surgery: a meta-analysis of cohort studies. *Int. J. Cardiol.* 258: 67–73.

10 Rodgers-Smith, E., Hammerton, R., Mathis, A. et al. (2020). Twelve previously healthy non-geriatric dogs present for acute kidney injury after general anesthesia for non-emergency surgical procedures in the UK. *J. Small Anim. Pract.* 61: 363–367.

11 Lopes, J.A. and Jorge, S. (2013). The RIFLE and AKIN classifications for acute kidney injury: a critical and comprehensive review. *Clin. Kidney J.* 6: 8–14.

12 Cowgill L. 2016. Grading of acute kidney injury. Available at: http://www.iris-kidney.com/pdf/4_ldc-revised-grading-of-acute-kidney-injury.pdf (accessed 28 February 2021).

13 Letatti, S.A.M., El Dib, R., Legatti, E. et al. (2018). Acute kidney injury in cats and dogs: a proportional meta-analysis of case series studies. *PLoS One* 13 (1): e0190772.

14 Polzin, D.J. (2011). Chronic kidney disease in small animals. *Vet. Clin. North Am. Small Anim. Pract.* 41: 15–30.

15 Relford, R., Robertson, J., and Clements, C. (2016). Symmetric dimethylarginine: improving the diagnosis and staging of chronic kidney disease in small animals. *Vet. Clin. North Am. Small Anim. Pract.* 46: 941–960.

16 Ostermann, M., Cennamo, A., Meersch, M. et al. (2020). A narrative review of the impact of surgery and anaesthesia on acute kidney injury. *Anaesthesia* 75 (Suppl 1): e121–e133.

17 Molinari, L., Sakhuja, A., and Kellum, J.A. (2020). Perioperative renoprotection: general mechanisms and treatment approaches. *Anesth. Analg.* 131: 1679–1692.

18 Mohmand, H. and Goldfarb, S. (2011). Renal dysfunction associated with intra-abdominal hypertension and the abdominal compartment syndrome. *J. Am. Soc. Nephr.* 22: 615–621.

19 Brock, N. (1994). Acepromazine revisited. *Can. Vet. J.* 35: 458–459.

20 Monteiro, E.R., Rodrigues, A. Jr., Assis, H.M.Q. et al. (2009). Comparative study on the sedative effects of morphine, methadone, butorphanol or tramadol, in combination with acepromazine, in dogs. *Vet. Anaesth. Analg.* 36: 23–33.

21 Bostrom, I., Nyman, G., Kampa, N. et al. (2003). Effects of acepromazine on renal function in anesthetized dogs. *Am. J. Vet. Res.* 64: 590–598.

22 Stepien, R.L., Bonagura, J.D., Bednarski, R.M. et al. (1995). Cardiorespiratory effects of acepromazine maleate and buprenorphine hydrochloride in clinically normal dogs. *Am. J. Vet. Res.* 56: 78–84.

23 Rangel, J.P.P., Monteiro, E.R., Bitti, F.S. et al. (2020). Hemodynamic effects of incremental doses of acepromazine in isoflurane-anesthetized dogs. *Vet. Anesth. Analg.* 48: 167–173.

24 Congdon, J.M., Marquez, M., Niyom, S. et al. (2011). Evaluation of the sedative and cardiovascular effects of intramuscular administration of dexmedetomidine with and without concurrent atropine administration in dogs. *J. Am. Vet. Med. Assoc.* 239: 81–89.

25 Murrell, J.C. and Hellebrekers, L.J. (2005). Medetomidine and dexmedetomidine: a review of cardiovascular effects and antinociceptive properties in the dog. *Vet. Anaesth. Analg.* 32: 117–127.

26 Selmi, A.L., Mendes, G.M., Lins, B.T. et al. (2003). Evaluation of the sedative and cardiorespiratory effects of dexmedetomidine, dexmedetomidine-butorphanol, and dexmedetomidine-ketamine in cats. *J. Am. Vet. Med. Assoc.* 222: 37–41.

27 Akashi, N., Murahata, Y., Hosokawa, M. et al. (2020). Cardiovascular and renal effects of constant rate infusions of remifentanil, dexmedetomidine and their combination in dogs anesthetized with sevoflurane. *J. Vet. Med. Sci.* 83: 285–296.

28 Frendin, J.H., Bostrom, I.M., Kampa, N. et al. (2006). Effects of carprofen on renal function during medetomidine-propofol-isoflurane anesthesia in dogs. *Am. J. Vet. Res.* 67: 1967–1973.

29 Saleh, N., Anoki, M., Shimada, T. et al. (2005). Renal effects of medetomidine in isoflurane-anesthetized dogs with special

reference to its diuretic action. *J. Vet. Med. Sci.* 67: 461–465.

30 Rathmell, J.P. and Rosow, C.E. (2015). Intravenous sedatives and hypnotics. In: *Stoelting's Pharmacology & Physiology in Anesthetic Practice*, 5e (eds. P. Flood, J. Rathmell, S. Shafer and R.K. Stoelting), 160–203. Philadelphia: Wolters Kluwer Health.

31 Holt, N.F. (2018). Renal disease. In: *Stoelting's Anesthesia and co-Existing Disease*, 7e (eds. R.L. Hines and K.E. Marschall), 425–448. Philadelphia: Elsevier.

32 Ilkiw, J.E., Suter, C.M., Farver, T.B. et al. (1996). The behaviour of healthy awake cats following intravenous and intramuscular administration of midazolam. *J. Vet. Pharmacol. Ther.* 19: 205–216.

33 Kukanich, B. and Wiese, A. (2015). Opioids. In: *Veterinary Anesthesia and Analgesia: The Fifth Edition of Lumb and Jones* (eds. K.A. Grimm, L.A. Lamont, W.J. Tranquilli, et al.), 207–226. Ames: Wiley Blackwell Publishing.

34 Cowan, A., Doxey, J.C., and Harry, E.J.R. (1977). The animal pharmacology of buprenorphine, an oripavine agent. *Br. J. Pharmacol.* 60: 547–554.

35 Steagall, P.V.M., Monteiro-Steagall, B.P., and Taylor, P.M. (2014). A review of the studies using buprenorphine in cats. *J. Vet. Intern. Med.* 28: 762–770.

36 Steagall, P.V.M., Ruel, H.L.M., and Yasuda, T. (2020). Pharmacokinetics and analgesic effects of intravenous, intramuscular or subcutaneous buprenorphine in dogs undergoing ovariohysterectomy: a randomized, prospective, masked, clinical trial. *BMC Vet. Res.* 16: 154.

37 Danesh, S. and Walker, L.A. (1988). Effects of central administration of morphine on renal function in conscious rats. *J. Pharmacol. Exp. Ther.* 244: 640–645.

38 Kongara, K., Chambers, P., and Johnson, C.B. (2009). Glomerular filtration rate after tramadol, parecoxib and pindolol following anaesthesia and analgesia in comparison with morphine in dogs. *Vet. Anaesth. Analg.* 36: 86–94.

39 Williamson, A.J., Soares, J.H.N., Henao-Guerrero, N. et al. (2018). Cardiovascular and respiratory effects of two doses of fentanyl in the presence or absence of bradycardia in isoflurane-anesthetized dogs. *Vet. Anaesth. Analg.* 45: 423–431.

40 Machado, C.E.G., Dyson, D.H., and Maxie, M.G. (2006). Effect of oxymorphone and hydromorphone on the minimum alveolar concentration of isoflurane in dogs. *Vet. Anaesth. and Anal.* 33: 70–77.

41 Williamson, A.J., Soares, J.H.N., and Pavlisko, N.D. (2018). Isoflurane minimum alveolar concentration sparing effects of fentanyl in the dog. *Vet. Anaesth. Anal.* 44: 738–745.

42 Davies, G., Kingswood, C., and Street, M. (1996). Pharmacokinetics of opioids in renal dysfunction. *Clin. Pharmacokinet.* 31: 410–422.

43 Cummings, K. and Naguib, M.A. (2015). Opioid agonists and antagonists. In: *Stoelting's Pharmacology & Physiology in Anesthetic Practice*, 5e (eds. P. Flood, J. Rathmell, S. Shafer and R.K. Stoelting), 217–256. Philadelphia: Wolters Kluwer Health.

44 Chauvin, M., Sandouk, P., Scherrman, J.M. et al. (1987). Morphine pharmacokinetics in renal failure. *Anesthesiology* 66: 327–331.

45 Conway, B.R., Fogarty, D.G., Nelson, W.E. et al. (2006). Opiate toxicity in patients with renal failure. *Br. Med. J.* 32: 345–346.

46 Osborne, R.J., Joel, S.P., and Slevin, M.L. (1986). Morphine intoxication in renal failure: the role of morphine-6-glucuronide. *Br. Med. J.* 292: 1548–1549.

47 Stone, P.A., Macintyre, P.E., and Jarvis, D.A. (1993). Norpethidine toxicity and patient controlled analgesia. *Br. J. Anaesth.* 71: 738–740.

48 Szeto, H.H., Inturrisi, C.E., Houde, R. et al. (1977). Accumulation of normeperidine, an active metabolite of normeperidine, in patients with renal failure of cancer. *Ann. Intern. Med.* 86: 738–741.

49 Johnston, S.A. and Fox, S.M. (1997). Mechanism of action of anti-inflammatory medications used for the treatment of osteoarthritis. *J. Am. Vet. Med. Assoc.* 210: 1486–1492.

50 Livingston, A. (2000). Mechanism of action of nonsteroidal anti-inflammatory drugs. *Vet. Clin. North Am. Small Anim. Pract.* 30: 773–781.

51 Papich, M.G. and Messenger, K. (2015). Non-steroidal anti-inflammatory drugs. In: *Veterinary Anesthesia and Analgesia: The Fifth Edition of Lumb and Jones* (eds. K.A. Grimm, L.A. Lamont, W.J. Tranquilli, et al.), 227–243. Ames: Wiley Blackwell Publishing.

52 Yabuki, A., Mitani, S., Sawa, M. et al. (2012). A comparative study of chronic kidney disease in dogs and cats: induction of cyclooxygenases. *Res. Vet. Sci.* 93: 892–897.

53 Papich, M.G. (2008). An update on nonsteroidal anti-inflammatory drugs (NSAIDs) in small animals. *Vet. Clin. North Am. Small Anim. Pract.* 38: 1243–1266.

54 Kongara, K. and Chambers, J.P. (2018). Robenacoxib in the treatment of pain in cats and dogs: safety, efficacy, and place in therapy. *Vet. Med. (Auckl)* 9: 53–61.

55 Ko, J.C.H., Miyabiyashi, T., Mandsager, R.E. et al. (2000). Renal effects of carprofen administered to healthy dogs anesthetized with propofol and isoflurane. *J. Am. Vet. Med. Assoc.* 217: 346–349.

56 Lobetti, R.G. and Joubert, K.E. (2000). Effect of administration of nonsteroidal anti-inflammatory drugs before surgery on renal function in clinically normal dogs. *Am. J. Vet. Res.* 61: 1501–1506.

57 Bostrom, I.M., Nyman, G.C., Lord, P.F. et al. (2002). Effects of carprofen on renal function and results of serum biochemical and hematologic analysis in anesthetized dogs that had low blood pressure during anesthesia. *Am. J. Vet. Res.* 63: 712–721.

58 Crandell, D.E., Mathews, K.A., and Dyson, D.H. (2004). Effect of meloxicam and carprofen on renal function when administered to healthy dogs prior to anesthesia and painful stimulation. *Am. J. Vet. Res.* 65: 1384–1390.

59 Bostrom, I.M., Nyman, G., Hoppe, A. et al. (2006). Effects of meloxicam on renal function in dogs with hypotension during anesthesia. *Vet. Anaesth. Analg.* 33: 62–69.

60 Surdyk, K.K., Brown, C.A., and Brown, S.A. (2012). Evaluation of glomerular filtration rate in cats with reduced renal mass and administered meloxicam and acetylsalicylic acid. *Am. J. Vet. Res.* 74: 648–651.

61 Hernandez-Avalos, I., Valverde, A., and Ibancovichi-Camarillo, J.A. (2020). Clinical evaluation of postoperative analgesia, cardiorespiratory parameters, and changes in liver and renal function tests of paracetamol compared to meloxicam and carprofen in dogs undergoing ovariohysterectomy. *PLoS One* 15 (2): e0223697.

62 Kongara, K., Cave, N., and Weidgraaf, K. (2020). Effect of non-steroidal anti-inflammatory drugs on glomerular filtration rate and urinary N-acetyl-ß-D-glucosaminidase activity in cats after dental surgery. *Vet. Anaesth. Analg.* 47: 631–636.

63 Dyer, F., Diesel, G., Cooles, S. et al. (2010). Suspected adverse reactions, 2009. *Vet. Rec.* 167: 118–121.

64 Surdyk, K.K., Sloan, D.L., and Brown, S.A. (2012). Renal effects of carprofen and etodolac in euvolemic and volume-depleted dogs. *Am. J. Vet. Res.* 73: 1485–1490.

65 Luna, S.P., Basollio, A.C., Steagall, P.V.M. et al. (2007). Evaluation of adverse effects of long-term oral administration of carprofen, etodolac, flunixin meglumine, ketoprofen, and meloxicam in dogs. *Am. J. Vet. Res.* 68: 258–264.

66 Gowan, R.A., Lingard, A.E., Johnston, L. et al. (2011). Retrospective case-control study of the effects of long-term dosing with meloxicam on renal function in aged cats with degenerative joint disease. *J. Fel. Med. Surg.* 13: 752–761.

67 Rausch-Derra, L., Huebner, M., and Wofford, J. (2016). A prospective, randomized, masked, placebo-controlled multisite clinical study of grapiprant, an EP4 prostaglandin receptor antagonist (PRA), in dogs with osteoarthritis. *J. Vet. Int. Med.* 30: 756–763.

68 Rausch-Derra, L., Huebner, M., and Rhodes, L. (2015). Evaluation of the safety of long-term, daily oral administration of grapiprant, a novel drug for treatment of osteoarthritic pain and inflammation, in healthy dogs. *Am. J. Vet. Res.* 76: 853–859.

69 Warne, L.N., Beths, T., Carter, J.E. et al. (2015). A review of the pharmacology and clinical application of alfaxalone in cats. *Vet. J.* 203: 141–148.

70 Dehuisser, V., Bosmans, T., Devreese, M. et al. (2019). Alfaxalone total intravenous anaesthesia in dogs: pharmacokinetics, cardiovascular data and recovery characteristics. *Vet. Anaesth. Analg.* 46: 605–612.

71 Kim, B., Jang, M., Sohn, J. et al. (2019). Effects of intramuscular alfaxalone/acepromazine on echocardiographic, biochemical, and blood gas measurements in healthy cats. *J. Am. Anim. Hosp. Assoc.* 55: 70–77.

72 Miller, C., Hughes, E., and Gurney, M. (2019). Co-induction of anaesthesia with alfaxalone and midazolam in dogs: a randomized, blinded clinical trial. *Vet. Anaesth. Analg.* 46: 613–619.

73 Pypendop, B.H., Barter, L.S., Pascoe, P.J. et al. (2019). Hemodynamic effects of subclinical, clinical, and supraclinical plasma alfaxalone concentrations in cats. *Vet. Anaesth. Analg.* 46: 597–604.

74 Chang, J., Kim, S., Jung, J. et al. (2011). Evaluation of the effects of thiopental, propofol, and etomidate on glomerular filtration rate measured by the use of dynamic computed tomography in dogs. *Am. J. Vet. Res.* 72: 146–151.

75 Fusellier, M., Desfontis, J.C., Madec, S. et al. (2007). Influence of three anesthetic protocols on glomerular filtration rate in dogs. *Am. J. Vet. Res.* 68: 807–811.

76 De Gasperi, A., Mazza, E., Noe, L. et al. (1996). Pharmacokinetic profile of the induction dose of propofol in chronic renal failure patients undergoing renal transplantation. *Minerva Anestesiol.* 62: 25–31.

77 Motayaheni, N., Phan, S., Eshragi, C. et al. (2017). A review of anesthetic effects on renal function: potential organ protection. *Am. J. Nephrol.* 46: 380–389.

78 Ilkiw, J.E., Pascoe, P.J., Haskins, S.C. et al. (1992). Cardiovascular and respiratory effects of propofol administration in hypovolemic dogs. *Am. J. Vet. Res.* 53: 2323–2327.

79 Carlos, R., Calvo, R., and Erill, S. (1979). Plasma protein binding of etomidate in patients with renal failure or hepatic cirrhosis. *Clin. Pharmacokinet.* 4: 144–148.

80 Kohrs, R. and Durieux, M.E. (1998). Ketamine: teaching an old drug new tricks. *Anesth. Analg.* 87: 1186.

81 Priano, L.L. (1982). Alteration of renal hemodynamics by thiopental, diazepam, and ketamine in conscious dogs. *Anesth. Analg.* 61: 853–862.

82 Schenk, H.D., Radke, J., Ensink, F.B. et al. (1995). Interactions between renal and general hemodynamics in fentanyl, droperidol, ketamine, thiopental and in peridural anesthesia- animal studies. *Anaesthesiol. Reanim.* 20: 60–70.

83 Xiang, L., Calderon, A.S., and Klemcke, H.G. (2020). Fentanyl impairs but ketamine preserves the microciculatory response to hemorrhage. *J. Trauma Acute Care Surg.* 89 (Suppl 2): S93–S99.

84 Hanna, R.M., Borchard, R.E., and Schmidt, S.L. (1988). Pharmacokinetics of ketamine HCl and metabolite I in the cat: a comparison of IV, IM, and rectal administration. *J. Vet. Pharmacol. Therap.* 11: 84–93.

85 Gelman, S., Fowler, K.C., and Smith, L.R. (1984). Regional blood flow during isoflurane and halothane anesthesia. *Anesth. Analg.* 63: 557–565.

86 Merin, R.G., Bernard, J.M., Doursout, M.F. et al. (1991). Comparison of the effects of isoflurane and desflurane on cardiovascular dynamics and regional blood flow in the chronically instrumented dog. *Anesthesiology* 74: 568–574.

87 Flood, P. and Shafer, S. (2014). Inhaled anesthetics. In: *Stoelting's Pharmacology & Physiology in Anesthetic Practice*, 5e (eds. P. Flood, J. Rathmell, S. Shafer and R.K. Stoelting), 98–159. Philadelphia: Wolters Kluwer Health.

88 Iguchi, N., Kosaka, K., and Iguchi, Y. (2020). Systemic haemodynamics, renal perfusion and renal oxygenation responses to changes in inspired oxygen fraction during total intravenous or volatile anaesthesia. *Br. J. Anaesth.* 125: 192–200.

89 Crandell, W.B., Pappas, S.G., and Macdonald, A. (1966). Nephrotoxicity associated with methoxyflurane anesthesia. *Anesthesiology* 27: 591–607.

90 Martis, L., Lynch, S., Napoli, M.D. et al. (1981). Biotransformation of sevoflurane in dogs and rats. *Anesth. Analg.* 60: 186–191.

91 Gentz, B.A. and Malan, T.P. (2001). Renal toxicity with sevoflurane: a storm in a teacup? *Drugs* 61: 2155–2162.

92 Driessen, B., Zarucco, L., Steffey, E.P. et al. (2002). Serum fluoride concentrations, biochemical and histopathological changes associated with prolonged sevoflurane anesthesia in horses. *J. Vet. Med. A Physiol. Pathol. Clin. Med.* 49: 337–347.

93 Sondekoppam, R.V., Narsingani, K.H., Schimmel, T.A. et al. (2020). The impact of sevoflurane anesthesia on postoperative renal function: a systematic review and meta-analysis of randomized controlled trials. *Can. J. Anaesth.* 67: 1595–1623.

94 Bito, H. and Ikeda, K. (1994). Long-duration, low-flow sevoflurane anesthesia using two carbon dioxide absorbents: quantification of degradation products in the circuit. *Anesthesiology* 81: 340–345.

95 Higuchi, H., Adachi, Y., Arimura, S. et al. (2000). Compound a concentrations during low-flow sevoflurane anesthesia correlate directly with the concentration of monovalent bases in carbon dioxide absorbents. *Anesth. Analg.* 91: 434–439.

96 Eger, E.I., Gong, D., Koblin, D.D. et al. (1997). Dose-related biochemical markers of renal injury after sevoflurane versus desflurane anesthesia in volunteers. *Anesth. Analg.* 85: 1154–1163.

97 Mazze, R.I., Callan, C.M., and Galvez, S.T. (2000). The effects of sevoflurane on serum creatinine and blood urea nitrogen concentration: a retrospective, twenty-two-center, comparative evaluation of renal function in adult surgical patients. *Anesth. Analg.* 90: 683–688.

98 Dorsch, J.A. and Dorsch, S.E. (2008). The circle system. In: *Understanding Anesthesia Equipment*, 5e, 223–281. Philadelphia: Lippincott Williams & Wilkins.

99 Hill, G.E., Lunn, J.K., Hodges, M.R. et al. (1977). N_2O modification of halothane-altered renal function in the dog. *Anesth. Analg.* 56: 690–695.

100 Furukawa, S., Nagashima, Y., Hoshi, K. et al. (2002). Effects of dopamine infusion on cardiac and renal blood flows in dogs. *J. Vet. Med. Sci.* 64: 41–44.

101 McDonald, R.H. Jr., Goldberg, L.I., McNay, J.L. et al. (1964). Effects of dopamine in man: augmentation of sodium excretion, glomerular filtration rate, and renal plasma rate. *J. Clin. Invest.* 43: 1116–1124.

102 Olsen, N.V. (1998). Effects of dopamine on renal haemodynamics, tubular function and sodium excretion in normal humans. *Dan. Med. Bull.* 45: 282–297.

103 Chertow, G.M., Sayegh, M.H., Allgren, R.L. et al. (1996). Is the administration of dopamine associated with adverse of favorable outcomes in acute renal failure? *Am. J. Med.* 107: 49–53.

104 Jones, D. and Bellomo, R. (2005). Renal-dose dopamine: from hypothesis to paradigm to dogma to myth and, finally, superstition? *J. Intensive Care Med.* 20: 199–211.

105 Karthik, S. and Lisbon, A. (2006). Low-dose dopamine in the intensive care unit. *Semin. Dial.* 19: 465–471.

106 Lauschke, A., Teichgraber, U.K.M., Frei, U. et al. (2006). 'Low-dose' dopamine worsens renal perfusion in patients with acute renal failure. *Kidney Int.* 69: 1669–1674.

107 Marik, P.E. and Iglesias, J. (1999). Low-dose dopamine does not prevent acute renal failure in patients with septic shock and oliguria. NORASEPT II study investigators. *Pract. Anaesth.* 107: 392–395.

108 Schenarts, P.J., Sagraves, S.G., Bard, M.R. et al. (2006). Low-dose dopamine: a physiologically based review. *Curr. Surg.* 63: 219–225.

109 Schnermann, J., Todd, K.M., and Briggs, J.P. (1990). Effect of dopamine on the tubuloglomerular feedback mechanism. *Am. J. Phys* 258: F790–F798.

110 Heyman, S.N., Kaminski, N., and Brezis, M. (1995). Dopamine increases medullary blood flow without improving regional hypoxia. *Exp. Nephrol.* 3: 33–41.

111 Flournoy, W.S., Wohl, J.S., Albrecht-Schmitt, T.J. et al. (2003). Pharmacologic identification of putative D1 dopamine receptors in feline kidneys. *J. Vet. Pharmacol. Ther.* 26: 283–290.

112 Wiese, A.J., Barter, L.S., and Ilkiw, J.E. (2012). Cardiovascular and respiratory effects of incremental doses of dopamine and phenylephrine in the management of isoflurane-induced hypotension in cats with hypertrophic cardiomyopathy. *Am. J. Vet. Res.* 73: 908–916.

113 Pascoe, P.H., Ilkiw, J.E., and Pypendop, B.H. (2006). Effects of increasing infusion rates of dopamine, dobutamine, epinephrine, and phenylephrine in healthy anesthetized cats. *Am. J. Vet. Res.* 67: 1491–1499.

114 Licht, N., Rozanski, E.A., and Rush, J.E. (2018). Vasopressor use in 41 critically ill cats (2007-2016). *Can. Vet. J.* 59: 1175–1180.

115 McClellan, J.M., Goldstein, R.E., Erb, H.N. et al. (2006). Effects of administration of fluids and diuretics on glomerular filtration rate, renal blood flow, and urine output in healthy awake cats. *Am. J. Vet. Res.* 67: 715–722.

116 Behnia, R., Koushanpor, E., and Brunner, E.A. (1996). Effects of hyperosmotic mannitol infusion on hemodynamics of dog kidney. *Anesth. Analg.* 82: 902–908.

117 Segev, G., Stafford, C., Kirby, K. et al. (2019). Sequential changes in urine production, glomerular filtration rate, and electrolyte excretion after mannitol administration. *J. Vet. Intern. Med.* 33: 1362–1367.

118 Taggert, W.R., Thibodeau, G.A., and Swanson, R.N. (1968). Mannitol induced renal alterations in rabbits. *S. D. J. Med.* 21: 30–34.

119 Stuart, F.P., Torres, E., Fletcher, R. et al. (1970). Effects of single, repeated, and massive mannitol infusion in the dog: structural and functional changes in the kidney and brain. *Ann. Surg.* 172: 190–204.

120 Dorman, H.R., Sondheimer, J.H., and Cadnapaphornchai, P. (1990). Mannitol-induced acute renal failure. *Medicine (Baltimore)* 69: 153–159.

121 Visweswaren, P., Massin, E.K., and Dubose, T.D. Jr. (1997). Mannitol-induced acute renal failure. *J. Am. Soc. Nephrol.* 8: 1028–1033.

122 Shi, J., Quin, J., Li, H. et al. (2018). Renal tubular epithelial cells injury induced by mannitol and its potential mechanism. *Ren. Fail.* 40: 85–91.

123 Yang, B., Xu, K., Xu, F. et al. (2014). Intravascular administration of mannitol for acute kidney injury prevention: a systematic review and meta-analysis. *PLoS One* 9 (1): e85029.

124 Sampath, S., Moran, J.L., Graham, P.L. et al. (2007). The efficacy of loop diuretics in acute renal failure: assessment using

Bayesian evidence synthesis techniques. *Crit. Care Med.* 335: 2516–2524.

125 Bove, R., Bellitti, A., Putzu, A. et al. (2018). Intermittent furosemide administration in patients with or at risk for acute kidney injury: meta-analysis of randomized trials. *PLoS One* 13 (4): e0196088.

126 Zhao, G., Xu, C., Ying, J. et al. (2020). Association between furosemide administration and outcomes in critically ill patients with acute kidney injury. *Crit. Care* 24: 75.

127 Langston, C. (2012). Managing fluid and electrolyte disorders in renal failure. In: *Fluid, Electrolyte, and Acid-Base Disorders in Small Animal Practice*, 4e (ed. S.P. DiBartola), 544–556. St. Louis: Elsevier Saunders.

128 Hokamp, J.A. and Nabity, M.B. (2016). Renal biomarkers in domestic species. *Vet. Clin. Path.* 45: 28–56.

129 Clark-Price, S.C. and Grauer, G.F. (2015). Physiology, pathophysiology, and anesthetic management of patients with renal disease. In: *Veterinary Anesthesia and Analgesia: The Fifth Edition of Lumb and Jones* (eds. K.A. Grimm, L.A. Lamont, W.J. Tranquilli, et al.), 681–697. Ames: Wiley Blackwell Publishing.

130 Reidenberg, M.M. and Drayer, D.E. (1984). Alteration of drug-protein binding in renal disease. *Clin. Pharm.* 9: 18–26.

131 Langston, C. (2017). Managing fluid and electrolyte disorders in kidney disease. *Vet. Clin. Small Anim.* 47: 471–490.

132 DiBartola, S.P. and DeMorais, H.A. (2012). Disorders of potassium: hypokalemia and hyperkalemia. In: *Fluid, Electrolyte, and Acid-Base Disorders*, 4e (ed. S.P. DiBartola), 92–119. St. Louis: Saunders Elsevier.

133 El-Sherif, N. and Turitto, G. (2011). Electrolyte disorders and arrhythmogenesis. *Cardiol. J.* 18: 233–245.

134 Langston, C., Cook, A., Eatroff, A. et al. (2017). Blood transfusions in dogs and cats receiving hemodialysis: 230 cases (June 1997–September 2012). *J. Vet. Intern. Med.* 31: 402–409.

135 Acierno, M.J., Brown, S., Colemen, A.E. et al. (2018). ACVIM consensus statement: guidelines for the identification, evaluation, and management of systemic hypertension in dogs and cats. *J. Vet. Intern. Med.* 32: 1803–1822.

136 Colemen, A.E., Shepard, M.K., Schmiedt, C.W. et al. (2016). Effects of orally administered enalapril on blood pressure and hemodynamic response to vasopressors during isoflurane anesthesia in healthy dogs. *Vet. Anaesth. Analg.* 43: 482–494.

137 Hojo, T., Shibuya, M., Kimura, Y. et al. Refractory hypotension during general anesthesia despite withholding telmisartin. *Anesth. Prog.* 67: 86–89.

7

Urogenital Concerns

Carrie A. Davis

Animal Imaging, Irving, TX, 75039, USA

Introduction

Minimally invasive procedures and surgeries may be indicated for evaluation or treatment of congenital, acquired, and neoplastic conditions involving the urogenital tract. Patients may present in a critically ill state encompassing an array of shock states with fluid, acid–base, electrolyte, and renal disturbances, in addition to anemia or other metabolic derangements. Thus, the anesthetist should not only be familiar with the pathophysiology and expected clinicopathologic abnormalities of the various conditions in order to appropriately stabilize patients prior to anesthesia, but also be cognizant of the pharmacologic agents and procedural risks while preparing to manage complications. Discussion of anesthetic concerns involving acute and chronic renal disease is described elsewhere (see Chapter 6).

Urogenital Emergencies

Urinary-tract-associated emergencies are broadly classified as (i) obstructive to urine flow, or (ii) resulting in accumulation of urine within the peritoneal cavity or retroperitoneal space. Discussion of emergencies involving the genital tract will center on pyometra, while cesarean sections are discussed in Chapter 18.

Urogenital emergencies are commonly encountered in small-animal practice and present with, or have the potential of progressing to, a life-threatening crisis if not rapidly managed [1]. Although reestablishing urine flow, surgical repair of the urinary tract, or ovariohysterectomy may be required for resolution, patients that are metabolically and hemodynamically unstable are regarded as urgent medical emergencies. Subjecting such patients to immediate anesthesia or surgery would likely compromise the outcome [2, 3]; however, pain management is essential. Additionally, sedation is commonly necessary to obtain diagnostics or perform minor procedures that are paramount to patient survival and stabilization prior to anesthesia. Emergency procedures of the urinary tract may be required in the recently traumatized patient, and to appropriately prioritize patient care, a thorough examination is required for identification of concomitant injuries or conditions.

Urethral Obstruction

Feline urethral obstruction is a common urinary tract emergency with an incidence rate

Canine and Feline Anesthesia and Co-Existing Disease, Second Edition. Edited by Rebecca A. Johnson, Lindsey B. C. Snyder and Carrie A. Schroeder.

Companion website: www.wiley.com/go/johnson/canine

between 2% and 13% at veterinary teaching hospitals across North America [4]. The condition is most common in male cats that are predisposed to obstruction due to their long, narrow urethra (compared to females). Various causes have been identified and can be categorized as anatomical or physical (urethral plugs, obstructive idiopathic urethritis, urolithiasis, urethral stricture, and neoplasia) or functional (urethral spasm). Canine urethral obstruction is less common, and occurs most frequently in males due to urolithiasis, but can also result from urethral strictures or neoplasia. Calculi commonly lodge just behind the caudal aspect of the os penis, but also lodge at the ischiatic arch and prostatic urethra [5].

Although most patients with urethral obstruction present in stable condition permitting rapid restoration of urethral patency using techniques such as retropulsion, urethrotomy, or urethrostomy, prolonged urethral obstruction results in severe cardiovascular compromise and collapse due to life-threatening electrolyte and acid–base abnormalities. Therefore, patients presenting with urethral obstruction should be treated as a medical emergency with evaluation of clinical signs being performed simultaneously with diagnostic evaluations, patient stabilization, and treatment.

Clinical Signs and Physical Examination

Clinical signs of urethral obstruction depend on the severity and duration of the occlusion, but can include stranguria or dysuria, vocalization, frequent licking of the perineal area in cats or the penis in dogs, hematuria, pollakiuria, oliguria or anuria, vomiting, mild lethargy, profound weakness, obtundation, or collapse [1, 6].

The presence of a firm, nonexpressible urinary bladder, which usually elicits a painful response on palpation, often reveals the diagnosis [1]; radiographs or ultrasound may also be helpful. Bladder size varies based on duration of obstruction and gentle palpation is encouraged due to the likelihood of mucosal injury weakening the bladder wall. Nevertheless, the presence of urine flow does not rule out partial urethral obstruction, particularly if the rate or pressure of the stream is reduced compared to normal. Additionally, absence of a palpable bladder does not rule out urethral obstruction, as the bladder may have ruptured.

In canines, an examination per rectum to assess the prostate and intrapelvic urethra may reveal abnormalities such as urethral enlargement, a mass or a palpable urolithiasis. Discoloration of the penis tip in a cat or visualization of a urethral plug is possible. The patient may be hypothermic or hyperthermic, tachycardic or bradycardic, tachypneic, and may have poor pulse quality. The critical patient has clinical signs associated with systemic acid–base and electrolyte abnormalities including dehydration (prolonged skin turgor and tacky mucous membranes [MMs]), hypovolemia, bradycardia, arrhythmias, hypothermia, weak pulses, and possibly obtundation and collapse [1, 7, 8].

Bradycardia and other arrhythmias should alarm the clinician into immediate action, as hyperkalemia is typically the cause. Furthermore, a low normal heart rate (HR) that inappropriately matches the clinical situation should urge the clinician to investigate hyperkalemia. A retrospective study of cats with urethral obstruction reported moderate bradycardia (100–140 beats min^{-1}) in 6% of cats and severe bradycardia (<100 beats min^{-1}) in 5% [7]. Additionally, bradycardia (<120 beats min^{-1}) in combination with hypothermia (<95.0–96.6 F) was 98% specific for severe hyperkalemia (8 mEq l^{-1}) [7].

Initial Database and Clinicopathology

The urgent database includes electrocardiogram (ECG), electrolytes, venous blood gas, packed cell volume (PCV), total solids (TSs), blood urea nitrogen (BUN), creatinine, blood glucose (BG), lactate, and ionized calcium (iCa), followed by a complete blood count (CBC) and biochemical panel. Dehydration, hypovolemia, decreased tissue perfusion, azotemia, metabolic acidosis, hyperkalemia, hyperphosphatemia, and hypocalcemia are possible sequelae to urethral obstruction [6, 7].

Dehydration results from a lack of oral fluid intake and losses by nonrenal routes such as vomiting [7]. Therefore, severe dehydration and significant prerenal azotemia in addition to renal and postrenal azotemia may be present. Urine outflow obstruction induces pressure back on the kidneys which decreases glomerular filtration rate (GFR), resulting in azotemia and decreased phosphorus, potassium, and hydrogen ion secretion [7]. Phosphorus retention may cause chelation of calcium [7, 9]; thus, iCa concentrations may be decreased. Ionized hypocalcemia (<1.0 mmol l^{-1}) occurred in 20% of cats in one study [7], and up to 75% in another [10]. The mechanical and electrical dysfunction induced by such ionized hypocalcemia amplifies the cardiac effects of hyperkalemia [7, 11].

Metabolic acidosis may induce respiratory compensation including increased minute ventilation (V_E), clinically recognized as larger tidal volume (TV) and occasionally tachypnea [12]. However, patients with life-threatening hyperkalemia often have poor compensatory responses, and the resulting respiratory acidosis will exacerbate the existing metabolic acidosis. Additionally, a concurrent metabolic acidosis may amplify the hyperkalemia-induced cardiotoxicity [7, 13]. However, these effects usually do not occur unless severe acidemia (pH <7.1) occurs [11].

Hyperkalemia may result from several mechanisms including shifting of potassium from the intracellular space in exchange with hydrogen ions in response to acidemia, impaired GFR with resultant inability to excrete potassium, and reabsorption from the damaged bladder mucosa [7]. Hyperkalemia increases the resting membrane potential of cells, resulting in a reduced gradient between the resting membrane and threshold potential, causing an increase in cell membrane excitability [13]. Additionally, potassium ion concentration is altered, resulting in cells that are slower in reaching threshold potential with prolonged recovery and prolonged cardiac action potential duration [14]. Eventually, the resting membrane potential may become less negative than the threshold potential, making the cell unable to repolarize after depolarization [6]. Life-threatening cardiac arrhythmias can result, progressing from bradycardia to ventricular fibrillation or asystole. The ECG may reveal bradycardia, prolonged P-R interval, decreased or absent P waves, widened Q-R-S complexes, and/or spiked T waves, to even wide complex tachycardia or ventricular tachycardia. Establishing cardiovascular stability is imperative, particularly in the face of severe hyperkalemia. Therefore, after the baseline HR, pulse palpation, and rhythm evaluation, an ECG and arterial blood pressure (ABP) should be obtained, especially in patients with bradycardia, tachycardia, arrhythmias, obtundation, or collapse.

It is important to consider anemia in patients with chronic renal dysfunction, urinary bladder hemorrhage associated with urethral obstruction [15], and cases of recent repeat urethral obstruction, during which anemia may develop secondary to dilutional fluid therapy required to manage postobstructive diuresis. Additionally, cats and patients with underlying cardiac disease may be subject to fluid overload during this diuresis phase, and this should be considered prior to and during anesthesia. Anemia induces impaired oxygen-carrying capacity, and oxygen supplementation is imperative throughout stabilization. In some cases, a blood transfusion may be necessary to address this complication.

Additional patient-dependent diagnostics may occur once the patient is stabilized and may include urinalysis with sediment evaluation, urine culture, and abdominal radiographs and/or ultrasound. Radiographs may be obtained in the conscious or sedated patient to localize and identify a cause of obstruction prior to passing a urethral catheter. Contrast urethrography, if required, should be attempted only after stabilization, as it generally requires deep sedation or general anesthesia to prevent the animal from responding to manipulation, which may result in iatrogenic trauma. Details of anesthetic-related concerns during imaging are described in the following text (see the section titled "Urinary Tract Diagnostic Imaging"), and the sedation protocol should be based on the procedure and individual patient.

Preanesthetic Management and Initial Stabilization

While prompt return of urethral patency is a priority, patients with metabolic abnormalities have an increased risk of complications if anesthetized, including cardiopulmonary arrest [3]. Therefore, rapid preanesthetic stabilization is imperative and includes restoring circulating volume and correction of electrolyte and acid–base abnormalities (Table 7.1). The degree of hyperkalemia, ECG alterations, and bladder distention dictate treatment priority, and how promptly relief of urethral obstruction should occur.

Throughout the stabilization process, supplemental oxygen and serial hands-on monitoring are advised, particularly when an arrhythmia or bradycardia has been documented. Monitoring parameters should include HR and rhythm with continuous ECG monitoring, pulse quality, and ABP. Intravenous (IV) access is a priority in all patients; to facilitate catheter placement, consider the patient's temperament, stability, and discomfort, and provide sedation when necessary, to avoid distress. Additionally, because urethral obstruction is classified as being moderately painful [16], appropriate analgesics are required (Table 7.2).

Crystalloids, as balanced electrolyte solutions, are preferred for correcting acid–base imbalances and remedy hypovolemia and dehydration. There was no difference in the rate of decline of serum potassium, but there was a more rapid correction of acidemia in cats treated with lactated ringer's solution (LRS) or Normosol-R than those treated with 0.9% sodium chloride [17, 18]. Fluid rates depend on the individual patient; however, for shock or poor perfusion conditions, fluid rates should be tailored to reach endpoints of resuscitation. Increments of approximately 25% of a shock dose (approximately 20 ml kg^{-1} in dogs, approximately 12 ml kg^{-1} in cats) over 15–20 min with reevaluation of endpoints such as mentation, HR, capillary refill time (CRT), and ABP are advised prior to continuing with fluid boluses. Once volume expansion is deemed adequate, or if resuscitation is not necessary, the fluid rate is based on patient hydration status, adding the calculated replacement of dehydration to normal maintenance fluid requirements. In patients with cardiac disease or predisposed breeds, more cautious fluid therapy and closer monitoring are advised.

Although most cats with urethral obstruction are relatively stable without serious metabolic abnormalities, severe hyperkalemia is the most common life-threatening problem (approximately 12% of cats, serum potassium >8 mEq l^{-1}) [7, 19]. Interestingly, the severity of clinical signs does not necessarily correlate with serum potassium concentrations; therefore, monitoring the ECG is the quickest way to document a life-threatening hyperkalemia. ECG issues will resolve with appropriate stabilization of the cardiac membrane and treatment of hyperkalemia. While cardiac conduction disturbances vary based on potassium concentrations, there is no threshold potassium concentration that can predict arrhythmia development, but generalizations can be made (Table 7.3). Although ultimate resolution of hyperkalemia involves reestablishing urethral patency, concentrations of potassium greater than 7.0 mEq l^{-1} may induce irregular idioventricular rhythms.

Table 7.1 Immediate evaluation and stabilization options in urinary tract obstruction/uroabdomen.

Abnormality	Immediate stabilization/comments
Bradycardia or arrhythmia	• Immediate ECG evaluation (Table 7.3) • Measure serum potassium • Obtain IV access • Immediately stabilize myocardium with calcium gluconate, followed by other treatments for hyperkalemia (Table 7.4) • Oxygen support, if tolerated
Hyperkalemia	• Examine for bradycardia or arrythmia • ECG evaluation (Table 7.3) • Obtain IV access • IV fluid support, based on individual, consider 10–20 ml kg^{-1} h^{-1} balanced crystalloid • Treat hyperkalemia (Table 7.4) • Reestablish urine flow. Consider urine diversion when appropriate: ○ Urethral obstruction: catheterize urinary bladder, cystocentesis ○ Uroabdomen: catheterize urinary bladder (if possible), peritoneal urine drainage • Manage concurrent metabolic acidosis and hypocalcemia
Hypovolemia	• Obtain IV access • IV fluid support targeting endpoints of resuscitation based on individual, options: ○ Balanced crystalloid: ¼ shock dose increments (approximately 20 ml kg^{-1} dog, approximately 12 ml kg^{-1} cat); reassess before repeating ○ Hypertonic saline (7.5%) over 10 min (4–7 ml kg^{-1} dog, 3–4 ml kg^{-1} cat)
Metabolic acidosis	• Obtain IV access • IV fluid support FIRST ○ Balanced crystalloid • Sodium bicarbonate, *consider* in severe case not responding to fluid support and pH <7.0 (Table 7.4)
Ionized hypocalcemia	• Obtain IV access • IV fluid support • IV calcium gluconate (Table 7.4)
Discomfort/stress	• Based on individual patient, opioid ± benzodiazepine (Table 7.2) and avoid drugs listed in Table 7.5

ECG, electrocardiogram; IV, intravenous.

Therefore, if the serum potassium concentration is greater than 7.0 mEq l^{-1}, regardless of ECG findings, correction is advised to reduce the risk of cardiopulmonary arrest. In a perfect situation, potassium concentrations should be near normal (<5.5–6.0 mEq l^{-1}) before anesthesia. Management of hyperkalemia is ultimately focused on antagonizing the cardiotoxic effects on the myocardial cells, reducing serum potassium through dilution, and increasing its elimination and redistribution. Therapy options for hyperkalemia management

Table 7.2 Common analgesics, sedatives, and anesthetics for urogenital anesthesia.

Drug[a]	Agent/dose	Comment
Premedicant, sedative, analgesic		
Opioids		
Analgesia, always titrate to effect, possible bradycardia, minimal effects on cardiovascular system, reversible with naloxone		
Hydromorphone (full mu-agonist)	0.05–0.2 mg kg^{-1} SC, IM, IV	– May induce vomiting or pant – Repeat every 2–6 h
Morphine (full mu-agonist)	Cat: 0.1–0.5 mg kg^{-1} SC, IM, slowly IV Dog: 0.2–1.0 mg kg^{-1} SC, IM, slowly IV	– Repeat every 2–4 h – Histamine release when administered rapidly IV – Caution: active metabolites in dogs may have delayed elimination in renal insufficiency, prolonging effects. Clearance may be slower in affected cats. Consider low-dose or other opioids in significant renal disease
Fentanyl (full mu-agonist)	1–5 μg kg^{-1} IV bolus or loading dose	– One dose duration approximately 15–30 min, requires CRI for continued effect (see below)
Methadone (mu-agonist, N-methyl-D-aspartate (NMDA) antagonist)	Dog: 0.05–0.6 mg kg^{-1} SC, IM, IV Cat: 0.05–0.5 mg kg^{-1} SC, IM, IV	– Repeat every 2–6 h
Butorphanol (kappa-agonist/ mu-antagonist)	0.1–0.5 mg kg^{-1} SC, IM, IV	– Mild analgesia, favorable for sedation and antiemetic effects – Repeat every 1–4 h
Buprenorphine (partial mu-agonist)	0.005–0.03 mg kg^{-1} SC, IV, IM or 0.01–0.03 mg kg^{-1} OTM in cats	– Moderate analgesia, difficult to reverse – 30 min to full effect – Repeat every 6–12 h
Benzodiazepines		
Sedation and muscle relaxation, no analgesia, antagonized with flumazenil, alone may induce excitement		
Midazolam	0.2–0.5 mg kg^{-1} IV, IM	– Water-soluble
Diazepam	0.2–0.5 mg kg^{-1} IV	– Contains propylene glycol – Metabolized to active metabolites, may cause prolonged sedation
Neuroleptanalgesia		
Combine opioid and benzodiazepine	Benzodiazepine 0.1–0.5 mg kg^{-1} and opioid of choice, such as butorphanol 0.1–0.4 mg kg^{-1}, etc.	– Maintain cardiovascular stability – May permit minor procedures ± sacrococcygeal epidural to remove urethral obstruction

Table 7.2 (Continued)

Drug[a]	Agent/dose	Comment
Sedation option for relief of urethral obstruction		
Benzodiazepine, ketamine, and opioid	Ketamine 0.5–4.0 mg kg^{-1} and benzodiazepine 0.1–0.5 mg kg^{-1} and opioid of choice such as butorphanol 0.1–0.4 mg kg^{-1}, etc.	– Consider sacrococcygeal epidural – Selection based on patient stability – Avoid if underlying cardiac disease – Urethral obstruction removal may require inhalant general anesthesia
Anesthetic induction agents		
Propofol	2–6 mg kg^{-1} IV titrated slowly to effect	– Rapid-acting, short duration – Respiratory depression – Peripheral vasodilation – Myocardial depression
Alfaxalone	0.5–5 mg kg^{-1} IV titrated slowly to effect, reduced doses advised in critically ill	– Add sedative to improve recovery – Respiratory depression – Off-label IM use in combination with opioid ± benzodiazepine to aid in fractious patient sedation to permit IV catheterization
Etomidate	1–2 mg kg^{-1} IV titrated to effect	– Cardiovascular stability – Caution: induces adrenocortical suppression which may be contraindicated in septic patients who have adrenal insufficiency (possible in severe pyometra)
Ketamine	2–5 mg kg^{-1} IV Use in combination with propofol, alfaxalone, or benzodiazepine	– Prolonged effects in patients with renal insufficiency or inability to excrete urine – Reduce dose by adding coinduction agents – May be contraindicated with some underlying cardiovascular diseases, dysrhythmias, or tachycardia – Caution in critically ill patients with catecholamine depletion, since direct myocardial depressant effects may induce hypotension
Maintenance		
Inhalant anesthetics	Isoflurane 1–2% or sevoflurane 2–3% to effect	– Dose-dependent cardiovascular and respiratory depression
Adjuncts		
Opioid CRI	Fentanyl 2–20 μg kg^{-1} h^{-1} after loading dose IV	30–50% MAC reduction

(continued)

Table 7.2 (Continued)

Drug[a]	Agent/dose	Comment
Ketamine CRI	0.1–1.2 mg kg^{-1} h^{-1} after loading dose of 0.5 mg kg^{-1} IV	10–30% MAC reduction
Lidocaine CRI (dog only)	1–6 mg kg^{-1} h^{-1} after loading dose of 1–2 mg kg^{-1} IV	15–30% MAC reduction
Epidural anesthesia: Sacrococcygeal	2% lidocaine 0.1–0.2 mg kg^{-1}	See Table 7.6
Epidural anesthesia: Lumbosacral (LS)	Morphine 0.1 mg kg^{-1} Bupivacaine 0.5 mg kg^{-1} (each may be used alone or together)	– If morphine is used alone, dilute with 0.9% saline to make 0.1 ml kg^{-1} volume – LS epidural total volume should not exceed 0.25 ml kg^{-1} or a maximum volume 8 ml (use 0.9% sterile saline to make up to 0.25 ml kg^{-1} volume)
Postoperative analgesics		
Opioids	As mentioned above, intermittent dosing or CRI	
Ketamine CRI	As mentioned above	
Lidocaine CRI in dogs only	As mentioned above	

[a] Other agents and doses are possible. SC, subcutaneous; IM, intramuscular; IV, intravascular; OTM, oral transmucosal; CRI, constant rate infusion; MAC, minimum alveolar concentration.

Table 7.3 Hyperkalemia-induced electrocardiographic (ECG) changes.

Serum potassium concentration (mEq l^{-1})	Expected ECG abnormalities
>5.5	T wave: tall and tented
>6.5	P-R interval: prolonged Q-R-S complex: duration prolonged R wave: amplitude decreased S-T segment: depressed
>7.0	P wave: amplitude decreased; duration increased Q-T segment: prolonged
>8.5	P wave: may disappear (atrial standstill) Abnormal rhythm: sinoventricular
>10.0	Q-R-S complex: widened and biphasic Abnormal rhythms: ventricular flutter, fibrillation, or asystole

are listed in Table 7.4 and discussed in the following text.

Mild increases in serum potassium in the stable patient may be corrected with dilutional fluid therapy and relief of the obstruction. Rapid intravascular volume expansion results in dilution of plasma potassium within minutes, and elimination via increased GFR simultaneously occurs. However, cystocentesis or reestablishment of urethral patency is imperative to permit elimination of potassium and prevent exacerbation of urine volume. Therefore, consider the patient's bladder size when administering necessary fluid support in correlation with how rapid the restoration of urine flow will occur. Therapeutic cystocentesis should be considered, particularly in cases with maximally expanded bladders in the presence of hyperkalemia-induced ECG abnormalities that do not permit rapid relief of urethral

Table 7.4 Hyperkalemia treatment.

Drug	Dose	Mechanism	Comments
IV fluid therapy: crystalloid	Based on individual patient, consider 10–20 ml kg^{-1}	Dilutional: IV volume expansion Elimination: increasing GFR	Effective within minutes, relief of urinary obstruction or peritoneal drainage must coincide, not advised as sole method for severe or life-threatening hyperkalemia
Insulin and 50% dextrose	0.5 U kg^{-1} IV regular insulin and 2 g U^{-1} (4 ml U^{-1}) IV 50% dextrose diluted 1:3 with saline	Redistribution: stimulates Na^+-K^+-ATPase activity, glucose and potassium move into cells	Onset 30 min, serial blood glucose measurements and supplement dextrose to prevent continued hypoglycemia
50% dextrose alone	0.5–1 g kg^{-1} (1–2 ml kg^{-1}) IV diluted 1:3 with saline, slowly over 3–5 min	Redistribution: induces endogenous insulin release, see above	Onset within 1 h, not advised as sole treatment in severe or life-threatening hyperkalemia
Terbutaline	0.01 mg kg^{-1} IV slowly	Redistribution: stimulation of Na^+-K^+-ATPase activity, moving potassium intracellularly	Onset 20–40 min, not advised as sole agent therapy, option to use inhaled β_2-adrenergic agonists
Sodium bicarbonate	0.3 × base deficit × body weight (in kg) and give 1/3–1/2 dose IV slowly over 15–30 min OR 1–2 mEq kg^{-1} IV slowly over 15 min	Redistribution: improves extracellular acidosis, indirectly stimulates activity of Na^+-K+-ATPase resulting in exchange of potassium for hydrogen ions	Onset 15 min, other treatments are advised first, can result in CSF acidosis and cerebral edema if given overzealously, caution in ionized hypocalcemia
10% calcium gluconate	50–150 mg kg^{-1} (0.5–1.5 ml kg^{-1}) IV slowly over 5–10 min with ECG monitoring during infusion to recognize bradycardia or worsening of arrhythmia	Antagonism: decreases cardiac excitability via reestablishing a more normal gradient between resting membrane and threshold potentials	Effective immediately (3–5 min) with short-lived duration, but a life-saving measure, antagonizes the effect of hyperkalemia on myocardium, does NOT alter serum potassium, other treatments should be instituted simultaneously
Urinary diversion	Uroabdomen: urethral catheterization and peritoneal drainage Urethral obstruction: urethral catheterization, alternatively perform cystocentesis	Elimination: uroabdomen potassium-containing urine exits the body, no longer being reabsorbed. Urethral obstruction, relief permits elimination	Recommended stabilization procedures in uroabdomen. Cystocentesis stabilization option when relief of urethral obstruction is not immediately possible

IV, intravenous; GFR, glomerular filtration rate; CSF, cerebrospinal fluid.

obstruction. Decompressive cystocentesis aids in rapid stabilization, allowing improved GFR and reduction of bladder pressure, which may facilitate urethral catheterization and retrograde urohydropropulsion [20]. Additionally, cystocentesis appears to be safe, as the overall risk of bladder rupture is low [20–22]. An injectable opioid ± benzodiazepine combination (Table 7.2) may be administered prior to cystocentesis not only to prevent patient movement leading to iatrogenic trauma but also to ease the discomfort secondary to the obstruction and procedure.

Additional therapies are indicated in patients with moderate potassium increases. Potassium redistribution via dextrose and insulin administration is effective within 20–40 min. Regular insulin (0.5 U kg^{-1} IV) promotes cellular uptake of glucose with simultaneous cotransport of potassium. Dextrose prevents hypoglycemia following insulin administration and is provided as a bolus (50% dextrose solution: 1 ml kg^{-1}, diluted 1:3 due to hyperosmolarity), followed by an infusion (1.25–2.5% dextrose: cats 2–3 ml kg^{-1} h^{-1}, dogs 2–6 ml kg^{-1} h^{-1}, expected 4–6 h duration), adjusted based on frequent BG monitoring. Another approach is to administer only IV dextrose as a bolus to induce the endogenous secretion of insulin.

In the presence of moderate to severe hyperkalemia, life-threatening bradycardia, or arrhythmias, calcium administration is indicated for immediate stabilization of the myocardium. Calcium gluconate (10% solution: 0.5–1.5 ml kg^{-1}) should be administered slowly IV over 5–10 min while continuously monitoring the ECG. If bradycardia worsens or shortening of the Q-T interval occurs, the infusion should be stopped. The effects of calcium administration only last 20–30 min, but it may be a life-saving measure [13]. Calcium therapy does not reduce serum potassium concentrations; therefore, its administration should be promptly followed with therapies including insulin and dextrose administration.

Beta-2-adrenergic receptor agonists can be used to redistribute potassium intracellularly. These agents reduce the potassium concentration by activating the sodium–potassium-ATPase pump. However, beta-2-adrenergic receptor agonists are not recommended as the sole therapy for management of hyperkalemia.

Concurrent abnormalities such as metabolic acidosis and ionized hypocalcemia can exacerbate hyperkalemic effects on cardiac conduction [13]. IV fluid therapy is the initial treatment in the management of metabolic acidosis; sodium bicarbonate therapy should be reserved for use only when fluid therapy is not effective and in the face of severe acidemia (pH <7.0). Sodium bicarbonate raises the pH, driving potassium intracellularly in exchange for hydrogen ions. This therapy may be less effective than dextrose and insulin at reducing potassium and should be used with caution due to resultant cerebrospinal fluid (CSF) acidosis and cerebral edema with overzealous administration. Therefore, incremental dosing is advised to avoid oversupplementation and a resulting alkalosis [23]. Additionally, acid–base management with alkalization in the face of ionized hypocalcemia should be considered with caution. As the pH increases, calcium binds to negatively charged proteins in addition to intracellular movement, potentially exacerbating ionized hypocalcemia and cardiac dysfunction [7]. While hypocalcemia resolves rapidly after reestablishing urine flow as serum phosphorus concentrations decrease, associated cardiac disturbances or muscle twitching or seizures (less common) should be managed with an IV infusion of calcium gluconate.

Electrolyte and acid–base abnormalities should be reassessed every 30–60 min after the initial treatment to correct derangements. The results should be used to guide continued therapy until the patient is stable and laboratory parameters are deemed acceptable for anesthesia.

Sedation and Anesthesia

The treatment goal is to rapidly relieve the obstruction without traumatizing the urethra [3]. Therefore, once cardiovascular stability is ensured, analgesia with sedation or general anesthesia is necessary for reestablishing urethral patency. Appropriate fluid replacement and correction of acid–base and electrolyte abnormalities are likely more important to success versus the recommendation of a specific anesthetic protocol. Drug selection should be individualized according to the procedure and specific needs of the patient; however, short-acting, reversible agents that provide adequate sedation and analgesia are ideal (Table 7.2). Injectable or inhalational anesthetic agents added to produce neuroleptanalgesia (opioid and a sedative such as a benzodiazepine) may be indicated. Severely debilitated patients may require only minimal sedation for diagnostics and the unblocking procedure.

Mask or box induction with volatile anesthetics should be avoided whenever possible, since inhalant anesthetic drugs cause dose-dependent depression of the central nervous system (CNS), cardiovascular, and respiratory systems. Compromised animals may not tolerate the high concentrations (possibly an overdose) of volatile anesthetics required to induce anesthesia when no concurrent drugs are administered. Additionally, masking/boxing is dangerous to the staff secondary to environmental contamination.

The anesthetist should inquire about current medications used for long-term management of lower urinary tract conditions, including alpha-adrenergic receptor antagonists such as phenoxybenzamine and prazosin. These may result in vasodilation and hypotension, which may be exacerbated in anesthetized patients. To this end, drugs known to induce hypotension, cardiovascular compromise, or nephrotoxicity should be avoided if possible (Table 7.5). Animals with decreased renal perfusion of any cause, such as shock, hypovolemia, dehydration, or hypotension, may be susceptible to nonsteroidal anti-inflammatory drug (NSAID)-induced renal damage; therefore, use of NSAIDs is not advised until appropriate renal function has been confirmed and cardiovascular status is stabilized [24]. Although the sedative effects of acepromazine and promotion of urethral smooth muscle relaxation seem desirable, simultaneous vasodilation may lead to hypotension, even with low IV doses. Therefore, acepromazine use in patients with preexisting hypovolemia, dehydration, or hypotension is discouraged, and, if selected, close monitoring and maintenance of normotension are advised. Alpha-2-adrenergic receptor agonists such as dexmedetomidine should be used with caution or avoided in patients with unresolved urinary obstruction, considering their diuretic effect secondary to inhibition of arginine vasopressin (AVP) or a hyperglycemic osmotic diuresis due to insulin inhibition [25]. Additionally, the bradycardia, peripheral vasoconstriction, decreased cardiac output (CO), and potential arrhythmias [26] may exacerbate the cardiotoxic effects of hyperkalemia [13].

Premedication using neuroleptanalgesia is an ideal choice (Table 7.2). Opioids have minimal direct effects on the cardiovascular system and provide analgesia, sedation, and reversibility. Potential negative opioid effects include bradycardia, emesis (hydromorphone, etc.), and possibly histamine release (e.g., morphine administered rapidly IV). In the face of severe hyperkalemic bradycardia, anticholinergics may not be effective [27, 28]; therefore, the clinician should consider treatment with immediate cardioprotective mechanisms (i.e., calcium administration) and reduction of potassium (Table 7.4) prior to administration of opioids, which may worsen bradycardia. Benzodiazepines in combination with an opioid cause minimal depression of the cardiovascular system and provide reversibility and sedation, permitting minor treatments or diagnostics and may aid in urethral relaxation through their effects on striated muscle.

Table 7.5 Drugs to avoid or use with caution.

Drug or drug class	Comments
NSAIDs	• Ill-advised in presence of decreased renal perfusion such as shock, hypovolemia, dehydration, hypotension, or presence of azotemia • Consider only after renal function has been confirmed and cardiovascular status is stabilized
Alpha-2-adrenergic receptor agonists (dexmedetomidine)	• Reduced cardiac output, increased SVR, bradycardia, and potential to induce dysrhythmias, may exacerbate the cardiotoxic effects of concurrent hyperkalemia • Promotes diuresis in face of inability to void urine • May consider in a patient with a stable cardiovascular system with timely establishment of urine flow
Phenothiazines (acepromazine)	• Vasodilation-induced hypotension possible at any dose, use is discouraged in cases with preexisting hypovolemia, dehydration, or hypotension • Negative effects may be exacerbated when used with other drugs, inducing cardiovascular depression • Consider only after cardiovascular status is stabilized, 0.005–0.03 mg kg^{-1} IV
Etomidate	• While etomidate exerts minimal cardiovascular effects, it induces adrenocortical suppression which may be contraindicated in septic patients who have adrenal insufficiency (possible in severe pyometra)
Ketamine	• May be contraindicated with some underlying cardiovascular diseases, dysrhythmias, or tachycardia • Caution in critically ill patients with catecholamine depletion in which ketamine's direct myocardial depressant effects may induce hypotension • Liver metabolism to varying degrees based on species; metabolites depend on renal excretion. Prolonged drug effects possible in cats with renal insufficiency, inability to eliminate urine and uroabdomen (continuously resorbed from urine in abdomen) • When ketamine is used, consider reduced dose and avoidance of repeat doses or a CRI until urine elimination is restored (cats)
Lidocaine	• Systemic lidocaine infusions are not advised for balanced anesthesia in cats due to severe cardiovascular depression and lack of effect on thermal pain • Systemic lidocaine is contraindicated in patients with escape rhythms, absence of P waves/atrial standstill, and should be used cautiously in bradycardia

NSAIDs, nonsteroidal anti-inflammatory drugs; SVR, systemic vascular resistance; IV, intravenous; CRI, constant rate infusion.

However, benzodiazepines may induce excitation and dysphoria, particularly when used alone; fortunately, more reliable sedation is likely to occur in geriatric or sick patients, and when coadministered with opioids.

Depending on the patient, analgesia and injectable or inhalational maintenance anesthesia may be necessary to reestablish urethral patency using catheterization and retropulsion. Some patients may respond to neuroleptanalgesia with the addition of subanesthetic doses of propofol (0.25–1.0 mg kg^{-1}), possibly in combination with a sacrococcygeal epidural (Table 7.6). Propofol is desirable for its short duration of action and is advisable in stable patients, but caution is advised in debilitated patients due to potential dose-dependent vasodilation and hypotension. However, methods to reduce the dose of propofol including adequate sedation and use of a coinduction agent

Table 7.6 Sacrococcygeal epidural procedure.

A) Patient should be adequately sedated or under general anesthesia with appropriate monitoring
B) Place the patient in sternal recumbency
C) Locate the sacrococcygeal space while mobilizing the tail, or the space between the first two coccygeal vertebrae, either is acceptable
D) Clip and aseptically prepare the area
E) Use sterile techniques for the procedure
F) Relocate the sacrococcygeal space, or space between the first two coccygeal vertebrae
G) Use a 25-gauge 1-in. needle with the index finger near the insertion site on midline to guide placement
H) Direct the needle at a 45° angle and slowly advance. A palpable "pop" may occur when passing through the ligament.
I) The needle should enter the epidural space without resistance. If the needle is superficial to the spinal canal or advanced beyond the epidural space to the floor of the vertebral canal, bone will be encountered. If superficial, redirect, walking along the bone until the space is entered. If the needle placement is deep, back out slightly.
J) Once the needle is placed, attach a syringe, aspirate, ensuring no blood is encountered, followed by infusion of 0.1–0.2 ml kg^{-1} (average 0.5 ml per cat) of 2% lidocaine. Injection should encounter minimal resistance.
K) Successful block reveals tail and rectal relaxation, producing anesthesia to the perineum, penis, urethra, colon, and anus

(e.g., benzodiazepines, opioids, or ketamine) may attenuate these effects. Alfaxalone, when used at recommended doses, maintains cardiovascular parameters within normal limits in healthy animals, and doses of 1–2 mg kg^{-1} IV over 60 s provide acceptable induction in dogs considered to be a poor anesthetic risk [29]. However, it should be administered to an appropriately sedated patient to prevent muscle twitching or poor recovery. Additionally, similar to propofol, respiratory depression and apnea can occur with alfaxalone; therefore, its use requires supplemental oxygenation and the ability to intubate the airway. Intramuscular (IM) use of alfaxalone in combination with other drugs (opioids, benzodiazepines, ketamine) is an option for sedation in patients in which it is not initially possible to obtain IV access, avoiding mask or box induction with inhalational anesthetics.

A ketamine coinduction with a benzodiazepine after premedication with an opioid is also an option, with or without the addition of inhalational anesthesia. However, caution is advised in patients with underlying cardiovascular disease [30], arrhythmias, tachycardia, or hemodynamic instability. Additionally, ketamine is metabolized by the liver in most species and its metabolites depend on renal excretion. Cats rely more extensively on renal elimination [31, 32], which may result in accumulation and prolonged anesthesia in cases of urinary obstruction. However, ketamine can be used in obstructed patients, being cognizant that no antagonist is available and repeat doses are discouraged until patency is established.

In all cases, patient monitoring is necessary, as all patients have the potential to decline rapidly. Monitoring should include HR, respiratory rate (RR) and character, CRT, pulse oximetry (SpO_2) to determine hemoglobin (Hb) saturation with oxygen, ECG, ABP, capnography if intubated, and temperature. Airway management is crucial, and supplemental oxygen during the procedure maximizes delivery of oxygen (DO_2) to the tissues. Many patients have not been fasted, thus aspiration of regurgitate or vomitus is a risk. Therefore, consider intubating all anesthetized patients, and be prepared to intubate and ventilate patients in an emergency. Additionally, antiemetics and prokinetics may be considered. Hypothermia may contribute to bradycardia and is an urgent concern with concurrent hyperkalemia- or opioid-induced bradycardia; therefore, it is important to maintain normothermia [12]. Systemic hypotension has a direct effect on renal perfusion, and mean ABP (MAP) should be maintained above 60–70 mmHg. If anesthesia is maintained with inhalants, their adverse cardiovascular effects should be minimized by avoiding overdose through close monitoring of anesthetic depth and decreasing their required concentration by adding intermittent doses or a constant rate infusion (CRI) of an opioid. Additionally, ensure an adequate circulating volume with continued IV fluid therapy at a surgical rate (dogs: 5 ml kg^{-1} h^{-1}, cats: 3 ml kg^{-1} h^{-1}), maintain an adequate HR with anticholinergics, and consider inotropic drugs such as dopamine (5–10 μg kg^{-1} min^{-1}) or dobutamine (2–5 μg kg^{-1} min^{-1}) to support myocardial function in maintaining CO, ABP, and renal blood flow.

Adjunctive Anesthetic Techniques

Several protocols are available to aid the anesthetist during the procedure chosen to relieve the urinary obstruction that provide multimodal analgesia, reduce the requirement for additional drugs negatively affecting the cardiovascular system, and possibly shorten the anesthetic event and ease catheter placement (Table 7.7).

A sacrococcygeal epidural can be used to relieve urethral obstruction and aid in placement of a urinary catheter in cats [3]. Patients must be appropriately immobilized, either sedated or under general anesthesia prior to epidural, although severely obtunded patients may require little sedation. The technique (Table 7.6) produces anesthesia of the perineum, penis, urethra, colon, and anus by blocking the pudendal, pelvic, and caudal nerves, without loss of motor function to pelvic limbs [33]. Lidocaine (0.1–0.2 ml kg^{-1} of 2% lidocaine) into the epidural space results in anesthesia within 5 min, lasting up to 60 min [3]. A successful block results in relaxation of the tail and rectum with no response to subsequent tail pinch. Contraindications for epidurals include coagulation disorders, sepsis, pyoderma at site of injection, severe hypovolemia or hypotension, and anatomic abnormalities. The risks associated with injections

Table 7.7 Analgesic or anesthetic adjunct considerations to reestablish urethral patency.

Analgesic or anesthetic considerations[a]	Dose	Comments
Local anesthesia	Sterile lidocaine gel, or 0.25 ml of 2% lidocaine added to sterile gel	Some lidocaine will be absorbed systemically, attention to total dose of lidocaine is advised
Atracurium besylate	0.5 mg ml^{-1} solution infused into urethra for 5 min prior to retrograde flushing	NMBA, majority of urethra is striated muscle, may reduce time to obstruction relief
Sacrococcygeal epidural anesthesia	0.1–0.2 ml kg^{-1} of 2% lidocaine (0.5 ml total volume in average cat)	See Table 7.6 for procedure. Contraindicated in patient with coagulation disorders, sepsis, pyoderma at site of injection, severe hypovolemia or hypotension, and anatomic abnormalities. Possible complications include infection or abscess at site injection, failure of technique to provide analgesia and possible systemic absorption of lidocaine, although doses described are far below recommended dose for IV lidocaine

[a] Appropriate sedation or general anesthesia should be ensured, based on individual patient (Table 7.2). NMBA, neuromuscular blocking agent; IV, intravenous.

at the sacrococcygeal location are low; the spinal cord ends at approximately the first sacral space (S1) in cats, thus the risk of puncturing the cord or penetrating the subarachnoid space is unlikely [3]. Potential complications include infection or abscess, failure to provide analgesia, and possible systemic absorption of lidocaine, although the described dose is low. However, this technique only provides analgesia up to 1 h; therefore, further analgesia may be required, and administration of buprenorphine (partial mu-opioid agonist) may be considered after relief of obstruction.

In addition to a well-lubricated catheter, sterile lidocaine gel, or 0.25 ml of sterile 2% lidocaine (5 mg) added to sterile gel, provides local anesthesia of the urethra beneficial for approximately 1 h, and should make the catheter placement more tolerable for the patient. Some lidocaine will be absorbed systemically through the urethral wall; therefore, attention to the lidocaine dose should be considered (0.25–1 mg kg^{-1}, up to 2 mg kg^{-1} total dose). Additionally, lidocaine is contraindicated in patients with escape rhythms or absence of P waves/atrial standstill and used cautiously in animals with bradycardia; even topical use may be avoided in such situations.

In cats with urethral obstruction, more successful first attempt resolutions and reduced time to relief of obstruction have been achieved when using 4 ml of a solution of 0.5 mg ml^{-1} atracurium besylate infused into the urethral lumen for 5 min prior to retrograde flushing [34]. Atracurium besylate is a neuromuscular blocking agent and should be effective for this purpose, as most of the urethra is striated muscle, and only the proximal 1/3 of the penile urethra is smooth muscle.

Urethrotomy/Urethrostomy

Under general anesthesia, most urethral calculi can be retropulsed into the urinary bladder, reestablishing urine flow until definitive treatment can occur such as medical dissolution, voiding urohydropropulsion, cystoscopy retrieval, lithotripsy, cystotomy, or other management. However, if retrograde urohydropropulsion is unsuccessful or one is unable to feed the catheter past the obstruction, the anesthetist should first ensure an adequate anesthetic plane exists and local anesthetic techniques are used. If failure remains, repeat cystocentesis may be required until the patient is deemed stable for a more definitive procedure such as permanent urethrostomy. Alternatively, urethrotomy may be an option for temporary diversion of urine or removal of calculi, and in those cases, the anesthetists should infuse a local anesthetic (2% lidocaine, dog: 2–5 mg kg^{-1}) over the urethrotomy site in combination with a sacrococcygeal epidural and provide sedation or general anesthesia, as necessary [35]. Monitoring is routine, and the anesthetic protocol is dependent on the patient's condition as described in the preceding text (Table 7.2).

Permanent urethrostomy, although not commonly an emergency procedure, may be deemed necessary in a stable patient with an irresolvable distal urethral obstruction unreachable by urethrotomy, and should be performed under general anesthesia. Additionally, a sacrococcygeal epidural may be considered for any perineal procedure [3]. Careful patient positioning and padding should be used to protect the pelvic limbs from injury when hanging off the surgery table. Additionally, if the pelvis is elevated above the head, compression of the diaphragm is possible; therefore, it is important to ensure adequate ventilation, and monitor end-tidal carbon dioxide (ETCO2) or arterial blood gases, supplementing ventilation if required. A purse-string suture is frequently placed in the anus, and its removal should be ensured following surgery. Intraoperative complications include hemorrhage, for which the anesthetist should be prepared, particularly in the anemic patient. If castration is performed in intact animals, additional analgesia such as a testicular block may be considered.

Postoperative sedatives to reduce hemorrhage induced by excitement following recovery from a urethrotomy or urethrostomy are advised, and an Elizabethan collar should be in place prior to recovery to prevent self-trauma. Additionally, topical petroleum jelly should be applied to the incision to prevent urine scald, and a local anesthetic agent (5% xylocaine ointment) may be added [35].

Recovery and Postoperative Care

After achieving urethral patency, continued patient monitoring is required until resolution of metabolic abnormalities occurs. The urinary catheter often remains in place and quantifying urine output may aid in the management of fluid therapy in the face of postobstructive diuresis; evaluation for fluid overload, particularly in cats, is advised. Analgesia is based on the procedure and serial patient evaluation and pure or partial mu-opioid agonists may be selected, based on validated pain scoring systems. NSAIDs should be used with caution in postobstructive patients in the face of hypovolemia and decreased renal function. Acepromazine, phenoxybenzamine, and prazosin may be useful in permitting urethral smooth muscle relaxation via alpha-1-adrenergic receptor antagonism. Additionally, the sedative effects of acepromazine may be beneficial in reducing stress but may be contraindicated in some patients.

Upper Urinary Tract Obstruction

Etiologies of feline upper urinary tract (kidneys or ureters) obstruction include calculus, soft tissue plugs, fibrosis, inflammation, stricture, and ureter neoplasia [36, 37]. Ureteral obstruction is an uncommon cause of urinary obstruction and azotemia [1]; however, if the ureteral obstruction does not resolve within 24–48 h of medical management or if the patient has complete ureteral obstruction, worsening azotemia, or progressive hydronephrosis, surgical intervention is often required [36, 38]. Surgical intervention may include ureterotomy, ureteral reimplantation, ureteral stenting, or subcutaneous ureteral bypass (SUB). If these are not possible, a nephrostomy tube, intermittent hemodialysis, nephrectomy, or other interventional technique may be required. Preoperative management, urgency, and prognosis depend on the underlying condition, patient status, and procedure at hand.

Clinical Signs and Physical Exam

Clinical signs of ureteral obstruction are nonspecific and range from mild to severe depending on duration if one or both ureters are obstructed or if chronic renal compromise exists and may include anorexia, lethargy, vomiting, weight loss, halitosis, polydipsia, dysuria, oliguria or anuria, and hematuria [1, 38, 39]. Life-threatening cardiac disturbances and collapse secondary to acid–base, electrolyte, and fluid derangements similarly described in urethral obstruction may occur, particularly in bilateral ureteral obstruction or chronic obstruction. Abdominal palpation may reveal abdominal pain and asymmetric kidneys. If one kidney is small and irregular and the other is enlarged, firm, and painful, this is highly suggestive of ureteral obstruction. Pallor or a heart murmur may be associated with anemia [40].

Initial Database and Stabilization

Diagnosis is difficult based on physical exam alone; therefore, a variety of imaging procedures may be performed once the patient is medically stabilized which can include abdominal radiographs (Figure 7.1), ultrasound, and contrast radiography (see the section titled "Urinary Tract Diagnostic Imaging").

A review of ureteral obstructions revealed that many cats (48%) were anemic, and dogs (44%) may have neutrophilia associated with a

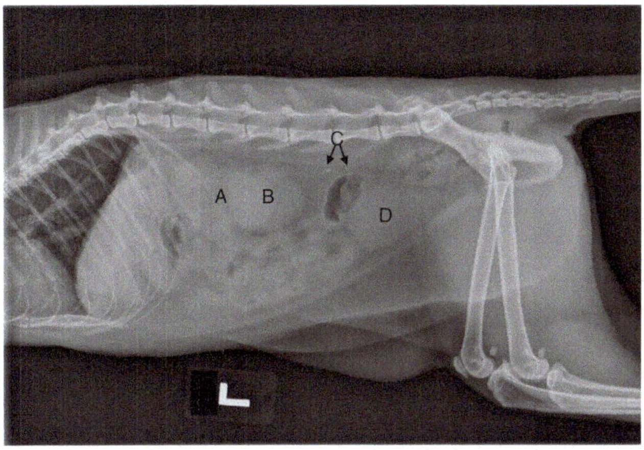

Figure 7.1 Lateral radiograph of a feline abdomen. The kidneys are asymmetric in size, with the left being smaller than the right. The left kidney is also misshapen. A few (approximately three) radiopaque calculi are identified in the caudodorsal abdomen at the level of lumbar vertebrae 5–6. These calculi were confirmed to be located within the ureter on ultrasonography. (A) Right kidney; (B) left kidney; (C) ureteral calculi; (D) urinary bladder.

pyelonephritis and thrombocytopenia that could be severe (<40 000 platelets). Azotemia was present in cats (83%) and dogs (50%), and hyperphosphatemia, hyperkalemia, and hypercalcemia or hypocalcemia may occur [40]. Urinary tract infections, hypovolemia, dehydration, and metabolic acidosis are also possible. Additionally, patients with chronic kidney disease may present with hypoalbuminemia and systemic hypertension (see Chapter 6) [41]. Therefore, blood gas analysis, CBC, biochemistry and coagulation panels, ABP measurements, urinalysis, and urine culture should be performed prior to anesthesia. Uremia impairs platelet adhesion and aggregation; therefore buccal mucosal bleeding time is recommended [42]. A crossmatch should be performed in any animal with coagulopathy or anemia, or if excessive intraoperative bleeding is likely. Unless an emergency exists making it necessary to intervene, dehydration, hypovolemia, electrolyte imbalances, metabolic acidosis, ABP abnormalities, anemia, coagulopathies, and uremia should be corrected prior to anesthesia.

Patient stabilization is identical to those with urethral obstruction (Table 7.1). Similarly, medical management of patients should be instituted prior to anesthesia. This may include aggressive IV fluid therapy, mannitol infusions, alpha-adrenergic receptor blockade, amitriptyline, and glucagon [40]. Additionally, many patients with underlying renal disease are treated with angiotensin-converting enzyme inhibitors (ACEIs). Consequently, preparation for alpha-adrenergic blockade or ACEI-induced hypotension exacerbated under anesthesia is advised. Careful evaluation of hydration status is paramount to avoid the possibility of fluid overload, congestive heart failure, or, in the case of anemic patients, hemodilution.

Anemia may result in decreased DO_2 to tissues due to decreased arterial oxygen content (CaO_2). Additionally, a shift of the oxyhemoglobin dissociation curve to the right is expected along with increased CO resultant to decreased blood viscosity. Oxygen support is imperative in these situations. Blood transfusion should be considered to avoid such consequences and based on the individual patient, transfusion is often advised prior to anesthesia if the Hb <7.0 g dl^{-1} (PCV <18–20%).

Hypoproteinemic patients may require oncotic support in which synthetic colloids (such as hydroxyethyl starch) may be an option for animals with low colloid osmotic pressure (COP); however, colloid administration could have clinically relevant adverse effects [43]. Synthetic starches are associated with increased risk of acute kidney injury in human patients. However, a direct correlation has not been established in veterinary patients, although similar risks are likely possible in critically ill animals. Additionally, synthetic starches interfere with coagulation and platelet function, decrease von Willebrand factor and factor VIII, and can prolong clotting times [43, 44]. Consequently, synthetic colloids are generally used with caution or avoided in patients with coagulopathies or renal impairment; however, clinical bleeding has not been reported in healthy animals receiving doses up to 20 ml kg^{-1} [43, 45]. Hydroxyethyl starch dosing may be limited to a maximum of 20 ml kg^{-1} day^{-1} in dogs and 10–20 ml kg^{-1} day^{-1} in cats [46], while others advise a CRI of up to 20–30 ml kg^{-1} day^{-1} [47]. It is important to note that there is no evidence-based consensus on the appropriate use of colloids in either human or veterinary medicine, and optimal use remains debatable, and at the discretion of the clinician. Additionally, intravascular volume status and concurrent diseases including hypertrophic cardiomyopathy may further complicate management with colloidal solutions.

Accurate assessment of intravascular volume and fluid responsiveness in the awake patient remains challenging with no single perfect monitoring tool. Placement of an intrathoracic jugular catheter (close to the right atrium) may be considered for central venous pressure (CVP) measurements. However, CVP has been shown to be unreliable in people and dogs to guide fluid therapy. Therefore, CVP measurements, despite being easy and cost-effective, should be used cautiously and never interpreted alone. They may be used in conjunction with physical exam parameters that evaluate CO, and trends in CVP measurements may be more important rather than isolated CVP values [48]. The amount of urine output compared to the amount of fluid administered along with serial body weights may be considered to guide fluid therapy in the preoperative and postoperative period, particularly when considered in clinical context and with other measured variables of volume status (vital signs, physical examination, and laboratory parameters). Advanced monitoring of volume status in the awake patient may also include serial echocardiographic assessments. Additionally, an arterial catheter may be considered during the perianesthetic period to permit direct blood pressure measurement, waveform analysis (detailed in the following text), and repeat blood gas evaluations. Placing a feeding tube during the anesthetic event will aid as an alternative therapeutic maneuver to reduce IV fluid volumes in the recovery period.

Sedation and Anesthesia

Anesthetic protocols vary based on the individual patient and the choice of protocol may be less important once the patient is stabilized; however, drugs known to induce hypotension or nephrotoxicity should be avoided (Table 7.5). Premedication should include a pure mu-opioid receptor agonist such as methadone, hydromorphone, or fentanyl, possibly with a benzodiazepine. Induction of anesthesia may occur with a variety of agents or combinations including propofol or alfaxalone; fentanyl combined with a benzodiazepine can be considered for induction in more critical patients. A ketamine coinduction may be selected; however, in cats, a moderate dose and avoidance of CRI until restoration of urine flow due to its dependence on renal clearance in this species resulting in possible prolonged recovery may be considered [31, 32]. Maintenance with an inhalant anesthetic in combination with a pure mu-opioid receptor agonist CRI (e.g., fentanyl) is recommended to provide analgesia and decrease the inhalant required, thereby reducing the associated cardiorespiratory depression and hypotension.

Local or regional anesthetic techniques will further reduce intraoperative anesthetic requirements and provide preemptive and postoperative analgesia. Examples include the use of a lumbosacral epidural (preservative-free bupivacaine 0.5 mg kg^{-1} and/or opioid such as 0.1 mg kg^{-1} morphine diluted with saline to a total volume of 0.1–0.2 ml kg^{-1}), incisional line block, and/or intraperitoneal infiltration of bupivacaine (cats 2 mg kg^{-1}, dogs 4.4 mg kg^{-1}) [49, 50]. Fascial plane blocks, such as the transversus abdominal plane (TAP), may be administered via ultrasound guidance as an alternative to an epidural as well. Techniques should be considered in combination, keeping track of total dose to avoid local anesthetic toxicity.

The most common intraoperative complication in cats undergoing surgery for correcting ureteral obstruction is hypothermia (87%) followed by hypotension (40.5%) and bradycardia (21.6%), in addition to hypertension and hypocapnia [36, 41]. It is important to monitor temperature and provide supplemental heat as needed because hypothermia can lead to arrhythmias, coagulopathies, decreased DO_2 to tissues, bradycardia, and decreased requirements for inhalational anesthetics. Intraoperative fluid therapy and noninvasive or invasive ABP monitoring are essential to maintain renal perfusion; the invasive method is ideal for immediate and more accurate assessment. Chronically hypertensive patients are expected to have an altered zone of autoregulation in which ABP should be maintained closer to their normal values to prevent hypoperfusion. Preoperative hypotension should be corrected prior to anesthesia and intraoperative hypotension prevented or intensively addressed in a timely manner. Management of hypotension via a combination of partial IV anesthesia (adjunct CRIs; Table 7.2) to decrease inhalant, adequate depth monitoring to prevent inhalant overdose, fluid support, maintenance of adequate HR with anticholinergics, and administration of inotropes (dopamine, dobutamine) and vasopressors is advised as necessary. CVP measurements have been shown to be unreliable and late indicators of changes in blood volume, fluid responsiveness, and fluid overload. Evaluation of volume status and fluid responsiveness remains challenging, but recent research encourages measurement with dynamic indices such as plethysmographic variability index (PVI), pulse pressure variation (PPV), systolic pressure variation (SPV), or stroke volume variation (SVV); however, their use is limited to patients that are mechanically ventilated with a known TV (8–10 ml kg^{-1}), without arrhythmias, and with no inspiratory effort [43]. Additionally, PPV and PVI were shown to predict fluid responsiveness more accurately than CVP [51]. Furthermore, PPV was shown to have better diagnostic accuracy to predict fluid responsiveness, but when invasive blood pressure is unavailable, PVI may predict fluid responsiveness in 70% of the population [52]. Intraoperative monitoring should additionally include SpO_2, capnometry, and ECG. Repeat blood gas evaluations along with continuous $ETCO_2$ monitoring are imperative to address and manage ventilation, acidosis, and electrolyte abnormalities.

Recovery and Postoperative Care

Postoperative complications in cats with SUB placement include pain, anorexia, nausea, hypertension, and urinary-tract-related issues [36], while cats with ureteral obstruction surgeries show persistent hypotension (40.5%), uroabdomen, and postobstructive diuresis [41]. Additionally, with a prevalence of over 40%, serial evaluations and management of pain in the postoperative period are a priority and highlight the importance of perioperative balanced anesthesia and multimodal analgesia including local anesthetic techniques [36]. The likelihood of postoperative hypertension and hypotension emphasizes the obligation of continued ABP monitoring and management including positive inotropes and vasopressor support. Management of postobstructive diuresis places patients at a high risk of fluid overload, particularly in cats. Continued monitoring of fluid status, never through an independent variable, rather by a combination of parameters, including serial vital signs, physical examination including serial body weight and urine output laboratory parameters, and possibly serial cardiac ultrasounds, is advised. In addition, enteral nutrition should be considered which necessitates placing a feeding tube during anesthesia.

Uroabdomen

Uroabdomen occurs secondary to a disruption of the urinary tract in which urine escapes into the peritoneal cavity, retroperitoneal cavity, or both. Uroperitoneum commonly develops from rupture of the lower urinary tract (distal ureters, bladder, or proximal urethra). In comparison, uroretroperitoneum results from injury to a kidney or proximal ureter with the peritoneum remaining intact [13]. The most common cause of uroperitoneum in dogs and cats is trauma to the abdomen or pelvis [2], and includes blunt, penetrating, and iatrogenic trauma. In cats, the bladder was the most common site of rupture secondary to blunt trauma, and the urethra was the most common site following catheterization [2]. Less common causes of uroperitoneum include bladder rupture secondary to neoplasia in dogs and urethral calculi or obstruction in cats [2, 12].

Consequences of uroabdomen include severe dehydration, hypovolemia, electrolyte derangements, metabolic acidosis, azotemia, and chemical peritonitis or septic peritonitis, ultimately leading to multiple metabolic imbalances and cardiac disturbances, which can be life-threatening if not addressed promptly [1, 13]. Therefore, rapid diagnosis and correction of derangements are imperative prior to advanced procedures/diagnostics, and anesthesia or surgery. The reported mortality rates for dogs and cats treated for uroabdomen are 21% [53] and 27.3% [2], respectively. Although associated injuries are responsible for most deaths, a delay in diagnosis of uroperitoneum increases the mortality rate [2]. Regardless of diagnosis timing, defects in the urinary tract are initially considered a medical emergency, requiring stabilization prior to repair.

Clinical Signs and Physical Exam

A thorough examination is essential, particularly in traumatized patients, to identify concomitant conditions and appropriately prioritize patient care. The incidence of urinary tract trauma that goes undetected is as high as 50% in dogs and 15.4% in cats [2, 12]. Such cases often present with other life-threatening conditions including hypovolemic shock, pulmonary contusions, fractures, or traumatic brain injuries. Initial diagnosis is often delayed due to quiescent clinical signs, and the lag time before clinical signs of azotemia and electrolyte abnormalities develops.

Clinical signs of uroabdomen vary depending on duration, underlying etiology, and derangements in electrolytes, acid–base status, and uremia [12]. Lethargy, anorexia, vomiting, stranguria, hematuria, restlessness, panting, abdominal guarding, hunched position, and abdominal distension with fluid wave are possible. If there is a concurrent urinary tract infection, septic peritonitis may result and clinical signs of septic shock and hypoperfusion may predominate [12]. Physical examination may reveal altered consciousness due to abdominal pain, uremia, or poor cardiovascular function, which intensify over time. Severe cases present with signs of dehydration (dry MM, decreased skin turgor, and increased PCV/TS), hypovolemia (pale MM, prolonged CRT, poor pulse quality), and hypovolemic shock [23]. Despite the presence of hypovolemia or shock, bradycardia may be identified; hyperkalemia should then be considered, although hypothermia or acid/base disturbances can contribute [12]. Cats may present differently than dogs, with bradycardia or tachycardia, pale MM, weak pulses and cool extremities, tachypnea, hypothermia, generalized weakness, and decreased mentation. Although anuria and dysuria are common, it is important to note that the ability to urinate or the presence of a palpable urinary bladder does not exclude rupture of the urinary tract and uroabdomen [2].

Initial Database and Clinicopathology

The most common laboratory abnormalities in patients with uroabdomen include hypovolemia, azotemia, metabolic acidosis, hyperkalemia, hyponatremia, hypocalcemia, and hyperphosphatemia [6, 13, 23]. An emergency blood screen should include PCV/TS, BG, venous or arterial blood gas, electrolytes, BUN, creatinine, and lactate; a full CBC and chemistry panel should be completed prior to advanced care. Urinary tract defects should be suspected based on history, physical exam, azotemia, hyperkalemia, and abdominal effusion. While survey radiographs may be obtained in an unsedated patient, they are rarely diagnostic [2]. Comparative tests between serum and abdominal effusion aid in diagnosis during the stabilization process which is described in the following text. Advanced imaging studies to definitively localize the source of urine leakage require sedation or anesthesia, which should be withheld until medical stabilization is ensured. Anesthetic concerns associated with positive-contrast radiography including excretory urography, cystography, and retrograde urethrography are discussed in the following text (see Figure 7.2 and the section titled "Urinary Tract Diagnostic Imaging").

Urine is high in potassium, hydrogen ions, and nitrogenous waste products, and low in sodium and chloride; therefore, as urine accumulates in the peritoneal space, these products are reabsorbed into the blood stream, resulting in severe hyperkalemia, metabolic acidosis, and azotemia [12]. The degree of reabsorption is

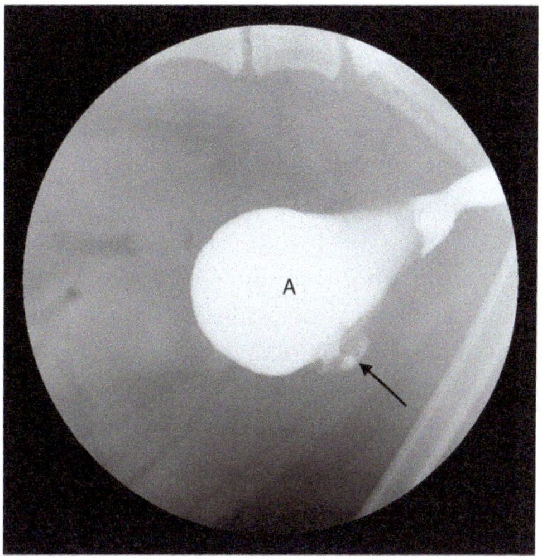

Figure 7.2 Retrograde positive-contrast cystogram, lateral radiograph. A = urinary bladder; arrow points to the leakage of iodinated contrast from the ventral wall of the urinary bladder consistent with a tear in the bladder wall.

dependent on the molecular size, which aids in diagnosis when comparing serum to abdominal effusion. Urea is a small molecule, rapidly equilibrating with the bloodstream and resulting in an increased serum BUN, yet there is little difference in concentrations between the blood and abdominal effusion. Creatinine is a larger molecule, unable to equilibrate as it diffuses slowly across the peritoneal membrane. Consequently, the concentration of creatinine in the abdominal effusion is significantly higher than in blood. Therefore, comparing creatinine concentrations of the peritoneal effusion to that of the serum creatinine supports the diagnosis of uroabdomen if the ratio is ≥2:1 [2, 13, 54]. Potassium is absorbed down the concentration gradient into the systemic circulation, resulting in hyperkalemia. The kidneys attempt to maintain homeostasis by increasing excretion of potassium [13], leading to even higher concentrations accumulating in the abdomen. Potassium cannot be absorbed across the peritoneal membrane as fast as it is excreted into the peritoneal cavity, resulting in concentrations in abdominal fluid higher than in peripheral blood [13, 55]. In dogs, a potassium ratio >1.4:1 is consistent with uroabdomen [13, 54], and a ratio >1.9:1 is diagnostic in cats [2]. However, it is imperative to collect serum and abdominal effusion samples at the same time.

Creatinine is also an osmotically active particle, creating a concentration gradient that draws fluid out of the intracellular and intravascular spaces into the peritoneal cavity [6] inducing hypovolemia, leading to hemodynamic compromise and hypovolemic shock [12]. Chemical peritonitis not only induces pain but also the resultant loss of protein into the abdomen decreases TS and exacerbates associated fluid shifts. The perceived volume depletion stimulates AVP secretion, resulting in water intake and retention by the kidneys, which dilutes plasma sodium, inducing hyponatremia. Additionally, since urine is usually sodium and chloride poor, sodium, chloride, and water move into the abdominal cavity due to the favorable concentration gradient and equilibrate rapidly across the peritoneal membrane [12]. The hypochloremia and hyponatremia are exacerbated if vomiting occurs [2, 12].

Concurrent dehydration and hypovolemia from fluid shifts exacerbate azotemia, metabolic acidosis, electrolyte derangements, and hypovolemic shock [7, 53]. Decreased GFR and inability to excrete urine may also lead to hyperphosphatemia, which may complex with calcium; therefore, iCa may be decreased. Hyperlactatemia occurs due to failure of oxygen delivery to the tissues either in the traumatized patient or in dehydration secondary to hypovolemia or cardiovascular compromise [12], exacerbating metabolic acidosis [53]. Respiratory compensation for metabolic acidosis may be manifested clinically by larger TV and occasionally by tachypnea [12].

Preanesthetic Management and Initial Stabilization

Treatment for uroabdomen ultimately depends on location and severity of damage to the urinary tract [2]. Although surgery is often necessary to repair the source of urine leakage, patients with concurrent trauma-related myocarditis, pulmonary contusions, or brain injuries or those with hypovolemia and acid–base and electrolyte abnormalities are poor anesthetic candidates. Uroabdomen is a medical emergency and prognosis improves after stabilization (Table 7.1), particularly in the absence of other injuries [13, 23]. Therefore, before surgical repair, the patient should be stable with respect to metabolic and electrolyte disturbances, cardiac stability, and renal function [13, 23, 55].

Uroabdomen patients are stabilized and monitored as described in the preceding text for urethral obstruction, and therapy is based on the individual patient's status. Although management of life-threatening hypovolemia and hyperkalemia is a priority, regardless of concomitant injuries or etiology, chemical peritonitis can be very painful [13]; therefore, pain management is imperative and initial analgesic drug choices are based on the patient's stability and concomitant conditions (Tables 7.2 and 7.5). Additionally, broad-spectrum antibiotic therapy should be administered early in septic patients; however, nephrotoxic choices should be avoided.

Fluid therapy and drainage of urine from the peritoneal cavity appear to be the most important factors in stabilization of patients with uroperitoneum [2] in addition to managing hyperkalemia (Table 7.4). IV fluids reestablish tissue perfusion and oxygen delivery, aid in reduction of hyperkalemia, and help resolve metabolic acidosis. Adequate venous access with multiple peripheral catheters is ideal. A balanced electrolyte solution such as Normosol-R or LRS in comparison to 0.9% sodium chloride may more rapidly improve acid–base status while not exacerbating preexisting acidosis [17, 18]. Sodium bicarbonate administration is reserved for cases exhibiting severe acidosis despite fluid therapy (Table 7.4). As previously detailed, fluid rate should be based on the patient needs, tailored to reach endpoints of resuscitation with concomitant conditions. As previously mentioned, increments of approximately 25% of a shock dose (approximately 20 ml kg^{-1} in dogs, approximately 12 ml kg^{-1} in cats) over 15–20 min and reevaluation of endpoints such as mentation, HR, CRT, ABP, and, ideally, urine output is advised prior to continued fluid boluses. Hypertonic (7.5%) saline solution (4–7 ml kg^{-1} in dogs, 3–4 ml kg^{-1} in cats) or synthetic colloids such as hydroxyethyl starch (5–10 ml kg^{-1} in dogs, 3–5 ml kg^{-1} in cats with normal capillary permeability) over 10 min may be considered for rapid volume expansion and maintenance of ABP in some cases. Large volumes of intraabdominal fluid may exert pressure on the diaphragm, which can compress the lungs, induce hypoxemia, and contribute to arrhythmias. Therefore, while fluid resuscitation is underway, ECG evaluation and laboratory diagnostics should be initiated in addition to oxygen supplementation, unless these procedures stress the patient. Although CVP has been shown to be an inaccurate method for evaluation of fluid responsiveness, in the awake patient or when dynamic monitoring devices are unavailable, trends in CVP may be considered when used in conjunction with other markers of resuscitation endpoints and CO. Additionally, the jugular catheter permits central venous access for assessment of global tissue oxygenation with central venous oxygen saturation ($S_{cv}O_2$). Although $S_{cv}O_2$ is a surrogate for mixed venous oxygen saturation (S_vO_2), they parallel each other, with a normal value of >70%. A reduction in $S_{cv}O_2$ may indicate reduced DO_2 or increases in oxygen uptake (VO_2) [56]. Furthermore, securing an arterial catheter provides minute-to-minute accurate blood pressure and waveform analysis.

Hyperkalemia is the likely cause of death in untreated uroperitoneum; therefore, if hyperkalemia is present, treatment must be focused on this life-threatening issue and any concurrent critical injuries [12]. Recall that hyperkalemia increases the resting membrane potential of the cell (making it less negative), which leads to a reduced gradient between the resting membrane and threshold potential, resulting in increased cell membrane excitability [13]. Deadly cardiac conduction disturbances can result, progressing from bradycardia to ventricular fibrillation or asystole (Table 7.3). Since the threshold potassium levels cannot predict the development of hyperkalemic-induced life-threatening arrhythmias, suspect uroabdomen patients should always undergo an ECG as part of their baseline diagnostics. Management of hyperkalemia is identical to that in urinary obstruction with calcium therapy for immediate life-saving stabilization of the myocardium, in addition to dilutional fluid therapy simultaneously increasing GFR, and in combination with methods of redistribution and elimination (Table 7.4). Concurrent abnormalities such as metabolic acidosis and hypocalcemia can exacerbate the effects of hyperkalemia on cardiac conduction and must also be corrected [13].

Urinary Diversion

Abdominal drainage expedites stabilization by reducing urine accumulation, therefore preventing continued resorption of electrolytes and waste products, and assisting with resolution of azotemia and hyperkalemia [2]. Peritoneal drainage can be accomplished with the aid of a local block and needle drainage or indwelling peritoneal drain with a closed collection system. Appropriate sedation to prevent movement and resultant iatrogenic trauma is advised (Table 7.2).

It is important to consider abdominal compartment syndrome and the risk of hemodynamic consequences secondary to rapid removal of abdominal fluid, including reperfusion injury. Even free-flow drainage could induce cardiovascular collapse or the vasovagal reflex. Therefore, it is suggested to drain the abdomen slowly to avoid consequences such as hypotension or arrhythmias. Additionally, a urinary catheter should be placed into the bladder, to not only quantify urine output, but to maintain bladder decompression, thereby reducing hydrostatic pressure and the possibility of leakage into the abdomen. In the case of unresolved urethral obstruction or urethral damage, cystocentesis may be an alternative to catheterization.

Sedation and Anesthesia

Anesthetic complications secondary to uncorrected dehydration, hypovolemia, electrolyte, or acid–base abnormalities, and abdominal compartment syndrome may occur; therefore, resolution of these abnormalities prior to anesthesia may be more important than anesthetic drug selection. In dogs with uroabdomen, 36% had intraoperative complications including hypotension, bradycardia, hemorrhage, regurgitation, and death [53]. Furthermore, 5% of dogs surgically managed had septic uroabdomen [53], emphasizing that anesthetic protocols should be selected for individual patients rather than a cookbook recipe for all patients within a disease category.

Drugs to be used with caution or to be avoided are listed in Table 7.5. The use of NSAIDs is not recommended due to the presence of hypovolemia and postrenal azotemia. Acepromazine-induced vasodilation is contraindicated with concurrent hypovolemia, dehydration, or hypotension. Alpha-2-adrenergic receptor agonist agents induce peripheral vasoconstriction, significant bradycardia, decreased CO, and may possibly induce arrhythmias especially with concurrent electrolyte disturbances, azotemia, or preexisting rhythm disturbances [13, 26]. Additionally, these agents induce diuresis, which may be contraindicated in patients with uroabdomen [13]. Ketamine is mainly metabolized by the liver and its metabolites excreted by the kidneys to varying degrees based on species; therefore, ketamine or its metabolites may constantly be resorbed with uroabdomen, possibly leading to prolonged anesthetic times [13]. Cats rely more heavily on renal excretion; therefore, effects may be exacerbated in this species. However, ketamine can be administered, perhaps at a reduced initial dosage, with repeat dosing or CRI only after urinary elimination is established or imminently pending. In cats, systemic lidocaine should be avoided or used with caution, since it has been shown to have no impact on thermal threshold [57] and is associated with cardiovascular depression [58].

Reversible drugs are ideal, avoiding those that may have negative effects on cardiac function and renal or gastrointestinal (GI) blood flow [13]. Analgesia provided by pure mu-opioid receptor agonists such as fentanyl (Table 7.2) is advised. Drugs that can induce vomiting, such as IM morphine or hydromorphone, should be used with caution, particularly in an unfasted, sedated, or mentally depressed patient. Additionally, antiemetic and/or promotility drugs should be considered. The dose of opioids should be decreased in the critically ill patient to decrease exacerbation of concurrent bradycardia, hypotension, or hypoventilation [13].

Anesthetic induction may occur with many protocols including ketamine coinduction with a benzodiazepine or propofol, keeping in mind that the negative cardiovascular effects of ketamine may be seen in a catecholamine-depleted patient. Debilitated patients may respond well to a combined fentanyl and benzodiazepine induction. Propofol is acceptable in a stable patient; however, it should be used with caution as a sole agent in debilitated patients due to potential dose-dependent vasodilation and hypotension. Hypotension may be decreased with volume loading, small doses of propofol titrated to effect, or adequate sedation and coinduction agents to reduce the dose. Alfaxalone may be selected in an appropriately premedicated patient; when used at recommended doses it maintains cardiovascular parameters within normal limits in healthy animals and is an acceptable induction agent at a dose of 1–2 mg kg^{-1} IV over 60 s in dogs considered to be a poor anesthetic risk [29]. As previously mentioned, similar to propofol, respiratory depression and apnea can occur with alfaxalone; therefore, its use requires supplemental oxygenation and the ability to intubate the airway.

Anesthetic maintenance with inhalational anesthetics is acceptable, although dose requirements are expected to be reduced in septic patients. In addition, these patients may also have significant vasodilation and hypotension. Managing hypotension includes reducing the vaporizer setting by implementing CRIs of opioids, ketamine, or lidocaine (only in canine patients) (Table 7.2), simultaneously ensuring appropriate intravascular volume, adequate HR with anticholinergics, and normothermia, and administering positive inotropes and vasopressors where appropriate. Serial measurements in dynamic indices such as PVI/PPV may assist in evaluating fluid responsiveness and need for additional therapies to manage hypotension. Lumbosacral epidural analgesics and/or anesthetics (Table 7.2) provide preemptive analgesia and decrease central sensitization, intraoperative inhalant levels, opioid requirements, and the need for postoperative rescue analgesia [33]. However, epidural anesthesia is contraindicated in patients that are septic, coagulopathic, and/or hypovolemic. Alternatively, consider a fascial plane block, such as a TAP block, with ultrasound guidance.

High volumes of intraabdominal fluid may induce abdominal compartment syndrome, which has progressive detrimental effects on the cardiovascular, respiratory, and CNS systems [59, 60] that may be exacerbated during sedation or anesthesia. Compression of the vena cava results in decreased venous return with resultant reduction in CO and hypotension. Diaphragmatic motions are decreased with ensuing compression of the lungs, decreased functional residual capacity (FRC), and impaired pulmonary function [59]. Dorsal recumbency exacerbates these changes. Hypoxemia may contribute to arrhythmias, and mask or flow-by oxygen during sedation procedures is recommended. Preoxygenation prior to anesthesia and intensive monitoring including RR and effort, SpO_2, $ETCO_2$, blood gases, ECG, lactate, and ABP should be performed. Additionally, positive end-expiratory pressure (PEEP) or higher peak inspiratory pressure (PIP) to recruit collapsed alveoli may not be effective in these situations and could be detrimental to venous return and CO, contributing to hypotension [61]. Release of pressure-inducing fluid from the abdomen during stabilization or in surgery may resolve these issues. However, it is advised to release fluid slowly, monitoring lung expansion and for cardiovascular collapse. Particularly if intraabdominal fluid remains at induction, intermittent positive pressure ventilation (IPPV) is advised. Other ventilation strategies may be indicated based on blood gas findings to avoid respiratory acidosis, considering the effects of pH on calcium, potassium, HR, respirations, blood vessels, and ABP.

Recovery and Postoperative Care

Postoperative complications occur in 53% of dogs with uroabdomen, and include death, regurgitation, persistent leakage of urine, aspiration pneumonia, disseminated intravascular coagulation (DIC), incisional infection leading to septic peritonitis, urinary incontinence, and anemia requiring blood transfusion [53]. Continued monitoring and cardiovascular support is imperative throughout the recovery period. Hands-on evaluation of HR and pulse quality, MM color, and CRT in addition to ECG, ABP, SpO_2, and $ETCO_2$ (until extubated) is advised. Continued fluid therapy, oxygen supplementation, inotrope or vasopressor support, and analgesics (Table 7.2) are expected, with selection based on individual patient needs. Blood gas evaluation, lactate, BG, PCV/TS, and coagulation panels should be considered to determine continued supportive care. The patient should remain intubated until the return of a strong gag or swallow, and until the patient can lift its head or remain in sternal recumbency. A nasogastric (NG) tube may be placed prior to anesthetic recovery to remove excess GI fluid and permit enteral support. An indwelling urinary catheter and possibly a cystostomy tube may be in place, necessitating the need for an Elizabethan collar.

Pyometra

Pyometra is an infectious and inflammatory condition of the uterus secondary to a bacterial infection, usually within 4 months post estrus; *Escherichia coli* is the most common pathogen. The pathogenesis involves hormonal factors in which progesterone plays a key role for establishment of infection with ascending opportunistic bacteria. The overall incidence in dogs is 199 per 10000 dog-years at risk [62]. Pyometra is not as common in cats; 2.2% are diagnosed before 13 years of age, with an incidence rate of 17 cats per 10000 cat-years at risk [63]. Surgical ovariohysterectomy is the safest and most effective treatment, as it removes the source of infection and prevents recurrence; however, medical management may be considered in select cases. Pyometra leads to generalized illness and, in severe cases, induces endotoxemia, sepsis [62], and systemic inflammatory response (SIRS). Therefore, immediate care is essential as patient status may deteriorate rapidly and early diagnosis, stabilization, and treatment increase the chances of survival. The mortality rate for pyometra is 3–20% [64]; however, if more severe systemic illness or complications (e.g., uterine rupture, peritonitis, or septic shock) develop, mortality is considerably higher. In fact, the mortality rate for queens with pyometra and uterine rupture is 57% [65].

Clinical Signs and Physical Exam

Clinical signs vary based on the severity of the disease and may include anorexia, weight loss, depression, lethargy, vomiting, diarrhea, polydipsia, polyuria, and mucopurulent to hemorrhagic vaginal discharge. If the cervix is closed, vaginal discharge will be absent and systemic illness is more severe [66]. Physical exam may reveal dehydration, tachycardia, tachypnea, weak pulse quality, pale, hyperemic, or toxic MM, fever, abdominal pain on palpation, and possibly an enlarged uterus. The abdomen should be palpated with care, as the uterus may be friable and subject to rupture [62].

Initial Database and Clinicopathology

Disease is easy to recognize in classic cases, but often challenging in cases with a closed cervix or obscure history. Diagnosis is based on clinical signs and physical examination, hematology and biochemistry panels, and diagnostic images revealing intrauterine fluid (Figure 7.3) [62]. A CBC, biochemical and coagulation panel, and blood gas should be performed. Leukocytosis, neutrophilia with a left shift, monocytosis, and normocytic, normochromic regenerative anemia are frequently seen in addition to hypovolemia or sepsis-induced liver and renal dysfunction [62]. Hyperproteinemia secondary to dehydration or hypoproteinemia secondary to sepsis-induced hypoalbuminemia may be seen. An initial hyperglycemia may progress to hypoglycemia in sepsis secondary to decreased gluconeogenesis, glycogen store depletion, and increased glucose utilization. Endotoxin is released into the circulation when bacteria lyse, induce local and systemic inflammation resulting in fever, lethargy, tachycardia, and tachypnea, and may induce fatal shock, DIC, and generalized organ failure [67]. Circulating inflammatory mediators and acute phase proteins may be increased, and a hypercoagulable state may exist. Approximately 60% of bitches and 86% of queens with pyometra suffer from sepsis [62, 68]. Therefore, pyometra is considered an emergency with surgery to promptly follow patient stabilization to remove the infection source. Medical treatment is not recommended in patients with serious illness, peritonitis, organ dysfunctions, or a closed cervix.

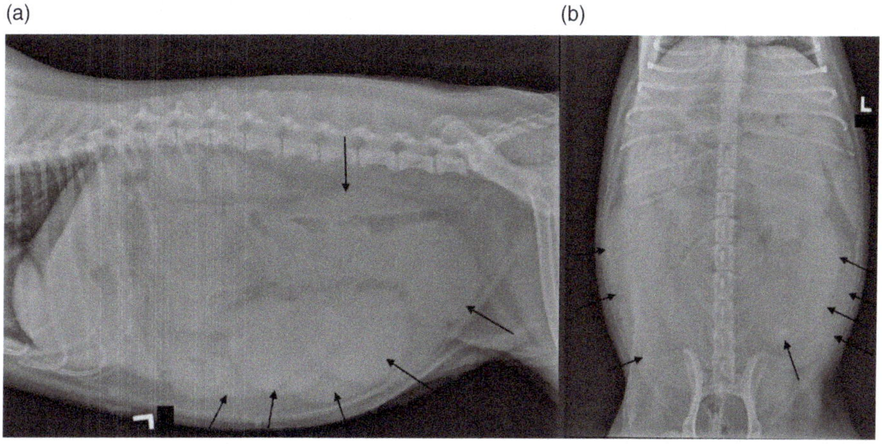

Figure 7.3 (a) Lateral and (b) ventrodorsal radiographic views of the abdomen. Multiple severely dilated soft tissue opaque tubular structures are identified within the mid to caudal abdomen (arrows), most consistent with an enlarged uterus. This patient was confirmed to have a pyometra.

Preanesthetic Management and Initial Stabilization

Removal of the infection is imperative due to the risk of endotoxemia and sepsis, but patients should be stabilized prior to surgery with adequate fluid therapy to correct hypotension, hypoperfusion, shock, dehydration, acid–base and electrolyte abnormalities, hypoglycemia, coagulation disturbances, and organ dysfunctions. Antibiotics should be administered early and selected to target the common pathogen; however, cases with sepsis should be administered antibiotics covering a wider range of pathogens while avoiding those with nephrotoxic properties [62]. While urgent stabilization is key, pain and stress during patient handling should be avoided, remedied with sedation and analgesia (Table 7.2), and considering individual patient needs.

Multiple, large-bore IV catheters should be placed to provide early goal-directed therapy with isotonic crystalloid fluids to restore circulating volume and tissue perfusion and normalize DO_2. Supplemental glucose should be provided as needed and adjusted based on serial evaluations. As stated earlier in this chapter, there is no evidence-based consensus on the most advantageous use of colloids in either human or veterinary medicine, and the optimal fluid choice and use of colloids remain debatable [44]. Hypertonic (7.5%) saline solution may be considered to maintain ABP and volume expansion. Blood products should be available for management of coagulopathy, and their effects on intravascular volume considered when calculating total fluid volume to be administered.

Serial lactate measurements can help gauge response to fluid therapy and endpoints of resuscitation, as hyperlactatemia is a cardinal sign of inadequate DO_2. In addition to supplemental oxygen, evaluation of serial ABP, temperature, HR and rhythm, MM color, continuous ECG, SpO_2 monitoring, and blood gas analysis is recommended throughout stabilization. Measuring CVP to aid in evaluation of fluid responsiveness is no longer recommended in humans or animals. However, central venous access may be obtained by a jugular catheter extending cranial to the right atrium to assess global tissue oxygenation with $S_{cv}O_2$ [56].

Arterial catheterization may be used for invasive ABP monitoring and blood gas sampling, although the benefits and risks in a patient with sepsis and clotting abnormalities should be weighed, particularly in felines. Patients in cardiovascular shock are vasodilated and may remain hypotensive despite volume resuscitation and may require vasopressors and/or inotropic support. Norepinephrine may be preferred in septic shock due to its actions on alpha-adrenergic receptors inducing vasoconstriction at clinically used doses, with the addition of vasopressin if norepinephrine is ineffective. iCa should be evaluated, and supplementation may be useful in the management of hypotension. Additionally, low-dose hydrocortisone may be considered if the patient is sympathetically exhausted; however, controversy and uncertainty exist with critical illness-related corticosteroid insufficiency; therefore, dosing regimen, duration of treatment, and tapering the protocol remain at the clinician's discretion [69].

Anesthesia and Monitoring

Monitoring is focused on maintaining hemodynamic function, cellular oxygenation, and pain management. Prior to induction, supplemental oxygen should be administered, and monitoring including ECG and ABP evaluation should be in place. Anesthetic protocols must be individualized according to the specific needs of each patient. Pyometra patients may be in shock, and the sympathetic nervous system (SNS) is stimulated to maintain DO_2. Many anesthetics blunt the response of the SNS, impair contractility, and induce vasodilation; therefore, a patient in compensatory shock may decompensate, particularly if not stabilized prior to anesthesia [30].

Septic animals often experience acid–base abnormalities, vasoplegia, altered pharmacokinetics and drug distribution, and hypoglycemia, all of which could contribute to reduced inhalant and systemic anesthetic requirements; therefore, reduced drug doses are expected. The IV administration route is preferred over IM or SC to permit drug titration, since the duration of action may be increased if abnormal hepatic and renal perfusions are present.

Cardiovascular and respiratory effects of agents in addition to their contraindications should be considered (Table 7.5). Premedication is indicated to provide adequate analgesia and sedation and reduce induction and maintenance drug requirements. Phenothiazine tranquilizers should be avoided in patients with cardiovascular instability or hypovolemia. Alpha-2-adrenergic receptor agonists are generally avoided in critical patients due to profound changes in CO and ABP. However, some data suggest that alpha-2-adrenergic receptor agonists lead to an improvement in microcirculation and reduce noradrenaline requirements in cases of septic shock, to which further investigation is required [70]. Benzodiazepines cause minimal cardiopulmonary depression; a small dose IV alone can induce profound sedation in critical patients and may be used as a coinduction agent. Opioid analgesics spare the cardiovascular system, but may induce vagally mediated bradycardia, which is managed with anticholinergic drugs. Opioids should be considered essential in a balanced anesthetic protocol, particularly in sick patients. Dose-dependent respiratory depression may occur; however, this is not a contraindication for use, but rather encourages attention to titration and monitoring. Fentanyl is recommended over IV administration of morphine and meperidine due to potential for histamine release with secondary vasodilation and hypotension, and IM administration of hydromorphone may induce vomiting, which is less likely with IV administration. GI protectants may be selected, particularly in the unfasted patient and those with vomiting or regurgitation.

Induction drugs should be administered with care, using the smallest dose, titrated slowly, to reach the desired effect to minimize their negative cardiovascular effects. Induction of unstable patients may be achieved with a combination of fentanyl and a benzodiazepine titrated IV to effect. Low-dose ketamine (0.5 mg kg^{-1} IV premedication, 0.6 mg kg^{-1} h^{-1} CRI intraoperatively, and 0.3 mg kg^{-1} h^{-1} CRI

24 h postoperatively) attenuates the inflammatory response and postoperative concentrations of serum C-reactive protein (CRP) in dogs with pyometra [71], and therefore should be considered. Ketamine, in combination with a benzodiazepine or propofol induction, may provide cardiovascular stability; however, awareness in critical patients with catecholamine depletion is advised due to ketamine's direct myocardial depressant effects potentially resulting in hypotension. Propofol decreases cardiac contractility and induces vasodilation and should be titrated slowly to effect and in combination with other agents (benzodiazepines, opioids, ketamine) to reduce the required dose. Additionally, alfaxalone administered at 1–2 mg kg^{-1} IV over 60 s is acceptable [29]. Septic patients may have relative adrenal insufficiency; therefore, etomidate should be used with caution or avoided due to its adrenocortical suppression [72].

Anesthetic maintenance with inhalant anesthetics creates a dose-dependent myocardial depression, hypotension, and respiratory depression. Monitoring depth is imperative to prevent anesthetic overdose particularly in septic patients who require a lower concentration of inhalants and have vasoplegia resulting in vasodilation and hypotension. Thus, inhalational anesthetic-sparing protocols are advised to ameliorate their effects on hypotension. Multimodal balanced anesthesia may be provided by a CRI of drugs such as fentanyl, ketamine, or midazolam. Additionally, lidocaine infusions may be used in dogs for the anesthetic-sparing [73], anti-inflammatory, anti-endotoxin [74, 75], and possible analgesic [76, 77] effects. Epidural morphine or local anesthetic administration may reduce intraoperative inhalant requirements; however, may be contraindicated in the face of sepsis, coagulopathy, or hypotension. Alternatively, fascial plane blocks such as an ultrasound-guided TAP block may be considered to provide perioperative regional analgesia to the abdominal wall [78]. Additionally, intraperitoneal or incisional bupivacaine (cats: 2 mg kg^{-1}, dogs: 4.4 mg kg^{-1}) following surgical completion may provide postoperative analgesia [49, 50].

Intraoperative monitoring and management of derangements including ECG, SpO_2, $ETCO_2$, HR, RR, and temperature should be routine, recalling that inhalant anesthetic requirements decrease with hypothermia. Anticholinergics should be available for management of vagally mediated bradycardia that can be induced upon handling of the abdominal organs. BG monitoring every 30–60 min with IV dextrose supplementation as needed is recommended in hypoglycemic and septic patients. IPPV to maintain PaO_2 and normocapnia with the aid of serial blood gas samples permits monitoring for acidosis and allows adjustments in ventilation. In the presence of hypovolemia or vasoplegia, positive pressure-induced hypotension may occur. Thus, lower TVs aimed at minimizing the impact on lung tissue, venous return, and CO should be used. Alternatively, a degree of permissive hypercapnia may be considered in hypotensive patients. Intraoperative fluid support should be customized to individual patient needs based on serial monitoring parameters including $S_{cv}O_2$, PVI/PPV or other dynamic indices, lactate, blood gases, invasive ABP, PCV/TS, HR, CRT, and MM color. Management of hypotension to maintain MAP above 60–70 mmHg may require inotropic (dopamine: 5–10 μg kg^{-1} min^{-1}, or dobutamine: 2–10 μg kg^{-1} min^{-1}; may be used concurrently), vasopressor (ephedrine 0.05–0.5 mg kg^{-1}, norepinephrine 0.1–1.0 μg kg^{-1} min^{-1}, vasopressin 0.01–0.01 μg kg^{-1} h^{-1}), and/or calcium support, in addition to anesthetic-sparing techniques mentioned in the preceding text. Hypotension that persists despite intense management may be remedied with discontinuation of inhalant anesthesia and transition to total IV anesthesia, and a CRI of agents such as fentanyl, ketamine, propofol, and lidocaine (canine patients) may be effective. Additionally, blood products should be available for management of concurrent of developing coagulopathy or intraoperative blood loss.

Recovery and Postoperative Care

Intensive postoperative monitoring is essential. Patients should be supported with external heat sources to normothermia. BG and ABP should be monitored with continued dextrose, inotropes, or vasopressors supplemented as needed. SpO_2 should continue to be evaluated with supplemental oxygen supplied until ventilating appropriately, verified with blood gas analysis. Continuous ECG, particularly in critical patients, is advised and lactate and urine output should be monitored to assist maintenance of circulating volume. Evaluation of MM color and CRT, PCV/TS, and clotting panels can help assess the need for blood products. Enteral nutrition may be considered to decrease IV fluid volumes and risk of fluid overload in the recovery period. Additionally, GI protectant and motility medications are recommended. Analgesics should be customized to the individual patient based on serial evaluations and commonly include a CRI (Table 7.2) of an opioid, ketamine, or lidocaine (canine patients).

Nonurgent Urogenital Procedures

Laparoscopic Urogenital Procedures

Laparoscopic assistance may be selected for management of many urogenital procedures and generally occur in a stable patient. The anesthetic protocol selection is based on the individual patient and procedure. Carbon dioxide (CO_2) is the preferred choice for insufflation, since it has a higher blood solubility than air, decreasing the risk of complications associated with venous emboli, and is nonflammable, therefore permitting simultaneous safe use of electrocautery. However, some potential complications exist. For example, hypercarbia may result in spontaneously breathing anesthetized patients secondary to absorption of CO_2 into the bloodstream; therefore, controlled ventilation may be required to maintain arterial CO_2 levels ($PaCO_2$) within normal parameters. Additionally, creation of a pneumoperitoneum and secondary increases in intraabdominal pressure have significant cardiovascular and respiratory consequences. Insufflation may result in displacement of the diaphragm cranially with compression of the lungs resulting in atelectasis, decreased FRC, and ventilation–perfusion mismatch resulting in hypoxemia and hypercarbia [79]. Additionally, the resultant decreased compliance potentiates the risk of barotrauma with IPPV. Therefore, ensuring an adequate fraction of inspired oxygen (FiO_2) is advised in addition to closely monitoring $ETCO_2$ and $PaCO_2$ values with cautious IPPV to prevent hypercapnia and barotrauma. Compression of the vena cava may reduce venous return to the heart with subsequent decreased CO and ABP; therefore, adequate volume support should be available, with inotropes or vasopressors administered as needed. Intraabdominal pressure should ideally be measured and kept well below approximately 20 mmHg [80].

Cystourethroscopy

Cystourethroscopy should be performed under general anesthesia to ensure patient comfort/relaxation and prevent movement, reducing the risk of iatrogenic trauma to the urinary tract. Many anesthetic protocols are appropriate and should be based on the individual patient. Incorporating benzodiazepines or acepromazine may be considered due to their actions on urethral (skeletal) muscle. Concurrent medications prescribed for their antispasmodic effects may have an impact on the anesthetic event, such as drugs with alpha-adrenergic receptor blocking actions (prazosin, phenoxybenzamine, and acepromazine). Alpha-adrenergic receptor blockade may result in vasodilation and hypotension, exacerbated in anesthetized patients; therefore, avoiding administration of additional alpha-adrenergic receptor blocking anesthetic drugs may be considered. Amitriptyline, an antidepressant drug, has alpha-adrenergic receptor blocking actions and anticholinergic effects and may be prescribed in patients with lower urinary tract disease; potential side effects include hypotension, tachycardia, arrhythmias, and sedation [79].

Following cystourethroscopy, patients show clinical signs of lower urinary tract discomfort for 2–5 days [81]. Therefore, methods to reduce discomfort include topical bupivacaine (2 mg kg^{-1} diluted 50:50 with saline) administered through the cystourethroscope as it is withdrawn. In addition, opioid analgesics such as buprenorphine, corticosteroids, or NSAIDs to reduce urethritis may be considered, based on the individual patient. Urethral antispasmodic drugs such as prazosin (1 mg per 15 kg^{-1} q 8 h in dogs and 0.25–0.5 mg total dose q 8–12 h in cats) are also an option [81].

Renal Biopsy

Renal disease is common in dogs and cats with varying degrees of abnormalities (see Chapter 6). Renal biopsies may be required to establish a definitive diagnosis in animals with renal disease and permit appropriate treatment. Studies reveal that immobilization is an important component for proper technique, and biopsies were more likely to be high quality if obtained while under general anesthesia [82]. Techniques may include percutaneous blind, percutaneous with ultrasound guidance, surgical or laparoscopic.

After careful consideration of the anesthetic protocol based on the individual patient (see Chapter 6), the anesthetist should be prepared to manage common complications of renal biopsy. Patients with renal compromise may have abnormalities including azotemia, uremic coagulopathy, hyperkalemia or hypokalemia, hypocalcemia, anemia, hypoalbuminemia, dehydration, hypertension, and metabolic acidosis, among other derangements. Recommended preoperative evaluation includes CBC, biochemistry and coagulation panels, blood gas evaluation, ABP measurement, and buccal mucosal bleeding times, as uremia is associated with abnormalities in platelet function [42]. While infrequent complications associated with renal biopsy occur in dogs (3.4%) and cats (8.5%), the most common was severe hemorrhage and this occurred in 9.9% of dogs and 16.9% of cats with complications [82]. Systemic hypertension or administration of NSAIDs within the previous five days may increase the risk of hemorrhage [82] in addition to azotemia, thrombocytopenia, or prolonged clotting times [42]. Therefore, blood typing and crossmatching are advised in animals with coagulopathy or anemia and blood products should be available.

Anesthetic protocols should be tailored to the individual patient and may include premedication with a combination of opioid and benzodiazepine, propofol or alfaxalone induction, and inhalant maintenance. Supplemental oxygen during the preanesthetic period and IV catheter placement is advised. Monitoring should be routine including temperature, SpO_2, ECG, capnometry, and ABP measurement. IV fluid supplementation rate is based on the individual patient. If hemorrhage occurs, blood products should be prepared and calculated for rapid response and administration.

Urinary Tract Diagnostic Imaging

Minimally invasive procedures for the diagnosis and treatment of congenital, acquired, and neoplastic conditions of the urinary tract are increasingly available and include routine radiography, ultrasound, fluoroscopy, and computed tomography (CT). Regardless of the imaging modality, radiation safety should be a priority for personnel. Furthermore, the anesthetist must ensure access to the patient for monitoring and to provide heat support, both of which must be achieved without interfering with the imaging procedures.

Excretory Urography

Excretory urography (Figure 7.4) involves the use of IV-administered iodinated contrast followed by one of several imaging modalities. Patient contraindications include dehydration, uncontrolled congestive heart failure, sensitivity to contrast material, and severe kidney failure [83]. As discussed in the preceding text, this procedure should be delayed until life-threatening metabolic derangements are stabilized. Patients should be appropriately sedated or under general anesthesia to optimize study quality and reduce radiation exposure to personnel. The use of nonionic organic iodides, such as iohexol, versus ionic agents is advised to reduce the frequency and severity of contrast agent reactions due to their lower osmolarity [84]. However, injection of systemic contrast media is not without risk, which may exacerbate renal injury and adverse effects may involve hemodynamic changes, including hypotension and anaphylactic shock. If an adverse reaction occurs, treatment is palliative and supportive. In addition to ensuring an adequate airway, oxygen, and hemodynamic support, severe anaphylactic shock and bronchospasms may require epinephrine, antihistamines, glucocorticoids, bronchodilators, vasopressors, or anticholinergics [79].

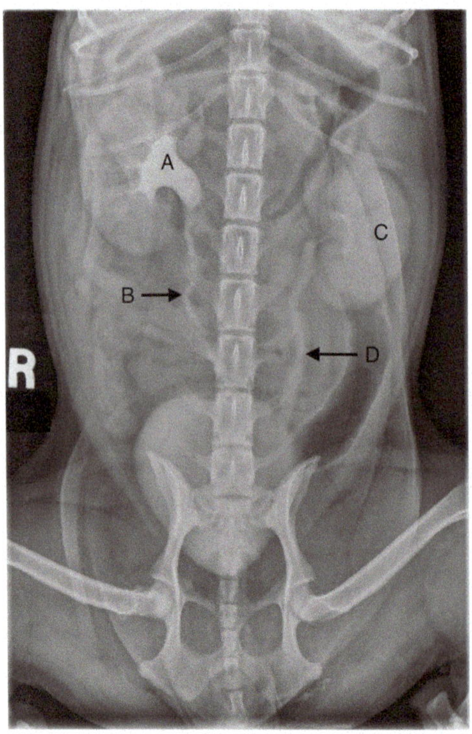

Figure 7.4 Excretory urography with positive (iodinated) contrast, ventrodorsal view. (A) Right hydronephrosis; (B) dilated right ureter (hydroureter); (C) left kidney with a mildly dilated renal pelvis; (D) dilated left ureter (hydroureter).

Cystography/Urethrography

Cystography and urethrography (Figure 7.5) involve instillation of a positive and/or negative contrast agent into the urinary bladder and/or urethra followed by one of several imaging modalities. Sedation or anesthesia is strongly recommended to minimize patient

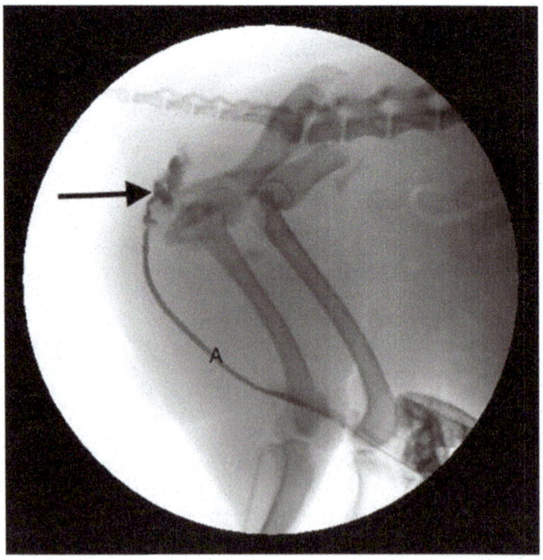

Figure 7.5 Fluoroscopic image, lateral view of the pelvis. Retrograde positive-contrast urethrogram in a male dog. (A) Normal penile urethra; arrow points to irregular, extravasated contrast at the level of the membranous urethra, consistent with a urethral tear. Note also the multiple pelvic fractures in this case, as the patient (1-year-old dog) had recent trauma.

pain and risk of iatrogenic trauma during urinary catheter placement, and additionally enhancing study quality and reducing radiation exposure to personnel. To ease urinary catheter placement and patient discomfort, sterile lidocaine gel may be applied to the catheter; however, attention to the dose in cats and small patients is advised, since systemic absorption may occur. This procedure should be delayed in patients with life-threatening metabolic derangements until deemed stable for sedation or anesthesia.

References

1 Balakrishnan, A. and Drobatz, K.J. (2013). Management of urinary tract emergencies in small animals. *Vet. Clin. North Am. Small Anim. Pract.* 43: 843–867.

2 Aumann, M., Worth, L.T., and Drobatz, K.J. (1998). Uroperitoneum in cats: 26 cases (1986-1995). *J. Am. Anim. Hosp. Assoc.* 34: 315–324.

3 O'Hearn, A.K. and Wright, B.D. (2011). Coccygeal epidural with local anesthetic for catheterization and pain management in the treatment of feline urethral obstruction. *J. Vet. Emerg. Crit. Care* 21: 50–52.

4 Lekcharoensuk, C., Osborne, C.A., and Lulich, J.P. (2001). Epidemiologic study of risk factors for lower urinary tract diseases in cats. *J. Am. Vet. Med. Assoc.* 218: 1429–1435.

5 McLoughlin, M.A. (2000). Surgical emergencies of the urinary tract. *Vet. Clin. North Am. Small Anim. Pract.* 30: 581–601.

6 Rieser, T.M. (2005). Urinary tract emergencies. *Vet. Clin. North Am. Small Anim. Pract.* 35: 359–373.

7 Lee, J.A. and Drobatz, K.J. (2003). Characterization of the clinical characteristics, electrolytes, acid-base, and renal parameters in male cats with urethral obstruction. *J. Vet. Emerg. Crit. Care* 13: 227–233.

8 Lee, J.A. and Drobatz, K.J. (2006). Historical and physical parameters as predictors of severe hyperkalemia in male cats with urethral obstruction. *J. Vet. Emerg. Crit. Care* 16: 104–111.

9 Burrows, C.F. and Bovee, K.C. (1978). Characterization and treatment of acid-base and renal defects due to urethral obstruction in cats. *J. Am. Vet. Med. Assoc.* 172: 801–805.

10 Drobatz, K.J. and Hughes, D. (1997). Concentration of ionized calcium in plasma from cats with urethral obstruction. *J. Am. Vet. Med. Assoc.* 211: 1392–1395.

11 Polzin, D.J., Osborne, C.A., and Bartges, J.W. (1996). Management of postrenal azotemia. *Vet. Clin. North Am. Small Anim. Pract.* 26: 507–513.

12 Costello, M.F. (2011). Urinary tract trauma. In: *Manual of Trauma Management in the Dog and Cat* (eds. K.J. Drobatz, M.W. Beal and R.S. Syring), 176–190. Chichester, UK: Wiley.

13 Stafford, J.R. and Bartges, J.W. (2013). A clinical review of pathophysiology, diagnosis, and treatment of uroabdomen in the dog and cat. *J. Vet. Emerg. Crit. Care* 23: 216–229.

14 Tag, T.L. and Day, T.K. (2008). Electrocardiographic assessment of hyperkalemia in dogs and cats. *J. Vet. Emerg. Crit. Care* 18: 61–67.

15 Beer, K.S. and Drobatz, K.J. (2016). Severe anemia in cats with urethral obstruction: 17 cases (2002-2011). *J. Vet. Emerg. Crit. Care* 26: 393–397.

16 Mathews, K.A. and Dyson, D.H. (2005). Analgesia and chemical restraint for the emergent patient. *Vet. Clin. North Am. Small Anim. Pract.* 35: 481–515.

17 Drobatz, K.J. and Cole, S.G. (2008). The influence of crystalloid type on acid-base and electrolyte status of cats with urethral obstruction. *J. Vet. Emerg. Crit. Care* 18: 355–361.

18 Cunha, M.G., Freitas, G.C., Carregaro, A.B. et al. (2010). Renal and cardiorespiratory effects of treatment with lactated ringer's solution or physiologic saline (0.9% NaCl) solution in cats with experimentally induced urethral obstruction. *Am. J. Vet. Res.* 71: 840–846.

19 Osborne, C.A., Lees, G.E., Polzin, D.J. et al. (1984). Immediate relief of feline urethral obstruction. *Vet. Clin. North Am. Small Anim. Pract.* 14: 585–597.

20 George, C.M. and Grauer, G.F. (2016). Feline urethral obstruction: diagnosis & management. *Today's Vet. Pract.*: 36–44.

21 Cooper, E.S. (2015). Controversies in the management of feline urethral obstruction. *J. Vet. Emerg. Crit. Care* 25: 130–137.

22 Hall, J., Hall, K., Powell, L.L. et al. (2015). Outcome of male cats managed for urethral obstruction with decompressive cystocentesis and urinary catheterization: 47 cats (2009-2012). *J. Vet. Emerg. Crit. Care* 25: 256–262.

23 Stilwell, C. (2017). Medical management of uroabdomen in cats. *Vet. Ireland J.* 7: 431–435.

24 KuKanich, B., Bidgood, T., and Knesl, O. (2012). Clinical pharmacology of nonsteroidal anti-inflammatory drugs in dogs. *Vet. Anaesth. Analg.* 39: 69–90.

25 Saleh, N., Aoki, M., Shimada, T. et al. (2005). Renal effects of medetomidine in isoflurane-anesthetized dogs with special reference to its diuretic action. *J. Vet. Med. Sci.* 67: 461–465.

26 Kennedy, M.J. and Johnson. R.A. (2015). Dexmedetomidine & atipamezole. NAVC Clin Brief 65–67.

27 Slade, T.J., Grover, J., and Benger, J. (2008). Atropine-resistant bradycardia due to hyperkalaemia. *Emerg. Med. J.* 25: 611–612.

28 Senthilkumaran, S., David, S.S., Manikam, R. et al. (2013). Atropine resistant bradycardia and hyperkalemia: our experiences. *Am. J. Emerg. Med.* 31: 1415.

29 Psatha, E., Alibhai, H.I.K., Jimenez-Lozano, A. et al. (2011). Clinical efficacy and cardiorespiratory effects of alfaxalone, or diazepam/fentanyl for induction of anaesthesia in dogs that are a poor anaesthetic risk. *Vet. Anaesth. Analg.* 38: 24–36.

30 Campbell, V.L. (2005). Anesthetic protocols for common emergencies. *Vet. Clin. North Am. Small Anim. Pract.* 35: 435–453.

31 Hanna, R.M., Borchard, R.E., and Schmidt, S.L. (1988). Pharmacokinetics of ketamine HCl and metabolite I in the cat: a comparison of i.v., i.m., and rectal administration. *J. Vet. Pharmacol. Ther.* 11: 84–93.

32 Waterman, A.E. (1983). Influence of premedication with xylazine on the distribution and metabolism of intramuscularly administered ketamine in cats. *Res. Vet. Sci.* 35: 285–290.

33 Garcia-Pereira, F. (2018). Epidural anesthesia and analgesia in small animal practice: an update. *Vet. J.* 242: 24–32.

34 Galluzzi, F., Fd, R., Menozzi, A. et al. (2012). Effect of intraurethral administration of atracurium besylate in male cats with urethral plugs. *J. Small Anim. Pract.* 53: 411–415.

35 Smeak, D.D. (2000). Urethrotomy and urethrostomy in the dog. *Clin. Tech. Small Anim. Pract.* 15: 25–34.

36 Luca, G.C., Monteiro, B.P., Dunn, M. et al. (2017). A retrospective study of anesthesia for subcutaneous ureteral bypass placement in cats: 27 cases. *J. Vet. Med. Sci.* 79: 992–998.

37 Hardie, E.M. and Kyles, A.E. (2004). Management of ureteral obstruction. *Vet. Clin. North Am. Small Anim. Pract.* 34: 989–1010.

38 Kyles, A.E., Hardie, E.M., Wooden, B.G. et al. (2005). Clinical, clinicopathologic, radiographic, and ultrasonographic abnormalities in cats with ureteral calculi: 163 cases (1984-2002). *J. Am. Vet. Med. Assoc.* 226: 932–936.

39 Snyder, D.M., Steffey, M.A., Mehler, S.J. et al. (2005). Diagnosis and surgical management of ureteral calculi in dogs: 16 cases (1990-2003). *N. Z. Vet. J.* 53: 19–25.

40 Berent, A.C. (2011). Ureteral obstructions in dogs and cats: a review of traditional and

new interventional diagnostic and therapeutic options. *J. Vet. Emerg. Crit. Care* 21: 86–103.

41 Garcia de Carellan Mateo, A., Brodbelt, D., Kulendra, N. et al. (2015). Retrospective study of the perioperative management and complications of ureteral obstruction in 37 cats. *Vet. Anaesth. Analg.* 42: 570–579.

42 Bigge, L.A., Brown, D.J., and Penninck, D.G. (2001). Correlation between coagulation profile findings and bleeding complications after ultrasound-guided biopsies: 434 cases (1993-1996). *J. Am. Anim. Hosp. Assoc.* 37: 228–233.

43 Fantoni, D. and Shih, A.C. (2017). Perioperative fluid therapy. *Vet. Clin. North Am. Small Anim. Pract.* 47: 423–434.

44 Wong, C. and Koenig, A. (2017). The colloid controversy: are colloids bad and what are the options? *Vet. Clin. North Am. Small Anim. Pract.* 47: 411–421.

45 Adamik, K.N., Yozova, I.D., and Regenscheit, N. (2015). Controversies in the use of hydroxyethyl starch solutions in small animal emergency and critical care. *J. Vet. Emerg. Crit. Care* 25: 20–47.

46 Davis, H., Jensen, T., Johnson, A. et al. (2013). AAHA/AAFP fluid therapy guidelines for dogs and cats. *J. Am. Anim. Hosp. Assoc.* 49: 149–159.

47 Glover, P.A., Rudloff, E., and Kirby, R. (2014). Hydroxyethyl starch: a review of pharmacokinetics, pharmacodynamics, current products, and potential clinical risks, benefits, and use. *J. Vet. Emerg. Crit. Care* 24: 642–661.

48 Hutchinson, K.M. and Shaw, S.P. (2016). A review of central venous pressure and its reliability as a hemodynamic monitoring tool in veterinary medicine. *Top Comp. Anim. Med.* 31: 109–121.

49 Carpenter, R.E., Wilson, D.V., and Evans, A.T. (2004). Evaluation of intraperitoneal and incisional lidocaine or bupivacaine for analgesia following ovariohysterectomy in the dog. *Vet. Anaesth. Analg.* 31: 46–52.

50 Benito, J., Monteiro, B., Lavoie, A.M. et al. (2016). Analgesic efficacy of intraperitoneal administration of bupivacaine in cats. *J. Feline. Med. Surg.* 18: 906–912.

51 Sano, H., Seo, J., Wightman, P. et al. (2018). Evaluation of pulse pressure variation and pleth variability index to predict fluid responsiveness in mechanically ventilated isoflurane-anesthetized dogs. *J. Vet. Emerg. Crit. Care* 28: 301–309.

52 Celeita-Rodriguez, N., Teixeira Neto, F.J., Garofalo, N.A. et al. (2019). Comparison of the diagnostic accuracy of dynamic and static preload indexes to predict fluid responsiveness in mechanically ventilated, isoflurane anesthetized dogs. *Vet. Anaesth. Analg.* 46: 276–288.

53 Grimes, J.A., Fletcher, J.M., and Schmiedt, C.W. (2018). Outcomes in dogs with uroabdomen: 43 cases (2006-2015). *J. Am. Vet. Med. Assoc.* 252: 92–97.

54 Schmiedt, C., Tobias, K.M., and Otto, C.M. (2001). Evaluation of abdominal fluid: peripheral blood creatinine and potassium ratios for diagnosis of uroperitoneum in dogs. *J. Vet. Emerg. Crit. Care* 11: 275–280.

55 Burrows, C.F. and Bovee, K.C. (1974). Metabolic changes due to experimentally induced rupture of the canine urinary bladder. *Am. J. Vet. Res.* 35: 1083–1088.

56 Noel-Morgan, J. and Muir, W.W. (2018). Anesthesia-associated relative hypovolemia: mechanisms, monitoring, and treatment considerations. *Front. Vet. Sci.* 5: 53.

57 Pypendop, B.H., Ilkiw, J.E., and Robertson, S.A. (2006). Effects of intravenous administration of lidocaine on the thermal threshold in cats. *Am. J. Vet. Res.* 67: 16–20.

58 Pypendop, B.H. and Ilkiw, J.E. (2005). Assessment of the hemodynamic effects of lidocaine administered IV in isofluraneanesthetized cats. *Am. J. Vet. Res.* 66: 661–668.

59 Nielsen, L.K. and Whelan, M. (2012). Compartment syndrome: pathophysiology, clinical presentations, treatment, and prevention in human and veterinary medicine. *J. Vet. Emerg. Crit. Care* 22: 291–302.

60 An, G. and West, M.A. (2008). Abdominal compartment syndrome: a concise clinical review. *Crit. Care Med.* 36: 1304–1310.

61 Marolf, V., Mirra, A., Fouche, N. et al. (2018). Advanced atrio-ventricular blocks in a foal undergoing surgical bladder repair: first step to cardiac arrest? *Front. Vet. Sci.* 5: 5.

62 Hagman, R. (2018). Pyometra in small animals. *Vet. Clin. North Am. Small Anim. Pract.* 48: 639–661.

63 Hagman, R., Holst, B.S., Moller, L. et al. (2014). Incidence of pyometra in Swedish insured cats. *Theriogenol.* 82: 114–120.

64 Kenney, K.J., Matthiesen, D.T., Brown, N.O. et al. (1987). Pyometra in cats: 183 cases (1979-1984). *J. Am. Vet. Med. Assoc.* 191: 1130–1132.

65 Davidson, A.P., Feldman, E.C., and Nelson, R.W. (1992). Treatment of pyometra in cats, using prostoglandin-F2-alpha: 21 cases (1982-1990). *J. Am. Vet. Med. Assoc.* 200: 825–828.

66 Jutkowitz, L.A. (2005). Reproductive emergencies. *Vet. Clin. North Am. Small Anim. Pract.* 35: 397–420.

67 McAnulty, J.F. (1983). Septic shock in the dog: a review. *J. Am. Anim. Hosp. Assoc.* 19: 827–836.

68 Brady, C.A., Otto, C.M., Van Winkle, T.J. et al. (2000). Severe sepsis in cats: 29 cases (1986-1998). *J. Am. Vet. Med. Assoc.* 217: 531–535.

69 Creedon, J.M.B. (2015). Controversies surrounding critical illness-related corticosteroid insufficiency in animals. *J. Vet. Emerg. Crit. Care* 25: 107–112.

70 Geloen, A., Pichot, C., Leroy, S. et al. (2015). Pressor response to noradrenaline in the setting of septic shock: anything new under the sun-dexmedetomidine, clonidine? A minireview. *BioMed. Res. Int.* 2015: 863715.

71 Liao, P., Chang, S., Chen, K. et al. (2014). Decreased postoperative C-reactive protein production in dogs with pyometra through the use of low-dose ketamine. *J. Vet. Emerg. Crit. Care* 24: 286–290.

72 Jackson, W.L. (2005). Should we use etomidate as an induction agent for endotracheal intubation in patients with septic shock? *Chest* 127: 1031–1038.

73 Valverde, A., Doherty, T.I., Hernandez, J. et al. (2004). Effect of lidocaine on the minimum alveolar concentration of isoflurane in dogs. *Vet. Anaesth. Analg.* 31: 264–271.

74 Fletcher, J.R. and Ramwell, P.W. (1978). E-coli endotoxin-shock in dog-treatment with lidocaine or indomethacin. *Br. J. Pharmacol.* 64: 185–191.

75 Bellini, L. and Seymour, C.J. (2016). Effect of intraoperative constant rate infusion of lidocaine on short-term survival of dogs with septic peritonitis: 75 cases (2007-2011). *J. Am. Vet. Med. Assoc.* 248: 422–429.

76 Ortega, M. and Cruz, I. (2011). Evaluation of a constant rate infusion of lidocaine for balanced anesthesia in dogs undergoing surgery. *Can. Vet. J.* 52: 856–860.

77 Smith, L.J., Bentley, E., Shih, A. et al. (2004). Systemic lidocaine infusion as an analgesic for intraocular surgery in dogs: a pilot study. *Vet. Anaesth. Analg.* 31: 53–63.

78 Schroeder, C.A., Snyder, L.B.C., Tearney, C.C. et al. (2011). Ultrasound-guided transversus abdominis plane block in the dog: an anatomical evaluation. *Vet. Anaesth. Analg.* 38: 267–271.

79 Robertson, S.A. (1999). Newer diagnostic and surgical techniques and their impact on anesthesia. *Vet. Clin. North Am. Small Anim. Pract.* 29: 665–682.

80 Gross, M.E., Jones, B.D., Bergstresser, D.R. et al. (1993). Effects of abdominal insufflation with nitrous oxide on cardiorespiratory measurements in spontaneously breathing isoflurane-anesthetized dogs. *Am. J. Vet. Res.* 54: 1352–1353.

81 Morgan, M. and Forman, M. (2015). Cystoscopy in dogs and cats. *Vet. Clin. North Am. Small Anim. Pract.* 45: 665–701.

82 Vaden, S.L., Levine, J.F., Lees, G.E. et al. (2005). Renal biopsy: a retrospective study of methods and complications in 283 dogs and 65 cats. *J. Vet. Intern. Med.* 19: 794–801.

83 Rademacher, N. (2019). Diagnostic imaging of the urinary tract. *Vet. Clin. North Am. Small Anim. Pract.* 49: 261–286.

84 Pollard, R.E. and Pascoe, P.J. (2008). Severe reaction to intravenous administration of an ionic iodinated contrast agent in two anesthetized dogs. *J. Am. Vet. Med. Assoc.* 233: 274–278.

8

Perioperative Fluid, Electrolyte, and Acid–Base Disturbances

Carolyn L. Kerr

Department of Clinical Studies, Ontario Veterinary College, Guelph, Ontario, N1H 2W1, Canada

Introduction

Alterations in body fluid volume, distribution, and composition, including disturbances in osmolality, electrolytes, and acid–base status, are not uncommon in veterinary patients presenting for anesthesia, particularly in the emergency setting. This chapter focuses on some of the most common disturbances in body fluid volume and composition, their etiologies, and the impact of their change on clinical management of patients before, during, and immediately after anesthesia. Additional literature addressing body fluid regulation physiology and pathophysiology and acid–base balance should be consulted for comprehensive reviews on this subject [1–4].

In general, perturbations in a patient's hydration, intravascular fluid volume, electrolyte composition, and/or acid–base status may be a manifestation of a disorder that has overwhelmed the body's ability to compensate for losses or additions in its content, or it may be indicative of a failure in regulatory mechanisms responsible for maintaining fluid and electrolyte balance. Disease processes involving the gastrointestinal, urological, and endocrine systems are the most common causes of fluid, electrolyte, and acid–base disturbances in patients requiring therapeutic interventions requiring anesthesia. A thorough patient history, physical examination, and blood electrolyte and gas analysis provide essential information during the assessment of body fluid disturbances. More in-depth diagnostics including urine specific gravity, urine electrolyte composition, thoracic radiography, and abdominal ultrasound will be required in select cases. Consequences of abnormalities in body fluid volume and composition most commonly include alterations in central nervous system (CNS), cardiac, and neuromuscular functions, all of which may alter the patient's response to drugs used in the perianesthetic period. Large multicenter studies have demonstrated an increase in perioperative mortality in human patients with alterations in serum electrolyte and acid–base status [5–9]. In veterinary medicine, several investigations on anesthetic-related morbidity and mortality have shown a negative impact of increasing American Society of Anesthesiologists (ASA) status on outcome [10–13]. While underlying conditions resulting in a patient being assigned an ASA status of III and IV are likely to be associated with fluid, electrolyte, and acid–base disturbances, specific details regarding patient hydration, intravascular volume, and

Canine and Feline Anesthesia and Co-Existing Disease, Second Edition. Edited by Rebecca A. Johnson, Lindsey B. C. Snyder and Carrie A. Schroeder.

Companion website: www.wiley.com/go/johnson/canine

acid–base and electrolyte status specifically on anesthetic outcome in clinical veterinary patients remain largely unknown. Current recommendations for patient management at this time are therefore primarily based on clinician experiences, data from human trials, and experimental investigations in veterinary species rather than from prospective or retrospective studies in veterinary patient populations. In general, recommendations regarding the management of a patient's water, electrolyte, and acid–base disturbances in the perianesthetic period are heavily influenced by the severity of the disturbance, as well as the nature of the underlying and concurrent conditions. At this time, studies evaluating patient outcome with various hemostatic alterations, as well as the response to specific goal-directed therapies, are appearing in the literature and will help to inform future strategies, as will be discussed.

In the normal animal, body fluid volume and composition, including water and electrolytes, are regulated by several overlapping mechanisms (Table 8.1). Disturbances in a patient rarely occur in isolation; however, for purposes of discussion, the chapter has been organized to address alterations in hydration, intravascular fluid volume, electrolytes, and acid–base disturbances.

Body Fluids

Body fluids are composed of water and dissolved solutes. Water makes up approximately 60% of the total body weight of domestic animal species, with two-thirds located in the intracellular space (approximately 40% of total body weight) and one-third located in the extracellular space (approximately 20% of total body weight). Of the extracellular water,

Table 8.1 Major physiologic factors that regulate body water and electrolytes [1–3].

Variable	Regulatory mechanism	Primary stimulus	Primary effect
Water	ADH	Serum osmolality	Increase water reabsorption in kidney
	Thirst	Serum osmolality	Increase water intake
Sodium	Aldosterone	Hyperkalemia, angiotensin II, adrenocorticotropic hormone (ACTH)	Increase Na^+ reabsorption in kidney
	Epinephrine	Sympathetic nervous system stimulation	Increase Na^+ reabsorption in kidney
	Angiotensin II	Renal perfusion	Increase Na^+ reabsorption in kidney
	ADH	Serum osmolality	Alter water reabsorption in kidney
Chloride	Kidney	Sodium, acid–base status	Alter sodium and chloride reabsorption
Potassium	Aldosterone	Hyperkalemia, angiotensin II	Decrease K^+ reabsorption in kidney
	Epinephrine	Sympathetic nervous system stimulation	Increase intracellular K^+ movement
	Insulin	Serum glucose	Increase intracellular K^+ movement
Calcium	Parathyroid hormone	Serum-ionized calcium	Increase Ca^{2+} reabsorption in kidney Increase Ca^{2+} mobilization from bone Increase calcitriol synthesis
	Calcitriol	Parathyroid hormone	Increase Ca^{2+} intestinal absorption
	Calcitonin	Serum-ionized calcium	Reduce Ca^{2+} mobilization from bone

roughly two-thirds is in the interstitial fluid space (approximately 15% of total body weight) and one-third in the intravascular space (approximately 5% of total body weight). Of note, the volume of water in the intravascular space constitutes approximately 50–60% of the total blood volume.

In general, there are major differences in solute concentrations, notably electrolytes and negatively charged proteins, between intracellular and extracellular spaces, whereas small differences exist between the interstitial and intravascular spaces (Table 8.2).

Varying solute concentrations play a key role in the oncotic and osmotic pressures and the net electrical potential in each space. Water and solutes move between different compartments via multiple mechanisms depending on the specific substance and the barrier separating the space. A semipermeable cell membrane, which is highly permeable to water but not solutes, separates the intracellular and extracellular spaces. Water moves between these latter two spaces through the cell membrane because of an osmotic pressure gradient created by differences in the number of osmotically active particles in each space. Solute movement between the intracellular and extracellular spaces occurs through channels in the cell membrane. In some cases, solutes can flow passively through channels. However, in other cases, they require active transport.

While the cell membrane separates the intracellular and extracellular spaces, the capillary endothelium separates the extracellular space into interstitial and intravascular fluid spaces. The classical description of transcapillary fluid movement is based on Starling's principle, whereby hydrostatic and oncotic forces that exist in the capillary and interstitial fluid are the major determinants of fluid fluxes across the capillary endothelium. Essentially, the hydrostatic pressure in the capillary and the oncotic forces in the interstitium are proposed to force water out of the capillary at the arteriolar end of the capillary, while oncotic pressure in the capillary pulls fluid back into the capillary at the venular end. While this fluid movement theory has guided the basic principles of fluid therapy for many decades, recent research has shifted the understanding regarding fluid and solute movement through fenestrated capillaries. A revised Starling's equation of fluid movement takes into consideration the endothelial glycocalyx layer, a membrane bound layer composed of glycoproteins and proteoglycans, as well as the endothelial basement membrane and the extracellular matrix [14]. The classic and revised Starling equations are illustrated in Table 8.3. Key principles in the current understanding of fluid dynamics between the interstitial and

Table 8.2 Approximate electrolyte content in intracellular, interstitial, and intravascular fluid spaces [3].

	Intracellular fluid (skeletal muscle cell; mmol l^{-1})	Interstitial fluid (mmol l^{-1})	Intravascular fluid (plasma; mmol l^{-1})
Na^+	12	145	142
K^+	140	4	4.3
Ca^{2+}	4.0	2.4	2.5
Mg^{2+}	34	1.1	1.1
Cl^-	4	117	104
HCO_3^-	12	27	24
HPO_4^{2-}, $H_2PO_4^-$	40	2	2
$Proteins^-$	50	0	14

Table 8.3 Classic and revised Starling's equation [14].

Classic Starling equation	Revised Starling equation
Net filtration = $K_fS\,[(P_{cap} - P_i) - \sigma\,(\pi_{cap} - \pi_i)]$	Net filtration = $K_fS\,[(P_{cap} - P_{sg}) - \sigma\,(\pi_{cap} - \pi_{sg})]$
K_fS = filtration coefficient	K_fS = filtration coefficient
P_{cap} = capillary hydrostatic pressure	P_{cap} = capillary hydrostatic pressure
P_i = interstitial hydrostatic pressure	P_{sg} = sub-glycocalyx hydrostatic pressure
π_{cap} = capillary oncotic pressure	π_{cap} = capillary oncotic pressure
π_i = interstitial oncotic pressure	π_{sg} = sub-glycocalyx oncotic pressure

intravascular spaces in the nondisease state relevant to the veterinary clinician include:

- The presence of an endothelial glycocalyx. This layer contributes to intravascular fluid volume and the oncotic forces within the capillary. The endothelial glycocalyx also acts as the barrier for fluid movement from the capillaries through the endothelial channels located in the sub-glycocalyx layer. Various disease states can result in endothelial glycocalyx dysfunction and a resultant increase in endothelial permeability [15].
- Unidirectional fluid movement into the capillary lumen from the interstitial space. Traditionally, bidirectional fluid movement was believed to occur between the capillary and interstitial space. It is now understood that minimal fluid movement back through fenestrated endothelial cells from the interstitial space occurs. Fluid that filters out of fenestrated capillaries returns to the circulation via the lymphatic system and cannot be "pulled back" into the vasculature through increasing oncotic pressure.
- Important forces in fluid movement out of capillaries are the transendothelial pressure difference and the plasma to sub-glycocalyx colloidal oncotic pressure.

In addition to fluid shifts between the various body compartments, body water intake and loss are regulated primarily by thirst and the impact of antidiuretic hormone (ADH), also known as arginine vasopressin (AVP), on the kidney. In the healthy animal, an increase in serum osmolality results in stimulation of osmoreceptors in the anterior hypothalamus, which increases thirst, and the release of AVP from the posterior pituitary. AVP, acting on collecting duct receptors of the kidney, promotes water reabsorption, resulting in a serum osmolality decrease. Alternatively, a decrease in serum osmolality results in a reduction in AVP secretion, decreasing the water reabsorption from the urine. In addition to serum osmolality, other factors can also influence AVP release from the posterior pituitary, including a decrease in blood volume or blood pressure. Several drugs, including morphine, phenothiazines, and barbiturates can also increase AVP section and alter body fluid dynamics. In humans and dogs, anesthesia and surgery increase serum AVP concentrations, a response attributed to shifts in intravascular fluid volumes and pressures [16, 17]. Although changes in serum AVP levels were not measured, urine output in dogs was reduced and total body water increased during anesthesia with routine intravenous (IV) fluid strategies using crystalloids with or without surgery [17–19]. The clinical significance of the typical body fluid increase in normal animals during anesthesia with routine fluid therapy is not known; however, the clinician should be aware that urine output alone is not a good indicator of body water volume status in the anesthetized patient.

Dehydration and Intravascular Volume Deficits

Dehydration occurs when body fluid losses are in excess of gains. Depending on the relative loss of water to electrolytes, the losses can result in hypertonic, hypotonic, or isotonic dehydration, based on the tonicity of the remaining body fluids [20]. Dehydration is typically quantified by the percent deficit of total body volume. For example, a patient is 10% dehydrated when the total body fluid deficit in liters is equivalent to [0.1] × [body weight in kg]. Clinical signs of dehydration will depend on the type of dehydration and the concurrent electrolyte changes, but, in general, signs attributed to dehydration >5% include dry mucous membranes, decreased skin elasticity, dull mentation, and increased heart rate. As the degree of dehydration progresses, the quality of peripheral pulses decreases and enophthalmos develops. With >12% dehydration, significant cardiovascular consequences including inadequate tissue perfusion secondary to intravascular volume deficits occur, and shock develops [21].

In a clinical study evaluating preoperative factors associated with hypotension in healthy dogs undergoing desexing, urine specific gravity was negatively associated with mean arterial pressure, suggesting preoperative hydration may contribute to lower blood pressure during anesthesia [22]. While there are limited large clinical trials specifically evaluating patient preoperative hydration status on outcomes in the veterinary literature, preoperative dehydration increases postoperative morbidity and mortality in large clinical trials involving humans [23]. Anesthetic drugs and ventilatory support measures may alter preload, afterload, and myocardial contractility, and therefore contribute to a significant reduction in cardiac output at surgical anesthetic planes compared to the awake state in normal veterinary patients. Fortunately, such changes are generally well tolerated in normal patients due to a substantial cardiovascular reserve. However, if a patient is dehydrated during anesthesia, the reduction in stroke volume and cardiac output will be exacerbated and the resultant cardiac output may be inadequate. In addition to addressing the underlying dehydration etiology, volume-deficit treatment is required to improve the patient's hemodynamic stability prior to anesthesia. As described by the Frank–Starling law of the heart, stroke volume increases with increasing end-diastolic volume or preload within normal physiologic ranges, assuming other factors, such as myocardial contractility, remain constant.

Recommended treatment regimens for fluid volume replacement generally include calculating fluid deficits, ongoing losses, and maintenance requirements. The fluid administration rate to correct dehydration should depend on severity of the patient's clinical signs, their expected cardiovascular reserve, and urgency of the underlying condition. In the nonemergent situation, a patient's volume deficit should be replaced over 12–24 h; if this is not possible, it is ideal if anesthesia can be delayed until the patient's heart rate and arterial blood pressure are within normal ranges. General recommendations include replacing approximately 50% of the patient's volume deficit over 4–6 h prior to anesthesia with the remaining deficit replaced more slowly. For the patient presenting in shock, approximately 25% of the calculated deficit should be administered rapidly, and then the patient reassessed. If the patient remains hemodynamically unstable or no improvement is noted, an additional approximately 25% of the deficit can be replaced rapidly after which an alternative strategy, such as modifying the type of resuscitation fluid, or providing additional hemodynamic support including inotropes and vasoactive agents, should be considered. An example of initial fluid therapy plans for a patient with 10% dehydration is provided in Table 8.4.

Fluid choice to correct dehydration should be based on the patient's electrolyte, acid–base, and serum protein levels; however, a balanced electrolyte solution is generally the initial fluid of choice, with adjustments made based on the patient's response to treatment including repeated evaluation of packed cell volume (PCV), total solids, blood gases, and electrolytes. Rates up to 90 $\mathrm{ml\,kg^{-1}\,h^{-1}}$ in the dog or

Table 8.4 Initial fluid therapy strategy in cases with varying urgency.

	3-year-old Labrador Retriever	3-year-old Labrador Retriever
Case urgency	High: scheduled for surgery in 4 h	Low: scheduled for surgery in 12–24 h
% dehydration	8%	8%
Patient weight	30 kg	30 kg
Volume deficit	$= 0.08 \times 30\,\text{kg} = 2.4\,\text{l}$	$= 0.08 \times 30\,\text{kg} = 2.4\,\text{l}$
Intravenous fluid	Balanced electrolyte solution	Balanced electrolyte solution
Initial fluid plan	Replace 50% of deficit over 4 h = 300 ml h^{-1} for 4 h Replace remaining deficit related to dehydration over next 8 h = 150 ml h^{-1} for 8 h Maintenance fluid requirements and ongoing losses should be added to the volume calculated for dehydration correction	Replace 100% of deficit over 12 h = 200 ml h^{-1} for 12 h Maintenance fluid requirements and ongoing losses should be added to the volume calculated for dehydration correction

60 ml kg^{-1} h^{-1} in the cat can be administered in an urgent setting in patients with normal cardiovascular function; however, this rate should be administered using a titrated approach whereby the patient's hemodynamic response to 15–20 ml kg^{-1} (dog) or 10–15 ml kg^{-1} (cat) of fluid therapy is verified every 10–15 min. Rates should be reduced as soon as hemodynamic variables return to acceptable values. Patients in shock may benefit from a colloid solution if, after replacement of approximately 50% of the calculated deficits, there is no improvement of clinical signs. A colloid may also be used in conjunction with a balanced electrolyte solution, either initially or during rehydration, in patients with total solids <3.5 g dl^{-1} or albumin <1.5 g dl^{-1}. Synthetic colloids, including dextrans, gelatins, and hydroxylethyl starch (HES) solutions, offer a convenient and accessible alternative to natural colloids such as fresh frozen plasma or albumin; however, synthetic products have been linked to complications including interference with coagulation, allergic reactions, and acute kidney injury in both human and veterinary patients [24–27]. Considerable geographic disparity exists regarding the availability of different products; however, current general recommendations include maintaining strict adherence to the individual product's maximum daily dose, and avoiding their use in patients with preexisting coagulopathies, kidney disease, or sepsis. In the case of HES solutions, the maximum daily doses in dogs and cats are approximately 20 and 15 ml kg^{-1}, respectively. In patients with specific electrolyte disturbances, details regarding recommended fluid strategies are provided in the following text.

In addition to hypovolemia due to whole body dehydration, intravascular volume deficits secondary to blood loss are not uncommon in veterinary medicine. Blood loss may occur prior to presentation to the veterinary clinic, during anesthesia and surgery, or in the postoperative period. In many cases, it is challenging to determine the quantity of blood that has been lost and the clinician must rely on a patient's clinical signs. In the normal awake patient, an approximately 10% loss of blood volume can reduce cardiac output. However, up to a 30% blood volume loss can occur before a decrease in arterial blood pressure is observed [28]. As heart rate and blood pressure are generally the only hemodynamic variables measured in awake veterinary patients, the clinician may not recognize the severity of the vascular volume loss prior to anesthesia. In the anesthetized patient, however, hemodynamic alterations, including a decrease in blood pressure, can occur with as little as approximately 10% blood volume loss. Intraoperatively, fluid collection systems can help quantify the quantity of blood lost if volume measurements are included on the collection device (Figure 8.1). To correct for fluids used to lavage a surgical site, the PCV of the collected fluid can be measured and the quantity of blood loss calculated according to Eq. (8.1):

$$\text{Blood loss}\,(\text{ml}) = \left[(\text{PCV in jar}) \times (\text{ml in jar})\right] / \text{patient PCV} \quad (8.1)$$

Traditional therapeutic goals following blood loss or during active hemorrhage include maintaining indicators of perfusion, such as blood pressure, heart rate, urine output, and body temperature within normal ranges, maintaining oxygen delivery capacity by keeping the PCV above 20% (Hb>6 $g\,dl^{-1}$), and preventing coagulopathies associated with excessive dilution of platelet and coagulation factors. Replacement of mild intravascular fluid losses with a balanced electrolyte solution is generally used in the perioperative period in patients with normal hemodynamic variables. Due to crystalloid redistribution throughout the body fluid spaces, administration volume should be approximately three times the estimated intravascular volume loss, at least initially. Administration of 15–20 $ml\,kg^{-1}$ of a balanced electrolyte solution at a rate up to 90 $ml\,kg^{-1}\,h^{-1}$ in the dog or 10–15 $ml\,kg^{-1}$ of a balanced electrolyte solution at a rate up to 60 $ml\,kg^{-1}\,h^{-1}$ in the cat can be used initially in an emergency situation with repeated volume administration based on the response to treatment; however, if a patient is hemodynamically unstable due to primary blood loss, alternatives to crystalloids should be sought. Specifically, if a patient is estimated to have lost greater than 20–25% of their blood volume, or they present with a high heart rate, low peripheral vascular pressures, and the primary cause is likely due to blood loss secondary to trauma or internal bleeding, the patient has likely lost greater than 30% of their blood volume. In such cases, colloids are highly recommended, as patient outcome may be negatively affected if fluid therapy is restricted to crystalloids [29, 30]. The individual patient and clinical situation will dictate the specific colloid required. In patients that are suitable candidates for synthetic colloids, the maximum daily dose should not be exceeded. Replacement fluids containing red cells such as packed red cells, combined with fresh frozen plasma, or fresh whole blood are indicated with major blood loss (>30%), particularly if a coagulopathy or preexisting anemia exists. In patients with uncontrolled hemorrhage, limiting the volume of crystalloid fluid administration while transitioning to fresh whole blood is currently recommended [30]. Standard transfusion practices, including crossmatching and

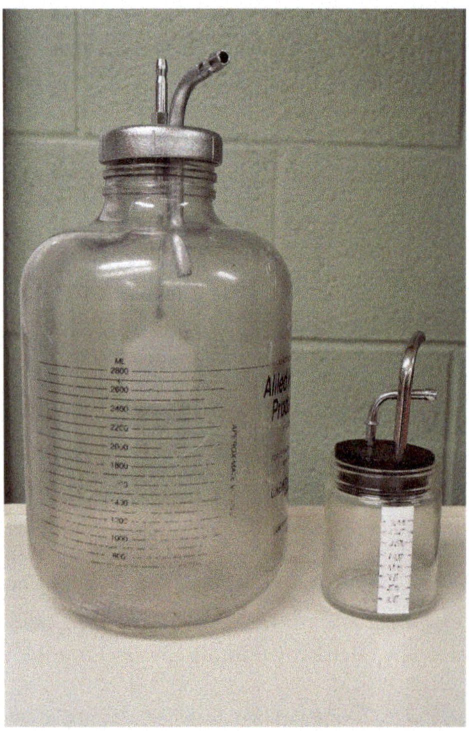

Figure 8.1 Example of a fluid collection system with numerical increments to quantify fluid/blood loss intraoperatively.

test dosing, should be followed. While the latter recommendations provide the clinician with guidelines, the individual patient's requirements will vary considerably and therapy should be individualized based on preexisting conditions, clinical response to treatment, and availability of suitable blood products. Use of antifibrinolytics, such as tranexamic acid, on outcomes of veterinary patients with massive blood loss remains to be determined [31, 32].

In humans, both perioperative patient overhydration and underhydration lead to increased morbidity; therefore, achieving euvolemia is a critical anesthetic goal [33, 34]. Goal-directed fluid therapy, in which individualized therapy is administered to achieve desired hemodynamic outcomes such as improvements in pulse pressure variation (PPV), stroke volume response to fluid challenge, and systolic pressure variation, is currently recommended to guide fluid therapy in humans undergoing major surgery [35, 36]. Preoperatively, patient mentation, core and peripheral body temperature, heart rate, blood pressure, urine output, and acid–base status can provide insight into rehydration adequacy in veterinary patients. Traditionally, arterial blood pressure, heart rate, urine output, repeat PCV/total solids measurement, and acid–base status have guided fluid administration rate intraoperatively. While these indices may provide an adequate guide to intravascular volume status of a patient, they are relatively nonspecific and insensitive. Ultimately, the goal is to provide intravascular volume expansion such that preload, or end-diastolic volume, results in a desired level of cardiac output. In veterinary medicine, assessment of fluid responsiveness in mechanically ventilated canine patients using real-time direct arterial pressure or plethysmographic (from the pulse oximeter) waveform analyses has shown promise (Figure 8.2) [37, 38]. For example, PPV≥13%, measured from the arterial pressure waveform, reasonably predicted fluid responsiveness in approximately 83% of dogs [37]. In addition, the noninvasive plethysmograph variability index (PVI), measured from the pulse oximeter, effectively predicted the PPV threshold value with high sensitivity and specificity [37].

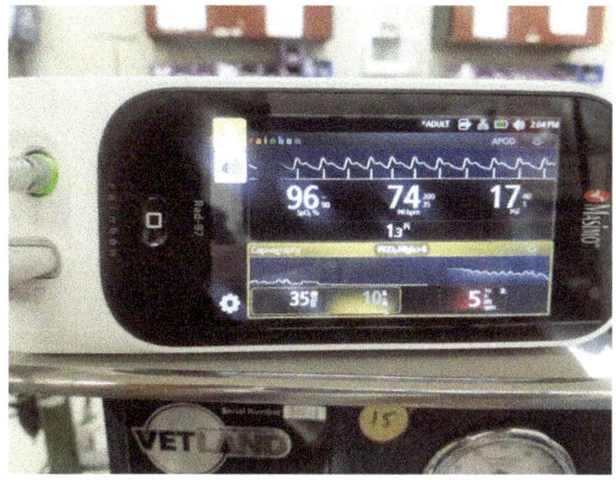

Figure 8.2 Example of a pulse oximeter which displays the plethysmograph variability index (PVI) used to determine fluid responsiveness in mechanically ventilated dogs. *Source*: Photo courtesy of Dr. R. Johnson, University of Wisconsin–Madison.

For hypovolemic patients requiring anesthesia, preoxygenation for 3–5 min is highly recommended prior to anesthetic induction to compensate for a potentially reduced cardiac output and/or reduced oxygen-carrying capacity secondary to decreased hemoglobin levels. Cardiopulmonary monitoring with an electrocardiogram (ECG), blood pressure monitor, and pulse oximeter should ideally start preoperatively and continue throughout the entire anesthetic period. Capnography and blood gas analysis should be added to the monitoring regimen during anesthesia. While no specific anesthetic regimen is contraindicated in the hypovolemic or dehydrated patient, sedative/anesthetic doses will be reduced. For example, propofol and ketamine doses, when used in combination with diazepam, were approximately 50% lower in hypovolemic compared with normal dogs [39]. In the critically ill patient, a combination of an opioid and benzodiazepine, such as hydromorphone (0.1 mg kg^{-1}) and diazepam/midazolam (0.2 mg kg^{-1}), is a suitable premedication and will induce less hemodynamic changes relative to other injectable techniques [39, 40]. The minimum alveolar concentration (MAC) of isoflurane is also reduced and inhalant delivery should be carefully titrated to effect [41]. The clinician should also be prepared to use constant rate infusions of opioid and nonopioid analgesics and, if feasible, locoregional blocks to reduce the inhalant anesthetic requirements and improve hemodynamic stability during anesthetic maintenance. Additional hemodynamic support measures such as inotrope and vasopressor infusions including dopamine and norepinephrine will also likely be required in these patients.

Alveolar hypoventilation and the associated increase in arterial carbon dioxide ($PaCO_2$) are not uncommon in compromised patients under general anesthesia and ventilatory support is frequently required. The increase in intrathoracic pressure during inspiration associated with positive pressure ventilation most notably reduces right ventricular preload and increases left ventricular afterload [42]. In some patients, this can result in a significant decrease in cardiac output, systemic arterial pressure (as noted with PPV and PVI), and overall oxygen delivery. The magnitude of these changes is dependent on the ventilatory strategy used and the patient's hemodynamic status. Therefore, if ventilatory support measures are required during anesthesia of the hypovolemic patient, strategies that utilize a low tidal volume and a long expiratory pause are recommended.

Electrolytes

Sodium

Most of the total body sodium is located within the extracellular space, with only low quantities located in the intracellular space, a relationship that is maintained by the cell membrane's Na^+-K^+-ATPase pump. Dietary intake is the sodium source for the body with sodium losses primarily occurring via the kidney in the normal dog and cat. In the kidney, sodium is freely filtered at the glomeruli, with reabsorption occurring to varying degrees in the renal tubules. Aldosterone is the major endogenous substance that controls the net quantity of sodium reabsorption (Table 8.1). Factors that increase the production and release of aldosterone and, therefore, the reabsorption of sodium include angiotensin II (which is increased secondary to a decrease in renal perfusion and activation of the renin–angiotensinogen–angiotensin I pathway), hyperkalemia, and adrenocorticotropic hormone. Factors that inhibit aldosterone release include atrial natriuretic factor and dopamine. Although possessing a less significant effect than aldosterone on sodium reabsorption in the kidney, catecholamines, and angiotensin II also directly impacts sodium excretion. Specifically, catecholamines increase sodium reabsorption at the proximal tubule via alpha-1-adrenergic-receptor-mediated effects and through stimulation of renin. Angiotensin II also directly promotes renal sodium reabsorption.

Serum (or plasma or whole blood) sodium concentrations are strictly a reflection of the quantity of sodium relative to the amount of water in the extracellular space and do not reflect total body sodium levels. Measured sodium levels result from factors that impact not only its own excretion and reabsorption, but also factors that influence water homeostasis in the body. Sodium, being the most plentiful ion in the extracellular fluid space, contributes most of the effective osmoles in serum. Thus, changes in serum sodium concentration impact serum osmolality and water homeostasis indirectly as described in the preceding text. The clinician needs to consider the patient's serum osmolality, hydration, and total body water status when presented with a hyponatremic or hypernatremic patient to devise a therapeutic plan as discussed in the following text. Overall, mismanagement of patients with abnormalities in serum sodium can lead to a delayed recovery or even deleterious outcomes; clinicians are encouraged to review sodium and water regulation physiology and the management of their disturbances prior to initiating therapy. Common causes of sodium abnormalities in the dog and cat are outlined in Table 8.5.

Table 8.5 Common causes of sodium disorders in dogs and cats [2, 43].

<table>
<tr><th></th><th>Hyponatremia</th><th>Hypernatremia</th></tr>
<tr><td>Altered losses</td><td>Increased Na⁺ loss[a]
Gastrointestinal loss (hypovolemic, hypoosmolality)
• Vomiting, diarrhea
Renal loss (hypovolemic, hypoosmolality)
• Hypoadrenocorticism
• Diuretics
Vascular loss (hypovolemic, hypoosmolality)
• Hemorrhage
Cutaneous loss (hypovolemic, hypoosmolality)
• Burns

Decreased water loss (gain of free water)
Drugs (hypervolemic, hypoosmolality)
Congestive heart failure (hypervolemic, hypoosmolality)
Liver disease (hypervolemic, hypoosmolality)
Renal disease (hypervolemic, hypoosmolality)
Psychogenic polydipsia (normovolemia, hypoosmolality)
Syndrome of inappropriate antidiuretic hormone secretion (normovolemia, hypoosmolality)</td><td>Increased water loss relative to Na⁺
Gastrointestinal loss (hypovolemic)
• Vomiting, diarrhea
Renal loss (hypovolemic or normovolemic)
• Diuresis (diabetes mellitus, postobstructive, mannitol)
• Renal disease
• Diabetes insipidus (central or nephrogenic)
Cutaneous loss (hypovolemic)
• Burns
Respiratory loss (hypovolemic)
• Panting
Fever (hypovolemic)
Decreased Na⁺ loss
Hyperadrenocorticism (hypervolemic)</td></tr>
<tr><td>Translocation</td><td>Greater Na⁺ movement relative to water
Third-space loss (hypovolemic, hypoosmolality)
• Peritonitis
• Ascites
• Ruptured bladder
Movement of water from intracellular fluid (ICF) into extracellular fluid (ECF)
Solute addition to ECF (hyperosmolality)
• Hyperglycemia
• Drugs: Mannitol</td><td>Greater water movement relative to Na⁺
Third-space loss (hypovolemic)
• Peritonitis
• Ascites
• Ruptured bladder</td></tr>
<tr><td>Altered intake or input</td><td>Decreased intake
Rare situation</td><td>Decreased water intake
Water deprivation (hypovolemic)
Increased Na⁺ intake
Salt poisoning (hypervolemic)
Hypertonic fluid or Na⁺ bicarbonate administration</td></tr>
</table>

[a] Sodium loss is generally an isotonic sodium loss with compensatory mechanisms to restore hypovolemia, resulting in hyponatremia.

Hyponatremia

Hyponatremia is generally defined as serum sodium concentrations <140 mmol l^{-1} in dogs, and 149 mmol l^{-1} in cats. Some authors define hyponatremia as a measured sodium concentration below the reference range, recognizing that values may vary according to analyzer type and nature of sample (whole blood versus serum) [43–45]. Common in hospitalized human patients, hyponatremia has been associated with an increase in morbidity and mortality, independent of the inciting cause [46, 47]. Furthermore, perioperative mortality in adult humans and pediatrics is elevated even when corrected for comorbidities [5, 6]. While no large multicenter prospective studies have been completed in veterinary medicine to date, hyponatremia has been associated with an increase in case fatality rate in both dogs and cats in a large retrospective study [48].

In veterinary patients requiring anesthesia, hyponatremia is most frequently associated with low plasma osmolality. However, it is possible for a patient to be hyponatremic and hyperosmolar if receiving mannitol or if severely hyperglycemic [48, 49]. Serum osmolality can be measured using an osmometer and it can be calculated using the following formulae (Eqs. (8.2) and (8.3)). Normally, the difference between the measured and calculated osmolality is 10 mOsm l^{-1}. An increase in this difference reflects an increase in unmeasured osmoles, such as mannitol or ethylene glycol:

$$\text{Calculated osmolality} = 2\left[\text{Na}^+\left(\text{mmol l}^{-1}\right)\right] + \text{glucose}\left(\text{mmol l}^{-1}\right) + \text{urea}\left(\text{mmol l}^{-1}\right) \tag{8.2}$$

or

$$\text{Calculated osmolality} = 2\left[\text{Na}^+\left(\text{mmol l}^{-1}\right)\right] + \left[\text{glucose}\left(\text{mg dl}^{-1}\right)/18\right] + \left[\text{urea}\left(\text{mg dl}^{-1}\right)/2.8\right] \tag{8.3}$$

Although rare, hyponatremic patients can also have a normal osmolality if they are hyperlipemic or severely hyperproteinemic. Generally, the clinical context, including patient history, physical examination, and awareness of concurrent medication, such as diuretics and glucocorticoids, in conjunction with standard preoperative diagnostics including serum biochemistry, provides the clinician with the most likely etiology and associated osmolality of the hyponatremia. In more complex cases, or cases with moderate to severe hyponatremia, urine electrolyte content and osmolality should be measured prior to initiation of therapy.

In addition to varying states of osmolality, patients can have different hydration states associated with low serum sodium levels. Hyponatremia with low plasma osmolality can be associated with hypovolemia, hypervolemia, or normovolemia, depending on the underlying etiology [44, 50]. A thorough preoperative assessment of patient hydration is also crucial to manage the patient appropriately in the perioperative period. The primary disturbances resulting in hypovolemic, hypoosmolar, hyponatremia are rarely associated with primary sodium loss; rather they are generally associated with isotonic or hypoosmolar fluid losses. Hyponatremia in these cases results from the compensatory mechanisms aimed at restoring blood volume including increased water intake and renal tubular reabsorption of water. In dogs, gastrointestinal or third-space losses are the most common extrarenal etiologies of hyponatremia, while in cats, urologic diseases, gastrointestinal, and third-space losses are the most common (Table 8.5) [48].

Clinical signs associated with hyponatremia are relatively nonspecific. Gastrointestinal signs such as vomiting and diarrhea are not uncommon and CNS signs can develop as a result of water shifting from the extracellular to the intracellular space due to the osmolality gradient. Neurons can compensate if the changes occur slowly by shifting other solutes out of the cell to minimize water accumulation. However, if the changes occur rapidly or are excessive, CNS signs such as lethargy, disorientation, ataxia, coma, and seizures can develop. Clinical signs of CNS dysfunction tend to occur with sodium levels $<120\,\text{mmol}\,l^{-1}$ or if the rate of decrease is $>0.5\,\text{mmol}\,l^{-1}\,h^{-1}$. Unfortunately, clinical signs associated with hyponatremia or excessive correction rates will be masked with sedation and anesthesia; therefore, the anesthetist will need to rely on repeat serum sodium measurements to guide ongoing therapy if the condition is not corrected fully prior to anesthesia.

The major concerns in the perioperative period for patients with hyponatremia relate to effects on the patient's CNS and volume status. The therapeutic approach before anesthesia depends on clinical sign severity and disorder chronicity. If possible, even mild hyponatremia and volume disturbances should be corrected prior to anesthesia based on the current association of hyponatremia with poor outcomes. The patient's clinical signs and disease chronicity should guide the rate and volume of IV therapy. Ideally, treatment of the primary cause can be initiated in addition to correction of the electrolyte disturbances. For example, patients with hypoadrenocorticism should receive mineralocorticoid replacement therapy in addition to fluid therapy to correct electrolyte disturbances prior to anesthesia. In urgent situations, correction of the hyponatremia should be started prior to anesthesia and continued throughout the anesthetic period and into recovery. The optimal treatment regimen for hyponatremic veterinary patients has yet to be determined; however, experts in critical care and internal medicine report consistent recommendations regarding the rate of change in serum sodium concentrations as discussed in the following text.

In the "severely symptomatic hypoosmolar hyponatremic patient" (for example, presenting with seizures or markedly abnormal behavior), treatment with small boluses ($2\,\text{ml}\,\text{kg}^{-1}$) of 3% NaCl to increase serum sodium by $4\text{–}6\,\text{mmol}\,l^{-1}$ is recommended [43]. Improvement in clinical signs attributed to the hyponatremia occurs when serum sodium reaches $125\,\text{mmol}\,l^{-1}$, at which point treatment should be adjusted according to the chronicity of the disease and the patient's overall volume status as described in the following text.

In the "acutely (<48 h) dehydrated hypovolemic hyponatremic" veterinary patient requiring anesthesia, administration of a balanced electrolyte solution such as lactated Ringer's solution, Plasma-Lyte A, Plasma-Lyte 148, or Normosol-R, to replace volume deficits, is recommended [44]. Correction of the volume deficit generally resolves the hyponatremia and volume replacement can occur relatively rapidly to reestablish extracellular fluid status. Changes in patient serum sodium concentrations at a rate of $1\text{–}2\,\text{mmol}\,l^{-1}\,h^{-1}$ are considered acceptable.

In the "hypovolemic dehydrated" patient with "chronic hyponatremia," serum sodium should be increased by $0.5\,\text{mmol}\,l^{-1}\,h^{-1}$ or $10\text{–}12\,\text{mmol}\,l^{-1}\,d^{-1}$ at maximum to avoid the risk of adverse neurological outcomes, including intracranial hemorrhage or osmotic demyelination [51–54]. Careful consideration of the patient's measured or calculated osmolality with consideration of the impact of other solutes such as glucose is required before initiation of treatment. For most cases, a balanced electrolyte solution is recommended to correct the hypovolemia with serial hourly serum sodium measurements used to guide fluid administration rate. Differences in sodium and osmolality exist among the various isotonic balanced electrolyte solutions. Of the balanced electrolyte solutions, lactated Ringer's solution is preferable for patients with chronic hyponatremia, as it has a lower osmolality and sodium content relative to the other solutions in this category. If the patient's rate of serum sodium increase is excessive following therapy initiation with a balanced electrolyte solution, further assessment of the patient's sodium deficit and infusion rate for correction is required. It is recommended that further resources with an in-depth discussion related to the treatment of hyponatremia are consulted in the nonurgent situation [44].

In the "normovolemic" or "hypervolemic chronically hyponatremic" patient who requires anesthesia, management will be heavily dependent on the underlying cause of the electrolyte disturbance and the nature and severity of the symptoms associated with hyponatremia. In some cases, individualized fluid therapy administration, using a variety of tailor-made fluids and possibly diuretic administration, will be necessary to correct both the sodium deficit and hypervolemic state [44].

Serum hypoosmolality has been shown to decrease halothane MAC in dogs [55]. Although the impact of hyponatremia on other anesthetic agents has not been determined, the clinician should select agents that can be titrated to effect to avoid overdose and adverse hemodynamic consequences. Intraoperatively, in patients with the potential for significant intravascular volume losses during surgery, a separate colloid infusion may be considered to replace intraoperative intravascular losses. If a synthetic colloid is used, selection of a product with sodium levels close to physiologic values should avoid excessive change in sodium concentration. As hyponatremic patients, particularly those with intravascular volume deficits, may also be prone to hypotension, the anesthetist should be prepared to use vasopressors and/or inotropes during anesthesia. Serum sodium and hydration status monitoring should continue during anesthesia and into the postoperative period. The syndrome of inappropriate antidiuresis or syndrome of inappropriate antidiuretic hormone (SIADH) secretion is not uncommon in critically ill human patients and may occur in the postoperative period. The condition, although rare, has been reported in both dogs and cats [44]. A decreased urine output despite normovolemia should trigger further diagnostic investigation to prevent iatrogenic hypervolemia from excessive fluid administration.

Hypernatremia

Hypernatremia is defined as serum sodium concentrations >160 $mmol\,l^{-1}$ in dogs, and 175 $mmol\,l^{-1}$ in cats. Hypernatremia is always associated with hyperosmolality. It is relatively rare in patients with normal mentation and free access to water but can be observed in the perioperative period in critically ill patients. As with hyponatremia, patients can be hypovolemic, normovolemic, or hypervolemic depending on the primary cause (Table 8.5). In one large retrospective study, gastrointestinal fluid losses, losses associated with diabetes insipidus, and fever were the most common pathophysiologic factors associated with hypernatremia in dogs, while in cats, kidney disease (acute and chronic) and gastrointestinal factors were the most common [56]. In this same study, the primary conditions resulting in hypernatremia were neurological and neoplasia in dogs and urological and neurological in cats. In terms of potential iatrogenic-acquired hypernatremia, hypernatremia associated with hypertonic saline or sodium bicarbonate administration is generally transient in the awake patient if unrestricted water intake is possible or if it is followed with appropriate balanced electrolyte solutions in the anesthetized patient. A recent study demonstrated hypernatremia following a single dose of activated-charcoal-containing sorbitol in dogs, a result believed to be secondary to loss of water via the gastrointestinal tract [57].

Clinical signs associated with hypernatremia generally occur with serum sodium levels exceeding 170 $mmol\,l^{-1}$ and include anorexia, lethargy, vomiting, muscular weakness, disorientation, ataxia, seizures, coma, and death. If patients have concurrent hypovolemia or hypervolemia, they may show cardiovascular changes such as tachycardia or pulmonary edema, respectively.

As with hyponatremia, hypernatremia should be corrected slowly over at least 48 h. If the patient is acutely (<48 h) hypernatremic and hypovolemic, the plasma volume deficit can be replaced with a balanced electrolyte solution over several hours followed by a slower correction of the hyperosmolality with the administration of hypotonic IV solutions such as 0.45% saline or 5% dextrose [44]. In cases of chronic hypernatremia, the serum sodium concentration should be decreased by no more than 1.0 $mmol\,l^{-1}\,h^{-1}$ due to the risk of neurologic complications. In cases of hypervolemia, loop diuretic administration may facilitate sodium excretion; however, if renal dysfunction is present, alternative therapies such as hemodialysis will be required.

During the anesthetic period, the clinician should continue to correct the hypernatremia as described previously. In the experimental setting, hypernatremia is associated with an increase in the MAC of inhalant anesthetics; it is possible that there will be increased inhalant anesthetic requirements [55, 58]. As discussed previously, a patient's intravascular volume status will also likely affect anesthetic requirements, and anesthetic depth should be monitored and delivery of anesthetics adjusted based on the basis of the individual animal assessment.

Chloride

Chloride is the major anion in the extracellular fluid and contributes significantly to maintaining extracellular osmolality. Intracellular chloride concentrations vary depending on the cell type; however, intracellular concentrations are consistently considerably lower than plasma levels. As with sodium, dietary intake is the main chloride source for the body with losses primarily occurring via the kidney and gastrointestinal tract. Plasma chloride regulation occurs in the kidney with acid–base and sodium concentrations being the major factors that influence chloride reabsorption or excretion [59].

Alterations in serum chloride may reflect a primary disorder of chloride, sodium, or total body water balance. Alternatively, they may be the consequence of a compensatory response in a patient with primary changes in acid–base status (see the section titled "Acid–Base Homeostasis and Disturbances"). Common causes of abnormalities in serum chloride in the dog and cat are outlined in Table 8.6.

Clinical signs related to serum chloride alterations are generally nonspecific and are associated with the concurrent alterations in osmolality/total body water or acid–base status. As such, consideration of these factors is required for appropriate patient management.

To correct for disturbances in total body water balance on measured plasma chloride, the effect of body water changes on serum chloride should first be determined by calculating a corrected chloride concentration. This can be achieved by using measured sodium relative to normal sodium concentrations as a correction factor according to the following equations (Eqs. (8.4) and (8.5)). If the corrected chloride values fall within normal values, the primary etiology of the abnormal measured chloride reflects abnormalities in total body water, and therapy should be directed accordingly:

$$\text{Canine}: \left[\text{Cl}^-\right]\text{corrected} = \left[\text{Cl}^-\right]\text{measured} \times 146 \big/ \left[\text{Na}^+\right]\text{measured} \tag{8.4}$$

$$\text{Feline}: \left[\text{Cl}^-\right]\text{corrected} = \left[\text{Cl}^-\right]\text{measured} \times 156 \big/ \left[\text{Na}^+\right]\text{measured} \tag{8.5}$$

Hypochloremia

Hypochloremia is defined as a serum-corrected chloride concentration <107 $mmol\,l^{-1}$ in dogs and 117 $mEq\,l^{-1}$ in cats. The most common causes of corrected hypochloremia relate to excessive loss of chloride relative to sodium via the gastrointestinal or renal systems (Table 8.6) [59, 60]. Corrected hypochloremia results in metabolic alkalosis due to an increase in the strong ion difference (see the section titled "Acid–Base Homeostasis and Disturbances"). A corrected hypochloremia can occur as a compensatory response to a chronic respiratory acidosis.

Clinical signs specifically attributed to hypochloremia have not been reported and abnormalities in patient health status associated with corrected hypochloremia primarily

Table 8.6 Common causes of chloride disorders in dogs and cats [59].

	Hypochloremia-corrected	Hyperchloremia-corrected
Altered losses	**Increased Cl^- loss** *Gastrointestinal loss* • Vomiting, diarrhea *Renal loss* • In response to chronic elevation in $PaCO_2$ (compensation for chronic respiratory acidosis) • Hyperadrenocorticism • Glucocorticoids • Diuretics	**Decreased Cl^- loss** *Renal retention* • Renal disease • Hypoadrenocorticism • Diabetes mellitus • In response to chronic reduction in $PaCO_2$ (compensation for chronic respiratory alkalosis) • Hypoalbuminemia **Increased Na^+ loss relative to Cl^-** *Gastrointestinal* • Diarrhea
Translocation	**Greater Cl^- movement relative to Na^+** *Peritonitis* *Ascites* *Ruptured bladder*	*Rare*
Altered intake or input	**Decreased intake** *Rare* **Increased Na^+ input relative to Cl^-** *Na^+ bicarbonate supplementation*	**Increased input** *IV fluid therapy with excessive Cl^- relative to Na^+* • (0.9% NaCl, hypertonic saline, KCl, NH_4Cl)

result from the metabolic alkalosis and concurrent electrolyte and water disorders. Treatment strategies should be aimed at correcting the underlying cause and supportive therapy should be directed at correcting the strong ion difference. Intravenous fluid therapy with 0.9% NaCl is the treatment of choice for the dehydrated hypovolemic hypochloremic patient. Serum potassium levels should be monitored and supplemental KCl added, if necessary, to treat hypokalemia (see the section titled "Potassium"). In normovolemic patients, chloride can be administered as KCl or NH_4Cl; however, this is rarely required in the patient with normal kidney function if the primary cause of the hypochloremia is addressed. Ideally, hypochloremia and its associated acid–base alterations are corrected prior to anesthesia. However, if this is not possible, therapy can be continued throughout the perianesthetic period.

Hypochloremia with a normal corrected chloride concentration is often referred to as an artificial hypochloremia and is associated with a concurrent hyponatremia [59]. It is associated with either a gain in body water or a third-space loss of both sodium and chloride.

Hyperchloremia

Hyperchloremia is defined as a serum chloride concentration >113 $mmol\,l^{-1}$ in dogs and 123 $mmol\,l^{-1}$ in cats. The most common causes of corrected hyperchloremia relate to excessive loss of sodium relative to chloride, greater retention of chloride relative to sodium, or an excessive gain of chloride (Table 8.6). Corrected hyperchloremia is associated with a nonrespiratory acidosis due to a decrease in the strong ion difference.

As with corrected hypochloremia, there are no specific clinical signs related to corrected hyperchloremia; signs are likely a reflection of a nonrespiratory acidosis and concurrent electrolyte disorder. Removal of the underlying cause should be attempted. If the patient is dehydrated, IV fluid therapy with a balanced electrolyte solution should be initiated with sodium bicarbonate added to the fluid therapy if plasma pH is less than 7.2 [59]. Ideally, at a minimum, the patient's volume status should be normalized before anesthesia.

Hyperchloremia with normal corrected chloride levels is generally associated with pure water loss or hypotonic loss. Bromide, a common therapy for idiopathic epilepsy, can cause interference with the measurement of chloride and can result in a false hyperchloremia [61]. Hyperchloremia in a normovolemic patient with a normal acid–base status and a negative anion gap should trigger further exploration of potential interference of chloride measurement by other ions such as bromide.

Potassium

While sodium is the major extracellular cation in the body, potassium is the major intracellular cation, with the extracellular levels representing <5% of total body potassium stores. The Na^+-K^+-ATPase pump located in the cell membrane maintains the relationship of intracellular to extracellular potassium and sodium by actively pumping sodium out of the cell and potassium into the cell. The relationship of intracellular to extracellular potassium is crucial to the cell's normal homeostasis, volume, and resting membrane potential. In particular, serum potassium levels heavily influence muscle and cardiac cell excitability, as the relative distribution of potassium across the cell membrane affects resting membrane potential and the subsequent ease of cellular depolarization and repolarization.

Serum potassium levels are influenced by oral potassium intake through dietary sources, output via urinary and gastrointestinal routes, and translocation between the intracellular to extracellular space. In nutritional studies evaluating potassium-restricted diets in humans and dogs, resting serum potassium levels correlate with total body and muscle cell potassium content, respectively [62, 63]. In disease states or when the body is under stress such as extreme exercise, serum potassium levels may not correlate with total body stores of potassium, an important consideration when considering the treatment of measured abnormalities in serum potassium.

Animals on commercial diets generally have an adequate intake of potassium to maintain both total body stores and normal serum potassium levels. The major factors that influence potassium translocation between the intracellular and extracellular spaces include insulin, epinephrine, and pH. Endogenous insulin and epinephrine, acting at beta-2-adrenergic receptors, increase potassium movement into cells from the extracellular space. Glucose reduces serum potassium indirectly by stimulating insulin release. Extracellular pH can also impact serum potassium levels acutely through cellular translocation. The degree of change in serum potassium is dependent on the specific acid–base alteration. In general, acidosis increases potassium movement from the intracellular to extracellular space, thereby increasing serum potassium levels. The degree of change reported is somewhat variable; however, in humans with nonrespiratory acidosis, serum potassium was reported to increase by 0.17 to 1.67 $mmol\,l^{-1}$ per 0.1 unit decrease in pH, whereas nonrespiratory alkalosis decreased serum potassium by 0.1 $mmol\,l^{-1}$ for each 0.1 unit increase in pH [64]. With respiratory acidosis, the reported change is also relatively small, with a 0.14 $mmol\,l^{-1}$ increase in serum potassium per 0.1 unit decrease in pH. In normal anesthetized dogs, respiratory alkalosis decreased serum potassium by 0.4 $mmol\,l^{-1}$ for each 0.1 unit increase in pH [65].

Serum potassium levels can be dramatically changed by alterations in urinary excretion of potassium. Briefly, potassium is freely filtered at the glomerulus, with approximately 80–90%

being reabsorbed back into the blood in the proximal tubule and ascending loop of Henle. In the distal nephron, further potassium reabsorption or secretion occurs. It is at this location that aldosterone impacts potassium homeostasis by reducing its reabsorption. Reductions in renal blood flow can reduce urinary potassium excretion, while changes in renal function can result in either an increase or decrease in serum potassium levels.

In clinical cases with complex disorders, it is important to recognize all factors that influence the measured serum levels of potassium including potassium intake, the relative potassium distribution in the body, as well as its level of excretion. Alterations in serum potassium rarely happen in isolation of alterations in body fluid status, and when therapies are initiated, shifts in serum levels may occur rapidly. For example, in a patient with severe hypovolemia and hypokalemia secondary to gastrointestinal fluid loss, further reductions in serum potassium may occur with correction of the patient's volume status despite potassium supplementation. Common causes of abnormalities in serum potassium in the dog and cat are outlined in Table 8.7.

Hypokalemia

Hypokalemia is defined as a serum potassium level of $<3.5\,\text{mmol}\,\text{l}^{-1}$ in both the dog and cat. As previously mentioned, normal animals generally consume their dietary potassium requirements [66]. In the chronically anorexic patient, however, low dietary intake can contribute to hypokalemia. Anorexic patients receiving prolonged fluid therapy with IV replacement solutions that have low quantities of potassium ($3\text{–}5\,\text{mmol}\,\text{l}^{-1}$) relative to daily body metabolic needs may also develop hypokalemia [66]. Insulin, glucose, and beta-2-adrenergic receptor agonist administration can reduce potassium levels secondary to intracellular transfer of potassium. Hyperglycemia and alkalosis can also reduce serum potassium levels secondary to intracellular transfer of potassium [70]. Potassium losses via the gastrointestinal tract or kidney are relatively common causes of significant hypokalemia [66, 67, 70]. Primary kidney disease, mineralocorticoid excess, or diuretic therapy can all result in hypokalemia (Table 8.7).

Clinical signs of hypokalemia include muscle weakness and dysrhythmias, both of which occur due to resting cell membrane potential shifts in muscle and cardiac cells to a more hyperpolarized state [67]. Not uncommonly, specific signs are not detected on physical examination, but are identified on diagnostic workup of a patient with concurrent disease. With hypokalemia, cats have more severe clinical signs compared to dogs. Muscle weakness and cardiac conduction disturbances are usually not detected until potassium levels are $<2.5\,\text{mmol}\,\text{l}^{-1}$. Cats may demonstrate cervical ventroflexion, forelimb hypermetria, and a broad-based hindlimb stance in addition to muscle weakness. Animals may present with bradyarrhythmias or tachyarrhythmias [66]. ECG changes associated with hypokalemia include supraventricular and ventricular arrhythmias [66, 68].

Hypokalemia treatment prior to anesthesia depends on clinical signs attributable to hypokalemia, the degree of serum potassium depletion, the underlying cause, and the urgency of the situation. In general, if not emergent, it is ideal to correct or improve a patient's serum potassium levels before anesthesia by the enteral compared with the parenteral route due to the relative risk of producing iatrogenic hyperkalemia. If the patient is symptomatic, or the enteral route is not feasible, potassium should be administered IV. It is highly recommended that if the IV route is chosen for supplemental potassium administration, an infusion pump be utilized for its administration, continuous ECG monitoring be performed, and serum potassium levels be monitored, the frequency of which is dependent on the rate of correction. In general, the rate of exogenous potassium administration via the IV route should not exceed $0.5\,\text{mmol}\,\text{kg}^{-1}\,\text{h}^{-1}$. To avoid vascular irritation at the site of

Table 8.7 Common causes of potassium disorders in dogs and cats [66–69].

	Hypokalemia	Hyperkalemia
Altered losses	**Increased loss** *Gastrointestinal loss* • Vomiting, diarrhea *Renal loss* • Diuretics • Postobstructive diuresis • Hyperthyroidism • Mineralocorticoids • Glucocorticoids • Na^+ bicarbonate • Excessive intake of Na^+	**Decreased loss** *Decreased renal/urinary excretion* • Renal disease • Urethral obstruction • Uroabdomen • Select gastrointestinal and diseases involving third-space accumulation of fluid (chylothorax, pleural, or peritoneal effusion) • Hypoadrenocorticism • Hypothyroidism • Ace inhibitor • Potassium-sparing diuretics • Non-steroidal anti-inflammatory drugs (NSAIDs)
Translocation	**Translocation** *Extracellular to intracellular* • Alkalemia • Hyperglycemia • Insulin/glucose administration • Catecholamines (beta-agonists) • Hypothermia	**Translocation** *Intracellular to extracellular* • Acidemia • Tissue trauma (cell lysis) • Insulin deficiency • Beta-blockers • Anesthesia-associated acute hyperkalemia
Altered intake or input	**Decreased intake** *Low dietary intake combined with urinary acidifiers* *IV fluid therapy with inadequate K^+ content*	**Increased intake** *IV fluid therapy with excessive K^+ content*

administration, concentrated potassium solutions such as potassium chloride ($2\,mmol\,K^+\,ml^{-1}$) or potassium phosphate ($4.36\,mmol\,K^+\,ml^{-1}$) can be mixed with ongoing replacement or maintenance IV fluid therapy to supplement potassium. Thorough fluid mixing must be performed to ensure consistent potassium delivery, as inconsistent mixing can lead to lethal consequences [71]. Guidelines for IV fluid supplementation with potassium based on the patient's potassium level are outlined in Table 8.8. It is important to consider the original potassium concentration in the fluid bag that the potassium is being added to, as well as the required final bag concentration; the maximum rate of potassium infusion should be no greater than $0.5\,mmol\,kg^{-1}\,h^{-1}$ [68].

During anesthesia, it is important not to cause further decreases in serum potassium in the patient with preexisting hypokalemia. A balanced electrolyte solution should be chosen over a potassium-free crystalloid fluid such as 0.9% sodium chloride for replacement fluid therapy. As discussed previously, further supplementation of IV fluids with potassium chloride can be performed if the patient is symptomatic; however, it is highly recommended that a second IV catheter be placed for replacement fluid administration to avoid exceeding the recommended rates due to

Table 8.8 Recommended potassium concentration in IV fluid therapy for the hypokalemic patient.

Serum potassium concentration ($mmol\,l^{-1}$)	Recommended potassium chloride concentration in IV fluid[a] ($mmol\,l^{-1}$)	Maximal fluid infusion rate[b] ($ml\,kg^{-1}\,h^{-1}$)
<2.0	80	6
2.0–2.5	60	8
2.6–3.0	40	12
3.1–3.5	28	18
3.6–5.0	20	25

[a] Amount added to fluid will depend on original concentration of potassium in fluid being administered. With replacement IV fluids with no potassium, the concentration represents the quantity of potassium to add to 1 l of fluid. These concentrations should be adjusted accordingly if original fluid already contains potassium.
[b] Maximum rate based on principle of not exceeding 0.5 $mmol\,kg^{-1}\,h^{-1}$. *Source:* Adapted from: http://www.aaha.org/globalassets/02-guidelines/fluid-therapy/fluid-therapy_tipsheet.pdf.

inadvertent IV fluid boluses. As in the conscious patient, when potassium is given IV at concentrations above normal serum plasma concentrations, it is recommended that fluid pump be utilized, continuous ECG monitoring be performed, and serum potassium levels be monitored. Agent administration such as insulin, beta-adrenergic receptor agonists, bicarbonate, and diuretics such as furosemide can further reduce potassium serum levels and should be avoided in the hypokalemic patient, if possible. Patient ventilation can also impact serum potassium level, as respiratory alkalosis will result in the intracellular movement of potassium. As such, if ventilatory support is instituted during anesthesia, arterial or end-tidal carbon dioxide levels should be monitored and maintained at normal or above normal levels unless the latter is contraindicated due to coexisting conditions. During anesthetic recovery, the impact of hypokalemia on respiratory muscle strength should be considered and ventilation adequacy aggressively monitored before removal of mechanical ventilation and/or oxygen supplementation.

Hyperkalemia

Hyperkalemia is defined as a serum potassium level > 5.5 $mmol\,l^{-1}$ in both dogs and cats. In general, hyperkalemia is present most frequently secondary to impaired excretion or translocation from the intracellular to extracellular space. Iatrogenic hyperkalemia secondary to excessive IV potassium supplementation can occur in the hospitalized patient. Renal disease, urethral obstruction, hypoadrenocorticism, and drug-associated impairment of potassium excretion are a few of the more common causes of hyperkalemia in small-animal patients (Table 8.7). Malignant hyperthermia is a relatively rare condition, but is of particular significance to anesthetists, as patients may be phenotypically normal prior to anesthesia, but develop severe hyperkalemia acutely in the perianesthetic period [72]. Acute hyperkalemia during general anesthesia of unknown etiology has also been reported in Greyhounds and a variety of other canine breeds [69, 73]. In Greyhounds, the condition may have a genetic association; however, the specific defect resulting in the hyperkalemia remains to be determined. Hyperkalemia of unknown etiology associated with anesthesia has also been reported in large nondomestic cats [74]. In humans, horses, and swine, hemolysis is associated with hyperkalemia; however, this is not the case in dogs. Interestingly, a small fraction of dogs (most commonly Akita, Shiba Inu, and English Springer Spaniel breeds) have erythrocytes with high potassium levels. However, hemolysis, in vivo or during sample handling, is unlikely to cause a clinically significant increase in measured serum potassium levels in these animals. Potassium levels in stored canine or feline blood also do not typically increase significantly. Canine and feline patients with severe thrombopathies or leukocytosis can have falsely elevated potassium due to storage artifact, as platelets and leukocytes have high levels of potassium, which may contaminate a serum sample if sample processing is not rapid [75].

Clinical signs associated with hyperkalemia primarily relate to the musculoskeletal and cardiovascular systems. Resting membrane potential is increased and is closer to the threshold potential for cellular depolarization, which initially makes cells hyperexcitable. Severity of signs is somewhat dependent on the rapidity of onset of the hyperkalemia with chronic elevations in potassium tolerated to a greater extent than acute elevations. Muscle weakness is generally present when serum potassium levels exceed 8.0 mmol l^{-1}. ECG changes include high, peaked, or deep T waves, prolonged P-R intervals, prolonged Q-R-S complexes, absent P waves, atrioventricular heart blocks, bradycardia, atrial standstill, ectopic beats, sine wave complexes, or ventricular fibrillation (see Chapter 6) [66, 68]. The latter changes are reported based on results of experimental studies in otherwise healthy animals. In this situation, ECG changes were evident with potassium levels >5.5 mmol l^{-1} and progressed to fibrillation or standstill with levels >10.1 mmol l^{-1}. In a clinical study involving 37 dogs and cats with potassium levels >5.5 mmol l^{-1}, 20 animals had arrhythmias and 17 had normal sinus rhythms despite potassium levels ranging from 5.5 to >10 mmol l^{-1} [76]. In addition, 68% of dogs and 47% of cats presenting to a referral hospital with serum potassium levels >6 mmol l^{-1} in which an ECG was obtained had ECG abnormalities which included spiked T waves, absent P waves, widened Q-R-S complexes, premature ventricular complexes, and ventricular tachycardia [66]. In this study, 35% of dogs and 14% of cats were categorized as having a bradyarrhythmia, while 7.5% of dogs and 8% of cats were considered tachycardic on hospital admission. Concurrent abnormalities including other electrolyte disturbances, hydration status, and varying levels of sympathetic stimulation likely contribute to the heterogeneity in clinical signs.

Ideally, anesthesia should be delayed until the patient can be stabilized and serum potassium levels reduced below 5.5 mmol l^{-1} to minimize potential dysrhythmias and further impairment in cardiovascular performance with anesthetic drug administration. This is, unfortunately, often not feasible in the emergent setting. ECG monitoring during treatment is highly recommended. Treatment focus prior to or during anesthesia should be aimed at reducing potassium administration, decreasing myocardial sensitivity to the elevated extracellular potassium concentrations, encouraging potassium movement from the extracellular to the intracellular space, and increasing potassium excretion when whole body potassium levels are thought to be elevated. If IV fluids containing potassium levels >5.0 mmol l^{-1} are being administered, they should be stopped and replaced with a balanced electrolyte solution. While physiologic saline (0.9%) was historically recommended over solutions containing potassium, the acidifying effect of 0.9% saline solution makes it less optimal, even in the hyperkalemic patient. In cats with experimentally induced urethral obstruction, as well as cats with naturally occurring urethral obstruction and hyperkalemia, IV administration of a balanced electrolyte solution resulted in a more optimal resuscitation compared to 0.9% saline solution with concurrent reestablishment of urinary output [77, 78]. Overall, consideration of the patient's hydration status, severity of the hyperkalemia, acid–base status, volume status, and concurrent electrolyte abnormalities should guide fluid therapy. Synthetic colloid use in critically ill patients remains controversial and, if renal disease is suspected, alternatives should be chosen for volume resuscitation in this group of patients [27]. Frequent monitoring of electrolyte and acid–base status should be used to dictate fluid therapy choices over time.

Calcium can be administered to raise the threshold potential of cardiac cells, thereby increasing the difference between the resting and threshold membrane potentials. While calcium does not have a direct effect on potassium levels, administration can provide greater cardiac stability by normalizing the difference between resting and threshold potentials, returning membrane excitability to normal. Calcium supplementation can be achieved with either calcium gluconate 10% (0.5–1.5 $ml\,kg^{-1}$) or calcium chloride 10% (0.2–0.5 $ml\,kg^{-1}$) administered over 5–10 min. Intravenous administration of insulin (0.5 $U\,kg^{-1}$ of regular insulin) and glucose (0.5–1.0 $g\,kg^{-1}$ or 1–2 $ml\,kg^{-1}$ of 50% dextrose) can also be administered to treat severe hyperkalemia. Insulin can be administered first followed immediately by glucose; they can be administered together as an infusion, or separately as infusions. Irrespective of administration method, serum glucose levels, in addition to potassium, should be monitored to avoid hyperglycemia. Correction of nonrespiratory acidosis by addressing the underlying etiology will also shift potassium to the intracellular space and help reduce serum potassium levels. In an emergency setting, sodium bicarbonate (1–2 $mmol\,kg^{-1}$) can be administered to adjust pH. However, it should not be administered immediately after calcium, as it may impact the effectiveness of calcium on the myocardium. If excessive body stores of potassium are likely, diuretics such as furosemide (1–2 $mg\,kg^{-1}$) can be administered to facilitate potassium excretion.

Other than succinylcholine, which is not routinely used in veterinary anesthesia, there are no specific contraindications in the hyperkalemic patient to any drugs currently used to achieve balanced anesthesia. As previously mentioned, however, hypoventilation should be avoided throughout the anesthetic period in the hyperkalemic patient. As monitoring the adequacy of ventilation is difficult prior to intubation and following extubation, avoiding high doses of opioids in combination with sedatives prior to induction of anesthesia (i.e., premedication) and during recovery is recommended to avoid undetectable or uncontrollable hypoventilation. During the anesthetic period, ventilation should be aggressively monitored and ventilatory support provided, if necessary, to ensure normocapnia.

Calcium

Most of the calcium is maintained in the skeleton, where it is present in the relatively poorly exchangeable form, hydroxyapatite, or in the more readily available form, calcium phosphate. Although present in relatively small amounts (approximately 1%), the remaining calcium, present in both the intracellular and extracellular spaces, is critical to normal body homeostasis. Enzymatic reactions, intracellular messaging, membrane transport, muscle contraction, and nerve conduction are a few of the major activities that are dependent on normal serum calcium levels [79, 80].

Within the extracellular space, ionized calcium is the most biologically active form of calcium. However, it is also present bound to proteins or complexed to other substances such as phosphorous, bicarbonate, sulfate, citrate, or lactate. While not biologically active, both bound and complexed calcium are important, as they equilibrate with the ionized fraction and provide a readily available source of calcium when the ionized fraction is reduced [79]. Changes in the extracellular pH can shift the relationship of ionized calcium to complexed or protein-bound factions. Most notably, a moderate to marked nonrespiratory acidosis increases ionized calcium fraction. As with other electrolytes, dietary intake is the source of calcium for the body with losses primarily occurring via the kidney and gastrointestinal tract. The skeleton can act as a calcium source when calcium absorption and reabsorption from the intestine and kidney are inadequate to maintain serum calcium levels.

In the normal patient, the serum-ionized calcium fraction is regulated primarily by parathyroid hormone, calcitriol (a metabolite of vitamin D), and calcitonin. In response to low ionized serum calcium levels, parathyroid hormone levels increase which increases renal tubular reabsorption of calcium, increases mobilization of calcium from bone, and stimulates calcitriol synthesis, which subsequently increases intestinal calcium absorption. Normal and elevated serum-ionized calcium levels inhibit parathyroid synthesis and secretion, decrease calcitriol synthesis, and stimulate calcitonin's secretion from the thyroid gland, thus reducing bone reabsorption by osteoclasts. Total serum calcium measurements include the ionized, complexed, and protein-bound fractions [79]. Ionized calcium concentration measurement is superior to assess patient calcium status; ionized calcium estimates taken from the total calcium measurement are not recommended [79, 81]. Several factors influence the ionized calcium fraction measurement including the type of sample (serum versus whole blood), the specific anticoagulant used, the volume of the sample relative to anticoagulant, exposure of the sample to air (with subsequent change in pH), and the analytic method used to measure calcium. Due to the potential variability, values should be compared to normal ranges reported for each laboratory that is specific to the methodology used to collect and store the sample [79]. Common causes of abnormalities in serum calcium in the dog and cat are outlined in Table 8.9.

Hypocalcemia

Hypocalcemia is defined as a "serum-ionized" calcium level $<1.25\,\text{mmol}\,\text{l}^{-1}$ in dogs and $1.1\,\text{mmol}\,\text{l}^{-1}$ in cats. In terms of "total" serum calcium concentrations, levels used to define hypocalcemia are $<2.0\,\text{mmol}\,\text{l}^{-1}$ in dogs and $<1.75\,\text{mmol}\,\text{l}^{-1}$ in cats. Although hypoalbuminemia is one of the most common causes of hypocalcemia based on the measurement of total serum calcium, the presence of hypocalcemia based on this measurement cannot be extrapolated to ionized calcium levels. When there are clinical signs or concurrent diseases in which abnormal calcium levels are possible, ionized calcium should be measured [81–83].

Mechanisms responsible for a decrease in serum-ionized calcium include an increased renal calcium loss, lack of calcium absorption from the gastrointestinal tract, or calcium redistribution from the ionized state to the bound or chelated state in the extracellular space. Acute and chronic renal failure, hyperphosphatemia, puerperal tetany, and pancreatitis are some of the more common medical causes of hypocalcemia [79, 84]. Hypocalcemia following surgical interventions can also occur due to hypoparathyroidism [85–88]. Parathyroid hormone has a very short serum half-life (3–5 min), and most dogs and cats develop hypocalcemia early in the postoperative period (days 2–4) following bilateral parathyroidectomy or thyroid and parathyroid lobectomy, although hypocalcemia can develop up to 21 days postoperatively [85–90]. In addition, clinical hypocalcemia can be reported postoperatively in dogs following tumor resection such as apocrine gland anal sac adenocarcinoma [91]. Dogs with soft-tissue trauma and both dogs and cats with sepsis can have reductions in serum-ionized calcium, a negative prognostic indicator [92–94]. Massive transfusion with blood products containing citrated anticoagulants also causes hypocalcemia [95]. Although uncommon, alkalosis can increase the protein binding of calcium in the extracellular space and result in significant hypocalcemia. Ionized calcium levels decrease in healthy dogs and cats undergoing general anesthesia and elective surgery, although values do not go below normal reference ranges and the decrease is not clinically significant [96].

Hypocalcemia lowers the threshold potential of excitable cells, thereby facilitating membrane depolarization, an effect that is

Table 8.9 Common causes of calcium disorders in dogs and cats [79].

	Hypocalcemia	Hypercalcemia
Altered losses	**Increased loss** *Renal loss* • Renal failure *Gastrointestinal loss* • Phosphate enemas • Protein-losing enteropathy *Other loss* • Puerperal tetany	**Decreased loss** *Renal loss* • Chronic renal disease • Hypoadrenocorticism • Hyperparathyroidism
Translocation	**Third-space loss** *Sepsis* *Peritonitis* *Pancreatitis* *Soft-tissue trauma* **Chelation/precipitation** *Blood product administration (citrate)* *Ethylene glycol toxicosis* *Na^+ bicarbonate therapy*	**From bone** *Malignancy (humoral hypercalcemia of malignancy)* *Hyperparathyroidism* *Bone disease* *Granulomatous disease*
Altered intake or input	**Decreased intake** *Unbalanced diet* *Decreased gastrointestinal absorption (high phosphorous diet)* *Hypoparathyroidism (idiopathic, post-bilateral thyroidectomy)* *IV fluid therapy without calcium (prolonged)*	**Increased intake** *Dietary*

potentiated by hyperkalemia and hypomagnesemia. Onset rate and severity of the ionized calcium deficit influence the degree of clinical signs, including muscle tremors and fasciculation, facial rubbing, muscle cramping, stiff gait, seizures, and behavioral changes. Acute severe hypocalcemia can result in hypotension, dysrhythmias, and decreased myocardial contractility [79]. ECG changes include prolongation of the Q–T interval and ventricular tachycardia [79]. Clinical sign severity is exacerbated by concurrent hypomagnesemia and hyperkalemia.

In the patient with chronic hypocalcemia with no clinical signs, specific treatment may not be necessary. However, if the patient has any symptoms related to hypocalcemia or if there is potential for further calcium reductions, therapy with calcium gluconate or calcium chloride should be initiated. Ideally, treatment would occur prior to anesthesia; however, a similar therapeutic approach can be applied at any point during the anesthetic period if symptoms related to hypocalcemia develop. A treatment regimen consisting of calcium gluconate (10%, 1–1.5 ml kg^{-1}), administered over 20–30 min followed by an infusion over 24 h containing 5–10 ml kg^{-1} administered with physiologic saline or a balanced electrolyte solution, is recommended for the symptomatic patient. It is advisable to monitor the ECG and arterial blood pressure during therapy. During anesthesia, alkalosis secondary to excessive ventilation or bicarbonate administration should be avoided, as this will result in further reductions in ionized calcium. In patients requiring massive whole blood transfusions (>90 ml kg^{-1}) intraoperatively, ionized calcium should be monitored and treatment instituted if hypocalcemia develops. In the patient undergoing parathyroid or thyroid surgery in which the parathyroid glands may be disrupted, ionized calcium should be monitored postoperatively, and hypocalcemia treated. Oral calcitriol has been explored as a possible perioperative treatment to increase intestinal absorption of calcium in dogs and cats undergoing parathyroidectomy [87, 89]. To date, it has not been shown to have a definitive positive outcome on the subsequent development of hypocalcemia in the immediate postoperative period and its use for this purpose remains equivocal [87, 89].

Hypercalcemia

Hypercalcemia is defined as an "ionized" serum calcium level >1.5 mmol l^{-1} in adult dogs and 1.4 mmol l^{-1} in adult cats. In terms of "total" serum calcium concentrations, levels used to define hypercalcemia are values >3.0 mmol l^{-1} in dogs and 2.75 mmol l^{-1} in cats. Dogs and cats up to 2 years old have ionized calcium levels that are 0.025–0.1 mmol l^{-1} higher than adults.

In dogs, hypercalcemia associated with malignancy (lymphoma, anal sac adenocarcinoma), renal failure, hyperparathyroidism, or hypoadrenocorticism is common, while idiopathic hypercalcemia, renal failure, malignancy, and hyperparathyroidism are the most frequent causes of hypercalcemia in the cat [97–99].

Hypercalcemia raises the threshold membrane potential in excitable cells, decreasing cell excitability. At high concentrations, calcium impairs cell function and can result in cell death. Clinical signs related to hypercalcemia are primarily associated with the CNS, gastrointestinal tract, heart, and kidneys. Polydipsia, polyuria, anorexia, lethargy, weakness, vomiting, prerenal azotemia, and chronic renal failure are common. Cardiac arrhythmias, seizures, or twitching can also occur with hypercalcemia, but are less common than when the patient is hypocalcemic.

The presence of clinical signs related to hypercalcemia is regarded as the primary indication to initiate aggressive treatment directed at lowering serum calcium levels rather than specific serum calcium levels [79]. The primary treatment goal for the hypercalcemic patient is removal of the underlying cause, which frequently requires general anesthesia. In the perianesthetic period, IV fluid therapy should be administered with the goal of correcting volume deficits and metabolic acidosis. Unless contraindicated because of underlying cardiopulmonary disease, the rate of fluid administration should result in correction of dehydration within 4–6 h. Physiologic saline is the recommended fluid of choice in the hypercalcemic patient, as the relatively high sodium concentration facilitates calcium excretion in the urine. If the patient has concurrent nonrespiratory acidosis, sodium bicarbonate can be added to the ongoing fluid therapy [79]. Balanced electrolyte solutions have also been shown to reduce ionized serum calcium levels, likely through volume expansion and dilution of serum calcium, and can be used in place of saline when treating mild hypercalcemia. After volume deficit correction, if the patient is still severely hypercalcemic, calciuresis can be attempted with continued aggressive fluid therapy with the addition of furosemide (2–4 mg kg^{-1} IV, every 8 or 12 h) to facilitate renal excretion of calcium. In such cases, the patient will need to be monitored for signs of volume overload and electrolytes monitored to prevent hypernatremia or hypokalemia. Glucocorticoids, including prednisolone or dexamethasone, are effective at lowering hypercalcemia associated with malignancy, hypervitaminosis D, cholecalciferol rodenticide toxicity, and granulomatous disease. Additional therapies reported to offer benefit in the ongoing management of the hypercalcemic patients include drugs aimed at reducing bone reabsorption, such as calcitonin and bisphosphates [79]. During anesthesia, ventilation should be aggressively monitored, and ventilation instituted when necessary to prevent respiratory acidosis.

Acid–Base Homeostasis and Disturbances

Acid–base disturbances alter the relative concentrations of hydronium and hydroxyl in the body, with acidemia defined as a pH (negative logarithm of the hydrogen ion concentration) of arterial blood <7.35 and alkalemia defined as a pH>7.45. Despite the constant generation of carbon dioxide (volatile acid) and nonvolatile acids (H^+) as a byproduct of oxidative metabolism, the hydrogen ion concentration in the body is maintained within a narrow range through intracellular and extracellular buffers with byproducts being excreted via the lungs (CO_2) or kidney (H^+) [4]. The CO_2 partial pressure in the blood is regulated primarily by chemoreceptors in the medulla, which sense its partial pressure in cerebrospinal fluid and alter the degree of alveolar ventilation. Peripheral chemoreceptors in the aortic and carotid bodies also sense changes in hydrogen ion concentration and stimulate alveolar ventilation. The kidneys preferentially control the excretion of Na^+ and Cl^- to influence H^+ and HCO_3^- excretion into and reabsorption from the urine. Normal respiratory and kidney functions are essential to maintain acid–base homeostasis in the body.

There are two different methods used to describe and characterize a patient's acid–base status, the traditional and the Fencl-Stewart approaches [4, 100, 101]. The former approach is based on the Henderson–Hasselbalch equation and relates the pH of blood to the hydrogen ion concentration and arterial partial pressure of CO_2 ($PaCO_2$) and classifies disturbances into respiratory and nonrespiratory (metabolic) disorders. With this approach, nonrespiratory disorders are further characterized based on the presence or absence of an anion gap. The Fencl–Stewart approach provides a more thorough, mechanistic approach to acid–base alterations and can explain the measured changes in a patient with complex acid–base alterations. This system classifies abnormalities into disorders in $PaCO_2$, strong ion difference, and the total plasma concentration of nonvolatile weak acids (primarily albumin and phosphorous), referred to as Atot. When compared to the traditional approach, the Fencl–Stewart approach requires knowledge of more variables including electrolytes, albumin, and phosphates. The traditional approach is therefore more easily applied and remains useful particularly during the anesthetic period if its limitations are recognized. The approach to the patient in the clinical setting should be to first determine the primary disturbance, followed by assessment of the expected compensation and secondary changes to determine if more than one disturbance is present. If a nonrespiratory acidosis is present, the anion gap is calculated.

The most common causes of primary acid–base disturbances are listed in Tables 8.10 and 8.11. The secondary changes in $PaCO_2$, pH, and HCO_3 in response to simple acid–base disturbances in dogs are provided in Table 8.12. Unfortunately, the anticipated changes in cats are not well-characterized, but the changes observed in the dog can be used as guidelines. A review of the primary acid–base disturbance categories will be followed by a stepwise approach to the assessment of a patient's acid–base status. The latter will be limited to patients with relatively common noncomplex abnormalities and normal plasma proteins and serum phosphorous levels. For a thorough review of mixed acid–base disorders, the reader is referred to several excellent reviews [102, 103].

Respiratory Acidosis

Primary respiratory acidosis results from an increase in $PaCO_2$ associated with a decrease in alveolar ventilation. The increase in $PaCO_2$ decreases pH and increases plasma bicarbonate secondary to increased quantities of dissolved carbonic acid. In the traditional approach to acid–base status, the increase in bicarbonate that occurs secondary to increases in $PaCO_2$ is considered a compensatory response, while the Fencl–Stewart approach

Table 8.10 Common causes of respiratory acidosis and alkalosis in dogs and cats.

	Respiratory acidosis	Respiratory alkalosis
Ventilatory drive	*Decreased ventilatory drive* • Drugs • CNS disease • Nonrespiratory alkalosis	*Increased ventilatory drive* • Hypoxemia • Respiratory disease • Sepsis • Pain • Hyperthermia • Nonrespiratory acidosis
Ability to ventilate	*Decreased ability to ventilate* • Upper airway obstruction • Neuromuscular disease • Extrapulmonary disease • Intrapulmonary disease	
CO_2 production	*Increased CO_2 production* • Malignant hyperthermia	*Decreased CO_2 production* • Pending cardiopulmonary arrest
Iatrogenic	• Inappropriate ventilator settings • Anesthetic equipment malfunction • Expired carbon dioxide absorbent	• Inappropriate ventilator settings

Table 8.11 Common causes of nonrespiratory acidosis and alkalosis in dogs and cats as categorized by the traditional and Fencl–Stewart approaches [100, 101].

Nonrespiratory acidosis	Nonrespiratory alkalosis
Increased anion gap/decreased SID[a], increased UMA[b] • Lactic acidosis • Diabetic ketoacidosis • Toxins: salicylate, ethylene glycol, metaldehyde • Uremic acidosis (increased Atot[c])	*Increased SID[a], chloride deficit* • Vomiting • Diuretics
Normal anion gap/decreased SID[a], increased Cl^- • Diarrhea • Renal tubular acidosis • Carbonic anhydrase inhibitors (acetazolamide) • NaCl fluid therapy	*Increased SID[a], increased Na^+* • Alkali administration ($NaHCO_3$) • Hyperaldosteronism • Hyperadrenocorticism
Dilutional acidosis, decreased SID[a], decreased Na^+	*Decreased Atot[c]* • Hypoalbuminemia

[a] SID = strong ion difference [b] UMA = unmeasured anions [c] Atot = sum of nonvolatile weak acids

identifies the compensatory response to elevations in $PaCO_2$ as an increase in urinary excretion of chloride ions, with changes in bicarbonate occurring secondarily [101]. Nonetheless, the expected changes in pH and bicarbonate resulting from elevations in $PaCO_2$ (Table 8.12) should be considered when interpreting the patient's overall acid–base status, as unexpected alterations may reflect concurrent abnormalities.

Table 8.12 Primary disturbances and expected secondary changes associated with acid–base disturbances in the dog [102].

	Secondary changes		
Primary disturbance	**pH**	**$PaCO_2$**	**HCO_3^-**
Respiratory acidosis • acute	Decreases by 0.05 for every 10 mmHg increase in $PaCO_2$		Increases by 1.5 mEq l^{-1} for every 10 mmHg increase in $PaCO_2$
Respiratory acidosis • chronic	Decreases by 0.07 for every 10 mmHg increase in $PaCO_2$		Increases by 3.5–5.5 mEq l^{-1} for every 10 mmHg increase in $PaCO_2$
Respiratory alkalosis • acute	Increases by 0.1 for every 10 mmHg decrease in $PaCO_2$		Decreases by 2.5 mEq l^{-1} for every 10 mmHg decrease in $PaCO_2$
Respiratory alkalosis • chronic	Increases by 0.15 for every 10 mmHg decrease in $PaCO_2$		Decreases by 5.5 mEq l^{-1} for every 10 mmHg decrease in $PaCO_2$
Nonrespiratory acidosis (decrease in SID[a], increase in Atot[b])		Decreases by 0.7–1 mmHg for each 1 mEq l^{-1} decrease in HCO_3^-	
Nonrespiratory alkalosis (increase in SID[a], decrease in Atot[b])		Increases by 0.7 mmHg for each 1 mEq l^{-1} increase in HCO_3^-	

[a] SID = strong ion difference
[b] Atot = sum of nonvolatile weak acids

Common causes of hypoventilation and subsequent respiratory acidosis (Table 8.10) include conditions that decrease ventilatory drive, a decreased ability to ventilate, an increase in carbon dioxide production, and other iatrogenic causes. In the perianesthetic period, opioids, particularly pure mu-opioid receptor agonists when used in combination with sedatives, and most anesthetic agents including inhalants and injectable agents result in mild to moderate alveolar hypoventilation and respiratory acidosis [104]. Clinical signs specific to respiratory acidosis may be small relative to signs related to the primary disorder resulting in hypoventilation. In particular, the patient's inspired oxygen content will dramatically alter the manifestation of respiratory acidosis, as marked hypoventilation in a patient breathing room air will result in hypoxemia and its associated signs while a patient receiving oxygen supplementation (inspired oxygen levels >30%) will usually not experience a reduction in oxygenation due to hypoventilation alone. Increases in $PaCO_2$ without concurrent hypoxemia result in sympathetic nervous system stimulation with increases in heart rate and cardiac output [105]. However, chronic respiratory acidosis without hypoxemia in the anesthetized, ventilated dog results in a decrease in heart rate and cardiac output [106]. Overall, the severity and duration of hypercapnia, as well as the specific anesthetic agents used, likely influence elevations in $PaCO_2$ during anesthesia. Respiratory acidosis diagnosis is by arterial blood gas analysis; in an intubated patient, end-tidal carbon dioxide levels can be used to estimate or evaluate trends in the severity of hypoventilation. The method of measurement, patient size, and the breathing circuit can all influence the relationship of the measured end-tidal carbon dioxide to $PaCO_2$; however, in general, end-tidal carbon dioxide is approximately 4–6 mmHg lower than $PaCO_2$ in normal cats and dogs, with greater differences seen with concurrent disease [107, 108].

If primary respiratory acidosis is present prior to anesthesia, an IV catheter should be placed and supplies to secure the patient's airway and provide ventilatory support should be prepared before proceeding with sedative, analgesic, or anesthetic drug administration. When possible, the underlying etiology should be discerned and removed if possible. For example, fluid or air within the thoracic space should be removed by thoracocentesis prior to anesthetic induction. Concurrent conditions including dehydration, electrolyte abnormalities, and hypoxemia should be corrected or at least improved prior to anesthesia with IV fluid and electrolyte therapy and oxygen supplementation. When feasible, monitoring of the ECG, blood pressure, and hemoglobin saturation should be initiated prior to induction. The degree of hypercapnia is likely to increase with anesthetic induction; a rapid induction and tracheal intubation, with aggressive monitoring of ventilation using capnometry immediately after intubation, is highly recommended. The specific degree of hypercapnia at which to institute ventilatory support has not been determined. However, during anesthesia, if pH is <7.2 or $PaCO_2$ is >60 mmHg, ventilatory support is generally recommended [109]. When pH is <7.1, cardiac contractility is decreased, and hemodynamic stability may be impaired [105]. Aggressive ventilatory monitoring is indicated in patients with preexisting respiratory acidosis both intraoperatively and during recovery from anesthesia. Oxygen supplementation and possibly prolonged ventilatory support may be required in the postanesthetic phase depending on the underlying condition.

Respiratory acidosis developing during general anesthesia with oxygen supplementation is not uncommon in healthy small-animal patients, as all anesthetics produce dose-dependent respiratory depression [104]. The degree of hypoventilation is dependent on the specific anesthetic protocol used, the anesthetic depth required, patient positioning, and the surgical intervention. Dogs and cats typically tolerate moderate increases in carbon dioxide and ventilatory support is generally not indicated until $PaCO_2$ levels exceed 60 mmHg, assuming other acid–base and electrolyte disturbances are not present. Equipment malfunctions, expired carbon dioxide absorbent, or inappropriate ventilator settings can all lead to elevations in $PaCO_2$ and should be considered, particularly when they are not consistent with the patients perceived degree of alveolar ventilation.

Respiratory Alkalosis

Primary respiratory alkalosis occurs because of hyperventilation, resulting in a decrease in $PaCO_2$ and an increase in pH. Plasma bicarbonate decreases secondary to the decrease in dissolved carbonic acid, and, while the change in bicarbonate is explained as a compensatory change in the traditional approach, it is now understood that the kidneys compensate for respiratory alkalosis by actively reducing chloride excretion in the urine with bicarbonate changes occurring secondarily (Table 8.12).

Primary respiratory alkalosis is not as common in the perioperative period as respiratory acidosis. However, it can occur secondary to an increase in ventilatory drive or a decrease in carbon dioxide production (Table 8.10). Hypoxemia, pain, exercise, and hyperthermia are more common causes of increased ventilatory drive leading to hypocapnia and respiratory alkalosis. Iatrogenic hyperventilation in small-animal patients is a common side effect of positive pressure ventilation which can be prevented with monitoring of end-tidal carbon dioxide levels. Acute, severe reductions in $PaCO_2$ may be indicative of a reduction in peripheral blood flow and impending cardiopulmonary arrest. There are very few clinical signs specifically related to respiratory alkalosis in the conscious patient; however, $PaCO_2$ levels <20 mmHg in the anesthetized animal reduce cerebral blood flow, myocardial perfusion, cardiac output, and systemic arterial blood pressure [110]. Treatment of respiratory alkalosis should be aimed at treating the underlying cause.

Nonrespiratory Acidosis

Primary nonrespiratory acidosis is characterized by a decrease in pH and a decrease in plasma bicarbonate. In the traditional approach, etiologies of nonrespiratory acidosis are grouped into those with a normal (hyperchloremic) or abnormal anion gap. The anion gap, a measurement of unmeasured anions minus unmeasured cations, can be calculated using the following formula (Eq. (8.6)):

$$\text{Anion gap} = \left[\left(\text{Na}^+ + \text{K}^+\right) - \left(\text{Cl}^- + \text{HCO}_3^-\right)\right] \tag{8.6}$$

The normal anion gap is 12–25 mmol l^{-1} in dogs and 13–31 mmol l^{-1} in cats [100, 111]. An increase in anion gap is associated with an increase in either endogenous or exogenous anions such as lactate (Table 8.11). A nonrespiratory acidosis without an increase in anion gap is associated with an increase in serum chloride in proportion to the reduction in HCO_3^-, and is also referred to as a hyperchloremic nonrespiratory acidosis. Common situations associated with this include diarrhea and renal failure. Hypoalbuminemia results in a decrease in the anion gap and the impact of this variable should be considered when evaluating the anion gap in the hypoproteinemic patient [112]. If albumin and phosphorous levels are available and they fall outside of normal ranges, a corrected anion gap can be calculated using Eqs. (8.7)–(8.10):

Dog

$$\begin{aligned}\text{Anion gap}&(\text{adjusted for albumin})\\ &= \left[\left(\text{Na}^+ + \text{K}^+\right) - \left(\text{Cl}^- + \text{HCO}_3^-\right)\right]\\ &+ \left[(0.42) \times \left(3.77 - \text{albumin in g dl}^{-1}\right)\right]\end{aligned} \tag{8.7}$$

$$\begin{aligned}\text{Anion gap}&(\text{adjusted for phosphorous})\\ &= \left[\left(\text{Na}^+ + \text{K}^+\right) - \left(\text{Cl}^- + \text{HCO}_3^-\right)\right]\\ &+ \left[(2.52) - \left(0.58 \times \text{phosphorous in mg dl}^{-1}\right)\right]\end{aligned} \tag{8.8}$$

Cat

$$\begin{aligned}\text{Anion gap}&(\text{adjusted for albumin})\\ &= \left[\left(\text{Na}^+ + \text{K}^+\right) - \left(\text{Cl}^- + \text{HCO}_3^-\right)\right]\\ &+ \left[(0.41) \times \left(3.3 - \text{albumin in g dl}^{-1}\right)\right]\end{aligned} \tag{8.9}$$

$$\begin{aligned}\text{Anion gap}&(\text{adjusted for phosphorous})\\ &= \left[\left(\text{Na}^+ + \text{K}^+\right) - \left(\text{Cl}^- + \text{HCO}_3^-\right)\right]\\ &+ \left[(2.52) - \left(0.58 \times \text{phosphorous in mg dl}^{-1}\right)\right]\end{aligned} \tag{8.10}$$

In the Fencl–Stewart approach, nonrespiratory acidosis is attributed to a decrease in the strong ion difference or an increase in the total plasma concentration of nonvolatile weak acids. Most strong ion difference abnormalities result in an acidosis from an increase in Cl^- or unmeasured anions, or a decrease in Na^+. In response to a nonrespiratory acidosis, alveolar hyperventilation occurs, $PaCO_2$ decreases, and pH returns toward normal (Table 8.12).

Clinical signs of acidosis are primarily dependent on the underlying cause and the rapidity of onset of the change in pH. However, in general, a pH <7.2 is associated with a decrease in enzymatic reactions throughout the body, an impairment of normal cell functions, and a reduction in myocardial contractility, cardiac output, and systemic arterial pressures, and predisposes to ventricular arrhythmias [102]. Correction of nonrespiratory acidosis should ideally be performed prior to anesthesia by addressing the underlying disturbance, although complete correction may not be feasible without a surgical intervention. In the case of an increased anion gap associated with a lactic acidosis, fluid therapy is the cornerstone of treatment with the goal of correcting fluid deficits and improving tissue perfusion. Ketoacidosis should be corrected with IV fluid and insulin therapy. Sodium bicarbonate addition to the treatment regime in the patient with lactic acidosis or ketoacidosis remains controversial; however, in the patient with uremic acidosis, fluid therapy with the addition of $NaHCO_3$ is recommended if the pH is below 7.2 [113]. In the patient with acidosis and a normal anion gap, fluid deficits should be corrected prior to anesthesia and, if the pH is below 7.2, $NaHCO_3$ therapy initiated. While the traditional approach to acid–base interpretation attributes the improvement in pH with $NaHCO_3$ therapy to the HCO_3^- component, the current understanding is that the Na^+ is responsible for the improvement in the patient's status by increasing in the strong ion difference, expanding the extracellular space, and increasing urine production [100].

Major preanesthetic considerations in the patient with nonrespiratory acidosis include the impact of the underlying condition on the patient's cardiovascular status and reserve, presence of concurrent electrolyte disturbances, choice of IV fluid and its administration rate, the need for additional treatments such as $NaHCO_3$, potential changes in the pharmacokinetics of drugs, and the need to support ventilation to prevent significant increases in $PaCO_2$, which would further contribute to reductions in pH. In the hemodynamically unstable patient, an ECG and invasive blood pressure monitoring should be used to assist with the optimization of fluid and inotrope therapy. The specific anesthetic protocol chosen should be guided by the patient's cardiovascular status; using a technique that permits drug titration to effect will minimize the risk of inadvertent drug overdose. A balanced electrolyte solution is generally the fluid of choice with the administration rate guided by the patient's hydration status. If $NaHCO_3$ is indicated as discussed in the preceding text, it can be mixed with the replacement fluid. However, it will increase the tonicity of the fluid. If hypertonicity is contraindicated, $NaHCO_3$ can be diluted with sterile water (1.5 ml of 1 mEq l^{-1} $NaHCO_3$ with 8.5 ml of sterile water) to achieve an isotonic solution [114].

The quantity of $NaHCO_3$ administered over the first few treatment hours is estimated by Eq. (8.11).

$$\mathrm{NaHCO_3}^-\left(\mathrm{mmol}\right) = 0.3 \times \text{body weight}\left(\mathrm{kg}\right) \times \text{bicarbonate deficit}\left(\mathrm{mmol\,l^{-1}}\right) \tag{8.11}$$

Blood gas analysis should be used to guide follow-up $NaHCO_3$ treatments, with the goal being to return pH to approximately 7.2. Complete correction of pH to normal is not recommended to avoid iatrogenic alkalosis. To prevent a concurrent respiratory acidosis with anesthetic induction, the anesthetist should be prepared to support ventilation immediately following intubation. Ideally, the adequacy of alveolar ventilation should be monitored with intermittent arterial blood gas analysis and/or capnometry.

Nonrespiratory Alkalosis

Primary nonrespiratory alkalosis is characterized by an increase in pH and plasma bicarbonate. The most common causes of nonrespiratory alkalosis in the dog and cat relate to excessive loss of chloride via the gastrointestinal tract secondary to vomiting or via the kidney due to diuretic administration (Table 8.10). In response to the alkalosis, alveolar hypoventilation occurs, $PaCO_2$ increases, and pH returns toward normal (Table 8.11). Clinical signs in patients with nonrespiratory alkalosis are primarily related to underlying conditions and associated electrolyte changes. Of particular significance is the effect of an increase in pH on serum potassium and ionized calcium, both of which decrease with the decrease in H^+ concentration [64, 65, 79]. Treatment goal is to address the underlying cause and correct volume and chloride deficits, with concurrent serum potassium monitoring recommended, as patients often have whole body deficits that result in hypokalemia when the pH returns toward normal. Intravenous fluid therapy with a balanced electrolyte solution or sodium chloride (0.9%) and potassium supplementation based on the individual patient is recommended. If possible, any volume deficits should be corrected prior to anesthesia. The choice of induction technique should be based on the individual patient's concurrent disease. Guidelines for potassium supplementation during anesthesia are provided in the preceding text.

Stepwise Approach to Acid–Base Status Assessment

Correct acid–base status assessment is heavily dependent on blood gas sample quality and blood gas analyzer accuracy. The approach taken in the following text is based on interpretation of an arterial blood gas sample with a blood gas analyzer with the ability to report electrolytes (Na^+, K^+, Cl^-).

1) Evaluate sample quality by assessing all the values reported. Sample dilution or improper mixing will result in an artificial reduction in measured hemoglobin, while contamination with air will falsely lower PCO_2 and elevate PO_2.
2) Evaluate the pH. If pH is <7.35, the patient is acidemic, if the pH is >7.45, the patient is alkalemic.
3) Consider pH and $PaCO_2$. If the direction of change is opposite, the primary disorder is respiratory in origin. If the direction of change is the same, the primary disorder is nonrespiratory in origin.
4) If the primary disorder is respiratory and the $PaCO_2$ is >45 mmHg, respiratory acidosis is present. If the primary disorder is respiratory and $PaCO_2$ is <30 mmHg, respiratory alkalosis is present. Consider if the expected change in pH and HCO_3^- is appropriate for the change in $PaCO_2$ (Table 8.12). If the changes are outside of anticipated range, more than one process may be present.
5) If the primary disorder is nonrespiratory, calculate the expected change in $PaCO_2$. If the change is outside of the anticipated range, more than one process may be present.
6) If the patient has a nonrespiratory acidosis, calculate the anion gap to determine most likely etiologies and the appropriate treatment approach. Consider the patient's serum phosphorous and albumin levels and their impact on the assessment of the anion gap.
7) If the patient has a nonrespiratory alkalosis, assess serum Na^+, Cl^-, and protein levels to determine the etiology of the alkalosis.

Stepwise Approach to the Anesthetic Management of the Patient with an Acid–Base Disorder

1) Following characterization of the acid–base disorder(s), consider the underlying etiology and concurrent abnormalities.
2) Initiate measures to address abnormalities in hydration and/or electrolyte disturbances.
3) Perform a thorough assessment of the cardiovascular system, including cardiac rhythm evaluation with an ECG and blood pressure, if indicated based on physical examination findings. Ensure secure IV access and attempt hemodynamic stabilization prior to preanesthetic medication.
4) Assess respiratory function and respiratory effort. If compromised, consider performing therapeutic measures such as thoracocentesis with local anesthesia prior to anesthetic induction. Oxygen supplementation should be initiated in patients with reduced PaO_2 or SpO_2 levels prior to premedication.
5) Consider monitoring devices and support measures such as fluid therapy, positive pressure ventilation, or inotrope administration that will likely be required during the anesthetic period and prepare accordingly.
6) The specific anesthetic protocol used should be based on the individual animal's condition. A balanced anesthetic approach using an opioid analgesic for premedication, injectable anesthetic induction agents

that are suitable for administration by titration such as alfaxalone, propofol, or an opioid/benzodiazepine combination, and a maintenance regime that incorporates locoregional anesthetic techniques and systemic analgesics to reduce general anesthetic requirements is preferable. In cases with severe respiratory acidosis, opioid premedication can be delayed until after anesthetic induction and ventilator support initiated.

7) Supportive measures including fluid, electrolyte, oxygen, and ventilatory support should be continued into the recovery until it is deemed unnecessary based on assessment of the individual patient.

References

1 Verlander, J.W. (2020). Water balance. In: *Cunningham's Textbook of Veterinary Physiology*, 6e (ed. B.G. Klein), 501–508. St. Louis: Elsevier.

2 Nelson, R.W. (2015). Water metabolism and diabetes insipidus. In: *Canine and Feline Endocrinology*, 4e (eds. E.C. Feldman, R.W. Nelson, C.E. Reusch and J.C.R. Scott-Moncrieff), 1–36. St. Louis: Elsevier Sanders.

3 Wellman, M.L., DiBartola, S.P., and Kohn, C.W. (2012). Applied physiology of body fluids in dogs and cats. In: *Fluid, Electrolyte, and Acid-Base Disorders in Small Animal Practice*, 4e (ed. S.P. DiBartola), 2–25. St. Louis: Elsevier.

4 DiBartola, S.P. (2012). Introduction to acid-base disorders. In: *Fluid, Electrolyte, and Acid-Base Disorders in Small Animal Practice*, 4e (ed. S.P. DiBartola), 231–252. St. Louis: Elsevier.

5 Benzon, H.A., Bobrowski, A., Suresh, S. et al. (2019). Impact of preoperative hyponatraemia on paediatric perioperative mortality. *Br. J. Anaesth.* 123: 618–626.

6 Madsen, C.M., Jantzen, C., Lauritzen, J.B. et al. (2016). Hyponatremia and hypernatremia are associated with increased 30-day mortality in hip fracture patients. *Osteoporos. Int.* 27: 397–404.

7 McCausland, F.R., Wright, J., and Waikar, S.S. (2014). Association of serum sodium with morbidity and mortality in hospitalized patients undergoing major orthopedic surgery. *J. Hosp. Med.* 9: 297–302.

8 McCluskey, S.A., Karkouti, K., Wijeysundera, D. et al. (2013). Hyperchloremia after noncardiac surgery is independently associated with increased morbidity and mortality: a propensity-matched cohort study. *Anesth. Anal.* 117: 412–421.

9 Moller, M., Adamsen, S., Thomsen, R.W. et al. (2010). Preoperative prognostic factors for mortality in peptic ulcer perforation: a systematic review. *Scand. J. Gastroenterol.* 45: 785–805.

10 Brodbelt, D.C., Blissitt, K.J., Hammond, R.A. et al. (2008). The risk of death: the confidential enquiry into perioperative small animal fatalities. *Vet. Anaesth. Anal.* 35: 365–373.

11 Brodbelt, D.C., Hammond, R.A., Tuminaro, D. et al. (2006). Risk factors for anaesthetic-related death in referred dogs. *Vet. Rec.* 158: 563–564.

12 Dyson, D.H., Maxie, M.G., and Schnurr, D. (1998). Morbidity and mortality associated with anesthetic management in small animal veterinary practice in Ontario. *J. Am. Anim. Hosp. Assoc.* 34: 325–335.

13 Guenheid, M., Aarnes, T.K., McLoughlin, M.A. et al. (2018). Risk of anesthesia-related complications in brachycephalic dogs. *J. Am. Vet. Med. Assoc.* 253: 301–306.

14 Woodcock, T.E. and Woodcock, T.M. (2012). Revised Starling equation and the glycocalyx model of transvascular fluid exchange: an improved paradigm for prescribing intravenous fluid therapy. *Br. J. Anaesth.* 108: 384–394.

15 Salmon, A.H. and Satchell, S.C. (2012). Endothelial glycocalyx dysfunction in disease: albuminuria and increased microvascular permeability. *J. Pathol.* 226: 562–574.

16 Desborough, J.P. (2000). The stress response to trauma and surgery. *Br. J. Anaesth.* 85: 109–117.

17 Hauptman, J.G., Richter, M.A., Wood, S.L. et al. (2000). Effects of anesthesia, surgery, and intravenous administration of fluids on plasma antidiuretic hormone concentration in healthy dogs. *Am. J. Vet. Res.* 61: 1273–1276.

18 Boscan, P., Pypendop, B.H., Siao, K.T. et al. (2010). Fluid balance, glomerular filtration rate, and urine output in dogs anesthetized for an orthopedic surgical procedure. *Am. J. Vet. Res.* 71: 501–507.

19 Ethier, M.R., Mathews, K.A., Valverde, A. et al. (2008). Evaluation of the efficacy and safety for use of two sedation and analgesia protocols to facilitate assisted ventilation of healthy dogs. *Am. J. Vet. Res.* 69: 1351–1359.

20 DiBartola, S.P. (2012). Disorders of sodium and water: hypernatremia and hyponatremia. In: *Fluid, Electrolyte, and Acid-Base Disorders in Small Animal Practice*, 4e (ed. S.P. DiBartola), 45–79. St. Louis: Elsevier.

21 Rudloff, E. (2017). Assessment of hydration. In: *Small Animal Critical Care Medicine*, 2e (eds. D.C. Silverstein and K. Hopper), 307–310. St. Louis: Elsevier.

22 Costa, R.S., Raisis, A.L., Hosgood, G. et al. (2015). Preoperative factors associated with hypotension in young anaesthetized dogs undergoing elective desexing. *Aust. Vet. J.* 93: 99–104.

23 Moghadamyeghaneh, Z., Phelan, M.J., Carmichael, J.C. et al. (2014). Preoperative dehydration increases risk of postoperative acute renal failure in colon and rectal surgery. *J. Gastrointest. Surg.* 18: 2178–2185.

24 Hartog, C. and Reinhart, K. (2009). Contra: hydroxyethyl starch solutions are unsafe in critically ill patients. *Intensive Care Med.* 35: 1337–1342.

25 Hayes, G., Benedicenti, L., and Mathews, K. (2016). Retrospective cohort study on the incidence of acute kidney injury and death following hydroxyethyl starch (HES 10% 250/0.5/5:1) administration in dogs. *J. Vet. Emerg. Crit. 3Care* 26: 35–40.

26 Boyd, C.J., Claus, M.A., Raisis, A.L. et al. (2019). Evaluation of biomarkers of kidney injury following 4% succinylated gelatin and 6% hydroxyethyl starch 130/0.4 administration in a canine hemorrhagic shock model. *J. Vet. Emerg. Crit. Care* 29: 132–142.

27 Wong, C. and Koenig, A. (2017). The colloid controversy. Are colloids bad and what are the options? *Vet. Clin. North Am. Small Anim. Pract.* 47: 411–421.

28 Schadt, J.C. and Ludbrook, J. (1991). Hemodynamic and neurohumoral responses to hypovolemia in conscious mammals. *Am. J. Physiol.* 260: H305–H318.

29 Crystal, M.A. and Cotter, S.M. (1992). Acute hemorrhage: a hematologic emergency in dogs. *Comp. Cont. Ed.* 60: 60–67.

30 Palmer, L. (2017). Fluid management in patients with trauma. Restrictive versus liberal approach. *Vet. Clin. North Am. Small Anim. Pract* 47: 397–410.

31 Sigrist, N., Olgiati, L., and Jud Schefer, R.S. (2018). Effect of tranexamic acid on intra- and postoperative haemorrhage in dogs with surgically treated hemoperitoneum. *Schweiz. Arch. Tierheilkd.* 160: 305–312.

32 Fletcher, D.J., Blackstock, K.J., Epstein, K. et al. (2014). Evaluation of tranexamic acid and epsilon-aminocaproic acid concentrations required to inhibit fibrinolysis in plasma of dogs and humans. *Am. J. Vet. Res.* 75: 731–738.

33 Corcoran, T., Rhodes, J.E., Clarke, S. et al. (2012). Perioperative fluid management strategies in major surgery: a stratified meta-analysis. *Anesth. Anal.* 114: 640–651.

34 Makaryus, R., Miller, T.E., and Gan, T.J. (2018). Current concepts of fluid management in enhanced recovery pathways. *Br. J. Anaesth.* 120: 376–383.

35 Weinberg, L., Banting, J., Churilov, L. et al. (2017). The effect of surgery-specific cardiac output-guided haemodynamic algorithm on outcomes in patients undergoing pancreaticoduodenectomy in a high-volume centre: a retrospective comparative study. *Anaesth. Intensive Care* 45: 569–580.

36 Asklid, D., Segelman, J., Gedda, C. et al. (2017). The impact of perioperative fluid therapy on short-term outcomes and 5-year survival among patients undergoing colorectal cancer surgery-a prospective cohort study within an ERAS protocol. *Eur. J. Surg. Oncol.* 43: 1433–1439.

37 Drozdzynaka, M.J., Chang, Y.M., Stanzani, G. et al. (2018). Evaluation of the dynamic predictors of fluid responsiveness in dogs receiving goal-directed fluid therapy. *Vet. Anaesth. Anal.* 45: 22–30.

38 Celeita-Rodriguez, N., Teixeira-Neto, F.J., Garofalo, N.A. et al. (2019). Comparison of the diagnostic accuracy of dynamic and static preload indexes to predict fluid responsiveness in mechanically ventilated, isoflurane anesthetized dogs. *Vet. Anaesth. Analg.* 46: 276–288.

39 Fayyaz, S., Kerr, C.L., Dyson, D.H. et al. (2009). The cardiopulmonary effects of anesthetic induction with isoflurane, ketamine-diazepam or propofol-diazepam in the hypovolemic dog. *Vet. Anaesth. Analg.* 36: 110–123.

40 Machado, C.G., Dyson, D.H., and Mathews, K.A. (2005). Evaluation of induction by use of a combination of oxymorphone and diazepam or hydromorphone and diazepam and maintenance of anesthesia by use of isoflurane in dogs with experimentally induced hypovolemia. *Am. J. Vet. Res.* 66: 1227–1237.

41 Mattson, S.F., Kerr, C.L., Dyson, D.H. et al. (2006). The effect of hypovolemia due to hemorrhage on the minimum alveolar concentration of isoflurane in the dog. *Vet. Anaesth. Analg.* 33: 296–301.

42 Pinsky, M.R. (2005). Cardiovascular issues in respiratory care. *Chest* 128: 592S–597S.

43 Burton, A.G. and Hopper, K. (2019). Hyponatremia in dogs and cats. *J. Vet. Emerg. Crit. Care* 29: 463–471.

44 Guillaumin, J. and DiBartola, S.P. (2017). Disorders of sodium and water homeostasis. *Vet. Clin. North Am. Small Anim. Pract.* 47: 293–312.

45 Guillaumin, J. and DiBartola, S.P. A quick reference on hyponatremia. *Vet. Clin. North Am. Small Anim. Pract.* 47: 213–217.

46 Waikar, S.S., Mount, D.B., and Curhan, G.C. (2009). Mortality after hospitalization with mild, moderate, and severe hyponatremia. *Am. J. Med.* 122: 857–865.

47 Holland-Bill, L., Christiansen, C.F., Heide-Jorgensen, U. et al. (2015). Hyponatremia and mortality risk: a Danish cohort study of 279508 acutely hospitalized patients. *Eur. J. Endocrinol.* 173: 71–81.

48 Ueda, Y., Hopper, K., and Epstein, S.E. (2015). Incidence, severity and prognosis associated with hyponatremia in dogs and cats. *J. Vet. Intern. Med.* 29: 801–807.

49 Clabots, M.F., Gaillard, E., and Aumann, M. (2019). Acute kidney injury, seizures, and hypertonic hyponatremia secondary to mannitol intoxication in a dog. *J. Vet. Crit. Care* 29: 680–685.

50 Drobatz, K.J. and Mandell, D.C. (2000). Differential diagnosis of laboratory abnormalities in critical care settings. In: *Kirk's Current Veterinary Therapy XIII Small Animal Practice* (ed. J.D. Bonagura), 106. Philadelphia: W.B. Saunders.

51 Brady, C.A., Vite, C.H., and Drobatz, K.J. (1999). Severe neurologic sequelae in a dog after treatment of hypoadrenal crisis. *J. Am. Vet. Med. Assoc.* 215: 222–225.

52 Churcher, R.K., Watson, A.D., and Easton, A. (1999). Suspected myelinolysis following rapid correction of hyponatremia in a dog. *J. Am. Anim. Hosp. Assoc.* 35: 493–497.

53 MacMillan, K.L. (2003). Neurologic complications following treatment of canine hypoadrenocorticism. *Can. Vet. J.* 44: 490–492.

54 O'Brien, D.P., Kroll, R.A., Johnson, G.C. et al. (1994). Myelinolysis after correction of hyponatremia in two dogs. *J. Vet. Intern. Med.* 8: 40–48.

55 Quasha, A.L., Eger, E.I., and Tinker, J.H. (1980). Determination and applications of MAC. *Anesthesiology* 53: 315–334.

56 Ueda, Y., Hopper, K., and Epstein, S.E. (2015). Incidence, severity and prognosis associated with hypernatremia in dogs and cats. *J. Vet. Intern. Med.* 29: 794–800.

57 Mix, K.A., Stafford, J., and Hofmeister, E. (2019). Effect of single dose administration activated charcoal containing sorbitol on serum sodium concentration and hydration status in dogs. *J. Vet. Emerg. Crit. Care* 29: 616–621.

58 Tanifuji, Y., Eger, E.I., and Terrell, R.C. (1978). Brain sodium, potassium, and osmolality: effect on anesthetic requirement. *Anesth. Analg.* 57: 404–410.

59 de Morais, H.A. and Biondo, A.W. (2012). Disorders of chloride: hyperchloremia and hypochloremia. In: *Fluid, Electrolyte, and Acid-Base Disorders in Small Animal Practice*, 4e (ed. D.B. SP), 80–91. St. Louis: Elsevier.

60 Bohn, A.A. and de Morais, H.A. (2017). A quick reference on chloride. *Vet. Clin. North Am. Small Anim. Pract.* 47: 219–222.

61 Piperisova, I., Neel, J.A., and Papich, M.G. (2009). What is your diagnosis? Marked hyperchloremia in a dog. *Vet. Clin. Pathol.* 38: 411–414.

62 Paterson, M.E., Kintzer, P.P., Cavanagh, P.G. et al. (1983). Natural history of potassium-deficiency myopathy in the dog: role of adrenocorticosteriod in rhabdomyolysis. *J. Lab. Clin. Med.* 102: 565–576.

63 Sterns, R.H., Cox, M., Feig, P.U. et al. (1981). Internal potassium balance and the control of the plasma potassium concentration. *Medicine* 60: 339–354.

64 Adrogue, H.J. and Madias, N.E. (1981). Changes in plasma potassium concentration during acute acid base disturbances. *Am. J. Med.* 71: 456–467.

65 Muir, W.W., Wagner, A.E., and Buchanan, C. (1990). Effects of acute hyperventilation on serum potassium in the dog. *Vet. Surg.* 19: 83–87.

66 Hoehne, S.N., Hopper, K., and Epstein, S.E. (2019). Retrospective evaluation of the severity of and prognosis associated with potassium abnormalities in dogs and cats presenting to an emergency room (January 2014–August 2015). *J. Vet. Emerg. Crit. Care* 29: 653–661.

67 Kogika, M.M. and de Morais, H.A. (2017). A quick reference on hypokalemia. *Vet. Clin. North Am. Small Anim. Pract.* 47: 229–234.

68 Dibartola, S.P. and de Morais, H.A. (2012). Disorders of potassium: hypokalemia and hyperkalemia. In: *Fluid, Electrolyte, and Acid-Base Disorders in Small Animal Practice*, 4e (ed. S.P. DiBartola), 92–119. St. Louis: Elsevier.

69 Taylor, P., Prymak, C., Hird, J. et al. (2018). Surgical complications: unanticipated hyperkalaemia. *Vet. Rec.* 182: 84.

70 Ha, Y.S., Hopper, K., and Epstein, S.E. (2013). Incidence, nature, and etiology of metabolic alkalosis in dogs and cats. *J. Vet. Intern. Med.* 27: 847–853.

71 Dhein, C.R. and Wardrop, K.J. (1995). Hyperkalemia associated with potassium chloride supplementation in a cat. *J. Am. Vet. Med. Assoc.* 206: 1565–1566.

72 Brunson, D.B. and Hogan, K.J. (2004). Malignant hyperthermia: a syndrome not a disease. *Vet. Clin. North Am. Small Anim. Pract.* 34: 1419–1433.

73 Jones, S.J., Mama, K.R., Brock, N.K., and Couto, C.G. (2019). Hyperkalemia during general anesthesia in two greyhounds. *J. Am. Vet. Med. Assoc.* 254: 1329–1334.

74 Reilly, S., Dessighi, M.R., Steeil, J.C. et al. (2014). Selected clinical, biochemical and electrolyte alterations in anesthetized captive tigers. *J. Zoo Wildl. Med.* 45: 328–334.

75 Reinmann, K.A., Knowlen, G.G., and Tvendten, H.W. (1989). Factitious hyperkalemia in dogs with thrombocytosis. The effect of platelets on serum potassium concentration. *J. Vet. Intern. Med.* 3: 47–52.

76 Tag, T.L. and Day, T.K. (2008). Electrocardiographic assessment of hyperkalemia in dogs and cats. *J. Vet. Emerg. Crit. Care* 81: 61–67.

77 Drobatz, K.J. and Cole, S.G. (2008). The influence of crystalloid type on acid-base and electrolyte status of cats with urethral obstruction. *J. Vet. Emerg. Crit. Care* 18: 355–361.

78 Cunha, M.C., Freitas, G.C., Carregaro, A.B. et al. (2010). Renal and cardiorespiratory effects of treatment with lactated Ringer's solution or physiologic saline (0.9% NaCl) solution in cats with experimentally induced urethral obstruction. *Am. J. Vet. Res.* 71: 840–846.

79 Schenek, P.A., Chew, D.J., Nagode, L.A. et al. (2012). Disorders of calcium: hypercalcemia and hypocalcemia. In: *Fluid, Electrolyte, and Acid-Base Disorders in Small Animal Practice*, 4e (ed. S.P. DiBartola), 120–194. St. Louis: Elsevier.

80 Rosol, T.J., Chew, D.J., Nagode, L.A. et al. (1995). Pathophysiology of calcium metabolism. *Vet. Clin. Pathol.* 24: 49–63.

81 Sharp, C.R., Kerl, M.E., and Mann, F.A. (2009). A comparison of total calcium, corrected calcium, and ionized calcium concentrations as indicators of calcium homeostasis among hypoalbuminemic dogs requiring intensive care. *J. Vet. Emerg. Crit. Care* 19: 571–578.

82 Schenck, P.A. and Chew, D.J. (2010). Prediction of serum ionized calcium concentration by serum total calcium measurement in cats. *Can. J. Vet. Res.* 74: 209–213.

83 De Bitro Calvae, J.F., Schenck, P.A., and Chew, D.J. (2017). A quick reference on hypocalcemia. *Vet. Clin. North Am. Small Anim. Pract.* 47: 249–256.

84 Coady, M., Fletcher, D.J., and Goggs, R. (2019). Severity of ionized hypercalcemia and hypocalcemia is associated with etiology in dogs and cats. *Front. Vet. Sci.* 6: 276.

85 Milovancev, M. and Schmiedt, C.W. (2013). Preoperative factors associated with postoperative hypocalcemia in dogs with primary hyperparathyroidism that underwent parathyroidectomy: 62 cases (2004–2009). *J. Am. Vet. Med. Assoc.* 242: 507–515.

86 Arbaugh, M., Smeak, D., and Monnet, E. (2012). Evaluation of preoperative serum concentrations of ionized calcium and parathyroid hormone as predictors of hypocalcemia following parathyroidectomy in dogs with primary hyperparathyroidism: 17 cases (2001–2009). *J. Am. Vet. Med. Assoc.* 241: 233–236.

87 Armstrong, A.J., Hauptman, J.G., Stanley, B.J. et al. (2018). Effect of prophylactic calcitriol administration on serum ionized calcium concentrations after parathyroidectomy: 78 cases (2005–2015). *J. Vet. Intern. Med.* 32: 99–106.

88 Singh, A., Giuffrida, M.A., Thomson, C.B. et al. (2019). Perioperative characteristics, histological diagnosis, and outcome in cats undergoing surgical treatment of primary hyperparathyroidism. *Vet. Surg.* 48: 367–374.

89 Feldman, E.C. (2015). Hypercalcemia and primary hyperparathyroidism. In: *Canine and Feline Endocrinology*, 4e (eds. E.C. Feldman, R.W. Nelson, C. Reusch and J.C.R. Scott-Moncrieff), 579–624. St Louis: Elsevier Saunders.

90 Tuohy, J.L., Worley, D.R., and Withrow, S.J. (2012). Outcome following simultaneous bilateral thyroid lobectomy for treatment of thyroid gland carcinoma in dogs: 15 cases (1994–2010). *J. Am. Vet. Med. Assoc.* 241: 95–103.

91 Olsen, J.A. and Sumner, J.P. (2019). Clinical hypocalcemia following surgical resection of apocrine gland anal sac adenocarcinomas in 3 dogs. *Can. Vet. J.* 60: 591–595.

92 Kellett-Gregory, L.M., Boller, E.M., Brown, D.C. et al. (2010). Ionized calcium concentrations in cats with septic peritonitis: 55 cases (1990–2008). *J. Vet. Emerg. Crit. Care* 20: 398–405.

93 Luschini, M.A., Fletcher, D.J., and Schoeffler, G.L. (2010). Incidence of ionized hypocalcemia in septic dogs and its association with morbidity and mortality: 58

cases (2006–2007). *J. Vet. Emerg. Crit. Care* 20: 406–412.

94 Holowaychuk, M.K. and Monteith, G. (2011). Ionized hypocalcemia as a prognostic indicator in dogs following trauma. *J. Vet. Emerg. Crit. Care* 21: 521–530.

95 Jutkowitz, L.A., Rozanski, E.A., Moreau, J.A. et al. (2002). Massive transfusion in dogs: 15 cases (1997–2001). *J. Am. Vet. Med. Assoc.* 220: 1664–1669.

96 Brainard, B.M., Campbell, V.L., Drobatz, K.J. et al. (2007). The effects of surgery and anesthesia on blood magnesium and calcium concentrations in canine and feline patients. *Vet. Anaesth. Analg.* 34: 89–98.

97 Messinger, J.S., Windham, W.R., and Ward, C.R. (2009). Ionized hypercalcemia in dogs: a retrospective study of 109 cases (1998–2003). *J. Vet. Intern. Med.* 23: 514–519.

98 Savary, K.C. (2000). Hypercalcemia in cats: a retrospective study of 71 cases (1991–1997). *J. Vet. Intern. Med.* 14: 184–189.

99 De Brito Galvao, J.F., Schenck, P.A., and Chew, D.J. (2017). A quick reference on hypercalcemia. *Vet. Clin. North Am. Small Anim. Pract.* 47: 241–248.

100 de Morais, H.A. and Constable, P.D. (2012). Strong ion approach to acid-base disorders. In: *Fluid, Electrolyte, and Acid-Base Disorders in Small Animal Practice*, 4e (ed. S.P. DiBartola), 319–329. St. Louis: Elsevier.

101 Sirker, A.A., Rhodes, A., Ground, R.M. et al. (2002). Acid-base physiology: the 'traditional' and 'modern' approaches. *Anaesthesia* 57: 348–356.

102 Neligan, P. and Deutschman, C. (2010). Perioperative acid-base balance. In: *Miller's Anesthesia*, 7e (ed. R. Miller), 1557–1674. Philadelphia: Churchill Livingstone.

103 de Morais, H.A. and Leisewitz, H.A. (2012). Mixed acid-base disorders. In: *Fluid, Electrolyte, and Acid-Base Disorders in Small Animal Practice*, 4e (ed. S.P. DiBartola), 302–315. St. Louis: Elsevier.

104 McDonell, W.C. and Kerr, C.L. (2015). Respiratory system. In: *Veterinary Anesthesia and Analgesia. The Fifth Edition of Lumb and Jones* (eds. K.A. Grimm, L.A. Lamont, W.J. Tranquilli, et al.), 529–558. Ames: Blackwell.

105 Walley, K.R., Lewis, T.H., and Wood, L.D.H. (1990). Acute respiratory acidosis decreases left ventricular contractility but increases cardiac output in dogs. *Circ. Res.* 67: 628–635.

106 Ramirez, J., Totapally, B.R., Hon, E. et al. (2000). Oxygen-carrying capacity during 10 hours of hypercapnia in ventilated dogs. *Crit. Care Med.* 28: 1918–1923.

107 Teixeira Neto, F.J., Carregaro, A.B., Mannarino, R. et al. (2002). Comparison of a sidestream capnograph and a mainstream capnograph in mechanically ventilated dogs. *J. Am. Vet. Med. Assoc.* 221: 1582–1585.

108 Hightower, C.E., Kiorpes, A.L., Butler, H.C. et al. (1980). End-tidal partial pressure of CO_2 as an estimate of arterial partial pressure of CO_2 during various ventilator regimes in halothane-anesthetized dogs. *Am. J. Vet. Res.* 41: 610–612.

109 Hammond, R. (2007). Automatic ventilators. In: *BSAVA Manual of Canine and Feline Anaesthesia and Analgesia*, 2e, 50. Gloucester: British Small Animal Veterinary Association.

110 Little, R.C. and Smith, C.W. (1964). Cardiovascular response to acute hypocapnia due to overbreathing. *Am. J. Physiol.* 206: 1025–1030.

111 Vanova-Uhrikova, I., Rauserova-Lexmaulova, L., Rehakova, K. et al. (2017). Determination of reference intervals of acid-base parameters in clinically healthy dogs. *J. Vet. Emerg. Crit. Care* 27: 325–332.

112 Artero, C.T. (2017). A quick reference on anion gap and strong ion gap. *Vet. Clin. North Am. Small Anim. Pract.* 47: 191–196.

113 Muir, W.W. (2015). Acid-base physiology. In: *Veterinary Anesthesia and Analgesia. The Fifth Edition of Lumb and Jones* (eds. K.A. Grimm, L.A. Lamont, W.J. Tranquilli, et al.), 357–371. Ames: Blackwell.

114 Pascoe, P.J. (2012). Perioperative management of fluid therapy. In: *Fluid, Electrolyte, and Acid-Base Disorders in Small Animal Practice*, 4e (ed. D.B. SP), 405–435. St. Louis: Elsevier.

9

Endocrine Disease

Berit L. Fischer

Crown Veterinary Specialists, Lebanon, NJ, 08833, USA

Introduction

Endocrine disease has largely been ignored in the veterinary literature up to this point regarding its impact on anesthesia. Many would argue that this is due to the uncommon development of severe complications and the fact that many of these patients perform well despite their disease(s). This chapter presents the pathophysiology associated with veterinary endocrinopathies and how it relates to patient management in the perianesthetic period.

Thyroid Disease

Thyroid Gland Anatomy and Physiology

The thyroid gland in dogs and cats is bilobed and sits just lateral to the trachea and medial to the common carotid arteries at the level of the thyroid cartilage [1]. Synthesis and secretion of thyroid hormones are dictated by the hypothalamic–pituitary–thyroid axis. Thyrotropin-releasing hormone (TRH) from the hypothalamus acts on the anterior pituitary to stimulate the release of thyrotropin-stimulating hormone (TSH). This then acts on the thyroid follicular cells to stimulate triiodothyronine (T3) and thyroxine (T4) synthesis and release into the circulation where they act on organs throughout the body. Thyroid hormones autoregulate their release by providing negative feedback on the pituitary and hypothalamus, thereby decreasing TSH and TRH release, respectively [1].

Thyroid Hormone Effects

Thyroid hormones, especially T3, work at the cellular level to elicit a broad range of biologic effects, which directly influence metabolic rate, protein synthesis, and normal fetal development [1, 2]. Of particular interest to the anesthesiologist are their chronotropic and inotropic effects on the heart, action on the respiratory centers of the brain to maintain sensitivity to hypercarbia and hypoxemia, and role in thermoregulation [1, 3].

Hypothyroidism

Canine Hypothyroidism

Thyroid hormone deficiency, through disruption of the hypothalamic–pituitary–thyroid axis, results in hypothyroidism. It is a relatively common endocrinopathy in dogs with a prevalence similar to that of humans between 0.2% and 0.8% [2, 4]. The etiology is primary in

Canine and Feline Anesthesia and Co-Existing Disease, Second Edition. Edited by Rebecca A. Johnson, Lindsey B. C. Snyder and Carrie A. Schroeder.

Companion website: www.wiley.com/go/johnson/canine

origin 95% of the time with destruction via autoimmune lymphocytic thyroiditis and idiopathic atrophy being most common. It tends to affect middle-aged to older dogs (mean approximately 7 years) with English Setters, Golden Retrievers, Giant Schnauzers, Dobermans, Boxers, Shetland Sheepdogs, and Cocker Spaniels being overrepresented [1, 4]. No gender predisposition has been identified.

Feline Hypothyroidism

Spontaneously occurring hypothyroidism in cats is rare [3]. It is most often encountered in cats which have been previously treated via radioiodine therapy or thyroidectomy for hyperthyroidism [1, 5]. Cats develop similar clinical signs as their canine counterparts including lethargy, weight gain, decreased grooming, and poor coat quality [1, 3].

Because it is a rare condition, many of the complications reported in humans and dogs have not been reported in cats. However, cats which become hypothyroid iatrogenically have an increased risk of developing azotemia and chronic kidney disease (CKD) [5]. Those that develop azotemia also have significantly shorter survival times when compared to their euthyroid, azotemic counterparts (456 vs. 728 days, respectively) [5].

Clinical Signs and Symptoms

Clinical signs are varied with multiple organ systems being affected (Table 9.1). Dermatologic abnormalities and signs associated with decreased metabolic rate are most common, presenting in 60–80% and 50% of hypothyroid dogs, respectively [3]. Although uncommon, cardiovascular and neuromuscular signs can be significant and are a source of perianesthetic morbidity.

Table 9.1 Clinical signs and physical exam findings of hypothyroidism in dogs and cats [1, 3, 4].

Decreased metabolic rate	*Cardiovascular*	*Neuromuscular*
Lethargy[a]	Sinus bradycardia[a]	*CNS*
Weakness	Weak apex beat	Seizures
Weight gain[a]	Decreased peripheral pulses	Ataxia
Exercise intolerance	Diastolic hypertension	Head tilt
Hypothermia[a]	Decreased left ventricular pump function	Positional nystagmus
Mental dullness		Strabismus
Decreased appetite[a]	Low QRS voltage	Decreased facial sensation
Dermatologic	Inverted T waves	
	Cardiac arrhythmias	*PNS*
Endocrine alopecia	AV block	
Dull, brittle haircoat[a]	Atrial fibrillation	Generalized weakness
Poor regrowth of hair[a]		Knuckling
Hyperpigmentation	*Gastrointestinal*	Dragging of limbs
Poor wound healing	Constipation	Paraparesis
Bruising	Diarrhea	Quadriparesis
Myxedema (puffy face)[a]	Delayed gastric emptying	Paralysis
Decreased grooming[a]		Lameness
Recurrent bacterial infections		Exercise intolerance
		Muscle atrophy
		Myopathy
		+/– Larngeal paralys
		+/– Megaesophagus

[a] Clinical signs reported in cats.

Clinicopathologic Findings

Changes seen in the CBC and biochemical profile are not pathognomonic for the disease and may not always be present. In 28–44% of dogs with hypothyroidism, a mild normocytic, normochromic, nonregenerative anemia is present [1, 4, 6]. This represents decreased erythropoiesis and bone marrow response from thyroid hormone deficiency. This anemia is rarely of concern for anesthesia but may need to be addressed in patients where significant blood loss is expected.

The most common abnormalities seen on the biochemical profile are hypercholesterolemia and hypertriglyceridemia [1, 3]. These result from impaired lipid metabolism and can be associated with atherosclerosis of blood vessels. There is a positive correlation with and increased prevalence of atherosclerosis in dogs diagnosed with hypothyroidism [7]. Although atherosclerosis is rare in dogs (0.5% prevalence), patients affected by it are 51 times more likely to be hypothyroid than not [7]. Other less common findings include mild to moderate increases in alkaline phosphatase (ALKP or ALP), alanine aminotransferase (ALT), aspartate aminotransferase (AST), and creatinine kinase, as well as mild hypercalcemia and hypoglycemia [1, 8, 9]. By contrast, cats may have a low ALKP, likely caused by decreased bone turnover [5].

Abnormalities are not typically found in the urinalysis of hypothyroid dogs. However, it is important to evaluate renal function in the hypothyroid patient undergoing anesthesia. Hypothyroidism is associated with decreased glomerular filtration rate (GFR) in both dogs and cats, attributed to both vasoconstriction of the afferent and efferent arterioles via impaired nitric oxide release from endothelial cells, and decreased cardiac output from a lowered metabolic rate [5, 10]. The reduced GFR could be exacerbated in the perianesthetic period by hypotension and decreased renal perfusion resulting in additional postoperative morbidity.

Diagnosis

Diagnosis is based on the presence of clinical signs and appropriate biochemical testing. The gold standard includes determination of free thyroxine (FT4) serum levels via modified equilibrium dialysis [1, 3]. Without clinical evidence of hypothyroidism, a low serum level of T4 is not diagnostic. Breed, age, certain drugs including barbiturates and corticosteroids, and the presence of chronic disease or critical illness may falsely decrease serum T4 [1, 11]. Accurate diagnosis often requires a thyroid panel including baseline TSH concentration, free T4, and possible autoantibody tests [1].

Treatment

Treatment consists of oral levothyroxine (T4) administration. Patients are often euthyroid within 4–6 weeks of treatment at an appropriate dose [1, 11]. Intravenous formulations of levothyroxine are available, but are only indicated in situations of myxedema coma, a rare manifestation of severe hypothyroidism characterized by obtundation, hypothermia, hypotension, hypoventilation, bradycardia, and nonpitting edema of the face [1, 2].

Anesthetic Management

Because hypothyroidism is a common canine endocrinopathy, it is important for the anesthetist to be aware of the pathophysiology it causes and how it can be managed in the perianesthetic period. The presence of mild or subclinical hypothyroidism is not an absolute contraindication for anesthesia. However, it is ideal that patients be treated and rendered euthyroid prior to undergoing anesthesia for elective procedures [2]. Similar anesthetic practices should be utilized for the hypothyroid feline patient as well, taking care to recognize the increased risk of renal morbidity when untreated [5, 12].

Preanesthetic Physical Exam

Patients with a history of hypothyroidism or where there is a high index of suspicion based on clinical signs should have a thorough preanesthetic workup including physical exam, blood work (complete blood count [CBC], biochemical profile), urinalysis, and recent serum FT4 level. Numerous organ systems are affected by thyroid hormone deficiency making a systematic preanesthetic physical exam especially important.

Overall body condition should be assessed, since many clinically hypothyroid patients are overweight resulting from lowered metabolic rate. Overweight or obese patients can be more difficult to manage under anesthesia [12]. Decreased thoracic compliance and compression atelectasis from increased organ weight can lead to hypoventilation and ventilation–perfusion mismatch [6, 12]. This could be exacerbated by decreased sensitivity and poor response to hypercarbia and hypoxemia, as well as altered diffusion of oxygen across the alveolar capillary membrane [2].

Careful cardiovascular evaluation should be performed because hypothyroidism leads to decreased numbers and affinity of beta-adrenergic receptors and a decreased catecholaminergic response [1]. Hypothyroid patients can present with bradyarrhythmias, poor peripheral pulses, and a weak apex beat from impaired myocardial contractility, decreased cardiac output, and poor peripheral perfusion [1, 3]. Although this decrease in contractility may be mild in most situations, severe cases of systolic dysfunction resulting in congestive heart failure have been reported in the dog [13].

Thoracic radiographs with or without an echocardiogram should be strongly considered in patients where physical exam findings suggest reduced cardiac function, and are essential in patients where a murmur, arrhythmia, or evidence of congestive heart failure (i.e., jugular pulses, coughing, exercise intolerance) is present. In patients with arrhythmias, an electrocardiogram (ECG) should be evaluated. Sinus bradycardia with decreased QRS amplitude and inverted T waves is most common. However, first- and second-degree atrioventricular blocks, ectopic beats, and, rarely, atrial fibrillation may be identified because of coronary artery atherosclerosis and subsequent myocardial hypoxia [1, 3, 7].

Blood pressure readings may reveal mild diastolic hypertension because of increased systemic vascular resistance (SVR) [2, 10, 14]. Hypertension does not usually require treatment, but the anesthetist should be aware that this could decrease circulating blood volume. When combined with the profound response hypothyroid patients often have to anesthetic drugs, significant hypovolemia and hypotension could result [2, 6]. An attempt to avoid this should be made by correcting any fluid deficits before anesthesia.

Neuromuscular system evaluation is important because thyroid hormones play a vital role in axon growth and transport [3]. Peripheral neuropathies and myopathies causing generalized weakness, ataxia, and knuckling, progressing to paresis and paralysis, may develop in hypothyroid patients [3, 4, 15]. Cranial nerves may also be affected, leading to decreased facial sensation, facial nerve paralysis, and vestibular disease. Despite being mentioned in concert with hypothyroidism, a causal relationship with laryngeal paralysis and megaesophagus has not been established [1, 3, 15]. Although not common, seizures, disorientation, and circling can occur in hypothyroid dogs as a result of cerebral hypoxia originating from atherosclerosis of cerebral vessels [3, 7, 16, 17]. In such cases, further impairment could occur following anesthesia [17].

Thyroid neoplasia is an uncommon cause of hypothyroidism in dogs; however, examination of the cervical region should be performed. Thyroid carcinomas or squamous cell carcinomas can be large enough to cause upper airway obstruction. Affected dogs may drool, cough, have a history of voice change, or have respiratory distress [1, 12]. Preparation for a difficult airway intubation including tracheostomy setup should be performed.

Preanesthetic Period

Hypothyroid patients may have altered anesthetic drug responses. Although a true sensitivity may not exist, the combination of lowered cardiac output, decreased circulating blood volume, hepatic metabolism, and renal excretion of drugs results in more profound changes in depth and hemodynamic parameters than expected in the euthyroid patient [2, 6]. Because inhalant anesthesia decreases metabolic rate, it is difficult to ascertain how hypothyroidism specifically influences minimum alveolar concentration (MAC) reduction. However, this is thought to be negligible [18]. Certainly, decreased thermoregulatory ability and cardiac output alone can significantly lower inhalant requirements in these patients [14, 18].

The untreated hypothyroid patient may respond to anesthesia with greater hemodynamic instability. It is advisable to choose anesthetic drugs that are relatively short-acting and titratable to minimize negative cardiovascular effects. The phenothiazine tranquilizer, acepromazine, is long-acting and causes vasodilation through antagonism of alpha-1-adrenergic receptors [19]. In hypothyroid patients who are volume-contracted and have decreased metabolic capabilities, it is best avoided. Ketamine has been promoted in human literature because of its ability to increase cardiac output and blood pressure in patients with an intact sympathetic nervous system [2]. Caution is advised in those hypothyroid patients who have arrhythmias or suspected myocardial dysfunction, since increases in myocardial oxygen demand could result in greater hemodynamic instability [1].

Decreased gastric-emptying time and ileus have been documented in humans with hypothyroidism and are suspected to occur in veterinary patients as well [1, 2, 6]. A full stomach could result in regurgitation and aspiration of gastric contents, as well as impair ventilation. Administration of gastroprotectants and prokinetics is recommended prior to anesthesia in humans and may be of use in veterinary patients as well [2, 6].

Hypothermia is a significant concern in the hypothyroid patient and results from impaired hypothalamic thermoregulation [2]. Hypothermia can be difficult to prevent and treat, and, when severe, can lead to impaired coagulation, decreased inhalant MAC, impaired response to adrenergic drugs, bradycardia, and refractory hypotension [2, 6]. Patient prewarming using a convective heat source for 20–30 min before anesthetic induction prevents hypothermia in healthy humans and dogs [6, 20]. Although it has not been evaluated in veterinary patients with hypothyroidism, prewarming is suggested to prevent hypothermia.

Because they tend to have minimal effects on the cardiovascular and respiratory systems, a combination of an opioid and benzodiazepine is favorable for premedication in the hypothyroid patient. Induction using propofol or alfaxalone allows titration to effect; however, rapid administration may lead to apnea and profound hypotension from vasodilation. Ketamine, as stated earlier, may benefit the otherwise healthy, hypothyroid patient because it indirectly stimulates the sympathetic nervous system to help support cardiac output, heart rate, and blood pressure. Either isoflurane or sevoflurane can be used for maintaining anesthesia.

Before anesthetic induction, the patient should be preoxygenated for 3–5 min, as reduced functional residual capacity (FRC) from increased body weight and possible airway obstruction from swollen pharyngeal tissues could lead to rapid desaturation [2, 12]. Induction and establishment of a patent airway should be rapid to avoid hypoxemia and hypoventilation, as well as aspiration of gastric contents.

Intraoperative Period

Monitoring Standard monitoring including blood pressure, capnometry, pulse oximetry, ECG, and temperature should be used. Direct or indirect methods of blood pressure monitoring can be used depending on the invasiveness of the procedure and American Society of Anesthesiologists (ASA) physical status of the patient. In patients in whom cardiovascular dysfunction is suspected, direct blood pressure monitoring is indicated.

If hypotension occurs, a systematic approach to treatment should be sought. Bolus administration of a crystalloid (5–10 $ml\,kg^{-1}$) along with a reduction in inhalant anesthetic concentration can help to minimize vasodilation and maintain adequate venous return to the heart. Bradyarrhythmias can be treated through anticholinergic administration and decreased myocardial contractility may benefit from positive inotropic support [2, 12]. Commonly used positive inotropes in veterinary medicine include dopamine (3–10 $\mu g\,kg^{-1}\,min^{-1}$) or dobutamine (1–10 $\mu g\,kg^{-1}\,min^{-1}$). In humans, hypothyroidism can lead to a concomitant decrease in adrenal cortical function and decreased circulating cortisol levels. If hypotension is refractory to treatment using the abovementioned methods, a physiologic dose of corticosteroids could be considered [2].

Prevention and aggressive treatment of hypothermia with active methods for warming including intravenous fluid warmers, circulating warm water blankets, and convective air warmers should be used. Assisted ventilation is often required because of decreased thoracic compliance and decreased sensitivity to hypercarbia and hypoxemia [12].

Locoregional Anesthesia and Analgesia

Locoregional anesthetic techniques are an important component of balanced anesthesia when indicated. In patients in whom a peripheral neuropathy is present, caution should be used because neurologic deficits may be exacerbated after regional anesthesia [21]. If additional hair clipping is required for locoregional anesthesia, it is advisable to inform the owner that hair regrowth may be slow or not occur [1].

Anesthetic Recovery

Monitoring should continue into the postanesthetic period. Recovery is often prolonged because of decreased hepatic metabolism and renal excretion of anesthetic drugs [2, 12]. Esophageal suctioning prior to recovery may prevent aspiration of gastric contents if silent regurgitation occurred during anesthesia. Respiratory depression may lead to postoperative hypoventilation with subsequent hypoxemia. Administration of supplemental oxygen via mask, prongs, or nasal catheter should occur after extubation if hemoglobin oxygen saturation decreases below 94%.

Hyperthyroidism

Feline Hyperthyroidism

Just as thyroid hormone deficiency results in multisystem dysfunction, excessive thyroid hormone also creates a montage of effects throughout the body. Hyperthyroidism is the most common endocrinopathy in cats older than 8 years with a mean age of 13 years [22]. The etiology is primary in origin and typically caused by multinodular adenomatous goiter or adenomatous hyperplasia like humans. No secondary or tertiary causes have been identified in cats, nor has a breed or gender predisposition been found [22].

Canine Hyperthyroidism

Hyperthyroidism in dogs is uncommon. It is often the result of a functional thyroid carcinoma which occurs only in approximately 10% of dogs with thyroid neoplasia [23]. Affected dogs are typically older than 8 years and more than half have distant metastases to the lung, regional lymph nodes, or liver at the time of diagnosis [23]. Another cause of canine hyperthyroidism includes excessive levothyroxine administration to dogs being treated for hypothyroidism. In dogs identified with hyperthyroidism, anesthetic precautions and preparation are like that of cats.

Clinical Signs and Symptoms

Thyroid hormones influence all tissues throughout the body by increasing gene transcription [22, 24, 25]. Excess thyroid hormone results in an overall increase in basal metabolic rate, which increases energy needs and oxygen consumption [22, 24]. The most common clinical signs in cats are weight loss and polyphagia (Figure 9.1) [22]. Affected cats also exhibit hyperactivity and aggression and may be difficult to restrain for physical exam and blood sampling. Gastrointestinal signs of vomiting and diarrhea may be present. Diarrhea likely results from decreased ororectal transit time and malabsorption. The cause of vomiting has not been fully elucidated but may result from thyroid hormone activity on the chemoreceptor trigger zone and altered motility of the esophagus, stomach, and duodenum [22]. Because hyperthyroidism is one of many causes of "endocrine hypertension," signs associated with high blood pressure including blindness or seizures could be present [24–27]. Panting, tachypnea, and dyspnea may occur from hyperthermia, respiratory muscle weakness, increased metabolic oxygen requirements, and cardiac failure [22, 26].

Thyroid neoplasia in the dog can have signs attributable to a cervical space-occupying mass including dysphagia, drooling, voice change, and varying amounts of respiratory distress [23]. Proper preparation for emergency airway management is imperative in these cases.

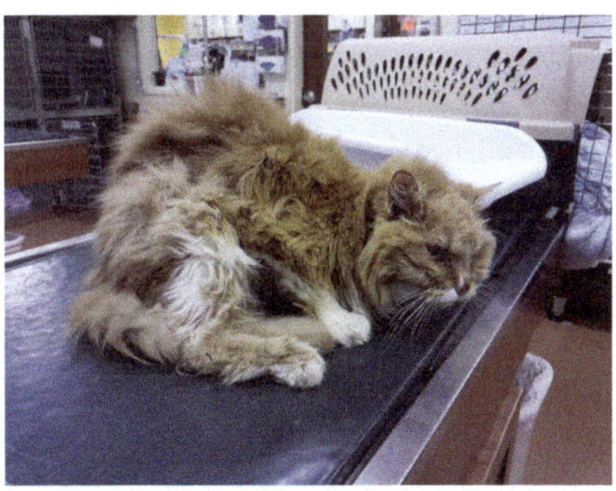

Figure 9.1 A hyperthyroid cat. Note the thin body condition and unkempt appearance.

Clinicopathologic Findings

Like hypothyroidism, there are no pathognomonic hematologic or biochemical changes associated with hyperthyroidism. The most common hematologic finding in cats is a mild increase in packed cell volume (PCV) reflective of the stimulatory effects thyroid hormones have on erythropoiesis [22]. Moderate increases in ALT and ALKP from a combination of increased bone turnover and decreased hepatic perfusion are seen in approximately 75% of hyperthyroid cats [22]. The presence or absence of azotemia should be interpreted with caution. Both increases in GFR from the high cardiac output state and decreased muscle mass result in lower serum concentrations of creatinine potentially masking CKD. Additional testing utilizing the renal biomarker, symmetric dimethylarginine (SDMA), and urine specific gravity (USG) may be more useful to the anesthetist when evaluating for underlying renal disease. Suggested cutoffs of $>10\,\mu g\,dl^{-1}$ and <1.030 for SDMA and USG, respectively, may improve sensitivity in detecting masked CKD in hyperthyroid cats [28].

Hypernatremia, hypokalemia, and hypercalcemia can also occur [22]. Potassium should be monitored carefully, as hypokalemia can be severe and cause muscle weakness. Hypercalcemia can be paraneoplastic in the dog or reflective of increased bone turnover [23]. Elevated serum calcium when combined with a heart that is already sensitized to catecholamines can result in myocardial irritability and arrhythmia formation [22, 29].

Hypercoagulability occurs in hyperthyroid humans and cats and could contribute to significant morbidity in the perianesthetic period [22, 29, 30]. Proposed mechanisms include increases in Factor VIII, Factor IX, fibrinogen, and altered metabolism of vitamin K. Although anticoagulant therapy has been used in preparation for human surgery, its use is controversial [22, 26, 29, 30]. Consideration for postoperative antithrombotic treatment may be advisable, particularly in cats already at risk for thrombosis from concurrent cardiac dysfunction.

Diagnosis

Diagnosis is usually straightforward in the face of appropriate clinical signs and an elevated T4 level. Additional diagnostics including cervical ultrasonography and scintigraphy can be used to confirm diagnosis should the T4 concentration not be supportive or where concurrent disease may falsely decrease thyroid hormone levels [22].

Treatment

There are multiple treatment options for hyperthyroidism in cats. Definitive treatments, such as thyroidectomy or radioiodine therapy, require the patient to be anesthetized or heavily sedated. Patients should be medically managed and euthyroid prior to anesthesia for elective procedures to avoid significant complications that can accompany uncontrolled hyperthyroidism [2, 31, 32]. This is done through the administration of methimazole, or, in Europe, carbimazole [22, 25, 32, 33]. Both are thioureylenes, which inhibit the synthesis of thyroid hormones, but do not influence thyroid hormones already in circulation. It is expected that cats treated via oral or transdermal routes are euthyroid with a decrease in clinical signs after 2–4 weeks of therapy [33]. T4 levels may respond within 1 week, so cases where there is a greater sense of urgency should be checked at that time [22, 25]. In patients where treatment with thioureylenes or other definitive means is not possible, the use of a commercial low iodine diet has also been used successfully to treat hyperthyroidism with normalization of total T4 concentrations being observed as early as 4 weeks of exclusive feeding [34]. Definitive treatment for functional thyroid carcinomas in dogs is thyroidectomy and requires similar medical management prior to anesthesia [23].

Anesthetic Management

Anesthetic management of the hyperthyroid patient can present a myriad of complications. While mild hypothyroidism may not overtly affect anesthesia, even mild hyperthyroidism can be of concern to the anesthetist. As with hypothyroidism, a thorough preanesthetic physical exam, considering the pathophysiology of hyperthyroidism, should be performed along with appropriate imaging and clinicopathologic testing.

Weight loss can be dramatic, and many patients present with cachexia. Although hyperthermia may be present in the awake state, the absence of body fat and the peripheral vasodilation from T3-induced relaxation of vascular smooth muscle can lead to rapid loss of core body heat in the anesthetized patient [1, 29]. Similarly, there is equal risk of hyperthermia, as patients may respond rapidly to warming measures or could potentially develop a thyrotoxic crisis caused by excessive release of thyroid hormones [2, 26, 31, 35].

The cardiovascular system is greatly affected by excess thyroid hormone necessitating a full cardiac workup before anesthesia. T3 acts directly on myocardial sodium, potassium, and calcium channels, as well as on α-myosin chains to increase contractility [36]. It also directly relaxes vascular smooth muscle causing peripheral vasodilation. The resulting decrease in SVR causes activation of the renin–angiotensin–aldosterone system (RAAS) leading to increased plasma volume and a 50–400% increase in cardiac output [22, 32, 36]. In addition, the number and affinity of beta-adrenergic receptors increase leading to increased myocardial sensitivity to catecholamines. These cardiovascular changes increase the work and oxygen demand of the heart causing progressive left ventricular hypertrophy and subsequent cardiac failure [22, 36]. Thus, patients often present with tachyarrhythmias and bounding peripheral pulses. Auscultation may reveal a systolic murmur, gallop rhythm, and adventitious pulmonary sounds consistent with cardiac failure [22, 26].

Systolic hypertension is present in approximately 17–87% of hyperthyroid cats and can also be found in dogs, necessitating blood pressure measurements in the preanesthetic evaluation [22, 24, 37]. Its presence can be associated with retinopathies or encephalopathies resulting in blindness, seizures, ataxia, and altered mental status. Hypertension may require treatment prior to anesthesia with antihypertensive drugs, such as amlodipine. Beta-adrenergic antagonists can be effective for decreasing heart rate but are only effective in decreasing blood pressure in approximately 30% of affected cats [24].

Cardiomegaly may not be seen on thoracic radiographs. Pleural effusion or pulmonary edema may be present if heart failure has occurred or in the rare situation of pulmonary hypertension. In dogs, radiographs may reveal metastasis that could impair oxygenation and ventilation under anesthesia [23].

Thyrotoxic cardiomyopathy is present in many affected cats but may vary in severity. Therefore, even if cardiomegaly is not present, echocardiography is recommended if a murmur is auscultated. Plasma levels of the N-terminal prohormone of brain natriuretic peptide (proBNP), a biomarker upregulated in the presence of myocardial stretch, can be used to help identify cats with potentially moderate to severe cardiac dysfunction when echocardiography is unavailable [38]. The anesthetist should be aware, however, that proBNP can be falsely elevated in the presence of azotemia.

Common ECG findings in hyperthyroidism include increased R-wave amplitude, sinus tachycardia, atrial fibrillation, supraventricular tachycardia, and atrial or ventricular premature contractions, all reflective of increased catecholamine sensitivity and/or myocardial hypoxia [22, 26].

Preanesthetic Period

Before surgery, a minimum database of PCV, total solids, electrolytes, and acid–base status should be performed with any aberrations identified and treated. Owners should be instructed to continue antithyroid medications the day of anesthesia because all have relatively short half-lives like that of humans [6, 31].

Increased metabolic rate, cardiac output, and hyperthermia caused by untreated hyperthyroidism lead to altered pharmacokinetics and pharmacodynamics of numerous anesthetic drugs. For example, in humans, hyperthyroid patients require increased fentanyl and propofol doses, and propofol clearance and volume of distribution are significantly increased [39]. Pharmacokinetics of the benzodiazepine, oxazepam, in rodents with hyperthyroidism also show increased dosing requirements to achieve effects similar to those in euthyroid rats [40]. Because of the variable drug responses and dramatic hemodynamic changes, it is best to use short-acting and reversible agents such as opioids and benzodiazepines at standard doses, administering additional drug only if adequate sedation is not achieved.

Drugs that promote activation of the sympathetic nervous system should be avoided, including ketamine at large induction doses [2, 6, 12]. Indirect catecholamine release could further increase oxygen demands of the heart, leading to myocardial hypoxia and malignant arrhythmias. Likewise, anticholinergics should be used with discretion [2, 6, 12]. Acepromazine has been advocated in the past because it desensitizes the myocardium to catecholamines [12]. However, with the advent of short-acting, antihypertensive agents, and concerns over rapid drops in preload associated with acepromazine, it should be used cautiously. Thiopental was also long advocated for use in hyperthyroidism due to its ability to block peripheral conversion of T4 to T3 [6, 12]. However, it is not available in the United States, making propofol or alfaxalone acceptable alternatives.

Preoxygenation should be performed before anesthetic induction because of increased oxygen demand of the tissues and the increased likelihood of developing hypoxemia [12]. This allows increased time for an airway to be established before hemoglobin desaturation.

Intraoperative Period

Anesthesia can be maintained safely in the hyperthyroid patient with inhalant or injectable anesthetics (total intravenous anesthesia [TIVA]) [12, 39]. Although the MAC of inhalants does not increase, the required doses of injectable drugs needed to maintain an adequate anesthetic plane may be higher than expected [12, 39]. Stress minimization during anesthesia avoids excessive catecholamine release and associated cardiovascular responses [6]. A constant rate infusion (CRI) of fentanyl (5–42 $\mu g\,kg^{-1}\,h^{-1}$) or locoregional block, if necessary, may assist in reducing the stress response and provides analgesia during anesthesia.

Monitoring In hyperthyroid patients who require anesthesia, extensive hemodynamic monitoring should be used including invasive blood pressure monitoring, ECG, capnometry, and pulse oximetry. Temperature monitoring is vital to monitor for hypothermia or hyperthermia. Because CO_2 production can be increased from the elevated basal metabolic rate, a rebreathing circuit is advised to ensure adequate CO_2 removal [12]. Intermittent positive pressure ventilation (IPPV) may also benefit the patient, since muscle weakness can predispose them to hypoventilation, hypercapnia, and subsequent indirect stimulation of the sympathetic nervous system [41].

Cautious fluid use is advised in the face of cardiac dysfunction and objective means of monitoring volume status should be used whenever possible. Sudden upward trends in central venous pressure may also help identify the onset of cardiac failure and volume overload. However, it is less useful in identifying low volume states and in guiding intraoperative fluid therapy. The use of dynamic fluid indices such as pulse pressure variation or plethysmography variance index, while still in their infancy in veterinary medicine, may prove to be better determinants of volume responsiveness [42].

Because hyperthyroid patients have higher metabolic oxygen requirements, tissue oxygen delivery is important to assess intraoperatively. In addition to monitoring hemodynamics and arterial oxygen partial pressure (PaO_2), the anesthetist may also consider the use of serial lactate concentrations, base deficits, and venous–arterial PCO_2 differences to further identify poor oxygen delivery and track response to therapy [43].

Thyroid Storm

Thyroid storm is a rare, life-threatening manifestation of uncontrolled hyperthyroidism well-described in humans [26, 29, 35]. It results from the sudden release of thyroid hormones into the circulation caused by a precipitating event such as stress, anesthesia, infection, trauma, or illness [26, 35]. Since there is no correlation between circulating hormone levels and the development of thyroid storm, it is difficult to ascertain which patients are at risk [26, 39]. Acute thyrotoxicosis, which presents similarly, can occur in veterinary species [26]. Clinical signs include exacerbation of those associated with hyperthyroidism, including tachyarrhythmias, hypertension, hyperthermia, congestive heart failure, and cardiac arrest (Table 9.2) [26]. Treatment targets decreasing thyroid hormone synthesis and secretion, blocking thyroid hormone actions at their effector sites, providing supportive care, and eliminating the precipitating cause [26, 29, 35].

Methimazole is the drug of choice to decrease synthesis of thyroid hormones. However, in situations of thyroid storm, methimazole is administered in combination with an iodine compound, such as potassium iodate, to prevent preformed thyroid hormone secretion [26]. While the immediate preanesthetic administration of methimazole to untreated hyperthyroid cats has not been investigated in terms of its effects on a thyrotoxic crisis, it appears reasonable that pretreatment may minimize severity when combined with other systemic treatments and is the current recommendation in thyrotoxic humans faced with emergent anesthesia [2].

Tachyarrhythmias and hypertension are in part caused by increased sensitivity to catecholamines and can be combated by

Table 9.2 Clinical manifestations of thyrotoxicosis [26, 27, 34].

Cardiac arrhythmias[a]
Tachycardia
Gallop rhythm
Atrial fibrillation
Ventricular premature contractions
Hypertension[a]
Retinopathies
Sudden blindness
Encephalopathies
Tachypnea
Hyperthermia[a]
Increased CO_2 production[a]
Panting
Bucking ventilator[a]
Dyspnea
Pulmonary edema
Muscle weakness
Congestive heart failure
Cardiac arrest[a]

[a] Manifestations observed under anesthesia.
Source: Adapted with permission from reference [26].

administration of a beta-adrenergic antagonist. Under anesthesia, the most rapid-acting, titratable agent available is the selective beta-1-antagonist, esmolol (0.05–0.15 mg kg^{-1} slow IV bolus followed by a CRI of 10–200 µg kg^{-1} min^{-1}) [19, 26]. Severe hypertension can also be treated with sodium nitroprusside or magnesium sulfate similar to patients with pheochromocytoma [19, 44]. Caution should be used with antihypertensive drugs, as patients with acute thyrotoxicosis are already maximally vasodilated and volume depleted. Indiscriminate use could lead to rapid cardiovascular collapse [24].

Supporting therapy should include goal-directed replacement of circulating volume with crystalloids and colloids, as well as treatment of hyperthermia with active cooling methods such as ice packs [26, 29]. Dextrose and potassium supplementation may be needed because of increased energy requirements [2]. Mechanical ventilation should be instituted to help eliminate excessive carbon dioxide produced in the pyrexic state. Cardiac failure and pulmonary edema may necessitate administration of diuretics to improve oxygenation and ventilation [26].

Postanesthetic Management

Monitoring should continue during recovery because thyroid storm in humans can occur up to 48 h after anesthesia [29]. Supplemental oxygen should be available to fulfill elevated metabolic oxygen requirements and prevent hypoxemia. Frequent blood pressure monitoring and telemetry can help identify the development of hypertension and arrhythmias in the immediate postoperative period. Patients undergoing surgery should receive appropriate multimodal analgesia to minimize pain and stress, as well as continued antithyroid drug administration.

Adrenal Disease

Adrenal Gland Anatomy and Physiology

Adrenal glands represent another integral component of the endocrine system, playing a vital role in fluid balance, the stress response, and sympathetic nervous system activation [6, 45]. They are paired, ovoid structures lying near the cranial pole of the kidneys and are composed of a cortex and medulla. The cortex has three layers: the zona glomerulosa secretes aldosterone to stimulate sodium and water retention, and the zona fasciculata and zona reticularis function together to produce cortisol and androgens. The medulla is functionally separate, producing catecholamines [45].

Hyperadrenocorticism (HAC; Cushing's Disease)

Cortisol is normally secreted from the adrenal cortex under the regulation of the hypothalamic–anterior pituitary–adrenal axis [45]. The hypothalamus secretes corticotropin-releasing hormone (CRH) to act on the anterior pituitary. It subsequently releases adrenocorticotropic hormone (ACTH) to stimulate secretion of cortisol from the adrenal cortex [45].

Canine Hyperadrenocorticism

Other than hypothyroidism, HAC is the most common endocrinopathy seen in middle-aged to older dogs [45]. Hyperadrenocorticism is caused by excessive circulating glucocorticoids, namely, cortisol, and can be caused by a primary functional adrenocortical tumor (AT) or be secondary to an ACTH-secreting pituitary adenoma (pituitary-dependent hyperadrenocorticism; PDH). Iatrogenic HAC from overzealous administration of glucocorticoids is also reported [45].

PDH is cited as the cause of HAC in approximately 80–85% of dogs [27, 45, 46]. Mean age of affected dogs is approximately 11 years with very little difference between PDH and AT. Common breeds include Poodles, Terriers, Beagles, and Dachshunds with females being overrepresented [45, 46].

Feline Hyperadrenocorticism

Hypoadrenocorticism is rare in cats and the etiology is most commonly pituitary in origin [47, 48]. Middle-aged to older cats are primarily affected with a median age of 10 years. No sex or breed predilection has been identified [47, 48].

Clinical Signs

Cortisol, like other endocrine hormones, has a wide scope of target organs and effects, including stimulation of hepatic gluconeogenesis, lipolysis, and protein catabolism. It can also impact erythropoiesis, vascular tone, kidney function, and acts as a "safety net" in times of stress to maintain homeostasis [45].

Compared to other endocrinopathies, the clinical presentation of HAC can be strikingly different between dogs and cats, since cats are considerably less responsive to the effects of glucocorticoids [48]. Dogs commonly present with polyuria/polydipsia from cortisol inhibition of antidiuretic hormone (ADH) release, and polyphagia, a presenting complaint not witnessed in other species [45]. Panting, pendulous abdomen, muscle weakness, and endocrine alopecia can help diagnose canine Cushing's disease (Figure 9.2) [12, 45, 46]. Clinical signs of HAC in cats tend to be more elusive and may not occur until other concurrent disease, such as diabetes mellitus, manifests [47, 48]. Cats demonstrate muscle weakness, poor haircoat, tachypnea, and thin, fragile skin [47, 48]. Rarely, both species may present with encephalopathies or retinopathies from atherosclerosis, pituitary tumor impingement, or secondary hypertension [45, 47–50].

Clinicopathologic Changes

Cortisol causes neutrophilia, monocytosis, lymphopenia, and eosinopenia [45]. This "stress leukogram" is seen commonly in dogs, whereas cats may show few hematologic changes [48]. Polycythemia can be caused by cortisol-induced erythropoiesis, increased circulating half-lives of red blood cells, or may signal the presence of a chronic hypoxic state from alveolar hypoventilation [45].

Changes in the biochemical profile can differ between dogs and cats, but increased ALT

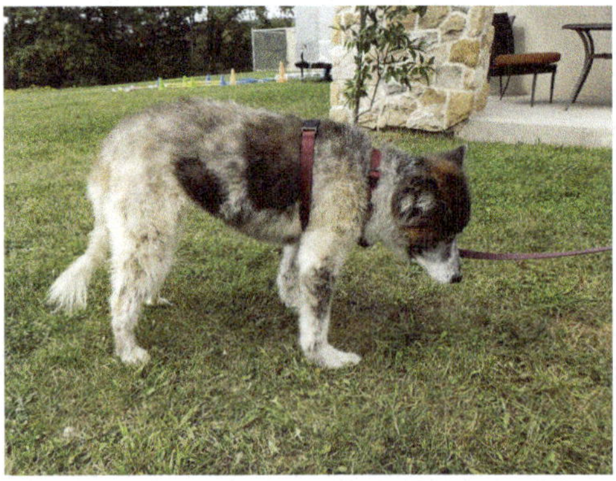

Figure 9.2 A dog diagnosed with hyperadrenocorticism caused by a functional adrenocortical tumor after presenting for polyuria, polydipsia, and muscle weakness. Note the thin, patchy haircoat.

from hepatocyte damage and impaired hepatic perfusion as well as hypercholesterolemia from increased lipolysis are seen in both species [45]. Both may also demonstrate mild to moderate hyperglycemia from increased gluconeogenesis and impaired insulin sensitivity [45, 48]. Dogs alone see dramatic elevations in ALKP from induction of a steroid-responsive ALKP isozyme not present in other species [45, 48]. Cortisol prevents ADH from binding to receptors on the renal tubules causing diuresis and a subsequent decrease in blood urea nitrogen (BUN) in dogs [45]. This is not observed in cats due to decreased renal glucocorticoid receptors [48].

Urinalysis is valuable in interpreting the effects of HAC. Dogs will typically have dilute urine with a specific gravity (SG) $<$1.020, whereas cats frequently maintain concentrating ability. If the urine is dilute in an affected cat, underlying renal disease should be suspected. Urinalysis may also reveal proteinuria from concurrent hypertension or infection, or glycosuria from diabetes mellitus [45, 48].

Blood gas analysis may occasionally identify alveolar hypoventilation and hypoxemia from respiratory muscle weakness and organomegaly [45]. Hypoxemia may also be present in patients who develop pulmonary thromboembolism (PTE) [51]. Excess cortisol is associated with a state of hypercoagulability and development of thromboembolic disease, as it increases production of coagulation factors II, V, VII, IX, X, and XII and decreases production of antithrombin III [45, 48].

Diagnosis

Diagnosis of HAC is not necessarily straightforward and should only be made considering clinical signs [45]. A multitude of tests are available; however, sensitivity is species-specific and cats and dogs differ with regard to reliable testing. In dogs, a low-dose dexamethasone suppression test is considered most diagnostic but is much less sensitive in cats [48]. A full explanation of tests and testing methods is outside the scope of this text and the reader is directed to additional sources [45].

Treatment

Medical treatment of PDH usually includes administration of either mitotane (o,p'-dichlorodiphenyldichloroethane; Lysodren®, Bristol Myers Squibb, Princeton, NJ) or trilostane (Vetoryl®, Dechra, Overland Park, KS). Mitotane is an adrenocorticolytic drug used in dogs which requires a loading period [45]. During this time, there is rapid destruction of adrenal cortical tissue making patients susceptible to developing adverse effects such as vomiting, diarrhea, lethargy, and Addisonian crisis. Until this phase is over, and the patient is regulated, anesthesia for elective procedures is discouraged.

Surgical options for patients with PDH include transsphenoidal hypophysectomy or bilateral adrenalectomy [4, 48, 52]. For patients undergoing hypophysectomy, the reader should also refer to the chapter addressing anesthesia and coexisting neurologic disease (see Chapter 3). For functional adrenocortical tumors (AT), unilateral adrenalectomy is often curative [53].

Anesthetic Management

Prior to anesthesia, a thorough physical exam, along with appropriate imaging and clinicopathologic testing, can pinpoint areas of concern and assist the anesthetist in preparing for anesthesia. The main actions of cortisol, as stated earlier, include gluconeogenesis, protein catabolism, and lipolysis [2, 45, 48]. The by-products of these processes, when in excess, have detrimental effects on the body with the cardiovascular system being particularly susceptible.

Hypertension from HAC occurs in approximately 50–86% of dogs, more than 80% of humans, and has been reported in cats [27, 45, 47, 49, 54]. Several factors contribute to hypertension including lipolysis-induced elevations of interleukin-6 (IL-6) and adiponectin and the development of hyperinsulinism and insulin resistance from increased gluconeogenesis [55].

Hyperinsulinism causes thickening of the vascular endothelium and increased vessel stiffness [55]. Cortisol causes vasoconstriction and increased SVR by decreasing endothelial nitric oxide, increasing levels of endothelin-1, and potentiating the vasoconstrictive effects of norepinephrine and angiotensin II [27, 54]. Additionally, hypercholesterolemia and hypertriglyceridemia cause the deposition of atherosclerotic plaques within the vessel walls [7]. These combined abnormalities cause hypertension and decreased perfusion of vital organs [44, 54, 55].

Organomegaly, muscle weakness, and truncal obesity decrease FRC, causing compression atelectasis and preventing adequate CO_2 removal [6, 41]. Hypoventilation can subsequently cause respiratory acidosis, venous admixture, and chronic hypoxemia, all of which are exacerbated under anesthesia. Pulmonary interstitial or bronchial calcium deposition may also contribute to impaired oxygenation [45].

Increased hematocrit, blood flow slowing, and hypercoagulability pose the threat of PTE formation which can dramatically affect both the cardiovascular and pulmonary systems. The resultant ventilation–perfusion mismatch may trigger hypoxic pulmonary vasoconstriction leading to increased pulmonary vascular resistance and development of right heart failure [45, 51].

Renal cortisol effects vary depending on species and the presence or absence of preexisting kidney disease. Dogs are the only species with HAC that develop polyuria and polydipsia via inhibition of ADH leading to a subsequent elevation in GFR [45, 48, 49, 52]. Over time, in combination with hypertension, this could result in glomerulosclerosis and renal failure. Dogs with HAC also develop increased renal vascular resistance and decreased renal blood flow which altogether could result in increased renal morbidity of patients [49].

The anesthetist should also pay close attention to the patient's integument. Cats are particularly vulnerable to tearing of the skin due to decreased keratin and loss of subcutaneous tissue [48]. Restraint for catheters and blood draws should be minimal to avoid skin damage. Sedative administration prior to handling should be considered if fragile skin syndrome is suspected [45, 48].

Preanesthetic Period

Prior to anesthesia, endocrine testing, a CBC, biochemical profile, blood gas, and urinalysis should be performed. Although patients with HAC frequently have one or more biochemical markers associated with hypercoagulability, no individual or combination of tests consistently identifies individuals at risk for thromboembolic disease. This makes recommendation of a particular test(s) difficult, as they can be costly with minimal interpretive benefit [56].

Hydration status should be determined, and fluid deficits corrected prior to induction. Because cortisol causes vasoconstriction, patients may have a contracted blood volume, resulting in decreased venous return and profound hypotension during anesthesia. Fluids can also be used to decrease hematocrit and sludging of blood, thus potentially reducing risk of thromboembolism and improving perfusion of capillary beds.

Before restraint for blood draws or catheter placement, blood pressures should be taken in accordance with the 2018 American College of Veterinary Internal Medicine (ACVIM) guidelines and hypertension documented [57]. The presence of hypertension may indicate a rightward shift in autoregulation of renal perfusion pressure (Figure 9.3). This necessitates maintenance of a higher mean arterial pressure during anesthesia to avoid decreased renal perfusion [58].

Thoracic radiographs are essential in patients who present with tachypnea or coughing and may reveal neoplasia, pulmonary or bronchial mineralization, congestive heart failure, or hyperlucency associated with PTE formation [45]. Likewise, they may show no evidence of disease; however, this does not

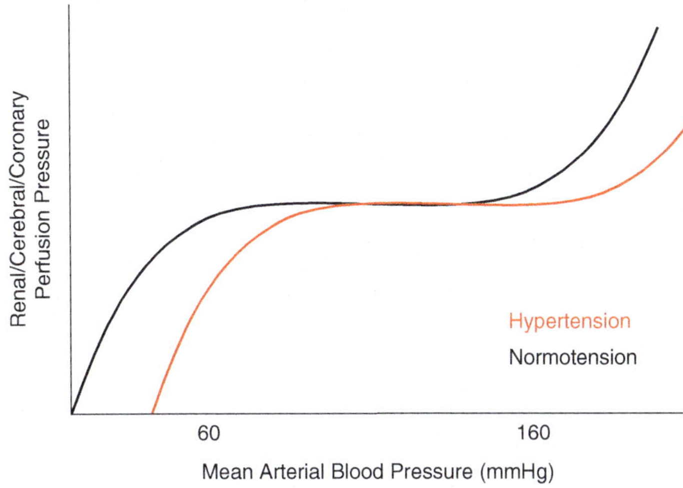

Figure 9.3 Schematic demonstrating the wide range of arterial blood pressures over which renal, cerebral, and coronary circulations can maintain steady perfusion pressure. In patients who are hypertensive, this curve shifts to the right [6, 56].

rule out PTE and should be interpreted in conjunction with an arterial blood gas.

Because patients with HAC are at risk for hypoventilation, short-acting, reversible drugs should be used, and excessive sedation avoided. Opioids and benzodiazepines are often well-tolerated. Low doses of the alpha-2-adrenergic agonist, dexmedetomidine ($1\,\mu g\,kg^{-1}$ IV or $3\,\mu g\,kg^{-1}$ IM), can be considered in patients with HAC without evidence of concurrent cardiovascular instability. After premedication, patients should be monitored and preoxygenated since many anesthetic drugs increase muscle relaxation and exacerbate respiratory depression. In addition, increased abdominal weight lowers FRC, decreasing the time it takes for hemoglobin desaturation [6].

Intraoperative Period

Anesthetic induction should be rapid to achieve an airway quickly and allow the anesthetist to assist ventilation. The induction agent etomidate inhibits 11-beta-hydroxylase, the enzyme necessary to produce cortisol, causing adrenocortical suppression for up to 24 h [59]. Although etomidate infusion is used before anesthesia to decrease cortisol levels in humans, its benefit as a one-time induction agent in veterinary patients is unknown [9]. Because cortisol can potentiate the actions of norepinephrine, anesthetic induction using ketamine could exacerbate hypertension and tachycardia and is therefore not advised in patients with impaired cardiac function or increased oxygen demand [27].

IPPV is often indicated because inhalant anesthetics are potent respiratory depressants and decrease sensitivity and response to elevated CO_2 levels similar to opioids [12]. Some patients with HAC rely on hypoxic drive for ventilation due to chronic elevations in CO_2 [6]. Thus, when administered 100% oxygen, the drive to ventilate in these patients may disappear making IPPV necessary.

Balanced anesthetic technique should be employed to minimize negative side effects and excessive sedation from any one drug. Multimodal analgesia utilizing a combination of systemic medications and locoregional techniques may minimize sedation in the postoperative period and prevent prolonged postanesthetic recumbency, a major risk factor in the development of PTE.

Treatment of hypertension is often not required in the perianesthetic period. Rapid, intermittent fluctuations in blood pressure, such as those seen in hyperthyroidism or pheochromocytoma, are typically not observed; however, large pulse pressure differences can be present. Although it is debatable whether treatment with antihypertensives, such as alpha-1-adrenergic antagonists, several days before undergoing anesthesia may be beneficial to improve circulating blood volume in those patients who have contracted volume from persistent hypertension, this practice may improve hemodynamic stability under anesthesia.

Monitoring Capnometry, pulse oximetry, ECG, temperature, and invasive or noninvasive blood pressure should be part of a standard monitoring protocol. When a neuromuscular blocking agent is used, train-of-four monitoring is necessary because muscle weakness can be profound. The anesthetist should pay close attention to temperature, as many of these patients are obese and at risk of hyperthermia. Arterial catheter placement for intermittent blood gas analysis allows oxygenation and ventilation to be monitored and addressed both during anesthesia and in the recovery period, especially in patients in whom PTE formation is suspected.

Severe PTE may be identified by a rapid decrease in end-tidal CO_2, hemoglobin desaturation, and cardiovascular collapse, and should be confirmed with blood gas analysis [51, 60]. PTE management is aimed at providing an oxygen-rich environment and administering anticoagulant therapy.

Preoperative antithrombotic therapy may be indicated in surgical patients with HAC. Rationale for use should include concurrent disease states, severity of surgical procedure, and associated risk of therapy [61]. Clopidogrel, an adenosine diphosphate inhibitor that prevents platelet aggregation, has been used as a prophylactic antithrombotic in at-risk populations. At standard doses, it can take 3–5 days to reach therapeutic efficacy. Recommendations indicate that a loading dose of 4–10 $mg\,kg^{-1}$ followed by 1–3 $mg\,kg^{-1}$ every 24 h may shorten this time frame. In patients where PTE already exists, anticoagulation therapies with a shorter onset of action, such as low-molecular-weight heparin or factor Xa inhibitors (xabans), can be considered in the postoperative period [62].

Recovery

Hypoventilation is the main concern in the immediate postanesthetic period. Patients who are unable to maintain a pulse oximetry reading of >93% on room air should be administered supplemental oxygen via mask, prongs, or nasal catheter [12]. Excessive sedation should be avoided and assisted mobilization should be instituted as soon as possible after recovery from anesthesia to prevent prolonged recovery and thrombus formation. If the patient is unable to be mobile, frequent changes in position and passive range of motion exercises are also acceptable.

Hypoadrenocorticism (Addison's Disease)

Hypoadrenocorticism is a disease characterized by insufficient plasma concentrations of cortisol and the mineralocorticoid, aldosterone [63]. The actions of cortisol are previously described, but its importance in regulation of vascular tone and blood pressure should be emphasized here. Aldosterone, part of the RAAS, plays a critical role in maintaining vascular volume and acid–base balance by stimulating sodium and water reabsorption and potassium and hydrogen ion excretion in the renal tubules [64].

Canine Hypoadrenocorticism

Hypoadrenocorticism is an uncommon endocrinopathy in dogs with an incidence of 0.06–0.33%. The most common etiology is immune-mediated destruction of the adrenal cortex with secondary causes occurring rarely. Iatrogenic hypoadrenocorticism following treatment for HAC, as well as after abrupt withdrawal of corticosteroids following long-term administration can also occur [63].

Affected dogs are typically female and younger with a mean age of 4 years. There are several breed predilections with Standard Poodles, Nova Scotia Duck Tolling Retrievers, and Portuguese Water Dogs demonstrating an autosomal recessive mode of inheritance. Atypical presentations, where only a glucocorticoid deficiency is present, are also possible [63, 64].

Feline Hypoadrenocorticism

Primary hypoadrenocorticism arising from immune-mediated destruction of the adrenal gland has been described in cats. It is rare, with only 40 cases described in the literature, and demonstrates no sex, breed, or age predilection [65, 66].

Clinical Signs

Clinical signs are often vague and resemble diseases of other organ systems, such as the gastrointestinal tract and kidney, making diagnosis difficult. The most common signs include intermittent anorexia, lethargy, vomiting, diarrhea, tremors, and polyuria/polydipsia [63, 67].

Clinicopathologic Changes

Patients with hypoadrenocorticism have several hematologic and biochemical abnormalities. Cortisol deficiency can result in the absence of a stress leukogram in an otherwise stressed patient, a normocytic, normochromic, nonregenerative anemia from suppression of erythropoiesis, or hypoglycemia from impaired gluconeogenesis. Aldosterone deficiency leads to hyponatremia, hypochloremia, hyperkalemia, metabolic acidosis, and changes associated with fluid loss and hypoperfusion such as prerenal azotemia, hypercalcemia, and hyperlactatemia [63, 67].

Clinical signs in cats with hypoadrenocorticism may present differently than those expected in canine patients. Cats are more likely to present with anorexia and are less likely to have vomiting and diarrhea. Notable biochemical differences may include severe hyponatremia with or without hyperkalemia [66].

Diagnosis and Treatment

Diagnosis can be difficult due to the overlap of clinical signs and clinicopathologic changes with other disease processes. While many patients with hypoadrenocorticism have low baseline cortisol concentrations, definitive diagnosis requires an ACTH stimulation test [67].

Treatment involves lifelong glucocorticoid and mineralocorticoid supplementation. Mineralocorticoid supplementation is achieved either through administration of the long-acting injectable drug desoxycorticosterone pivalate (DOCP) or via twice daily administered oral fludrocortisone. Because of fludrocortisone's glucocorticoid activity, patients treated with it may require minimal or no additional glucocorticoid [67].

Anesthetic Management

Most Addisonian patients presenting for elective surgery are well-regulated. Clear communication with the owner regarding what medications the patient is receiving to manage its hypoadrenocorticism, including dose, frequency, and when last administered, is important. At a minimum, the patient should undergo a complete physical exam and baseline blood tests to assess hydration, acid–base status, blood glucose, and electrolyte balance prior to anesthesia. Where there is concern about poor regulation, blood pressure measurement and ECG are also warranted.

Anesthesia, surgery, trauma, and illness can all cause increases in cortisol concentrations, in healthy patients. Therefore indicating Addisonian patients will likely require additional corticosteroid supplementation in these instances. Studies examining appropriate glucocorticoid supplementation preoperatively in dogs and cats with hypoadrenocorticism are lacking. Guidelines in humans have attempted to stratify need based on procedure invasiveness; however, Hsu et al (2012) demonstrated a significant rise in cortisol concentration regardless of sedation, anesthesia, or procedure in healthy patients [68].

Based on this, it is likely that Addisonian veterinary patients require additional glucocorticoid suppementation prior to anesthesia, surgery, or other stressful procedures. Owners should be advised to administer the prescribed dose of glucocorticoid at a minimum the morning before surgery. Doubling this dose may assure that adequate glucocorticoid is available in the face of mounting stress. If the anesthetist determines that additional supplementation is needed, dexamethasone sodium phosphate 0.1–0.25 $mg\,kg^{-1}$ IV or prednisolone sodium succinate 2 $mg\,kg^{-1}$ IV can be administered preoperatively and continue into the postoperative period until the patient is able to restart their oral medications [69]. In patients undergoing major surgery or prolonged hospitalization, additional supplementation, either IV or PO, should be continued until discharge and then slowly tapered.

In well-regulated Addisonian patients, a wide array of anesthetic and analgesic drugs, as well as locoregional techniques, are acceptable for use. Many drugs, including dexmedetomidine and opioids, may demonstrate the ability to prevent or blunt increases in plasma cortisol and ACTH concentrations. Propofol alone might not achieve this; therefore, the provision of appropriate analgesia is especially important. Etomidate, unlike other anesthetic drugs, blocks endogenous cortisol synthesis up to 24 h by inhibiting the enzyme 11-beta-hydroxylase and is not recommended in patients with hypoadrenocorticism [59].

Monitoring

Monitoring should be tailored to each individual based on surgical procedure, operative risk, and ASA status. Standard monitoring including capnography, arterial blood pressure, pulse oximetry, ECG, and temperature monitoring is advised. Ensuring adequate anesthetic depth and avoiding hypothermia help to minimize stress on the body. Placement of an arterial catheter for the purpose of monitoring invasive blood pressure may be warranted since hypotension can be more common in these patients. Fluid therapy should be goal-directed and in a well-regulated Addisonian is not expected to be different than that of a healthy patient.

Addisonian Crisis

Emergent surgical diseases can cause Addisonian crisis in patients with previously undetected or otherwise well-controlled hypoadrenocorticism if cortisol levels are insufficient for the increased demand. Patients may present in hypovolemic shock, with concurrent metabolic acidosis, hypoglycemia, hyperkalemia, and hyponatremia. Stabilization prior to anesthesia should include goal-directed fluid resuscitation with either scratch isotonic crystalloids or colloids and correction of life-threatening hyperkalemia (see Chapter 8). Early intervention with inotropic or vasopressor support may be indicated. If it is a known Addisonian patient, dexamethasone sodium phosphate 0.25 $mg\,kg^{-1}$, prednisolone sodium succinate 2 $mg\,kg^{-1}$, or hydrocortisone 0.5–0.625 $mg\,kg^{-1}$ IV with or without DOCP 2.2 $mg\,kg^{-1}$ IM or SC should be administered [69].

Critical-Illness-Related Corticosteroid Insufficiency (CIRCI)

While not Addisonian patients by definition, it seems relevant to mention a subset of critically ill patients who develop relative corticosteroid insufficiency as a result of decreased production, altered metabolism, and impaired response to circulating cortisol concentrations [70]. As a result, they often have severe hypotension, refractory to fluid and vasopressor support. Critical-illness-related corticosteroid insufficiency has been identified in humans as well as veterinary patients with septic shock, severe trauma, and gastric dilatation–volvulus (GDV) [71]. Diagnosis in people requires an ACTH stimulation test with a change in cortisol concentration $<9\,\mu g\,dl^{-1}$ [70]. In critically ill anesthetized patients, the anesthetist should have a high index of suspicion of CIRCI in patients who are minimally responsive to vasopressor therapy and fluid resuscitation. Administration of corticosteroids in these patients may prove beneficial in helping reestablish homeostasis.

Recovery

Minimizing stress in the postanesthetic period is of utmost importance in the Addisonian patient. Ensuring appropriate analgesia, providing external convective heat sources, and a quiet environment can help achieve this. Continued blood pressure monitoring to identify hypotension in the immediate postanesthetic period is recommended. Parenteral corticosteroid therapy should continue until the patient is able to eat. At that time, oral therapy can be restarted and tapered following discharge.

Pheochromocytoma

Pathophysiology

Pheochromocytomas are uncommon neoplasms that arise from the chromaffin cells of the adrenal medulla [72]. Chromaffin cells are responsible for synthesis and secretion of epinephrine and norepinephrine, which, in turn, act on adrenergic receptors. The adrenal medulla behaves as a sympathetic postganglionic nerve fiber and releases catecholamines under neural control to preserve homeostasis of the autonomic nervous system and during times of "fight or flight." Pheochromocytomas release catecholamines independent of neural control causing uncontrolled stimulation of adrenergic receptors resulting in hypertension and tachyarrhythmias [2, 72].

Pheochromocytomas account for a very small percentage of all neoplasia in dogs and only five cases have been reported in cats [72–74]. Other species in which pheochromocytomas have been documented include horses, cattle, elephants, rhinoceros, rats, and river otters [31, 75–77]. Patients are middle-aged to older animals with no sex or breed predilection [75]. Mean age of affected dogs is approximately 10.6 years and affected cats have ranged in age from 7 to 22 years [72, 74].

Pheochromocytomas mainly arise from the adrenal gland(s), although an extra-adrenal origin has been reported in a dog [72]. In humans and dogs, pheochromocytomas are more commonly found on the right adrenal gland [78]. However, over a 4-year period (2008–2012), pheochromocytomas were primarily left-sided at the author's practice (75%, n = 15; unpublished observations), suggestive of selection bias where right-sided adrenal masses may have a higher likelihood of referral to a tertiary facility and hence, publication, due to their invasiveness and difficult removal [78]. Bilateral disease also occurs in approximately 10% of patients [72].

These tumors often occur concurrently with other diseases including other endocrinopathies such as HAC and diabetes mellitus [53, 78]. Pheochromocytomas can occur with other adrenocortical tumors in the dog such that 13 out of 61 (21%) dogs with adrenal tumors had both a functional adrenocortical tumor and pheochromocytoma [75]. Likewise, one of the five documented cases in cats also had a cortisol-secreting tumor, suggesting that a diagnosis of HAC is not one of exclusion for pheochromocytoma [74].

Approximately 25–50% of pheochromocytomas are malignant and locally invasive into nearby vasculature [53, 75]. Distant metastases occur in 13–28% of cases with the spleen, liver, lung, lymph nodes, and bone being most affected [75]. When metastasis is not present, surgery is often curative resulting in long-term survival [53, 75].

Catecholamine levels produced by healthy chromaffin cells are 60–80% epinephrine, with the remainder being norepinephrine [72]. In humans, catecholamine secretion is altered in pheochromocytomas with neoplastic chromaffin cells secreting predominantly norepinephrine most of the time with a much smaller percentage secreting epinephrine, or, in rare instances, dopamine [72, 79, 80]. The secretion pattern of pheochromocytomas in dogs and cats has not been fully elucidated; however, the presence of higher concentrations of normetanephrine, the metabolite of norepinephrine, versus metanephrine, the metabolite of epinephrine, may indicate that norepinephrine is the primary catecholamine in veterinary patients as well [73, 80].

Clinical Signs

Pheochromocytomas can present with any number of clinical signs, none of which are pathognomonic for the disease. Clinical signs only occur in 30–50% of patients and are related to either sympathetic nervous system activation or extensive thrombosis of associated vasculature (Table 9.3) [72, 75].

Physical exam findings related to catecholamine surge may include hypertension, tachyarrhythmias, pale mucous membranes, poor femoral pulses, weakness, seizures, blindness, collapse, and sudden death (Table 9.4) [72, 78, 80]. If the surrounding vasculature is invaded by tumor, partial occlusion of the affected vessels may cause hindlimb edema, ascites, and abdominal pain [72]. Pheochromocytomas often present with concurrent diseases including other neoplasms; the clinical signs present may be reflective of these other disease processes.

Table 9.3 Clinical signs of pheochromocytoma [27, 53, 70, 71, 79].

None	Seizures
Anxiety	Acute blindness
Pacing	Epistaxis
Panting	Hindlimb edema
Dyspnea	Distended abdomen/ascites
Weakness	Abdominal pain
Anorexia	Collapse
Diarrhea	Sudden death
Vomiting, polyuria/polydipsia	

Table 9.4 Physical exam findings in pheochromocytoma [70, 76, 78].

Normal physical exam	Retinal hemorrhage
Hypertension	CNS signs
Tachycardia	Hindlimb edema
Arrhythmias	Abdominal pain
Weak femoral pulses	Ascites/fluid wave
Pale or hyperemic mucous membranes	

Clinicopathologic Findings

Hematologic and biochemical changes, like clinical signs, tend to be mild and nondescript and may reflect those of concurrent diseases. Hematologic abnormalities include mild anemia, leukocytosis, and lymphopenia [72]. Biochemical abnormalities may include azotemia, hyperglycemia, and elevated levels of the hepatic enzymes ALT and ALKP [72, 75].

Diagnosis

Diagnosis is difficult since clinical signs can be vague and nonspecific. Abdominal ultrasound, computed tomography, and magnetic resonance imaging are able to visualize larger tumors but are unable to differentiate pheochromocytomas from tumors of adrenocortical origin (Figure 9.4) [72]. Diagnostic testing, therefore, has focused on quantifying catecholamine levels or their metabolites within the

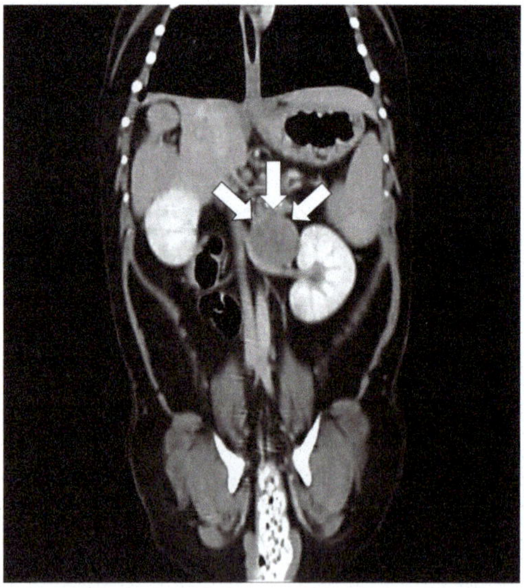

Figure 9.4 Computed tomography image of a dog with a right-sided pheochromocytoma (white arrows). Note its close association with the renal vasculature and caudal vena cava. *Source:* Photo courtesy of Veterinary Specialty Center, Buffalo Grove, IL.

urine or plasma. The caveat remains that dogs and cats in hospital settings are stressed, and they are likely to already have elevated levels of catecholamines and metanephrines even with nonadrenal disease, resulting in false positive readings [73]. To improve test specificity, studies have focused on validating testing protocols and establishing normal ranges [73, 81]. Plasma-free normetanephrine and/or plasma normetanephrine:creatinine ratio measurements via high-performance liquid chromatography are the most appropriate and can be considered diagnostic if the values exceed four times the high end of the documented range for dogs [73, 80–82].

Other diagnostic methods include radiolabeled meta-iodobenzylguanidine (MIBG) with I-131 or I-123, or positron emission tomography (PET) using p-[^{18}F]fluorobenzylguanidine, both of which are taken up into the neoplastic chromaffin cells and visualized [83, 84]. However, these methods are expensive, require special equipment, and are currently limited in their availability for routine veterinary use.

Treatment

Adrenalectomy via laparoscopy or laparotomy is the treatment of choice, since patients that survive the perioperative period generally have good long-term survival [75]. Tumors that are deemed nonresectable or where metastasis is already present are managed medically using alpha- and beta-adrenergic antagonists (see in the following text) [72]. Chemotherapy has been used with relatively poor results. However, use of molecular-targeted therapies, such as tyrosine kinase receptor antagonists, has shown promise [85].

Anesthetic Management

There are four major anesthetic goals for pheochromocytoma resection including: (i) adequate patient preparation, (ii) stress minimization in the perioperative period, (iii) controlling hemodynamic instability intraoperatively until the blood supply to the tumor has been ligated, and (iv) managing the postexcisional effects of antihypertensive therapies.

Patient Preparation

Preoperative management of patients with pheochromocytomas begins well before the scheduled surgery. Paroxysmal activation of alpha-1-adrenergic receptors by norepinephrine results in vasoconstriction, hypertension, and reduced vascular volume [72, 78]. Because catecholamines are sporadically released by the tumor, blood pressure measurements identify hypertension in <50% of canine patients [75, 86]. Therefore, normal blood pressure in the presence of an adrenal tumor does not exclude pheochromocytoma as a diagnosis nor bypasses the need for preanesthetic treatment with alpha-adrenergic receptor antagonists. Administration of alpha-adrenergic receptor antagonists for 1–4 week prior to anesthesia allows gradual vasodilation and reestablishment of vascular volume [79]. Use of phenoxybenzamine, a noncompetitive, nonselective alpha-adrenergic antagonist, began in the early 1950s and led to a significant decrease in human mortality from 40–60% to <6% [78, 79]. Similarly, dogs pretreated with phenoxybenzamine had significantly less mortality than those who had not (13% vs. 48%) [78].

While phenoxybenzamine has been the gold standard in veterinary medicine for pheochromocytoma resection preparation, its utility has become somewhat controversial and cost-prohibitive in recent years. Prazosin is a readily available selective alpha-1-adrenergic antagonist that can be used as an alternative. No direct studies comparing the preoperative alpha blocking effects of phenoxybenzamine and prazosin have been performed in veterinary medicine. However, studies in humans have had variable results, and, therefore, no consensus on the superiority of one treatment over the other regarding intraoperative stability and postoperative need for vasopressor support has been achieved [87, 88].

Prior to beginning alpha-adrenergic receptor antagonist therapy, patients should undergo an ECG for the arrhythmia detection, an ophthalmic exam, and serial blood pressure measurements as described by the American College of Veterinary Internal Medicine consensus statement on hypertension [57]. A CBC, biochemical profile, electrolytes, and urinalysis should be evaluated to look for underlying disease. Thoracic radiographs to identify metastasis or other pulmonary and cardiac changes should be performed.

If beginning patients on phenoxybenzamine, it is recommended to start at a dose of 0.5 mg kg^{-1} twice daily with repeated blood pressure measurements and ECG every 3–5 days. [86]. Systolic and diastolic blood pressures should be consistently <160 and 100 mmHg, respectively, during treatment [54]. The phenoxybenzamine dose may be doubled at each blood pressure check to a maximum dose of 2 mg kg^{-1} PO every 12 h until surgery or until the patient demonstrates signs of hypotension, such as weakness, ataxia, or syncope. Because of phenoxybenzamine's long-lasting effects, it may be advisable to discontinue treatment 24 h prior to surgery. Most patients on this regimen are adequately prepared for surgery within 10–14 d; however, some may require up to 4 weeks of therapy.

The antihypertensive effects of prazosin can have a faster onset of action and are associated with a greater incidence of orthostatic hypotension in humans [88]. The extra label dose for hypertension is 0.5–2 mg per dog orally every 8–12 h and 0.25–0.5 mg per cat orally every 24 h [19]. Because of the variable effect, it is recommended to start at the lowest dose and carefully titrate upward, following the same monitoring pattern as described for phenoxybenzamine.

If alpha-adrenergic blockade has been established and the patient continues to have tachycardia or other dysrhythmias, administration of a beta-adrenergic antagonist, such as atenolol, may also be indicated [79, 89]. The need for beta-blockade in humans is decreased in patients given a selective rather than a nonselective alpha-1-adrenergic antagonist. Since presynaptic alpha-2-adrenergic receptors are responsible for negative feedback inhibition of norepinephrine release from the nerve terminal, their blockade by phenoxybenzamine may allow continued release, thus leaving the patient susceptible to dysrhythmias [79, 90].

Prior to surgery, intravenous crystalloids should be administered to address fluid deficits. Blood pressures and ECG should be repeated and a minimum database of PCV, total solids, electrolytes, and acid–base status should be performed.

All handling and restraint should be performed with minimal stress to the patient, since stress is one of the triggers for a pheochromocytoma crisis (Table 9.5); [72, 91].

Table 9.5 Triggers for pheochromocytoma crises [2, 77].

Stress
Anesthesia induction
Increased intraabdominal pressure
Bladder expression
Abdominal insufflation
Histamine release
Morphine
Meperidine
Atracurium
Elevated PCO_2
Tumor manipulation
Drugs causing sympathetic nervous system (SNS) stimulation
Ketamine
Halothane
Ephedrine
Nitrous oxide
Metoclopramide
Glucagon
Succinylcholine

Preanesthetic Management

Patients should be premedicated to allow easy handling and catheter placement for direct blood pressure measurement and venous access. Combinations including a pure mu-opioid agonist (such as hydromorphone or methadone) and benzodiazepine are recommended, since they are short-acting, titratable, and do not cause histamine release (vs. morphine). Although acepromazine is an alpha-1 receptor antagonist and could be useful in preventing hypertensive crises, its use is not advised because its long duration of action and irreversibility may exacerbate hypotension following tumor removal.

Following sedation, preoxygenation via face mask is advisable if the patient is not stressed by its administration. Since anesthetic induction can trigger a catecholamine surge, it is important to monitor invasive blood pressure and ECG throughout induction if possible [79]. Additionally, antihypertensive and antiarrhythmic drugs should be readily available. No ideal induction protocol has been identified for pheochromocytoma removal. Both propofol and etomidate have been used safely with various coinduction agents like fentanyl [53]. One could assume, based on pharmacodynamic similarities to propofol, that alfaxalone would be suitable as well; however, no studies to date have examined this. Ketamine is usually avoided for induction, since it causes indirect stimulation of the sympathetic nervous system and induction doses could trigger a crisis [79]. Mask or chamber induction is not recommended due to poor monitoring ability and undue patient stress. Sufficient induction agent levels should be used to ensure that intubation is smooth with minimal laryngeal stimulation. Several different techniques for anesthetic maintenance during pheochromocytoma removal have been reported. A balanced approach utilizing agents that minimize rapid hemodynamic changes during tumor removal as well as the profound hypotension following ligation of the tumor blood supply is desirable. The combination of an inhalant anesthetic and a CRI of short-acting opioid, such as fentanyl and remifentanil, is well-described [92]. These agents decrease sympathetic nervous system outflow through various mechanisms, reducing catecholamine release during anesthesia. Patients may also benefit from a CRI of lidocaine due to the increased risk for ventricular arrhythmias. More recent literature describes the use of intraoperative dexmedetomidine infusions in humans. Its action on presynaptic alpha-2-adrenergic receptors inhibits norepinephrine release from the nerve terminal, thereby decreasing sympathetic outflow [19, 93]. In dogs, dexmedetomidine reduces plasma norepinephrine concentrations by approximately 80%, but can be accompanied by transient hypertension and decreased cardiac output due to effects on peripheral alpha-2-adrenergic receptor activation on vascular smooth muscle [86]. This contrasts with humans where the action is primarily antihypertensive with hypertension only occurring at high doses. In healthy dogs, infusion rates of $0.5\,\mu g\,kg^{-1}\,h^{-1}$ following a loading dose of $0.5\,\mu g\,kg^{-1}$ IV result in an approximately 18% reduction of isoflurane MAC without significant alterations in heart-rate and blood pressure [94]. While its anecdotal use has been reported, there are currently no clinical studies examining the cardiovascular effects of low dose dexmedetomidine CRIs in veterinary patients undergoing resection of a pheochromocytoma. Its benefit in veterinary medicine, therefore, remains to be determined.

Locoregional techniques can also be employed for pheochromocytoma removal. Epidural opioid administration and local anesthetics can reduce sympathetic nervous system stimulation and subsequent catecholamine release associated with skin incision, but do not affect catecholamine release associated with tumor manipulation [79]. The use of a quadratus lumborum block, which provides both somatic and visceral antinociception of the abdomen, has been recently reported in human literature for laparoscopic pheochromocytoma excision [95]. This novel block is described in the dog; however, its utility in this subset of patients is unknown [96].

Intraoperative Period

Monitoring Invasive hemodynamic monitoring (e.g., arterial blood pressure) is essential, since rapid fluctuations can occur. Placement of a central line to help assess vascular volume, and for the administration of vasoactive drugs intraoperatively and postoperatively, is advised. As with hyperthyroidism, the use of dynamic measures to assess volume status may provide the anesthetist with more objective means for identifying patients that will benefit from additional fluid support. IPPV is often required to avoid hypoventilation, since hypercarbia can stimulate catecholamine release [41]. Detection and characterization of arrhythmias via ECG monitoring allow treatment with appropriate antiarrhythmic agents.

Arrhythmia/Hypertension Management

Tumor manipulation frequently causes a catecholamine surge with paroxysmal hypertension and tachycardia even in patients where alpha-adrenergic blockade has been established [91]. Breakthrough hypertension and tachycardia occur from incomplete blockade with massive catecholamine release and via release of other vasoconstrictive mediators such as neuropeptide Y causing hypertension through nonadrenergic mechanisms [97].

Hypertensive crises require immediate intervention. Systolic blood pressure can quickly surmount 250 mmHg leading to cerebral encephalopathy, stroke, retinal detachment, multiple organ failure, and cardiac arrest [54]. Treatment should be instituted as systolic blood pressure reaches 180 mmHg, since this degree of hypertension directly correlates with target organ damage [27, 54].

Previous methods of treating hypertension have included administration of low doses of acepromazine and increasing inhalant concentration. However, the use of rapid-onset, short-acting hypotensive drugs has become the preferred method for maintaining hemodynamic stability (Table 9.6). Sodium nitroprusside is a potent arteriolar and venodilator that can be administered as a CRI to control hypertension. Although its duration of action is <5 min, it can rapidly cause profound hypotension due to significant decreases in venous return [79]. Magnesium sulfate ($MgSO_4$) has also shown promise in treatment of pheochromocytoma crisis by reducing blood pressure through direct inhibition of catecholamine receptors, inhibition of catecholamine release from both the adrenal medulla and nerve terminal, and direct arteriolar vasodilation [92, 98, 99]. It has a wide therapeutic range and does not typically cause profound hypotension seen with sodium nitroprusside. Clevidipine, an ultra-short-acting intravenous calcium channel antagonist, is showing promise for treatment of intraoperative hypertension in humans [100]. It is a vasoselective arteriolar dilator that is delivered as a CRI. Because it does not cause venodilation, venous return is minimally affected, resulting in better hemodynamic stability than nitroprusside [70, 98, 100]. The cost of clevidipine has decreased over time, which may make its use in veterinary medicine a viable option in the future for intraoperative management of pheochromocytoma.

Supraventricular tachycardia which may also accompany sudden release of catecholamines is frequently treated with the selective beta-1-adrenergic receptor antagonist, esmolol. Esmolol has a quick onset and short duration of action and is administered as a bolus or as a CRI to decrease heart rate, myocardial contractility, and atrioventricular (AV) node conduction [19].

While tachycardia and hypertension are expected findings during anesthesia, the anesthetist should be aware that third-degree atrioventricular block and other cardiac conduction disturbances have been observed in both dogs and humans (personal observation) [101]. These can arise during the perianesthetic

Table 9.6 Antihypertensive and antiarrhythmic drugs used in pheochromocytoma anesthetic management [19, 84, 97, 98].

Drug name	*Mechanism of action*	*Notes*	*Dose*
Sodium nitroprusside	Arteriolar and venodilator via nitric oxide release	Short-acting decreases in preload and afterload, can cause profound hypotension, cyanide metabolite	1–10 $\mu g\,kg^{-1}\,min^{-1}$ Do not exceed 0.5 $mg\,kg^{-1}\,h^{-1}$
Esmolol	Selective beta-1-adrenergic antagonist, decreases heart rate, contractility, AV node conduction	Short-acting, metabolized by esterases, can be administered as a CRI	Bolus: 100–500 $\mu g\,kg^{-1}$ CRI: 10–200 $\mu g\,kg^{-1}\,min^{-1}$
$MgSO_4$	Directly inhibits catecholamine receptors and release from nerve terminals, vasodilator	Wide therapeutic safety margin	Bolus: 30–50 $mg\,kg^{-1}$ over 15 min CRI: 15–25 $mg\,kg^{-1}\,h^{-1}$
Clevidipine	Blocks L-type Ca^{++} channels to produce selective arteriolar vasodilation	Short-acting, rapid onset, metabolized by esterases, expensive, CRI only	1–5 $\mu g\,kg^{-1}\,min^{-1}$ Start at low dose and titrate to effect[a]
Dexmedetomidine	Activates presynaptic alpha-2-adrenergic receptors to decrease NE release from nerve terminals	Used as an antihypertensive in humans; its use in veterinary species has not been evaluated	Loading dose: 0.5 $\mu g\,kg^{-1}$ CRI: 0.5–1 $\mu g\,kg^{-1}\,h^{-1}$

[a] Personal communication regarding use of clevidipine for treatment of hypertensive crisis in dogs with pheochromocytoma. CRI, constant rate infusion; NE, norepinephrine.

period and may be the result of myocardial ischemic damage and fibrosis from chronic sympathetic stimulation.

Emergency Adrenalectomy

While most adrenalectomies can be planned and properly prepared for, some require immediate surgery due to rupture. These patients typically present in hypovolemic shock and require stabilization with fluids and/or blood products. Mortality in patients where alpha-adrenergic blockade has not been established is higher than in those with blockade due to contracted vascular volume and poor perfusion from chronic vasoconstriction [78]. Short-acting antihypertensive agents and antiarrhythmics, such as those described previously, can be used intraoperatively to minimize hemodynamic instability. However, institution of beta-adrenergic blockade should not be done prior to alpha-adrenergic receptor blockade, as uninhibited, intense vasoconstriction could result [79].

Postoperative Period

Following tumor blood supply ligation, patients can become rapidly hypotensive from sudden cessation of sympathetic stimulation, adrenergic receptor downregulation, and long-lasting effects from alpha- and beta-adrenergic receptor antagonists [79, 89, 98]. Goal-directed fluid resuscitation with crystalloids along with inotropic or vasopressor support is often necessary to increase cardiac output. Use of adrenergic agonists, such as norepinephrine and phenylephrine, may be unrewarding in this manner because of receptor downregulation and pharmacologic adrenergic receptor antagonism. However, vasopressin (CRI of 0.001–0.004 $U\,kg^{-1}\,min^{-1}$), via activation of vascular V-1 receptors, may help by causing vasoconstriction not mediated through adrenergic mechanisms [19, 101]. Additionally, vasopressin is effective in the presence of hypoperfusion and metabolic acidosis, both of which may occur in the postoperative pheochromocytoma patient [101, 102].

Intense monitoring should continue in the postoperative period including telemetry, central venous pressure, and direct arterial blood pressure. While hypotension tends to occur most often, patients can continue to be hypertensive for several days and should continue to receive phenoxybenzamine until normotensive [79, 89]. If significant arrhythmias are present, oxygen supplementation is advised.

Diabetes Mellitus

Diabetes mellitus results from deficient serum insulin levels or decreased sensitivity of peripheral tissues to its effects, otherwise known as "insulin resistance." It is a common pancreatic endocrinopathy of humans, dogs, and cats with an incidence between 1 in 100 and 1 in 500, respectively [103]. Diabetes mellitus is designated as either type I, where destruction of the pancreatic beta cells leads to absolute hypoinsulinemia, or type II, where a combination of impaired insulin secretion and decreased tissue insulin sensitivity leads to elevated serum glucose levels [102].

Canine Diabetes Mellitus

Type I diabetes mellitus is most found in dogs and is usually caused by immune-mediated destruction of the pancreatic beta cells. It affects dogs between the ages of 4 and 14 years but is most frequently diagnosed in dogs between 7 and 10 years of age. Keeshonds and females are overrepresented [103].

Feline Diabetes Mellitus

By contrast, 80–95% of cats with diabetes mellitus are type-II diabetics, and, of these, approximately 70% require exogenous insulin administration [104, 105]. Cats are usually middle-aged at presentation with a peak incidence between 10 and 13 years. Male cats are affected more frequently than females and Burmese may be predisposed [104, 105].

Clinical Signs and Symptoms

Four classic clinical signs associated with diabetes mellitus in both cats and dogs include polyuria, polydipsia, polyphagia, and weight loss [103, 105]. Clinical signs are directly related to increased serum osmolarity caused by hyperglycemia, and the catabolic state from impaired glucose utilization by the tissues. Other symptoms can manifest from chronic hyperglycemia including blindness from cataract formation, and plantigrade stance in cats with diabetic neuropathy [103, 105, 106].

Clinicopathologic Changes

Minimal changes are seen on the CBC, but may reflect dehydration (polycythemia), or the presence of infection (leukocytosis) [103]. One consistent biochemical abnormality in an uncontrolled diabetic is persistent hyperglycemia. Increased lipolysis causes hypercholesterolemia, hypertriglyceridemia, and higher levels of circulating fatty acids. Other changes are often reflective of complications arising from diabetes and include azotemia, elevated amylase and lipase, mild to moderate increases in ALT and ALKP, hyponatremia, and hypokalemia [103].

Glycosuria is found as glucose levels surpass the renal tubular threshold (200 mg dl^{-1} in dogs and 250–300 mg dl^{-1} in cats). Osmotic diuresis from hyperglycemia decreases urine concentration producing a specific gravity between 1.025 and 1.035 [103]. Proteinuria often results from persistent hypertension and resultant glomerulopathy or urinary tract infection [102]. Poorly controlled diabetics may have ketonuria [104, 105].

Table 9.7 Complications of diabetes mellitus [7, 21, 106, 107, 109–112].

Complication	Anesthetic concerns
Atherosclerosis	Decreased organ blood flow Ischemia
Hypertension	Retinal hemorrhage Hypertensive encephalopathy Impaired autoregulation of renal, cerebral, and coronary circulation Renal failure
Retinopathy	Representative of cerebral vascular impairment
Nephropathy	Hypertension Renal failure
Peripheral neuropathy	Prolonged locoregional block Prolonged or shortened neuromuscular block Increased risk of further nerve injury
Autonomic neuropathy	Gastroparesis Hypotension Poor vasomotor tone Respiratory depression Impaired thermoregulation Cardiac failure/arrest

Diagnosis

Diabetes mellitus is confirmed with persistent fasting hyperglycemia and concurrent glycosuria. Cats can have sporadic serum glucose elevations from stress and often need serial glucose measurements or fructosamine concentration to help establish the diagnosis [104, 105].

Treatment

Treatment for most diabetic dogs and cats involves the administration of various insulin preparations which are beyond the scope of this chapter. However, diet, activity level, treatment of concurrent diseases, and avoidance of drugs that promote insulin resistance, such as glucocorticoids, all help to control diabetes mellitus [103, 105].

Anesthetic Management

In humans and dogs, anesthesia and surgery in the diabetic patient are associated with higher complication rates, mortality rates, and longer hospital stays [31, 105, 106]. Higher perianesthetic issues are attributed to impaired glucose homeostasis on the cardiovascular system, the central and peripheral nervous systems, the autonomic nervous system, the kidneys, and the eyes [103, 105, 107–109]. Many deleterious effects are caused by damage to vascular endothelium throughout the body (Table 9.7) [103, 107, 108].

Hypertension is present in approximately 46% of diabetic dogs and, to a much lesser extent, cats, and is attributed to atherosclerosis from increased lipolysis, impaired vasodilation, electrolyte abnormalities, and thickening of the vascular endothelium in response to elevated levels of the glucose by-products, sorbitol and advanced glycation end-products (AGEs) [7, 26]. Hypertension subsequently increases cardiac work with eventual myocardial dysfunction and remodeling [110]. With other forms of endocrine hypertension, blindness, renal failure, encephalopathy, stroke, and cardiac arrest are possible outcomes, and, if uncontrolled, affected diabetic patients are at greater risk of hemodynamic instability under anesthesia [26].

Since both the central and peripheral nervous systems are affected by diabetes mellitus, hyperglycemia and vascular damage can impair cerebral vasodilation in response to increasing carbon dioxide levels [106]. This, combined with atherosclerosis of the cerebral vessels, may result in decreased cerebral perfusion and ischemia. In anesthetized patients, this can be even more detrimental, as impaired autoregulation may require higher mean arterial blood pressure to maintain brain oxygen delivery [111, 112].

Peripheral neuropathy occurs in approximately 50% of diabetic humans, approximately 10% of diabetic cats, and less frequently in dogs [106, 107, 113]. Affected patients present with hindlimb weakness, ataxia, proprioceptive deficits, decreased tendon reflexes, muscle atrophy, and decreased muscle tone [106, 113]. Cats in particular may present with a plantigrade stance and neuropathic pain due to vascular changes, ischemia, axonal degeneration, and demyelination causing to sensorimotor deficits [103, 107].

Autonomic neuropathy is a serious manifestation of diabetes mellitus associated with altered parasympathetic tone, leading to tachycardia, delayed gastric-emptying time, orthostatic hypotension, altered respiratory responses to hypoxia, impaired thermoregulation, and cardiac failure [106, 108, 112, 114]. Although not commonly reported in veterinary species, cardiac autonomic neuropathy has been documented in diabetic dogs [114].

Humans with diabetes mellitus are commonly affected by diabetic nephropathy from vascular changes induced by hyperglycemia [108]. Damaged glomeruli leak protein into the urine leading to glomerulosclerosis, decreased GFR, and eventual renal failure [108]. In veterinary patients, renal changes and proteinuria are more frequently attributed to hypertension and care should be taken to ensure adequate renal perfusion during the perianesthetic period [26].

Diabetic Ketoacidosis (DKA)

Diabetic ketoacidosis causes severe hyperglycemia, dehydration, metabolic acidosis, obtundation, and cardiovascular collapse, and can occur with uncontrolled disease, as well as following severe illness, infection, or increased stress from anesthesia and surgery [103, 104]. Proper patient stabilization includes administration of intravenous fluids, potassium supplementation, insulin, and occasionally sodium bicarbonate [103].

Preanesthetic Period

Most important in the anesthetic management of diabetic patients are the goals of minimizing hyperglycemia and avoiding hypoglycemia. Anesthetic drugs and the stress of anesthesia and surgery affect blood glucose levels [109]. It is strongly recommended that newly diagnosed diabetics and those that are poorly controlled be regulated prior to undergoing anesthesia for elective procedures; newly diagnosed human diabetics have the highest complication rates and mortality when compared to controlled diabetics and nondiabetics [106].

Prior to anesthesia, a thorough physical exam should be performed to evaluate all organ systems and assess hydration. Neurologic evaluation may suggest peripheral neuropathy, and fundoscopic exam may reveal changes in retinal vessels, suggesting hypertension [113, 115]. Vascular changes in the retina may be reflective of abnormalities of the cerebral vessels as well [113]. Fasting in diabetics can lead to altered insulin requirements. Recent preoperative guidelines for diabetic human patients only missing one meal recommend the continuation of long-term insulin at 50% of the dose the morning of surgery with evaluation and additional supplementation of insulin as a variable rate intravenous insulin infusion (VRIII) and/or dextrose if needed [116]. In cats, overnight fasting does not significantly affect morning blood glucose concentration. It is therefore considered acceptable to similarly advise owners to withhold food, not water, and administer 50% of the normal insulin dose the morning of anesthesia [117].

In dogs, established recommendations are lacking. Commonly used insulin preparations tend to be intermediate in duration and may have an earlier nadir than the long-lasting formulas used in cats. This may result in unintended hypoglycemia if given to a fasted patient. In this case, the administration of 50% of the usual dose of insulin may be given with a small meatball of easily digestible food. Alternatively, if the dog is scheduled for anesthesia early in the day, it may be advisable to instruct owners to withhold the morning insulin dose and evaluate blood glucose concentration immediately upon arrival at the hospital where insulin requirements can be adjusted and monitored [12].

In patients where blood glucose concentrations are $<100\,\mathrm{mg\,dl^{-1}}$, it is advised to not administer insulin and start a 2.5–5% dextrose infusion [104]. Likewise, if blood glucose is $>300\,\mathrm{mg\,dl^{-1}}$, 50% of the patient's usual insulin dose can be administered subcutaneously or an infusion of regular insulin (0.025–$0.05\,\mathrm{U\,kg^{-1}\,h^{-1}}$) along with dextrose and potassium chloride can be started depending on when the patient is scheduled for induction [19, 104, 112]. Blood glucose levels should be checked every 30–60 min to avoid hypoglycemia and direct continued therapy [109, 112].

Electrolytes, acid–base status, PCV, total solids, BUN, creatinine, and lactate should also be evaluated [109]. Urine should be checked for glucose, ketones, and protein. Ketonuria is cause for concern, even if the patient is not acidotic since hyperglycemic surges from stress could push a diabetic patient into DKA and elective procedures should be postponed until no ketones are present [109]. Acidemia and hyperlactatemia may indicate poor tissue perfusion and hypovolemia and should be corrected prior to anesthesia.

Osmotic diuresis leads to dehydration, loss of sodium and potassium, and decreased circulating blood volume [2]. Preoperative intravenous fluids should be administered to help prevent hemodynamic instability following anesthesia induction [106]. Because diabetic patients may have increased risk of regurgitation and aspiration from delayed gastric emptying, the anesthetist should also consider the use of gastroprotectant and prokinetic therapies [6, 106].

Decreasing surgical stress using appropriate analgesic techniques is imperative to minimize alterations in glucose. Opioids inhibit sympathetic nervous system activation and cortisol secretion and do not impair glucose homeostasis [106, 118]. Alpha-2-adrenergic receptor agonist administration is controversial. They inhibit insulin secretion through activation of alpha-2A-adrenergic receptors on the pancreatic beta cells and therefore may exacerbate hyperglycemia [119]. However, Restitutti et al demonstrated dexmedetomidine in healthy dogs does not exacerbate hyperglycemia and the decrease in insulin secretion was balanced by the decrease in sympathetic nervous system activity from presynaptic alpha-2-adrenergic receptor activation [120]. In addition, dexmedetomidine decreases lipolysis and reduces cortisol levels in stressed animals. Thus, dexmedetomidine may benefit the diabetic patient, but warrants further examination [121].

The induction agents, propofol, alfaxalone, and etomidate, do not adversely affect glucose homeostasis and can be used in the diabetic patient [106, 117, 120]. However, ketamine indirectly stimulates the sympathetic nervous system which could indirectly worsen hyperglycemia [6, 12]. Volatile anesthetics significantly affect glucose homeostasis by inhibiting insulin release in response to hyperglycemia. However, whether this can affect outcomes of diabetic veterinary patients is not fully elucidated [106, 118].

Intraoperative Period

Anesthetic induction should be smooth and rapid with inflation of the pilot balloon occurring while the patient is still in sternal recumbency to protect the airway from possible regurgitation and aspiration. Most important during the intraoperative period is monitoring blood glucose every 30–60 min for the duration of the procedure [103, 104]. Although there is no standard as to how tight glycemic control should be in veterinary patients, an acceptable goal is to maintain blood glucose between 150 and 200 mg dl^{-1}. Although lower glucose concentrations between 80-120 mg dl^{-1} are associated with a decrease in anesthetic morbidity in humans, the risk of post-operative hypoglycemia and resultant mortality is higher [112]. Therefore, this tighter therapeutic target range is not recommended [112].

Locoregional Anesthesia and Analgesia

Locoregional anesthesia and analgesia can be beneficial in diabetic patients, since it reduces stress and release of counterregulatory hormones (epinephrine, glucagon, and cortisol) [109]. However, its use is controversial in patients with diabetic peripheral neuropathy because of suspected reductions in nerve blood flow, increased ischemic damage in the presence of local anesthetics, and exacerbation of neurologic deficits in the postanesthetic period [21]. Demyelination, axon degeneration, and sensory and motor blockade prolongation are observed in diabetic rodent models after injection of 0.5% ropivacaine into the sciatic notch. The neurotoxic effects were exacerbated when dexmedetomidine (20 μg ml^{-1}) was added to the ropivacaine, with motor and sensory blockade lasting >60 h [121]. Risk:benefit ratios should therefore be considered prior to utilizing these techniques.

Neuromuscular Junction Blockade

The duration of the neuromuscular blocking agent vecuronium is significantly longer in diabetic versus nondiabetic humans, possibly related to changes in the neuromuscular junction and motor nerve conduction. However, the opposite has been observed in diabetic dogs where the duration of both vecuronium and rocuronium is significantly decreased in comparison to nondiabetic dogs [122, 123]. Thus, train-of-four monitoring should be used to assess return of function considering the variable effects on muscle function blockade by these drugs.

Complications

Diabetic patients are at risk of greater hemodynamic instability under anesthesia and may have impaired responses to anesthetic drugs [106]. Severe hypotension is more common in anesthetized diabetic dogs than nondiabetic dogs and frequently requires fluid and inotropic support [124].

Monitoring

Monitoring needs should be related to the invasiveness of the procedure and ASA physical status. Uncontrolled or unstable diabetic patients should have invasive blood pressure monitoring. Objective methods to assess circulating blood volume should be utilized and addressed as necessary. Temperature, capnometry, ECG, and pulse oximetry are standard. Diabetic patients may have altered thermoregulation putting them at greater risk for hypothermia; aggressive prevention and treatment should be pursued using circulating warm water blankets and convective heat sources [108].

Recovery

Glucose monitoring should continue every 30–90 min until the patient is eating. This duration can be shortened by avoiding excessive sedation in the postoperative period. It is important to recognize that the stress of surgery and release of inflammatory mediators may lead to increased insulin requirements following anesthesia [112]. Dextrose and insulin administration tailored to patient needs and a multimodal approach to provide adequate analgesia can minimize stress while maintaining glucose homeostasis [103, 104].

Summary

Endocrine disease adversely affects homeostasis and, as such, can impact anesthesia. Patients presenting for elective procedures should be treated beforehand and have stable disease. Although major complications resulting from these diseases are uncommon, when present, they can be significant. For those patients who are unable to be stabilized prior to anesthesia, a full understanding of the pathophysiology of the disease and what complications should be expected can prepare the anesthetist for the challenges they impose.

References

1 Scott-Moncrieff, J.C. (2014). Hypothyroidism. In: *Canine and Feline Endocrinology*, 4e (eds. E.C. Feldman, R.W. Nelson, C.E. Reusch and J.C. Scott-Moncrieff), 77–135. St. Louis: Saunders.

2 Wall, R.T. (2008). Endocrine disease. In: *Stoelting's Anesthesia and Co-Existing Disease*, 5e (eds. R.L. Hines and K.E. Marschall), 365–406. Philadelphia: Churchill Livingstone.

3 Scott-Moncrieff, J.C. (2007). Clinical signs and concurrent diseases of hypothyroidism in dogs and cats. *Vet. Clin. North Am. Small Anim. Pract.* 37: 709–722.

4 Mooney, C.T. (2011). Canine hypothyroidism: a review of aetiology and diagnosis. *New Zealand Vet. J.* 59: 105–114.

5 Williams, T.L., Elliott, J., and Syme, H.M. (2010). Association of iatrogenic hypothyroidism with azotemia and reduced survival time in cats treated for hyperthyroidism. *J. Vet. Intern. Med.* 24: 1086–1092.

6 Morgan, G.E., Mikhail, M.S., and Murray, M.J. (2006). Anesthesia for patients with endocrine disease. In: *Clinical Anesthesiology*, 4e (eds. G.E. Morgan, M.S. Mikhail and M.H. Murray), 802–816. New York: McGraw-Hill.

7 Hess, R.S., Kass, P.H., and Van Winkle, T.J. (2003). Association between diabetes mellitus, hypothyroidism or hyperadrenocorticism, and atherosclerosis in dogs. *J. Vet. Intern. Med.* 17: 489–494.

8 Hofer-Inteeworn, N., Panciera, D.L., Monroe, W.E. et al. (2012). Effect of hypothyroidism on insulin sensitivity and glucose tolerance in dogs. *Am. J. Vet. Res.* 73: 529–538.

9 Lobetti, R.G. (2011). Hypercalcemia in a dog with primary hypothyroidism. *South Afr. Vet.* 82: 242–243.

10 Panciera, D.L. and Lefebvre, H.P. (2009). Effect of experimental hypothyroidism on glomerular filtration rate and plasma creatinine concentration in dogs. *J. Vet. Intern. Med.* 23: 1045–1050.

11 Scott-Moncrieff, J.C. (2012). Thyroid disorders in the geriatric veterinary patient. *Vet. Clin. North Am. Small Anim. Pract.* 42: 707–725.

12 Adams, J.F., Figueiredo, J.P., and Graves, T.K. (2015). Physiology, pathophysiology, and anesthetic management of patients with gastrointestinal and endocrine disease. In: *Veterinary Anesthesia and Analgesia. The Fifth Edition of Lumb and Jones* (eds. K.A. Grimm, L.A. Lamont, W.J. Tranquilli, et al.), 641–681. Ames: Wiley-Blackwell Publishing.

13 Flood, J.A. and Hoover, J.P. (2009). Improvement in myocardial dysfunction in a hypothyroid dog. *Can. Vet. J.* 50: 828–834.

14 McMurphy, R.M., Hodgson, D.S., Bruyette, D.S. et al. (1996). Cardiovascular effects of 1.0, 1.5, and 2.0 minimum alveolar concentrations of isoflurane in experimentally induced hypothyroidism in dogs. *Vet. Surg.* 25: 171–178.

15 Rossmeisl JH. 2010. Resistance of the peripheral nervous system to the effects of

chronic canine hypothyroidism. J Vet Intern Med. 24: 875–881.

16 Pancotto, T., Rossmeisl, J.H. Jr., Panciera, D.L. et al. (2010). Blood-brain-barrier disruption in chronic canine hypothyroidism. *Vet. Clin. Pathol.* 39: 485–493.

17 Blois, S.L., Poma, R., Stalker, M.J. et al. (2008). A case of primary hypothyroidism causing central nervous system atherosclerosis in a dog. *Can. Vet. J.* 49: 789–792.

18 Babad, A.R. and Eger, E.I. (1968). The effects of hyperthyroidism and hypothyroidism on halothane and oxygen requirements in dogs. *Anesthesiology* 29: 1087–1093.

19 Education Concepts, LLC (2018). Plumb's Veterinary Drugs (version 2020.5) [Mobile application software]. Retrieved from http://play.google.com/google-play.

20 Read MR, Hutchinson A, Berard B, et al. (2012). Preinduction warming prevents hypothermia in anesthetized dogs. Paper presented at: WCVA 2012. Proceedings of the 11th World Congress of Veterinary Anaesthesiology; Sept 23–27; Cape Town, South Africa.

21 Candido, K.D. (2009). Regional anesthesia and the patient with preexisting neuropathy. *Anesthesiol. News* 35: 1–8.

22 Scott-Moncrieff, J.C. (2014). Feline hyperthyroidism. In: *Canine and Feline Endocrinology*, 4e (eds. E.C. Feldman, R.W. Nelson, C.E. Reusch and J.C. Scott-Moncrieff), 136–195. St. Louis: Saunders.

23 Scott-Moncrieff, J.C. (2014). Canine thyroid tumors and hyperthyroidism. In: *Canine and Feline Endocrinology*, 4e (eds. E.C. Feldman, R.W. Nelson, C.E. Reusch and J.C. Scott-Moncrieff), 196–212. St. Louis: Saunders.

24 Henik, R.A., Stepien, R.L., Wenholz, L.J. et al. (2008). Efficacy of atenolol as a single antihypertensive agent in hyperthyroid cats. *J. Feline Med. Surg.* 10: 577–582.

25 Hoffman, G., Marks, S.L., Taboada, J. et al. (2003). Transdermal methimazole treatment in cats with hyperthyroidism. *J. Feline Med. Surg.* 5: 77–82.

26 Ward, C.R. (2007). Feline thyroid storm. *Vet. Clin. North Am. Small Anim. Pract.* 37: 745–754.

27 Reusch, C.E., Schellenberg, S., and Wenger, M. (2010). Endocrine hypertension in small animals. *Vet. Clin. North Am. Small Anim. Pract.* 40: 335–352.

28 Peterson, M.E., Varela, F.V., Rishniw, M. et al. (2018). Evaluation of serum symmetric dimethylarginine concentration as a marker for masked chronic kidney disease in cats with hyperthyroidism. *J. Vet. Intern. Med.* 32: 295–304.

29 Klubo-Gwiezdzinska, J. and Wartofsky, L. (2012). Thyroid emergencies. *Med. Clin. North Am.* 96: 385–403.

30 Cui, Y., Heuser, K., Bauer, N. et al. (2019). Coagulation parameters in hyperthyroid cats before and after radioiodine treatment compared with healthy controls. *J. Feline Med. Surg.* 21: 1134–1140.

31 Kohl, B.A. and Schwartz, S. (2009). Surgery in the patient with endocrine dysfunction. *Anesthesiol. Clin.* 27: 687–703.

32 Langley, R.W. and Burch, H.B. (2003). Perioperative management of the thyrotoxic patient. *Endocrinol. Metab. Clin. North Am.* 32: 519–534.

33 Rutland, B.E., Nachreiner, R.F., and Kruger, J.M. (2009). Optimal testing for thyroid hormone concentration after treatment with methimazole in healthy and hyperthyroid cats. *J. Vet. Intern. Med.* 23: 1025–1030.

34 Loftus, J.P., DeRosa, S., Struble, A.M. et al. (2019). One-year study evaluating efficacy of an iodine-restricted diet for the treatment of moderate-to-severe hyperthyroidism in cats. *Vet. Med. (Auckl.)* 10: 9–16.

35 Hirvonen, E.A., Niskanen, L.K., and Niskanen, M.M. (2004). Thyroid storm prior to induction of anaesthesia. *Anaesthesia* 59: 1020–1022.

36 Epstein FH. 2001. Thyroid hormone and the cardiovascular system. N Engl J Med. 344(7): 501–509.

37 Simpson, A.C. and McCown, J.L. (2009). Systemic hypertension in a dog with a functional thyroid gland adenocarcinoma. *J. Am. Vet. Med. Assoc.* 235: 1474–1479.

38 Harris, A.N., Beatty, S.S., Estrada, A.H. et al. (2017). Investigation of an N-terminal prohormone of brain natriuretic peptide point-of-care ELISA in clinically normal cats and cats with cardiac disease. *J. Vet. Intern. Med.* 31: 994–999.

39 Tsubokawa, T., Yamamoto, K., and Kobayashi, T. (1998). Propofol clearance and distribution volume increase in patients with hyperthyroidism. *Anesth. Analg.* 87: 195–199.

40 Walker, J.S., Klockowski, P.M., and Levy, G. (1989). Kinetics of drug action in disease states. Effect of experimental hyperthyroidism on the hypnotic activity of a benzodiazepine (oxazepam) in rats. *Pharm. Res.* 6: 404–407.

41 McDonnell, W.N. and Kerr, C.L. (2015). Physiology, pathophysiology, and anesthetic management of patients with respiratory disease. In: *Veterinary Anesthesia and Analgesia. The Fifth Edition of Lumb and Jones* (eds. K.A. Grimm, L.A. Lamont, W.J. Tranquilli, et al.), 513–555. Ames: Wiley-Blackwell Publishing.

42 Sano, H., Seo, J., Wightman, P. et al. (2018). Evaluation of pulse pressure variation and pleth variability index to predict fluid responsiveness in mechanically ventilated isoflurane-anesthetized dogs. *J. Vet. Emerg. Crit. Care* 28: 301–309.

43 Boller, E. and Boller, M. (2015). Assessment of fluid balance and the approach to fluid therapy in the perioperative patient. *Vet. Clin. North Am. Small Anim. Pract.* 45: 895–915.

44 Lord, M.S. and Augoustides, J.G.T. (2012). Perioperative management of pheochromocytoma: focus on magnesium, clevidipine, and vasopressin. *J. Cardiothorac. Vasc. Anesth.* 26: 526–531.

45 Behrend, E.N. (2014). Canine hyperadrenocorticism. In: *Canine and Feline Endocrinology*, 4e (eds. E.C. Feldman, R.W. Nelson, C.E. Reusch and J.C. Scott-Moncrieff), 377–451. St. Louis: Saunders.

46 deBruin, C., Meij, B.P., Kooistra, H.S. et al. (2009). Cushing's disease in dogs and humans. *Horm. Res.* 71: 140–143.

47 Feldman, E.C. (2014). Hyperadrenocorticism in cats. In: *Canine and Feline Endocrinology*, 4e (eds. E.C. Feldman, R.W. Nelson, C.E. Reusch and J.C. Scott-Moncrieff), 452–484. St. Louis: Saunders.

48 Cross, E., Moreland, R., and Wallack, S. (2012). Feline pituitary-dependent hyperadrenocorticism and insulin resistance due to a plurihormonal adenoma. *Top. Companion Anim. Med.* 27: 8–20.

49 Novellas, R., de Gopegui, R., and Espada, Y. (2008). Determination of renal vascular resistance in dogs with diabetes mellitus and hyperadrenocorticism. *Vet. Rec.* 163: 592–596.

50 Smith, R.R., Mayhew, P.D., and Berent, A.C. (2012). Laparoscopic adrenalectomy for management of a functional adrenal tumor in a cat. *J. Am. Vet. Med. Assoc.* 241: 368–372.

51 West, J.B. (2003). Vascular diseases. In: *Pulmonary Pathophysiology: The Essentials*, 6e (ed. J.B. West), 101–122. Philadelphia: Lippincott Williams & Wilkins.

52 Smets, P.M.Y., Lefebvre, H.P., Meij, B.P. et al. (2012). Long-term follow-up of renal function in dogs after treatment for ACTH-dependent hyperadrenocorticism. *J. Vet. Intern. Med.* 26: 565–573.

53 Lang, J.M., Schertel, E., Kennedy, S. et al. (2011). Elective and emergency surgical management of adrenal gland tumors: 60 cases (1999-2006). *J. Am. Anim. Hosp. Assoc.* 47: 428–435.

54 Brown, A.L., Beatty, J.A., Lindsay, S.A. et al. (2012). Severe systemic hypertension in a cat with pituitary-dependent hyperadrenocorticism. *J. Small Anim. Pract.* 53: 132–135.

55 Cabrera Blatter, M.F., del Prado, B., Miceli, D.D. et al. (2012). Interleukin-6 and insulin increase and nitric oxide and adiponectin decrease in blind dogs with pituitary-dependent hyperadrenocorticism. *Res. Vet. Sci.* 93: 1195–1202.

56 Pace, S.L., Creevy, K.E., Krimer, P.M. et al. (2013). Assessment of coagulation and potential biochemical markers for hypercoagulability in canine hyperadrenocorticism. *J. Vet. Intern. Med.* 27: 1113–1120.

57 Acierno, M.J., Brown, S., Coleman, A.E. et al. (2018). ACVIM consensus statement: guidelines for the identification, evaluation, and management of systemic hypertension in dogs and cats. *J. Vet. Intern. Med.* 32 (6): 1803–1822.

58 Racasan, S., Joles, A., Boer, P. et al. No dependency of RBF and autoregulation in the spontaneously hypertensive rat. *Am. J. Physiol. Renal Physiol.* 285: F105–F112.

59 Dabbagh, A., Sa'adat, N., and Heidari, Z. (2009). Etomidate infusion in the critical care setting for suppressing the acute phase of cushing's syndrome. *Anesth. Analg.* 108: 238–239.

60 Morgan, G.E., Mikhail, M.S., and Murray, M.J. (2006). Anesthesia for patients with respiratory disease. In: *Clinical Anesthesiology*, 4e (eds. G.E. Morgan, M.S. Mikhail and M.H. Murray), 571–584. New York: McGraw-Hill.

61 Goggs, R., Blais, M.C., Brainard, B.M. et al. (2019). American College of Veterinary Emergency and Critical Care (ACVECC) consensus on the rational use of antithrombotics in veterinary critical care (CURATIVE) guidelines: small animal. *J. Vet. Emerg. Crit. Care.* 29: 12–36.

62 Blais, M., Bianco, D., Goggs, R. et al. (2019). American College of Veterinary Emergency and Critical Care (ACVECC) consensus on the rational use of antithrombotics in veterinary critical care (CURATIVE) guidelines: defining antithrombotic protocols. *J. Vet. Emerg. Crit. Care* 29: 60–74.

63 Scott-Moncrieff, J.C. (2014). Hypoadrenocorticism. In: *Canine and Feline Endocrinology*, 4e (eds. E.C. Feldman, R.W. Nelson, C.E. Reusch and J.C. Scott-Moncrieff), 485–520. St. Louis: Saunders.

64 Klein, S.C. and Peterson, M.E. (2010). Canine hypoadrenocorticism: part I. *Can. Vet. J.* 51: 63–69.

65 Sicken, J. and Neiger, R. (2013). Addisonian crisis and severe acidosis in a cat: a case of feline hypoadrenocorticism. *J. Feline Med. Surg.* 15: 941–944.

66 Woolcock, A.D. and Ward, C. (2015). Successful treatment of a cat with primary hypoadrenocorticism and severe hyponatremia with desoxycorticosterone pivalate (DOCP). *Can. Vet. J.* 56: 1158–1160.

67 Van Lanen, K. and Sande, A. (2014). Canine hypoadrenocorticism: pathogenesis, diagnosis, and treatment. *Top. Companion Anim. Med.* 29: 88–95.

68 Hsu, A.A., von Elten, K., Chan, D. et al. (2012). Characterization of the cortisol stress response to sedation and anesthesia in children. *J. Clin. Endocrinol. Metab.* 97: 1830–1835.

69 Lathan, P. and Thompson, A.L. (2018). Management of hypoadrenocorticism (Addison's disease) in dogs. *Vet. Med. (Auckl.)* 9: 1–10.

70 Annane, D., Pastores, S.M., Rochwerg, B. et al. (2017). Guidelines for the diagnosis and management of critical illness-related corticosteroid insufficiency (CIRCI) in critically ill patients (part I): Society of Critical Care Medicine (SCCM) and European Society of Intensive Care Medicine (ESICM) 2017. *Intensive Care Med.* 43: 1751–1763.

71 Martin, L.G., Groman, R.P., Fletche, D.J. et al. (2008). Pituitary-adrenal function in dogs with acute critical illness. *J. Am. Vet. Med. Assoc.* 233: 87–95.

72 Reusch, C.E. (2014). Pheochromocytoma and multiple endocrine neoplasia. In: *Canine and Feline Endocrinology*, 4e (eds. E.C. Feldman, R.W. Nelson, C.E. Reusch and

J.C. Scott-Moncrieff), 521–554. St. Louis: Saunders.

73 Wimpole, J.A., Adagra, C.F.M., Billson, M.F. et al. (2010). Plasma free metanephrines in healthy cats, cats with non-adrenal disease and a cat with suspected phaeochromocytoma. *J. Feline Med. Surg.* 12: 435–440.

74 Calsyn, J.D.R., Green, R.A., Davis, G.J. et al. (2010). Adrenal pheochromocytoma with contralateral adrenocortical adenoma in a cat. *J. Am. Anim. Hosp. Assoc.* 46: 36–42.

75 Barthez, P.Y., Marks, S.L., Woo, J. et al. (1997). Pheochromocytoma in dogs: 61 cases (1984-1995). *J. Vet. Intern. Med.* 11: 272–278.

76 Bertelsen, M.F., Steele, S.L., Grondahl, C. et al. (2011). Pheochromocytoma in a white rhinoceros (ceratotherium simum). *J. Zoo Wildlife Med.* 42: 521–523.

77 Schlanser, J.R., Patterson, J.S., Kiupel, M. et al. (2012). Disseminated pheochromocytoma in a north American river otter (*Lontra canadensis*). *J. Zoo Wildlife Med.* 43: 407–411.

78 Herrera, M.A., Mehl, M.L., Kass, P.H. et al. (2008). Predictive factors and the effect of phenoxybenzamine on outcome in dogs undergoing adrenalectomy for pheochromocytoma. *J. Vet. Intern. Med.* 22: 1333–1339.

79 Kinney, M.A.O., Narr, B.J., and Warner, M.A. (2002). Perioperative management of pheochromocytoma. *J. Cardiothorac. Vasc. Anesth.* 16: 359–369.

80 Quante, S., Boretti, F.S., Kook, P.H. et al. (2010). Urinary catecholamine and metanephrine to creatinine ratios in dogs with hyperadrenocorticism or pheochromocytoma, or in healthy dogs. *J. Vet. Intern. Med.* 24: 1093–1097.

81 Gostelow, R., Bridger, N., and Syme, H.M. (2013). Plasma-free metanephrine and free normetanephrine measurement for the diagnosis of pheochromocytoma in dogs. *J. Vet. Intern. Med.* 27: 83–90.

82 Kook, P.H., Grest, P., Quante, S. et al. (2010). Urinary catecholamine and metadrenaline to creatinine rations in dogs with a phaeochromocytoma. *Vet. Rec.* 166: 169–174.

83 Bommarito, D.A., Lattimer, J.C., Selting, K.A. et al. (2011). Treatment of a malignant pheochromocytoma in a dog using 131-I metaiodobenzylguanidine. *J. Am. Anim. Hosp. Assoc.* 47: 188–194.

84 Berry, C.R., DeGrado, T.R., Nutter, F. et al. (2002). Imaging of pheochromocytoma in 2 dogs using p-[18F]fluorobenzylguanidine. *Vet. Radiol. Ultrasound* 43: 183–186.

85 Ye, L., Santarpia, L., and Gagel, R.F. (2010). The evolving field of tyrosine kinase inhibitors in the treatment of endocrine tumors. *Endocr. Rev.* 31: 578–599.

86 Williger, H.M., Prinzen, F.W., and Roekaerts, P. (2006). The effects of esmolol and dexmedetomidine on myocardial oxygen consumption during sympathetic stimulation in dogs. *J. Cardiothorac. Vasc. Anesth.* 20: 364–370.

87 Bruynzeel, H., Feelders, R.A., Groenland, T.H.N. et al. (2010). Risk factors for hemodynamic instability during surgery for pheochromocytoma. *J. Clin. Endocrinol. Metab.* 95: 678–685.

88 Agrawal, R., Mishra, S.K., Bhatia, E. et al. (2014). Prospective study to compare peri-operative hemodynamic alterations following preparation for pheochromocytoma surgery by phenoxybenzamine or prazosin. *World J. Surg.* 38: 716–723.

89 Bajwa, S.S. and Bajwa, S.K. (2011). Implications and considerations during pheochromocytoma resection: a challenge to the anesthesiologist. *Indian J. Endocr. Metab.* 15: 337–344.

90 Zhu, Y., Hong-chao, H., Su, T. et al. (2010). Selective a1-adrenoceptor antagonist (controlled release tablets) in preoperative management of pheochromocytoma. *Endocrinology* 38: 254–259.

91 Kline, J.P. (2010). Use of clevidipine for intraoperative hypertension caused by an undiagnosed pheochromocytoma: a case report. *AANA J.* 78: 288–290.

92 Domi R and Laho H. 2012. Management of pheochromocytoma: old ideas and new drugs. Nig J Clin Prac. 15(3): 253-257.

93 Neukirchen, M. and Kienbaum, P. (2008). Sympathetic nervous system: evaluation and importance for clinical general anesthesia. *Anesthesiology* 109: 1113–1131.

94 Pascoe, P.J., Raekallio, M., Kuusela, E. et al. (2006). Changes in minimum alveolar concentration of isoflurane and some cardiopulmonary measurements during three continuous infusion rates of dexmedetomidine in dogs. *Vet. Anaesth. Analg.* 33: 97–103.

95 Giordano, C., Bassoricci, E., Fusco, P. et al. (2019). Ultrasound-guided quadratus lumborum block type 2 associated to continuous intravenous infusion of dexmedetomidine for anesthesiologic management in laparoscopic adrenalectomy for pheochromocytoma: could it be a safe strategy [letter to the editor]. *Minerva Anesthesiol.* 85: 919–920.

96 Garbin, M., Portela, D.A., Bertolizio, G. et al. (2020). Description of ultrasound-guided quadratus lumborum block technique and evaluation of injectate spread in canine cadavers. *Vet. Anaesth. Analg.* 47: 249258.

97 Senanayake, P., Denker, J., Bravo, E.L. et al. (1995). Production, characterization, and expression of neuropeptide Y by human pheochromocytoma. *J. Clin. Invest.* 96: 2503–2509.

98 Lord MS and Augoustides JGT. 2012. Perioperative management of pheochromocytoma: focus on magnesium, clevidipine, and vasopressin. J Cardio Vasc Anesth 26(3): 526–531.

99 Bryskin, R. and Weldon, B.C. (2010). Dexmedetomidine and magnesium sulfate in the perioperative management of a child undergoing laparoscopic resection of bilateral pheochromocytomas. *J. Clin. Anesth.* 22: 126–129.

100 Prlesi, L. and Cheng-Lai, A. (2009). Clevidipine: a novel ultra-short-acting calcium antagonist. *Cardiol. Rev.* 17: 147–152.

101 Mak, G. and Allen, J. (2013). Simultaneous pheochromocytoma and third-degree atrioventricular block in 2 dogs. *J. Vet. Emerg. Crit. Care* 23: 610–614.

102 Udeh, C.I., Diaz-Gomez, J.L., Satyapriya, A. et al. (2012). Recent advances in perioperative anesthetic management update on the role of vasopressin and its effects on outcomes. *Curr. Pharm. Des.* 18: 6308–6313.

103 Nelson, R.W. (2014). Canine diabetes mellitus. In: *Canine and Feline Endocrinology*, 4e (eds. E.C. Feldman, R.W. Nelson, C.E. Reusch and J.C. Scott-Moncrieff), 213–257. St. Louis: Saunders.

104 Reusch, C.E. (2014). Feline diabetes mellitus. In: *Canine and Feline Endocrinology*, 4e (eds. E.C. Feldman, R.W. Nelson, C.E. Reusch and J.C. Scott-Moncrieff), 258–314. St. Louis: Saunders.

105 Rand, J.S. and Marshall, R.D. (2005). Diabetes mellitus in cats. *Vet. Clin. North Am. Small Anim. Pract.* 35: 211–224.

106 Kadoi, Y. (2010). Anesthetic considerations in diabetic patients. Part I: preoperative considerations of patients with diabetes mellitus. *J. Anesth.* 24: 739–747.

107 Estrella, J.S., Nelson, R.N., Sturges, B.K. et al. (2008). Endoneurial microvascular pathology in feline diabetic neuropathy. *Microvasc. Res.* 75: 403–410.

108 Fowler, M.J. (2008). Microvascular and macrovascular complications of diabetes. *Clin. Diabetes* 26: 77–82.

109 Robertshaw, H.J. and Hall, G.M. (2006). Diabetes mellitus: anaesthetic management. *Anaesthesia* 61: 1187–1190.

110 Benedicto, H.G., Bombonato, P.P., Macchiarelli, G. et al. (2011). Structural arrangement of the cardiac collagen fibers of healthy and diabetic dogs. *Microsc. Res. Tech.* 74: 1018–1023.

111 Morgan, G.E., Mikhail, M.S., and Murray, M.J. (2006). Neurophysiology and anesthesia. In: *Clinical Anesthesiology*, 4e (eds. G.E. Morgan, M.S. Mikhail and M.J. Murray), 614–630. New York: McGraw-Hill.

112 Kadoi, Y. (2010). Anesthetic considerations in diabetic patients. Part II. Intraoperative and postoperative management of patient with diabetes mellitus. *J. Anesth.* 24: 748–756.

113 Morgan, M.J., Vite, C.H., Radhakrishnan, A. et al. (2008). Clinical peripheral neuropathy associated with diabetes mellitus in 3 dogs. *Can. Vet. J.* 49: 583–586.

114 Kenefick, S., Parker, N., Slater, L. et al. (2007). Evidence of cardiac autonomic neuropathy in dogs with diabetes mellitus. *Vet. Rec.* 161: 83–88.

115 Landry, M.P., Herring, I.P., and Panciera, D.L. (2004). Funduscopic findings following cataract extraction by means of phacoemulsification in diabetic dogs: 52 cases (1993-2003). *J. Am. Vet. Med. Assoc.* 225: 709–716.

116 Barker, P., Creasey, P.E., Dhatariya, K. et al. (2019). Peri-operative management of the surgical patient with diabetes 2015. *Anaesthesia* 70: 1427–1440.

117 Sparkes, A.H., Cannon, M., Church, D. et al. (2015). ISFM consensus guidelines on the practical management of diabetes mellitus in cats. *J. Feline Med. Surg.* 17: 235–250.

118 Tanaka, K., Kawana, T., Tsutsumi, Y.M. et al. (2011). Differential effects of propofol and isoflurane on glucose utilization and insulin secretion. *Life Sci.* 88: 96–103.

119 Munoz, K.A., Robertson, S.A., and Wilson, D.V. (2017). Alfaxalone alone or combined with midazolam or ketamine in dogs: intubation dose and select physiologic effects. *Vet. Anaesth. Analg.* 44: 766–774.

120 Restitutti, F., Raekallio, M., Vainionpaa, M. et al. (2012). Plasma glucose, insulin, free fatty acids, lactate and cortisol concentrations in dexmedetomidine-sedated dogs with or without MK-467: a peripheral α-2 adrenoceptor antagonist. *Vet. J.* 193: 481–485.

121 Yu, Z.Y., Geng, J., Li, Z.Q. et al. (2019). Dexmedetomidine enhances ropivacaine-induced sciatic nerve injury in diabetic rats. *Br. J. Anaesth.* 122: 141–149.

122 Clark, L., Leece, E.A., and Brearley, J.C. (2012). Diabetes mellitus affects the duration of action of vecuronium in dogs. *Vet. Anaesth. Analg.* 39: 474–479.

123 Haga, H.A., Bettembourg, V., and Lervik, A. (2019). Rocuronium infusion: a higher rate is needed in diabetic than nondiabetic dogs. *Vet. Anaesth. Analg.* 46: 28–35.

124 Oliver, J.A.C., Clark, L., Corletto, F. et al. (2010). A comparison of anesthetic complications between diabetic and nondiabetic dogs undergoing phacoemulsification cataract surgery: a retrospective study. *Vet. Ophthal.* 13: 244–250.

10

Nutritional Disease

Lindsey B. C. Snyder

Department of Surgical Sciences, School of Veterinary Medicine, University of Wisconsin–Madison, Madison, WI, 53706, USA

Introduction

The World Health Organization defines *obesity* is an abnormal or excessive fat accumulation in adipose tissue to the extent that health is impaired [1–3]. Excess adipose tissue occurs when the caloric intake surpasses the caloric expenditure [4, 5]. Owing to the prevalence of obesity in the human population, the World Health Organization has classified obesity into simple obesity (body mass index [BMI] 30–34.9 kg m^{-2}), severe obesity (BMI 35–39.9 kg m^{-2}), morbid obesity (BMI 40–49.9 kg m^{-2}), and super morbid obesity (BMI ≥40 kg m^{-2}) [6]. Although it is unknown what the actual increase in anesthetic risk is due to excessive body weight, it is generally believed that the likelihood of anesthetic complications will be greater in the overweight animal.

Pathophysiology

Obesity is the most common medical condition in companion animals and is associated with several comorbidities [2]. Approximately 55% of dogs and 53% of cats in the USA are overweight or obese [7]. Worldwide, 22–40% of dogs are obese [2, 5, 8, 9]. Even higher percentages are observed in dogs and cats between 5 and 10 years of age [5]. Coincidently, with obesity in humans comes an increase in morbidity, such as diabetes and musculoskeletal conditions [7]. The criteria for obesity are not as clear-cut in veterinary patients as with human patients, as optimal body weights have not been established for our species and varying breeds. However, it is still concluded that when a patient's weight is 15% above normal for its breed, it is "overweight," and when a patient's weight is 30% above normal, it is "obese" [2]. Body condition scoring (BCS) has been established as a validated method to assess body composition (see the section titled "Ideal Body Weight") [10].

Risk factors for the development of obesity in veterinary patients have been identified. There is a link between certain breeds and their genetic predisposition for obesity. Cairn Terriers, West Highland White Terriers, Scottish Terriers, Shetland Sheepdogs, Basset Hounds, Cavalier King Charles Spaniels, Dachshunds, Beagles, Cocker Spaniels, and Labrador Retrievers are genetically predisposed to obesity. Likewise, particular breeds appear to be resistant to obesity, such as the Sighthound group [2]. Aging is associated with

Canine and Feline Anesthesia and Co-Existing Disease, Second Edition. Edited by Rebecca A. Johnson, Lindsey B. C. Snyder and Carrie A. Schroeder.

Companion website: www.wiley.com/go/johnson/canine

an increase in the likelihood of obesity. With aging, the lean body mass decreases, resulting in a decrease in the total daily energy needs of the animal. In conjunction with a decrease in total daily energy needs, the animal's voluntary activity is typically decreased, possibly because of comorbidities of aging, such as osteoarthritis. The decrease in total daily energy needs combined with a decrease in activity can lead to weight gain if caloric intake is not decreased as well [2].

Excessive weight can have a major impact on the overall health of the animal. In humans, morbid obesity (BMI of ≥40–44.9 $kg\,m^{-2}$) is associated with an increased likelihood of diabetes mellitus [11], respiratory failure, hypertension, left ventricular hypertrophy, atherosclerosis, myocardial ischemia, and some forms of cancer compared to nonobese patients [4]. Mild to moderate hypertension is described in up to 60% of obese human patients, whereas 5–10% of obese human patients have severe hypertension. With time, hypertension can lead to left ventricular dilation, increased left ventricular wall stress, compensatory left ventricular hypertrophy, and left ventricular diastolic dysfunction [4]. Overweight animals are expected to have a shorter life span and increased incidence of osteoarthritis, diabetes mellitus, cardiovascular disease, pancreatitis, mammary tumors, and renal disease [5, 8]. Studies suggest that 31% of diabetes mellitus and 34% of lameness could be abolished if overweight and obese cats were at an ideal body weight [5].

An increase in body adipose tissue alters cardiopulmonary physiology, leading to an increase in cardiac output (CO), oxygen consumption, and closing capacity, and a decrease in functional residual capacity (FRC). In humans, these alterations can cause the associated pathologies of hypertension, coronary artery disease [1], and obstructive sleep apnea [11]. With morbid obesity in humans, the excessive body tissue decreases the FRC, expiratory reserve volume, and total lung capacity. The FRC decreases exponentially with increasing BMI in humans. When the FRC decreases to the range of the closing capacity, small airway closure takes place, leading to ventilation–perfusion mismatch, right to left shunting, and arterial hypoxemia [3]. Finally, with increasing body weight, there is an increase in blood volume proportional to the body surface area (BSA). This increase in blood volume contributes to an increase in preload and an increase in resting CO. Ultimately, increased left heart diastolic filling and left ventricular hypertrophy can occur (Table 10.1) [1].

Obesity results in restrictive lung disease due to the presence of excessive visceral fat, adding pressure to abdominal organs and increasing the inhalational efforts of the animal. Ventilation is subsequently limited by the adipose tissue and breathing is easily compromised by placing the animal in a recumbent position. Dorsal recumbency is the worst position, as it puts the largest portion of the lung in a dependent position [8]. Ventilation should be supported in all obese patients. This can be accomplished with manual ventilation or with a mechanical ventilator. Monitoring of the patient's arterial CO_2 and O_2 levels is used to determine the rate and volume of ventilation needed by the animal.

Adipose tissue is a major source of inflammatory mediators, and obesity is, therefore, linked to chronic low-grade inflammation [12].

Table 10.1 Physiologic changes associated with obesity.

Hypertension
Left ventricular hypertrophy
Restrictive pulmonary disease
Increased intraabdominal pressure
Decreased chest wall compliance
Decreased lung volumes
Exercise intolerance
Increased atelectasis
Increased ventilation/perfusion mismatching
Increased volume of distribution
Musculoskeletal conditions
Increased blood volume

Research suggests a mechanism for the link between excess body weight and many diseases. Adipose tissue, once thought to be physiologically inert, is an active producer of hormones such as leptin and resistin, and numerous cytokines [5]. The chronic inflammation observed in obese humans is thought to be one of the significant links between obesity and cardiovascular disease [12]. Additional physiologic alterations associated with obesity include increases in tubular reabsorption, which initiates volume expansion of the extracellular volume. In humans, the total extracellular volume is increased; however, the circulating blood volume on a volume/weight basis is decreased [4]. Finally, splanchnic blood flow is approximately 20% higher in obese as compared to lean individuals. Cerebral and renal blood flows are near normal in the face of obesity [4].

Anesthetic Management of the Obese Patient

Induction

Anesthetic induction is a demanding period regardless of the patient's BMI. With an obese patient, morbidity causes induction to be even more delicate. With induction and intubation, obese humans have a proportionately greater decrease in cardiac index (CI) than lean individuals. CI decreases 17–33% in obese patients compared to 4–11% in controls. This decrease in CI continues postoperatively in obese individuals, whereas it returns to baseline in nonobese control patients [1, 13].

The physiologic changes induced by obesity, such as the decrease in CI, can significantly affect the distribution, binding, and elimination of anesthetic drugs. The alterations in pharmacokinetics can lead to severe adverse events if dosing is based solely on the actual body weight [4]. However, systemic absorption of oral drugs does not seem to be significantly affected by obesity, although some studies report a delay in gastric emptying in the overweight patient [4].

When evaluating the alterations of pharmacokinetics on the drug propofol, obese children require significantly less propofol for loss of lash reflex than do lean children; obese children are given a lower dose of propofol on the basis of actual body weight than their nonobese peers [14]. Clearance of propofol appears to be linearly related to lean body weight rather than to total body weight [6]. It is recommended that the dose of propofol for both induction and maintenance of anesthesia should be based on actual body weight in obese individuals analogous to their lean counterparts [4]. In obese humans, both the volume of distribution and the clearance of propofol were significantly correlated to total body water. Therefore, there is a concurrent increase in the volume of distribution, as well as clearance, with the elimination half-life being similar in obese and lean patients. There were no signs of propofol accumulation or prolonged duration of action when propofol was administered on actual body weight in obese humans [4].

In veterinary patients, overweight dogs were found to need a lower intravenous propofol dose per kilogram of total body weight for endotracheal intubation compared to normal body conditions dogs. This suggests that a dosing on lean body weight might be more beneficial in overweight dogs [15]. However, when obese dogs are dosed for propofol based on a lean body weight adjustment, the dose of propofol administered was higher than for ideal body condition score dogs. The differences in doses may conclude that fat interferes in the pharmacokinetics and pharmacodynamics of propofol and raises the question of whether it should be excluded or not when calculating the propofol dosage in induction of anesthesia in obese dogs (Table 10.2) [16].

Thiopental, however, has a significantly longer elimination half-life when administered on actual body weight in obese individuals owing to the increased volume of distribution. The dose of thiopental for

Table 10.2 Drug dosing in the obese patient.

Propofol	Actual or lean body weight
Thiopental	Lean body weight
Midazolam	Actual body weight
Diazepam	Actual body weight
Opioids	Dependent on lipophilic nature of drug
Highly lipophilic	Lean body weight
Minimally lipophilic	Actual body weight

induction of anesthesia of obese patients can be based on lean body mass to avoid prolongation of effects [4].

Whether used for sedation or part of an induction protocol, the dose of benzodiazepine should be adjusted in the overweight patient. Benzodiazepines are highly lipophilic drugs and are highly affected by excess adipose tissue. With obesity comes a significant increase in volume of distribution and elimination half-life of benzodiazepines. Regardless of the benzodiazepine being used, the dose should be increased in obese patients in proportion to the total body weight owing to increases in volume of distribution and distribution in the excess fat [4].

Despite the growing obese population, clinical studies have, thus far, unsuccessfully defined a universal size descriptor suitable for use in the obese population. For this reason, titration to clinical end points or the use of the bispectral index remains prudent [17]. Because induction agent doses are typically titrated to clinical effect, some may argue that new dosing recommendations are unnecessary for the human or veterinary populations [6].

Maintenance

Concern with anesthetizing an obese patient focuses on the physiologic alterations associated with excess adipose tissue as opposed to alterations in pharmacodynamics. Obesity is linked with restrictive pulmonary disease caused by increased intraabdominal pressure and decreased chest wall compliance due to the increased weight of the chest wall [4, 18], resulting in a decrease in static and dynamic lung volumes, expiratory reserve volume, and total lung capacity [19]. In addition, the mass effect of intraabdominal adipose tissue contributes to the decrease in respiratory compliance [1]. These changes are further affected by anesthesia and surgical procedures [4]. Changes in ventilation such as a reduction in the FRC, expiratory reserve volume, and total lung capacity are frequent observations of the clinically obese [20]. The FRC exponentially decreases with increasing total body weight [1]. Under anesthesia, lean people have a decrease in FRC by 20%, whereas obese people have a 50% decrease in FRC [1]. The low FRC and expiratory reserve volume contribute to rapid desaturation with apnea (as is often seen on anesthetic induction) or hypoventilation and air trapping with poor lung function [19]. The reduced FRC causes portions of the lung to have premature airway closure and atelectasis, resulting in ventilation–perfusion mismatch [1].

Anesthesia further complicates the respiratory pathophysiology observed in obese individuals. The reduced lung volumes and increased ventilation–perfusion mismatching significantly increase the likelihood of hypoxemia during and after anesthesia [4]. During inhalant anesthesia, morbidly obese human patients experience more atelectasis than lean patients. In addition, the atelectasis can remain for up to 24 h after the end of anesthesia [17], where complete resolution occurs more immediately in nonobese patients [18]. The application of 10 cm H_2O of positive end-expiratory pressure (PEEP) increases oxygenation in obese human patients and is associated with better oxygenation and a longer duration of apnea before hypoxia develops [1]. This effect is related to recruitment of alveoli [17]. However, the improvement of arterial oxygenation by the addition of PEEP does so at the expense of CO and oxygen delivery [4].

Barotrauma during ventilation is not uncommon in obese individuals [19, 21]. It is postulated that perhaps clinicians overestimate the lung size of obese patients and choose tidal volume based on actual body weight rather than lean body weight [21]. The mode of ventilation is highly important in obese patients. In comparing pressure-controlled ventilation to volume-controlled ventilation, in obese human patients (BMI>35) undergoing laparoscopic gastric banding, pressure-controlled ventilation was associated with an increase in pH, PaO_2, and oxygen saturation, while $PaCO_2$ was decreased. Because there is higher inspiratory flow with pressure-controlled ventilation, increases in alveolar recruitment may lead to a decrease in ventilation–perfusion mismatching [19].

Epidural anesthesia is a common adjunct to inhalant anesthesia for general anesthesia maintenance. Epidural anesthesia is more difficult in the obese patient for multiple reasons. Most obvious, the landmarks are more difficult to find in obese patients, making epidurals more technically difficult [4]. In obese patients, fatty infiltration of the epidural space, in addition to an increase in blood volume secondary to increased intraabdominal pressure, may reduce the volume of the space, making epidurals more difficult to perform and spread of the drug less predictable [4]. Since the epidural space is reduced in obese animals, the volume of epidural drug administered will not increase as the animals become overweight. As a rule, epidural drugs should be dosed on the lean animal's weight. Despite the downsides, epidurals are extremely useful to reduce the respiratory depression and secondary complications from the respiratory depression caused by other systemic drugs [4]. Ultrasound guidance of epidural injection has been used in obese dogs. Ultrasound imaging identified the point of needle insertion for lumbosacral injection in seven obese Labrador Retrievers. Epidural injection was successfully achieved in obese dogs with the assistance of ultrasound imaging mitigating the difficulties experienced with overweight patients [22].

The highly lipophilic drug sufentanil has been found to have a markedly prolonged elimination half-life in obese people. The increase is relative to that in the volume of distribution and possible accumulation of drug in excess fatty tissue [4]. Dosing of highly lipophilic drugs should be altered in obese patients. Conversely, the administration of the hydrophilic drug atracurium has no difference in recovery times between obese and nonobese individuals. The lower lipid solubility of desflurane and sevoflurane makes them the volatile anesthetics of choice in obese individuals [4].

Administration route depends on how the specific agent is dosed and depends on the pharmacologic mechanism of action. For example, receptor-bound drugs obviously work at specific receptors on the cell membrane. For the most part, receptor numbers are not specifically associated with the animal's weight and the dose does not necessarily need to be increased [8].

Monitoring the overweight animal can be more challenging, since normal physiologic parameters seen in ideal-weight patients are frequently altered. For example, the normal heart rate of the obese animal may be higher due to the increased cardiac work [8]. Ventilation will often be faster, but shallower than for the lean animal due to reduced tidal volume associated with excessive weight; end-tidal or arterial CO_2 analysis are excellent methods of assessing the adequacy of ventilation in all patients but are especially imperative in obese patients. Blood pressure should be similar to animals of normal weight, but caution should be taken to ensure that all parts of the animal are well-perfused, since some areas may experience additional pressure due to excess fat. Checking pulses in each leg and the tongue aids in the assessment of blood flow to all areas.

Postoperative Care

In the postoperative period, the depressant effects of analgesic and anesthetic drugs on the respiratory system can negatively impact patient safety. The work of breathing is greatly increased postoperatively because of the increase in body mass required to move while breathing [4]. The risk of postoperative hypoxia is high in obese patients [4]. Furthermore, oxygen demand increases by up to 50% in the immediate postoperative time, requiring a significant increase in both CO and oxygen delivery to tissues. The CO needs to increase to meet the increased oxygen demand even in the face of a decreased FRC. If CO is unable to cope, the patient is much more likely to develop postoperative complications [1]. Recovery times have been found to be comparable in obese and lean humans after anesthetic procedures lasting from 2–4 h. Although there is a delay in recovery due to fat accumulation of lipid-soluble drugs, the reduced blood flow to adipose reduces the tissue uptake of these drugs [4]. Therefore, the blood gas solubility, rather than fat solubility, may be the leading force influencing time to recovery in morbidly obese patients [11].

In obese patients, there is a higher rate of postoperative infection and delayed wound healing because of obesity on the immune system. Obesity impairs cell-mediated immune responses and decreases lymphocyte immune function and the natural killer cell activity [3].

Anesthetic recovery for the overweight animal is one of the critical aspects of anesthetic management. Make sure the animal is well-padded and is positioned to prevent pressure points on the nerves and muscles. Positioning the patient to facilitate ventilation is also important. Remember that the overweight animal may not have normal respiratory muscle strength and may need more assistance in regaining sternal recumbency as well as normal ventilatory efforts. Drug elimination and metabolism, as well as any respiratory depressant effects, will likely be prolonged in the overweight animal, so timely discontinuation of the gas anesthetics should be performed.

Additional Concerns

In addition, drug injection site and needle length should be chosen to ensure that the drugs are injected into muscle rather than fat. Injections into fat will be absorbed more slowly than drugs administered intramuscularly. The slower onset can also result in longer duration of effect than is expected in the lean animal. In addition, the chosen muscle may also affect the speed and depth of sedation achieved [23].

The overweight animal also has more difficulty dissipating body heat, resulting in hyperthermia; monitoring of body temperature is critical to prevent overheating. However, hypothermia can also be a problem and rewarming of the animal can be difficult [8]. Some breeds are classically associated with obesity. Bulldogs, Pugs, and Boston Terriers have frequently been associated with brachycephalic airway [24] which can worsen with excessive weight. Extra care should be taken to assure a patent airway is maintained in these animals.

Additional Nutritional Concerns

Boutique Diets (Grain-Free Diets, Novel Protein Diets, All-Meat Diet)

Grain-free diets have become a popular trend among pet owners in the past several years. In July 2018, the United States Food and Drug Administration (FDA) released a statement on its investigation of a possible link between diet and dilated cardiomyopathy (DCM). The FDA reported on cases of DCM in dogs eating pet foods containing a high percentage of peas, lentils, other pulses (beans, lentils, chickpeas), or potatoes, many of which were labeled grain-free. None of the reported cases of DCM in dogs being fed a grain-free diet had any genetic predisposition to DCM [25]. Historically, low-protein diets designed for the management of urate stones have been associated with DCM. This is postulated to be due to low-protein diets being low in essential and nonessential amino acids or vital precursors for carnitine and taurine synthesis. Supplementing these diets with taurine and L-carnitine reversed the DCM in these patients [26]. The possible association between grain-free or legume-based diets and the development of DCM has led some veterinary cardiologists to recommend pet owners switch their dogs to grain-based diets without exotic protein sources and avoiding boutique brands. However, others state that there is insufficient evidence-based research on whether there is a definitive link between grain-free diets and DCM [26]. Interestingly, evidence has shown that in 23 of 24 dogs diagnosed with taurine deficiency and DCM were fed diets that were either grain-free, legume-rich, or a combination of these, and 23 of 24 dogs had significant improvement in their echocardiographic parameters, including resolution of congestive heart failure and normalization of taurine concentrations following diet change and taurine supplementation [27]. Dogs with a history of a grain-free diet, or other boutique diet, should be evaluated for DCM prior to anesthesia. Specific recommendations for anesthetizing a patient with DCM can be found in Chapter 1.

Although varied from the grain-free diet, the bones and raw food (BARF) diet has potential concerns as well, such as the zoonotic potential of bacterial transmission to humans. The BARF diet, consisting of high amounts of animal components such as meat, offal, and raw meaty bones combined with small amounts of plant components such as vegetables and fruits, contributes to changes in the fecal microbiome compared to dogs on a commercial diet. Fecal samples of dogs fed the BARF diet had higher concentrations of *Clostridium*, *Enterobacteriaceae*, and *Fusobacterium* [28]. These findings do not have a known direct impact on anesthesia at this time but play an important part in malnutrition of the patient and zoonotic disease transmission to humans [28, 29]. The use of a meat-based diet has been linked to surgical-site infection. The presence of *Salmonella* spp. in the surgical site of a dog following dorsal laminectomy at the L7-S1 intervertebral disc space and in the dog's diet is concerning for the dog and for public health [30]. Strict vigilance to avoid cross-contamination of disease-causing organisms on anesthetic equipment and monitors is necessary when anesthetizing patients eating an all-meat diet.

Ideal Body Weight

As stated previously, the criteria for obesity are not as clear-cut in veterinary patients as with human patients, as optimal body weights have not been established for our species and varying breeds. However, it is still concluded that when a patient's weight is 15% above normal for its breed, it is "overweight," and when a patient's weight is 30% above normal, it is "obese" [2]. Therefore, an ideal body weight can be hard to determine for a particular patient. The patient's breed and age play into this determination. Aging is associated with an increase in the likelihood of obesity. With aging, the lean body mass decreases, resulting in a decrease in the total daily energy needs of the animal [2]. The method most associated with determining an ideal body weight for a patient is the use of a body condition score.

BCS is a common, validated method to assess body composition in companion animals based on a 9-point scale. Dogs and cats that score an 8–9/9 are considered obese. There is a direct relationship between the BCS and body fat percentage (BF%). Each unit increase in the BCS is equivalent to a 5% increase in BF%. A patient with an ideal score of 5/9 has a BF% of 20–25%. Therefore, obese patients with a BCS of 8/9 have a BF% more than 35%. BCS tools can be found at http://www.wsava.org/nutrition-toolkit. Additionally, with each increase in the BCS over 5/9, there is a 10% increase in the ideal weight [10]. Therefore, a patient with a BCS of 7/9 would be considered 20% overweight. This information can be used to calculate an ideal weight for patients when adjustments to anesthetic drugs are necessary in the face of obesity.

An alternative to using the ideal body weight versus total body weight confusion is to calculate drug dosages based on the BSA. These calculations can be more accurate and provide a better method for accurate dosing (Table 10.3).

Table 10.3 Sample body weight–body surface area conversions.

Dogs		Cats	
Body weight (kg)	BSA (m^2)	Body weight (kg)	BSA (m^2)
1.0	0.101	0.5	0.063
5.0	0.295	1.0	0.100
10.0	0.469	2.0	0.159
15.0	0.614	3.0	0.208
20.0	0.744	4.0	0.252
25.0	0.864	5.0	0.292
30.0	0.975	6.0	0.330
35.0	1.081	7.0	0.366
40.0	1.181	8.0	0.400
45.0	1.371	9.0	0.433
50.0	1.371	10.0	0.464
55.0	1.461		

Body surface area (BSA) in square meters = K × body weight in grams$^{2/3} \times 10^{-4}$.
K = constant (10.1 for dogs, 10.0 for cats).

Cachexia

In addition to obesity, cachexia is another significant nutritional concern that can impact anesthesia. Information on anesthetizing a cachexic patient can be found in Chapter 17.

References

1 Donohoe, C.L., Feeney, C., and Carey, M.F. (2011). Perioperative evaluation of the obese patient. *J. Clin. Anesth.* 23: 575–586.

2 Byers, C.G., Wilson, C.C., Stephens, M.B. et al. (2011). Exploring the causes and consequences of canine obesity. *Vet. Med.* 1: 1–7.

3 Cheah, M.H. and Kam, P.C.A. (2005). Obesity: basic science and medical aspects relevant to anesthetists. *Anaesthesia* 60: 1009–1021.

4 Casati, A. and Putzu, M. (2005). Anesthesia in the obese patient: pharmacokinetic considerations. *J. Clin. Anesth.* 17: 134–135.

5 Laflamme, D.P. (2006). Understanding and managing obesity in dogs and cats. *Vet. Clin. North Am. Small Anim. Pract.* 36: 1283–1295.

6 Green, B. and McLeay, S. (2011). Anesthetizing the obese. *Anesth. Analg.* 113: 1–3.

7 de Godoy, M.R. and Swanson, K.S. (2013). Nutrigenomics: using gene expression and molecular biology data to understand pet obesity. *J. Anim. Sci.* 91: 2949–2964.

8 German, A.J. (2006). The growing problem of obesity in dogs and cats. *J. Nutr.* 136: 1940S–1946S.

9 Gossellin, J., Wren, J.A., and Sunderland, S.J. (2007). Canine obesity – an overview. *J. Vet. Pharmacol. Therap.* 30: 1–10.

10 Love, L. and Cline, M.G. (2015). Perioperative physiology and pharmacology in the obese small animal patient. *Vet. Anaesth. Analg.* 42: 119–132.

11 Arain, S.R., Barth, C.D., Shankar, H. et al. (2005). Choice of volatile anesthetic for the morbidly obese patient: sevoflurane or desflurane. *J. Clin. Anesth.* 17: 413–419.

12 Chung, M.Y., Hong, S.J., and Lee, J.Y. (2011). The influence of obesity on postoperative

inflammatory cytokine levels. *J. Int. Med. Res.* 39: 2370–2378.

13 Agarwal, N., Shibutani, K., SanFilippo, J.A. et al. (1982). Hemodynamic and respiratory changes in surgery of the morbidly obese. *Surgery* 92: 226–234.

14 Olutoye, O.A., Yu, X., Govindan, K. et al. (2012). The effect of obesity on the ED_{50} of propofol for loss of consciousness in children and adolescents. *Anesth. Analg.* 115: 147–153.

15 Boveri, S., Brearley, J.C., and Dugdale, A.H.A. (2013). The effect of body condition on Propofol requirement in dogs. *Vet. Anaesth. Analg.* 40: 449–454.

16 Devito, F.C., Patricia, G.C.F., Flor, P.B. et al. (2020). Comparative study of anaesthesia induction in obese dogs using propofol dosages based on lean body weight or total body weight. *Vet. Animal Sci.* 10: 100131.

17 Corrie, K.R., Chillstone, S., and Hardman, J.G. (2011). The effect of obesity and anesthetic maintenance regimen on postoperative pulmonary complications. *Anesth. Analg.* 113: 4–6.

18 Eichenberger, A.S., Proietti, S., Wicky, S. et al. (2002). Morbid obesity and postoperative pulmonary 14 atelectasis: an underestimated problem. *Anesth. Analg.* 95: 1788–1792.

19 Pedoto, A. (2012). Lung physiology and obesity: anesthetic implications for thoracic procedures. *Anesthesiol. Res. Pract.* 2012: 1–7.

20 Cortinez, L.I., Gambus, P., Troconiz, I.F. et al. (2011). Obesity does not influence the onset and offset of sevoflurane effect as measured by the hysteresis between sevoflurane concentration and bispectral index. *Anesth. Analg.* 113: 70–76.

21 Jaber, S., Coisel, Y., Chanques, G. et al. (2012). A multicentre observational study of intra-operative ventilator management during general anaesthesia: tidal volumes and relation to body weight. *Anaesthesia* 67: 999–1008.

22 da Silva, L.C.B.A., Pacheco, P.F., Sellera, F.P. et al. (2020). The use of ultrasound to assist epidural injection in obese dogs. *Vet. Anaesth. Analg.* 47: 137–140.

23 Carter, J.E., Lewis, C., and Beths, T. (2013). Onset and quality of sedation after intramuscular administration of dexmedetomidine and hydromophone in various muscle groups in dogs. *J. Am. Vet. Med. Assoc.* 243: 1569–1572.

24 Lodato, D.L. and Hedlund, C.S. (2012). Brachycephalic airway syndrome: management. *Compend. Contin. Educ. Vet.* 34: E1–E6.

25 Freid, K.J., Freeman, L.M., Rush, J.E. et al. (2021). Retrospective study of dilated cardiomyopathy in dogs. *J. Vet. Intern. Med.* 35: 58–67.

26 McCauley, S.R., Clark, S.D., Quest, B.W. et al. (2020). Review of canine dilated cardiomyopathy in the wake of diet-associated concerns. *J. Anim. Sci.* 98: 1–20.

27 Kaplan, J.L., Stern, J.A., Fascetti, A.J. et al. (2018). Taurine deficiency and dilated cardiomyopathy in golden retrievers fed commercial diets. *PLoS One* 13 (12): 1–19.

28 Schmidt, M., Unterer, S., Suchodolski, J.S. et al. (2018). The fecal microbiome and metabolome differs between dogs fed bones and raw food (BARF) diets and dogs fed commercial diets. *PLoS One* 13 (8): 1–20.

29 Davies, R.H., Lawes, J.R., and Wales, A.D. (2019). Raw diets for dogs and cats: a review, with particular reference to microbiological hazards. *J. Sm. Anim. Pract.* 60: 329–339.

30 Kent, M., Boozer, L., Glass, E.N. et al. (2017). Post-operative salmonella surgical site infection in a dog. *Can. Vet. J.* 58: 936–940.

11

Genetic Disease

Tania Perez Jimenez

Veterinary Clinical Sciences, College of Veterinary Medicine, Program in Individualized Medicine (PrlMe), Washington State University, Pullman, WA, 99164, USA

Introduction

Genetic factors have been described to affect an individual's response to anesthetic drugs in humans for more than 50 years [1]. Some of these responses have been attributed to either gender, comorbidities, size, previous drug use, drug interactions, or the characteristics of the procedure being performed [2]. Findings associated with the recent advancements in genome sequencing and genetic mapping have revealed that genetic differences and interindividual variability play an important part in drug response. This has brought us to the era of individualized medicine, which has opened the door to a rapid and vast knowledge base regarding congenital malformations, inherited diseases, and the genetic implication of treatment, either drug- or nondrug-related. Genetic inheritance is a very important component of anesthesia practice. Providing this primer on pharmacogenetics and clinical genetics will provide us with the tools and basic knowledge necessary to understand the implications of genetics on anesthesia practice.

Pharmacogenetics

The basic definition of pharmacogenetics encompasses the individual's response to a medication based on their genetic makeup. The main principle of pharmacogenetics is based on the identification of these genetic variants (polymorphisms) that affect the individual's response to medications and drugs, a significant number of which are used in anesthesia practice. Some of the drugs that have been described are codeine, tramadol, inhalant anesthetics, local anesthetics, and muscle relaxants, among others [3]. The altered response to these drugs can be due in part to issues with the drug interacting with its target (effect) and drug disposition (metabolizing enzymes, transporters, and receptors) [4]. Pharmacogenetics has the possibility to make drug therapy individualized, to decrease or completely avoid the occurrence of adverse drug reactions (ADRs) and toxicity, and to improve drug efficacy by tailoring the treatment to the patient's genotype [5]. In veterinary medicine, significant discoveries have been made due to observations by practicing clinicians worldwide, and some others will be made in part with the development of the canine genome [6].

Canine and Feline Anesthesia and Co-Existing Disease, Second Edition. Edited by Rebecca A. Johnson, Lindsey B. C. Snyder and Carrie A. Schroeder.

Companion website: www.wiley.com/go/johnson/canine

We have determined the existence of breed-related differences in drug response in companion and production animals. Some examples in small animals are propofol and thiopental use in Greyhounds, acepromazine in boxers, and drug effects in herding breeds [7]. These few examples bring another relationship, which is not just drug metabolism and disposition, but, more specifically, the difference in breeds and the incidence of specific diseases that also become a challenge for the anesthetist.

Genetically Related Diseases

Breed-Related Differences

The wide variety of breeds and the genetic variation within them can affect drug pharmacokinetics and pharmacodynamics. There can be an inconsistency in dosages and response across multiple breeds. The impact of this in pharmacokinetic and pharmacodynamic studies can be significant, since the results obtained in one breed can be inapplicable in another and have inconsistent effects. The consequences can be important in new drug development when trying to identify a dosage of a medication in veterinary practice. It is important to remember that some of these differences can be metabolic and physiologic [8].

Drug Metabolism and Disposition

Enzymes responsible for the metabolism and disposition of many drugs, xenobiotics, and other compounds are the cytochrome P450 enzymes. In humans, some members of this group are polymorphic, with some significant differences found according to race/ethnic population [9]. One of these enzymes, which is responsible for metabolizing many medications, is the CYP2D6 in humans, with its canine ortholog (equivalent) CYP2D15. CYP2D15 has been investigated in the dog, and five polymorphisms have been described [10]; the impact of these on drug metabolism has not been fully elucidated. There are only a few studies that look into drugs metabolized by CYP2D15 in small animals. One describes the pharmacokinetics of celecoxib in a population of laboratory Beagles [11], where two phenotypes could be differentiated by their elimination capacity (the extensive metabolizer [EM] and the poor metabolizer [PM] phenotypes). This showed a predominant role of CYP2D15 and variants in celecoxib metabolism, with slightly over 50% of the 242 dogs in the study being in the PM group, which will ultimately impact drug effect and help guide additional or alternative therapy for nonsteroidal anti-inflammatory drugs (NSAID)-related analgesia. Related to the possibility of this variability causing alterations on other drugs, work with tramadol has shown that the active metabolite, O-desmethyltramadol (M1), is formed exclusively by CYP2D15 in the dog [12]. It is possible then that CYP2D15 polymorphisms could potentially affect the analgesic properties of tramadol, with less analgesia in the population with the PM phenotype. The effect of these variants on other drugs metabolized by the same enzyme is unknown at the moment in veterinary medicine.

One clear example where a polymorphism that affects metabolism has been described in detail is that found in CYP2B11, the enzyme responsible for hydroxylating propofol in dogs, among other drugs. Remarkably, there is a decrease in the clearance and a lower liver metabolism of propofol overall in Greyhounds [13], and when Greyhounds are compared to mixed-breed dogs [14, 15] and Beagles [15]. The metabolism of other anesthetic drugs is also affected in Greyhounds, such as the thiobarbiturates (thiopental) [16]. This decrease in clearance and lower liver metabolism ultimately cause delayed and prolonged recoveries. This enzyme polymorphism might not only affect Greyhounds, but has been extrapolated to other members of the Sighthound family (Irish Wolfhound, Afghan

Hound, borzoi, saluki, etc.). Another anesthetic drug that has also shown prolonged recoveries in Greyhounds is alfaxalone [17]. Following premedication with morphine and acepromazine, Greyhounds induced with alfaxalone had a duration of anesthesia up to five times longer than dogs not premedicated, with a prolonged elimination half-life, even though the clearance is still small. However, this difference may be due in part to the transient decrease in blood pressure and hepatic blood flow caused by the acepromazine/morphine combination and not solely genetic differences in this breed.

Anesthetic Recommendations

In addition to abnormalities in drug disposition as described, Sighthounds tend to present with high hematocrits (>50%) and low serum proteins (mostly low albumin), which can affect drug binding and free fractions of drugs, increasing the active portion [18]. Furthermore, their lean bodies (low amount of fat) can affect drug redistribution (lipophilic drugs will have a lower volume of distribution) [8] and thermoregulation [18]. When anesthetizing a Greyhound or any member of the Sighthound family, attention should be paid not just to the drug administered, but also to the dosage used. For anesthetic induction, anesthetic agents should be administered to effect to titrate the minimum amount of drug necessary. To this end, premedications should be encouraged to avoid stress and decrease the required amount of induction agent. When deciding which premedication agents to use, preference should be given to drugs that can be reversed in the event of a prolonged recovery, such as alpha-2-adrenergic receptor agonists, opioids, and benzodiazepines.

Transporters

One of the most clinically important drug (efflux) transporters (pumps) is the P-glycoprotein (P-gp). They belong to the family of adenosine triphosphate (ATP)-binding cassette (ABC) transporters. Polymorphisms on this transporter, specifically ABCB1, are well-studied in veterinary medicine. They are expressed on cell membranes in many tissues (brain, intestine, kidney, and liver), and the main function is to limit systemic and organ uptake of drug and contribute to their excretion [19]. There is a genetic mutation that encodes for this protein, the MDR1 gene in dogs [20] and cats [21]; the mutation is referred as ABCB1-1Δ. There are three phenotypes described in dogs: homozygous (mutant), intermediate (heterozygous), and the wild type. Dogs affected by this mutation include a variety of breeds classified under the herding breed category (Collies, Border Collies, Australian, English, and German Shepherds, Old English and Shetland Sheepdogs, etc.), with more than 75% of Collies and 50% of Australian and English Shepherds carrying at least one mutant allele [22]. The ABCB1-1Δ has been identified in some Sighthounds (Longhaired Whippet) with a somewhat high frequency (30–50%) and in some mixed-breed dogs with a lower frequency (≤1%). In cats, approximately 4% carry the polymorphism. Particularly important is the loss of function of the P-gp on the brain since this protein is a component of the blood–brain barrier. It is then expected that drug penetration is increased, and these animals would be sensitive to the neurological toxicity caused by some of the substrates. Anesthetic drugs that are substrates of this transporter are acepromazine, butorphanol, loperamide, vecuronium [23, 24], verapamil, diltiazem, morphine, and fentanyl [25]. Additionally, some drugs may act as inhibitors of the P-gp efflux activity, such as the antimicrobial agents erythromycin and ketoconazole, the antidepressants fluoxetine and paroxetine, the opioids methadone and pentazocine, and the cardiac drugs verapamil, amiodarone, carvedilol, quinidine, and nicardipine [25].

Anesthetic Recommendations

Caution is warranted when administering some of the drugs mentioned previously to patients that have been diagnosed or are suspected of having the mutant allele (Collies). Doses should be carefully chosen (likely decreased) and close monitoring should be performed for any untoward signs. For example, with acepromazine, sedation is increased and prolonged when administered at dose of $0.04\,mg\,kg^{-1}$ IV [26]. Other drugs commonly administered with acepromazine, such as the opioids morphine, butorphanol, fentanyl, and methadone (known P-gp substrates), may also affect the degree of sedation. Particular attention should be paid to the coadministration of substrates of P-gp and inhibitors (Table 11.1). Careful consideration when selecting antimicrobials, opioids, and cardiac drugs is warranted.

Malignant Hyperthermia

Malignant hyperthermia (MH) is a rare pharmacogenetic disorder in dogs. Onset is due to exposure to a triggering agent such as depolarizing neuromuscular blockers (NMBs; succinylcholine) or inhalant anesthetics (halothane, isoflurane, sevoflurane). Clinical signs associated with this syndrome include hypercapnia, which is the most prominent clinical sign in dogs, muscle rigidity, increased body temperature (which lags behind the hypercapnia), hyperkalemia, metabolic acidosis, tachycardia, rhabdomyolysis, and disseminated intravascular coagulation [27, 28]. Death will rapidly ensue if signs are not detected early, and treatment is started. No specific breed has been associated with this disorder; reports in the literature include Pointer, Greyhound, Labrador Retriever, Saint Bernard, and Springer Spaniel breeds [29].

This syndrome can be explained by a mutation in the gene that encodes for the ryanodine receptor (RyR1), which is a skeletal muscle calcium release channel (Figure 11.1). It is transmitted in dogs as an autosomal-dominant trait [30]; therefore, only one copy of the mutation is needed to produce offspring with MH. There could also be other genes involved and associated with the RyR1 receptor, such as CACNA1S, the α-subunit of the L-type voltage-gated dihydropyridine (DHP) receptor [31]. The result is an increase in sensitivity of the channel to open, triggered by anesthetic medications. About 10 cases have been reported through the years in the literature, 4 of which were Greyhounds; this suggests a possible breed predisposition.

The diagnosis of MH is usually based on clinical signs without a specific diagnostic test (contracture testing muscle biopsies or gene sequencing). Often it occurs in healthy animals that present for anesthesia and have no history of anesthesia-related complications. One of the first indications seen by the anesthetist is the marked increase in end-tidal ($ETCO_2$) or arterial carbon dioxide levels without an alternative explanation [29]. Genetic sequencing is available for dogs that looks for and verifies the presence of the dominant MH mutation through a buccal swab, blood, or dewclaw sample. It can be tested on any breed [32].

This syndrome as such has not been diagnosed in cats. There are three reports in the literature that describe very similar clinical findings to the dog: changes in heart rate, arrhythmias, and increases in body temperature and limb rigidity. All three cats died during cardiopulmonary resuscitation (CPR) attempts. MH was presumed but not confirmed [33].

Anesthetic Recommendations

If there is no familial or any other history of an anesthetic adverse event, it is difficult to say with any degree of certainty which animals can develop MH. Early recognition of symptoms and avoidance of the possible causative agent should prevent most episodes of MH. An anesthetic protocol free of triggering agents (succinylcholine and volatile anesthetics) should be chosen.

A safe protocol could include benzodiazepines (diazepam, midazolam), phenothiazines (acepromazine), alpha-2-adrenergic

Table 11.1 Selected P-glycoprotein substrates and inhibitors [25].

Substrates	Inhibitors
Anticancer drugs	**Antidepressants**
Doxorubicin	Fluoxetine
Docetaxel	St. John's wort
Vincristine	Paroxetine
Vinblastine	
Etoposide	**Antimicrobial agents**
Mitoxantrone	Erythromycin
Actinomycin D	Itraconazole
	Ketoconazole
Steroid hormones	
Aldosterone	**Opioids**
Cortisol	Methadone
Dexamethasone	Pentazocine
Methylprednisolone	
	Cardiac drugs
Antimicrobial agents	Verapamil
Erythromycin	Amiodarone
Ketoconazole	Carvedilol
Itraconazole	Quinidine
Tetracycline	Nicardipine
Doxycycline	Cardiac drugs
	Verapamil
Opioids	
Loperamide	**Immunosuppressants**
Morphine	Cyclosporine
	Tacrolimus
Cardiac drugs	
Digoxin	**Miscellaneous**
Diltiazem	Bromocriptine
Verapamil	Chlorpromazine
Talinolol	Tamoxifen
	Grapefruit juice
Immunosuppressants	
Cyclosporine	
Tacrolimus	
Miscellaneous	
Ivermectin	
Amitriptyline	
Terfenadine	
Ondansetron	
Domperidon	
Phenothiazines	
Vecuronium	

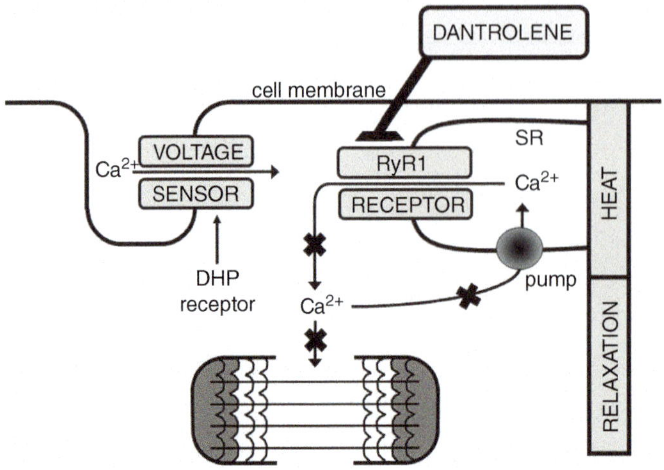

Figure 11.1 Dantrolene is an intracellular muscle relaxant that decreases excitation–contraction coupling by antagonizing the ryanodine (RyR1) receptor within the sarcoplasmic reticulum (SR). This results in an inhibition of the calcium release necessary for muscle contraction, thus causing relaxation. *Source:* Illustration courtesy of Caroline Baer.

receptor agonists (dexmedetomidine), etomidate, propofol, alfaxalone, opioids, dissociative agents (ketamine, Telazol), nitrous oxide, non-depolarizing NMBs (atracurium, cis-atracurium, vecuronium, rocuronium, etc.) and local anesthetics. Protocols with total intravenous anesthesia (TIVA) and or local/regional anesthesia techniques can be used successfully. The doses do not change from any other patient for any of the drugs mentioned in the preceding text.

Mechanical ventilation and oxygen administration free of traces of volatile anesthetic agents should be available when anesthetizing an animal either suspected or confirmed for MH. Anesthetic monitoring must include $ETCO_2$ measurement, since increases in CO_2 are one of the first signs encountered in a MH episode in dogs. Other measurements that should be monitored are heart rate, blood pressure, pulse oximetry, electrocardiography (ECG), and core body temperature.

Before treating for MH, a combination of signs should include at least three of the following to diagnose the syndrome: hypercapnia, elevation in body temperature, cardiac arrhythmias, acidosis, and muscle rigidity. The first step should be to stop any possible triggering agent (inhalants or depolarizing NMB); the anesthesia machine should be flushed with 100% oxygen to eliminate any residual inhalant in the circuit; IV fluid therapy should be started and blood should be drawn to run laboratory tests (blood gas, creatinine kinase, glucose, electrolytes, acid–base status, lactate). Since the most likely cause of death in these cases is hyperkalemia-induced cardiac arrhythmias, the animal should be ventilated with 100% oxygen to treat hypercapnia and accompanying respiratory acidosis, and a combination of insulin (0.25–0.5 U kg^{-1} regular insulin) together with 0.5 ml kg^{-1} of 50% dextrose will promote the movement of potassium into the cells. If dantrolene is going to be used (see in the following text), the administration of calcium channel blockers (verapamil, diltiazem) is contraindicated, since these medications can affect potassium concentrations and worsen the hyperkalemia [34]. If severe metabolic acidosis is present, $NaHCO_3$ may also be administered at 1–2 mEq kg^{-1}. Monitoring of $ETCO_2$, core body temperature, and blood gases should continue to assess the effectiveness of the therapy.

The administration of dantrolene, a postsynaptic muscle relaxant and intracellular calcium antagonist, is life-saving and specific for MH (Figure 11.1). It should be administered as soon as possible as a single dose (3 mg kg^{-1} IV); additional doses might be required (up to 10 mg kg^{-1}) to stop the hypermetabolic episode. Dantrolene comes in a vial as a lyophilized powder and needs to be reconstituted in 60 ml of sterile water. Dantrolene is highly irritating, so it is best to administer it as a fast IV infusion and through a large-bore IV catheter. Hypotension and hypovolemia can present in advanced MH episodes; an aggressive fluid therapy protocol should be initiated. Normal saline (0.9% NaCl), Plasma-Lyte, or 5% dextrose in water (D5W) are acceptable choices; try to avoid solutions with added calcium (lactated Ringer's solution). ECG and blood pressure should be monitored constantly. The placement of an arterial line not only helps to monitor blood pressure but also gives direct access to blood sampling. The use of lidocaine or procainamide (1–2 mg kg^{-1}) is warranted in the case of significant ventricular arrhythmias. If the rhythm persists, constant rate infusions are recommended.

Since rhabdomyolysis could also be present, a urinary catheter should be placed to measure urine output and kidney function, and to check for the presence of myoglobin. The use of osmotic or loop diuretics might be necessary to prevent kidney damage due to the accumulation of myoglobin or protein. Monitoring and ongoing care (fluid therapy, temperature control) should be continued for at least 24–48 h after the incident, to ensure there is no recurrence of symptoms.

Opioid Receptors

A single-nucleotide polymorphism (SNP) has been described in the canine mu-opioid receptor gene [35]. These SNPs seem to be specific to dogs and cannot be compared to the SNPs present in humans. A higher allelic prevalence (77%) in Alaskan Malamute, Siberian Husky, and Labrador Retriever breeds was found for one of the SNPs [35]. Effects seen in dogs with this mutation are more related to side effects such as dysphoria after the administration of a mu-opioid agonist. It has not been determined if this SNP has any other effect in opioid response under anesthesia.

Anticholinergic Response

Breed differences in the dose–response relationship to anticholinergics have also been reported. Even though anticholinergics are mainly used for the treatment of sinoatrial or incomplete atrioventricular block caused by increases in vagal tone due to medications, disease, or surgical stimulation, their effects are also significant in other organ systems.

Atropine and glycopyrrolate were tested on Beagles and Labrador Retrievers to evaluate the duration these drugs had on gastric motility [36]. In Beagles, low dosages of atropine (0.02 mg kg^{-1} IM) and glycopyrrolate (0.005 mg kg^{-1} IM) completely inhibited gastric motility for at least 30 min, while doubling the doses caused a complete cessation of motility for more than 3 h. In Labrador Retrievers, the effects of glycopyrrolate and atropine lasted over 6 and 3 h, respectively, regardless of the dose used. This alteration in motility could be worrisome in patients that already suffer from gastrointestinal (GI) disturbances where the presence of ileus can be detrimental to the recovery.

Brachycephalic Airway Obstruction Syndrome (BAOS)

Brachycephalic syndrome results from alterations that encompass morphological and functional characteristics that affect the upper and lower airways; other systems such as the GI tract may be involved. Some of the dog breeds most affected are Pugs, Boston Terriers, English and French Bulldogs, Pekingese, Shih Tzu, Cavalier King Charles Spaniels, Boxers, and Bullmastiffs, and cat breeds such as

Himalayan, Persian, and Scottish Fold, among others [37].

The most notable characteristic of this group is the presence of a shorter, wider skull, believed to be related to a discrete genetic mutation without a reduction in the size of the associated soft tissues. This results in an excess of tissues causing an increase in upper airway resistance [38]. Brachycephalic airway obstruction syndrome consists of anatomic defects and effects that develop secondary to prolonged respiratory abnormalities and increases in airway resistance.

Abnormalities associated with this syndrome also include stenotic nares, elongated soft palate, small nasal passages, everted saccules, laryngeal collapse, and tracheal hypoplasia. Other abnormalities have been described in specific breeds such as nasopharyngeal turbinates in Pugs and English Bulldogs and malformed nasal conchae in French and English Bulldogs [39]. Common secondary GI signs are frequent episodes of vomiting, regurgitation, and ptyalism [39], and, in some cases, hiatal hernia [40]. Brachycephalic dogs with BAOS are susceptible to heat stress because their anatomical malformations make it difficult for them to lose heat through panting.

Anesthetic Recommendations

A thorough and accurate history is important in brachycephalic animals. Special attention should be paid to a history of exercise intolerance, snoring, heat intolerance, stertor/stridor, gagging/retching, regurgitation, vomit, cyanosis, and episodes of syncope; the historical presence of these clinical signs can provide valuable information as to the significance of underlying problems and allows for preparation for potential complication during anesthetic induction, maintenance, and recovery [41].

On presenting clinical exam, the patient should be evaluated for evidence of respiratory signs such as dyspnea, tachypnea, and decreased airflow through the nose. Stertorous and stridorous noise coming from the upper airway might be obvious especially if the patient is stressed during the exam.

Management of the GI signs before anesthesia can decrease the incidence of complications and improve the prognosis. Administration of omeprazole ($1\,\text{mg}\,\text{kg}^{-1}$ at least 4 h before induction of anesthesia) has been shown to improve the decreases in esophageal pH (likely associated with gastroesophageal reflux) in patients under anesthesia [42]. If gastroesophageal reflux occurs during anesthesia, there is an increased risk of aspiration pneumonia, esophagitis, pharyngeal irritation, and possible esophageal stricture [43]. If regurgitation is noticed at the nares/mouth, then the tip of the head should be lowered with the nose pointing downward to improve drainage and the area of the larynx should be gently flushed with lukewarm water and suctioned. It is also recommended to also lavage and suction the esophagus [44].

Premedication is beneficial, since it provides sedation, decreases anxiety, facilitates the placement of an IV catheter, reduces the amount of total drug needed for induction, and provides analgesia. There are no perfect anesthesia protocols for patients with BAOS. The selection of a drug over another depends on the temperament of patient, presence of underlying disease, procedure to be performed, drugs available at the practice, and how familiar the clinician is with the different drugs and combinations.

Acepromazine in the preanesthetic period is commonly used in combination with an opioid; it produces reliable sedation/anxiolysis and has minimal ventilatory effects in dogs [45]. However, it may worsen upper airway obstruction in brachycephalic animals due to pharyngeal relaxation. If more sedation is needed, dexmedetomidine can be used with caution and in low dosages to avoid excessive sedation and the development of upper airway obstruction or hypoventilation. Sedated patients should be monitored closely for signs of upper airway obstruction (increased respiratory effort, stridor/stertor).

Body temperature should be kept within the normal range until the patient is discharged, since hypothermia can induce shivering, and this will increase oxygen demand. Hyperthermia should also be avoided, since it can worsen respiratory distress [46].

Preoxygenation should be performed with a mask if the patient allows via the anesthetic circuit with 100% oxygen for a minimum of 3 min before anesthetic induction (Figure 11.2). This increases the time to hemoglobin desaturation during periods of hypoventilation or apnea following administration of induction agents [47]. Endotracheal intubation can be challenging in this population. A variety of endotracheal tube sizes and lengths should be readily available in addition to a laryngoscope with a good light source, a stylet in case visualization of the larynx is difficult, and suctioning equipment

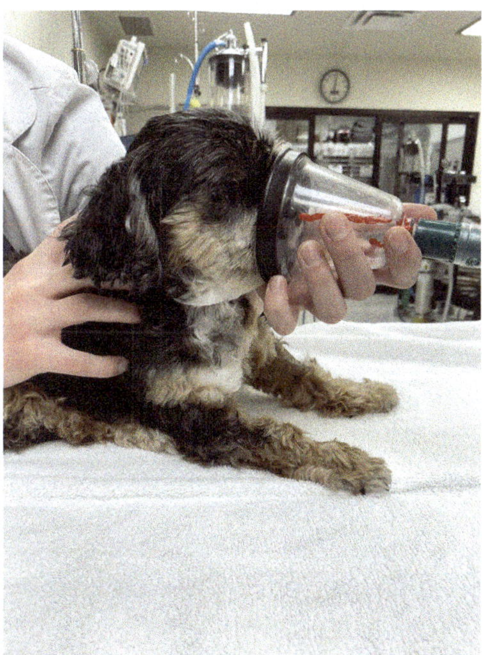

Figure 11.2 Preoxygenation of a brachycephalic dog before induction of general anesthesia with 100% oxygen and oxygen mask.

in case of regurgitated material in the airway/larynx (Figure 11.3).

Hypoventilation and hypercapnia are common and are generally a dose-dependent anesthetic consequence. Other factors that can contribute are opioid adjuncts, patient positioning, and obesity. Additionally, the small trachea and the small endotracheal tube needed to secure the airway increase airway resistance and the work of breathing. The use of capnography/capnometry to monitor $ETCO_2$ helps to recognize significant hypoventilation, which might require the use of positive pressure ventilation.

The use of multimodal analgesia is important in patients with respiratory disease. The presence of pain and stress can worsen hypoventilation (airway obstruction, increased work of breathing, increased oxygen consumption and demand). The protocols should include NSAIDs, opioids, ketamine, and local anesthesia techniques [48].

von Willebrand Disease (VWD)

Bleeding experienced in patients with VWD is caused by functional and quantitative deficiencies in the von Willebrand factor (VWF), a large plasma glycoprotein that is important in primary hemostasis with two important functions: (i) supporting platelet adhesion at sites of vascular injury and (ii) promotion of platelet aggregation under high shear conditions. In addition, VWF is important in fibrin formation, since it acts as carrier for factor VIII in the circulation, maintaining normal levels by decreasing its clearance [49]. VWF circulates when active as molecules of different sizes that make up multimers from 500 to 200 000 kDa. VWD is one of the most common hereditable bleeding disorders, being reported in more than 50 dog breeds. The methods of transmission are autosomal incomplete dominant and recessive inheritance patterns [50]. In breeds such as the Doberman Pinscher (up to 73%), most of the dogs tested have decreased plasma-circulating concentrations of VWF.

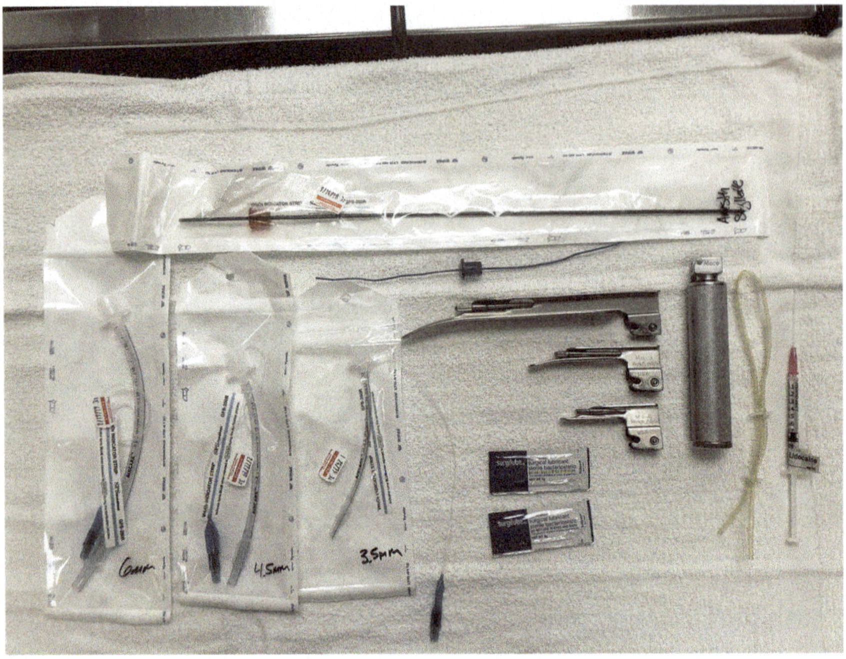

Figure 11.3 Endotracheal tubes in different sizes, a stylet, sterile lube, lidocaine syringe, and laryngoscope with different blade sizes. Materials needed for intubation of a brachycephalic dog.

VWD is categorized into three types. Type 1 is the most common form of VWD; its principal characteristic is a low concentration of VWF, but normal function of the protein. Clinical signs seen in Type 1 are mild and initially occur with trauma or deciduous tooth loss. There is a possibility of life-threatening hemorrhage [51]. The degree to which a patient is affected is correlated to the level of VWF activity, with the low levels correlated to the clinical signs. Patients are classified as normal if their VWF is 70–80%, borderline if 50–69%, and abnormal if <50%. Patients heterozygous to the VWD mutation and are Type 1 have less than half the normal concentration of VWF, and homozygous patients produce no VWF protein [52]. Type 2 VWD presents with a low concentration of VWF and a significant deficiency of the high-molecular-weight multimers; platelet adhesion becomes less effective. In Type 3, there is a complete absence of all multimers.

Anesthetic Recommendations

Preparation should be made in advance if a patient is either confirmed or is suspicious of having VWD requires anesthesia. Due to the high breed prevalence, all Doberman Pinschers should be tested. If the surgery is an emergency, a buccal mucosal bleeding time (BMBT) is recommended but not specific for VWD (normal for dogs should be 2–4 min). In VWD, the BMBT will be prolonged and different depending on the type (Type 1: 5–12 min; Type 2: >12 min; Type 3: >12 min). BMBT should be performed together with a platelet functional analysis test (for example, PFA 100) and a low plasma VWF:Ag ratio [53].

BMBT is usually performed in dogs under sedation. Common sedatives such as acepromazine or dexmedetomidine have been investigated to determine their platelet aggregation or clot formation. Acepromazine can cause a transient reduction in platelet aggregation [54], but the effect of this in a patient with VWD is unknown. Alpha-2-adrenergic agonists have receptors on the platelets (250–300) and conflicting results have been found in human medicine. in vitro, dexmedetomidine can enhance platelet aggregation. The effect changes when an antagonist (yohimbine) is administered, and platelet aggregation is suppressed [55].

Agents to promote hemostasis and blood products should be readily available. Antiplatelet drugs and NSAIDs should be stopped or weaned off before the procedure. Antifibrinolytic agents such as tranexamic acid or aminocaproic acid are reasonable and cost-efficient alternatives for stopping bleeding after minor surgical procedures, gingival bleeds (dental prophylaxis), or epistaxis (rhinoscopies). They can be used alone or in combination with desmopressin [56]. Other blood products that can be used in patients with VWD are fresh frozen plasma (10–20 ml kg^{-1}), frozen plasma (10–20 ml kg^{-1}), and cryoprecipitate (1 unit per 10 kg).

The use of desmopressin acetate (DDAVP) has been recommended in patients with VWD. Desmopressin is a vasopressin analog that can induce the release of preformed, high-molecular-weight multimers of VWF from endothelial cells. Administration results in improvement in the hemostatic function, with minimal increases in the concentration of VWF [57]. The recommended dosage is 1 μg kg^{-1} SC or IV and it should be administered 30 min prior to surgery. Intranasal or conjunctival sac administration in dogs is common; however, the evidence supporting the efficacy through this route is lacking.

Summary

Pharmacogenomics and personalized medicine are becoming an important field in veterinary medicine and anesthesia, since a significant number of drugs described to cause variability are widely use in our daily practice. Interindividual variation in drug response is as common in dogs just as in humans. Veterinary medicine is still behind our human counterparts, but even behind, very significant discoveries in the field have been made in the last 20 years. We should be moving from a single-gene approach to a whole-genome approach to better understand the variability on the response to drugs by some individuals.

References

1 Searle, R. and Hopkins, P. (2009). Pharmacogenomic variability and anaesthesia. *Br. J. Anaesth.* 103 (1): 14–25.

2 Ama, T., Bounmythavong, S., Blaze, J. et al. (2010). Implications of pharmacogenomics for anesthesia providers. *AANA J.* 78 (5): 393–399.

3 Galinkin, J., Demmer, L., and Yaster, M. (2010). Genetics for the pediatric anesthesiologist: a primer on congenital malformations, pharmacogenetics, and proteomics. *Anesth. Analg.* 111 (5): 1264–1274.

4 Morgan, B., Aroke, E., and Dungan, J. (2017). The role of pharmacogenomics in anesthesia pharmacology. *Annu. Rev. Nurs. Res.* 35 (1): 241–256.

5 Weinshilboum, R. (2003). Inheritance and drug response. *N. Engl. J. Med.* 348 (6): 529–537.

6 Ostrander, E. and Wayne, R. (2005). The canine genome. *Genome Res.* 15 (12): 1706–1716.

7 Mealey, K., Martinez, S., Villarino, N. et al. (2019). Personalized medicine: going to the dogs? *Hum. Genet.* 138 (5): 467–481.

8 Fleischer, S., Sharkey, M., Mealey, K. et al. (2008). Pharmacogenetic and metabolic differences between dog breeds: their impact

on canine medicine and the use of the dog as a preclinical animal mode. *AAPS J.* 10 (1): 110–119.

9 McGraw, J. and Waller, D. (2012). Cytochrome P450 variations in different ethnic populations. *Expert Opin. Drug Metab. Toxicol.* 8 (3): 371–382.

10 Roussel, F., Duignan, D., Lawton, M. et al. (1998). Expression and characterization of canine cytochrome P450 2D15. *Arch. Biochem. Biophys.* 357 (1): 27–36.

11 Paulson, S., Engel, L., Reitz, B. et al. (1999). Evidence for polymorphism in the canine metabolism of cyclooxygenase 2 inhibitor, celecoxib. *Drug Metab. Dispos.* 27 (10): 1133–1142.

12 Perez Jimenez, T., Mealey, K., Grubb, T. et al. (2016). Tramadol metabolism to O-desmethyltramadol (M1) and N-desmethyl tramadol (M2) by dog liver microsomes: species comparison and identification of responsible canine cytochrome P450s. *Drug Metab. Dispos.* 44 (12): 1963–1972.

13 Hay-Kraus, B., Grenblatt, D., Venjatakrishnan, K. et al. (2000). Evidence for propofol hydroxylation by cytochrome P4502B11 in canine liver microsomes: breed and gender differences. *Xenobiotica* 30 (6): 575–588.

14 Zoran, D., Riedesel, D., and Dyer, D. (1993). Pharmacokinetics of propofol in mixed-breed dogs and greyhounds. *Am. J. Vet. Res.* 54 (5): 755–760.

15 Court, M., Hay-Kraus, B., and Hill, D. (1999). Propofol hydroxylation by dog liver microsomes: assay development and dog breed differences. *Drug Metab. Dispos.* 27 (11): 1293–1299.

16 Sams, R. and Muir, W. (1988). Effects of phenobarbital on thiopental pharmacokinetics in greyhounds. *Am. J. Vet. Res.* 49 (2): 245–249.

17 Pasloske, K., Sauer, B., Perkins, N. et al. (2009). Plasma pharmacokinetics of alfaxalone in both premedicated and unpremedicated greyhound dogs after single, intravenous administration of Alfaxan at a clinical dose. *J. Vet. Pharmacol. Ther.* 32 (5): 510–513.

18 Court, M. (1999). Anesthesia of the sighthound. *Clin. Tech. Small Anim. Pract.* 14 (1): 38–43.

19 Mealey, K., Greene, S., Bagley, R. et al. (2008). P-glycoprotein contributes to the blood-brain, but not blood-cerebrospinal fluid, barrier in a spontaneous canine p-glycoprotein knockout model. *Drug Metab. Dispos.* 36 (6): 1073–1079.

20 Mealey, K., Bentjen, S., Gay, J. et al. (2001). Ivermectin sensitivity in collies is associated with a deletion mutation of the mdr1 gene. *Pharmacogenetics* 11 (8): 727–733.

21 Mealey, K. and Burkc, N. (2015). Identification of a nonsense mutation in feline ABCB1. *J. Vet. Pharmacol. Ther.* 38 (5): 429–433.

22 Mealey, K. and Meurs, K. (2008). Breed distribution of the ABCB1 delta (multidrug sensitivity) polymorphism among dogs undergoing ABCB1 genotyping. *J. Am. Vet. Med. Assoc.* 233 (6): 921–924.

23 Mealey, K. (2013). Adverse drug reactions in veterinary patients associated with drug transporters. *Vet. Clin. N. Am. Small Anim. Pract.* 43 (5): 1067–1078.

24 Mealey, K. (2004). Therapeutic implications of the MDR-1 gene. *J. Vet. Pharmacol. Therap.* 27 (5): 257–264.

25 Mealey, K. (2006). Adverse drug reactions in herding-breed dogs: the role of P-gp. *Compendium* 28 (1): 23–33.

26 Deshpande, D., Hill, K., Mealey, K. et al. (2016). The effect of the canine ABCB1-Delta mutation on sedation after intravenous administration of acepromazine. *J. Vet. Intern. Med.* 30 (2): 636–641.

27 Kirmayer, A., Klide, A., and Puvance, J. (1984). Malignant hyperthermia in a dog: case report and review of the syndrome. *J. Am. Vet. Med. Assoc.* 185: 978–982.

28 Nelson, T. (1991). Malignant hyperthermia in dogs. *J. Am. Vet. Med. Assoc.* 198 (6): 989–994.

29 Brunson, D. and Hogan, K. (2004). Malignant hyperthermia: a syndrome not a disease. *Vet. Clin. N. Am. Small Anim. Pract.* 34 (6): 1419–1433.

30 Roberts, M., Mickelson, J., Patterson, E. et al. (2001). Autosomal dominant canine malignant hyperthermia is caused by a mutation in the gene encoding the skeletal muscle calcium release channel (RYR1). *Anesthesiology* 95 (3): 716–725.

31 Stewart, S., Hogan, K., Rosenberg, H. et al. (2001). Identification of the Arg1086His mutation in the alpha subunit of the voltage-dependent calcium channel (CACNA1S) in a north American family with malignant hyperthermia. *Clin. Genet.* 59 (3): 178–184.

32 Available at: https://www.animalgenetics.us/canine/Genetic_Disease/MH.asp. Accessed February 25, 2020.

33 Thomson, S., Burton, C., and Armitage-Chan, E. (2014). Intra-operative hyperthermia in a cat with a fatal outcome. *Vet. Anaesth. Analg.* 41 (3): 290–296.

34 Miller, S. (2015). Sympatholytics. In: *Stoelting's Pharmacology and Physiology in Anesthetic Practice*, 5e (eds. P. Flood, J. Rathmell and S. Shafer), 474–500. Philadelphia, PA: Wolters Kluwer Health.

35 Hawley, A. and Wetmore, L. (2010). Identification of single nucleotide polymorphisms within exon 1 of the canine mu-opioid receptor gene. *Vet. Anaesth. Analg.* 37 (1): 79–82.

36 Burger, D., Wiestner, T., Hubler, M. et al. (2006). Effect of anticholinergics (atropine, glycopyrrolate) and prokinetics (metoclopramide, cisapride) on gastric motility in beagles and Labrador retrievers. *J. Vet. Med. A Physiol. Pathol. Clin. Med.* 53 (2): 97–107.

37 Meola, S. (2013). Brachycephalic airway syndrome. *Top. Comp. Anim. Med.* 28 (3): 91–96.

38 Pollinger, J., Bustamante, C., Fledel-Alon, A. et al. (2005). Selective sweep mapping of genes with large phenotypic effects. *Genome Res.* 15 (12): 1809–1819.

39 Ginn, J., Kumar, M., McKiernan, B. et al. (2008). Nasopharyngeal turbinates in brachycephalic dogs and cats. *J. Am. Anim. Hosp. Assoc.* 44 (5): 243–249.

40 Poncet, C., Dupre, G., Freiche, V. et al. (2005). Prevalence of gastrointestinal tract lesions in 73 brachycephalic dogs with upper respiratory syndrome. *J. Small Anim. Pract.* 46 (6): 273–279.

41 Lodato, D. and Hedlund, C. (2012). Brachycephalic airway syndrome: pathophysiology and diagnosis. *Compend. Contin. Educ. Pract. Vet.* 34 (7): E1–E5.

42 Panti, A., Bennett, R., Corletto, F. et al. (2009). The effect of omeprazole on oesophageal pH in dogs during anaesthesia. *J. Small Anim. Pract.* 50 (10): 540–544.

43 Wilson, D. and Walshaw, R. (2004). Postanesthetic esophageal dysfunction in 13 dogs. *J. Am. Anim. Hosp. Assoc.* 40 (6): 455–460.

44 Wilson, D. and Evans, A. (2007). The effect of topical treatment on esophageal pH during acid reflux in dogs. *Vet. Anaesth. Analg.* 34 (5): 339–343.

45 Popovic, N., Mullane, J., and Yhap, E. (1972). Effects of acetylpromazine maleate on certain cardiorespiratory responses in dogs. *Am. J. Vet. Res.* 33 (9): 1819–1824.

46 Mosing, M. (2016). General principles of preoperative care. In: *BSAVA Manual of Canine and Feline Anaesthesia and Analgesia*, 3e (eds. T. Duke-Novakowski, M. de Vries and C. Seymour), 13–23. Glouchester: British Small Animal Veterinary Association.

47 McNally, E., Robertson, S., and Pablo, L. (2008). Comparison of time to desaturation between preoxygenated and nonpreoxygenated dogs following sedation with acepromazine maleate and morphine and induction of anesthesia with propofol. *Am. J. Vet. Res.* 70 (11): 1333–1338.

48 Downing, F. and Gibson, S. (2018). Anaesthesia of brachycephalic dogs. *J. Small Anim. Pract.* 59 (12): 725–733.

49 De Meyer, S.F., Deckmyn, H., and Vanhoorelbeke, K. (2009). Von Willebrand factor to the rescue. *Blood* 113 (21): 5049–5057.

50 Moser, J., Meyers, K., and Russon, R. (1996). Inheritance of von Willebrand factor deficiency in Doberman Pinschers. *J. Am. Vet. Med. Assoc.* 209 (6): 1103–1106.

51 Brooks, M. and Catalfamo, J. (2010). Von Willebrand disease. In: *Schalm's Veterinary Hematology*, 6e (eds. D. Weiss and K. Wardrop), 612–618. Ames: Wiley.

52 Brooks, M. (1992). Management of canine von Willebrand's disease. *Probl. Vet. Med.* 4 (4): 636–646.

53 Brooks, M. and Catalfamo, J. (2010). Immune-mediated thrombocytopenia, Von Willebrand disease and platelet disorders. In: *Textbook of Veterinary Internal Medicine*, 7e (eds. S. Ettinger and E. Feldman), 772–783. St. Louis: Saunders Elsevier.

54 Barr, S., Ludders, J., Looney, A. et al. (1992). Platelet aggregation in dogs after sedation with acepromazine and atropine and during subsequent general anesthesia and surgery. *Am. J. Vet. Res.* 53 (11): 2067–2070.

55 Kawamoto, S., Hirakata, H., Sugita, N. et al. (2015). Bidirectional effects of dexmedetomidine on human platelet functions *in vitro*. *Eur. J. Pharmacol.* 766: 122–128.

56 Seligsohn, U. (2012). Treatment of inherited platelet disorders. *Haemophilia* 18 (suppl 4): 161–165.

57 Callan, M. and Giger, U. (2002). Effect of desmopressin acetate administration on primary hemostasis in Doberman Pinschers with type-1 von Willebrand disease as assessed by a point-of-care instrument. *Am. J. Vet. Res.* 63 (12): 1700–1706.

12

Anesthesia for Ophthalmic Patients

Philip Lerche

Department of Veterinary Clinical Sciences, College of Veterinary Medicine, The Ohio State University, Columbus, OH, 43210, USA

Introduction

Animals presenting for ophthalmic surgery pose several challenges to the anesthetist, including the effects of anesthetic drugs on intraocular pressure (IOP) and tear production, patient positioning, reflexes that may occur during intraoperative manipulation of the eye, the effect of topically or systemically administered ophthalmic drugs, and, in many older animals, coexisting disease. Additionally, procedures that require the globe to be positioned centrally within the orbit for optimal surgical access (e.g., cataract removal and extensive conjunctival surgery) frequently require the use of neuromuscular blocking agents (NMBAs) and mechanical ventilation.

Intraocular Pressure

IOP is a function of the relationship between aqueous humor production and its drainage, the majority of which occurs in cats and dogs via the trabecular meshwork of the anterior chamber angle [1]. This relationship can be quantified as follows:

$$\text{IOP} = (\text{aqueous humor formulation rate}/\text{aqueous humor outflow rate}) + \text{episcleral venous pressure} \qquad (12.1)$$

Ocular perfusion pressure determines the blood supply to the retina and optic nerve and is defined as the difference between mean arterial blood pressure and IOP. Thus, an increase in IOP can lead to a decrease in optic nerve function, leading to a potential loss of vision if not recognized and treated. A major goal when anesthetizing animals that present with preexisting glaucoma for both ophthalmic and nonophthalmic surgeries is to prevent unwanted increases in IOP. It is also imperative to prevent sudden increases in IOP in patients that present with partial or imminent loss of globe integrity (e.g., descemetocele, trauma, deep corneal ulcer) to prevent complete rupture. The physical, physiologic, and pharmacologic causes of increased IOP are presented in Table 12.1.

There are several factors that may increase IOP via increased central venous pressure (CVP). Physical restraint of a struggling patient as well as inadvertent pressure on the jugular veins may cause increased CVP and IOP. Vomiting, straining, and coughing all increase IOP by temporarily increasing CVP [2].

Canine and Feline Anesthesia and Co-Existing Disease, Second Edition. Edited by Rebecca A. Johnson, Lindsey B. C. Snyder and Carrie A. Schroeder.

Companion website: www.wiley.com/go/johnson/canine

Table 12.1 Factors causing an increase in IOP.

Physical	Physiologic	Pharmacologic
Pressure on eyelids (e.g., face mask)	Vomiting Coughing	Succinylcholine Etomidate[a]
Endotracheal intubation	Preexisting glaucoma	Ketamine[b]
Excessive restraint and struggling	Hypoxemia Hypercapnia	Nitrous oxide
Pressure on the jugular veins		
Head below body		
Cataract surgery		

[a] If myoclonus occurs
[b] High dosage or as sole agent

Coughing or gagging during stimulation of the larynx and pharynx during endotracheal intubation transiently increases IOP [3]. Thus, in patients with increased IOP, intubation during very light planes of anesthesia should be avoided. The use of topical lidocaine applied to the glottis or the administration of intravenous lidocaine ($2\,mg\,kg^{-1}$ IV) to decrease stimulation during intubation is also prudent [4]. The presence of preexisting glaucoma and the development of hypercarbia and/or hypoxemia all lead to increases in IOP [5]. As with all anesthetic patients, it is important to carefully monitor ventilatory status as well as oxygenation and supplement oxygen and offer ventilatory support as needed. However, oxygen supplementation should be delivered with caution, as any pressure applied to the eyes via the eyelids such as digital compression or placement of a face mask causes a direct increase in IOP. Elevating the head above the rest of the body will tend to decrease IOP, while, conversely, lowering the head below the body (i.e., Trendelenburg position) may elevate IOP. In the postanesthetic period, measures to avoid acute increases in IOP must continue to be considered. It is important to note that increases in IOP have been shown to occur in approximately 20% of dogs following cataract surgery [6]. It is therefore prudent to maintain intravenous access for administration of diuretics or for sedation if anterior chamber paracentesis is needed to relieve high IOP after anesthetic recovery.

Many anesthetic drugs directly decrease or do not change IOP; however, side effects such as vomiting (opioids, alpha-2-adrenergic receptor agonists), hypercapnia (propofol, alfaxalone, opioids, alpha-2-adrenergic receptor agonists, inhalants), or myoclonus (etomidate) may cause IOP to increase. Ketamine and succinylcholine have also been shown to increase IOP [7]. Both propofol and alfaxalone when given as a single IV bolus caused an initial small, transient increase in IOP 2 min after administration to dogs followed by a significant decrease in IOP for 25 min [8]. In another study, alfaxalone administration increased IOP in healthy dogs, and the highest IOP recorded was associated with intubation [9].

Tear Production

In dogs, atropine given subcutaneously and topically is correlated with a decrease in tear production [10, 11]. Similarly, general anesthesia has been found to decrease tear production for up to 24 h after general anesthesia; anesthetic events lasting more than 2 h had a significantly greater impact on postoperative tear production than shorter procedures [12]. Conversely, a different study demonstrated that tear production returned to normal immediately after short (1 h) and long (4 h) anesthetic episodes when either isoflurane or desflurane was used as the sole anesthetic agent [13]. Conflicting results of these studies may be due to a difference in methods, as multiple drugs (premedication, injectable induction agents) were used in the former study, including atropine, which may account for the different findings. Alfaxalone and propofol have been shown to reduce tear production [8]. General anesthesia with sevoflurane after administration of morphine, acepromazine, or after no premedication also reduced tear production [14]. Tear production was decreased in cats after acepromazine and xylazine sedation [15]. Yet another study reported that, in the intensive care unit setting, tear production was reduced by approximately 50% in dogs with no history of eye disease and no recent anesthetic episodes [16]. This should be taken into consideration when hospitalizing dogs prior to surgery for disease management (e.g., diabetes mellitus or chronic renal disease). In cases of unilateral ocular surgery, the unaffected eye should be protected and treated with a topical artificial tear ointment or gel. In cats, application of an eye gel caused less postoperative irritation, as identified by reduced blepharospasm, compared to an ointment [17]. Tear production was decreased after surgery regardless of treatment type. Tear production was decreased in cats anesthetized with a medetomidine–ketamine combination, and within 15 min of atipamezole administration returned to normal [18].

Patient Positioning

The head of the patient is typically somewhat distant to the anesthetist during ophthalmic surgery, resulting in several challenges (Figure 12.1). First, it is not possible to assess anesthetic depth using the palpebral reflex, globe position within the orbit, or jaw tone. The anesthetist must rely on cardiovascular and respiratory monitoring and feedback from the surgeon about response to surgery as indicators of anesthetic depth change. Second, the endotracheal tube, endotracheal tube connector, and patient end of the breathing system are not visible or easily accessed. This makes it more difficult to detect accidental extubation (especially if capnometry is not utilized), the presence of leaks, and disconnections. Third, it may not be possible to place or access monitoring equipment on the tongue (pulse oximeter), in the esophagus (temperature probe, stethoscope), or connected to the breathing system (capnometry) depending on the distance from the anesthetic monitor to the patient's head. Finally, movement of the surgery table or patient by the anesthetist during surgery may make it challenging for the ophthalmologist, particularly when an operating microscope is being used, as small movements will be greatly magnified in the surgeon's field of vision.

Oculocardiac Reflex (Aschner Reflex)

Pressure or traction on the globe or nearby extraocular tissues during surgery may induce an oculocardiac reflex (OCR) via the trigeminal (cranial nerve V, afferent limb) and vagal (cranial nerve X, efferent limb) nerves that results in the development of dysrhythmias. The most common dysrhythmia noted is bradycardia; however, ventricular ectopy and asystole may also occur. The presence of hypercarbia increases the likelihood of OCR occurring [19]. Initial management involves communicating the occurrence of OCR to the surgeon, who should stop manipulating the eye immediately. If the OCR persists or is severe, treatment with an anticholinergic may be necessary. Commencement of cardiopulmonary resuscitation should immediately be initiated in the case of asystole. In a retrospective study of 145 dogs undergoing enucleation, OCR occurred in approximately 5% of cases [20]. Age, breed, and preoperative anticholinergic treatment were not associated

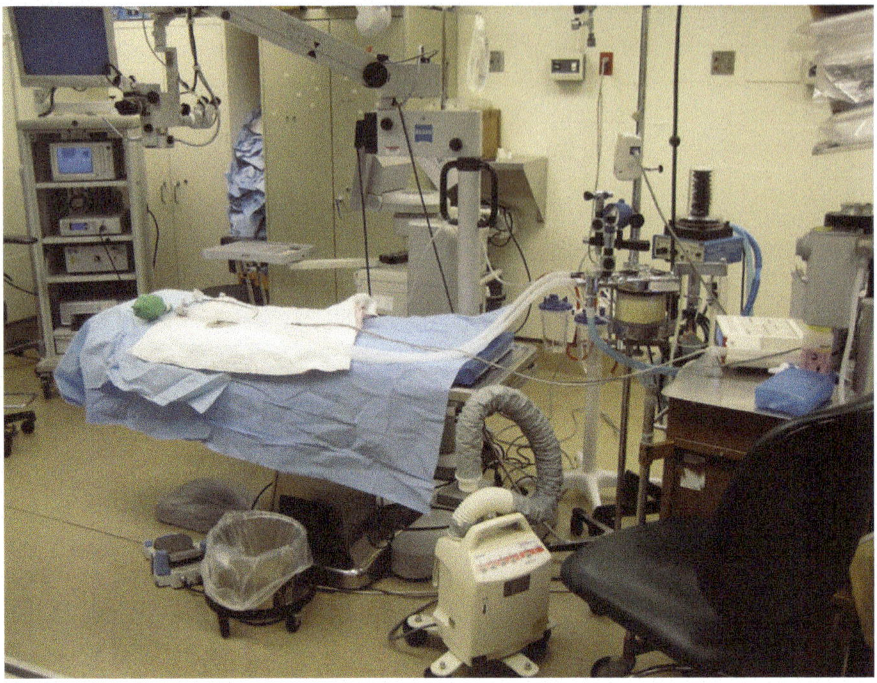

Figure 12.1 Typical setup of an ophthalmology operating room, with the animal's head placed distant from the anesthesia machine and the anesthetist.

with an increase in the prevalence of OCR, whereas retrobulbar nerve block decreased the chance of OCR occurring.

Ophthalmic Drugs

Many patients that present for ophthalmic surgery have received ophthalmic drugs prior to surgery. Thus, it is important to understand their potential physiologic impact. Systemically administered drugs are much more likely to result in side effects; however, systemic absorption of topically applied drugs can occur. It is important to recognize the potential for side effects of ophthalmic drugs administered by any route, so that when they occur, they can be managed appropriately.

Drugs Used to Treat Glaucoma

Cholinergic agents (e.g., pilocarpine) increase the rate of aqueous humor outflow. If absorbed systemically, unwanted parasympathetic effects such as bradydysrhythmias and bronchoconstriction may be seen [1]. Topically applied adrenergic agonist drugs (e.g., epinephrine and phenylephrine) may lead to systemic hypertension and tachycardia [21]. Adrenergic antagonists (e.g., timolol) will have the opposite effect if absorbed (i.e., bradycardia).

Inhibition of carbonic anhydrase (CA) by systemic administration of acetazolamide leads to a decrease in aqueous humor formation [22]. The CA enzyme is also present in the kidney, and its inhibition interferes with renal electrolyte exchange mechanisms resulting in a decrease in bicarbonate reabsorption. This leads to hyperchloremia, hypokalemia, and metabolic acidosis. Topical CA inhibitors such as brinzolamide have generally superseded the systemic use of acetazolamide, as they have minimal side effects.

Diuretic use (e.g., mannitol) may lead to an initial volume expansion, which, in patients with moderate to severe cardiovascular disease, may cause pulmonary overload and edema, or congestive heart failure [23]. Ultimately dehydration, hyponatremia, and metabolic acidosis may occur.

Topical Corticosteroids

Prolonged corticosteroid drop use may depress the adrenal cortex and possibly result in hypoadrenocorticism, thus decreasing an animal's ability to respond appropriately to the stress of anesthesia and surgery [24]. Hypoadrenocorticism usually results in hyponatremia, hyperkalemia, and dehydration, as well as lethargy and inappetence (see Chapter 9). A patient presenting for nonurgent ophthalmic surgery with clinical symptoms and blood work that are suspicious of hypoadrenocorticism should undergo further diagnostics and treatment. In the case of a patient where hypoadrenocorticism is suspected that needs urgent or emergency ophthalmic procedures, every effort should be made to correct hydration and electrolyte status prior to anesthesia. It may be necessary to administer supplemental corticosteroids prior to anesthesia (e.g., prednisolone 1–2 $mg\,kg^{-1}$ IV).

Drugs Used to Dilate the Pupil

Topical atropine drops may result in tachydysrhythmias and bronchodilation if absorbed into the systemic circulation [25]. If abnormal cardiac rhythms are detected during the preanesthetic physical examination, an electrocardiogram should be performed to document and identify the arrhythmias. If possible, surgery can be postponed so that treatment of a dysrhythmia can be initiated prior to anesthesia (see Chapter 1). The electrocardiogram should be closely monitored during surgery in the case of atropine being applied topically.

The Presence of Coexisting Disease

Patients presenting for ophthalmic surgery range in age, and older animals often have coexisting diseases of other body systems. Renal, cardiovascular, and endocrine diseases are more common in older patients and should be managed appropriately (see corresponding chapters in this book). For example, the incidence of cataract formation in diabetic dogs is high, and these patients often present for anesthesia to remove sclerotic lenses and replace them with prosthetics. It is important to monitor blood glucose frequently in these patients because withholding food and the unavoidable stress associated with the perioperative period (being in the unfamiliar environment of the veterinary clinic) may lead to unexpected hyperglycemia or hypoglycemia, and both may occur within the same anesthetic episode. The anesthetist should be prepared to treat hypoglycemia by adding dextrose to IV fluids (2.5–5% solutions, as needed, are usually adequate). Severe hyperglycemia (blood glucose >450 $mg\,dl^{-1}$) can be treated with regular insulin intraoperatively [26]. Serial blood glucose measurement is useful to determine the current trend of blood glucose, as well as response to any treatment. Hypoglycemia is generally easier to manage than hyperglycemia, and it has been shown that inhalant anesthesia has an anti-insulin effect in rabbits [27]. Although it is not clear whether this occurs in cats and dogs, it may be prudent to delay or postpone nonemergent ophthalmic surgery in patients with a blood glucose that is >450 $mg\,dl^{-1}$ until treatment results in stable and declining levels.

Neuromuscular Blockade and Ventilation

During general anesthesia, the globe of the eye rotates away from a central position, typically in a ventromedial or ventrolateral direction. This position is not ideal for performing intraocular and some keratoconjunctival surgeries. The use of nondepolarizing NMBAs to relax the extraocular muscles allows the eye to maintain a central position, which greatly facilitates surgery (Figure 12.2).

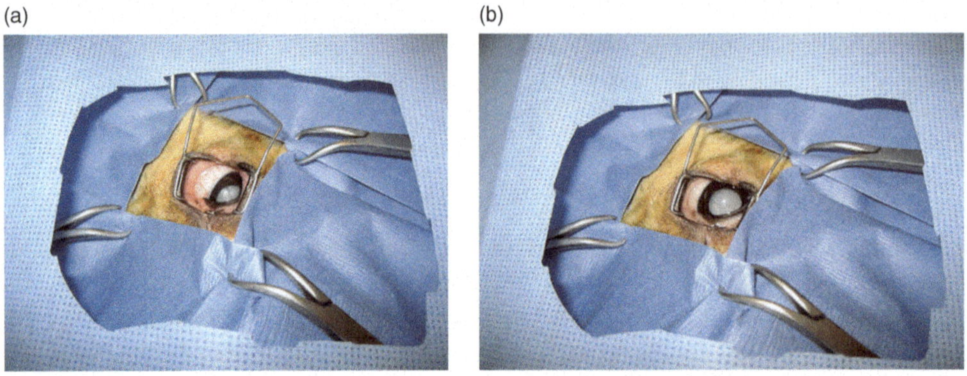

Figure 12.2 (a) The eye prior to administration of a neuromuscular blocking agent (NMBA) for cataract surgery. The globe is rotated ventrally such that the sclera is prominent, and the cornea partially covered by the lower eyelid. (b) The same eye after NMBA administration. The globe has returned to a more central position, with more of the cornea visible to the surgeon.

Table 12.2 Commonly used neuromuscular blocking agents [28].

Drug	Metabolism	Effects
Atracurium	Primarily extrahepatic: Hofmann elimination and ester hydrolysis	Block may be prolonged by acidosis and hypothermia Possibility of histamine release resulting in hypotension
Cisatracurium	Primarily extrahepatic: Hofmann elimination	Block may be prolonged by acidosis and hypothermia Does not cause histamine release
Vecuronium	Hepatic metabolism and renal elimination	Cardiovascular stability Prolonged action with renal insufficiency
Rocuronium	Hepatic metabolism and renal elimination	Cardiovascular stability

Nondepolarizing NMBAs exert their action on the neuromuscular junction by competitively antagonizing acetylcholine (ACh) at the postjunctional ACh receptors. Various short-acting NMBAs that have an onset of action of 1–5 min and a duration lasting up to 30 min are available for clinical use. Their pharmacologic and side effects are contrasted in Table 12.2. In addition to the details mentioned under each drug, neuromuscular blockade can be prolonged by concurrent antibiotic administration, hypothermia, electrolyte and acid–base disturbances, and the use of inhalational anesthetic agents.

The degree of neuromuscular blockade can be monitored using a nerve stimulator (Figure 12.3). The common fibular (peroneal) nerve running over the distal aspect of the lateral thigh is more accessible than the radial nerve during ophthalmic surgery. The most well-known technique used to determine degree of blockade is the train-of-four (TOF). In this technique, four supramaximal stimuli are applied at 2 Hz. The twitches of the limb produced by the first stimulus (T1) and the last (T4) were traditionally compared visually or by touch by the anesthetist to provide a T4/T1 ratio. Prior to NMBA administration, the ratio

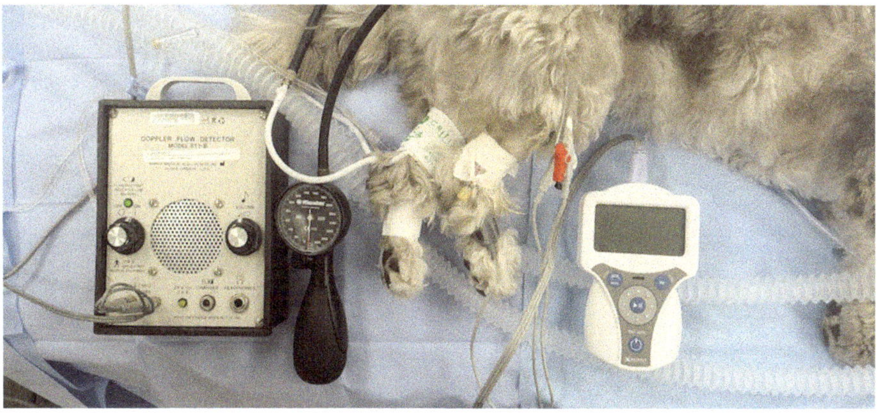

Figure 12.3 Hind limb of a dog showing placement of clips on the skin over the common fibular (peroneal) nerve, intravenous catheter, Doppler crystal, and noninvasive blood pressure cuff.

should be 1.0 (i.e., all twitches are of the same magnitude). If the NMBA occupies 70% or more of the receptors, then the twitches will become weaker, or "fade," with T4 fading first, followed by T3 and T2. Return of T4 such that the T4/T1 ratio is greater than 0.9 represents clinical recovery from blockade. At this level of recovery from blockade, the patient has competent laryngeal and respiratory function, and is no longer at high risk for aspirating gastric contents. It has been shown that anesthesiologists cannot reliably detect subtle changes in twitch strength between T1 and T4 once the ratio is above 0.4, thus it is recommended that an objective assessment of blockade is used [29]. More modern nerve stimulators that incorporate a visual representation of twitch strength based on accelerometry, shown as twitch height graphically, are helpful in this regard (Figure 12.4). An alternative technique, double burst stimulation, applies two stimuli at 50 Hz. The ratios of the two evoked twitches are then compared in a similar manner to T4/T1. Guided by these methods of monitoring neuromuscular blockade, in addition to surgical requirements, additional doses of NMBA may be needed for longer surgeries to maintain an optimal surgical position of the eye. Typically, the dose required to maintain neuromuscular block is one-third to one-half of the dose initially used.

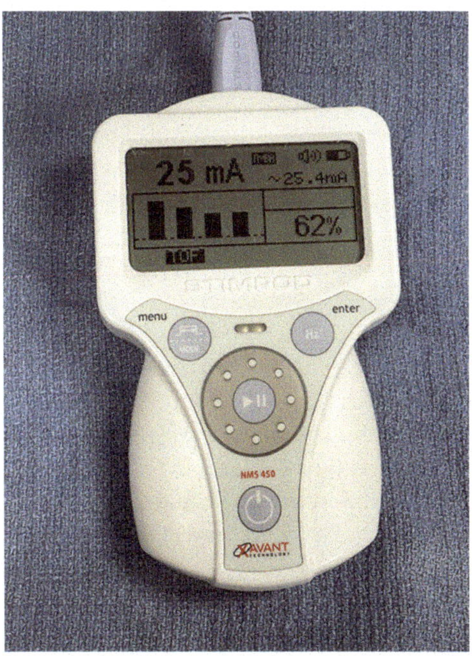

Figure 12.4 Peripheral nerve stimulator with a graphic representation of the twitches obtained using the train-of-four technique. In this case, the T4/T1 ratio is 0.62, or 62%.

Manual or mechanical ventilation is mandatory following NMBA administration. Mechanical ventilation provides consistent tidal volume and respiratory rate and allows the anesthetist's hands to be free for other tasks; it is thus preferred over manual ventilation when neuromuscular

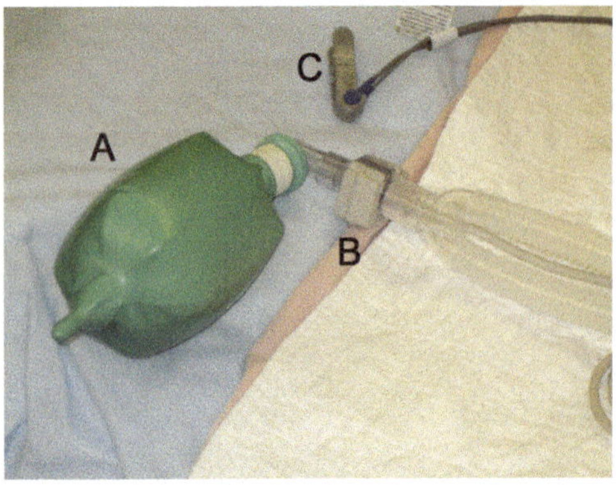

Figure 12.5 Prior to anesthesia, the ventilator should be checked to make sure it is working correctly. This is achieved by placing an (a) anesthetic breathing bag on the patient end of the anesthetic breathing circuit to act as a "lung." The ventilator can then be cycled to ensure proper function. Note also that a mainstream (b) end-tidal CO_2 analyzer is attached to the breathing system, and a (c) pulse oximeter probe is ready to be attached to the patient.

blockade is performed. The anesthetist should be familiar with the mechanical ventilator being used, and the ventilator should be checked to ensure that it is in working order prior to connecting a patient to it (Figure 12.5).

At the end of the procedure, it is essential to determine whether residual neuromuscular blockade is present. Monitoring with a nerve stimulator is used to determine if reversal of neuromuscular blockade is required (see the preceding text). Blockade reversal with neostigmine ($0.04\,mg\,kg^{-1}$) or edrophonium ($0.5\,mg\,kg^{-1}$) must be preceded by anticholinergic treatment to avoid bradycardia, bronchoconstriction, and diarrhea. It is possible for recurarization to occur in patients (the effects of paralysis return either totally or partially) even after reversal, and postoperative observation for several hours is warranted.

Pain Management

The eye has a well-developed network of sensory nerve fibers, with the cornea having abundant nociceptors that are sensitive to external injury (corneal ulcer, laceration, or foreign body). Pain from within the eye (uveitis, acute glaucoma) is most likely transmitted via stimulation of nociceptors in the ciliary body and iris [30]. Surgery of the eyelids and other periorbital tissues will also induce a pain response. As with any other surgery, analgesia for ophthalmic surgery should follow the basic principles of pain management. The aim should be to make the patient as comfortable as possible by providing preemptive (administering analgesics prior to the start of surgery) and multimodal (using drugs that act via different receptor mechanisms) analgesia where appropriate.

Local Anesthetics

Local anesthetics abolish nociceptive transmission, and, together with a low incidence of systemic side effects when administered appropriately, can provide effective intraoperative and short-term analgesia for ophthalmic surgery. Topical local anesthetics will provide relief for keratoconjunctival pain and, although they work rapidly, they may cause pain when first administered. Tetracaine and proparacaine have a short duration of action of up to 15 min. This class of drugs has classically not been recommended for long-term topical pain management due to purported delayed healing of the cornea; however, a review of the literature in human ophthalmology concluded that when administered at lower concentrations, given at the appropriate dose, for a short time (typically less than 3 days), healing of corneal abrasions was not impaired [31]. Intraocular local anesthetic has been investigated in dogs, with intracameral injection of preservative-free lidocaine producing no adverse effects on IOP or corneal thickness [32]. Intravenous lidocaine infusion ($25\,\mu g\,kg^{-1}\,min^{-1}$ following a $1\,mg\,kg^{-1}$ bolus) provided comparable analgesia to morphine infusions in dogs undergoing intraocular surgery with no side effects reported [33].

Multiple local anesthetic techniques have been described to provide anesthesia to the eye. Sensory loss to the globe and eyelids as well as akinesia (globe immobility) can be achieved via retrobulbar local anesthetic administration (Figure 12.6) [34]. Side effects of this technique include retrobulbar hemorrhage, damage to the optic nerve, and intrathecal injection, so should be performed by a trained individual. Peribulbar anesthesia has been used in dogs. This technique avoids some of the complications of retrobulbar drug administration by placing the needle such that an extraconal injection is performed, depositing a volume of local anesthetic approximately two to four times that necessary for retrobulbar blockade [35]. Local anesthetic can be deposited in the episcleral space (i.e., between the sclera and Tenon's membrane), and is referred to as *sub-Tenon's block*. A blunt cannula is used to perform the technique, avoiding the complications of techniques requiring a sharp needle. In dogs, administration of 1–2 ml of 2% lidocaine using this technique produces akinesia and mydriasis [36]. Complications include chemosis and ecchymoses. An auriculopalpebral nerve block can be performed to facilitate surgery of the upper eyelid and closely associated structures [37]. Local anesthetic is deposited subcutaneously dorsal to the zygomatic arch at its caudal one-third. In a review of techniques for ophthalmic locoregional anesthesia in small animals, it was noted that since few controlled, prospective clinical studies that compare local anesthetic techniques exist, one technique cannot be recommended over another [38]. The focus should be on understanding the limits and potential side effects of each technique.

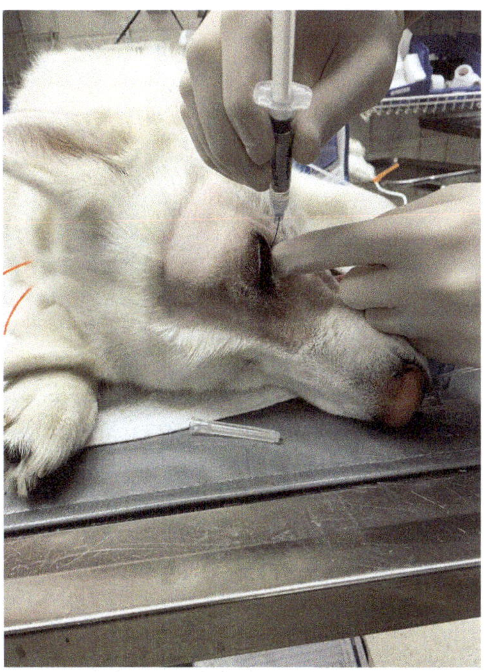

Figure 12.6 Retrobulbar injection of bupivacaine. Source: Photo courtesy of Dr. Carrie Schroeder.

Opioids

While topical administration of morphine (1% solution) relieved pain associated with corneal ulcers in dogs without affecting healing [39], systemic administration of opioids is frequently required, and is often included with a sedative to provide neuroleptanalgesia prior to induction of general anesthesia.

Maropitant administration 1 hour prior to premedication with hydromorphone, an opioid with mu-agonist activity, has been shown to decrease the incidence of opioid-induced vomiting [40]. As vomiting may significantly increase IOP, consideration should therefore be given to including maropitant as part of the preanesthetic regimen in any patient with increased IOP or concern for corneal perforation.

Opioids are classified according to their receptor activity: mu-opioid receptor agonists (e.g., morphine, methadone, hydromorphone, meperidine, fentanyl); partial mu-opioid receptor agonists (e.g., buprenorphine); and opioid receptor antagonist–agonists (e.g., butorphanol). The degree of analgesia provided, as well as the incidence of side effects encountered, is highest with mu-opioid receptor agonists. The anesthetist must weigh the pros and cons when choosing an opioid for ophthalmic patients. For example, IOP was increased after sedation with acepromazine and meperidine compared to acepromazine and butorphanol [41]. Hypercarbia due to hypoventilation and vomiting are common with mu-opioid receptor agonists, and both side effects can increase IOP [5]. Methadone has a decreased incidence of vomiting as compared to the intramuscular administration of hydromorphone and morphine and may be more appropriate in cases where IOP is increased. Alternatively, opioids can be given after induction. Intraoperative pain can be treated by IV boluses (e.g., hydromorphone) or constant rate infusions of opioids (e.g., fentanyl). Postoperative vomiting is rare in cats and dogs; however, if patients require opioids to control pain after surgery, they should be observed for vomiting and/or retching. If this occurs, opioid administration should be decreased.

Nonsteroidal Anti-Inflammatory Drugs

Nonsteroidal anti-inflammatory drugs (NSAIDs) decrease inflammation by inhibiting cyclooxygenase in the arachidonic acid pathway, leading to inhibition of prostaglandins. Topical and systemic NSAIDs are effective at treating ocular pain and may decrease unwanted sequelae of ocular inflammation such as glaucoma. Systemic absorption of topical NSAIDs is minimal, and they are commonly used with topical corticosteroid drops [42]. Caution should be used when administering systemic NSAIDs to patients with renal disease, coagulopathy, hypovolemia, hypotension, and gastrointestinal disease. Concomitant use with systemic corticosteroids should be avoided.

Anesthetic Management

All drugs and equipment needed for the anesthetic episode should be gathered and checked prior to use. This includes anesthetic induction drugs, NMBAs and reversal drugs as needed, monitoring equipment, and, if NMBAs are to be used, a peripheral nerve stimulator and mechanical ventilator.

Animals should be gently restrained for administration of premedication and for catheter placement and anesthetic induction. If struggling occurs or if excessive pressure around the neck (i.e., pressure on the jugular veins) is necessary, IOP will be increased. Administration of additional sedation is preferred in these cases.

Drug choices in patients that are not at risk for globe rupture and have normal IOP depend on a risk assessment based on the patient's systemic health status and any behavioral considerations. In animals with glaucoma, ocular foreign bodies, deep corneal ulcers, or partial prolapse of the vitreous, it is essential to prevent further increases in IOP, which may lead to loss of vision or globe rupture. Drugs that may cause vomiting or retching should be avoided in these patients, administered IV, or administered after anesthetic induction as mentioned in the preceding text (opioids, alpha-2-adrenergic receptor agonists in cats). The administration of antiemetics (e.g., maropitant) should be strongly considered prior to the sedation or administration of opioid analgesics.

Intravenous catheter placement in a hind limb will give the anesthetist better access for drug administration during surgery (Figure 12.3). Fluid administration set extensions can be used to facilitate access if a catheter is placed in a forelimb; however, drugs will take longer to enter the circulation. This may be problematic if emergency drugs need to be given; a small fluid bolus may be administered to ensure complete drug delivery to the patient. Intravenous anesthetic induction should be performed with the goal of smoothly and rapidly intubating the animal. Intubation should not be performed under a very light plane of anesthesia, as this is more likely to result in gagging and a short-lived increase in IOP.

During surgery, the anesthetist must focus on changes in heart rate and blood pressure as well as respiratory rate and pattern (if the patient is not being ventilated mechanically) as indicators of anesthetic depth. As the head is away from the anesthetist and covered with drapes, it is also important to be sure that the patient-to-breathing system connection is maintained. A deflated anesthetic breathing bag, a ventilator that cannot produce adequate peak inspiratory pressure, and a report of the smell of inhalant by the surgeon are all indicators that there is a circuit leak and intervention is required. An elbow connector between the patient and the breathing system is useful to facilitate surgical access to the patient and reduce the incidence of kinking of or drag on the endotracheal tube (Figure 12.7). Reinforced or guarded endotracheal tubes are available that, while expensive, are resistant to kinking.

During surgery, adequacy of ventilation, circulation, and oxygenation should be monitored. Capnography is an extremely useful tool to assess adequacy of ventilation during spontaneous as well as mechanical ventilation. It is also useful to help detect partial or complete disconnection of the endotracheal tube from the breathing system. Heart rate, blood pressure, and the electrocardiogram should be used to assess cardiovascular function. Pulse oximetry is useful to measure oxygenation. Probes placed on the tongue can easily become dislodged, leading to false alarms and erroneous readings. Pulse oximeter probes can be placed on the prepuce, vulva, skin folds, or toes as an alternative. If neuromuscular blockade is to be performed, a nerve stimulator should also be used to assess degree of blockade (see the section titled "Neuromuscular Blockade and Ventilation").

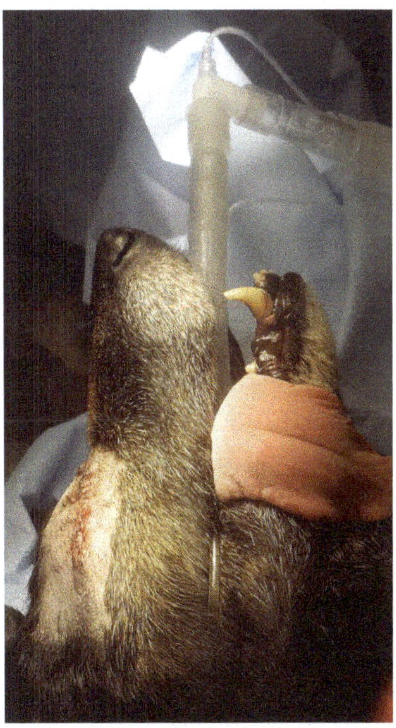

Figure 12.7 An elbow connector placed between the endotracheal tube and breathing system to reduce the likelihood that the endotracheal tube will become kinked.

Anesthetic Recovery

Patients should not be allowed to repeatedly gag on or make multiple attempts to cough out the endotracheal tube; the tube should be removed after the first reaction to prevent increases in IOP associated with coughing against a closed glottis. It is essential that both eyes be protected during recovery. If both eyes have been operated on, the patient should be recovered in sternal recumbency. Emergence delirium and excitement should be treated with sedation as needed, for example, acepromazine, dexmedetomidine, or, in the case of thrashing, propofol. Many animals will try to scratch at their eyes following surgery, and placement of an Elizabethan collar is often necessary to protect surgical incisions and the surface of the eye (Figure 12.8). Care must be taken not to increase IOP during restraint. It may be better to sedate a postsurgical ophthalmic patient rather than trying to perform physical restraint.

In cases where NMBAs have been administered, reversal should be administered prior to ending anesthesia, with the goal of the TOF to reach a T4/T1 ratio of at least 0.9 (see the section titled "Neuromuscular Blockade and Ventilation"). Patients should be observed closely to ensure adequate ventilation and oxygenation. If a patient begins to desaturate

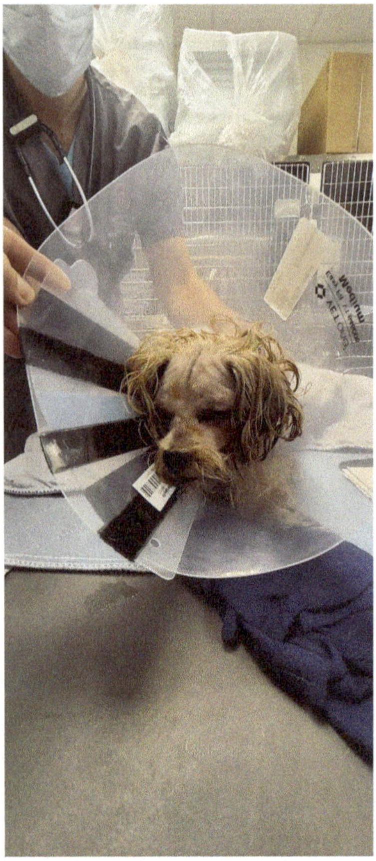

Figure 12.8 A patient in recovery following surgery to remove bilateral cataracts. The dog is in sternal recumbency and has an Elizabethan collar.

or appears to be dyspneic or cyanotic, supplemental oxygen should be provided until the cause is established and treated. Oxygen delivered via face mask may be useful in situations where the patient is no longer intubated, but a face mask should not be applied to an animal's face in a way that places undue pressure on the eyes. If the cause of the problem is not elicited, it may be necessary to reinduce anesthesia and reintubate the patient in order to maintain oxygenation. It may be necessary to administer an additional dose of neostigmine or edrophonium if residual neuromuscular blockade is suspected.

Postoperative Care

Comorbidities aside, an intravenous catheter should remain in place for several hours in cases of cataract surgery, in animals with glaucoma, in diabetic animals, and in cases where NMBAs have been used. In glaucoma patients and after cataract surgery, steps may need to be taken to reduce IOP, such as administering mannitol. Diabetic patients may need glucose supplementation or insulin administration until their normal routine is reestablished, and following the use of NMBAs, patients may require additional reversal.

References

1 Collins, B.K., Gross, M.E., Moore, C.P. et al. (1995). Physiologic, pharmacologic, and practical considerations for anesthesia of domestic animals with eye disease. *J. Am. Vet. Med. Assoc.* 207: 220–230.

2 Cunningham, A.J. and Barry, P. (1986). Intraocular pressure – physiology and implications for anaesthetic management. *Can. Anaesth. Soc. J.* 33: 195–208.

3 Keating, S.C.J., Sage, A.M., Ambrisko, T.D. et al. (2020). The effect of midazolam or lidocaine administration prior to etomidate induction of anesthesia on heart rate, arterial pressure, intraocular pressure and serum cortisol concentration in healthy dogs. *Vet. Anaesth. Analg.* 47: 160–167.

4 Panti, A., Cafrita, I.C., and Clark, L. (2016). Effect of intravenous lidocaine on cough response to endotracheal intubation in propofol-anaesthetized dogs. *Vet. Anaesth. Analg.* 43: 405–411.

5 Karadag, R., Sen, A., Golemez, H. et al. (2008). The effect of short-term hypobaric hypoxic exposure on intraocular pressure. *Curr. Eye. Res.* 33: 864–867.

6 Chahory, S., Clerc, B., Guez, J. et al. (2003). Intraocular pressure development after cataract surgery: a prospective study in 50

dogs (1998–2000). *Vet. Ophthalmol.* 6: 105–112.

7 Gross, M.E. and Pablo, L.S. (2015). Ophthalmic patients. In: *Lumb & Jones' Veterinary Anesthesia*, 5e (eds. K.A. Grimm, L.A. Lamont, W.J. Tranquilli, et al.), 963–982. Ames: Wiley.

8 Costa, D., Leiva, M., Moll, X. et al. (2015). Alfaxalone versus propofol in dogs: a randomised trial to assess effects on peri-induction tear production, intraocular pressure and globe position. *Vet. Rec.* 176: 73.

9 Bauer, B.S. and Ambros, B. (2016). The effects of intravenous alfaxalone with and without premedication on intraocular pressure in healthy dogs. *Can. J. Vet. Res.* 80: 156–161.

10 Ludders, J.W. and Heavner, J.E. (1979). Effect of atropine on tear formation in anesthetized dogs. *J. Am. Vet. Med. Assoc.* 175: 585–586.

11 Hollingsworth, S.R., Canton, D.D., Buyukmichi, N.C. et al. (1992). Effect of topically administered atropine on tear production in dogs. *J. Am. Vet. Med. Assoc.* 200: 1481–1484.

12 Herring, I.P., Pickett, J.P., Champagne, E.S. et al. (2000). Evaluation of aqueous tear production in dogs following general anesthesia. *J. Am. Anim. Hosp. Assoc.* 36: 427–430.

13 Shepard, M.K., Accola, P.J., Lopez, L.A. et al. (2011). Effect of duration and type of anesthetic on tear production in dogs. *Am. J. Vet. Res.* 72: 608–612.

14 Mouney, M.C., Accola, P.J., Cremer, J. et al. (2011). Effects of acepromazine maleate or morphine on tear production before, during, and after sevoflurane anesthesia in dogs. *Am. J. Vet. Res.* 72: 1427–1430.

15 Ghaffari, M.S., Malmasi, A., and Bokaie, S. (2010). Effect of acepromazine or xylazine on tear production as measured by Schirmer tear test in normal cats. *Vet. Ophthalmol.* 13: 1–3.

16 Chandler, J.A., van der Woerdt, A., Prittie, J.E. et al. (2013). Preliminary evaluation of tear production in dogs hospitalized in an intensive care unit. *J. Vet. Emerg. Crit. Care* 23: 274–279.

17 Peche, N., Köstlin, R., Reese, S. et al. (2015). Postanesthetic tear production and ocular irritation in cats. *Tierarztl. Prax. K. Kleintiere Heimtiere* 43: 75–82. (Abstract in English, article in German).

18 Di Pietro, S., Macrì, F., Bonarrigo, T. et al. (2016). Effects of a medetomidine-ketamine combination on Schirmer tear test I results of clinically normal cats. *Am. J. Vet. Res.* 77: 310–314.

19 Blanc, V.F., Hardy, J.F., Milot, J. et al. (1983). The oculocardiac reflex, a graphical and statistical analysis in infants and children. *Can. Anaesth. Soc. J.* 30: 360–369.

20 Vézina-Audette, R., Steagall, P.V.M., and Gianotti, G. Prevalence of and covariates associated with the oculocardiac reflex occurring in dogs during enucleation. *J. Am. Vet. Med. Assoc.* 255: 454–458.

21 Pascoe, P.J., Ilkiw, J.E., Stiles, J. et al. (1994). Arterial hypertension associated with topical ocular use of phenylephrine in dogs. *J. Am. Vet. Med. Assoc.* 205: 1562–1564.

22 Rose, R.J. and Carter, J. (1979). Some physiological and biochemical effects of acetazolamide in the dog. *J. Vet. Pharmacol. Ther.* 2: 215–221.

23 Gilroy, B.A. (1986). Intraocular and cardiopulmonary effects of low-dose mannitol in the dog. *Vet. Surg.* 15: 342–344.

24 Glaze, M.B., Crawford, M.A., Nachreiner, T.F. et al. (1988). Ophthalmic corticosteroid therapy: systemic effects in the dog. *J. Am. Vet. Med. Assoc.* 192: 73–75.

25 Chua, W.H., Balakrishnan, V., Chan, Y.H. et al. (2006). Atropine for the treatment of childhood myopia. *Ophthalmol.* 113: 2285–2291.

26 Moitra, V.K. (2015). Drugs that alter glucose regulation. In: *Stoelting's Anesthesia and co-Existing Disease*, 5e (eds. P. Flood, J.P. Rathmell and S. Shafer), 748–754. Philadelphia: Wolters Kluwer Health.

27 Tanaka, K., Kawano, T., Tomino, T. et al. (2009). Mechanisms of impaired glucose tolerance and insulin secretion during isoflurane anesthesia. *Anesthesiol.* 111: 1044–1051.

28 Brull, S.J. and Meistelman, C. (2020). Pharmacology of neuromuscular blocking drugs. In: *Miller's Anesthesia* (eds. M.A. Gropper, R.D. Miller, N.H. Cohen, et al.), 792–831. Philadelphia: Elsevier.

29 Naguib, M., Brull, S.J., Kopman, A.F. et al. (2018). Consensus statement on perioperative use of neuromuscular monitoring. *Anesth. Analg.* 127: 71–80.

30 Belmonte, C. and Tervo, T.T. (2013). Pain in and around the eye. In: *Wall and Melzack's Textbook of Pain*, 6e (eds. S.B. McMahon, M. Koltzenburg, I. Tracey and D.C. Turk), 843–860. Philadelphia: Elsevier, Saunders.

31 Swaminathan, A., Otterness, K., Milne, K. et al. (2015). The safety of topical anesthetics in the treatment of corneal abrasions: a review. *J. Emerg. Med.* 49: 810–815.

32 Gerding, P.A., Turner, T.L., Hamor, R.E. et al. (2004). Effects of intracameral injection of preservative-free lidocaine on the anterior segment of the eyes in dogs. *Am. J. Vet. Res.* 65: 1325–1330.

33 Smith, L.J., Bentley, E., Shih, A. et al. (2004). Systemic lidocaine infusion as an analgesic for intraocular surgery in dogs: a pilot study. *Vet. Anaes. Analg.* 31: 53–63.

34 Bartholomew, K.J., Smith, L.J., Bentley, E. et al. Retrospective analysis of complications associated with retrobulbar bupivacaine in dogs undergoing enucleation surgery. *Vet. Anesth. Anlag.* 47: 588–594.

35 Watagatsuma, J.T., Deschk, M., Floriano, B.P. et al. (2014). Comparison of anesthetic efficacy and adverse effects associated with peribulbar injection of ropivacaine performed with and without ultrasound guidance in dogs. *Am. J. Vet. Res.* 75: 1040–1048.

36 Ahn, J.S., Jeong, M.B., Park, Y.W. et al. (2013). Comparison of systemic atracurium, retrobulbar lidocaine, and sub-Tenon's lidocaine injections in akinesia and mydriasis in dogs. *Vet. J.* 196: 103–108.

37 Park, S.A., Lee, I., Lee, L. et al. (2009). Combination auriculopalpebral nerve block and local anesthesia for placement of a nictitating membrane-to-superotemporal bulbar conjunctival flap in dogs. *J. Anim. Hosp. Assoc.* 45: 164–167.

38 Shilo-Benjamini, Y. (2019). Review of ophthalmic local and regional anesthesia in dogs and cats. *Vet. Anaesth. Analg.* 46: 14–27.

39 Stiles, J., Honda, C.N., Krohne, S.G. et al. (2003). Effect of topical administration of 1% morphine sulfate solution on signs of pain and corneal wound healing in dogs. *Am. J. Vet. Res.* 64: 813–818.

40 Hay Kraus, B.L. (2013). Efficacy of maropitant in preventing vomiting in dogs premedicated with hydromorphone. *Vet. Anaesth. Analg.* 40: 28–34.

41 Tamura, E.Y., Barros, P.S., Cortopassi, S.R. et al. (2002). Effects of two preanesthetic regimens for ophthalmic surgery on intraocular pressure and cardiovascular measurements in dogs. *Vet. Ther.* 3: 81–87.

42 Giuliano, E.A. (2004). Nonsteroidal anti-inflammatory drugs in veterinary ophthalmology. *Vet. Clin. North Am. Small Anim. Pract.* 34: 707–723.

13

Oral and Maxillofacial Disorders

Christopher J. Snyder and Jason W. Soukup

Department of Surgical Sciences, School of Veterinary Medicine, University of Wisconsin–Madison, Madison, WI, 53706, USA

Introduction

The prevalence of periodontal disease is reported to impact 30–80% of dogs and cats older than 3 years [1–4]. In addition, oral diseases are among the most common diagnoses made in small-animal general practices [2]. Proper control and minimization of periodontal disease potentially reduces periodontal-disease-related bacteremia [5, 6] and systemic inflammatory factors (C-reactive protein) [7], both of which may serve as risk factors for other systemic disorders. An association between periodontal disease and histologic changes in renal, hepatic, and the myocardial tissue has been proposed [8]. These changes could theoretically be linked to abnormal organ function, changes in anesthetic drug metabolism, and reduced drug effectiveness. In addition, the chronic pain and inflammation associated with periodontal disease can negatively impact an animal's quality of life and their ability to heal.

Non-anesthesia dental (NAD) procedures are dental techniques performed on conscious dogs and cats. Currently there is a lack of peer-reviewed literature supporting that NAD procedures are safe or are as effective as anesthetized cleanings and oral examinations [9]. NAD procedures do not allow subgingival cleaning, periodontal probing, or radiographic evaluation. Performing dental procedures in this manner puts both the pet and operator at risk of being bitten or injured by sharp instruments. The American Veterinary Dental College [10], American College of Veterinary Anesthesia and Analgesia [11], and American Animal Hospital Association [12] all have positions or policy statements against NAD procedures. Without general anesthesia, a thorough and complete oral examination cannot be performed, and intraoral radiographs cannot be taken. Safe and judicious use of sedatives and anesthetics is necessary to facilitate appropriate assessment, diagnostics, and treatment of patients.

Fundamentally, periodontal disease itself will not directly affect sedative and anesthetic drug metabolism. However, chronic pain and inflammation associated with periodontal disease or other oral conditions may result in "wind-up" pain. These patients may exhibit signs of central or peripheral nervous system sensitization and may require a higher analgesic dosing with multimodal analgesics owing to their heightened state of sensitivity. The severity or chronicity of oral disease may also impact the effectiveness of local anesthetic drugs due to the pathologic changes such as

Canine and Feline Anesthesia and Co-Existing Disease, Second Edition. Edited by Rebecca A. Johnson, Lindsey B. C. Snyder and Carrie A. Schroeder.

Companion website: www.wiley.com/go/johnson/canine

acidic pH of inflamed tissues altering uptake and action of these drugs.

Locoregional Anesthetic/ Analgesic Agents

A variety of drugs are used in local and regional anesthesia for procedures involving the oral cavity. Appropriately placed regional anesthetic blocks in the oral cavity have been shown to reduce the amount of inhalant anesthetic by as much as 23% [13]. Of the sodium channel blockers used in local and regional anesthesia, the amide family of drugs, which includes lidocaine and bupivacaine, is the most common. Toxic or maximum doses should always be considered when deciding how much local anesthetic to administer [14].

There has been a trend in the anesthesia and pain management of human patients to combine drugs with differing mechanisms of action to enhance or prolong the anesthetic or analgesic potential of local or regional blocks. The addition of opioids and alpha-2-adrenergic receptor agonists with a local anesthetic appears to demonstrate the best potential for enhancing pain relief. For example, chronic nociceptive stimulation results in the upregulation of mu-opioid receptors in the peripheral nervous system [15]. In human patients, mixing an opioid with the local anesthetic extends the duration of postoperative analgesia [16, 17]. Although not statistically significant, one study in dogs suggests that buprenorphine mixed with local anesthetic in regional dental blocks may extend the block duration over bupivacaine alone [18]. Clinically, buprenorphine mixed with the local anesthetic and administered in local and regional blocks may be used. The use of alpha-2-adrenergic receptor agonists, such as dexmedetomidine, combined with local anesthetics or administered as a local anesthetic may also benefit patients [19]. When alpha-2-adrenergic receptor agonists are used as a local anesthetic in humans, pain management occurs at the local level without evidence of hemodynamic side effects from systemic absorption [20]. More chronic conditions may have the additional recruitment of peripheral mu receptors [21] and, therefore, benefit the most from synergy between the locally administered opioid, alpha-2-adrenergic receptor agonists, and local anesthetics. The combination of epinephrine and a local anesthetic is commercially available and may improve the local anesthetic duration due to vasoconstrictive effects slowing tissue clearance of the local anesthetic, as well as epinephrine demonstrating primary antinociceptive activity [19].

While a longer local anesthetic duration may be desirable in many situations to encourage a smooth recovery and extend surgical site anesthesia, the presence of intraoral sutures and lack of sensation at a maxillary surgery site may result in complications with healing. In maxillary procedures, such as resections or oronasal fistula repair, excessive tongue pressure against the surgery site may be disadvantageous and the use of longer-acting local anesthetics may be undesirable. In theory, since the surgical site is blocked by local anesthetics, and the tongue that maintains sensation can feel the sutures, the animal may be preoccupied with the abnormal feeling of foreign material in the oral cavity. The tongue may continue to rub and/or put pressure on the surgical site longer when long-acting local anesthetics are used, potentially increasing the risk of surgical closure dehiscence to a greater degree than with short-acting local anesthetics. In particular, in major oral surgery cases with associated chronic discomfort, the addition of buprenorphine to a short-acting local anesthetic may improve analgesia through the interaction with peripheral mu receptors while not prolonging local anesthesia [15]. In major oral surgery where postoperative pain management with regional anesthesia is desirable, surgical disruption of the normal anatomy may be so extensive that reliable and predictable delivery of regional anesthetic nerve blocks is not possible. A recently available formulation of bupivacaine liposome injectable suspension is available and designed to provide postoperative pain relief for 72 h when infiltrated into surgical site tissues [22]. Further data are needed to determine whether this drug delivers safe and effective pain management when delivered as a peripheral nerve block for dental procedures [23].

Locoregional Agent Administration

Regional and local anesthetic use in humans is widely accepted as beneficial. Complications associated with inferior alveolar nerve blocks, including prolonged paresthesia or paralysis, have been reported to occur in 0.00013–0.01% of human dental patients [24]. Local and regional anesthesia in humans permits procedures including extraction and root canal therapy to be performed on an outpatient basis. One potential complication that generates much anxiety among veterinarians is inadvertent anesthesia of the tongue and subsequent patient responses to the anesthetized tongue during recovery. However, peripheral nerve paresthesia and subsequent self-mutilation involving the tongue of both veterinary and human patients are only anecdotally reported.

Injection and placement of local anesthetic may cause physiologic responses, even in the anesthetized patient, because many commercial products have an acidic pH. If an increase in heart rate, respiratory rate, or physical reaction is present, this may be loosely interpreted as confirmation that the local anesthetic has been administered in the correct location. However, the absence of a reaction does not correlate to the local anesthetic being placed in the incorrect location, as the patient may be in a deep anesthetic plane that renders them unresponsive.

When considering needle placement and injection, some resources recommend needle bevel placement in a particular orientation when performing nerve blocks with local anesthetics. With accurate placement approximated to the target nerve, bevel direction may be less important. Placing the local anesthetic in areas over the periosteum adjacent to the foramen out of which the nerve emerges will help to distribute the anesthetic once the needle is removed and digital pressure is applied. A variety of different needle types have been used in human patients with varying results. Standard short bevel needles used in veterinary patients are sufficient for placing regional dental and oral surgical blocks. Once the needle penetrates mucosa, it should be advanced slowly to minimize the risk of nerve or vessel penetration. However, unless the vessel or nerve is confined, the neurovascular structures should be displaced by the bevel rather than penetrated [25]. Some resources advocate the use of very-small-gauge needles. Although the physical tissue injury would be much smaller, human anesthesiologists exerted more digital plunger pressure during local anesthetic injection than they realized, translating to faster velocity and greater tissue injury with a smaller-gauge needle [25]. With the small volumes used in the administration of veterinary dental blocks, 25- to 27-gauge, $1\text{–}1^{1}/_{2}$-in. needles are commonly used in canine and feline patients undergoing oral surgery to minimize this trauma.

A wide variety of local anesthetic dosage volumes for dental patients have been reported in the literature without substantial evaluation of these volumes versus clinical effectiveness or duration of action. Dye perfusion studies have reported use of volumes in cadavers ranging from 0.4 ml (inferior alveolar block) to volumes of 1–3 ml [26] for a maxillary block using the modified infraorbital approach (through the infraorbital canal described in the following text) [27]. Delivering small volumes with accurate placement to achieve clinical effect may minimize the risk for accidental anesthesia of unintended structures such as the tongue.

When performing local or regional anesthetic blocks, aspirating ("drawing back") negative pressure to avoid intravascular delivery is essential. Because of the beveled orientation of the needle tip, spinning the syringe barrel 90° along the long access and reaspirating should, at some point, draw the bevel off the vessel wall and result in blood drawn into the syringe if it is intravascular. If blood is drawn into the syringe, advance the needle slightly forward or backward and reaspirate. If repeated attempts result in aspiration of blood, remove the needle and try positioning it again. Medication should be administered with the needle placed on the periosteum for the middle mental and caudal mandibular blocks. Even if the bevel is not directly over the nerve, by injecting on the periosteum, the local anesthetic will cover more surface area and increase the chance that the nerve will be contacted. Once the local anesthetic has been administered, the needle should be withdrawn and digital pressure applied for 1 min to provide adequate time for prevention of hematoma formation. Injection should not be continued as the needle is withdrawn because inadvertent intravascular injection may result if the vessel was perforated during needle placement.

Commonly reported local anesthetics used for nerve blocks include lidocaine, bupivacaine, lidocaine/bupivacaine combinations, ropivacaine, mepivacaine, and combinations including epinephrine. Bupivacaine and lidocaine appear to be the most frequently reported local anesthetics used in dentistry and oral surgery patients with ropivacaine being a commonly used substitute for bupivacaine. Some variability exists regarding the reported time to onset and duration of activity of these medications; however, general expectations regarding onset of action and duration of action are illustrated in Table 13.1. Because the total maximum dose varies between bupivacaine and lidocaine, careful calculations must be made before mixing these medications. Mixing lidocaine with bupivacaine for infraorbital blocks in dogs showed an increased duration of activity as compared to lidocaine alone [29]. However, onset times were not specifically evaluated and the duration of action of bupivacaine only was not reported. Some pharmacists caution the mixing of lidocaine with bupivacaine fearing that the solution pH and pKa will render the bupivacaine partially unavailable. Any potential shorter duration of onset for anesthesia with lidocaine should be carefully weighed against decreased duration of effectiveness of bupivacaine if this mixture is going to be used.

Bupivacaine or ropivacaine are commonly used in local and regional anesthesia for patients undergoing oral surgery because they have a longer duration of activity than lidocaine [28, 30]. The use of bupivacaine provides ample time to deliver oral systemic pain medications before the local anesthetic wears off. Bupivacaine's 6–10 min onset of action is considered intermediate. The duration of action may reach 4–6 h when placed in areas predominately involving soft tissue or 6–8 h when placed in a foramen [30]. Whichever drug is chosen, careful attention should be made to the drug concentration listed on the bottle, as bupivacaine is available in many concentrations including 0.25%, 0.5%, and 0.75% solutions.

Maxillofacial Locoregional Techniques

When performing the middle mental or major palatine nerve blocks, the needle should not be threaded into the foramen. Placing the needle into the foramina risks transecting or lacerating the nerve. Krug and Losey (2011) reported that the actual penetration of the local anesthetic medication into the middle mental foramen was questioned, as well as its clinical effectiveness [31]. Thus, innervation to the teeth, oral cavity soft and hard tissues, and soft tissues of the face may be an intricate assortment of contributions from branches of multiple cranial nerves [31]. Because few measures of clinical areas of desensitization exist in veterinary patients, regional anesthetic blocks should be administered as a component of multimodal pain management, not a sole source of anesthesia and pain management.

Table 13.1 Local anesthetic drugs.

Drug	Lidocaine	Bupivacaine	Ropivacaine
Time to onset	1–2 min	6–10 min	5–10 min
Duration of activity	1.5–2 h	4–10 h	3–8 h
Total maximum dosages	5 mg kg^{-1} (dog); 1 mg kg^{-1} (cat)	2 mg kg^{-1} (dogs and cats)	3 mg kg^{-1} (dogs) [28]

Table 13.2 Anatomic coverage associated with specific nerve blocks.

Anesthetic block location	Anatomy covered
Dental	
Intraosseous	Tooth-specific—periodontal ligament, alveolar bone, gingiva, mucosa, and pulp
Intraligamentary	Tooth-specific—periodontal ligament, gingiva, and pulp
Mandible	
Caudal mandibular (inferior alveolar)	I1–M3, lower lip from the caudal mental foramen rostral
Middle mental	I1–PM2, lower lip from middle mental foramen rostral
Maxilla	
Caudal maxillary	I1–M2, palatal mucosa, upper lip from infraorbital canal rostral
Infraorbital	I1–PM3, upper lip from infraorbital canal rostral
Major palatine	Ipsilateral palatal mucosa

I, incisor; M, molar; PM, premolar.

In cases where surgical manipulation will approach midline, as in extracting the first or second incisors or biopsy near the palatal midline, consideration should be given to the potential for crossover innervation to occur [32, 33]. Likewise, one should also consider the surgical manipulation associated not only with extraction, but also with closure. In addition, patients may not be adequately anesthetized by an infraorbital regional block when palatal tissues are undermined during extraction of canine or premolar teeth. In most situations, the caudal maxillary block or inferior alveolar blocks may provide more complete regional anesthesia (Table 13.2).

Intraosseous and intraligamentary anesthesia techniques have been described (Table 13.2) [34, 35]. Veterinary patients commonly require multiple intraoral procedures to be performed. Rather than multiple intraligamentary or intraosseous anesthetic blocks for adequate regional anesthesia, a single regional anesthetic injection may anesthetize an entire quadrant of the mouth. Local anesthetic administration using intraligamentary or intraosseous techniques may successfully anesthetize focal areas of the mouth, but may require the use of specialized needles and injection ports [34]. These blocks are performed by placing the needle into the intraligamentary space in several areas around the affected tooth. This technique targets the sensory fibers of the tooth's pulp. Very small volumes of local anesthetic are used in both intraosseous and intraligamentary local anesthesia.

Specific Regional and Local Blocks

Intraligamentary and Intraosseous Blocks

Intraligamentary and intraosseous local anesthetic blocks provide the most focal form of local anesthesia. These techniques are not performed as commonly in veterinary medicine because they often require the use of special syringes, needles, and dosing cartridges.

However, veterinary dental patients often have multiple locations within the oral cavity and within the same quadrant where a single regional block will provide anesthesia. The effectiveness of a local block of a specific tooth may be difficult to assess in veterinary patients; these techniques may be more appropriate to address pulpal innervation, an assessment not commonly performed in general practice. As opposed to regional anesthetic blocks, local anesthetic techniques may be less effective at providing anesthesia when soft tissue flaps are created, and osteotomies are performed to facilitate tooth removal. The periodontal ligament space and root anatomy may also offer challenges, as the density of alveolar bone is greater in veterinary patients than it is in humans [35].

Intraligamentary injections are performed by injecting 0.2 ml of local anesthetic per root at various locations around the root surface into the periodontal ligament space (Figure 13.1). A special dosing syringe is necessary, and, in cases of severe periodontal disease, the pH of the inflamed environment may decrease the lipophilicity and efficacy of the anesthetic. Intraosseous anesthetic delivery requires an intraosseous delivery needle, which is inserted into the interproximal bone for anesthetic delivery. A unique injection port remains in place for additional anesthetic delivery [35].

Infraorbital Block

The infraorbital block is performed by administering the local anesthetic within the infraorbital canal. Signal transmission is blocked at the level of the infraorbital nerve. Ramifications in the floor of the infraorbital canal course through the alveolar bone and are responsible for innervating the ipsilateral maxillary incisors, canine tooth, first, second, and third premolar teeth, buccal mucosa, portions of the ipsilateral lip, and soft tissues of the rostral cheek (Figure 13.2). Local anesthetic placement in this location may not reliably anesthetize the palatal mucosa and fourth premolar tooth, and may not completely anesthetize the central incisors because of crossover innervation. Small volume delivery with accurate placement may be best to achieve clinical effect with dosing varying from 0.1 mL in small dogs and cats up to 0.5 ml in large-breed dogs.

The upper lip should be reflected dorsally and the neurovascular bundle digitally palpated. The infraorbital canal and neurovascular bundle should be palpable at the level of the maxillary third premolar distal root. After palpating these structures, the needle can be

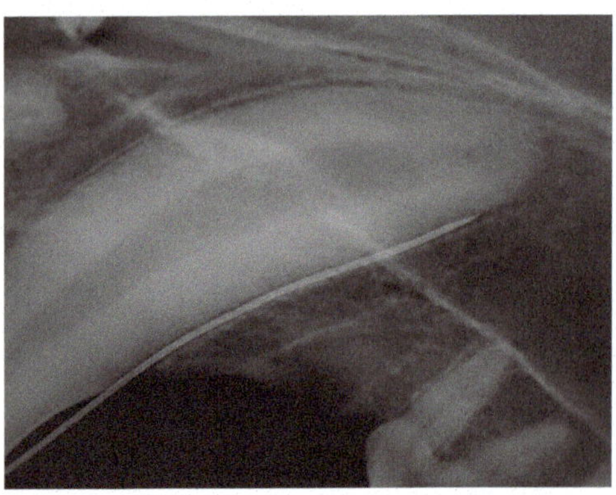

Figure 13.1 Intraligamentary local anesthetic delivery utilizes a small-gauge flexible needle that is threaded into the periodontal ligament space. Source: Image courtesy of Thoulton W. Surgeon, DVM, FAVD, DAVDC.

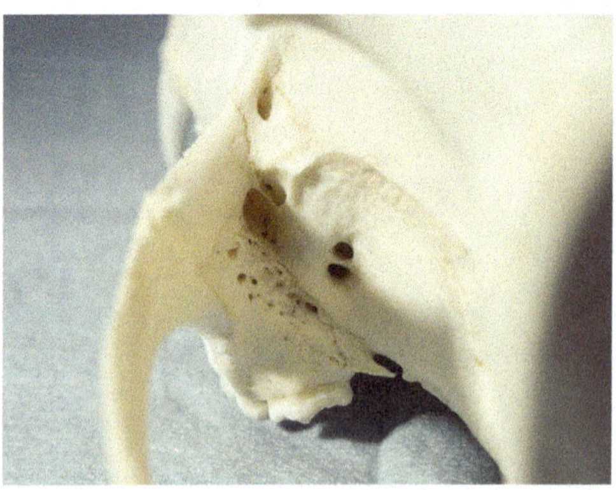

Figure 13.2 Ramifications in the floor of the infraorbital canal provide the canals for neurovascular supply to the apices of the maxillary teeth. Placement of the infraorbital regional anesthetic block provides sodium channel blockade of the nerves at this level.

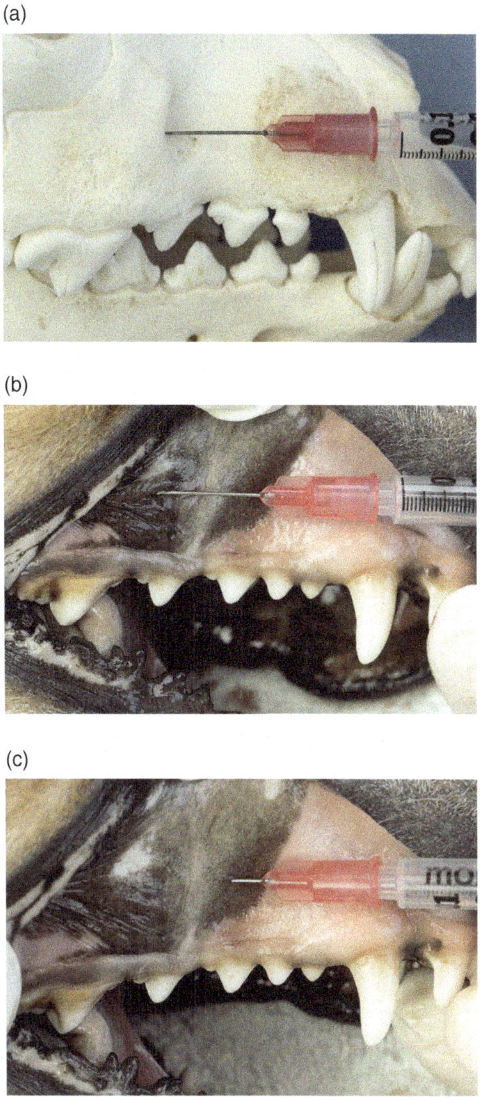

Figure 13.3 (a) The infraorbital artery/vein/nerve can be palpated emerging immediately dorsal to the mesial roots of the fourth premolar and distal root of the third premolar in dogs (Note: This patient has a supernumery first premolar tooth). The vessel can be isolated through digital palpation and digitally retracted in large-breed dogs. (b) The needle bevel should enter mucosa several millimeters rostral to the canal opening/neurovascular bundle to permit the needle to be redirected into the canal opening. (c) The needle should be advanced far enough to ensure intracanal placement. Note that the needle and syringe are parallel to the hard palate.

inserted through the mucosa and directed along the neurovascular bundle and into the canal (Figures 13.3 and 13.4). To reduce traumatizing the globe, maintain the syringe parallel to the hard palate. Once the needle is advanced through soft tissues to the infraorbital canal opening, it is important to aspirate with the syringe in order to ensure the needle bevel is not intravascular. Digital pressure should be applied for 1 min after withdrawal of the needle to prevent leakage of the local anesthetic and reduce the likelihood for hematoma development as a result of inadvertent vessel puncture.

Caudal Maxillary Block

Proper placement of the caudal maxillary nerve block will anesthetize the maxillary teeth in the ipsilateral quadrant, lip, hard/soft palatal mucosa, and buccal soft tissues. While ultrasound-guided techniques provide accurate and precise local anesthetic placement at the level of the trigeminal nerve for major caudal maxillectomy procedures, conventional anatomic landmark-based delivery of local anesthetics commonly occurs in practice [36]. By guiding the needle through the infraorbital canal and into the suborbital soft tissues, the needle tip should approximate the course of the maxillary branch of the facial nerve at the level of the sphenopalatine nerve (Figure 13.5). The local anesthetic should be administered when the needle tip has been advanced to a point immediately caudal to the last molar tooth (Figure 13.6). Successful block in large-breed dogs may require the use of a 3-in. spinal needle, although 1½-in. needle length typically provides adequate clinical effect (Figure 13.7). It may help to overlie the needle on the mucosa prior to placement to predetermine the depth of necessary needle advancement into the canal for the needle tip to be located at the last molar tooth. Other variations to this technique have been described elsewhere [35]. By using the infraorbital canal to direct needle placement, the natural anatomy is used to guide proper placement of the local anesthetic.

Needle placement and orientation are identical to the infraorbital nerve block except that

(a)

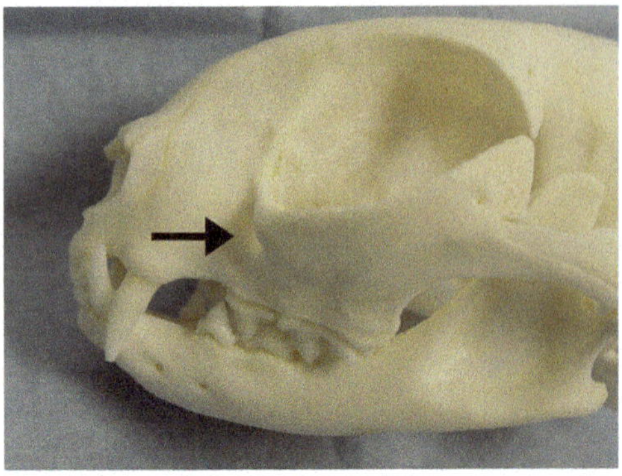

(b)

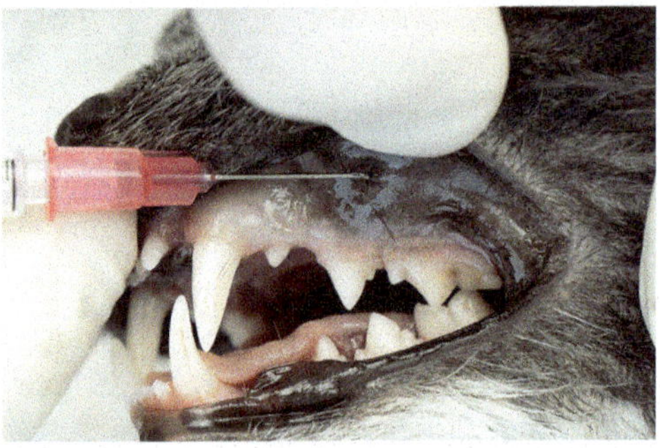

(c)

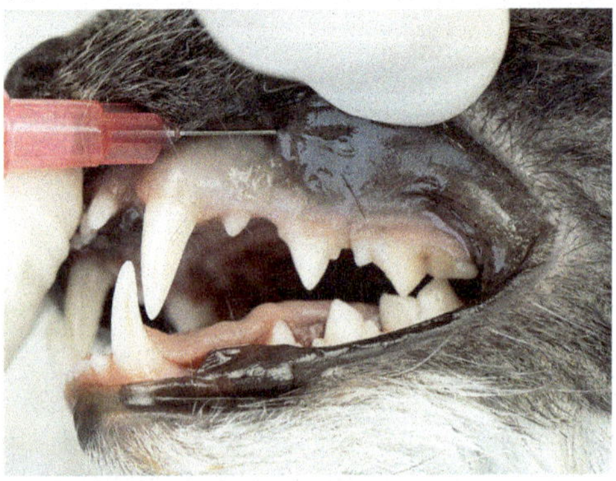

Figure 13.4 (a) The infraorbital canal in the feline rests 4–6 mm ventral from the medial canthus of the orbital rim and apical to the maxillary third premolar. (b) Needle placement should take place immediately rostral to the third premolar to permit redirection of needle into the infraorbital canal and location can be approximated by overlaying the needle on top of mucosa. (c). Needle penetration through mucosa can take place several millimeters in front of where the needle tip should end, and care should be taken to ensure that the syringe and needle are maintained parallel to the hard palate.

(a)

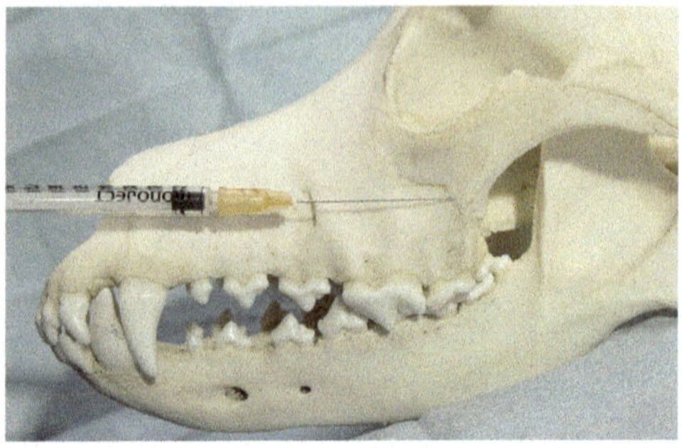

(b)

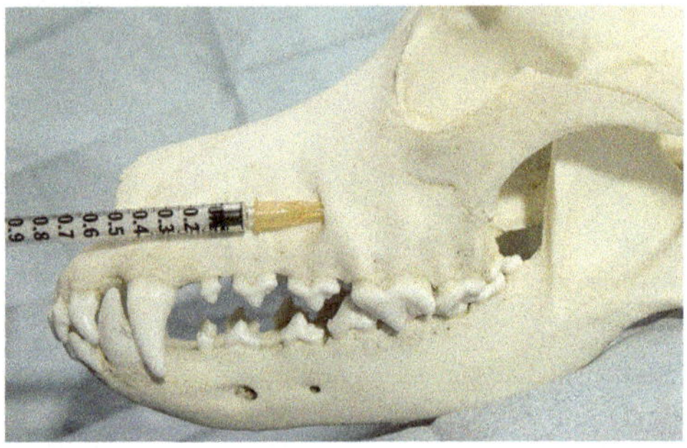

(c)

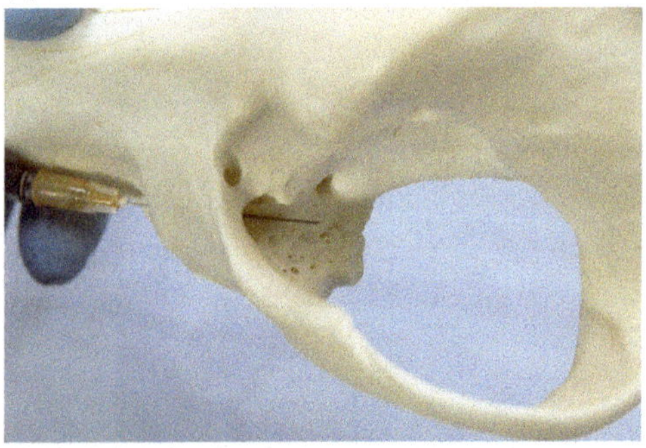

Figure 13.5 (a) Needle length can be evaluated by laying the needle along the alveolar mucosa and palpating the caudal aspect of the maxillary bone in dogs. (b) Advancement of the needle through the infraorbital canal and maintaining the parallel position to the roof of the mouth will direct the needle bevel toward the maxillary branch of the trigeminal nerve. (c) Placing the block in this location will also block transmission of the major palatine nerve responsible for innervation of the palate.

the needle is guided through the infraorbital canal. Care should be taken to maintain the needle parallel with the hard palate to reduce the risk of inadvertent globe penetration. This

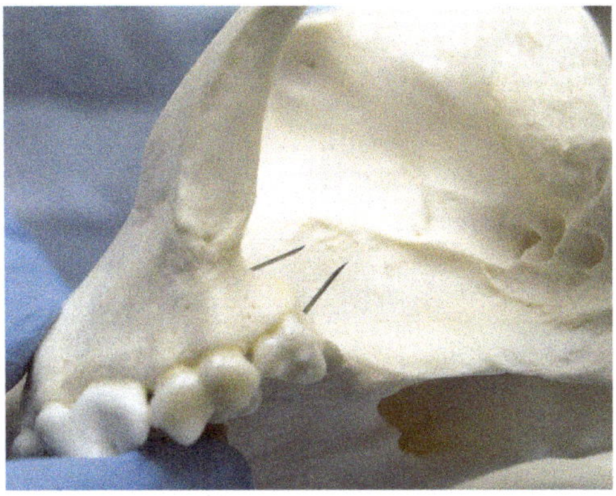

Figure 13.6 This image demonstrates the convergent nature of the infraorbital canal and major palatine foramen by placing needles through each foramen. By advancing the local block needle caudally through the infraorbital canal, a single regional block can be placed that will anesthetize both the infraorbital branch of the maxillary nerve and the major palatine branch of the maxillary nerve. Owing to the small size of the foramen, needles should not be advanced through the major palatine foramen.

regional nerve block is not recommended in buphthalmic or severely enophthalmic patients due to increased risk for globe penetration, and particular attention should be paid when performing this block in brachycephalic dogs and cats due to the shortened length of the infraorbital canal and increased risk for the needle to be misdirected and resulting in damage to the globe (Figure 13.8).

Major Palatine Block

The major palatine nerve is responsible for sensation of the palatal mucosa. This regional block may be used in conjunction with the infraorbital nerve block for desensitization of the ipsilateral teeth from the incisors to the third premolar. Solely, the major palatine block may provide complete coverage for biopsies of the palatal mucosa. In most clinical situations, performing a caudal maxillary block will desensitize the palatal mucosa, as well as the teeth and soft tissues on the ipsilateral side of the oral cavity, and the major palatine block is not needed.

(a)

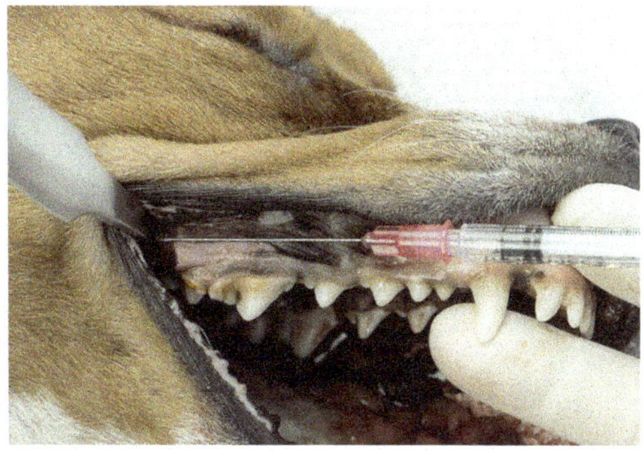

(b)

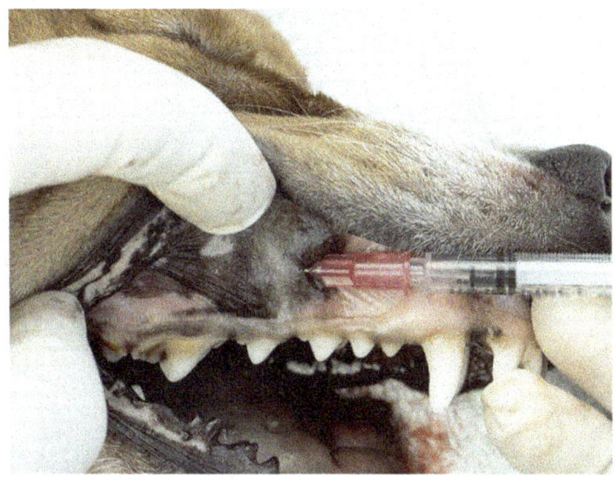

Figure 13.7 (a) It may be helpful to overlie the needle on mucosa in the location of the infraorbital canal to gauge the depth necessary to advance the needle (Note: This patient has a supernumery first premolar tooth). (b) In medium-sized and large-sized dogs, even the $1^1/_2$-in. needles will be inserted to approximately the hub. The caudal maxillary block is performed by threading the needle through the infraorbital canal and keeping the needle parallel with the hard palate. Note that this dog has a supernumerary first premolar tooth and that the landmark for the infraorbital canal is dorsal to the maxillary third premolar tooth.

The major palatine foramen rests between the palatal midline and the medial (palatal) aspect of the dentition. Because of anatomic variation, the foramen will be located between the mesial aspect of the first molar tooth and mesial aspect of the fourth premolar tooth, and variation may also exist between the right and left sides of the same patient (Figure 13.9). To ensure effective delivery as the nerve courses rostrally, the local anesthetic should be deposited closer to the rostral extent of these

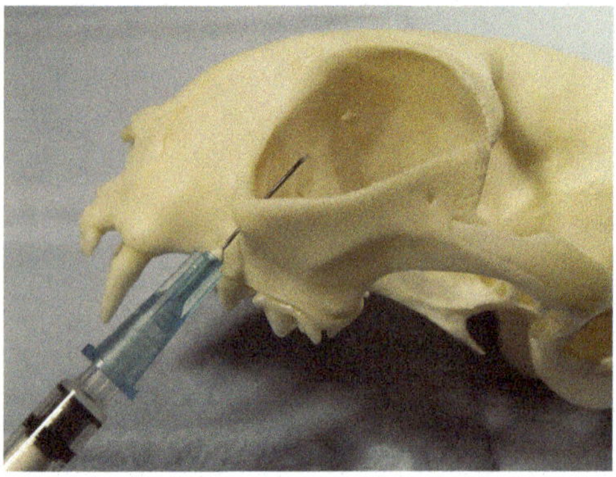

Figure 13.8 Brachycephalic canine and feline skull shapes have a short infraorbital canal. The shortened canal minimizes the natural restriction by the canal to prevent deflection of the needle toward the globe. Orienting the needle and syringe in this direction risks iatrogenic trauma to the globe.

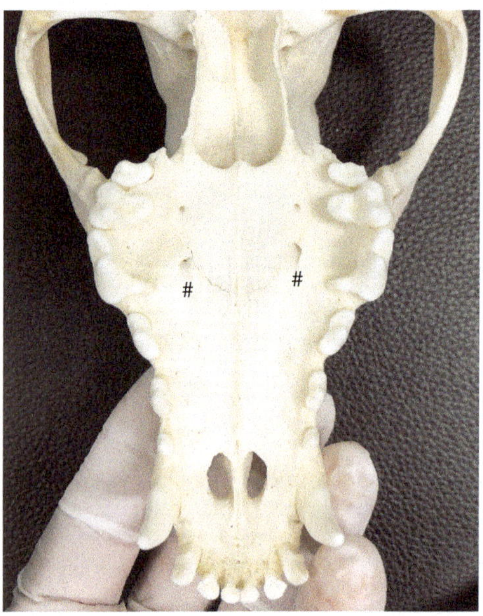

Figure 13.9 The major palatine foramina (#). The major palatine nerve is responsible for sensation associated with the palatal mucosa. Note the anatomic variation in the rostrocaudal direction of the right and left major palatine foramina within the same skull.

landmarks (Figure 13.10). Efforts to isolate and thread the needle into the major palatine foramen should be avoided to prevent nerve injury. In addition, directing the needle at a 45° angle to the palate and penetrating the palatal

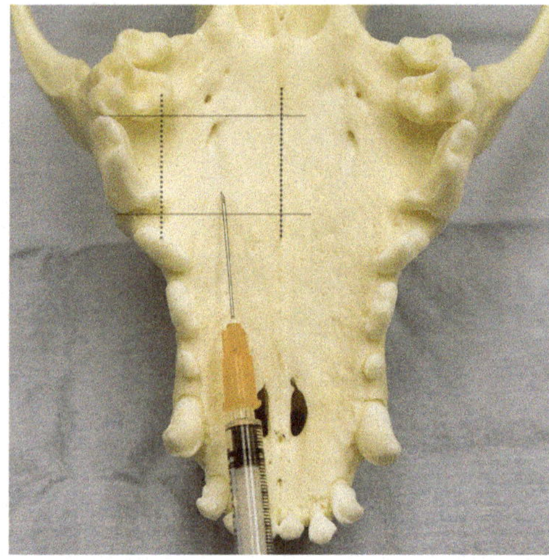

Figure 13.10 The dashed lines represent palatal midline and the palatal edge of the fourth premolar and first molar teeth. The solid lines represent the rostral and distal most landmarks between which the major palatine foramen lies. Placement of local anesthetic should err toward the rostral edge of this area to ensure that the major palatine nerve courses through the local anesthetic.

mucosa one to two rugal folds rostral from the desired location of local placement may help to avoid local anesthetic leakage immediately after withdrawal (Figure 13.11). By placing the local anesthetic against periosteum, the local anesthetic will disperse along tissue planes and, potentially, improve the likelihood of effective delivery of the local anesthetic.

Middle Mental Block

Ventral to the mesial root of the second premolar lies the middle mental foramen (Figure 13.12). The foramen is centered between the ventral cortex and the alveolar crest. A branch of the inferior alveolar nerve emerges through the middle mental foramen and is responsible for innervation of the ipsilateral rostral lip, mandibular incisors, and the first and second premolar teeth.

The needle should enter the rostral aspect of the labial frenulum and travel along the periosteum, directed toward the mesial root of the second premolar (Figure 13.13). Directing the needle through the labial frenulum allows for

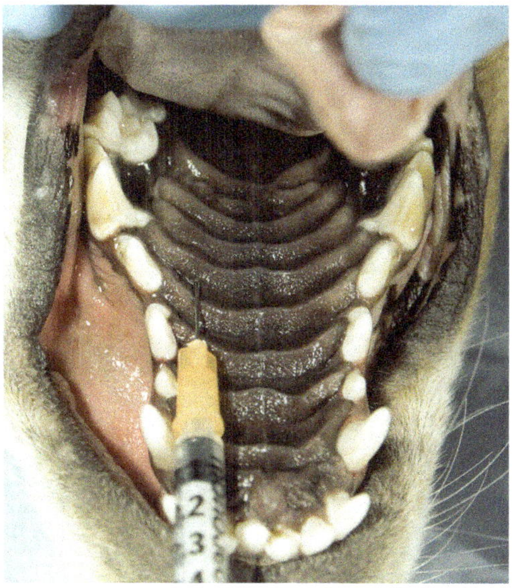

Figure 13.11 Needle placement for the major palatine nerve block. The needle should be placed and advanced through the palatal mucosa, with needle tip terminating at the rostral extent of the landmarks of the area where the major palatine may exist.

placement of the needle tip along the periosteum and will aid in the retention of the local anesthetic without leakage on needle removal. The foramen may be easily palpated in larger dogs. Threading the needle into the foramen is not advised because the compact space may result in traumatic nerve damage. Unilateral placement of this local anesthetic may be insufficient to anesthetize the central incisors because of crossover innervation, and bilateral use of this technique may be necessary. With close attention to accurate placement, small anesthetic volumes ranging from 0.1 (cats and small dogs) to 0.3 ml (large dogs) may sufficiently provide adequate regional anesthesia while minimizing inadvertent blockade to unintended structures such as the tongue.

Caudal Mandibular Block

There are two approaches for the placement of a caudal mandibular nerve block (discussed in the following text). The mandibular branch of the trigeminal nerve enters the mandibular foramen on the lingual aspect of the caudal mandible and continues in the mandibular canal as the inferior alveolar nerve. The inferior alveolar nerve is responsible for innervation of the mandibular molars, premolars, canine teeth, and incisors. The inferior alveolar nerve branches exit the mandible at the caudal, middle, and rostral mental foramina, which are responsible for sensory information from the alveolar mucosa, gingiva, and rostral lip. The mandibular foramen is identified using several prominent landmarks. In dogs and cats, the mandibular foramen rests approximately halfway between the third mandibular molar and the angular process on the lingual side of the mandible. Palpation of the depression in the caudal mandible immediately rostral to the angular process is frequently referred to as the ventral notch of the mandible. On the

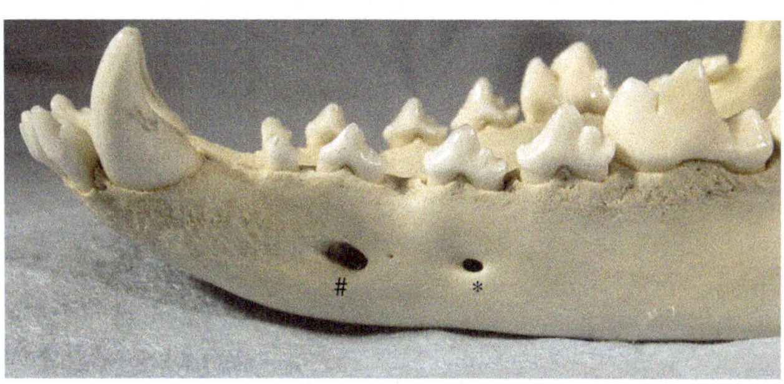

Figure 13.12 The middle mental (#) and caudal mental (*) foramina. The middle mental foramen is more prominent, located ventral to the mesial root of the second premolar. Placing the local anesthetic at the level of the middle mental foramen will create regional anesthesia for the ipsilateral lower lip, incisors 1–3, canine tooth, and the first and second premolars.

(a) (d) (b) (e) (c) (f)

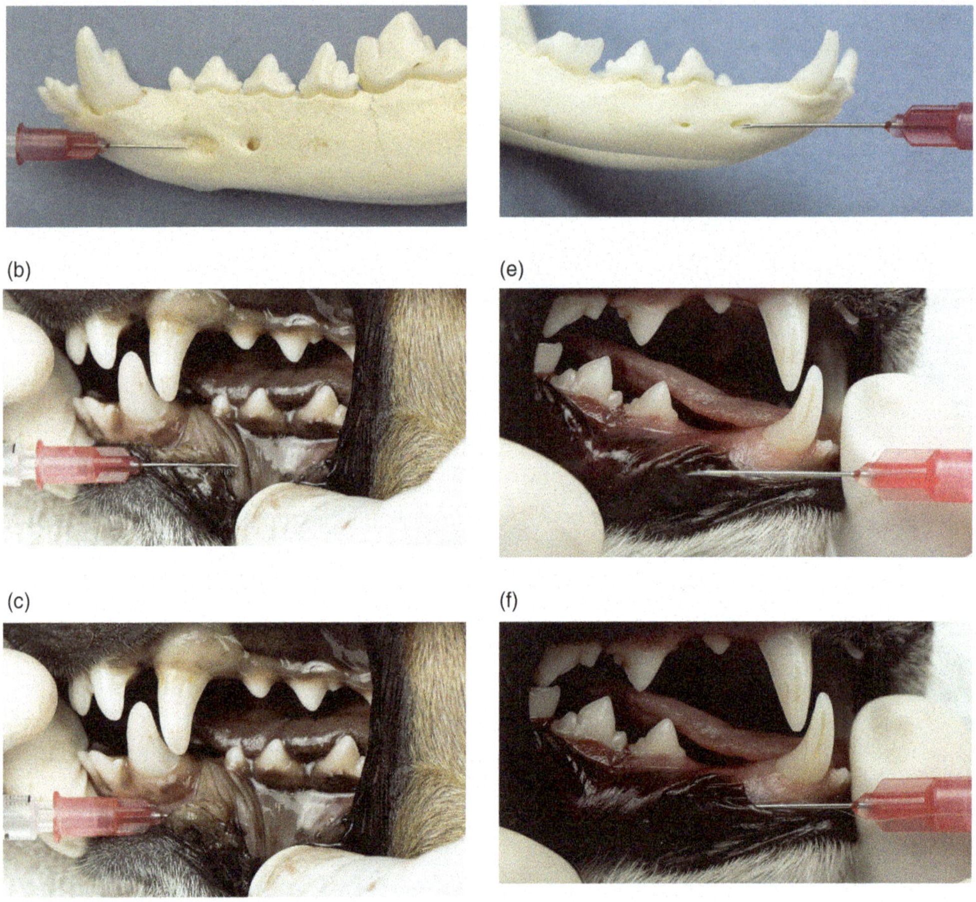

Figure 13.13 (a) The middle mental foramen can be blocked by advancing the needle along the periosteum beginning with the needle penetrating mucosa immediately rostral to the labial frenulum. Advancing the needle through the labial frenulum will help direct the needle toward the foramen, as well as to help retain the local anesthetic along the periosteum and prevent leakage of the local anesthetic once the needle is withdrawn. (b) Overlying the needle on mucosa to gauge the distance to advance the needle tip may be helpful for (c) accurate placement. (d) The absence of first and second premolar teeth in cats can make placement of this block somewhat blind; (e) the labial frenulum serves as the landmark beneath where the middle mental foramen is located and indicates how far the needle should be advanced (f).

lingual surface of the mandible, centered over the ventral notch is the mandibular foramen. The ventral notch may be subtle and difficult to palpate in feline patients. Using computed tomography (CT) contrast to measure the contact between contrast and the mandibular foramen as well as the distance or length of contact between dye and the inferior alveolar nerve demonstrated improved accuracy and precision using the intraoral versus the extraoral technique [37]. Small amounts of local anesthetic (0.1–0.3 ml) are sufficient for regional anesthesia when placed properly.

Intraoral Approach

The angular process and last mandibular molar serve as landmarks. Retract the lip with one hand and place the index finger on the angular process. Opening and closing the mouth should result in the angular process moving slightly. Incorrect placement of the index finger on the tympanic bulla will result

(a)

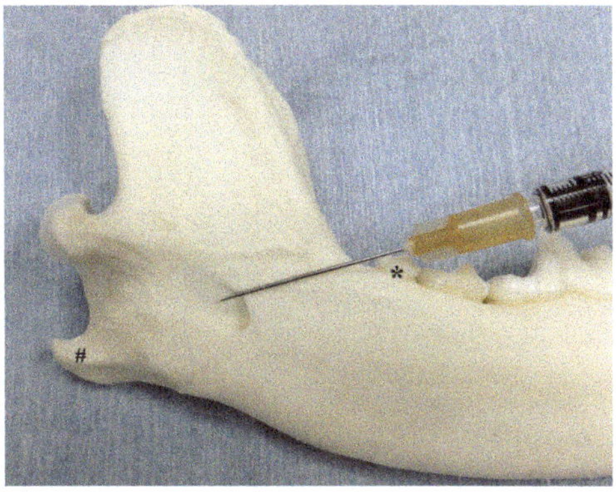

(b)

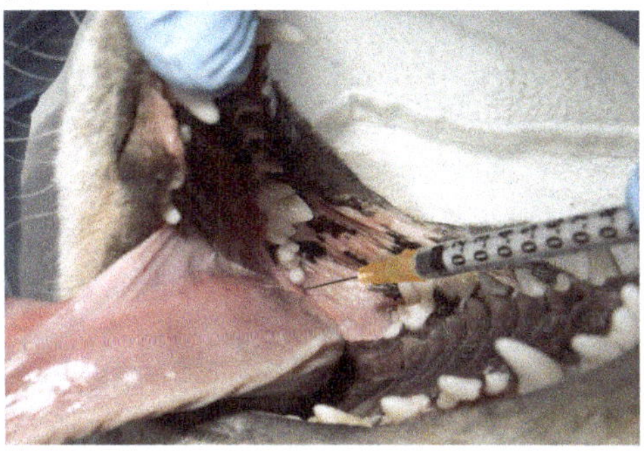

Figure 13.14 (a) The intraoral approach to local block placement relies on the skeletal landmarks of the angular process of the mandible (#) and the mandibular third molar (*). The angular process should be palpated a finger placed on the process to provide directional support. (b) The needle is placed caudal to the last molar and immediately adjacent to the periosteum on the lingual surface. Approximately half the distance between the last molar and the angular process will be the inferior alveolar foramen. By placing the local anesthetic along periosteum and providing digital pressure afterward, the local will be dispersed over a larger area ensuring coverage of the mandibular branch of the trigeminal nerve.

in no movement while placing the mandible through a range of motion. Maintaining the index finger on the angular process serves to help direct needle placement. The needle tip should be placed onto the gingiva immediately caudal and lingual to the last molar. The needle should be directed along periosteum and toward the angular process. Local anesthetic should be deposited half the distance between the point of needle entry and the tip of the angular process (Figure 13.14). By maintaining the needle along periosteum, the placement of the local anesthetic along the bone may help diffusion of the local anesthetic to aid in desensitizing the mandibular nerve. Close approximation of the needle to bone also serves to reduce the likelihood of inadvertent anesthesia of the lingual nerves, which may result in self-trauma of the tongue.

Extraoral Approach

The extraoral approach is dependent on the location and palpation of the ventral mandibular notch. This approach should not be attempted if there is evidence of dermatitis or other infection in the location of needle penetration. After palpation of the ventral mandibular notch, the needle and syringe are oriented perpendicular to the ventral cortical bone. The needle should pierce the skin and contact the ventral cortical bone. Small adjustments are made reorienting the needle off the medial edge of the bone. Advancing the needle along periosteum may help to ensure that local anesthetic placement is against bone to aid in diffusion and reduce the chance that lingual nerves will be affected. The needle tip should be advanced 1/4 cm in cats and up to 1 cm in large dogs (Figure 13.15). Some references recommend digitally palpating the mandibular nerve intraorally when directing the needle extraorally. Caution should be exercised to avoid an inadvertent needle stick when practicing this technique.

Complications and Contraindications

When placing the needle through the infraorbital canal, care must be taken to avoid contacting or penetrating the globe. Progression of intraocular disease culminating with enucleation has been reported in a cat [38]. Transient blindness following inadvertent intravitreal injection of bupivacaine in a dog has been reported [39]. While the specifics of which

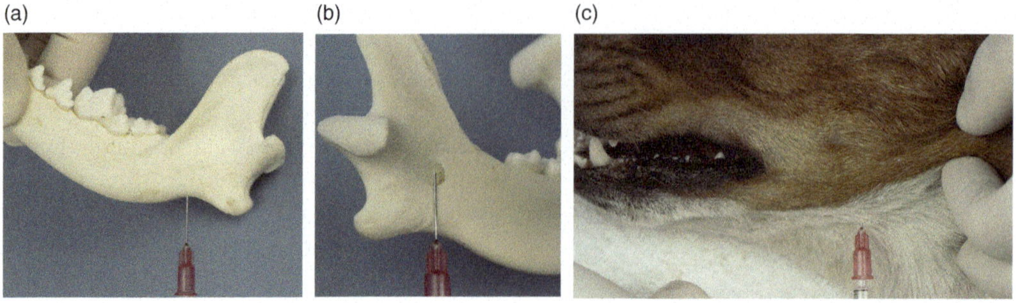

Figure 13.15 (a) The extraoral technique for the caudal mandibular nerve block involves palpating the ventral notch of the mandible. (b) On palpating the ventral notch and placing the needle directly onto the ventral cortical bone, (c) the needle can be "walked off" the bone (on the lingual side) and advanced to 0.5–1 cm depending on the size of the animal. Digital pressure can be applied in the mouth after injection to help disperse the local and prevent hematoma formation.

techniques were used for placement of maxillary blocks in these cases, safe administration avoiding the globe should be possible if the syringe and needle are oriented parallel with the hard palate. Retropulsion of the globe during needle placement or ophthalmic conditions such as buphthalmos may increase the risk for perforation. Care should be taken, and risks considered when performing these caudal blocks in these patients. Brachycephalic conformation and felines should not be at increased risk for globe penetration if the needle is maintained parallel to the hard palate.

Self-trauma due to inadvertent anesthesia of the tongue is anecdotally mentioned in the veterinary literature. Close attention and deliberate anesthetic placement along the periosteum of the lingual surface of the mandible should avoid this complication. Small volumes (maximum of 0.3–0.5 ml) of anesthetic accurately placed will also theoretically reduce the likelihood of this occurrence. In addition, anesthetic recovery in sternal recumbency may also help reduce this occurrence, since it encourages both gravity-dependent diffusion of the local anesthetic and normal anatomic placement of the tongue [40].

Care should be taken when performing or planning regional anesthesia for the collection of tissues for histologic evaluation. Risk of soft tissue or bony tumor seeding exists if the needle is placed in the vicinity of the suspected mass. In addition, the presence of a mass may alter the local anatomy, and predictability of local block placement may be decreased. Whenever risk exists for potentially seeding tumor cells, other means of multimodal pain management should be considered.

Inflammation and Local Anesthetic Efficacy

The most common indications for surgical intervention in the oral cavity of dogs and cats are chronic inflammatory conditions of the periodontium (periodontitis) and the endodontic system (pulpitis). Chronic oral inflammation, such as that seen with periodontal and endodontic disease, culminates in severe infection and inflammation. As a result, local tissue pH is lowered, which can reduce local anesthetic efficacy. The tissue acidity decreases the lipophilicity of the anesthetic by diminishing the available nonionized base that can penetrate the nerve sheath, ultimately resulting in reduced local anesthetic effectiveness [41].

Techniques to minimize inflammatory effects on local anesthetics include (i) delivering the anesthetic away from the area of inflammation to not only improve efficacy of the anesthetic but also to minimize the possibility of spreading the infection to an unaffected area, and, (ii) if within the safe dosage range, delivering a larger volume of anesthetic to effectively deliver more of the nonionized base that can diffuse through the nerve sheath and have an effect on nerve conduction [41].

Pathology Chronicity and Analgesic Needs

Patients will present for oral treatment in various states of chronicity. Pain management in acute conditions (e.g., recently fractured tooth) may be as simple as the usage of a local anesthetic immediately before treatment or, perhaps, a few days of postoperative nonsteroidal anti-inflammatory drugs (NSAIDs). However, many patients present with chronic conditions of the oral cavity (e.g., stomatitis/gingivostomatitis, chronic pulpitis/endodontic infection, oral cancer, dental caries, temporomandibular joint disorders, and tooth resorption), which often lead to a chronic pain state. Because normal animal behavior frequently masks pain, these oral conditions may be present for years before being appropriately addressed. Underappreciation and undertreatment of pain associated with these conditions by both the owner and the veterinary professional may confound the problem [42]. Oral and dental pain in cats are sometimes difficult to assess, which emphasizes the need for thorough assessment and aggressive management in this species [42, 43]. In some conditions (stomatitis/gingivostomatitis), quality oral hygiene implementation is crucial to successful management. To succeed in this endeavor, the patient must be on the precipice of being pain-free. A holistic approach to pain management is important, including the use of pharmaceutics and complementary therapies (e.g., acupuncture) [44]. Chronic pain leads to an alteration of the central nervous system and the way pain signals are processed (i.e., central sensitization) [44]. Thus, drug therapy should be multimodal (NSAIDs, opioids, N-methyl-D-aspartate (NMDA) antagonists [ketamine, amantadine], anticonvulsants [gabapentin], tricyclic antidepressants, and/or steroids), and analgesic pain management should be continuous [44]. As pain is minimized, appropriate oral hygiene can be implemented, and individual drugs can be removed from the treatment regimen in a stepwise manner.

Anesthetic Management of Other Oral and Maxillofacial Conditions

Oral and Maxillofacial Trauma

There are few circumstances when a maxillofacial fracture is a true emergency. Intractable bleeding (oral or nasal) would necessitate immediate anesthesia to address the bleeding or ligate major vascular supplies such as the carotid artery. Patients with maxillofacial trauma should be closely evaluated and screened for signs of head trauma. Pupillary light reflexes, nystagmus, and aberrant cranial nerve reflex responses should increase the suspicion of head trauma. Considerations for patients sustaining head trauma can be found in Chapter 3.

Other than being extremely painful, patients with maxillofacial trauma do not pose unique anesthetic risks or considerations beyond airway management. Airway management and jaw fracture pose obvious challenges, which may be reduced with extraoral methods of intubation. Anesthetic management should proceed as for any other patient with trauma (see Chapter 21).

Oral and Maxillofacial Surgery

The term "oral and maxillofacial surgery" encompasses a wide range of surgery types that may include, but is not limited to, nonsurgical extraction of a single rooted tooth, repair of an oronasal fistula, and wide surgical resection of a maxillary neoplasia. The degree of intraoperative and postoperative pain will vary greatly depending on, among many things, the procedure invasiveness and types of tissues that are manipulated. A nonsurgical incisor extraction may only cause minor discomfort, easily managed with an intraoperative local anesthetic, such as bupivacaine, and a postoperative NSAID. However, a more invasive procedure, such as a caudal maxillectomy, will require additional analgesics. Potential measures to improve both intraoperative and postoperative pain in major oral surgery should include multimodal techniques and are described in the following text.

Long-Acting Local Anesthetics–Bupivacaine

Bupivacaine may have a prolonged effect up to 8 h after administration [45]. Because of its intermediate onset of action, it should be administered soon after the patient is anesthetized, so that it takes effect while the patient is surgically prepped. In addition, the use of liposomal bupivacaine is being investigated as a formulation designed to extend the duration of the local anesthesia. Liposomal bupivacaine improves patient comfort in dogs following stifle surgery when infiltrated in the surgery site [46]. When used for brachial plexus blocks in rabbits and dogs, this formulation was well tolerated by tissues [23]. Currently, definitive investigations into the effects of liposomal bupivacaine for regional anesthesia in dentistry patients are lacking.

Buprenorphine Combined with Local Anesthetics

Although not completely determined in dogs or cats, multiple human studies show a prolonged analgesic effect of at least 28 h with a significantly lower requirement for rescue opioids due to uncontrolled pain when buprenorphine is added to local anesthetics [17]. In 75% of human patients, the addition of buprenorphine to bupivacaine provided complete analgesia that lasted 30 h beyond the duration provided by bupivacaine alone [17]. This technique may be similarly useful in veterinary oral surgery [18].

Local Anesthetic Redosing

If a shorter-acting local anesthetic such as lidocaine is used, an additional lidocaine injection at the end of the procedure may aid in postoperative pain control. If this technique is used, avoid exceeding the maximum allowable dose. Redosing local anesthetics through the use of wound-soaker catheters in major oral surgery sites has been described in a horse [47]; however, usefulness in small animals may also be considered due to successful application for other surgical conditions in dogs [48].

Intraoperative and Postoperative Continuous Rate Infusions

Continuous rate infusion (CRI) of opioids, such as fentanyl or morphine, with or without adjuncts such as lidocaine and/or ketamine can be a useful technique for intraoperative and postoperative pain management. For major oral surgery cases (mandibulectomy, maxillectomy, jaw fracture repair, etc.), fentanyl CRI or a CRI of morphine or fentanyl with lidocaine and ketamine (MLK/FLK) is frequently encountered.

Circumstances Requiring Unique Anesthetic Management Approaches

Airway Management

There are several situations when orotracheal intubation is either impractical or not possible in oral and maxillofacial patients. Several alternative techniques are available. The technique chosen depends on the peculiarities of each patient and their specific condition. However, the most common alternative technique is pharyngotomy intubation (Figure 13.16). Standard pharyngotomy intubation techniques are readily available in surgery textbooks [49]. Placement of the pharyngotomy endotracheal tube on the left side permits the placement of a pharyngostomy feeding tube into the esophagus through the same stoma before extubation if concern exists regarding the patient's willingness or ability to eat after surgery. Pharyngostomy feeding tubes may be associated with increased complications over esophagostomy feeding tubes, and clinical decision-making and clinician preference become important for postoperative supplemental feeding considerations.

An unobstructed assessment of occlusion can also be accomplished through general anesthetic delivery using the transmylohyoid intubation technique (Figure 13.17). As an alternative to pharyngotomy intubation, transmylohyoid intubation utilizes a caudal ventral mandibular surgical approach at the level of the mandibular first molar tooth. A combination of sharp and blunt dissection through skin, release of the transmylohyoid muscle attachment, and incising through lingual mucosal adjacent to the first molar tooth permits easy access to the caudal oral cavity for intubation [50]. This technique may be preferable if no indication exists for placement of a pharyngostomy feeding tube. Transmylohyoid intubation can be performed on the left or right side and may be the preferable technique for trauma patients, but may be less effective for patients requiring unobstructed surgical visualization of the caudal oral cavity such as cleft palate repair or oncologic resection.

(a)
(b)

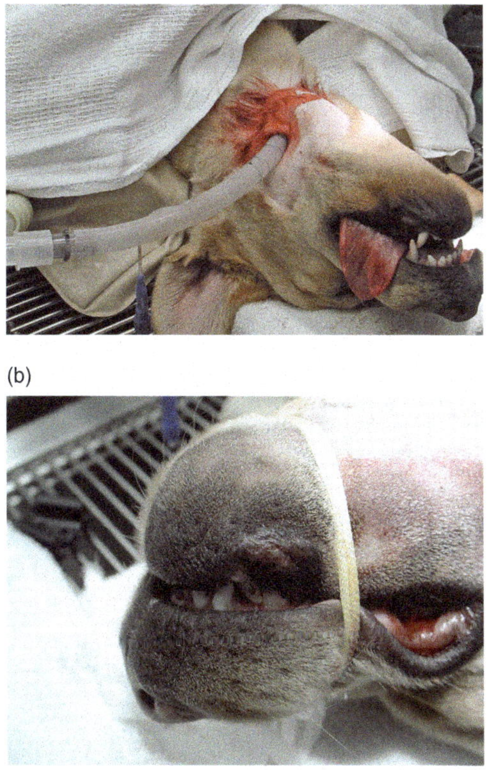

Figure 13.16 (a) This patient sustained a caudal mandibular fracture and was maintained on inhalant with a pharyngotomy intubation placement. (b) Intubation in this manner permitted the use of a gauze muzzle to maintain this patient in normal occlusion and the fracture to be approached with an extraoral surgical approach.

Occlusion Assessment

Early return to function and maintaining occlusion are fundamental principles unique to oral and maxillofacial trauma management. Often, the endotracheal tube exiting the oral cavity may obscure or interfere with evaluation of occlusion during repair. To evaluate occlusion during anesthesia, unique techniques exist to combat this challenge.

Once the patient is orotracheally intubated, if traditional intubation techniques are used, an identical-sized endotracheal tube can be used to evaluate the placement length, and an ideal length can be established. The tracheal tube adapter can be removed, the tracheal tube cut to length, and the adapter replaced. Modifications to tube length should not be so drastic that the pilot tube and associated cuff be disrupted. The goal should be to have an endotracheal tube with the adapter positioned

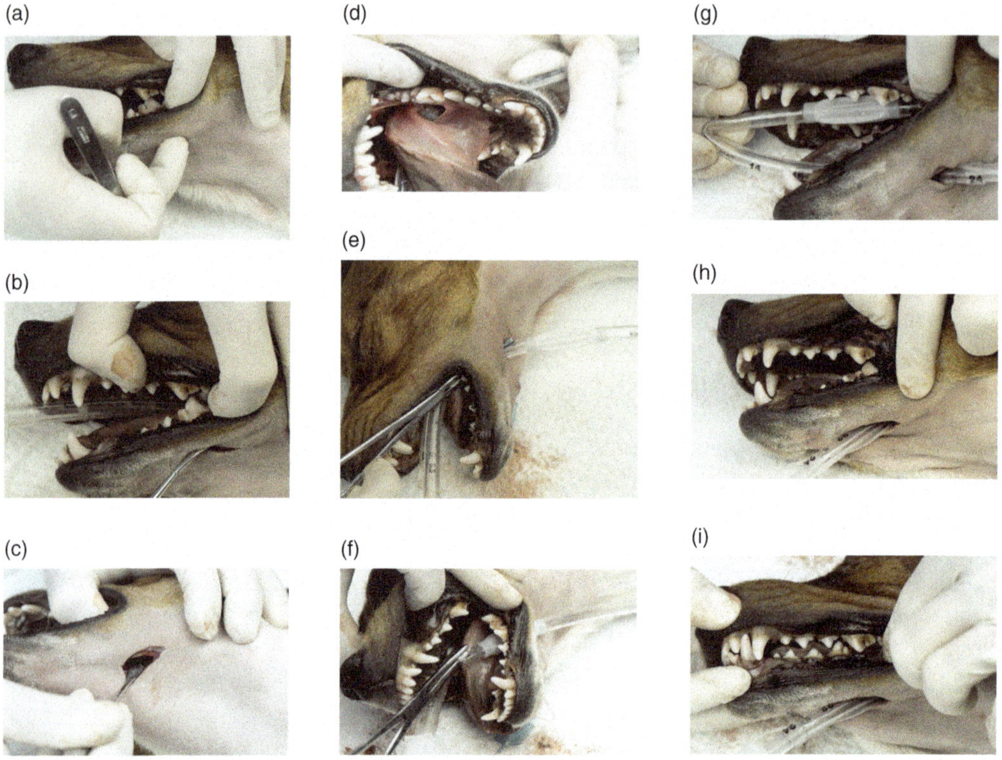

Figure 13.17 (a) With the patient fully anesthetized and instrumented, surgical access for placement of the endotracheal tube occurs at the level of the mandibular first molar tooth. (b) An incision is created through skin and subcutaneous tissues directly onto the ventral cortex at this location. (c) Blunt dissection permits undermining attachment of the mylohyoid muscle from the ventral mandible permitting elevation of soft tissues off lingual cortical bone at the level of this tooth. (d) An intraoral incision is created at the location of the periosteal elevation permitting placement of hemostats to grasp a second endotracheal tube to be advanced through the incision (e, f) alongside the lingual surface of the mandible. (g) Once in the oral cavity, the transmylohyoid endotracheal tube is bent, the orotracheal endotracheal tube removed, and the transmylohyoid endotracheal tube is advanced into the trachea. (h) As the transmylohyoid endotracheal tube is advanced in the trachea, the bend straightens, and the anesthetic monitoring unit should confirm accurate placement. (i) Transmylohyoid intubation permits easy assessment of occlusion for jaw fracture repair.

within the oral cavity. This location of the adapter will permit intermittent disconnection from the breathing circuit to assess occlusion and ensure that the fracture repair does not result in overcorrection or undercorrection, resulting in inappropriate tooth-on-tooth contact. Modifying endotracheal tube length may be safer than risking tracheal laceration or main stem bronchial intubation resulting from advancing the endotracheal tube deeper into the airway.

More practically, once the patient with maxillofacial trauma is anesthetically stable, a treatment plan is created that involves returning the patient to normal occlusion; converting the patient to a pharyngotomy or transmylohyoid intubation may make the repair and intraoperative evaluations of occlusion more efficient. With pharyngotomy or transmylohyoid intubation, the oral cavity is bypassed entirely, and occlusion can be more closely monitored. In many situations, after having the oral cavity completely free and unimpinged by the endotracheal tube, it becomes quite reasonable to place the patient's mouth into the pretrauma occlusion and use gauze or other restraint to maintain the mouth in that position. Once the patient's occlusion is returned to normal, the fracture fragments should be oriented in a position that will be conducive to maintaining that normal occlusion.

Maxillomandibular Fixation

Careful anesthetic consideration should be given if the selected method of fixation involves maxillomandibular fixation (MMF). When these repair techniques are used with composite or acrylic materials to bond teeth from the mandibular arcade to the maxillary arcade, a plan must be made to address how the patient will be intubated at the time of MMF removal. For example, once the induction agent is given, extension of the neck and use of a long laryngoscope blade with a light source or even a rigid or flexible endoscope may be necessary to visualize the larynx to facilitate intubation. A long stylet may also be utilized to facilitate passage of the endotracheal tube. Ketamine may be chosen for induction since apnea is less likely than if propofol or alfaxalone boluses are used. If apnea occurs or an airway cannot be established, it may be possible to quickly cut or remove the bonding material once the induction agent has been administered, and the patient immediately intubated for further evaluation.

Other Oral and Maxillofacial Surgery Techniques

Uninhibited access to the oral cavity is often crucial for successful major oral surgery such as maxillectomy, mandibulectomy, palatal defect repair, and glossectomy. Without having the endotracheal tube taking up valuable space in the oral cavity, surgery becomes more manageable and helps ensure a more positive outcome, with fewer intraoperative complications. In this situation, a pharyngotomy or transmylohyoid intubation may be more practical.

In addition, some neoplastic lesions in the caudal oral cavity may be large enough to either significantly compromise a patient's airway or interfere with orotracheal intubation. In such circumstances, it may be necessary to perform a temporary tracheostomy until the airway can be recovered.

Trismus

In a strict sense, trismus is defined as an inability to open the mouth due to spastic activity of the muscles of mastication [51]. However, it is commonly used generically to describe an inability to open the mouth from any potential cause, which may include the following: masticatory myositis, craniomandibular osteopathy, tetanus, retropharyngeal abscess, retrobulbar abscess, odontogenic infection, temporomandibular apparatus dysplasia, temporomandibular apparatus trauma, temporomandibular apparatus neoplasia, salivary gland disease, and postradiation fibrosis.

These conditions share a common denominator in that the diagnostic workup for these conditions typically requires general anesthesia for diagnosis and/or treatment. The degree to which a patient is affected by trismus can vary and may cause extreme difficulty intubating the patient through the oral cavity. When confronted with a patient with known trismus or a condition that could cause trismus, the anesthetist should be prepared for the implementation of tracheostomy intubation or for the use of an endoscope to aid with intubation. Pharyngotomy intubation is not an option in these situations, as it requires initial orotracheal intubation while the extraoral pharyngotomy approach is made. Premedications and induction agents that can cause vomiting should be avoided.

References

1 Gad, T. (1968). Periodontal disease in dogs. *J. Periodont. Res.* 3: 268–272.

2 Lund, E.M., Armstrong, P.J., Kirk, C.A. et al. (1999). Health status and population characteristics of dogs and cats examined at private veterinary practices in the United States. *J. Am. Vet. Med. Assoc.* 214: 1336–1341.

3 Golden, A.L., Stoller, N., and Harvey, C.E. (1982). A survey of oral and dental diseases in dogs anesthetized at a veterinary hospital. *J. Am. Anim. Hosp. Assoc.* 18: 891–899.

4 Harvey, C.E., Shofer, F.S., and Laster, L. (1994). Association of age and body weight with periodontal disease in North American dogs. *J. Vet. Dent.* 11: 94–105.

5 Harvey, C.E. and Hammond, B.F. (1993). Bacterial isolates from blood cultures of dogs undergoing dentistry. *Vet. Surg.* 22: 327–329.

6 Nieves, M.A., Hartwig, P., Kinyon, J.M. et al. (1997). Bacterial isolates from plaque and from blood during and after routine dental procedures in dogs. *Vet. Surg.* 26: 26–32.

7 Rawlinson, J.E., Goldstein, R.E., Reiter, A.M. et al. (2011). Association of periodontal disease with systemic health indices in dogs and the systemic response to treatment of periodontal disease. *J. Am. Vet. Med. Assoc.* 238: 601–609.

8 DeBowes, L.J., Mosier, D., Logan, E. et al. (1996). Association of periodontal disease and histologic lesions in multiple organs from 45 dogs. *J. Vet. Dent.* 13: 57–60.

9 Moser, S.A. (2013). Getting to the root of anesthesia-free veterinary dental care. *DVM360 Magazine* 11(1).

10 American Veterinary Dental College (2004). Companion animal dental scaling without anesthesia. Available at: https://www.avdc.org/PDF/Dental_Scaling_Without_Anesthesia.pdf (accessed 16 April 201)8.

11 American College of Veterinary Anesthesia and Analgesia (2013). Anesthesia free dentistry. Available at: http://acvaa.org/wp-content/uploads/2019/05/Anesthesia_Free_Dentistry.pdf (accessed 6 February 2020).

12 Bellows, J., Berg, M.L., Dennis, S. et al. (2019). 2019 AAHA dental care guidelines for dogs and cats. *J. Am. Anim. Hosp. Assoc.* 55: 49–69.

13 Snyder, C.J. and Snyder, L.B.C. (2013). Effect of regional mepivacaine anesthesia via an infraorbital nerve block on minimum alveolar concentration of isoflurane in clinically normal anesthetized dogs undergoing a modified form of dental dolorimetry. *J. Am. Vet. Med. Assoc.* 242: 199–204.

14 Martin-Flores, M. (2013). Clinical pharmacology and toxicology of local anesthetics and adjuncts. In: *Small Animal Regional Anesthesia and Analgesia* (eds. L. Campoy and M.R. Read), 25–40. Ames, IA: Wiley-Blackwell.

15 Stein, C., Millan, M.J., Shippenberg, T.S. et al. (1989). Peripheral opioid receptors mediating antinociception in inflammation. Evidence for involvement of mu, delta and kappa receptors. *J. Pharmacol. Exp. Ther.* 248: 1269–1275.

16 Candido, K.D., Winnie, A.P., Ghaleb, A.H. et al. (2002). Buprenorphine added to the local anesthetic for axillary brachial plexus block prolongs postoperative analgesia. *Reg. Anesth. Pain Med.* 27: 162–167.

17 Modi, M., Rastogi, S., and Kumar, A. (2009). Buprenorphine with bupivacaine for intraoral nerve blocks to provide postoperative analgesia in outpatients after minor oral surgery. *J. Oral Maxillofac. Surg.* 67: 2571–2576.

18 Snyder, L.B., Snyder, C.J., and Hetzel, S. (2016). Effects of buprenorphine added to bupivacaine infraorbital nerve blocks on isoflurane minimum alveolar concentration using a model for acute dental/oral surgical pain in dogs. *J. Vet. Dent.* 33: 90–96.

19 Förster, J.G. and Rosenberg, P.H. (2003). Clinically useful adjuvants in regional

anesthesia. *Curr. Opin. Anaesthesiol.* 16: 477–486.

20 Eisenach, J.C., De Kock, M., and Klimscha, W. (1996). Alpha (2) -adrenergic agonists for regional anesthesia. A clinical review of clonidine (1984–1995). *Anesthesiology* 85: 655–674.

21 Lamont, L.A. (2008). Multimodal pain management in veterinary medicine: the physiologic basis of pharmacologic therapies. *Vet. Clin. North Am. Small Anim. Pract.* 38: 1173–1186.

22 Lascelles, B.D. and Kirby Shaw, K. (2016). An extended release local anaesthetic: potential for future use in veterinary surgery patients? *Vet. Med. Sci.* 2: 229–238.

23 Richard, B.M., Newton, P., Ott, L.R. et al. (2012). The safety of EXPAREL® (bupivacaine liposome injectable suspension) administered by peripheral nerve block in rabbits and dogs. *J. Drug Deliv.* 2012: 1–10.

24 Hillerup, S. and Jensen, R. (2006). Nerve injury caused by mandibular block analgesia. *Int. J. Oral Maxillofac. Surg.* 35: 437–443.

25 Greensmith, J.E. and Bosseau Murray, W. (2006). Complications of regional anesthesia. *Curr. Opin. Anaesthesiol.* 19: 531–537.

26 Duke, T. (2000). Local and regional anesthetic and analgesic techniques in the dog and cat: part II, infiltration and nerve blocks. *Can. Vet. J.* 41: 949–952.

27 Fizzano, K.M., Claude, A.K., Lan-Hsin, K. et al. (2017). Evaluation of a modified infraorbital approach for a maxillary nerve block for rhinoscopy and nasal biopsy of dogs. *Am. J. Vet. Res.* 78: 1025–1035.

28 Castejón-González, A.C. and Reiter, A.M. (2019). Locoregional anesthesia of the head. *Vet. Clin. Small Anim. Pract.* 49: 1041–1061.

29 Pascoe, P.J. (2016). The effects of lidocaine or a lidocaine-bupivacaine mixture administered into the infraorbital canal in dogs. *Am. J. Vet. Res.* 77: 682–687.

30 Lantz, G.C. (2003). Regional anesthesia for dentistry and oral surgery. *J. Vet. Dent.* 20: 181–186.

31 Krug, W. and Losey, J. (2011). Area of desensitization following mental nerve block in dogs. *J. Vet. Dent.* 28: 146–150.

32 Rood, J.P. (1977). Some anatomical and physiological causes of failure to achieve mandibular analgesia. *Br. J. Oral Surg.* 15: 75–82.

33 Rood, J.P. (1978). The organization of the inferior alveolar nerve and its relation to local analgesia. *J. Dent.* 6: 305–310.

34 Rochette, J. (2005). Regional anesthesia and analgesia for oral and dental procedures. *Vet. Clin. North Am. Small Anim. Pract.* 35: 1041–1058.

35 Pascoe, P.J. (2012). Anesthesia and pain management. In: *Veterinary Dentistry and Oral Surgery* (eds. F.J. Verstraete and M. Lommer), 23–42. St. Louis: Elsevier.

36 Viscasillas, J. and Ter Haar, G. (2017). Ultrasound guided trigeminal nerve block as local anaesthetic technique for exenteration and excision of the zygomatic arch with partial caudal maxillectomy in a dog. *Vet. Anesth. Analg.* 44: 688–690.

37 Goudie-DeAngelis, E.M., Snyder, C.J., Raffe, M.R. et al. (2016). A pilot study comparing the accuracy of two approaches to the inferior alveolar nerve block in canine cadavers. *Intern. J. Appl. Res. Vet. Med.* 14: 49–58.

38 Perry, R., Moore, D., and Scurrell, E. (2015). Globe penetration in a cat following maxillary nerve block for dental surgery. *J. Feline Med. Surg.* 17: 66–72.

39 Alessio, T.L. and Krieger, E.M. (2015). Transient unilateral vision loss in a dog following inadvertent intravitreal injection of bupivacaine during a dental procedure. *J. Am. Vet. Med. Assoc.* 246: 990–993.

40 Beckman, B.W. (2006). Pathophysiology and management of surgical and chronic pain in dogs and cats. *J. Vet. Dent.* 23: 50–60.

41 Malamed, S.F. (2004). Local anesthetic considerations in dental specialties. In: *Handbook of Local Anesthesia*, 5e (ed. S.F. Malamed), 269–281. St. Louis: Elsevier.

42 Evangelista, M.C., Watanabe, R., Leung, V.S.Y. et al. (2019). Facial expressions of pain in cats: the development and validation of a Feline Grimace Scale. *Sci. Rep.* 9: 1–11.

43 Watanabe, R., Doodnaught, G., Proulx, C. et al. (2019). A multidisciplinary study of pain in cats undergoing dental extractions: a prospective, controlled clinical trial. *PLoS One* 14 (3): e0213195.

44 Lascelles, D.X. and Gaynor, J.S. (2011). Chronic pain management. In: *Essentials of Small Animal Anesthesia and Analgesia*, 2e (eds. K.A. Grimm, W.J. Tranquilli and L.A. Lamont), 147–157. Ames, IA: Wiley.

45 Muir, W.W., Hubbell, J.A., Skarda, R.T. et al. (2000). Local anesthetic drugs and techniques. In: *Handbook of Veterinary Anesthesia*, 3e (eds. W.W. Muir, J.A. Hubbell, R.T. Skarda and R.M. Bednarski), 41–56. St. Louis: Mosby.

46 Lascelles, B.D.X., Rausch-Derra, L.C., Wofford, J.A. et al. (2016). Pilot, randomized, placebo-controlled clinical field study to evaluate the effectiveness of bupivacaine liposome injectable suspension for the provision of post-surgical analgesia in dogs undergoing stifle surgery. *BMC Vet. Res.* 12: 168.

47 Carmalt, J.L. and Linn, K.A. (2013). Large segmental mandibulectomy for treatment of an undifferentiated sarcoma in a horse. *Vet. Surg.* 42: 433–439.

48 Armitage-Chan, E. (2013). Use of wound soaker catheters in pain management. *In Practice* 35: 24–29.

49 Harvey, C.E. (1993). Oral cavity: the tongue, lips, cheeks, pharynx, and salivary glands. In: *Textbook of Small Animal Surgery*, 2e (ed. D. Slatter), 510–530. Philadelphia: W.B. Saunders.

50 Soukup, J.W. and Snyder, C.J. (2015). Transmylohyoid orotracheal intubation in surgical management of canine maxillofacial fractures: an alternative to pharyngotomy endotracheal intubation. *Vet. Surg.* 44: 432–436.

51 Blood, D.C. and Studdert, V.P. (1999). *Saunders Comprehensive Veterinary Dictionary*, 2e, 1165. London: W.B. Saunders.

14

Hematologic Disorders

Molly Shepard[1] and Benjamin Brainard[2]

[1] MedVet Medical and Cancer Centers for Pets, 3305 N California Ave, Chicago, IL, 60618, USA
[2] Department of Small Animal Medicine & Surgery, College of Veterinary Medicine, University of Georgia, Athens, GA, 30602, USA

Introduction

Aerobic metabolism, the bedrock physiologic process accounting for 90% of all cellular metabolism in mammals, represents an essential step in the maintenance of cell integrity and systemic organ function. For aerobic metabolism to proceed and efficiently produce the energy substrates vital for these biologic processes, a perpetual balance must be maintained between the delivery and consumption of O_2 in tissues. The principal cardiovascular goal in the management of any anesthetic episode is the maintenance of oxygen delivery to tissues.

Oxygen delivery (DO_2) is the product of cardiac output (Q) and arterial oxygen content (CaO_2). Oxygen content comprises both dissolved and hemoglobin (Hb)-bound oxygen in the blood. The calculation of CaO_2 considers the arterial partial pressure of oxygen (PaO_2, in millimeters of mercury), the Hb concentration (in grams per deciliter of blood), and saturation of arterial Hb with oxygen (SaO_2, percentage expressed as a decimal). This relationship is described by Eq. (14.1) [1]:

$$CaO_2 = \left[\frac{1.34\,\text{ml}\,O_2}{\text{g}}\,\text{Hb} \times [\text{Hb}] \times SaO_2\right] + \left[\frac{\frac{0.003\,\text{ml}\,O_2}{\text{dl blood}}}{\text{mmHg} \times PaO_2}\right] \tag{14.1}$$

Because approximately 97% of total CaO_2 is bound to Hb in mammalian blood [2], the contribution of Hb concentration and SaO_2 to CaO_2 is much greater than that of PaO_2. As a result, disorders in oxygen-carrying capacity (e.g., anemia and dyshemoglobinemias) have a much greater impact on oxygen delivery to tissues compared to disorders of decreased dissolved oxygen stores, although low dissolved oxygen will adversely affect the Hb saturation (Table 14.1). Table 14.1 demonstrates the effects of anemia, hypoxemia, and dyshemoglobinemia (e.g., methemoglobinemia) on CaO_2 and subsequent DO_2. In general, mammalian CaO_2 is equal to 19.9 ml O_2 dl^{-1} blood under standard conditions (arterial partial pressure of CO_2 of 40 mmHg, 37 °C body temperature, pH 7.4, and [Hb] of 15 g dl^{-1}) [1]. While the severe hypoxemia (decreased PaO_2) shown in Table 14.1

Canine and Feline Anesthesia and Co-Existing Disease, Second Edition. Edited by Rebecca A. Johnson, Lindsey B. C. Snyder and Carrie A. Schroeder.

Companion website: www.wiley.com/go/johnson/canine

Table 14.1 Effects of anemia, hypoxemia, and methemoglobinemia on the oxygen content of arterial blood.

Patient status	[Hb] ($g\ dl^{-1}$)	SaO_2 (%)	PaO_2 (mmHg)	CaO_2 ($ml\ O_2\ dl^{-1}$)	DO_2 ($ml\ min^{-1}$) (assuming cardiac output approximately $2\ l\ min^{-1}$)
Normal	15	97.5	100	19.9	398
Hypoxemia	15	85	50	17.2	344
Anemia	7.5	97.5	100	10.1	202
Methemoglobinemia (33% MetHb)	10	97.5 (functional saturation)	100	13.3	266

A 50% reduction in hemoglobin concentration (e.g., severe anemia) causes a more profound decrease in oxygen delivery than a 50% reduction in dissolved oxygen (severe hypoxemia). Methemoglobinemia decreases the availability of normal hemoglobin, thereby decreasing oxygen delivery to tissues. Oxygen delivery in this table is calculated on the basis of a cardiac output of $2\ l\ min^{-1}$.

causes a relatively small decrease in overall CaO_2 ($17.2\ ml\ O_2\ dl^{-1}$ blood), severe reductions in oxygen-carrying capacity (anemia or methemoglobinemia) produce more profound reductions in CaO_2. Changes in cardiac output (increases in heart rate, stroke volume, or both) can compensate for low CaO_2 to a degree, but, at critical points, tissue oxygen delivery may be compromised.

Oxygen Content Monitoring in the Anesthetized Patient

Arterial oxygen content may be monitored by blood-gas analysis or may be estimated via oximetry and hematology tests, including packed cell volume (PCV), hematocrit (Hct), and Hb concentration. Blood-gas analysis quantifies the partial pressure of oxygen dissolved in arterial or venous blood (PaO_2, PvO_2) and the saturation of Hb with oxygen (SaO_2, SvO_2). Patients breathing room air (approximately 21% O_2) in the absence of pulmonary disease or other sources of poor gas exchange (e.g. low pulmonary perfusion), are expected to have a PaO_2 between 80 and 100 mmHg, PvO_2 of 42 ± 5 mmHg, SaO_2 of 98–100%, and SvO_2 of 75% [3]. Pulse oximetry provides a less invasive means of monitoring Hb–oxygen saturation within a specific peripheral capillary bed, yielding an "SpO_2" value.

The relationship between PaO_2 and SaO_2 (or SpO_2) is described by the oxyhemoglobin dissociation curve (Figure 14.1). In general, as PaO_2 increases, more oxygen is available to bind to Hb, to a maximum of 100% saturation. An SpO_2 value of 100% correlates with PaO_2 values $\geq$100 mmHg, whereas an SpO_2 of 95% correlates with a PaO_2 of approximately 80 mmHg. An SpO_2 value of 94% correlates with a PaO_2 of approximately 70 mmHg and is consistent with hypoxemia that merits further diagnostics and treatment.

Various physiologic changes affect the affinity of Hb for oxygen and may result in a shift of the oxyhemoglobin curve to the right (decreased affinity, favoring offloading of oxygen to the tissues) or to the left (increased affinity, favoring onloading of oxygen to Hb). In humans, the conditions that decrease affinity of Hb for oxygen include increased partial pressure of CO_2, increased body temperature, increased 2,3-diphosphoglycerate (2,3-DPG) concentration within the erythrocyte, and decreased blood pH. The conditions that increase affinity of Hb for oxygen include decreased blood CO_2 concentration, decreased body temperature, decreased 2,3-DPG, and increased pH (Figure 14.1).

Hemoglobin structure also influences its affinity for oxygen [4]. Normal Hb must be in the reduced, ferrous (Fe^{2+}) state to bind oxygen.

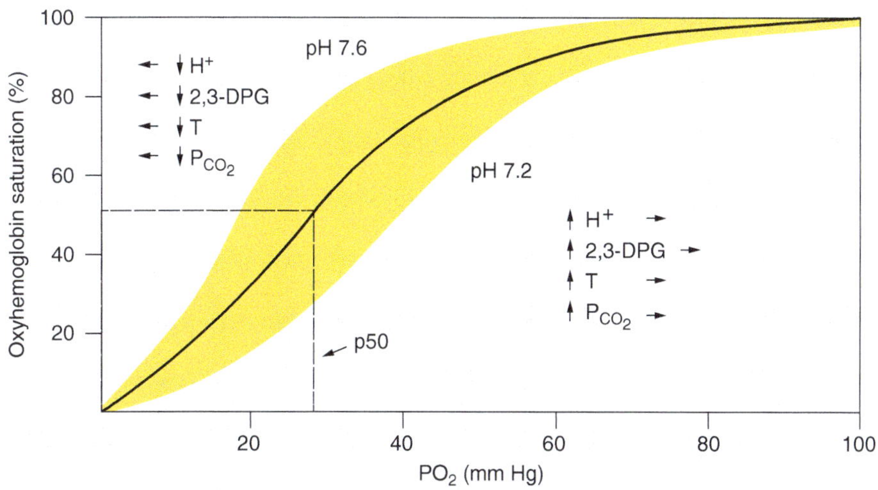

Figure 14.1 Oxyhemoglobin dissociation curve and regulating factors. Physiologic factors that shift the curve to the left, facilitating binding of oxygen to hemoglobin, include alkalemia (decreased circulating hydrogen ion concentration), decreased body temperature, decreased circulating partial pressure of CO_2, and decreased concentration of 2,3-diphosphoglycerate (2,3-DPG). Factors that shift the curve to the right, facilitating offloading of oxygen to the tissues, are acidemia, increased 2,3-DPG concentration, increased body temperature, and increased circulating partial pressure of CO_2.

Dyshemoglobinemias can be caused by the presence of methemoglobin (metHb) or carboxyhemoglobin (COHb). MetHb is an oxidation product of Hb that forms a reversible complex with oxygen and impairs offloading of oxygen to the tissues. There are congenital and acquired causes of methemoglobinemia, including toxicity from acetaminophen, nitrates, benzocaine, benzyl alcohol, and prilocaine. Feline Hb appears to be more sensitive to MetHb formation than canine Hb [5]. Carboxyhemoglobin (COHb) is formed when Hb is exposed to carbon monoxide. Carbon monoxide competitively binds to Hb with an affinity more than 200-fold greater than Hb's affinity for oxygen and is most commonly encountered in patients exposed to products of combustion (e.g., house fires) [6].

Oxygen-carrying capacity may be quantified by tests including Hct, PCV, red blood cell (RBC) count, and Hb concentration. Hct is the percentage of blood composed of RBCs. Centrifugal methods yield PCV, which accurately estimates Hct. Hct can be calculated by automated cell counters; however, because many hematology analyzers are designed for human blood and most domesticated mammalian species (except for dogs) have smaller erythrocytes than humans, this method of Hct calculation has more potential for error than PCV. Calculation of Hb concentration provides the most specific indicator of oxygen-carrying capacity but may be falsely high in the presence of hemolysis, lipemia, Heinz bodies, or synthetic Hb products. When erythrocytes are normal in size and intravascular hemolysis is not significant, Hb concentrations should equal approximately one-third of the Hct. For example, patients with a hemoglobin concentration of $10\,g\,dl^{-1}$ of blood are expected to have a concurrent hematocrit of approximately 30%.

Causes of anemia in companion animals can be generally classified into three categories, as follows (Table 14.2) [7]: (i) inadequate erythrocyte production (i.e., abnormal erythropoiesis), (ii) increased consumption or destruction (e.g., hemolysis), and (iii) loss (e.g., hemorrhage). Causes of decreased erythrocyte production include systemic disease (e.g., chronic kidney disease, neoplasia with myelophthisis),

Table 14.2 Pathophysiology of anemia.

Hemorrhage		Accelerated erythrocyte destruction		Abnormal erythropoiesis	
Acute	Chronic	Intravascular hemolysis	Extravascular hemolysis	Reduced erythropoiesis	Defective erythropoiesis
GI ulcers **Hemostasis defects** **Neoplasia** **Thrombocytopenia** **Trauma** **Surgery**	**Disseminated intravascular coagulation (DIC)** **Toxicities** • Rodenticide • Bracken fern • Sweet clover **Hemophilia A and B**	**Bacteria** • *Clostridium hemolyticum, C. novyi, C. perfringens* • *Escherichia coli* **RBC parasites** • *Babesia* spp. **Chemicals and plants** • Acetaminophen • *Brassica* spp. • Copper • Onions • Red maple **Immune-mediated** • Immune-mediated hemolytic anemia (IMHA) **Hypoosmolality** **Fragmentation** **Hypophosphatemia** **G6PD deficiency** **Glutathione (GSH) deficiency (sheep)** **Hepatic failure (horses)** **Phosphofructokinase deficiency (dogs)**	**RBC parasites** • *Anaplasma* spp. • *Cytauxzoon* spp. • *Hemobartonella* (*Mycoplasma*) spp. **Immune-mediated** • Hemolytic anemia • *Ehrlichia* spp. • Feline leukemia virus • Hemangiosarcoma • RBC parasites • *Sarcocystis* spp. **Intrinsic erythrocyte defects** **Fragmentation** • DIC • Heartworm • Hemangiosarcoma • Vasculitis **Hemophagocytic syndrome** **Hypersplenism** **Malignant histiocytosis**	**Anemia of chronic disorders** • Chronic inflammation • Neoplasia **Cytotoxic bone marrow damage** • Estrogen • Phenylbutazone • Cytotoxic cancer drugs • Radiation • Bracken fern **Reduced erythropoietin** • Chronic renal disease • Hypoadrenocorticism • Hypothyroidism • Hypoandrogenism **Immune-mediated** • Pure red cell aplasia **Infection** • *Ehrlichia* spp. • Feline leukemia virus • Feline panleukopenia virus • Parvovirus **Myelophthisis** • Lymphocytic leukemia • Metastatic neoplasia • Myelofibrosis • Myeloproliferative disorders	**Abnormal maturation** **Disorders of heme synthesis** **Disorders of nucleic acid synthesis**

Source: Adapted from: Brockus and Andreasen (2003).

or toxicities (e.g., estrogen). Hemolysis may develop secondary to immune-mediated mechanisms or toxicities, neoplasia, or infection with RBC parasites (e.g., *Babesia* spp.). Chronic hemorrhage in veterinary patients may frequently be subtle or subclinical, making signs such as melena or elevated blood urea nitrogen (BUN) (possible indicators of gastrointestinal bleeding) significant component of the preanesthetic workup. Hemorrhage may also be due to anticoagulant rodenticide toxicity, and vitamin K_1 therapy may be indicated before the patient undergoes any invasive procedures (see the following section). In patients presenting for anesthesia and surgery who may have clinical signs of anemia due to any of the aforementioned causes, at minimum, a platelet count and coagulation panel are indicated to better define the patient's hemostatic ability. It is also prudent to obtain a blood type on the patient before anesthesia, which may facilitate rapid transfusion during the procedure, if necessary.

The chronicity of a patient's anemia may influence the management of intraoperative hemorrhage. With chronic anemia, Hb gradually develops an increased relative ability to carry oxygen, due to an increase in 2,3-DPG. This physiologic change may partially compensate for the anemia-related oxygen delivery deficit [8]. Because of this physiologic adaptation, patients with chronic anemia may tolerate small intra-anesthetic decreases in Hct without requiring RBC transfusion. It bears consideration, however, that an unpredictable degree of drug-related vasodilation or splenic engorgement may occur during anesthesia, making even a small decrease in the circulating RBC mass a catastrophic event for animals with preexisting anemia. Adult patients with chronic hypoxemia also develop increased 2,3-DPG levels over time, shifting their oxyhemoglobin dissociation curve to the right, which favors offloading of oxygen to their tissues [9].

Intravenous crystalloid therapy may further exacerbate this anemia, reducing blood viscosity, precipitating edema, and potentially impairing O_2 delivery at the microvascular level. These special considerations for anemic patients thereby justify inclusion of monitoring which may suggest disturbances in tissue oxygen delivery (e.g., serial lactate quantification, mixed-venous SO_2 [as a surrogate of oxygen extraction], or tachycardia not attributable to hypercapnia, hypovolemia, chronotropic therapy, pain, or an inadequate plane of anesthesia).

Hydration status should be considered while interpreting Hct values—anemia in a dehydrated or hypovolemic patient may only reveal itself after replacement of the fluid deficit. Serum total protein, albumin, BUN, and creatinine concentrations may also be elevated in dehydrated patients, although serum protein concentrations and decreases in body weight have proven more useful than azotemia or elevated Hct as indicators of dehydration in otherwise healthy dogs [10]. Healthy horses are likewise expected to lose body weight and have elevated blood protein concentration in the face of water deprivation, with no reliable change in PCV [11]. Interpretation of PCV may be further confounded in species known to undergo splenic contraction during times of stress (e.g., horses and dogs). Azotemia should always be interpreted with respect to urine-specific gravity to differentiate renal, postrenal, and prerenal (dehydration or hypovolemia) causes. Hct should always be interpreted in conjunction with historical information, physical examination, and biochemistry findings in preparation for anesthetic management of individual patients.

Caution should be exercised in the interpretation of PCV values in the midst of acute hemorrhage. Due to splenic contraction, acute hemorrhage is frequently accompanied only by a decreased total protein with a normal to increased PCV; changes in PCV may not be seen until hemorrhage is severe or adequate volume resuscitation has been administered, thus uncovering the degree of blood loss.

Best practices in the emergent treatment of severe hemorrhage and hemorrhagic shock have evolved significantly, from a large-volume crystalloid-based approach to restricted and goal-oriented fluid therapy, now integrating earlier transfusion of blood products. The understanding of the endothelial glycocalyx has revolutionized medical awareness of vascular fluid and protein dynamics and has shifted the focus of resuscitation efforts from the macrocirculation to one more inclusive of microcirculatory factors [12–14].

While traditional approaches to intraoperative hemorrhage in dogs may have consisted of boluses of isotonic crystalloid fluids in the amount of two or three times the volume of blood lost, investigations of hemorrhagic shock therapy in humans supports lower-volume resuscitation (even using hypertonic crystalloid solutions [15, 16]) and earlier use of blood products, especially in cases of severe hemorrhage [17]. While natural and artificial colloids (e.g., albumin and hydroxyethyl starch (HES) solutions) can restore intravascular volume [18], the correlation in humans of artificial colloids with increased mortality risk, acute renal failure, and coagulopathy has deemphasized the use of hetastarches, especially in patients with sepsis or septic shock [19]. The significance of these concerns in veterinary patients is unknown [20–22]. With wider availability of canine albumin, however, this colloid may prove to be a useful adjunct to small-volume resuscitation in canine patients when used as a 5% solution.

An approach prioritizing the restoration of oxygen delivery to the microcirculation supports the earlier restoration of volume using blood products to replace shed RBCs, plasma, and platelets, ideally in a 1:1:1 ratio if there is massive hemorrhage, or at least earlier consideration of expanding the RBC mass in patients with intraoperative hemorrhage. Fresh or stored whole blood may be an optimal product to have on hand prior to surgeries where excessive hemorrhage is anticipated.

Much of the data supporting a 1:1:1 ratio of blood products, with limited crystalloid, for resuscitation is derived from the human trauma literature. Human patients with traumatic shock experience impaired perfusion, resulting in acidosis, and a hyperfibrinolytic coagulopathic condition ("acute coagulopathy of trauma and shock") caused by endothelial injury and hypothermia, all of which contribute to morbidity and mortality following shock [14]. In patients with ongoing hemorrhage following trauma, principles of low-volume or damage-control resuscitation advocate the maintenance of systemic hemodynamics while limiting additional hemorrhage until the source may be addressed. The techniques utilized to achieve these goals include permissive hypotension (systolic arterial pressure approximately 80–90 mmHg or mean arterial pressure approximately 60–65 mmHg), low-volume fluid resuscitation, and titration of agents to minimize microvascular hypoperfusion (normalize systemic vascular resistance) until hemostasis is reestablished. Once hemorrhage is controlled, more aggressive fluid therapy may be considered to address systemic ischemia before irreversible endothelial injury occurs. The use of fresh or stored whole blood or a 1:1:1 ratio of platelets:plasma:RBCs is advocated for these patients, and is expected to improve outcome.

Veterinary care centers face unique challenges to the implementation of low-volume resuscitation, and its relevance for intraoperative hemorrhage, where the source may be rapidly controlled (as opposed to human patients that encounter trauma and hemorrhage outside of the hospital environment), is unclear. Blood product availability may be limited (particularly concentrated platelet products), and the cost of resuscitation using blood products may be cost-prohibitive to pet owners. In the face of these challenges and current controversies regarding artificial colloids, the authors advocate consideration of the integration of natural colloids (fresh frozen plasma [FFP], albumin) and other blood products in the resuscitation of patients with hemorrhagic shock, in addition to careful consideration of the actual crystalloid fluid needs during procedures. Monitoring during anesthesia and resuscitation should include blood pressure, heart rate, and measures of perfusion and DO_2 such as serial lactate quantification and urine output.

Red Blood Cell Transfusions

The goal of RBC transfusions is to improve the oxygen-carrying capacity of the blood and, thus, the oxygen delivery to tissues in anemic patients. RBCs may be transfused in the form of fresh or stored whole blood or in prepared solutions of packed red blood cells (pRBCs). With the use of appropriate anticoagulants and nutrients (e.g., as from RBC preservative solutions), pRBCs from dogs and cats may be stored refrigerated up to 35 days, although storage lesions may occur in older units. Storage lesions include a decrease in RBC deformability (due to adenosine triphosphate loss), a depletion of 2,3-DPG, and a progressive acidosis within the unit. In humans, transfusion of RBC products stored for longer periods can result in limited improvement in tissue oxygen delivery and may be implicated in the development of transfusion-related acute lung injury (TRALI) [23]. No reports of TRALI have been published in the veterinary literature to date, although there is some evidence that leukoreduction of pRBC units may decrease transfusion-associated inflammation [24], and older RBC units may be more likely to cause transfusion reactions [25, 26]. The effects of different anticoagulant storage media have been described for canine, feline, and equine RBCs [27–29].

RBC transfusion is generally indicated for anesthetized or preanesthetic patients with Hb concentrations ≤ 5–$7\,\mathrm{g\,dl^{-1}}$ (corresponding to a PCV of approximately 15–20%), especially if the decrease has been acute. Hb concentrations below this threshold can lead to significant decreases in oxygen delivery to tissues, and if hemorrhage occurs in these patients, the reduction in oxygen delivery may be precipitous. Hemorrhage constituting >20% of a patient's blood volume, when accompanied by clinical signs indicating a sympathetic response to hypovolemia (e.g., tachycardia and hypotension), may also justify transfusion of RBC, in addition to volume stabilization with isotonic crystalloids and colloids. Approximate blood volumes of various species are listed in Table 14.3.

Another indicator for transfusion in anemic patients may be hyperlactatemia (blood lactate $> 2.0\,\mathrm{mmol\,l^{-1}}$), which suggests inadequate tissue oxygen delivery. Lactic acid is produced during anaerobic glycolysis and is indicative of a situation wherein the oxygen demand of the tissues exceeds the oxygen delivered [30]. Blood lactate concentration reflects the balance of lactate production by body tissues and the liver's ability to metabolize it, which is rarely the limiting step (except for significant hepatic hypoperfusion). The blood lactate should be evaluated with respect to the patient, as it may be influenced by other factors including vessel selection (central versus peripheral venous sample), struggle during venipuncture of a peripheral vein, hypoxemia, or prolonged venous occlusion during venipuncture. Hyperlactatemia may support the decision to transfuse an anemic patient, in addition to hematology results and clinical signs indicating a sympathetic response to hypovolemia or hemorrhage (e.g., tachycardia, hypotension, and pale mucous membranes).

Before transfusion of a patient with whole blood or pRBCs, the blood type of canine and

Table 14.3 Approximate blood volumes for veterinary species.

Species	Approximate blood volume ($\mathrm{ml\,kg^{-1}}$)
Canine	86
Feline	55
Equine	76
Bovine	55
Murine	79

feline patients should be determined. In general, type-specific blood transfusions in small-animal patients that have not received prior blood transfusions do not require cross-matching. In emergent scenarios, dog erythrocyte antigen (DEA)-1-negative canine blood may be used in dogs without blood typing, but the possible presence of preexisting alloantibodies between feline blood types makes blood typing imperative before transfusion. In patients who have received prior transfusions or for whom more than 3 days have elapsed since a previous transfusion, cross-matching is recommended to decrease the chance of immunologic reactions to blood transfusion. Procedures for blood collection and cross-matching have been reviewed elsewhere [31].

Blood product dosing is based on the volume of RBCs required to raise the recipient's PCV to a desired value. An estimated volume for administration may be obtained using the following formula (Eq. (14.2)):

$$\begin{aligned}&\text{Volume of donor blood required}\left(\text{ml}\right)\\&\quad=\text{Recipient's blood volume}\\&\quad\times\left(\text{Desired PCV}-\text{Recipient PCV}\right)/\\&\qquad\text{PCV of donor blood}\end{aligned} \tag{14.2}$$

It is generally assumed that the PCV of pRBC is 60–80%, while the donor PCV of whole blood will vary with the donor. Short-hand calculations estimate a dose of $1\,\text{ml kg}^{-1}$ of pRBC or $3\,\text{ml kg}^{-1}$ of whole blood to raise the recipient PCV by 1%. A formula representing the total required volume of pRBC as 1.5 ml of pRBC × desired% PCV rise × kg body weight (BW) was also recently shown to be accurate [32]. Blood is typically supplied in aliquots of 500, 250, or 125 ml, and pRBCs are usually available in units of 250 or 125 ml. If sterile tubing welders are available, these bags may also be split into smaller volumes for administration to smaller patients. An opened (i.e., pierced with an IV administration set) bag of blood should be administered over a maximum of 4 h.

Despite compatibility testing, any blood transfusion recipient may develop a reaction, although acute hemolytic reactions are uncommon in dogs [25, 33]. Identification of a transfusion reaction in an anesthetized patient can be challenging: urticaria may be hidden under surgical drapes, and changes in heart rate, blood pressure, or body temperature may be confounded by the effects of surgical stimuli, heat loss from body cavities, and anesthetic drug effects. Transfusions should be initiated at low rates; for example, $1–2\,\text{ml kg}^{-1}\,\text{h}^{-1}$ for the first 15 min and then increased if no apparent reaction has developed. The duration of transfusion depends on the acuteness and severity of hemorrhage, although the transfusion should be complete by 4 h after initiation. Patients at greater risk for transfusion reaction may be administered intramuscular diphenhydramine, $2\,\text{mg kg}^{-1}$ body weight. Transfusion technique significantly influences survival of RBCs in canine patients. Compared to administration by gravity flow, RBCs administered by volumetric or syringe pump may undergo more shear stress, which may cause lysis or decreased survival of the transfused cells [34].

In emergent scenarios, blood may be given rapidly either using a pressure infusion bag or by attaching an inline three-way stopcock and 60-ml syringe to pull blood from the unit and then rapidly infusing it into the patient through an inline filter. In scenarios such as these, with severe hemorrhage, the replacement of coagulation factors with FFP is frequently indicated, and the plasma may be used along with crystalloid and colloid fluids to maintain intravascular volume. Fresh or stored whole blood contains both RBC and plasma components. Sequelae of massive hemorrhage in anesthetized patients include dramatically reduced drug requirement (including inhalant anesthetics), cardiovascular instability, and development of metabolic acidosis, in addition to potential coagulopathy from accelerated hypothermia or the dilutional effects of fluid resuscitation and loss of coagulation factors. Patients administered large doses of blood products may also develop hypocalcemia (ionized calcium <1.2 $mmol\,l^{-1}$) because of the citrate anticoagulant in blood products [35]. Hypocalcemia can precipitate cardiac arrhythmias and hypotension and exacerbate coagulopathy. Calcium may be supplemented intravenously as follows: 5–15 $mg\,kg^{-1}$ of elemental calcium or 50–150 $mg\,kg^{-1}$ of 10% calcium gluconate over a 10–20-min period, while monitoring heart rate and rhythm via electrocardiogram. Calcium infusion should be slowed or discontinued if evidence of cardiotoxicity such as bradycardia, sudden elevation of the S-T segment, or shortening of the Q-T interval occurs. Due to the citrate anticoagulant in blood products, the calcium must be administered through a separate or well-flushed catheter, and crystalloid fluids without calcium or magnesium should be used to flush the administration set of blood cells at the end of the transfusion.

Anesthetic Considerations for Patients with Anemia

Anesthetic management of anemic patients should include preoxygenation, careful quantification of hemorrhage, minimization of hemodilution, and drug protocols that have a minimal influence on circulating RBC availability. Preoxygenation for patients with decreased oxygen-carrying capacity will not greatly affect the proportion of Hb molecules bound with oxygen but will delay desaturation during anesthetic induction and may increase the oxygen transfer gradient at the level of the tissues (by increasing the amount of dissolved oxygen). In normal dogs premedicated with acepromazine and morphine and induced with propofol, 3 min of preoxygenation (100 $ml\,kg^{-1}\,min^{-1}$ of 100% oxygen) significantly delayed Hb desaturation, compared to dogs allowed to breathe room air prior to induction [36].

Maintenance of oxygen delivery in the face of anemia depends on hemodynamic as well as metabolic compensatory mechanisms. Anemia-related decreases in CaO_2 stimulate a sympathetic response, which includes an increase in cardiac output (increased stroke volume or heart rate), as well as an increase in tissue oxygen extraction. These compensatory changes occur to fulfill the energy substrate and oxygen requirements of aerobic metabolism. The oxygen extraction ratio, normally about 25–30%, can increase to about 60–70% before oxygen consumption (VO_2) is limited by oxygen delivery (Figure 14.2). Oxygen delivery in humans may remain normal in the face of Hb concentrations as low as 5 $g\,dl^{-1}$ (caused by isovolemic hemodilution) due to compensatory increases in cardiac output and oxygen extraction [37]. When oxygen delivery decreases below the point of maximal tissue oxygen extraction (the critical DO_2 point), tissue hypoxia ensues, and the tissues begin to use anaerobic metabolism for maintenance of cellular energy (Figure 14.2). Anaerobic metabolism can lead to a systemic lactic acidosis. Anesthetic agents that have minimal negative effects on cardiac output and vascular tone should be chosen for the patient with anemia, to preserve these intrinsic compensatory mechanisms as much as possible.

Anesthesia can obtund the mechanisms of compensation for anemia. Humans subjected to normovolemic hemodilution while anesthetized with a fentanyl/nitrous oxide/isoflurane in oxygen combination had much smaller increases in stroke volume (and thus cardiac index) than awake patients undergoing the same hemodilution. These anesthetized humans did show an increased oxygen extraction to compensate for the decrease in DO_2 [38]. From the perspective of anesthetic monitoring, hemodynamic responses to inappropriate hemodilution cannot be relied on for treatment decisions. Tachycardia, for example, may not occur in normovolemic patients as they approach their critical DO_2 point. Anemic, anesthetized patients are at greater risk of reduced tissue oxygen delivery and may have reduced capacity to activate the sympathetic compensatory mechanisms seen

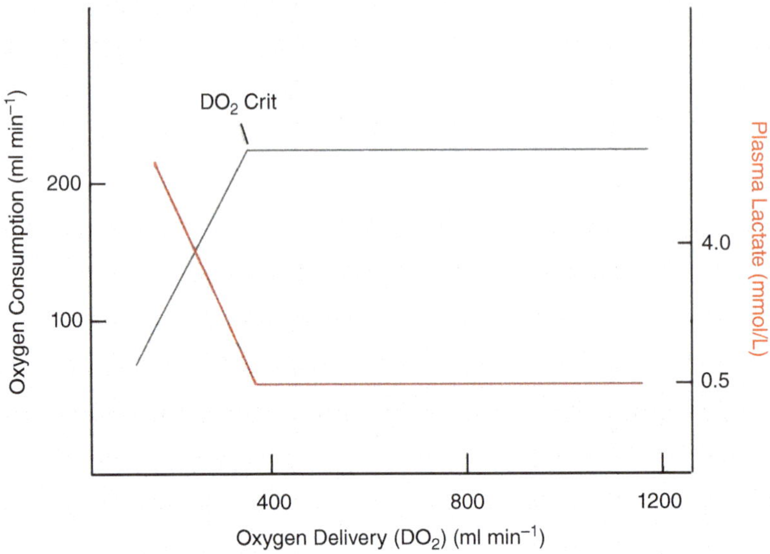

Figure 14.2 Relationship between oxygen delivery (DO_2) and consumption (VO_2). As flow (Q) or DO_2 decreases, oxygen extraction increases, and VO_2 remains stable. When DO_2 decreases below the level requiring maximal tissue oxygen extraction (the critical DO_2 point), VO_2 concurrently decreases, resulting in tissue hypoxia. *Source:* Used with permission from Muir MM. (2007). Cardiovascular system. In: Tranquilli et al. editors, Lumb and Jones' Veterinary Anesthesia and Analgesia, 4th edition, p. 109. Ames: Blackwell.

in conscious individuals. The anesthetist must be vigilant in monitoring vital signs, blood loss, and even serial measures of DO_2 indices, such as blood lactate concentration, to ensure adequate DO_2.

Injectable and inhalant anesthetic agents may significantly decrease circulating erythrocyte mass by causing RBC sequestration in the spleen. The spleen serves as an important reservoir for RBCs, sequestering up to 40% of the RBC mass at any one time [39]. Isoflurane can decrease Hct by >30% in healthy ferrets due to splenic sequestration of RBCs [40]. Significant reductions in Hct can also occur after administration of various injectable agents; the following drugs, alone or in combination, have been shown to result in a 5–20% decrease in canine PCV: acepromazine, thiopental, propofol, and ketamine/diazepam. Combinations using thiopental and acepromazine produced greater reductions in PCV than ketamine/diazepam [41]. For this reason, acepromazine and thiopental are relatively contraindicated in anemic patients, and other drugs that may promote vasodilation and splenic engorgement (e.g., propofol) should be used sparingly.

Injectable drugs known to cause significant hemolysis should be avoided in anemic patients. Formulations of etomidate and diazepam in propylene glycol may cause intravascular hemolysis due to the hyperosmolarity of the solution [42]. The administration of both of these drugs may be indicated in some compromised patients, given the relative cardiovascular stability associated with both drugs. Dilution of etomidate solution in 0.9% saline immediately before induction will decrease the osmolarity of the solution and may help to prevent hemolysis. Anesthetists concerned about hemolysis related to diazepam may select midazolam as an alternative, as it is water-soluble and does not contain propylene glycol. Application of a balanced, multimodal approach will also reduce the doses of each drug, thereby minimizing negative side effects attributable to each individual agent.

Red Blood Cell Disorders and Blood Viscosity

Abnormal Hct (high or low) can result in decreased oxygen delivery due to changes in blood viscosity and tissue blood flow. Hemoglobin concentration and blood viscosity for maximal relative oxygen delivery are $15\,g\,dl^{-1}$ and approximately 2 cP, respectively. Blood viscosity affects DO_2 by affecting the efficient movement of erythrocytes through capillaries. Decreases in blood viscosity can also lower DO_2 beyond the effects of the anemia alone (Figure 14.3). The most important determinant of blood viscosity is Hct; patients with polycythemia or anemia are especially susceptible to decreased DO_2. Polycythemia reduces RBC movement at the capillary level, creating a "sludging" effect, and prolongs capillary transit time. Inadequate blood viscosity, as seen in severely anemic patients, increases the likelihood of turbulent blood flow. This turbulence is recognized as physiologic cardiac murmurs in anemic patients.

Polycythemia or erythrocytosis describes an increased RBC number. Some canine breeds (e.g., Sighthounds) may have higher erythrocyte counts than other breeds, which should be taken into consideration when interpreting Hct data [43]. Polycythemia is characterized as either absolute, denoting an increased total RBC mass, or relative polycythemia, denoting a normal RBC mass but increased Hct due to decreased plasma volume (i.e., hemoconcentration). Absolute polycythemia is further categorized into primary (polycythemia vera) and secondary polycythemia, which results from conditions including chronic hypoxia. Chronic

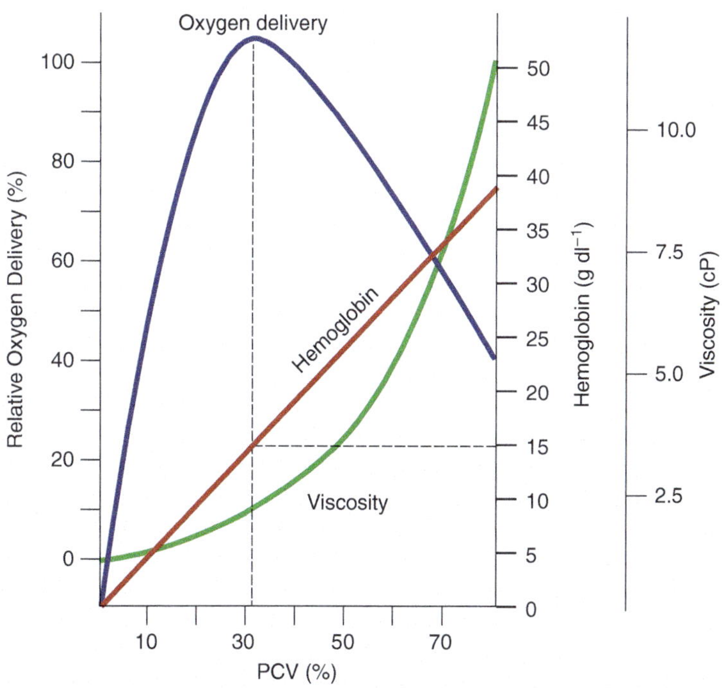

Figure 14.3 The effects of hemoglobin concentration and blood viscosity on relative oxygen delivery. Relative oxygen delivery is maximized at a hemoglobin concentration of $15\,g\,dl^{-1}$ and blood viscosity of approximately 9 cP. From this point, decreases or increases in hemoglobin concentration and blood viscosity result in significant decreases in relative oxygen delivery. *Source:* Used with permission from: Muir MM. (2007). Cardiovascular system. In: Tranquilli et al. editors, Lumb and Jones' Veterinary Anesthesia and Analgesia, 4th edition, p. 64. Ames: Blackwell.

hypoxia leading to increased release of erythropoietin and secondary proliferation of RBCs may occur as a physiologic response to high altitudes, intracardiac right-to-left shunting, or, less commonly, severe pulmonary disease. Relative polycythemia most commonly results from loss of body fluid and subsequent hemoconcentration. Clinical signs of polycythemia are attributable to hyperviscosity and decreased microcirculatory flow. Depending on the severity of the disease, patients may be at greater risk of tissue hypoxia and thrombosis. Hyperviscosity (caused by elevations of blood cells or plasma proteins) commonly manifests as neurologic abnormalities (seizures and collapse) secondary to compromised cerebral microcirculation.

Treatment guidelines for polycythemia depend on the pathogenesis of the disorder. Relative polycythemia should be treated with fluid therapy to replace intravascular volume, as well as directed therapy for the underlying disorder before anesthesia. Isotonic fluid therapy should be evaluated on a case-by-case basis regarding each patient's serum protein concentrations. For example, a combination of synthetic colloids and isotonic crystalloids may be considered for a polycythemic patient who has concurrent hypoalbuminemia, to minimize decreases in oncotic pressure. Intravenous fluids in cases of relative polycythemia due to hypovolemia should be administered to achieve physiologic endpoints, and, if possible, anesthesia should be delayed until the patient has stabilized.

Therapeutic phlebotomy is indicated for patients with primary polycythemia, with a target Hct <55% for dogs and <50% in cats [44]. Phlebotomy may be accomplished in an awake patient or may require sedation. Sedative options can include neuroleptic combinations such as butorphanol and midazolam in dogs and ketamine with midazolam for cats. Drugs known to cause significant splenic sequestration of RBCs (e.g., acepromazine) should be avoided. Removed blood volume should be replaced with a combination of crystalloid and synthetic or natural colloid. Alternatively, if the blood is collected into a sterile container with appropriate anticoagulant, it may be centrifuged for removal of the RBCs, so that the plasma portion may be returned to the patient.

Disorders of Hemostasis

Disorders of hemostasis encountered by the anesthetist can be generally characterized as those that predispose the animal to a hemorrhagic phenotype (hypocoagulability) and those that predispose the animal to thrombosis (hypercoagulability/thrombophilia). There are also some disorders (e.g., disseminated intravascular coagulopathy [DIC]) that form a spectrum between hypercoagulability and hypocoagulability and can present with a variable phenotype.

Hypocoagulable Disorders

Primary Hemostasis

Primary hemostasis refers to the interaction of the platelet with the vascular endothelium or subendothelium, resulting in platelet activation. The activated platelet releases several substances that recruit and activate additional platelets at the site of injury and experiences a change in the distribution of membrane phospholipids [45]. The exposure of phosphatidylserine (among others) on the platelet surface provides an anchor for assembly of the tissue factor (TF)/factor VIIa complex that will initiate secondary hemostasis, toward formation of fibrin. Disorders of primary hemostasis may be congenital or acquired and are usually problems of either platelet number or function.

Evaluation of Primary Hemostasis

A number of techniques exist to evaluate platelet function. In patients with thrombocytopenia, physical examination frequently reveals pinpoint hemorrhages (petechiae) that may be seen on the gums, the ear pinnae, the inguinal area, or on other glabrous skin. Patients with thrombocytopathia who have normal platelet counts will not necessarily have petechiae [46]. Presenting complaints in patients with abnormal primary hemostasis can range from hematuria and epistaxis to oral mucosal bleeding or gastrointestinal bleeding, which may be manifest as melena [47].

Important laboratory tests for evaluation of a patient with primary hemostatic dysfunction include an accurate platelet count. Machine counts should be verified with a blood smear to evaluate for platelet clumping, which can result in a spurious thrombocytopenia. The simplest test of the ability of platelets to adhere to areas of endothelial damage is the buccal mucosal bleeding time (BMBT) [47]. To perform the BMBT, the lip is folded up to expose the buccal mucosa and lightly secured in place with a gauze tie. Using a Surgicutt® device (Accriva Diagnostics Inc., San Diego, CA), a standard incision (5 mm long and 1 mm deep) is made in the buccal mucosa. Once the incision is made, the area is observed (and timed) for the cessation of bleeding. If necessary, blood may be blotted using a filter paper every 30 s if care is taken not to disturb the fragile platelet gel forming over the incision area. The bleeding time is the time until all bleeding has ceased and is generally between 3 and 5 min in a normal animal. In cats, because the buccal mucosa is not easily accessible, a modification (oral mucosal bleeding time) is performed by placing the cutting device above the upper canine tooth. Cats generally need to be sedated or anesthetized for this test. The BMBT will be abnormally prolonged if patients have either thrombocytopenia or thrombocytopathia [47, 48].

The PFA-100 (Siemens Healthcare, Tarrytown, NY) is a benchtop platelet function analyzer that simulates the shear stress encountered by platelets in blood flowing past a vascular defect. Using a vacuum, blood is aspirated through a small aperture coated with either collagen and adenosine diphosphate (ADP) or collagen and epinephrine. These substances will activate platelets and induce a platelet plug across the aperture. The time until the aperture is completely occluded by the plug is reported as the closure time, in seconds, with a maximum value of 300 s. The PFA-100 has been used to evaluate hemostasis in dogs and can rapidly identify platelet defects caused by von Willebrand disease (vWD) and nonsteroidal anti-inflammatory drug (NSAID) administration [49, 50].

Platelet aggregometry may be performed using either whole blood or platelet-rich plasma, and it tests the ability of platelets to aggregate in response to a discrete stimulus, such as ADP or collagen. This test is performed on specialized equipment under low shear conditions and investigates how platelets respond to specific agonists or how drugs affect platelet responses [51]. Aggregometry is primarily a research tool and not readily available to most practitioners, but many studies that assess drug effects and other platelet function abnormalities report aggregometry results. Flow cytometry has also been used in veterinary medicine to investigate platelet function and phenotype and has aided the diagnosis of specific platelet function defects [52–54].

Disorders of Primary Hemostasis

Thrombocytopenia is an absolute decrease in the number of circulating platelets. Normal platelet count in dogs and cats ranges between 250 and 500×10^3 platelets per microliter. Thrombocytopenias are generally considered $<150 \times 10^3$ platelets per microliter and may be as low as $5–10 \times 10^3$ per microliter. Due to the tendency of platelets to clump if they are activated by inflammation or a traumatic blood sampling, manual verification of a low platelet count by blood smear evaluation should be performed. At 100X power, one platelet represents 15×10^3 per microliter, so 10–15 platelets per field is considered normal. As a rule, spontaneous bleeding does not occur at platelet counts $>20 \times 10^3$ per microliter, although a more conservative cutoff for patients who are undergoing surgery is generally about 50×10^3 per microliter. Some breeds, notably the Cavalier King Charles Spaniel, can have a hereditary macrothrombocytopenia, where the platelets are fewer and larger than normal, but without identifiable abnormalities in platelet function or hemostasis [55].

One of the more common causes of thrombocytopenia in dogs is an immune-mediated thrombocytopenia (IMT). IMT is characterized by extremely low platelet counts ($<20 \times 10^3$ per microliter), and patients may experience spontaneous bleeding from mucosal surfaces. The cause of IMT is generally presumed to be idiopathic, although drugs (e.g., trimethoprim-sulfa) have been implicated in some cases [56, 57].

Mild to moderate thrombocytopenia ($40–100 \times 10^3$ per microliter) is frequently seen in animals with diseases that induce inflammation or DIC [58]. Some of these diseases include neoplasia, sepsis, pancreatitis, heartworm infection, or trauma with crush injury, and these patients may require emergent anesthesia and surgery for therapy of the primary cause. Infection with some of the tick-borne diseases (e.g., *Ehrlichia* spp.) can also be associated with mild to moderate thrombocytopenia. In addition, patients who are actively bleeding or who have experienced blood loss frequently have a modest decrease in platelet count.

Treatments in Preparation for Anesthesia

In human patients, recommendations for transfusions of platelet-containing products (platelet concentrate, platelet-rich plasma) are made in individuals with $<50 \times 10^3$ platelets per microliter who require invasive procedures. In veterinary medicine, blood products containing platelets alone are not readily available to most practitioners. The easiest and most practical way to administer platelets to a patient before surgery is via transfusion of fresh whole blood, although the number of platelets provided will vary depending on the platelet concentration of the donor and likely will not increase the platelet count significantly. The amount of blood to transfuse may be calculated on the basis of patient RBC needs (see the section titled "Red Blood Cell Transfusions") or may be empirically administered at 10–20 ml kg^{-1} if the patient is not anemic. Despite the lack of increase in platelet count, fresh whole blood may provide enough platelets to stop ongoing bleeding and provide some hemostatic support during surgery. With appropriate attention to surgical hemostasis and transfusions as indicated, surgery can be safely performed in patients with moderate to severe thrombocytopenia.

Frozen dimethylsulfoxide (DMSO)-stabilized canine platelet concentrate is available; however, the activity of these platelets is significantly diminished compared to fresh platelets [59]. Other available options include lyophilized platelet concentrate, although the efficacy of these for bleeding thrombocytopenic patients is still under investigation [53]. The options for platelet transfusions in veterinary medicine have been reviewed [60]. In patients who do not need emergent surgery, vincristine (0.02 mg kg^{-1} IV once) may be used to increase the number of circulating platelets, although an increase in circulating platelet number may not be evident for up to 4 days, and leukopenia may result [61].

Anesthetic concerns specifically related to animals with thrombocytopenia are applicable to any patient at risk for significant hemorrhage. Animals should be handled gently, and transport during and after anesthetic induction should be carefully planned and executed to avoid iatrogenic trauma and hemorrhage. Thrombocytopenic animals may develop hematomas at the site of intramuscular injections, and these should be minimized or avoided. Animals may also develop hematomas at the site of peripheral intravenous or intraarterial catheters; if necessary, these peripheral areas may have a pressure wrap placed to encourage hemostasis. Jugular venipuncture is contraindicated due to the inability to tamponade bleeding, and for the same reason, femoral arterial puncture is not recommended. The dorsal metatarsal site is preferred for arterial catheter placement in thrombocytopenic animals. In addition, animals are likely to bleed from disturbed mucosal areas, and catheters (e.g., intranasal and urinary), if necessary, should be placed with care, and rectal or esophageal temperature monitoring should be performed judiciously. Hemorrhage of the arytenoids or tracheal mucosa may occur from aggressive endotracheal intubation and may result in postoperative upper airway obstruction. Neuraxial analgesia and peripheral nerve block techniques are contraindicated in these patients due to the potential for catastrophic bleeding.

In addition to these practical aspects of patient care, the use of drugs that may impair platelet function should be avoided, and NSAIDs are contraindicated. The use of synthetic colloids (e.g., hetastarch) may be necessary for oncotic support during anesthesia; however, these drugs may also impair platelet function (see the following sections) and should be used judiciously. Transient impairment of platelet function after acepromazine administration has been described [62]. While the clinical importance in a healthy dog seems minimal, in thrombocytopenic patients, the effect, if any, may be magnified.

Thrombocytopathias

Thrombocytopathias, or platelet dysfunction, may be caused by some systemic diseases, but are more frequently a result of inherited traits or due to drug effects on the platelet. Clinical signs of thrombocytopathias are characterized by bleeding from mucosal surfaces. Milder forms are first diagnosed in patients who have prolonged bleeding after surgery for spay and neuter. Although patients may have cutaneous bruising, petechiae are rarely seen, as they result from an absolute decrease in platelet number. Patients usually have an adequate number of circulating platelets (although the total number may be lower if there has been hemorrhage) and a normal coagulation profile.

Platelet dysfunction has been reported in patients with moderate to severe uremia and may result from alterations in the platelet membrane or in the platelet response to some stimuli [48, 63]. Animals with hypothyroidism may have mild platelet dysfunction, but the origin of this change is unclear and of questionable clinical relevance [64–66]. In animals with severe uremia that require anesthesia, the same precautions listed previously for patients with thrombocytopenias are relevant. Additional anesthetic concerns for the uremic patient are discussed in Chapters 6 and 7.

The most common inherited thrombocytopathia in dogs is vWD. vWD describes a complex of diseases associated with malformation or absence of von Willebrand factor (vWF), necessary for tethering of activated platelets to areas of endothelial injury. Type I vWD is characterized by a lower total amount of functional vWF, although all sizes of vWF are present, and is the most common type of vWD seen in dogs, with Doberman Pinschers overrepresented. The clinical severity of Type I vWD depends on the quantitative degree of vWF activity present [46]. Type II vWD comprises a group of functional variants of vWF characterized by alterations in the size profile of circulating vWF (e.g., a lower amount of large-molecular-weight vWF) [46]. Type III vWD is characterized by complete lack of circulating vWF and is the most severe clinical presentation of vWD. vWD may be diagnosed by functional assays (e.g., BMBT or PFA) [67], or the actual amount of functional vWF can be measured. The latter is reported as a percentage of activity, with normal activity between 65% and 150%. Animals affected with clinically important vWD frequently have activities of ≤40% [46].

Prophylactic therapy to prevent bleeding in patients with vWD includes cryoprecipitate, which is also indicated if the patient is actively bleeding. Cryoprecipitate is made from FFP and contains a concentrated amount of vWF and coagulation factor VIII (fVIII). Cryoprecipitate is available in frozen and lyophilized forms and is usually administered at a dose of 3–5 $ml\,kg^{-1}$ [68]. Desmopressin acetate (DDAVP) has been used in humans and dogs with vWD, and in humans with Type I vWD it results in a twofold to fourfold increase in circulating vWF and coagulation fVIII [69]. Dogs with Type I vWD showed an improvement of clinical signs (decreased mucosal bleeding time and shortened PFA closure time) and an increase in circulating vWF after DDAVP therapy [67]. The recommended dosage for DDAVP is 1 $\mu g\,kg^{-1}$, administered subcutaneously or as a subconjunctival drop. In Doberman Pinschers with an unknown vWF titer presenting for emergent surgery, DDAVP is routinely administered, and transfusion products should be available for intraoperative and postoperative transfusion.

Other inherited platelet function defects that have been reported in veterinary species include Glanzmann thrombasthenia, reported in Great Pyrenees, Otterhounds, and several horses and characterized by dysfunction in the platelet fibrinogen receptor [70]. Several dog breeds and Simmental cattle have a heritable thrombocytopathia distinguished by an intracellular signaling defect in the platelet that prevents activation of the fibrinogen-binding site. Scott syndrome, a lack of platelet procoagulant activity, has been reported in German Shepherds and is characterized by an inability of platelets to support secondary hemostasis, leading to hemorrhage [71]. Frequently, these defects manifest themselves as spontaneous bleeding or as excessive bleeding after surgeries for spay or neuter or after ear crop, tail dock, or dew claw removal. Patients with these and other platelet defects who require anesthesia and surgery are at an increased risk for bleeding intraoperatively and postoperatively. Before surgery, dogs should be blood-typed, and adequate plasma and RBCs should be available. The administration of platelet rich plasma (PRP) or platelet concentrates can also be considered for these dogs before elective surgery; if surgery is emergent and platelet products are not available, fresh whole blood remains a good option for transfusion needs during surgery, and the animals may require continued transfusion care into the postoperative period.

Many commonly used pharmaceuticals can alter platelet function and may result in impaired platelet aggregation or adhesion. NSAIDs can affect platelet aggregation by impairing the production of platelet thromboxane A_2 (TXA2) by the cyclooxygenase (COX) enzyme. TXA_2 is a proaggregatory substance and helps to activate additional platelets at areas of vascular damage. It also results in vasoconstriction at the site, which may help to mitigate blood loss. Aspirin is the archetypical NSAID and significantly decreases platelet aggregation to collagen in patients who are sensitive to TXA_2 [72]. Dogs have been identified that are insensitive to the platelet effects of NSAIDs due to a presumed decreased sensitivity to TXA_2 [73]. Feline platelets may also be relatively resistant to inhibition of TXA_2 release, as measured by aggregometry [74]. While ASA causes an irreversible inhibition of COX, the other commonly used veterinary NSAIDs (e.g., carprofen and meloxicam) have reversible binding and cause only a transient decrease in platelet function, if at all [75]. Because most COX in circulating platelets is presumed to be the COX-1 isoform (which may or may not be correct) [76], drugs that specifically target the COX-2 isoform (e.g., deracoxib and firocoxib) are not expected to alter platelet function, even in sensitive dogs [72]. The use of ketoprofen has also been associated with decreases in platelet aggregation [75]. In general, there are no contraindications to the performance of local or neuraxial analgesic techniques in patients receiving NSAIDs.

Synthetic colloids are commonly used for volume support of critically ill patients in the perioperative period. These colloids (hetastarch, tetrastarch, and dextran) are usually a 6% solution in an isotonic crystalloid. Smaller molecular weight colloids (e.g., tetrastarch) are excreted more rapidly and may be amenable to a higher total daily dose. The impact of colloids on coagulation indices is well documented, and they have effects on both platelet function and clot strength that may be problematic in patients with bleeding tendencies. Hetastarches can bind to circulating vWF/fVIII complexes, resulting in increased clearance and impairing platelet adhesion to sites of vascular injury [77]. Hetastarches can also cause an increase in fibrinolysis and a weaker clot strength because they can become integrated into the clot. The effect of HES solutions on coagulation varies with the molecular composition of the product and carrier solution; products with higher molecular weights and molar substitution ratios are more likely to interfere with coagulation, due primarily to a longer duration in circulation and slower breakdown kinetics [78, 79], and products in a balanced electrolyte solution might have less effect on coagulation than those in normal saline [80]. It is generally accepted that doses up to 24 ml kg^{-1} d^{-1} of hetastarch (670/0.75) and up to 50 ml kg^{-1} d^{-1} of tetrastarch (130/0.45) will cause minimal perturbations of platelet function and coagulation, and patients who receive more than this amount should be monitored for adverse effects. These effects may be more pronounced in patients with preexisting defects in primary hemostasis or thrombocytopenia.

Clopidogrel irreversibly inhibits platelet activation by antagonism at the ADP $P2Y_{12}$ receptor. Its pharmacokinetics and pharmacodynamics have been described in cats, dogs, and horses [51, 81, 82]. Few adverse events have been described in veterinary patients; however, clopidogrel does impair platelet aggregation, and the use of additional anticoagulant (e.g., heparins) or analgesic (e.g., NSAIDs) medications in these patients should be considered carefully in the context of their underlying disease. Clopidogrel is metabolized to an active metabolite by the hepatic CYP3A4/3A5 enzyme system and may affect metabolism (or be affected by metabolism) of drugs used for anesthesia that are processed in a similar manner [51]. Most notably, proton-pump inhibitor drugs (e.g., ondansetron) may affect the metabolism of clopidogrel to the active metabolite, decreasing antiplatelet effects [83]. The anesthesiologist must consider the disease that merited initial use of antiplatelet agents, and anesthetic choices will be more dictated by this condition than by concurrent drug therapy. These drugs may, however, lead to an increase in surgical bleeding, although the literature evaluating human patients recommends that antiplatelet agents not be discontinued before anesthesia and surgery in patients with an increased risk for the development of thrombosis (e.g., patients with coronary artery disease) [84]. Other authors have recommended that clopidogrel be discontinued for 5 days before surgeries where bleeding might be catastrophic (ocular surgery, neurosurgery, urological surgery, or major vascular surgery) [85]. Other publications with human patients have recommended a 7–10-day period without clopidogrel before surgery [85]. Recommendations for discontinuation of antiplatelet agents in veterinary species mirror this advice [86]. Adverse effects of neuraxial analgesia in human patients receiving antiplatelet medication have been reported [87]. Each case should be evaluated individually, and if platelet function testing is available, the return of ADP sensitivity in platelets may be monitored and can help guide surgical timing, as well as the use of neuraxial techniques.

As noted previously, acepromazine may be associated with a transient decrease in platelet function, and if a clinical effect does exist, it may not be apparent unless acepromazine is administered with a more potent platelet antagonist, although this has not been studied. Although platelets do have alpha-2-adrenergic receptors, the effect of dexmedetomidine and related drugs on platelet function has not been described, although a weak agonist effect (similar to epinephrine) might be expected, at least in canine platelets. Isolated articles have described antiplatelet effects of ketamine [88], midazolam [89], propofol [90], halothane, and sevoflurane [91], but the clinical relevance is unclear. Opioid drugs, barbiturates, and etomidate appear to have little effect on aggregation of human platelets [91].

In any animal with decreased platelet function due to disease, heritability, or drugs, the anesthetist must carefully weigh the benefits of neuraxial analgesia with the risk of bleeding. If the patient has a transient platelet dysfunction or a low platelet number due to systemic disease, a postponement of surgical procedures may be indicated if feasible until the platelet numbers can rebound or at least until appropriate transfusion products may be obtained.

Secondary Hemostasis

Secondary hemostasis refers to the aspects of coagulation that consist of the coagulation cascade, a series of serine proteases (the factors) that are sequentially activated, culminating in the formation of fibrin monomers, which are subsequently cross-linked by factor XIIIa. Although the measurement of the prothrombin time (PT) and activated partial thromboplastin time (aPTT) provides a framework for understanding the coagulation effect of the various factors in the coagulation cascade, most of the coagulation in vivo occurs by activation of the TF pathway (extrinsic pathway), which produces a small amount of thrombin (initiation) [92]. The small amount of thrombin produced by the extrinsic pathway has a strong agonist effect on the intrinsic pathway, and the majority of thrombin generated during coagulation is generated via this pathway (amplification and propagation). Initiation of coagulation requires an appropriate cell surface for the assembly of the TF–factor VIIa complex, which is provided by the activated platelet, among other surfaces [92].

Evaluation of Secondary Hemostasis

Secondary hemostasis is evaluated by monitoring the formation of fibrin in blood or plasma after exposure to an activating substance. This is the basis of the activated clotting time (ACT), the PT, aPTT, and the thrombin time (TT), which corresponds to fibrinogen concentration. The ACT is performed on whole blood added to diatomaceous earth (a strong contact activator), while the other tests are performed on citrated plasma with appropriate activators. Samples for coagulation testing should be acquired via a clean direct venipuncture and placed immediately into a plastic or siliconized glass tube containing sodium citrate (usually 3.2%) to a ratio of 1:9 citrate to blood (v:v). Some point-of-care coagulation analyzers can analyze PT and aPTT on citrated whole blood or on native (uncitrated) whole blood [93]. The normal values for dogs and cats will vary with the machine and technique. Prolongation of clotting times usually requires a factor to have an activity <30% of normal.

Disorders of Secondary Hemostasis

Animals with ineffective secondary hemostasis may present with hypovolemic shock due to hemorrhage. Physical examination findings can include pale to white mucous membranes, tachycardia, and weak pulses. In animals without hemorrhage, physical examination will be essentially normal with regard to the underlying disease. Common sites for hemorrhage include the peritoneal cavity, pleural space, retroperitoneum, pericardium, and joints (hemarthrosis). Performing surgery on patients with significant abnormalities of secondary hemostasis can result in catastrophic hemorrhage. Fresh frozen plasma contains all coagulation factors and is an effective way to replace clotting factors and slow or stop hemorrhage from factor deficiency. Stored plasma lacks coagulation factors V and VIII and may be less useful in the context of severe hemorrhage but does contain all of the vitamin-K-dependent coagulation factors and may help to correct coagulopathies in patients with specific deficiencies (e.g., due to ingestion of anticoagulant rodenticides). Fresh whole blood also contains all coagulation factors, while stored whole blood may experience degradation of some factors; these products are indicated to treat anemia due to hemorrhage. In animals with hemorrhagic shock, rapid replacement of intravascular volume is indicated, and transfusion products containing RBCs (pRBC and fresh whole blood) are likely indicated.

Coagulation factor deficiencies may be congenital or acquired. Acquired factor deficiencies may result from toxicities or systemic disease. The liver is the source of circulating coagulation factors in the body, and hepatic dysfunction may result in a coagulopathy. Animals with hepatic disease, especially if undergoing invasive procedures, must have a coagulation profile performed and treatment for coagulopathy if indicated. Coagulopathies are particularly common in cats with hepatic lipidosis, which is also a population that frequently requires anesthesia for hepatic biopsy or aspirate and placement of feeding tubes. At least part of the coagulopathy associated with hepatic lipidosis may be due to malabsorption of vitamin K and parenteral supplementation is indicated before invasive procedures [94]. In many cats, intestinal disease contributes to the malabsorption, although cholestasis in any species may contribute to decreased absorption of vitamin K. If vitamin K therapy does not improve the coagulation profile, additional therapies (e.g., FFP) are indicated before anesthesia and surgery. Primary hepatic disease may also result from ingestion of toxins (e.g., xylitol and mushrooms) in dogs and may result in fulminant hepatic failure with coagulopathy. In addition to primary hepatic disease, systemic diseases can prolong clotting times due to factor depletion. Diseases such as sepsis, pancreatitis, neoplasia, and heartworm disease are associated with the development of the systemic inflammatory response syndrome (SIRS) and DIC. If the consumptive coagulopathy of DIC is severe, coagulation abnormalities will result from factor consumption (see the following text) [58]. Anesthetic choices in these patients are driven more by the underlying disease rather than the coagulation status; however, if invasive procedures are necessary, transfusion of FFP (at least $10\,\mathrm{ml\,kg^{-1}}$) is indicated to normalize coagulation parameters [95]. For patients with defects of primary hemostasis, the benefits of local or neuraxial blockade should be carefully weighed with the risks of uncontrollable hemorrhage. Anesthesia for patients with hepatic disease is covered in Chapter 4.

Toxins or drugs can directly affect the coagulation system. The most common toxins with these effects are the anticoagulant rodenticides. There are many generations of anticoagulant rodenticides, and newer generation formulations generally last longer than the earlier ones. Examples of first-generation rodenticides include warfarin, while brodifacoum and bromadiolone are second-generation products. Warfarin is occasionally used in clinical patients, but is uncommon. Patients with acute rodenticide intoxication rarely require anesthesia; however, occasionally, anesthesia is needed to place thoracic drains for hemothorax or to remove bleeding organs from the abdomen. It is more likely (although still relatively unlikely) that a patient with rodenticide toxicosis will present for anesthesia and surgery, with the owner unaware that their coagulation function is impaired, which may result in excessive surgical and postoperative hemorrhage. In the acute scenario, if a patient is experiencing hemorrhage due to vitamin K antagonism, FFP or stored plasma is the treatment of choice, but continued treatment (and preferred treatment in the absence of hemorrhage) is administration of vitamin K_1 (phytonadione), orally or subcutaneously (intravenous injection may result in anaphylaxis). Depending on the degree of factor depletion, vitamin K administration will rapidly correct coagulation abnormalities in a patient without hemorrhage. Before anesthesia and surgery, at least 2–3 days of therapy (2.5–5 mg kg^{-1} orally, every 12–24 h) should result in normalization of coagulation times, but a repeat coagulation panel is indicated before elective procedures.

Unfractionated heparin (UFH) is a drug that can cause an acquired defect in secondary hemostasis. UFH accelerates the inactivation of coagulation factors II and X by antithrombin (AT). It is frequently used in critically ill patients who are thought to be at risk for thrombosis or thromboembolism or in those whom anticoagulation is essential to therapy (e.g., animals receiving hemodialysis). UFH has variable pharmacodynamics that are not only dose-dependent, but also unpredictable to a certain degree [96, 97]. The coagulation effects of a single (250 U kg^{-1}) subcutaneous dose of UFH (as monitored by coagulation testing) wane 9–12 h after the dose, but coagulation effects are more persistent after prolonged dosing. The maximum anticoagulant effect of a single UFH subcutaneous injection is about 4 h after the injection. The effect of UFH may be monitored by measuring the anti-factor Xa activity in the plasma or may be estimated by evaluating the aPTT, which prolongs with heparin therapy [96]. The anesthetist should assess the coagulation status of patients before anesthesia. In patients receiving heparin therapeutically, coagulation times are expected to be only moderately prolonged (approximately twice normal), and the danger of uncontrollable hemorrhage is not as great as in those patients with profound prolongations of coagulation times. Low-molecular-weight heparins (LMWH) are smaller heparin molecules that are as useful for thromboprophylaxis as UFH but have been associated with a lower incidence of hemorrhage in humans. LMWH do not prolong any coagulation test, and so plasma levels must be estimated by measuring the anti-factor Xa activity.

In anesthesia of human patients, recommendations for neuraxial analgesia/anesthesia in individuals receiving heparin therapy during or after surgery have been made [98, 99]. The American Society of Regional Anesthesia and Pain Medicine recommendations include the following: avoiding neuraxial analgesia in patients with known coagulopathies, delaying surgery (and heparin administration) if the epidural puncture is traumatic, delaying the time from epidural puncture to systemic heparinization for at least 60 min, judiciously using heparin with reversal when indicated, and, finally, removing epidural catheters when normal coagulation is restored (or at the nadir of heparin effect), with postoperative monitoring for signs of epidural hematoma [99]. It has also been recommended to place indwelling epidural catheters up to 24 h before surgery in elective cases [99]. The American College of Chest Physicians has published guidelines for perioperative management of anticoagulated patients [85]. In those patients who receive chronic vitamin K antagonist therapy (e.g., warfarin) that cannot be discontinued, it is recommended to use "bridging therapy" with either UFH or LMWH for the perioperative period until dangers of hemorrhage related to surgery are over (usually 12–24 h after surgery). If vitamin K antagonist therapy can be interrupted without the need for bridging therapy, recommendations are to stop therapy approximately 5 days before surgery to allow normalization of coagulation times (and to verify normal coagulation times before surgery). In human patients receiving therapy with IV UFH, recommendations are to stop this therapy 4 h before surgery, whereas if a patient is receiving subcutaneous LMWH therapy, the final dose should be 24 h before surgery (this may be different in animals where the pharmacokinetics of these drugs does not necessarily support once-daily dosing) [100]. The resumption of heparin therapy may occur at variable intervals depending on the severity of the surgery and the relative chance of postoperative bleeding. In patients who are receiving antiplatelet therapy such as aspirin or clopidogrel, the consensus recommends stopping these drugs 5–7 days before surgery if possible, although in patients at high risk for thrombosis, therapy can be continued up to and through the procedure. Minor surgeries (e.g., dental prophylaxis or dermatologic procedures) generally do not require the interruption of anticoagulant therapy [86]. For emergent surgeries on patients receiving anticoagulant or antiplatelet drugs, the availability of vitamin K or FFP is necessary for patients treated with warfarin, while UFH may be reversed with protamine (see the following section) if necessary. In patients receiving antiplatelet therapies, DDAVP (1 $\mu g\,kg^{-1}$ subcutaneously) may be given before surgery [68], and fresh whole blood, PRP, or platelet concentrate may be helpful to prevent bleeding due to platelet inhibition. The use of activated factor VII has not been extensively described in the surgical management of anticoagulated small animals but may provide an emergent therapy for excessive surgical bleeding [101].

Protamine is a drug that may be used to reverse the anticoagulant effects of UFH; it works by binding free heparin and allows the complex to be cleared without causing additional anticoagulation. Protamine can also act as an anticoagulant, however, and may lead to anticoagulation if more drug is given than heparin is present to bind. For this reason, the dosing recommendations for protamine are scaled. The initial dose is 1 mg of protamine for every 100 U of heparin to be inactivated. This dose of protamine is decreased by half for every 30 min elapsed since the heparin administration. Protamine should be diluted in sterile 0.9% saline and administered slowly IV. Protamine is frequently used to reverse heparin effects where UFH is used in large doses, such as cardiopulmonary bypass or hemodialysis.

Viscoelastic Coagulation Monitoring

Newer viscoelastic tests of coagulation such as thromboelastography (TEG, Haemonetics, Braintree, MA), rotational thromboelastometry (ROTEM, TEM International, Munich, Germany), or Sonoclot (Sienco Inc., Morrison, CO) evaluate aspects of both primary and secondary hemostasis, in addition to fibrinolysis. These tests graph the change in viscosity, as liquid blood forms into a clot and can describe hypocoagulable and possibly hypercoagulable states [102]. Numerous reports in the veterinary literature have described the evaluation of these techniques in dogs, cats, and horses, although there is currently a wide variability in techniques that makes comparison across centers difficult [103–105].

The values derived from viscoelastic coagulation devices are related to the different phases of coagulation that the blood undergoes. The initial period, before the liquid blood starts to clot, is represented by the R time (TEG), computed tomography (CT) (ROTEM), or ACT (Sonoclot) (Figure 14.4). This value approximates traditional plasmatic coagulation testing (e.g., PT, aPTT), and abnormalities in this value are generally attributed to coagulopathy. The R time value is sensitive to the activator used in the test (generally tissue factor/phospholipids, kaolin, ellagic acid, or none), and technique-specific reference intervals should be generated for each testing center [104]. The K (TEG) or clot formation time (CFT; ROTEM) value is primarily a measure of the speed of clot formation, and is the time to achieve a tracing width of 10 mm. The alpha angle (TEG and ROTEM) or the clot rate (CR, Sonoclot) is a measure of the speed of clot formation once coagulation starts. This parameter reflects the rapidity of fibrin formation and in particular, the association of fibrin with platelets to increase the strength and stability of the forming clot; it is dependent on both fibrinogen concentration and platelet number (see Figure 14.5 for illustrations of a tracing from a thrombocytopenic dog). The maximum amplitude (MA; TEG) or maximum clot firmness (MCF; ROTEM) is an indicator of the plasma fibrinogen concentration, but also requires the integration of platelets to create the final clot strength. Alterations in the various parts of the tracings can help guide transfusion decisions, specifically if

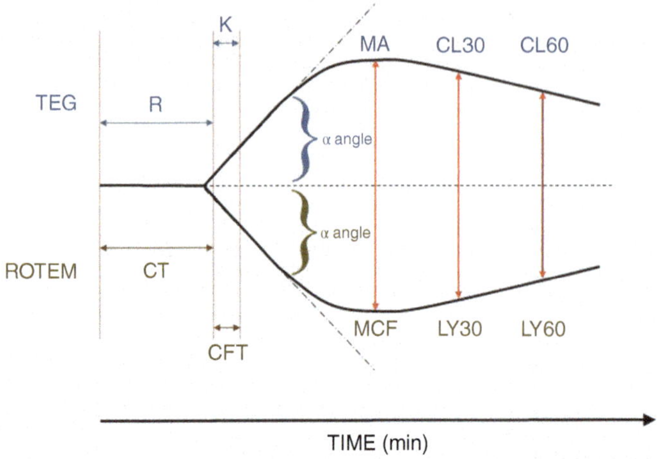

Figure 14.4 Typical TEG (top) and TEM (ROTEM) (bottom) tracings. R, reaction time; K, kinetics; α angle, slope between R and K (TEG), or slope of tangent at 2 mm amplitude (TEM); MA, maximum amplitude; CL30, clot lysis at 30 min; CL60, clot lysis at 60 min; CFT, clot formation time; MCF, maximal clot firmness; LY30, lysis at 30 min; LY60, lysis at 60 min. *Source:* Adapted from: Srivastava A, Kelleher A. 2012. Point-of-care coagulation testing. *Contin Educ Anesthesia Crit Care Pain* 13:12–6.

platelet, plasma, or cryoprecipitate (i.e., fibrinogen) may help normalize coagulation. This may be particularly valuable for patients undergoing cardiopulmonary bypass, due to the extreme coagulation alterations that occur during the process. Among the parameters, the MA appears to be the most reliable to determine the presence of hypercoagulability in human medicine [106, 107], although endpoints and cutoff values for predicting hypercoagulable states in veterinary medicine are yet to be determined [108].

In addition to the procoagulant parameters measured by TEG and ROTEM, these tests can also assess fibrinolysis, or clot breakdown. Fibrinolysis measures are determined by comparing the amplitude of the tracing at 30 and 60 min following the MA or MCF (LY30 and LY60, or CL30 and CL60 for both). Dogs do not show strong fibrinolysis in routine viscoelastic testing, and newer techniques using the addition of exogenous tissue plasminogen activator (tPA) have been described [109]. These techniques have been applied to identify animals with hyperfibrinolysis [110].

Disseminated Intravascular Coagulopathy

DIC is an acquired condition that is generally induced by an underlying systemic inflammatory state. DIC is characterized by a consumptive coagulopathy, where clot formation is initiated systemically. The result of systemic activation of coagulation is a gradual decrease in platelet numbers (as they are integrated into the forming clots) and a gradual prolongation of coagulation times, as the soluble factors are used up. In addition, fibrinolysis is also triggered, which can lead to a systemic fibrinolytic state. Circulating microthrombi may lodge in the microvasculature of organs and contribute to organ dysfunction or failure. Additionally, macrothrombosis (e.g., portal vein thrombus) may also be triggered by DIC. Cross talk between inflammation and activation of coagulation is supported by the production of thrombin (which also serves to sustain systemic inflammation through interaction with white blood cells) and tissue-factor-bearing monocytes, which are stimulated by inflammatory cytokines to display tissue factor, a

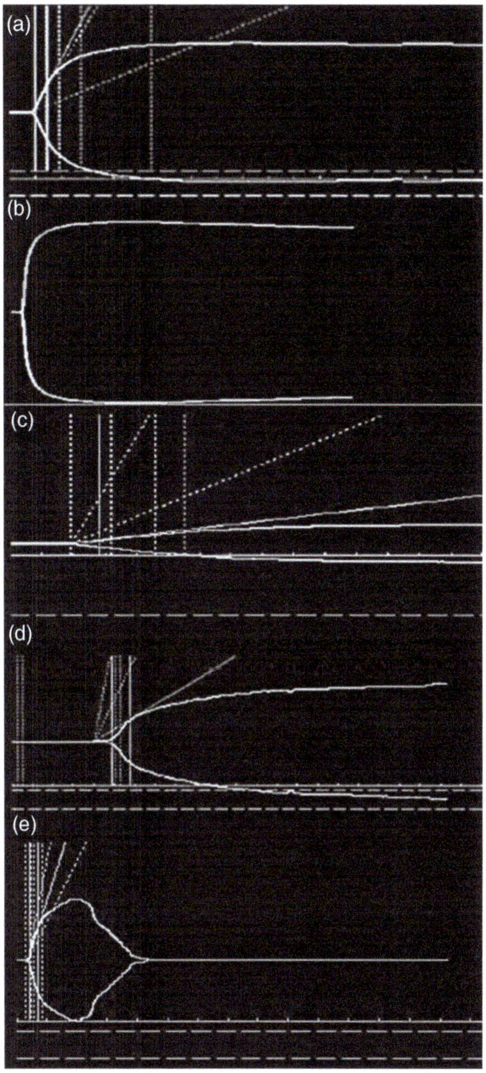

Figure 14.5 TEG (activated with tissue factor) tracings from (a) a normal dog, (b) a dog with hypercoagulability, (c) thrombocytopenia, (d) anticoagulant rodenticide exposure, and (e) hyperfibrinolysis.

strong activator of the extrinsic coagulation pathway.

As a consumptive coagulopathy starts, the body is initially able to compensate for the changes in coagulation, and overt clinical changes (e.g., hemorrhage) are not apparent, although physical examination can be consistent with SIRS (see Chapter 21). This compensated state is called nonovert DIC and is diagnosed in animals with clinical signs of inflammation and specific changes in coagulation parameters. Specifically, animals with nonovert DIC have a decreased platelet count (usually between 60 and 120 × 10^3 platelets per microliter) and may have normal fibrinogen concentration, PT, and aPTT. As the nonovert syndrome progresses toward overt DIC, gradual prolongations in aPTT are seen (while PT stays within normal range). The combination of a low platelet count, slightly (1.5–2 times normal) aPTT, and normal PT should immediately alert the clinician to nonovert DIC, and an effort should be made to identify and treat the source of inflammation.

Overt DIC occurs because of continued consumption of platelets and coagulation factors and is characterized by the presence of both hemorrhage and thrombosis, as the coagulation system becomes more dysfunctional. This is the phenotype associated with classic DIC and is more difficult to treat. Laboratory tests for animals with overt DIC usually display moderate to low platelet count (40–100 × 10^3 per microliter) and prolongations in both PT and aPTT, with low fibrinogen concentrations.

The most common causes of DIC in companion animals include diseases associated with inflammation, hypoperfusion, or both [111]. Many types of neoplasia, sepsis, infective endocarditis, pancreatitis, snake envenomation, heat stroke, trauma, gastric dilatation–volvulus syndrome, and hemolytic disease (immune-mediated as well as toxic or infectious) have all been associated with the development of DIC in dogs and cats [111]. Since hypoxia and hypoperfusion may serve as additional inflammatory stimuli, care should be taken during anesthesia of patients with predisposing conditions to mitigate any possible secondary injury that could trigger DIC.

The treatment of DIC is controversial, although the resolution of the inciting cause should be the primary objective for clinicians. This may include surgery, as for drainage of an abscess, or medical therapy. It is preferable to resolve the underlying condition prior to anesthesia, if possible. In animals with overt DIC, therapy for hypocoagulability and anemia may consist of transfusions with plasma products, packed RBCs, or whole blood to support oxygen delivery and hemostasis. The possibility for hemorrhage should be anticipated and, if an animal is receiving anticoagulant medications to treat thrombosis, may be more likely. The discontinuation of anticoagulant medications prior to invasive procedures is case-specific and should be based on the balance between the relative risk of thrombosis and the relative danger of hemorrhage during the procedure [86].

Hypercoagulable States

In recent years, increased attention has been paid to diseases in veterinary medicine that may result in a hypercoagulable phenotype, indicating animals that are prone to the development of thrombosis or thromboembolism [112]. A working knowledge of these diseases and therapies is necessary for the anesthetist because it may affect case management, and animals receiving therapeutic anticoagulant therapy may experience increased bleeding during surgical procedures. Common diseases that have been associated with an increased tendency to form clots include immune-mediated hemolytic anemia (IMHA) [112], protein-losing nephropathies [113], hypertrophic cardiomyopathy, sepsis, heartworm disease, and some forms of neoplasia [114]. In addition, therapy with prednisone increases TEG indices that are consistent with hypercoagulability [115], and the natural response to both surgery and pregnancy induces a relative hypercoagulable state. In one study of patients who developed necropsy-confirmed thromboembolism or thrombosis, the presence of a jugular vein catheter was associated with thrombosis, as was a diagnosis of hyperadrenocorticism (HAC) [116]. The veterinary literature is divided regarding the prevalence of a hypercoagulable presentation in patients with HAC [117, 118]. Disseminated intravascular coagulation is associated with an initial hypercoagulable phase before the more commonly recognized hypocoagulable phase; when animals are hypercoagulable, both microthromboses and macrothromboses can occur and impair tissue oxygen delivery.

Laboratory results that may be suggestive of hypercoagulability include viscoelastic testing indices, as well as markers of the activation of coagulation, such as thrombin–antithrombin (TAT) complexes. A PT or aPTT that is shorter than the reference range is not necessarily associated with hypercoagulability [119], but other measures, such as an elevated fibrinogen concentration, are more associated with this trait. In patients with protein-losing disease (enteropathy or nephropathy), the loss of AT may predispose to hypercoagulability [120]. Antithrombin activity can be measured in citrated plasma. In patients in whom a clot may have already formed, elevations in plasma d-dimers indicate that fibrinolysis is occurring. In patients suspected of having thrombosis, imaging of the vasculature, either using ultrasonography or CT angiography, may confirm the presence of clots.

Rudolf Virchow suggested some underlying characteristics that may indicate a predisposition to thrombosis in susceptible patients [112]. These include the presence of a hypercoagulable state, occurrence of endothelial damage, and the presence of altered blood flow in the vasculature [112]. In some patients, more than one of these factors may be present. From an anesthesia standpoint, the best practice is to limit catheter placements (and thus endothelial damage) to those that are necessary for the procedure. During anesthetic procedures, the maintenance of adequate blood pressure and tissue oxygen delivery is important, and anesthetic protocols should be chosen that minimize hemodynamic instability. If patients are suspected of thrombosis or hypercoagulability, therapy with either antiplatelet drugs or anticoagulant medications may have been instituted before anesthesia, and the precautions listed previously for these scenarios should be followed.

Disorders of Fibrinolysis

Hyperfibrinolysis in veterinary medicine is most frequently associated with DIC but has also been described as an idiosyncratic response to surgery or inflammation in some Sighthounds (specifically Greyhounds) [121, 122]. In addition, dogs with acute hemoperitoneum (generally secondary to neoplasia) displayed hyperfibrinolysis that was positively correlated to the degree of shock (using blood lactate concentration as a surrogate) [110]. An increase in fibrinolysis can be detected by an increased number of circulating fibrin fragments, either fibrin(ogen) degradation products (FDPs) or d-dimers. D-dimers can only be formed after fibrin cross-linking has occurred in a mature clot and so are indicative of fibrinolysis of an actual thrombus. FDPs are less specific and can represent particles of fibrin that have broken down from clots or pieces of fibrinogen that have been broken down in circulation, without ever forming a clot. The hyperfibrinolytic aspect of DIC is not treated specifically, but transfusions of FFP or cryoprecipitate can replenish fibrinogen that has been consumed. Delayed (2–3 days) postoperative bleeding in retired racing Greyhounds has been reported and has been posited to be caused by hyperfibrinolysis [95, 96]. It is not possible to predict which dogs will experience delayed bleeding, but it is wise to closely monitor Sighthounds in the postoperative period. Drugs such as epsilon-aminocaproic acid [109] or tranexamic acid [123] may be useful to mitigate hyperfibrinolysis in some cases.

References

1 Lumb, A.B. (2000). Oxygen. In: *Nunn's Applied Respiratory Physiology*, 5e (ed. A.B. Lumb), 188. Boston: Butterworth Heinemann.

2 Guyton, A.C. and Hall, J.E. (2006). Transport of oxygen and carbon dioxide in blood and tissue fluids. In: *Textbook of Medical Physiology*, 11e (eds. A.C. Guyton and J.E. Hall), 505. Philadelphia: Elsevier Saunders.

3 Silverstein, D.C. and Hopper, K. (2015). *Small Animal Critical Care Medicine*, 2e, 27, 28, 82. St. Louis: Saunders Elsevier.

4 Cambier, C., Wierinckx, M., Clerbaux, T. et al. (2004). Haemoglobin oxygen affinity and regulating factors of the blood oxygen transport in canine and feline blood. *Res. Vet. Sci.* 77: 83–88.

5 Nash, S.L., Savides, M.C., Oehme, F.W. et al. (1984). The effect of acetaminophen on methemoglobin and blood glutathione parameters in the cat. *Toxicology* 31: 329–334.

6 Ashbaugh, E.A., Mazzaferro, E.M., McKiernan, B.C. et al. (2012). The association of physical examination abnormalities and carboxyhemoglobin concentrations in 21 dogs trapped in a kennel fire. *J. Vet. Emerg. Crit. Care (San Antonio)* 22: 361–367.

7 Brockus, C.W. and Andreasen, C.B. (2003). Erythrocytes. In: *Duncan and Prasse's Veterinary Laboratory Medicine Clinical Pathology* (eds. K.S. Latimer, E.A. Mahaffey and K.W. Prasse), 29–37. Ames: Iowa State Press.

8 Torrance, J., Jacobs, P., Restrepo, A. et al. (1970). Intraerythrocytic adaptation to anemia. *N. Engl. J. Med.* 283: 165–169.

9 Oski, F.A., Gottlieb, A.J., Miller, W.W. et al. (1970). The effects of deoxygenation of adult and fetal hemoglobin on the synthesis of red cell 2,3-diphosphoglycerate and its in vivo consequences. *J. Clin. Invest.* 49: 400–407.

10 Hardy, R.M. and Osborne, C.A. (1979). Water deprivation test in the dog: maximal normal values. *J. Am. Vet. Med. Assoc.* 174: 479–483.

11 Carlson, G.P., Rumbaugh, G.E., and Harrold, D. (1979). Physiologic alterations in the horse produced by food and water deprivation during periods of high environmental temperatures. *Am. J. Vet. Res.* 40: 982–985.

12 Eick, B.G. and Denke, N.J. (2018). Resuscitative strategies in the trauma patient: the past, the present and the future. *J. Trauma Nurs.* 25: 254–263.

13 Palmer, L. (2017). Fluid management in patients with trauma. *Vet. Clin. North Am. Small Anim. Pract.* 47: 397–410.

14 Bjerkvig, C.K., Strandenes, G., Eliassen, H.S. et al. (2016). "Blood failure" time to view blood as an organ: how oxygen debt contributes to blood failure and its implications for remote damage control resuscitation. *Transfusion* 56: S182–S189.

15 Lavu, H., Sell, N.M., Carter, T.I. et al. (2014). The HYSLAR trial: a prospective randomized controlled trial of the use of a restrictive fluid regimen with 3% hypertonic saline versus lactated ringers in patients undergoing pancreaticoduodenectomy. *Ann. Surg.* 260: 445–453.

16 Duchesne, J.C., Guidry, C., Hoffman, J.R. et al. (2012). Low-volume resuscitation for severe intraoperative hemorrhage: a step in the right direction. *Am. Surg.* 78: 936–941.

17 Dutton, R. (2006). Fluid management for trauma: where are we now? *Contin. Educ. Anaesth. Crit. Care Pain* 6: 144–147.

18 McBride, D., Raisis, A.L., Hosgood, G. et al. (2017). Hydroxyethyl starch 130/0.4 compared with 0.9% NaCl administered to greyhounds with haemorrhagic shock. *Vet. Anaesth. Analg.* 44: 444–451.

19 Schick, M.A., Baar, W., Bruno, R.R. et al. (2015). Balanced hydroxyethylstarch (HES 130/0.4) impairs kidney function in-vivo without inflammation. *PLoS One* 10: e0137247.

20 Boyd, C.J., Claus, M.A., Raisis, A.L. et al. (2019). Evaluation of biomarkers of kidney injury following 4% succinylated gelatin and 6% hydroxyethyl starch 130/0.4 administration in a canine hemorrhagic shock model. *J. Vet. Emerg. Crit. Care* 29: 132–142.

21 Zersen, K.M., Mama, K., and Mathis, J.C. (2019). Retrospective evaluation of paired plasma creatinine and chloride concentrations following hetastarch administration in anesthetized dogs (2002–2015): 244 cases. *J. Vet. Emerg. Crit. Care* 29: 309–313.

22 Diniz, M.S., Teixeira-Neto, F.J., Goncalves, D.S. et al. (2018). Effects of 6% tetrastarch or lactated Ringer's solution on blood coagulation in hemorrhaged dogs. *J. Vet. Intern. Med.* 32: 1927–1933.

23 Sachs, U.J. (2011). Recent insights into the mechanism of transfusion-related acute lung injury. *Curr. Opin. Hematol.* 18: 436–442.

24 McMichael, M.A., Smith, S.A., Galligan, A. et al. (2010). Effect of leukoreduction on transfusion-induced inflammation in dogs. *J. Vet. Intern. Med.* 24: 1131–1137.

25 Maglaras, C.H., Koenig, A., Bedard, D.L. et al. (2017). Retrospective evaluation of the effect of red blood cell product age on occurrence of acute transfusion-related complications in dogs: 210 cases (2010–2012). *J. Vet. Emerg. Crit. Care* 27: 108–120.

26 Hann, L., Brown, D.C., King, L.G. et al. (2014). Effect of duration of packed red blood cell storage on morbidity and mortality in dogs after transfusion: 3,095 cases (2001–2010). *J. Vet. Intern. Med.* 28: 1830–1837.

27 Wardrop, K.J. (1995). Selection of anticoagulant-preservatives for canine and feline blood storage. *Vet. Clin. North Am. Small Anim. Pract.* 25: 1263–1276.

28 Wardrop, K.J., Owen, T.J., and Meyers, K.M. (1994). Evaluation of an additive solution for preservation of canine red blood cells. *J. Vet. Intern. Med.* 8: 253–257.

29 Mudge, M.C., Macdonald, M.H., Owens, S.D. et al. (2004). Comparison of 4 blood storage methods in a protocol for equine pre-operative autologous donation. *Vet. Surg.* 33: 475–486.

30 Pang, D.S. and Boysen, S. (2007). Lactate in veterinary critical care: pathophysiology and management. *J. Am. Anim. Hosp. Assoc.* 43: 270–279.

31 Hohenhaus, A.E. (2006). Blood transfusion and blood substitutes. In: *Fluid, Electrolyte* *and Acid-Base Disorders in Small Animal Practice*, 3e (ed. S.P. DiBartola), 567–583. St. Louis: Saunders Elsevier.

32 Short, J.L., Diehl, S., Seshadri, R. et al. (2012). Accuracy of formulas used to predict post-transfusion packed cell volume rise in anemic dogs. *J. Vet. Emerg. Crit. Care* 22: 428–434.

33 Prittie, J.E. (2003). Triggers for use, optimal dosing, and problems associated with red cell transfusions. *Vet. Clin. North Am. Small Anim. Pract.* 33: 1261–1275.

34 McDevitt, R.I., Ruaux, C.G., and Baltzer, W.I. (2011). Influence of transfusion technique on survival of autologous red blood cells in the dog. *J. Vet. Emerg. Crit. Care* 21: 209–216.

35 Jutkowitz, L.A., Rozanski, E.A., Moreau, J.A. et al. (2002). Massive transfusion in dogs: 15 cases (1997–2001). *J. Am. Vet. Med. Assoc.* 220: 1664–1669.

36 McNally, E.M., Robertson, S.A., and Pablo, L.S. (2009). Comparison of time to desaturation between preoxygenated and non-preoxygenated dogs following sedation with acepromazine maleate and morphine and induction of anesthesia with propofol. *Am. J. Vet. Res.* 70: 1333–1338.

37 Weiskopf, R.B., Viele, M.K., Feiner, J. et al. (1998). Human cardiovascular and metabolic response to acute, severe isovolemic anemia. *JAMA* 279: 217–221.

38 Ickx, B.E., Rigolet, M., and Van Der Linden, P.J. (2000). Cardiovascular and metabolic response to acute normovolemic anemia. Effects of anesthesia. *Anesthesiology* 93: 1011–1016.

39 Merin, R.G., Hoffman, W.L., and Kraus, A.L. (1977). The role of the canine spleen in cardiovascular homeostasis during halothane anesthesia. *Circ. Shock.* 4: 241–246.

40 Marini, R.P., Callahan, R.J., Jackson, L.R. et al. (1997). Distribution of technetium 99m-labeled red blood cells during isoflurane anesthesia in ferrets. *Am. J. Vet. Res.* 58: 781–785.

41 Wilson, D.V., Evans, A.T., Carpenter, R.A. et al. (2004). The effect of four anesthetic protocols on splenic size in dogs. *Vet. Anaesth. Analg.* 31: 102–108.

42 Doenicke, A., Roizen, M.F., Hoernecke, R. et al. (1997). Haemolysis after etomidate: comparison of propylene glycol and lipid formulations. *Br. J. Anaesth.* 79: 386–388.

43 Campora, C., Freeman, K.P., Lewis, F.I. et al. (2011). Determination of haematological reference intervals in healthy adult greyhounds. *J. Small Anim. Pract.* 52: 301–309.

44 Polycythemia, H.A. (2005). *Textbook of Veterinary Internal Medicine*, 6e (eds. S.J. Ettinger and E.C. Feldman), 215–218. St. Louis: Elsevier.

45 Boudreaux, M.K. and Catalfamo, J.L. (2010). Platelet biochemistry, signal transduction, and function. In: *Schalm's Veterinary Hematology* (eds. D.J. Weiss and K.J. Wardrop), 569–575. Ames: Wiley-Blackwell.

46 Brooks, M.B. and Catalfamo, J.L. (2010). Von Willebrand disease. In: *Schalm's Veterinary Hematology* (eds. D.J. Weiss and K.J. Wardrop), 612–618. Ames: Wiley-Blackwell.

47 Brooks, M. and Catalfamo, J. (1993). Buccal mucosa bleeding time is prolonged in canine models of primary hemostatic disorders. *Thromb. Haemost.* 70: 777–780.

48 Jergens, A.E., Turrentine, M.A., Kraus, K.H. et al. (1987). Buccal mucosa bleeding times of healthy dogs and of dogs in various pathologic states, including thrombocytopenia, uremia, and von Willebrand's disease. *Am. J. Vet. Res.* 48: 1337–1342.

49 Callan, M.B. and Giger, U. (2001). Assessment of a point-of-care instrument for identification of primary hemostatic disorders in dogs. *Am. J. Vet. Res.* 62: 652–658.

50 Mischke, R. and Keidel, A. (2003). Influence of platelet count, acetylsalicylic acid, von Willebrand's disease, coagulopathies, and haematocrit on results obtained using a platelet function analyser in dogs. *Vet. J.* 165: 43–52.

51 Brainard, B.M., Kleine, S.A., Papich, M.G. et al. (2010). Pharmacodynamic and pharmacokinetic evaluation of clopidogrel and the carboxylic acid metabolite SR 26334 in healthy dogs. *Am. J. Vet. Res.* 71: 822–830.

52 Sharpe, K.S., Center, S.A., Randolph, J.F. et al. (2010). Influence of treatment with ultralow-dose aspirin on platelet aggregation as measured by whole blood impedance aggregometry and platelet P-selectin expression in clinically normal dogs. *Am. J. Vet. Res.* 71: 1294–1304.

53 Brooks, M.B., Randolph, J., Warner, K. et al. (2009). Evaluation of platelet function screening tests to detect platelet procoagulant deficiency in dogs with Scott syndrome. *Vet. Clin. Pathol.* 38: 306–315.

54 Boudreaux, M.K., Panangala, V.S., and Bourne, C. (1996). A platelet activation-specific monoclonal antibody that recognizes a receptor-induced binding site on canine fibrinogen. *Vet. Pathol.* 33: 419–427.

55 Davis, B., Toivio-Kinnucan, M., Schuller, S. et al. (2008). Mutation in beta1-tubulin correlates with macrothrombocytopenia in Cavalier King Charles Spaniels. *J. Vet. Intern. Med.* 22: 540–545.

56 Lewis, D.C., Meyers, K.M., Callan, M.B. et al. (1995). Detection of platelet-bound and serum platelet-bindable antibodies for diagnosis of idiopathic thrombocytopenic purpura in dogs. *J. Am. Vet. Med. Assoc.* 206: 47–52.

57 Lavergne, S.N. and Trepanier, L.A. (2007). Anti-platelet antibodies in a natural animal model of sulphonamide-associated thrombocytopaenia. *Platelets* 18: 595–604.

58 Brainard, B.M. and Brown, A.J. (2011). Defects in coagulation encountered in small animal critical care. *Vet. Clin. North Am. Small Anim. Pract.* 41: 783–803.

59 Guillaumin, J., Jandrey, K.E., Norris, J.W. et al. (2010). Analysis of a commercial dimethyl-sulfoxide-stabilized frozen canine platelet concentrate by turbidimetric aggregometry. *J. Vet. Emerg. Crit. Care* 20: 571–577.

60 Callan, M.B., Appleman, E.H., and Sachais, B.S. (2009). Canine platelet transfusions. *J. Vet. Emerg. Crit. Care* 19: 401–415.

61 Rozanski, E.A., Callan, M.B., Hughes, D. et al. (2002). Comparison of platelet count recovery with use of vincristine and prednisone or prednisone alone for treatment for severe immune-mediated thrombocytopenia in dogs. *J. Am. Vet. Med. Assoc.* 220: 477–481.

62 Barr, S.C., Ludders, J.W., Looney, A.L. et al. (1992). Platelet aggregation in dogs after sedation with acepromazine and atropine and during subsequent general anesthesia and surgery. *Am. J. Vet. Res.* 53: 2067–2070.

63 Mischke, R. and Schulze, U. (2004). Studies on platelet aggregation using the born method in normal and uraemic dogs. *Vet. J.* 168: 270–275.

64 Avgeris, S., Lothrop, C.D. Jr., and McDonald, T.P. (1990). Plasma von Willebrand factor concentration and thyroid function in dogs. *J. Am. Vet. Med. Assoc.* 196: 921–924.

65 Panciera, D.L. and Johnson, G.S. (1994). Plasma von Willebrand factor antigen concentration in dogs with hypothyroidism. *J. Am. Vet. Med. Assoc.* 205: 1550–1553.

66 Sullivan, P., Gompf, R., Schmeitzel, L. et al. (1993). Altered platelet indices in dogs with hypothyroidism and cats with hyperthyroidism. *Am. J. Vet. Res.* 54: 2004–2009.

67 Callan, M.B., Giger, U., and Catalfamo, J.L. (2005). Effect of desmopressin on von Willebrand factor multimers in Doberman pinschers with type 1 von Willebrand disease. *Am. J. Vet. Res.* 66: 861–867.

68 Stokol, T. and Parry, B. (1998). Efficacy of fresh-frozen plasma and cryoprecipitate in dogs with von Willebrand's disease or hemophilia a. *J. Vet. Intern. Med.* 12: 84–92.

69 Michiels, J.J., van Vliet, H.H., Berneman, Z. et al. (2009). Managing patients with von Willebrand disease type 1,2 and 3 with desmopressin and von Willebrand factor-factor VIII concentrate in surgical settings. *Acta Haematol.* 121: 167–176.

70 Boudreaux, M.K. (2012). Inherited platelet disorders. *J. Vet. Emerg. Crit. Care* 22: 30–41.

71 Brooks, M.B., Catalfamo, J.L., Brown, H.A. et al. (2002). A hereditary bleeding disorder

of dogs caused by a lack of platelet procoagulant activity. *Blood* 99: 2434–2441.

72 Brainard, B.M., Meredith, C.P., Callan, M.B. et al. (2007). Changes in platelet function, hemostasis, and prostaglandin expression after treatment with nonsteroidal anti-inflammatory drugs with various cyclooxygenase selectivities in dogs. *Am. J. Vet. Res.* 68: 251–257.

73 Johnson, G.J., Leis, L.A., and King, R.A. (1991). Thromboxane responsiveness of dog platelets is inherited as an autosomal recessive trait. *Thromb. Haemost.* 65: 578–580.

74 Cathcart, C.J., Brainard, B.M., Reynolds, L.R. et al. (2011). Lack of inhibitory effect of acetylsalicylic acid and meloxicam on whole blood platelet aggregation in cats. *J. Vet. Emerg. Crit. Care* 22: 99–106.

75 Lemke, K.A., Runyon, C.L., and Horney, B.S. (2002). Effects of preoperative administration of ketoprofen on anesthetic requirements and signs of postoperative pain in dogs undergoing elective ovariohysterectomy. *J. Am. Vet. Med. Assoc.* 221: 1268–1275.

76 Thomason, J., Lunsford, K., Mullins, K. et al. (2011). Platelet cyclooxygenase expression in normal dogs. *J. Vet. Intern. Med.* 25: 1106–1112.

77 Van der Linden, P. and Ickx, B.E. (2006). The effects of colloid solutions on hemostasis. *Can. J. Anaesth.* 53: S30–S39.

78 Westphal, M., James, M.F., Kozek-Langenecker, S. et al. (2009). Hydroxyethyl starches: different products – different effects. *Anesthesiology* 111: 187–202.

79 Franz, A., Braunlich, P., Gamsjager, T. et al. (2001). The effects of hydroxyethyl starches of varying molecular weights on platelet function. *Anesth. Analg.* 92: 1402–1407.

80 Wierenga, J.R., Jandrey, K.E., Haskins, S.C. et al. (2007). in vitro comparison of the effects of two forms of hydroxyethyl starch solutions on platelet function in dogs. *Am. J. Vet. Res.* 68: 605–609.

81 Hogan, D.F., Andrews, D.A., Green, H.W. et al. (2004). Antiplatelet effects and pharmacodynamics of clopidogrel in cats. *J. Am. Vet. Med. Assoc.* 225: 1406–1411.

82 Brainard, B.M., Epstein, K.L., LoBato, D. et al. (2011). Effects of clopidogrel and aspirin on platelet aggregation, thromboxane production, and serotonin secretion in horses. *J. Vet. Intern. Med.* 25: 116–122.

83 Douketis, J.D., Berger, P.B., Dunn, A.S. et al. (2008). The perioperative management of antithrombotic therapy: American College of Chest Physicians evidence-based clinical practice guidelines (8th edition). *Chest* 133: 299S–339S.

84 Brainard, B.M., Buriko, Y., Good, J. et al. (2019). Consensus on the rational use of antithrombotics in veterinary critical care (CURATIVE): domain 5-discontinuation of anticoagulant therapy in small animals. *J. Vet. Emerg. Crit. Care* 29: 88–97.

85 Tam, N.L., Pac-Soo, C., and Pretorius, P.M. (2006). Epidural haematoma after a combined spinal-epidural anaesthetic in a patient treated with clopidogrel and dalteparin. *Br. J. Anaesth.* 96: 262–265.

86 Chang, Y., Chen, T.L., Wu, G.J. et al. (2004). Mechanisms involved in the antiplatelet activity of ketamine in human platelets. *J. Biomed. Sci.* 11: 764–772.

87 Sheu, J.R., Hsiao, G., Luk, H.N. et al. (2002). Mechanisms involved in the antiplatelet activity of midazolam in human platelets. *Anesthesiology* 96: 651–658.

88 De La Cruz, J.P., Paez, M.V., Carmona, J.A. et al. (1999). Antiplatelet effect of the anaesthetic drug propofol: influence of red blood cells and leucocytes. *Br. J. Pharmacol.* 128: 1538–1544.

89 Kozek-Langenecker, S.A. (2002). The effects of drugs used in anaesthesia on platelet membrane receptors and on platelet function. *Curr. Drug Targets* 3: 247–258.

90 Monroe, D.M. and Hoffman, M. (2006). What does it take to make the perfect clot? *Arterioscler. Thromb. Vasc. Biol.* 26: 41–48.

91 Hyatt, R.C. and Brainard, B.M. (2016). Point of care assessment of coagulation. *Top. Companion Anim. Med.* 31: 11–17.

92 Epstein, K.L., Brainard, B.M., Lopes, M.A. et al. (2009). Thrombelastography in 26 healthy horses with and without activation by recombinant human tissue factor. *J. Vet. Emerg. Crit. Care* 19: 96–101.

93 Ralph, A.G., Brainard, B.M., Pittman, J.R. et al. (2012). Effects of rest temperature, contact activation, and sample technique on canine thrombelastography. *J. Vet. Emerg. Crit. Care* 22: 320–326.

94 Babski, D.M., Brainard, B.M., Ralph, A.G. et al. (2012). Sonoclot® evaluation of single-and multiple-dose subcutaneous unfractionated heparin therapy in healthy adult dogs. *J. Vet. Intern. Med.* 26: 631–638.

95 Pittman, J.R., Koenig, A., and Brainard, B.M. (2010). The effect of unfractionated heparin on thrombelastographic analysis in healthy dogs. *J. Vet. Emerg. Crit. Care (San Antonio)* 20: 216–223.

96 Chaney, M.A. (1997). Intrathecal and epidural anesthesia and analgesia for cardiac surgery. *Anesth. Analg.* 84: 1211–1221.

97 Horlocker, T.T., Wedel, D.J., Rowlingson, J.C. et al. (2010). Regional anesthesia in the patient receiving antithrombotic or thrombolytic therapy: American Society of Regional Anesthesia and Pain Medicine evidence-based guidelines (3rd edition). *Reg. Anesth. Pain Med.* 35: 64–101.

98 Alwood, A.J., Downend, A.B., Brooks, M.B. et al. (2007). Anticoagulant effects of low-molecular-weight heparins in healthy cats. *J. Vet. Intern. Med.* 21: 378–387.

99 Knudsen, T., Kristensen, A.T., Nichols, T.C. et al. (2011). Pharmacokinetics, pharmacodynamics and safety of recombinant canine FVIIa in a study dosing one haemophilia a and one haemostatically normal dog. *Haemophilia* 17: 962–970.

100 Ganter, M.T. and Hofer, C.K. (2008). Coagulation monitoring: current techniques and clinical use of viscoelastic point-of-care coagulation devices. *Anesth. Analg.* 106: 1366–1375.

101 Wiinberg, B. and Kristensen, A.T. (2010). Thromboelastography in veterinary medicine. *Semin. Thromb. Hemost.* 36: 747–756.

102 Goggs, R., Blais, M.C., Brainard, B.M. et al. (2019). American College of Veterinary Emergency and Critical Care (ACVECC) consensus on the rational use of antithrombotics in veterinary critical care (CURATIVE) guidelines: small animal. *J. Vet. Emerg. Crit. Care* 29: 12–36.

103 McCrath, D.J., Cerboni, E., Frumento, R.J. et al. (2005). Thromboelastography maximum amplitude predicts postoperative thrombotic complications including myocardial infarction. *Anesth. Analg.* 100: 1576–1583.

104 Thawley, V.J., Sánchez, M.D., Drobatz, K.J. et al. (2016). Retrospective comparison of thromboelastography results to postmortem evidence of thrombosis in critically ill dogs: 39 cases (2005–2010). *J. Vet. Emerg. Crit. Care* 26: 428–436.

105 Brown, J.C., Brainard, B.M., Fletcher, D.J. et al. Effect of aminocaproic acid on clot strength and clot lysis of canine blood determined by use of an in vitro model of hyperfibrinolysis. *Am. J. Vet. Res.* 77: 1258–1265.

106 Fletcher, D.J., Rozanski, E.A., Brainard, B.M. et al. (2016). Assessment of the relationships among coagulopathy, hyperfibrinolysis, plasma lactate, and protein C in dogs with spontaneous hemoperitoneum. *J. Vet. Emerg. Crit. Care* 26: 41–51.

107 Ralph, A.G. and Brainard, B.M. (2012). Update on disseminated intravascular coagulation: when to consider it, when to expect it, when to treat it. *Top. Companion Anim. Med.* 27: 65–72.

108 Sinnott, V.B. and Otto, C.M. (2009). Use of thromboelastography in dogs with immune-mediated hemolytic anemia: 39 cases (2000–2008). *J. Vet. Emerg. Crit. Care* 19: 484–488.

109 Donahue, S.M., Brooks, M., and Otto, C.M. (2011). Examination of hemostatic parameters to detect hypercoagulability in dogs with severe protein-losing nephropathy. *J. Vet. Emerg. Crit. Care* 21: 346–355.

110 Andreasen, E.B., Tranholm, M., Wiinberg, B. et al. (2012). Haemostatic alterations in a group of canine cancer patients are associated with cancer type and disease progression. *Acta Vet. Scand.* 54: 3.

111 Rose, L.J., Dunn, M.E., Allegret, V. et al. (2011). Effect of prednisone administration on coagulation variables in healthy beagle dogs. *Vet. Clin. Pathol.* 40: 426–434.

112 Palmer, K.G., King, L.G., and Van Winkle, T.J. (1998). Clinical manifestations and associated disease syndromes in dogs with cranial vena cava thrombosis: 17 cases (1989–1996). *J. Am. Vet. Med. Assoc.* 213: 220–224.

113 Klose, T.C., Creevy, K.E., and Brainard, B.M. (2011). Evaluation of coagulation status in dogs with naturally occurring canine hyperadrenocorticism. *J. Vet. Emerg. Crit. Care* 21: 625–632.

114 Jacoby, R.C., Owings, J.T., Ortega, T. et al. (2001). Biochemical basis for the hypercoagulable state seen in Cushing syndrome; discussion 1006–7. *Arch. Surg.* 136: 1003–1006.

115 Marín, L.M., Iazbik, M.C., Zaldivar-Lopez, S. et al. (2012). Retrospective evaluation of the effectiveness of epsilon aminocaproic acid for the prevention of postamputation bleeding in retired racing greyhounds with appendicular bone tumors: 46 cases (2003–2008). *J. Vet. Emerg. Crit. Care* 22: 332–340.

116 Song, J., Drobatz, K.J., and Silverstein, D.C. (2016). Retrospective evaluation of shortened prothrombin time or activated partial thromboplastin time for the diagnosis of hypercoagulability in dogs: 25 cases (2006–2011). *J. Vet. Emerg. Crit. Care* 26: 398–405.

117 Hall, R. and Mazer, C.D. (2011). Antiplatelet drugs: a review of their pharmacology and management in the perioperative period. *Anesth. Analg.* 112: 292–318.

118 Marin, L.M., Iazbik, M.C., Zaldivar-Lopez, S. et al. (2012). Epsilon aminocaproic acid for the prevention of delayed postoperative bleeding in retired racing greyhounds undergoing gonadectomy. *Vet. Surg.* 41: 594–603.

119 Center, S.A., Warner, K., Corbett, J. et al. (2000). Proteins invoked by vitamin K absence and clotting times in clinically ill cats. *J. Vet. Intern. Med.* 14: 292–297.

120 Goodwin, L.V., Goggs, R., Chan, D.L. et al. (2011). Hypercoagulability in dogs with protein-losing enteropathy. *J. Vet. Intern. Med.* 25: 273–277.

121 Newsome, L.T., Weller, R.S., Gerancher, J.C. et al. (2008). Coronary artery stents: II. Perioperative considerations and management. *Anesth. Analg.* 107: 570–590.

122 Snow, S.J., Ari Jutkowitz, L., and Brown, A.J. (2010). Trends in plasma transfusion at a veterinary teaching hospital: 308 patients (1996–1998 and 2006–2008). *J. Vet. Emerg. Crit. Care* 20: 441–445.

123 Osekavage, K.E., Brainard, B.M., Lane, S.L. et al. (2018). Pharmacokinetics of tranexamic acid in healthy dogs and assessment of its antifibrinolytic properties in canine blood. *Am. J. Vet. Res.* 79: 1057–1063.

15

Skin and Musculoskeletal Diseases

Paulo V. M. Steagall

Faculté de Médecine Vétérinaire, Université de Montréal, Saint-Hyacinthe, Québec, J2S 2M2, Canada

Introduction

This chapter presents a concise description of the pathophysiology, diagnosis, and treatment of the most relevant canine and feline skin and musculoskeletal diseases. An emphasis is given to the impact of these diseases on anesthetic and analgesic management of patients. In some instances, skin and musculoskeletal disease is presented as a secondary complication rather than the main clinical concern. Adequate preanesthetic patient assessment and monitoring are essential for the successful outcome of any case.

Burns

Skin burns are a result of thermal, chemical, electrical, or radiation injury [1–4]. In dogs, exposure to high ambient temperatures has been associated with severe burns with concomitant heatstroke; a condition known as dorsal thermal necrosis [5]. Patients with burns may constitute a life-threatening condition that requires intensive care and aggressive pain management. Burns have been classified as follows:

- *Superficial partial-thickness* (e.g., first-degree) burns involve only the epidermis and healing generally occurs within 5 days. Lesions are bright red, nonblistered, and painful.
- *Deep partial-thickness* (e.g., second-degree) burns involve all epidermal layers and variable depths of the dermis. They may appear dry or blistered and moist, usually resulting in the formation of scar tissue after a prolonged healing period (Figure 15.1).
- *Full-thickness* (e.g., third-degree) burns involve destruction of the entire dermis and may extend into the subcutaneous tissues. They are dry, leathery, and appear white or charred. These burns are expected to be insensate, and loss of function may result.

Characterization of injury severity is warranted for appropriate prognosis and treatment planning. The criterion has been adapted from the human literature and is described elsewhere [5]. Full-thickness burns can be initially numb; however, late nerve regeneration can be a significant cause of neuropathic pain in humans. It is also important to recognize that all burn stages can be present in the same patient, making pain assessment and treatment more challenging. For example, dogs with

Canine and Feline Anesthesia and Co-Existing Disease, Second Edition. Edited by Rebecca A. Johnson, Lindsey B. C. Snyder and Carrie A. Schroeder.

Companion website: www.wiley.com/go/johnson/canine

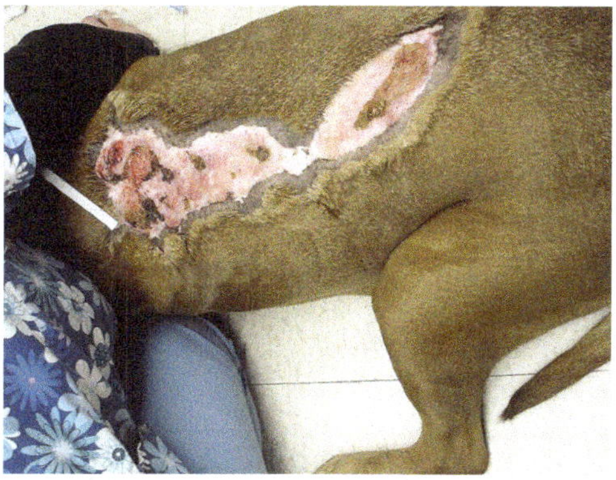

Figure 15.1 Dorsal aspect of a dog with thermal scald, deep partial-thickness burns.

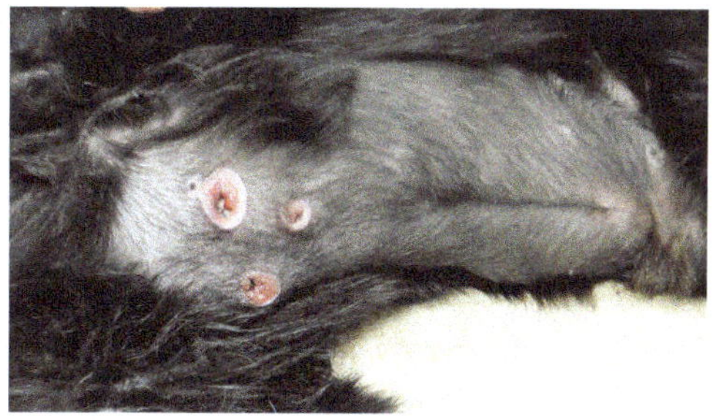

Figure 15.2 Accidental multifocal burns associated with the use of magnetic-resonance-imaging-compatible electrocardiogram patches in a dog. These burns were not noted until days later and are often called occult or heating pad burns.

"garden hose scalding syndrome" can present with thermal scald burns of different degrees after exposure to hot water from hoses lying in the sun in the Southern and Western regions of the United States [1].

Knowledge about burns in veterinary medicine is limited and is mostly related to personal experience, case reports, and review articles [1, 3, 4, 6, 7]. However, the prevalence of burns and associated injuries can be relatively high, especially after large fires (i.e., flame burns) in specific geographic regions. Radiation burns associated with radiation therapy treatment may also present a problem in veterinary oncology. Iatrogenic burns may occur in the perianesthetic period and may be associated with inappropriate monitoring in the magnetic resonance imaging (MRI) unit (Figure 15.2) or with the use of supplemental heat to treat or prevent hypothermia during general anesthesia (Figure 15.3). In the latter cases, occult burns are commonly overlooked until the injury is evident days later.

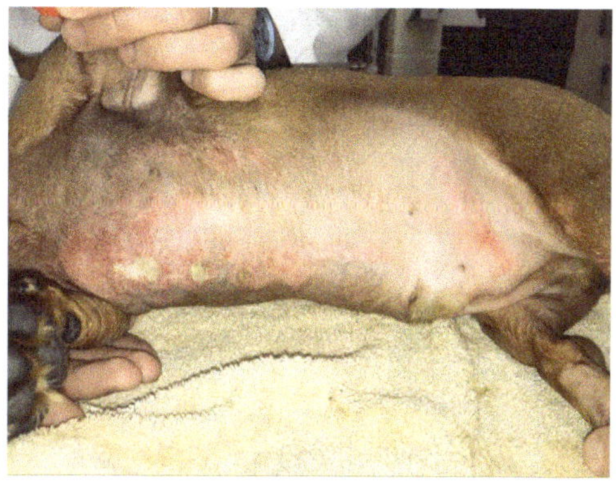

Figure 15.3 Accidental burns related with the use of polymer fiber resistive warming devices or adaptations to prevent or treat hypothermia such as beverage plastic bottles with hot water during anesthesia. These burns may happen due to faulty equipment, the use of high temperatures, equipment misuse, and direct contact between the conductive material and skin with pressure points creating "hot spots." Burns during general anesthesia are usually less common with forced-air warming devices. *Source:* Photo courtesy of Dr. Javier de Benito.

Metabolic Derangements and Systemic Effects

Euthanasia may be advisable if lesions extend to >50% of total body surface area (TBSA). After a burn injury affecting >20% of the patient's TBSA or if the wounds are of deep, partial, or full thickness, a systemic inflammatory response syndrome (SIRS) may develop within minutes of the injury, resulting in cardiovascular collapse and multiorgan system failure (Figure 15.4) [8]. Sepsis is another important consideration in burn patients and one major cause of death [9]. Wound-, respiratory-, and catheter-related infections may occur secondary to the compromised integrity of the natural barriers and subsequent free passage of bacteria

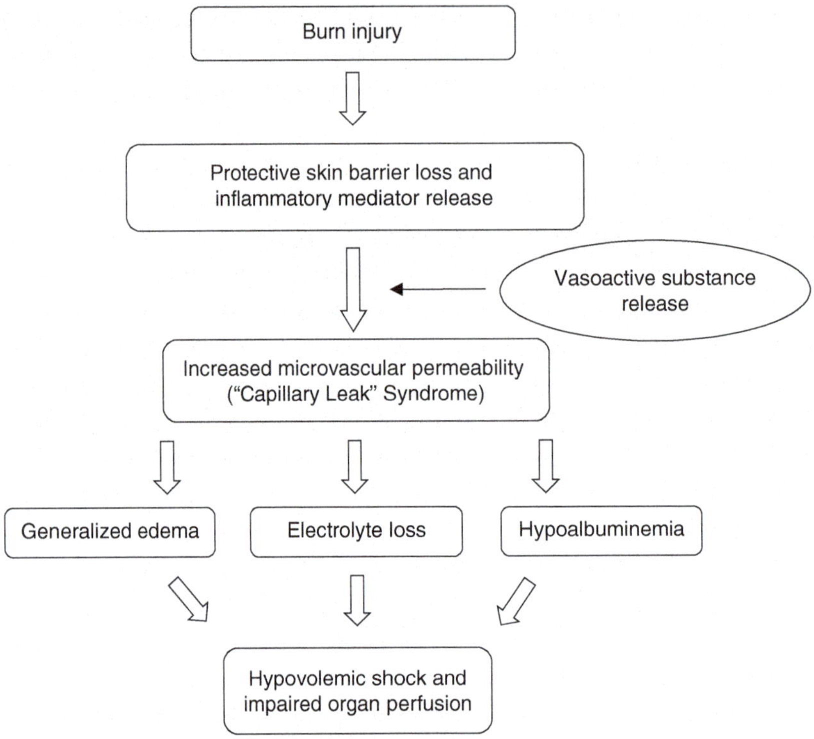

Figure 15.4 Algorithm of burn injury.

and endotoxins through the skin, contributing to the development of multiorgan failure. Humoral immunity and cell-mediated immunity are altered resulting in immunosuppression, which may further increase the prevalence of sepsis. Other signs may be present in sepsis, such as fever or hypothermia, tachycardia, bradycardia (more commonly in cats), tachypnea, altered mental status, hypoglycemia or hyperglycemia, edema, leukopenia or leukocytosis, hemodynamic instability, thrombocytopenia, ileus, hypocoagulability or hypercoagulability, and hyperlactatemia, among others [9]. A hypermetabolic response is typically observed until final resolution of the wounds and long after. This consists of a variety of disorders such as increased sympathetic stimulation, gluconeogenesis, protein catabolism, insulin resistance, and weight loss.

Smoke inhalation injury is of concern and constitutes an important aspect of increased morbidity. Direct thermal damage to respiratory epithelium leads to sloughing and edema of the upper airways that, in addition to the formation of cellular casts, may obstruct the airways [10]. The systemic inflammatory response, with the release of thromboxane, causes pulmonary vasoconstriction, hypertension, and hypercoagulability. Carbon monoxide (CO) poisoning frequently occurs in conjunction with inhalation injury, further contributing to tissue hypoxia. Carbon monoxide interferes with the oxygen transport function of blood by combining with hemoglobin to form carboxyhemoglobin; the latter has about 240 times the affinity of oxygen for hemoglobin leading to hypoxemia and high morbidity.

Treatment and Anesthetic Management

Wound care is paramount in the management of burn patients and has been described elsewhere [4]. Emergency treatment is often required with burns, since patients may be at high risk for metabolic derangements. However, many individuals are not presented to the veterinarian immediately after injury, especially in occult burns. The risk of hypoxemia should be minimized with 100% inspired oxygen administration via face mask or nasal cannula; gentle manipulation should minimize patient's fear and anxiety during oxygenation. Immediately following injury (within 2–4 h of burns), cool compresses aid in alleviating pain and stopping any ongoing burning trauma due to high skin temperatures. Careful attention to catheter-related infection must be made and aseptic technique should be practiced. Intraosseous catheterization is an alternative if intravenous (IV) access is limited. Antibiotic administration may be required in the presence of sepsis. Considerations for fluid therapy are presented in Figure 15.5 [11].

Direct myocardial depression leading to hypotension can be treated with infusion rates of dopamine (5–15 $\mu g\,kg^{-1}\,min^{-1}$ IV) or dobutamine (1–5 $\mu g\,kg^{-1}\,min^{-1}$ IV). If inhalation injury has occurred, systemic administration of beta-adrenergic receptor agonists such as terbutaline or inhaled albuterol can be used to treat bronchospasm. Supplemental oxygen should be provided for as long as deemed necessary according to blood gas analysis. However, long-term use (i.e., days) of high concentrations of oxygen (i.e., patients under ventilation in the intensive care unit) can lead to oxygen toxicity. Nutritional support may be required depending on the severity and location of skin burns. Hypothermia is usually observed in patients with burns due to rapid and excessive heat loss and should be prevented and treated accordingly. Individuals with burns are typically expected to develop excruciating pain and to have exceedingly high opioid requirements [12]. The prevalence of acute neuropathic pain in humans with burns can be up to 52% for years after the injury and is

- Crystalloid solutions are preferred during the first 24 h of treatment because of increased microvascular permeability, which tends to ameliorate after the first 24 h.
- Thereafter, the addition of colloids (1–3 $mL\,kg^{-1}\,h^{-1}$) for restoration of plasma volume is beneficial, especially if hypoalbuminemia is present. According to the Starling's law:

  Net filtration = $K_f\,[(P_{cap} - P_{if}) - (\pi_P - \pi_{if})]$.

where, K_f represents the net permeability of the capillary wall, P represents the hydrostatic pressure generated by the heart (P_{cap}) or tissues (P_{if}), and π represents the oncotic pressure generated by plasma proteins (π_P) or filtered proteins and mucopolysaccharides in the interstitium (π_{if})

- Therefore, severe hypoalbuminemia as observed in burns results in a reduction of oncotic pressure, which increases the net force favoring filtration of fluid out of the capillary, leading to generalized edema. When considering colloid therapy, the newer hetastarch products have lower molecular weights (~130 kDa) and a molar substitution ratio of four hydroxyethyl groups (HES 130/0.4). Clinically, these compounds do not remain in plasma as long as other larger starch products (e.g., HES 450/0.7). In addition, fewer alterations in coagulation are observed when compared to other colloids (e.g., HES 200/0.5).
- Colloid therapy may be advantageous by reducing the inflammatory response and protecting against vascular leakage while increasing vascular volume. According to the manufacturer, maximum HES 130/0.4 has been administered at 50 $mL\,kg^{-1}\,day^{-1}$ in human studies [7].
- Electrolytes and colloid osmotic pressure measurements can be monitored frequently and used as guidelines for choosing the appropriate fluid and electrolyte replacement therapy in a long-term basis.

Figure 15.5 Considerations for fluid therapy in the burn patient.

associated with an increased extent/percentage of body surface burns at presentation [13–15]. These patients are at high risk of developing chronic pain syndromes following healing [16]. An association between acute pain severity during hospitalization and the prevalence of persistent burn pain may exist and the same issue could exist in veterinary patients. Therefore, analgesic administration is imperative, and agents (Table 15.1) should be given in the emergency setting, especially if one considers that pain increases morbidity and the extent of protein catabolism, and delays healing. Analgesics can be administered as a constant rate infusion (CRI) to maintain long-term therapeutic plasma concentrations. For example, ultra-short-acting mu-opioid receptor agonists such as remifentanil or fentanyl in combination with ketamine, an N-methyl D-aspartate (NMDA) receptor antagonist, are recommended in the treatment of central sensitization [17]. In dogs, lidocaine may also provide additional analgesia administered either using an infusion or transdermal patch. The lidocaine patch is $10\times14\,cm^2$ and contains 700 mg of lidocaine in an aqueous base with other inactive ingredients. This formulation of lidocaine produces analgesia without blocking all the sensory and motor inputs [18] and can be used in cats as well [18]. However, it is not known if changes in skin permeability would change the safety and efficacy of lidocaine patches in burn patients. Lidocaine has also been shown to have free-radical scavenging and anti-inflammatory properties when administered systemically [19, 20]. Nonsteroidal anti-inflammatory drugs (NSAIDs) should be withheld until renal function is reestablished and should not be administered in combination with corticosteroids. Gabapentin has been used in cats with neuropathic injury due to burns [2]. The drug can be easily incorporated into the multimodal analgesic approach, although evidence-based information is lacking for patients with burns. It is not clear what dosages are effective for these cases, but

Table 15.1 Suggested analgesics for the management of pain in patients with burns.

Drug	Dosage	Comments
Remifentanil	2–8 $\mu g\,kg^{-1}\,h^{-1}$ IV infusion	Can be combined with ketamine
Fentanyl	1–4 $\mu g\,kg^{-1}\,h^{-1}$ IV infusion	Can be combined with ketamine
Ketamine	2–10 $\mu g\,kg^{-1}\,min^{-1}$ IV infusion	Can be combined with remifentanil or fentanyl
	1–2 $mg\,kg^{-1}$ bolus followed by 25–50 $\mu g\,kg^{-1}\,min^{-1}$ IV infusion	
Lidocaine	OR	IV use in dogs only
	Patch of $10\times14\,cm^2$ containing 700 mg of lidocaine (50 mg of lidocaine per gram of adhesive patch)	
Gabapentin	10–20 $mg\,kg^{-1}$ every 8 h PO	
Amantadine	3–5 $mg\,kg^{-1}$ every 24 h PO	
Nonsteroidal anti-inflammatory drugs	Follow label recommendations	Should be withheld until renal function is reestablished. Should not be administered in combination with corticosteroids

IV, intravenously; CRI, constant rate infusion; PO, orally.

gabapentin has been shown to produce perioperative pain relief in combination with opioids in dogs and cats [21, 22]. Amantadine is an orally administered NMDA antagonist that can be given as long as pain persists. Constant nursing and care contribute to the pain assessment and treatment and can improve animal welfare.

General anesthesia may be required for daily wound management or for escharotomies with skin graft coverage to attenuate the postburn hypermetabolic response. This is usually the case for full-thickness burns. Inhalant anesthetics should be reserved for cases where smoke inhalation injury is not present; sevoflurane is preferred for suppressing upper airway reactivity while being the least irritating/pungent anesthetic agent for inhalation [23]. Otherwise, total intravenous anesthesia (TIVA) with propofol (0.2–0.4 $mg\,kg^{-1}\,min^{-1}$) is recommended. Alfaxalone infusion (0.2–0.4 $mg\,kg^{-1}\,min^{-1}$) is also a potential alternative for TIVA; however, anesthetic recoveries can be protracted and of poor quality [24]. Ventilatory support can be provided with positive end-expiratory pressure (PEEP), but barotrauma is best avoided with the use of low peak airway pressures. Sterile endotracheal tubes (high-volume, low-pressure cuff) and lubricants should be used for patient intubation to decrease the risk of secondary infection. In humans, there is no conclusive evidence about the use of steroids for the management of severe upper airway edema [25, 26]. Overall, the patient should be evaluated on a case-by-case basis because shock, hyperdynamic circulation, decreased serum albumin concentration, increased alpha-1 acid glycoprotein concentration, and altered receptor sensitivity alter the response to various drugs. Anesthetic induction can be performed with any of the classic IV anesthetic agents such as propofol, alfaxalone, or ketamine combined with a benzodiazepine. The dosages and choice of anesthetic will depend on the physical status and preoperative evaluation of the patient and the use of other drugs with anesthetic-sparing effects. Etomidate or opioid/benzodiazepine (e.g., fentanyl with midazolam) induction can be used if cardiovascular collapse is present, especially in dogs. If serial anesthetic events for wound debridement are required, repeated use of etomidate should be avoided due to adrenocortical suppression. Overall, balanced anesthetic techniques are preferred; doses can be given "to effect."

Chronic Pain Syndrome after Feline Onychectomy

Onychectomy ("declawing" or phalangectomy) is the amputation of the third phalanx of each digit of cats [27]. This still occurs in the United States and parts of Canada, even considering that most owners are against this practice or think onychectomy is a painful procedure [28–31]. It involves surgical trauma and nerve damage. The surgical procedure is aggressive with many postoperative complications. Owners sometimes choose to declaw their cats to prevent property damage or personal injury from scratching. The discussion of the ethical issues involved with feline onychectomy is ongoing, but several state/province legislations have banned the procedure in North America.

Laser onychectomy should be the preferred over scalpel surgical approach due to significantly decreased hemorrhage and postoperative complications including pain [32]. Complications after feline onychectomy can be as high as 50% and include persistent postsurgical pain [33, 34]. Radiographic and clinical signs include lameness, back pain, protrusion of the second phalanx, muscle loss, flexor tendon contracture, reluctance to jump, inappropriate eliminating habits, licking and chewing at the digits, aversion to the feet being touched, bleeding, swelling, changes in weight-bearing, infection, neuropathies, chronic draining tracts, and regrowth of claws [32, 33, 35–39]. There is also a possible link between onychectomy and late onset osteosarcoma [40], hypothesized to result from chronic inflammation inducing neoplastic changes, as has been reported in cats with injection-site sarcomas [41]. Chronic pain syndrome after feline onychectomy is characterized by behavioral changes that may develop within the immediate postoperative period or years after the procedure. These changes can lead to suffering, reduced quality of life, and disability. Central sensitization after severe peripheral nociceptive input can result in allodynia and chronic pain, which involves the activation of NMDA receptors. Secondary hyperalgesia is expected due to the amplification of postoperative pain. The diagnosis of the syndrome is mostly based on clinical signs and behavioral changes after ruling out degenerative joint disease or other complications that could be surgically corrected.

Anesthesia and Perioperative Analgesia

Judicious perioperative anesthetic and analgesic management may avoid chronic pain development after feline onychectomy. The following analgesic principles and techniques should be used in these cases:

- Multimodal analgesia is characterized by the simultaneous use of two or more different classes of analgesics, where each class of analgesic acts at different levels of the nociceptive input pathway and has different onsets and durations of action.
- Analgesic doses may be reduced while minimizing the incidence of adverse effects.
- Postoperative pain attenuation usually occurs with preventive analgesic administration. Opioid and local anesthetic use is recommended to prevent central sensitization and reduce intraoperative analgesic requirements and anesthetic-induced cardiopulmonary depression due to their inhalant anesthetic-sparing effects [42–44].
- Preoperative NSAID administration improves postoperative analgesia in cats undergoing onychectomy [44]. For example, cats receiving meloxicam for 5 days had better outcomes than those receiving for only 3 days [45]. Additionally, long-term administration of NSAIDs might be required in some cases (see the section titled "Chronic Pain Syndrome Treatment").

Cats undergoing onychectomy are generally young and healthy at presentation and, therefore, minimal preoperative diagnostics are required before general anesthesia unless otherwise indicated. The patient's history and physical examination will guide the anesthetic plan. Table 15.2 shows the perioperative anesthetic management for cats undergoing onychectomy.

Table 15.2 Perioperative analgesic management for cats undergoing onychectomy.

- Premedication: dexmedetomidine (5–10 μg kg^{-1}) or acepromazine (0.03–0.05 mg kg^{-1}) + hydromorphone (0.05–0.1 mg kg^{-1}) or methadone (0.3–0.5 mg kg^{-1}) IM. The addition of ketamine (2–3 mg kg^{-1}) might be required in cats requiring chemical restraint.
- Induction: ketamine (5 mg kg^{-1}) + diazepam or midazolam (0.25 mg kg^{-1}), propofol (3–8 mg kg^{-1}), or alfaxalone (1–3 mg kg^{-1}) IV considering that these cats are usually healthy. Doses should be given to effect depending on the protocol and effects of premedication.
- NSAIDs: meloxicam (0.2 mg kg^{-1} SC after induction; then 0.05 mg kg^{-1} PO every 24 h for 3 days; this is "off-label use" in the United States, but not in Canada) or robenacoxib (1–2.4 mg kg^{-1} SC followed by PO for 3–5 days).
- Local blocks: 0.5% bupivacaine hydrochloride (2 mg kg^{-1} as a maximum dose). Therefore, the total volume should be divided depending on the number of limbs undergoing surgery. Dilution may be required when used in kittens (1:1 with saline). Doses for liposomal bupivacaine preparations are described in the text.
- Postoperative: buprenorphine at 0.24 mg kg^{-1} SC if veterinarians are using a high-concentrated formulation of buprenorphine (1.8 mg ml^{-1}) every 24 h for up to 3 days in the United States shortly after extubation. Otherwise, buprenorphine at 0.02 mg kg^{-1} can be administered IV every 4 h after hydromorphone administration, and then 0.02 mg kg^{-1} buccally every 8 h for 2–3 days as "home-medication." A second dose of hydromorphone or methadone can be administered IV or IM until therapy is switched to buprenorphine.

The veterinarian should be aware of NSAID label recommendations in cats, which can vary among countries. For example, in Europe, meloxicam is licensed for long-term use at $0.05\,mg\,kg^{-1}\,day^{-1}$. Treatment of acute and chronic pain after feline onychectomy may require off-label administration of NSAIDs such as robenacoxib and meloxicam, unless contraindicated (see the section titled "Chronic Pain Syndrome Treatment").

In the perioperative setting and under general anesthesia, blockade of the distal branches of the radial, ulnar, median, common peroneal, and tibial nerves can be performed with bupivacaine (Figure 15.6) [46]. An alternative four-point local anesthetic block has been also described in cats with precise anatomical landmarks and high success of nerve staining in cat cadavers [47]. Bupivacaine hydrochloride is preferred over lidocaine due to its long-acting anesthetic effects. In the United States, an injection of liposomal bupivacaine injectable suspension is approved for use in a peripheral nerve block to provide up to 72 h of regional postoperative pain after single administration in cats following onychectomy. The dose of liposomal bupivacaine injectable solution is $5.3\,mg\,kg^{-1}$ ($0.4\,ml\,kg^{-1}$) per forelimb. The administration technique and further details on handling of the suspension can be found on the manufacturer's website [48].

Local anesthetics are safe when appropriate doses and techniques are used. For this reason, toxic doses must be calculated, especially in kittens. Nonflammable antiseptic should be used around the local block sites if laser surgery is to be performed. Safety glasses must be used for protection of the eyes from any reflected beam during laser surgery [27].

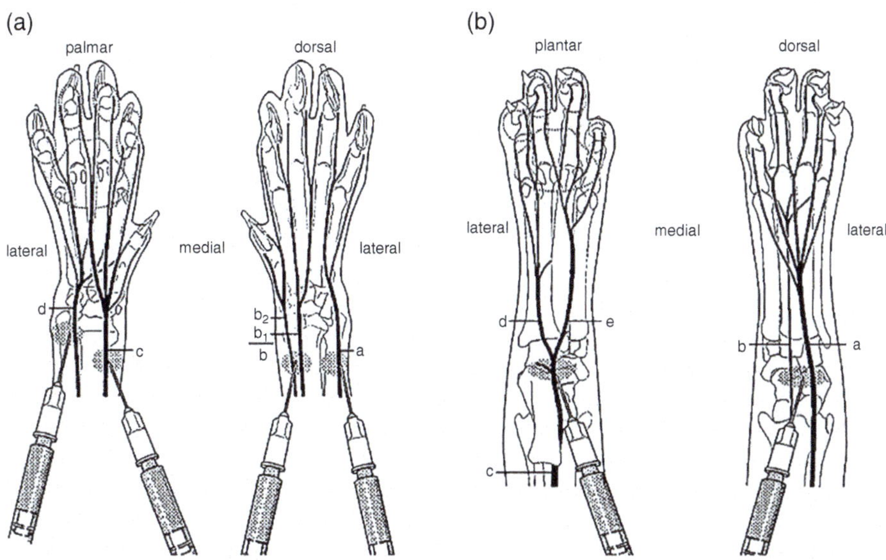

Figure 15.6 (a) In the thoracic distal limbs, on the dorsomedial aspect and proximal to the carpal joint, the superficial branches of the radial nerve are desensitized with local anesthetics. Proximal and lateral to the accessory carpal bone, the palmar and dorsal cutaneous branches of the ulnar nerve are desensitized with local anesthetics. The median nerve is blocked proximal to the median carpal pad. Alternatively, a four-point digital block or a ring block can be performed by injecting bupivacaine into the subcutaneous tissues distal to the carpal joints [46]. (b) In the pelvic distal limb, on the dorsomedial aspect and distal to the tarsus, the superficial branches of the common peroneal nerve are desensitized. Ventromedially and distal to the tarsal joints, the superficial branches of the tibial nerve are blocked. For these procedures, local anesthetics are administered at each site in the subcutaneous tissues using a 22-gauge 1-in. needle [46]. *Source:* Adapted from reference 46, with permission.

Chronic Pain Syndrome Treatment

Cats must be examined for any other source of pain when chronic pain after feline onychectomy is suspected; the feet must be evaluated for residual inflammation or underlying infection. Diagnostic imaging can determine the presence of any remaining bony fragments and claw regrowth. If the syndrome is confirmed, analgesia and treatment of central sensitization are therapeutic goals. A multimodal analgesic approach for long-term treatment with the combination of NMDA receptor antagonists, opioids, and NSAIDs is proposed in Table 15.3 [49]. Therapy is usually constituted by off-label administration of analgesics.

Ketamine is a dissociative anesthetic with NMDA receptor antagonistic properties that is commonly used in cats. Activation of NMDA receptors is involved with the transmission and exacerbation of nociceptive stimuli in the dorsal horn of the spinal cord, which plays a key role in neuropathic and chronic pain. Ketamine may prevent central sensitization and the development of chronic pain and is normally administered as a bolus (0.3–0.5 mg kg^{-1}) followed by an infusion (2–10 μg kg^{-1} min^{-1}) during hospitalization [17]. Amantadine (3–5 mg kg^{-1} PO every 12 or 24 h) is also an NMDA receptor antagonist that has been administered to cats as part of chronic pain treatment after feline onychectomy.

Table 15.3 Suggested treatments for feline chronic pain syndrome after onychectomy using off-label medications: an attempt to reverse central sensitization and allodynia.

- Amantadine: 3 mg kg^{-1} PO every 24 h for 21 days.
- Meloxicam: 0.05 mg kg^{-1} PO every 24 h for 4 days; then 0.025 mg kg^{-1} PO every 24 h for 4 days, then 0.05 mg per cat PO every 24 h for 4 days, and finally 0.05 mg per cat PO every 48 h for 5 days.
- Buprenorphine: 0.01–0.02 mg kg^{-1} every 8 h buccally for up to 5 days (2–3 days) or 0.24 mg kg^{-1} SC for up to 3 days of a high-concentration formulation of buprenorphine (1.8 mg kg^{-1}; in the United States).
- Gabapentin: 10–20 mg kg^{-1} PO every 8 h until resolution of clinical signs. Gabapentin should be tapered down over a 3-week period to avoid breakthrough pain.

Analgesic therapy involves opioid administration, such as buprenorphine, especially during breakthrough pain. A sustained-release formulation of buprenorphine has been advocated to provide analgesia for up to 5 days in cats [50]. Alternatively, a high-concentration buprenorphine formulation (1.8 mg ml^{-1}) can be administered at 0.24 mg kg^{-1} SC every 24 h. NSAID administration has been recommended at a progressively decreasing dosing schedule for up to 12 days. A full biochemical profile is mandatory before NSAID therapy is initiated. Cats must be carefully observed for the development of NSAID-induced adverse effects; immediate cessation of NSAID should occur if adverse effects arise.

Gabapentin is a calcium channel antagonist that can be used as an adjuvant in the treatment of hyperalgesia and allodynia. This drug has been widely used for neuropathic pain treatment in humans and rodents, although its mechanism of action is not fully elucidated. Gabapentin (10–20 mg kg^{-1} every 8–12 h PO) may be useful as part of a multimodal analgesic approach in the treatment of feline onychectomy pain syndrome. Shredded paper or compressed paper pallets should be used in the litter box until effective therapy becomes evident.

The advent of anti-nerve growth factor (NGF) monoclonal antibodies could represent a significant advantage in the treatment of persistent postsurgical pain such as chronic pain syndrome after feline onychectomy. In brief, NGF is pro-nociceptive and can contribute to peripheral and central sensitization. Species-specific antibodies that target NGF have been used in the treatment of feline osteoarthritis with promising results. Studies indicated adequate safety and efficacy for up to 6 weeks after a single subcutaneous injection in cats [51, 52].

Auricular Disease

The ear is a specialized extension of the integumentary system. Auricular diseases can be particularly painful, especially in the presence of chronic inflammation and neoplasia (Figure 15.7). Sedation and general anesthesia are occasionally required to perform an otic examination, diagnosis, and/or treatment. Ear infection or inflammation can induce neurological deficits due to the proximity of the facial nerve and sympathetic innervations of the eyes and ears. The classification of otitis is described in the following text:

- Otitis externa describes any inflammatory condition of the external ear canal. Clinical signs consist of head shaking, scratching, otic pain, variable accumulation of cerumen or exudates, and malodor.
- Otitis media may result from extension of otitis externa through the tympanic membrane, aspiration of pharyngeal contents up the auditory tube, or from hematogenous spread, neoplasia, trauma, and inflammatory polyps. However, otitis media may be a perpetuating factor for otitis externa.
- Otitis interna is usually an extension of otitis media or neoplasia of the middle ear. A careful neurological examination is required to locate the vestibular signs, as animals with otitis interna will present with nystagmus, circling, or falling toward the side of the lesion. If there is involvement of the labyrinth, animals may become nauseated and vomit. Horner's syndrome or deficits in cranial nerves may be observed with otitis media and/or interna [53].

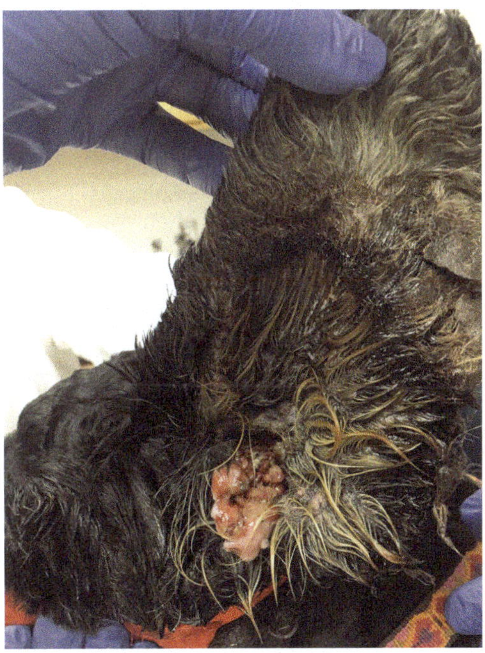

Figure 15.7 An invasive adenocarcinoma and chronic inflammation of the auricular canal in a dog. A secondary infection with *Pseudomonas* was diagnosed. Auricular disease can produce severe pain and impair the patient's quality of life. *Source:* Photo courtesy of Dr. Lucilene Bernardi de Souza.

Diagnosis

Skull radiography, computed tomography (CT), and MRI are commonly indicated for otic evaluation. These procedures normally involve general anesthesia and are employed to evaluate the integrity of the tympanic bulla and reveal the presence of underlying otitis media, neoplasia, polyps, foreign bodies, otitis interna, and central vestibular disease [54]. Advanced imaging helps in distinguishing the anatomic location of the disease process. CT is considered superior to MRI for bony changes, whereas MRI is better for detection of soft tissue abnormalities in both dogs and cats [55]. Cytologic and culture examinations are performed to detect endoparasite/ectoparasite infection, inflammatory processes, or neoplastic lesions. Auricular tumors are more common in cats than dogs and include squamous cell carcinoma, mast cell tumor, basal cell tumor, and fibrosarcoma. General anesthesia is also performed for a complete otoscopic examination in cases of severe otitis in which thorough cleaning of the ear is necessary for therapy and diagnosis [53].

If the tympanic membrane is intact in a dog with otitis media, a myringotomy is performed to obtain samples for culture and susceptibility testing and cytologic examination. Briefly, a spinal needle penetrates the tympanic membrane through the caudoventral aspect of the pars tensa. Suction is applied and samples collected. Ear flushing of external ear canal is usually required under the same anesthetic episode [54].

Brainstem auditory evoked response (BAER) is an objective hearing test that detects the presence or absence of hearing or progression of changes in hearing. Electrodes placed on standard head sites record responses to an auditory stimulus generated. The waves generated are evaluated, and each wave corresponds to a specific cranial nerve or portion of it, or an area of the central nervous system. Since there is conduction of impulses through the brainstem, the test is also valuable for diagnosis of brainstem lesions. Sedation is often required for uncooperative patients. Both sedation and anesthesia cause changes in wave latency [53].

Treatment

In addition to medical therapy, surgery is commonly performed in dogs and cats for the treatment of ear diseases. Aural hematoma repair due to self-induced trauma of head shaking or scratching is an example. In this case, blood accumulates within the fractured cartilage of the pinna, and swelling is most visible on the concave aspect. Treatment of otitis externa or other underlying cause is required to avoid recurrence of aural hematoma. Surgical incision, drainage, curettage, and closure with mattress sutures provide apposition of the cartilage edges.

The two most common surgical procedures for the treatment of otitis externa are lateral ear resection and total ear canal ablation (TECA) [56]. Opening the vertical ear canal with lateral ear resection in dogs improves aeration, decreases humidity, facilitates removal of cerumen or exudate, and improves the distribution of topical medication in the ear canal. TECA is the mainstay treatment of end-stage otitis and malignant otic neoplasia. The technique is always combined with bulla osteotomy to allow complete removal of all secretory epithelium and exudate associated with the external and middle ear. Severe secondary changes and proliferative disease are surgically removed with the ear canal. Finally, a lateral bulla osteotomy of the tympanic bulla allows complete exploration of the middle ear for the removal of secretory epithelium, exudates, and/or tumor. Surgical complications include facial nerve paralysis, hemorrhage, severe pain, and hearing loss [57]. Secondary complications may occur due to compressive bandage placement, especially in cats, causing obstruction of the airways with further hypoxemia, collapse, and death.

Anesthetic Management

Health status and differentiation of ear disease (i.e., primary or secondary disorder) are important for the anesthetic management. Endocrinopathies are a common cause of ear disease. Systemic glucocorticoid administration is usually the elective therapy for acute inflammation of the ear canal, chronic proliferative changes of the ear canal, and allergic otitis. Special attention should be paid to antibiotic therapy that could potentially involve drug-induced toxicity. Nephrotoxicity induced by aminoglycosides manifests clinically as nonoliguric renal failure, with a slow rise in serum creatinine and a hypo-osmolar urinary output developing days after initiation of therapy. Systemic aminoglycoside administration is nephrotoxic because a small but sizable proportion of the drug accumulates in the proximal tubules after glomerular filtration [58]. Therefore, the veterinarian should be aware of this potential nephrotoxic effect in animals treated with aminoglycosides.

If a ruptured eardrum is present, manipulation or flushing can cause material to drain through the Eustachian tube into the nasopharynx, resulting in aspiration. An appropriately sized, cuffed endotracheal tube is always required for these procedures.

Chronic ear conditions are associated with pain on palpation and may be exacerbated during the otoscopic examination (Figure 15.7). Pain on opening the mouth may be related to middle ear involvement because of inflammation, swelling, and pain within the bulla, located adjacent to the temporomandibular joint. The ears can be extremely sensitive and painful; anesthetic depth must be rapidly adjusted if head shaking is observed during surgery or otoscopy; a bolus of injectable anesthetic is usually preferred over increases in the concentration of inhalant anesthetics in these cases. Perioperative analgesia is imperative in the management of TECA and bulla osteotomy, as these surgical interventions are highly invasive and painful procedures. Multimodal analgesia with local anesthetic blocks, opioid, and anti-inflammatory drug administration should be the cornerstone in the treatment of perioperative pain associated with TECA. Premedication with a sedative combined with a mu-opioid receptor agonist (e.g., methadone [0.2–0.3 $mg\,kg^{-1}$ in the cat or 0.5–1.0 $mg\,kg^{-1}$ in the dog] or hydromorphone [0.025–0.05 $mg\,kg^{-1}$ in the cat or 0.1–0.2 $mg\,kg^{-1}$ in the dog]) is recommended. In the intraoperative and postoperative periods, fentanyl reduces inhalant anesthetic requirements, often resulting in less cardiopulmonary depression while providing reliable analgesia. Doses up to 42 $\mu g\,kg^{-1}\,h^{-1}$ have produced maximum reductions in the minimum alveolar concentrations of inhalant (approximately 63%) in dogs [59]. However, the use of lower doses will lessen the likelihood of opioid-induced dysphoria in the anesthetic recovery period. Lower doses of fentanyl (10–15 $\mu g\,kg^{-1}\,h^{-1}$ IV) may be combined with lidocaine (50 $\mu g\,kg^{-1}\,min^{-1}$ IV; in dogs only) and/or ketamine (10 $\mu g\,kg^{-1}\,min^{-1}$ IV) as part of a balanced anesthetic technique. In cats undergoing ovariohysterectomy, a combination of remifentanil (20 $\mu g\,kg^{-1}\,h^{-1}$ IV) and ketamine (30 $\mu g\,kg^{-1}\,min^{-1}$ IV) reduced isoflurane concentrations by approximately 48% when compared with saline infusions [60]. Remifentanil infusion alone reduced these requirements by only approximately 15% when compared with saline infusions. Therefore, the infusions of a mu-opioid receptor agonist and ketamine could potentially reduce inhalant anesthetic-induced adverse effects and provide smooth short-term anesthetic protocols in cats. Anesthetic recoveries were not protracted due to ketamine infusions [60].

Local and regional techniques can be utilized in addition to systemic analgesic agents. This approach usually minimizes the development of breakthrough pain and a high incidence of opioid-induced side effects (e.g., dysphoria, respiratory depression, or drug-induced hyperalgesia). A local anesthetic block has been described in dogs undergoing TECA. Under general anesthesia, bupivacaine is injected in a line from the wing of the atlas to the caudal aspect of the vertical ear canal to block the greater auricular nerve. The drug is administered between the caudodorsal aspect of the masseter muscle and rostral aspect of the vertical ear canal to desensitize the auriculotemporal nerve [61, 62]. Another method of analgesic administration has been described with the use of a local anesthetic delivery system that allows continuous delivery of local anesthetics via a fenestrated catheter (Figure 15.8) [63, 64]. An elastomeric bulb or syringe pump device is filled with drug to deliver a constant volume directly to the surgical site. However, results of these studies could not demonstrate a significant benefit in using local anesthetic blocks in dogs that underwent TECA when other multimodal analgesic techniques were employed. Despite the lack of significant differences among treatment groups, a benefit may exist, and failing to detect an advantage could be attributable to an inadequate dosage of the drug, technique error, inconsistent analgesia of all nerves, adequate effect of other systemic analgesics, and/or poor study design, including inappropriate methods for the recognition and evaluation of pain in animals.

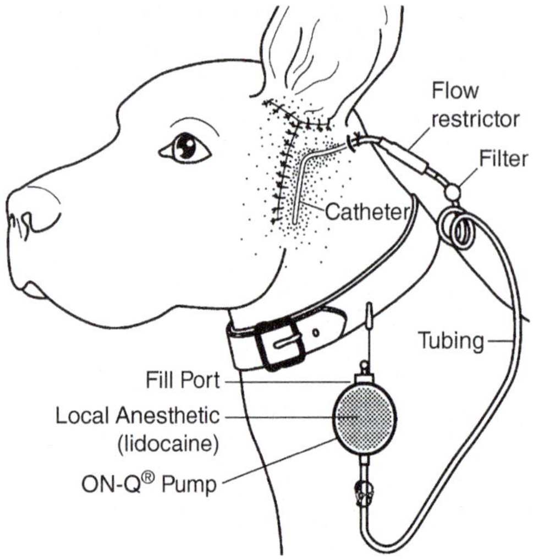

Figure 15.8 Application of a pain booster local anesthetic infusion system in a total ear canal ablation. *Source:* Adapted from reference 63, with permission.

Laryngeal Paralysis

Laryngeal paralysis (LP) is a well-recognized cause of upper respiratory stridor and dyspnea in dogs and more rarely in cats [65, 66]. The disease is characterized by laryngeal malfunction during abduction of the arytenoid cartilages, thus creating an inspiratory partial or full upper airway obstruction. Hereditary and acquired forms have been recognized in dogs and cats [67]. The hereditary form, less frequent than the acquired form, affects young dogs of many breeds such as Bouvier, Bull Terrier, Dalmatian, Rottweiler, and Siberian Husky. Mixed-breed dogs can be affected by both forms of the disease. The acquired form is most reported in middle-aged to older dogs; Labrador Retrievers are overrepresented [68, 69], but other breeds such as Golden Retrievers, Afghan Hounds, Irish Setters, Standard Poodles, and Saint Bernards have been affected [70].

Unilateral or bilateral LP can be a result of trauma or an intrathoracic or extrathoracic mass that could compress or stretch the recurrent laryngeal nerve [65, 67]. In addition, neuropathy of the recurrent laryngeal nerve, myopathy of the intrinsic laryngeal muscles, as well as neuromuscular disorders such as myasthenia gravis (MG), megaesophagus, or idiopathic myositis have been associated with LP. In addition, LP may be a manifestation of a generalized neuromuscular disorder from a peripheral neuropathy [67]. LP can be linked to esophageal dysfunction and generalized weakness [68], as well as to other clinical neurological deficits, electrodiagnostic, and/or pathologic abnormalities [69, 71]. In cats, LP is an uncommon cause of upper airway obstruction, although both forms have been observed. The acquired form has been reported after bilateral thyroidectomy, but no breed or sex predisposition has been identified in this species [66].

Clinical Signs

Clinical sign severity is dependent on the severity of LP and can manifest from altered barking, gagging, coughing, and mild exercise intolerance to severe respiratory distress. Inspiratory stridor or increased lung sounds cranially may be noted during thoracic auscultation. Dyspnea, collapse, cyanosis, and hyperthermia may occur in the emergency setting, possibly requiring general anesthesia and ventilatory support [67]. Vomiting, regurgitation, and inhalation of gastrointestinal contents into the respiratory tract (i.e., aspiration pneumonia) may occur. Clinical signs are usually progressive, and patients are presented for investigation late in the course of the disease. Other clinical signs include concurrent pelvic limb weakness with bilateral cranial tibial muscle atrophy, generalized weakness, and neurological deficits.

Diagnosis

Physical examination and laboratory findings may be unremarkable. The most used method for diagnosing LP is laryngoscopy (Figure 15.9). Failure of one or both of the arytenoid cartilages to abduct during inspiration may confirm the diagnosis.

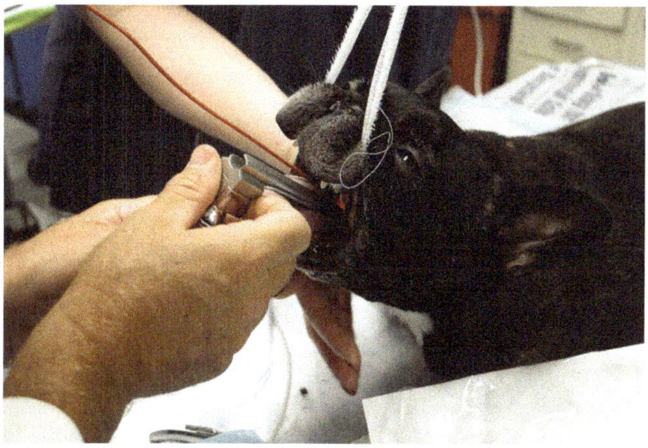

Figure 15.9 Laryngoscopy is the preferred method for the diagnosis of laryngeal paralysis. The procedure is performed via direct examination of the laryngeal function under sedation and a light depth of general anesthesia. Oxygen insufflation should be provided to prevent hypoxemia. *Source:* Photo courtesy of Dr. Giacomo Gianotti.

Treatment

The treatment of LP ultimately involves surgical management. Several interventions are described, but unilateral or bilateral arytenoid cartilage lateralization is usually the surgical treatment of choice in dogs due to a lower complication rate compared with other techniques [70]. Successful medical management has been described in cats with mild clinical signs.

Anesthetic Management

A thorough physical examination and auscultation along with thoracic radiography are recommended for the investigation of megaesophagus and aspiration pneumonia. During the preoperative assessment, the patient should be handled quietly and carefully to avoid stress- or fear-induced tachypnea that could potentially produce airway obstruction with subsequent increased work of breathing and acute respiratory distress. Partial airway obstruction with increased inspiratory effort and work of breathing may cause increased negative pressure, leading to pulmonary edema. Resistance to breathing is dictated by Hagen–Poiseuille law and can be severely increased during partial airway obstruction or with the use of inappropriately small endotracheal size tubes (Figure 15.10). Continuous oxygenation via face mask for 3 min before induction of anesthesia should be mandatory for these cases to prevent or treat hypoxemia. Stress-induced hyperthermia can be treated with controlled ice packing, alcohol application, or a cold-water bath and the administration of acepromazine. Acepromazine causes a decrease in respiratory rate in dogs at doses higher than 0.025 $mg\,kg^{-1}$ without changes in $PaCO_2$, pH, bicarbonate concentrations, or PaO_2 [72]. Because acepromazine produces mild sedation and has a relatively long duration of action, it is often used to calm anxious patients and is an appropriate choice for patients with LP. Appropriate sedation is accomplished with the combination of acepromazine (0.01–0.03 $mg\,kg^{-1}$) and butorphanol (0.2–0.3 $mg\,kg^{-1}$) or buprenorphine (0.01–0.02 $mg\,kg^{-1}$) IV. In addition, the use of acepromazine–butorphanol improves the quality of laryngeal examination [73].

Other preoperative secondary changes such as laryngeal and pulmonary edema can be addressed with the administration of corticosteroids (dexamethasone 0.2–1.0 $mg\,kg^{-1}$ every

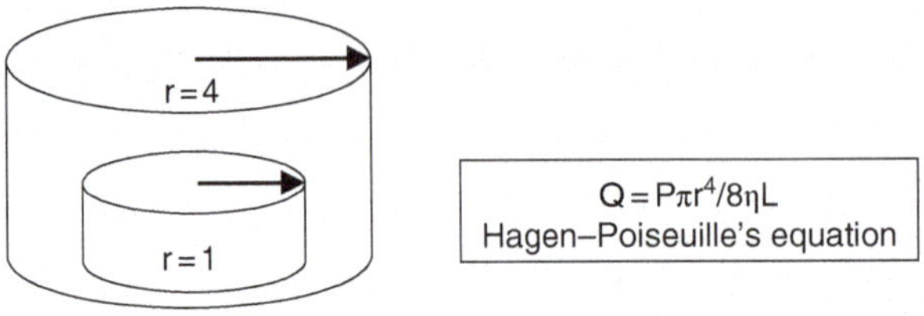

Figure 15.10 The Hagen–Poiseuille law applies when flow is laminar (linear relationship of flow to pressure). Resistance is directly proportional to flow rate (Q) during laminar flow. The internal diameter (r) of the airway is the most important factor determining the resistance to gas flow. The equation shows that doubling the length (L) of the airway only doubles the airway resistance, while halving the radius reduces the flow to 1/16 of its original value if the pressure (P) drop along the tube remains the same. The flow is proportional to the fourth power of the radius. For example, an airway has a radius of 1 and a flow of 1 ml min^{-1}. If the radius is increased by 4, the flow is increased to 256 ml min^{-1}. Changes in resistance (and therefore flow) tend to parallel changes in the work of breathing. η is the viscosity of fluid. In the figure, "1" and "4" are arbitrary numbers to demonstrate what happens when there is a fourfold increase in radius.

12 h as needed). However, steroids are usually reserved for postoperative administration when laryngeal edema and swelling, cyanosis, hypoxemia, and respiratory difficulties are observed after extubation. Tracheostomy is the last resource when other emergency treatments have failed to alleviate distress.

The use of opioids for LP examination is controversial. Opioids produce an antitussive effect through a central inhibition of the cough center that is mediated by both mu (μ)- and kappa (κ)-opioid receptor agonists [67]. Independent of their antitussive effects, agonists of mu-opioid receptors are known for causing dose-dependent, centrally mediated respiratory depression that could be clinically relevant in patients with LP. This effect can be exacerbated by concurrent use of other respiratory depressants such as some injectable and inhalant anesthetics. Therefore, dogs and cats should be closely monitored after opioid therapy, sedation, and recovery of anesthesia and 100% oxygen should be provided. Another important concern is that opioids may decrease esophageal sphincter pressure and increase the incidence of gastroesophageal reflux (GER) during anesthesia and the early postoperative period. In patients with LP, postanesthetic esophagitis, regurgitation, and possible aspiration pneumonia are of great concern. Some opioids, morphine in particular, may increase the incidence of GER during anesthesia compared with other drugs from the same class [74, 75]. The CRI of metoclopramide is commonly administered postoperatively in an attempt to increase lower esophageal sphincter tone and avoid postoperative regurgitation and aspiration [76]. However, high doses are required to achieve this clinical effect (bolus of 1 mg kg^{-1} followed by continuous infusion of 1 mg kg^{-1} h^{-1}) [76]. A CRI of the serotonin 5-HT_4 receptor agonist cisapride (1 mg kg^{-1} diluted into a 100 ml bag of 0.9% saline and administered at a beginning rate of 50 ml h^{-1} and increasing doses if no changes in vital parameters were noted) has been suggested to reduce postoperative aspiration pneumonia in dogs with LP [77]. Although definitive recommendations could not be made, cisapride infusion was well tolerated and a lower, but not significant, rate of aspiration pneumonia was recorded (i.e., one out of 50 dogs) in comparison with dogs not treated with cisapride (i.e., six out of 50 dogs). However, these dogs were sedated with acepromazine in combination with buprenorphine or butorphanol, and received maropitant IV, famotidine IV, and diphenhydramine IM before surgery [77]. Intravenous maropitant administration is commonly used to prevent vomiting in dogs undergoing unilateral or bilateral arytenoid cartilage lateralization. However, the drug did not prevent GER in a small population of anesthetized dogs premedicated with acepromazine–hydromorphone [78].

Buprenorphine, a partial mu-opioid receptor agonist that tends to cause less respiratory depression and dysphoria than full agonists (hydromorphone or morphine), may provide adequate sedation and pain management throughout surgery. Alternatively, pure mu-opioid receptor agonists may be used in the intraoperative period and either buprenorphine or an opioid agonist–antagonist (i.e., butorphanol) may be used in the postoperative period. If profound sedation and/or respiratory depression are observed, opioids can be reversed with the administration of an opioid antagonist (i.e., naloxone) or an agonist–antagonist [79]. A multimodal analgesic approach is beneficial with the addition of a NSAID.

Anticholinergics have been used to prevent vagal-induced bradycardia resulting from laryngeal manipulation and/or opioid administration and can be particularly useful in brachycephalic breeds. However, thick mucus can be produced, leading to increased fluid viscosity, airway obstruction, and increased work of breathing (increased breathing resistance; Figure 15.10).

For laryngoscopy, sedation followed by a light depth of anesthesia is required to perform the laryngeal examination without losing the laryngeal reflex (Figure 15.9). If anesthetic depth is excessive, arytenoid motion will be depressed or absent even in healthy dogs. In this scenario, the larynx should be patiently observed continuously as the animal awakes; doxapram should also be administered at this point (see the following text). Dogs and cats should be preoxygenated via face mask or flow-by oxygen, as well as throughout laryngoscopy. A tube (e.g., red rubber tube or flexible long urinary catheter) is placed close to the trachea for oxygen insufflation. The tube is connected to the oxygen line via a three-way stopcock that normally connects the anesthesia machine with the breathing system (Figure 15.11). Misdiagnosis of LP may be avoided by selecting anesthetic regimens, with the least effect on arytenoid motion. Nevertheless, there is currently no established universal protocol for the evaluation of laryngeal function in small animals.

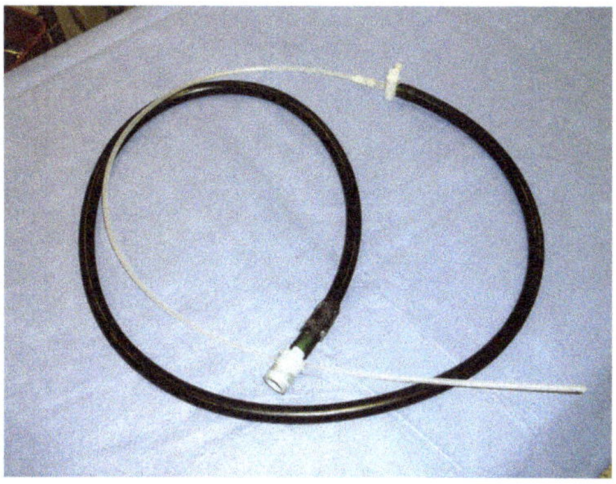

Figure 15.11 A flexible long urinary catheter is used to provide oxygen insufflation during laryngoscopy. The distal part of the catheter is placed close to the trachea. The tube is connected to the fresh gas flow output where normally the anesthetic machine is connected to the breathing system.

Doxapram hydrochloride is a central nervous stimulant that increases respiratory rate and tidal volume. The drug is often given during laryngoscopy because increased intrinsic laryngeal motion may be useful for differentiating normal dogs from those with LP [80–82]. However, complete airway occlusion is a risk, and endotracheal intubation may be potentially necessary with the use of doxapram.

Overall, induction and recovery phases of anesthesia are critical in dogs and cats with LP. On the other hand, maintenance of anesthesia is generally uneventful when pain is controlled, and the airways are secured. Standard monitoring should be adequate with the understanding that pulse oximetry is useful for monitoring early hypoxemia during laryngoscopy and anesthetic recovery. No significant difference was detected when thiopental, propofol, and diazepam–ketamine were compared during evaluation of laryngeal function in dogs [83]. On the contrary, arytenoid motion was significantly greater after thiopental administration when compared to propofol, ketamine–diazepam, acepromazine–thiopental, and acepromazine–propofol [84]. Other studies have shown that propofol, propofol–diazepam, thiopental, and alfaxalone are similarly useful for evaluation of laryngeal function as long as they are administered to effect and a light depth of anesthesia is maintained [85, 86]. Shorter evaluation times are usually achieved with the administration of propofol or thiopental and doxapram in acepromazine–butorphanol-sedated animals than with alfaxalone [87]. In the aforementioned studies, different dosage regimens and methodologies are used, likely accounting for the varying results. Additionally, propofol, thiopental, and alfaxalone are respiratory depressants, and slow and carefully titrated administration is advised to avoid apnea. In addition, ketamine has shown to cause mild decreases in respiratory rate, minute volume, and PaO_2. Laryngeal examination should be kept to a minimal period to avoid complications while attention is given to a rapid and smooth endotracheal intubation. Cats are prone to laryngospasm and desensitization of the arytenoids is recommended with a few drops of lidocaine before intubation and after laryngeal examination.

Dogs and cats are generally extubated during surgery for evaluation of airway diameter after arytenoid cartilage lateralization. Small boluses of propofol (0.3–0.5 $mg\,kg^{-1}$) are given, and a new endotracheal tube should be available for intubation. During anesthetic recovery in dogs, the endotracheal tube may be left partially inflated to avoid regurgitation entering the trachea and subsequent aspiration pneumonia. Extubation is performed when coughing is observed, and swallowing reflexes have returned. Sedation may be necessary for a stress-free recovery. Acepromazine (0.01–0.02 $mg\,kg^{-1}$ IV) or dexmedetomidine (0.5 $\mu g\,kg^{-1}$ IV) can be administered after extubation or if the patient is already showing signs of agitation and/or distress. However, it is important to avoid excessive sedation in a patient that may be prone to aspiration pneumonia. Reintubation can be performed when swelling and laryngeal edema are present. Pulmonary edema is not uncommon due to increased thoracic negative pressure and work of breathing. Furosemide (1 $mg\,kg^{-1}$) is administered in addition to corticosteroids. Monitoring the patient's ventilation status is of utmost importance. Ideally, animals should be hospitalized in the critical care unit after surgery. Postoperative complications include aspiration pneumonia, laryngeal edema, recurrence of clinical signs, and transient Horner's syndrome, among others [69]. Despite some degree of morbidity and common postoperative complications, surgery is the recommended treatment in dogs for the improvement of quality of life, especially if one considers the life-threatening nature of the disease [70, 71, 88]. In cats, unilateral arytenoid lateralization also appears to provide good prognosis [66, 89].

Malignant Hyperthermia

Malignant hyperthermia (MH) (also discussed in Chapter 11, Genetic Disease) is defined as a pharmacogenetic clinical syndrome characterized by skeletal muscle rigidity, rapid increases in core body temperature, hypercapnia, and metabolic acidosis. MH is associated with multiple genetic and environmental points of entry [90]. This syndrome is primarily caused by a mutation in the ryanodine receptor (RyR1) gene with an autosomal dominant inheritance pattern [91]. The ryanodine receptor, or calcium-release channel, is located in the sarcoplasmic reticulum membrane of skeletal muscle and is essential to control calcium movement during the excitation–contraction coupling process. Uncontrolled calcium release from the sarcoplasmic reticulum into the myoplasm may cause muscle rigidity and a hypermetabolic state, with release of cations and enzymes, and excessive heat and acid production.

MH is usually triggered by halogenated volatile anesthetics (e.g., halothane, isoflurane, and sevoflurane) and depolarizing muscle relaxants (e.g., succinylcholine); stress and other ion channelopathies have also been identified as important initiating factors [92]. MH-like syndromes have been reported in various dog breeds, including Greyhounds, Border Collies, Cocker Spaniels, Doberman Pinschers, Pointers, Siberian Huskies, and Saint Bernards [90, 91, 93–96]. No breed disposition has been identified; the anecdotal belief that Greyhounds were genetically susceptible to MH has not been confirmed [92]. Suspected MH has been rarely described in the cat [97].

Clinical Signs

Unlike MH in pigs, canine MH does not typically present with lactic acidosis or an early onset of muscle rigidity, but rather an increased production of carbon dioxide and oxygen consumption. Slow increases in core body temperature are observed, but lag behind the production of carbon dioxide and tachypnea. Ventricular premature contractions, ventricular bigeminy, fibrillation, and tachycardia have been reported in dogs and cats with MH-like syndromes [90, 93, 96, 97].

Diagnosis

MH episodes may occur in healthy animals without a previous history of anesthetic problems. Persistent and elevated increases in the concentrations of carbon dioxide despite aggressive ventilatory support should be viewed as potential positive MH cases. Other causes of hypercapnia, cardiac arrhythmias, metabolic acidosis, increased body temperature, and muscle rigidity must be ruled out. Tachypnea and tachycardia can be attributed to "light" anesthesia, which is easily addressed by proper anesthetic depth monitoring. Hyperthermia has been observed after heat stroke, iatrogenic overheating, or opioid administration.

MH-like syndromes have been documented in the literature, but an in vitro muscle contracture test (IVCT) was rarely performed to confirm the MH diagnosis. Therefore, the true MH incidence is unknown in veterinary medicine. Suspected MH animals could undergo the IVCT, in which a muscle sample is exposed to halothane and caffeine, and the sensitivity of contractive patterns to these triggering agents is measured. However, a negative test does not exclude an MH reaction. The test is sometimes cost-prohibitive, which makes the conclusive diagnostic impractical. Clinically, the end-tidal carbon dioxide and core body temperature monitoring are useful for early diagnosis and treatment of MH.

Treatment and Anesthetic Management

Clinical sign recognition and immediate elimination of known triggering factors may prevent and/or treat signs of MH (Figure 15.12). Discontinuation of inhalant anesthetic administration and depolarizing neuromuscular blocking drugs are key components in management of MH. Decontamination of the anesthetic machine by vaporizer removal and the replacement of parts in contact with an inhalant anesthetic are recommended. The gas-flow circuit should be flushed with fresh gas at a rate of $10 l min^{-1}$ for a minimum of 10 min. The use of gas analyzers that monitor end-tidal inhalant anesthetics identifies any residual anesthetic in the breathing system. Even a small fraction of volatile anesthetic can trigger the syndrome in MH-susceptible patients. It is recommended to replace the anesthetic machine in use with another one with an oxygen source and not commonly used for anesthesia. Excess carbon dioxide production can lead to rapid carbon dioxide absorber exhaustion. Drugs considered safe for administration include barbiturates, propofol, opioids, benzodiazepines, dexmedetomidine, ketamine, droperidol, and nondepolarizing neuromuscular blocking drugs. TIVA is considered if anesthesia cannot be terminated, yet may not prevent a MH-like syndrome from occurring [95].

Effective sedation and analgesia are important to minimize perioperative stress and pain, respectively, as these can be triggering factors. An opioid (morphine [0.5–1 $mg kg^{-1}$] or methadone [0.5 $mg kg^{-1}$] IM) can be given with

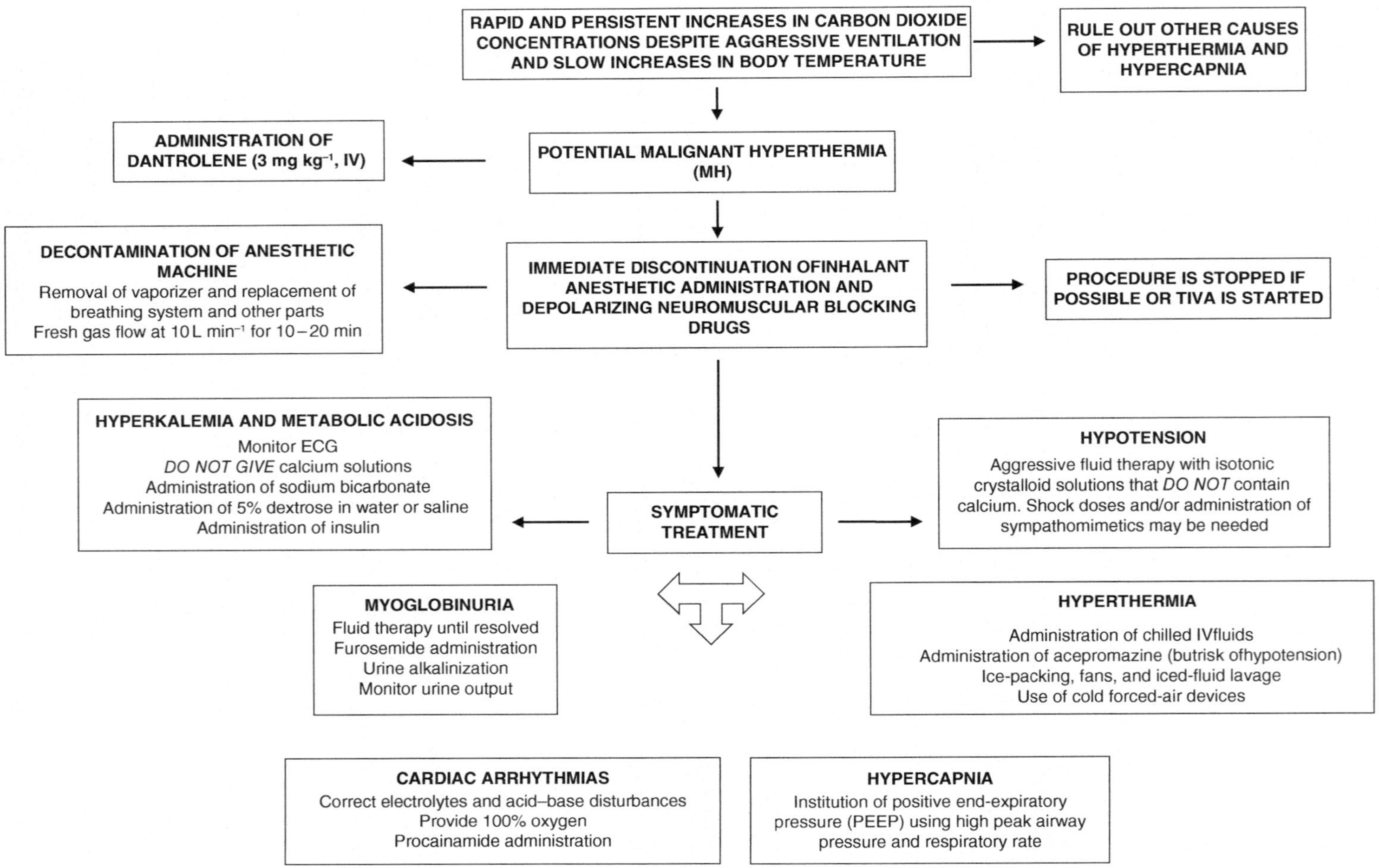

Figure 15.12 Algorithm for MH treatment.

midazolam (0.1–0.2 mg kg^{-1} IM), acepromazine (0.02–0.05 mg kg^{-1} IM), or dexmedetomidine (3–5 μg kg^{-1} IM). Anesthetic induction can be accomplished with any IV anesthetic agent. Monitoring of end-tidal carbon dioxide is essential for the early diagnosis of a MH episode. Hyperventilation and high peak airway pressure, with PEEP, are commonly needed to decrease carbon dioxide levels. Invasive blood pressure and electrocardiogram monitoring should be rapidly instituted to monitor for cardiac dysrhythmias and changes in blood pressure.

Aggressive fluid therapy with isotonic crystalloid solutions is sometimes needed due to hypotension. In this case, calcium-containing crystalloid solutions are not acceptable due to the pathogenesis of MH, and 5% dextrose in water, 0.9% saline, or balanced salt solutions are preferred. Acetated polyionic solutions are calcium free balanced electrolyte solutions that can be infused IV in cases of severe hypotension ("shock dose" is approximately 60–90 ml kg^{-1} h^{-1}). However, the latter contains less sodium than plasma, which could lead to greater loss of fluid into the intracellular compartment. Acetate is metabolized rapidly throughout the body, and the alkalinizing effect is readily available. 0.9% saline contains higher amounts of chloride than plasma and tends to decrease the strong ion difference, leading to hyperchloremic acidosis. Dextrose (5%) in water contains no electrolytes, and it is rarely indicated as the primary replacement solution. Only free water remains when dextrose is metabolized; high concentrations of glucose may be detrimental in both acute renal and cerebral injuries. In any crystalloid therapy, the volume retained in the vascular space is rapidly distributed into the interstitial space, producing only a short-term volume expansion. Hypertension and tachycardia may be observed due to sympathetic stimulation caused by severe hypercapnia. Fluid therapy might also be important to prevent acute renal injury associated with deposition of myoglobin in the renal tubules. The use of osmotic and loop diuretics and urine alkalinization should prevent rhabdomyolysis-induced kidney failure. Cool IV fluids may be preferred in the presence of hyperthermia [95]. Indeed, patient cooling can be accomplished with ice packing, fans, and iced fluid lavage. Heating blankets and convective heaters must be turned off. Acepromazine has been used as palliative therapy for hyperthermia. The drug induces hypothermia by acting in the thermoregulatory center of the hypothalamus and blocking alpha-1-adrenergic receptors, which ultimately results in peripheral vasodilation and loss of body heat [95].

Cardiac arrhythmias are best treated with the administration of procainamide during episodes of MH, as lidocaine has been documented to compromise the outcome by increasing myoplasmic calcium content leading to exacerbation of the hypermetabolic state [93].

Laboratory testing may include serum electrolytes, lactate and creatine kinase (CK) measurements, and blood gas analysis. The goal is to identify acid–base disturbances (acidemia) and to monitor progression of the treatment. Hyperkalemia-induced cardiac dysrhythmias are an important cause of death in these patients and should be addressed immediately. Metabolic acidosis potentiates hyperkalemia and may be treated with sodium bicarbonate (1–2 mEq kg^{-1} empirically or when bicarbonate deficiency is calculated, IV). Calcium solutions are contraindicated, and the prognosis may be compromised [96]. Intravenous glucose administration combined with insulin helps drive potassium into the cells and provides an exogenous energy source with which to replace depleted cerebral metabolic substrates. A urinalysis can be useful for the diagnosis of myoglobinuria.

Dantrolene is the recommended life-saving therapeutic agent. It is an intracellular calcium antagonist that has skeletal-muscle-relaxant properties [98]. A single dose of 3 mg kg^{-1} is administered immediately after the recognition of MH, but additional doses up to 10 mg kg^{-1} may be needed. The drug is provided as a lyophilized power (20 mg) with mannitol (3 g) added to improve solubility. Dantrolene should be mixed in water (60 ml) and administered via a large-bore catheter to avoid venous irritation [90]. Unfortunately, because of its high cost and the low incidence of MH as an anesthesia-related complication in veterinary medicine, dantrolene is not always available in all veterinary institutions, which may lead to a high prevalence of anesthetic death during the occurrence of MH cases [96]. The use of nondepolarizing neuromuscular blocking drugs has been suggested as an alternative to dantrolene because these drugs block acetylcholine from occupying binding sites at the neuromuscular junction and prevent muscle depolarization and contraction. Increases in CK may be followed as a rough guide for therapy. In case of death, complete rigor mortis occurs a few minutes after the onset of cardiac arrest, and necropsy findings are usually inconclusive.

Myasthenia Gravis

MG is a chronic autoimmune disorder caused by a decrease in functional nicotinic acetylcholine (ACh) receptors (AChR) at the neuromuscular junction due to their destruction or inactivation by circulating autoantibodies, typically of immunoglobulin G (IgG) class [99]. Acetylcholine is essential for muscle contraction at the neuromuscular junction. The defect in transmission resulting from AChR loss results in focal or generalized muscle weakness and exhaustion (Figure 15.13) [100, 101]. The condition is characterized by exhaustion of voluntary muscles with repetitive use or exercise followed by partial recovery or alleviation with rest. Two forms have been described: congenital and acquired. The congenital form results from an inherited deficiency of ACh receptors at the postsynaptic membranes in the skeletal muscle, which is presented in puppies and kittens aged about 3–8 weeks. In this case, breeds include English Springer Spaniel, Jack Russell Terrier, and Fox Terrier [102]. On the other hand, acquired MG is a common immune-mediated disorder that has been reported in German Shepherds, Golden and Labrador Retrievers, Chihuahuas, and Dachshunds; however, a high prevalence has also been found in Akitas [103]. Abyssinians and Somali are the most common cat breeds that are predisposed to the condition with relative risk increased after 3 years of age [104]. A description of the pathogenesis, classification of MG, and treatment have been reviewed in detail elsewhere [105].

Clinical Signs

Acquired MG has a wide spectrum of clinical presentations, which include paraneoplastic, focal, and appendicular myasthenic patients. The latter can be divided into acute fulminating or generalized MG [106]. The focal form shows facial (decreased palpebral blink), pharyngeal (decreased gag reflex), or laryngeal (vocalization changes, inspiratory stridor, and vocal fold abduction) dysfunction. Muscle weakness and fatigue in the presence of normal spinal reflexes and excessive salivation and regurgitation as a result of megaesophagus are normally observed in dogs and cats with generalized MG. Megaesophagus has been found in approximately 20% of cats, whereas the condition affects 30–40% of dogs with acquired MG. The incidence of megaesophagus and dysphagia is usually lower in cats due to the difference in distribution of skeletal muscle in the esophagus between the two species [102, 104]. Dysphagia, stiff and short-strided gait, muscle tremors, and/or persistent dilated pupils can be observed in both dogs and cats. Cats may be unable to retract their claws, and signs may progress to paresis, cervical ventroflexion, and weight loss [107]. These patients are at high risk of aspiration pneumonia that may lead to respiratory failure and necessitate euthanasia [106].

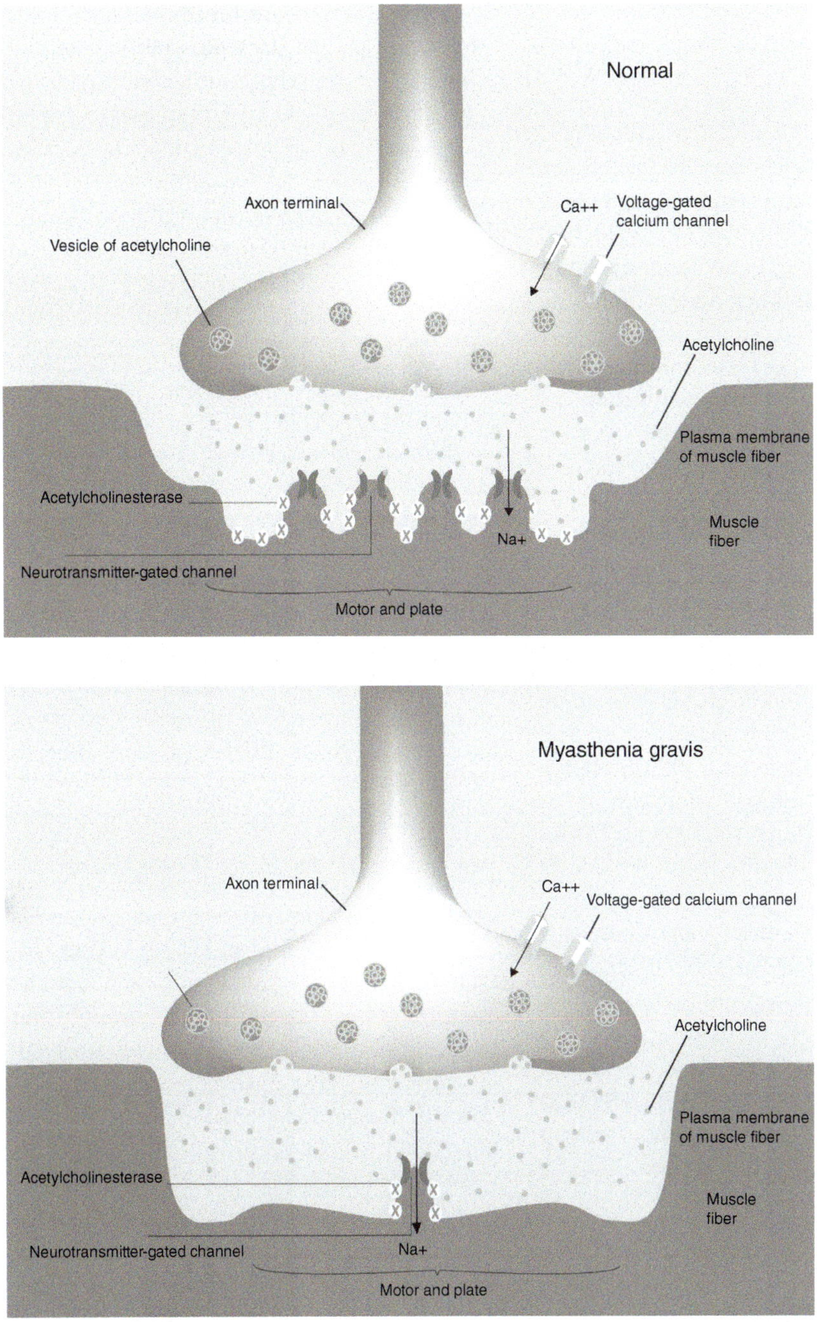

Figure 15.13 Neuromuscular junction of a normal or myasthenic individual. Myasthenia gravis results in simplified synaptic folds, widened synaptic spaces, and less acetylcholine receptors [100]. *Source:* Adapted from reference 100; courtesy of Jaqueline Steagall.

Diagnosis

The ultimate diagnosis is confirmed by the detection of serum antibodies against muscle AChR. The test is objective and quantitative and is the most reliable diagnostic technique for the diagnosis of acquired MG. Titers ≥0.3 and 0.6 nmol l^{-1} are positive for MG in cats and dogs, respectively [105]. In addition, a positive response to the administration of edrophonium has been used as a diagnostic tool. The administration of an anticholinesterase drug such as this will effectively increase the concentration of ACh in the synaptic cleft, optimizing the opportunities for successful interaction between ACh and its receptors. Most animals with MG will exhibit improving signs immediately after edrophonium administration, and these effects will last for approximately 5 min. However, the test is neither sensitive nor specific [104]. Finally, it may not be helpful in cases of focal MG in cats where the response may be unpredictable or in dogs with acute fulminating MG. In the latter, marked antibody-mediated destruction of AChR has occurred. Intercostal muscle biopsy may also be used to identify AChR antibodies at the neuromuscular junction. Electromyography may also confirm megaesophagus, especially important in MG patients that have a significant risk of aspiration pneumonia during general anesthesia. It is important to differentiate MG from other muscle disorders that cause weakness such as hyperthyroidism or hypothyroidism, and botulism, among others [103].

Treatment

Anticholinesterase drugs (e.g., neostigmine and pyridostigmine) are the first line of treatment for MG. These drugs inhibit the enzyme acetylcholinesterase (true cholinesterase), which is typically responsible for the hydrolysis of ACh into choline and acetic acid and thus increases the amount of neurotransmitter available at the preganglionic sympathetic and parasympathetic nerve endings and neuromuscular junction [101]. Pyridostigmine bromide (0.2–2 mg kg^{-1} PO every 8–12 h, or 0.01–0.03 mg kg^{-1} h^{-1} IV) has been used in dogs, and its syrup (5 mg kg^{-1} PO every 12 h, diluted 1:1 with water to decrease gastric irritation) has been given to cats. The doses should be tailored to the individual needs and according to clinical response. Systemic administration of neostigmine can be given (0.01–0.04 mg kg^{-1} IM every 6–8 h) to individuals with significant dysphagia and regurgitation in the emergency setting [105]. However, cholinergic crisis may result from an excess of ACh at the nicotinic and muscarinic receptors due to excessive administration of an anticholinesterase drug. Corticosteroids are commonly administered if muscle weakness is not controlled by the administration of anticholinesterase drugs due to their immunosuppressant effects. Therapy is initiated with a low dose (prednisone, 0.5 mg kg^{-1} day^{-1}), but it can be increased to immunosuppressant dosages (2–4 mg kg^{-1} day^{-1}).

Anesthetic and Analgesic Management

Myasthenic dogs and cats may undergo general anesthesia for different surgical interventions. The placement of a gastrostomy tube might be required to provide nutritional support until regurgitation and dysphagia have resolved. A tracheal or bronchoalveolar lavage is performed if aspiration pneumonia is present. Finally, a median sternotomy is indicated in cases of thymoma.

Perioperative considerations should include a thorough physical examination and thoracic radiographs for the assessment of megaesophagus and potential aspiration pneumonia (Figure 15.14). Other immune-mediated conditions should be identified and treated accordingly because there is usually more than one disorder involved in patients with MG. Fine-needle aspiration cytology is performed for a definite diagnosis of thymoma if a cranial mass in the mediastinum is identified. Thymectomy

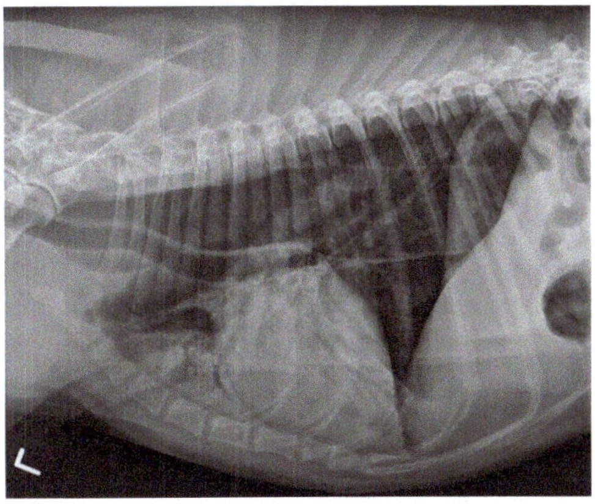

Figure 15.14 Left lateral thoracic image of a dog with generalized megaesophagus and aspiration pneumonia, which are commonly observed in myasthenia gravis. There is generalized gas dilatation of the esophagus and a ventrally located alveolar pattern of the right cranial and middle lung lobes. Note the prominent air bronchograms that are best seen superimposed with the cardiac silhouette. *Source:* Photo courtesy of Radiology Service, Department of Surgical Sciences, School of Veterinary Medicine, University of Wisconsin-Madison.

must be considered in these cases because many animals will have a dramatic resolution of their signs after surgery including a decrease in ACh antibody titer. Anesthetic management of patients with megaesophagus is mandatory, including appropriate therapy and concerns to prevent regurgitation and aspiration pneumonia.

Respiratory depression may be accentuated after opioid administration and other IV anesthetics; therefore, preoxygenation may be considered, and short-acting drugs may be chosen. Opioids (methadone [0.2–0.5 mg kg^{-1}], butorphanol [0.2–0.4 mg kg^{-1}, if pain is not involved], buprenorphine [0.01–0.02 μg kg^{-1}], or fentanyl [2–10 μg kg^{-1}] IV or IM) with or without midazolam (0.1–0.2 mg kg^{-1} IV or IM) is recommended. Morphine, hydromorphone, and dexmedetomidine should be used with caution due to the risk of vomiting and further aspiration. Propofol (1–4 mg kg^{-1} IV) or alfaxalone (1–3 mg kg^{-1} IV) in combination with diazepam or midazolam (0.1–0.2 mg kg^{-1} IV) can be an option for the induction of anesthesia. Balanced anesthesia using drugs such as fentanyl, lidocaine, and/or ketamine provides good cardiovascular stability by reducing inhalant agent requirements during anesthesia. In addition, the combination of these drugs with different pharmacologic mechanisms may provide a better analgesic protocol and even greater inhalant-sparing effect in animals undergoing surgery.

Hypotension due to compression of large intrathoracic vessels by the surgeons and the thymoma per se is expected and can be treated with the administration of crystalloids, colloids, and/or sympathomimetics such as dopamine (5–15 μg kg^{-1} min^{-1}). Aggressive pain management is required for dogs and cats undergoing median sternotomy with analgesic infusion, NSAID administration if no contraindications exist, and regional anesthetic blocks (e.g., intercostal and intrapleural blocks). The epidural administration of morphine (0.1 mg kg^{-1}) for treatment of postoperative is an adjuvant analgesic in patients undergoing thoracotomy. Other support therapy includes the prevention of hypothermia and provision of PEEP during chest opening. A detailed anesthetic management of patients with MG is described in a literature review [107].

An important aspect of anesthetic management of patients with MG is the increased sensitivity to nondepolarizing neuromuscular blockade agents. This sensitivity is dependent on the balance between active and nonfunctional AChR, but these agents can produce profound skeletal muscle weakness [99]. Therefore, an initial dose should be titrated to effect, whereas close monitoring of neuromuscular blockade is accomplished using a peripheral nerve stimulator. In humans with MG, the potency of atracurium and vecuronium is increased twofold compared to the response in normal patients. Both drugs were administered to two myasthenic dogs undergoing thymoma removal. The doses were reduced by approximately 66% (atracurium) and 20% (vecuronium) of the calculated dose for normal dogs. Neuromuscular blockade was reversed with the administration of neostigmine and an anticholinergic [108, 109]. Pyridostigmine inhibits the metabolism of mivacurium, and it may prolong its effect; therefore, the administration of mivacurium should be avoided in patients with MG. Animals should be monitored closely during the recovery period to ensure appropriate ventilation.

Myopathies

General clinical signs associated with myopathies include weakness with normal proprioception, normal to decreased myotatic reflexes, voice change, stiff gait, and ventral neck flexion (most commonly in the cat). Myopathies can be of inflammatory, infectious, metabolic, or inherited origin. Decreased energy supplies can lead to abnormal muscle oxidative metabolism and resultant weakness. Endocrine disturbances such as hypothyroidism or hyperthyroidism, or hypoadrenocorticism or hyperadrenocorticism, have been implicated in pathogenesis of some metabolic myopathies. Along the same lines, hypokalemia (hypokalemic myopathies) and hypocalcemia can result in severe muscle weakness and tetany, as both ions are important in the regulation of muscle ion channel and excitation–contraction coupling within the skeletal muscle. Masticatory muscle myositis (MMM) is an important type of inflammatory myositis and may present with trismus (see Chapter 13, Oral and Maxillofacial Disorders). Other inflammatory myopathies such as canine and feline idiopathic polymyopathies, dermatomyositis, protozoal myositis, and other inherited myopathies (hereditary Labrador Retriever myopathy and myotonia) are important to the well-being of the individual, but are uncommon in veterinary anesthesia and analgesia and will not be discussed in depth in this chapter.

Muscle biopsy may be a relevant diagnostic tool when electrodiagnostic testing cannot rule out a disease or be performed. Biopsy may reveal fiber-type grouping, group atrophy, degeneration, inflammation, or infiltration with fat and connective tissue. Myopathies generally affect fibers in a more random pattern, with muscle necrosis, regeneration, and inflammation. Infiltration with local anesthetics is considered part of the anesthetic plan, which is ultimately determined by the individual's health status. Depending on the behavior and physical status of the patient, small biopsies can be performed under heavy sedation with a combination of dexmedetomidine (5–10 μg kg^{-1} in dogs and 5–20 μg kg^{-1} in cats IM) and opioid analgesics (butorphanol 0.2–0.4 mg kg^{-1} or buprenorphine 0.02 mg kg^{-1} IM). Incisional anesthesia (i.e., infiltration of skin and subcutaneous) with local anesthetics may be considered (up to 2 mg kg^{-1} of 0.5% bupivacaine or 5 mg kg^{-1} of 2% lidocaine). Patients require vigilant monitoring using a "hands-on" approach with pulse oximetry when heavy sedation is used; atipamezole (100–200 μg kg^{-1} IM) can be given to reverse dexmedetomidine at the end of the procedure to shorten anesthetic recovery. More invasive biopsies that require surgical intervention are performed under general anesthesia with proper monitoring, fluid therapy, etc. The anesthetic protocol will be decided based on the age, breed, physical status of the patient, laboratory testing, imaging, etc.

Noninfectious Inflammatory Joint Diseases

Osteoarthritis (OA) is the most important joint disease in veterinary medicine. The other causes of noninfectious inflammatory joint diseases are relatively common in dogs, but rare in cats. These disorders are described as polyarthritis syndromes mediated by immune complex formation and deposition. The syndromes include systemic lupus erythematosus (SLE), rheumatoid arthritis (RA), and idiopathic and reactive polyarthritis. On radiographic evidence of joint destruction, these syndromes are classified as either erosive (RA and feline chronic progressive polyarthritis) or nonerosive.

Nonerosive, noninfectious polyarthritis in which a primary cause (SLE, reactive, or RA) cannot be identified is referred to as idiopathic, immune-mediated. Canine immune-mediated polyarthritis is a diagnosis of exclusion based predominantly on clinical signs, laboratorial examination including synovial fluid analysis, and failure to identify an infectious cause after culture of synovial fluid.

Osteoarthritis

OA is a complex disorder of movable joints characterized by deterioration of articular cartilage, osteophyte formation and bone remodeling, pathology of periarticular tissues including synovium, subchondral bone, muscle, tendon, and ligament, and/or an intermittent inflammatory process of variable degree. The pathogenesis is related to joint trauma from biomechanical stress, joint injury, or abnormal loading due to neuropathy, ligamentous injury including cranial cruciate ligament deficiency, or muscle atrophy. Osteoarthritic pain is described as a complex interplay between structural change, biochemical alterations, peripheral and central pain-processing mechanisms, and individual cognitive processing of nociception [110]. The pathophysiological changes of OA and mechanisms of OA-induced pain have been reviewed elsewhere [111–115]. These articles take into consideration the complexity and multifactorial pathogenesis of OA and the potential for central sensitization and neuropathic pain. Disability and changes in quality of life are commonly observed both in humans and animals.

Osteoarthritis is the most important cause of chronic pain in dogs, and the anesthetist may be consulted for questions regarding pain management of these animals. It tends to affect older, obese, and heavy-breed dogs; however, it can be observed in young dogs as well. Radiographic signs of degenerative joint disease range from 21% to 90% of the feline population. The condition is underdiagnosed, and the clinical relevance of OA is not known in this species [116]. Therefore, a large part of the canine and feline population undergoing general anesthesia could be affected by OA. Clinical signs include change of attitude, lameness, stiff posture/gait, partial weight-bearing, reluctance to move, vocalization on palpation with attempts to escape, and reduced activity. Cats are notorious for hiding signs of pain, but a decrease in grooming and signs of immobility and inability to jump into counters or even into their litter box have been associated with degenerative joint disease [117]. A review article has summarized the recent advances in clinical feline chronic pain assessment including OA [34].

From the anesthetist's perspective, OA per se has limited impact on anesthetic management, and the anesthetic plan should be chosen on a case-by-case basis where the physical status of the individual and the presence of other concomitant diseases/drug therapies are considered. Some patients with OA develop obesity, which can increase the percentage of fat tissue over the lean mass, increasing the volume of distribution for lipophilic drugs into tissues that are not metabolically active (see Chapter 10, Nutritional Disease). In these cases, doses should be reduced and/or calculated according to an estimation of lean body weight. Additionally, obesity can be related to other endocrine and cardiovascular diseases [118]. Inflammatory and possibly neuropathic pains are of concern because cartilage damage results in elevation and stretching of the richly innervated periosteum, which produces a direct stimulation of the joint capsule and bone receptors by cytokines, ligands of inflammatory origin, and physical stimulation of subchondral bone, muscle, tendons, and ligaments. Thus, osteoarthritic patients may show signs of central sensitization because of a prolonged and constant noxious stimulus input to the spinal cord produced by the degenerative process. Thereafter, some of these animals can feel extreme pain during the perioperative period, and careful manipulation of joints and positioning is recommended in combination with appropriate padding of all joints, with particular attention given to diseased joints.

Chronic pain management involves weight management and analgesic drug administration such as NSAIDs, tramadol, gabapentin, amantadine, and nutraceuticals, among others. For this reason, a high prevalence of adverse effects may be observed in the canine and feline population with OA after the administration of human analgesic products for pain management such as ibuprofen and aspirin. In addition, potential drug interactions may be appreciated. Strong evidence exists for the analgesic efficacy of carprofen, firocoxib, and meloxicam in the treatment of OA, but not for doxycycline, electrostimulated acupuncture, extracorporeal shockwave therapy, gold wire acupuncture, hyaluronan, pentosan polysulfate, P54FP (extract of turmeric), tiaprofenic acid, or tibial plateau leveling osteotomy in dogs [119]. However, the absence of evidence does not exclude the potential benefits of these therapies in the treatment of OA syndrome. New nondrug therapy modalities including physiotherapy and rehabilitation, therapeutic laser and heat, and (electro)acupuncture have been largely used in combination with analgesic administration for the treatment of OA in dogs and cats. Joint replacement surgery may be recommended when pain due to OA is persistent and disabling with significant limitation of joint function. Treatment options for maladaptive conditions in dogs and cats, including novel therapies for OA such as anti-NGFs, have been extensively reviewed elsewhere [120–122].

Systemic Lupus Erythematosus

SLE is a chronic, multisystemic, immune-mediated disease of unknown etiology; however, genetic factors are implicated in disease pathogenesis. In SLE, there is circulation of immune complexes that were formed by antinuclear antibody (ANA) production. These complexes will induce inflammation and vasculopathies that cause organ system dysfunction (e.g., glomerulonephritis) and the resultant clinical signs [123]. Breeds affected include Spitzes, Shetland Sheepdogs, Collies, German Shepherds, and Beagles, whereas reports of SLE are rare in the cat [124].

Systemic clinical signs will vary according to the organ involved and include intermittent fevers of unknown origin, polyarthritis, lymphadenopathy, erythematous skin lesions, hemolytic anemia with icteric mucous membranes, immune-mediated thrombocytopenia with petechiae and ecchymoses, myositis, and polyneuritis. Protein-losing nephropathy and hypoalbuminemia may result from glomerulonephritis, which can lead to ascites and peripheral edema. SLE-induced polyarthritis is the most common manifestation (70–90%) that may be confirmed by arthrocentesis. Reported clinical signs may include reluctance to walk, stiffness, lameness, joint swelling, and pain on palpation.

A complete blood count (CBC), platelet count, biochemistry profile, urinalysis, and urine protein/creatinine ratio should be performed to differentiate SLE from other causes of polyarthritis [123]. Radiographic examination of the joints is important to rule out erosive polyarthritis (RA). Synovial fluid analysis after arthrocentesis may reveal increases in white blood cell count, with neutrophils representing most of the inflammatory cells. Lupus erythematosus (LE) cells are rarely found after joint taps. Bone marrow aspiration shows nonregenerative anemia, neutropenia, and/or thrombocytopenia, and is used to rule out multiple myeloma [125]. The presumptive diagnosis includes the LE cell test and the ANA test. The diagnosis is suggestive for SLE when both tests are positive, and the animal has two or more of the clinical signs [126].

Therapy is based on symptomatic treatment with steroids, analgesics, and immunosuppressive drugs to achieve disease remission. Prednisone usually results in disease remission. Immunosuppressive doses (3–4 $mg\,kg^{-1}\,day^{-1}$)

may be initially used for the first 2 weeks and then decreased (1–2 mg kg^{-1} day^{-1}) for another 2 weeks. According to the clinical response, the dose can be reduced even more (1–2 mg kg^{-1} every 48 h) and tapered as needed. Synovial fluid must be reexamined routinely during therapy. Azathioprine is administered to dogs that are nonresponsive to steroid treatment but can cause myelosuppression; dogs are at an increased risk for developing pancreatitis when on it. Chondroprotective agents may also prove to be beneficial in some situations.

Anesthetic management will be based on the magnitude of organ system dysfunction and the toxicity profile of the chosen therapeutic agents (e.g., prolonged glucocorticoid therapy). Abrupt cessation of glucocorticoid therapy may result in an Addisonian crisis and an additional dose of steroids is given for such cases, especially during prolonged surgical interventions. However, long-term corticosteroid administration may cause polyuria, polydipsia, hyperglycemia, and hypercholesterolemia. Chest and abdominal radiographs may be useful to detect pleural and/or pericardial effusion and ascites, respectively, due to hypoalbuminemia. Table 15.4 shows the recommended guidelines for the perioperative management of SLE [126]. Even so, the impact of SLE on specific anesthetic techniques has not been investigated, and the lack of evidence combined with the heterogeneity of disease manifestations makes it difficult to establish definitive anesthetic management protocols [127]. Ultimately, the anesthetic plan will be chosen on a case-by-case basis where the physical status of the individual and the presence of other concomitant diseases are considered. For instance, colloid administration may be indicated for maintenance of oncotic pressure in cases of hypoalbuminemia, especially for long procedures. Preoxygenation is recommended for cases of severe hemolytic anemia. Some of these animals can feel extreme pain during the perioperative period, and careful manipulation of joints is recommended. Pain management is a crucial part of the treatment and should be considered as a long-term intervention. Opioids are usually administered as part of premedication, but NSAIDs are normally contraindicated due to chronic administration of corticosteroids. The use of sympathomimetics is recommended for cases where maintenance of cardiac output and blood pressure is a concern, especially when adequate renal perfusion is required.

Table 15.4 Key points in the perioperative management of animals with SLE [127].

- The history and physical examination should include a thorough review of disease activity and accrued organ damage.
- A CBC should be evaluated for anemia, thrombocytopenia, and leukopenia.
- Other complementary blood work should be performed to investigate serum electrolytes, creatinine, urea, and hepatic enzymes, among others. Glomerulonephritis or drug-induced hepatotoxicity should be monitored.
- Urinalysis may be important for monitoring elevated proteinuria, or the presence of red or white blood cells in the urine.
- Thoracic radiographs are crucial to evaluate pleural and pericardial effusions.
- Abdominal radiographs are recommended if ascites is suspected.
- During general anesthesia, the clinician should focus on renal protective strategies with maintenance of urine output while avoiding hypoperfusion and hypotensive states.
- Careful patient positioning is important, since these animals are predisposed to pain.
- Adverse effects of systemic analgesics and drug interactions must be considered in pain management.

Rheumatoid Arthritis

This condition is characterized by erosive polyarthritis and progressive joint degeneration of unknown origin. Canine RA resembles human RA where rheumatoid factors form immune complexes that are deposited in the synovium. By contrast, the pathogenesis of RA is different from feline chronic progressive polyarthritis where an erosive process of the joint is observed because of an infectious cause. In RA, granulation tissue results in cartilage erosion and joint swelling and may lead to ligament rupture. Clinical signs are similar to other joint inflammatory diseases; however, radiographic features in the late stages of RA reveal periarticular osteoporosis, loss of articular cartilage, and focal irregular areas of subchondral bone destruction. Luxation is a consequence of the erosive process; destruction of the joint by an erosive process differentiates RA from other nonseptic inflammatory joint diseases. RA is a much more destructive, progressive, and debilitating condition than osteoarthritis. The diagnosis is confirmed by detecting rheumatoid factor against denatured or immune-complexed IgG. A titer of 1:16 or higher is considered to be positive; nevertheless, false positives may be seen. Treatment relies on the use of immunosuppressive, analgesic, and chondroprotective drugs similar to SLE, but the long-term erosive process is not inhibited, and response to treatment is variable. Pain and limb function may be improved after arthroplasty, joint replacement, or arthrodesis. Pain management is a crucial part of the anesthetic protocol. Multimodal analgesia and balanced anesthetic techniques should be used for chronic pain management (i.e., gabapentin 10–20 mg kg^{-1} every 8–12 h PO and/or amantadine 3–5 mg kg^{-1} every 12–24 h PO). NSAIDs are contraindicated if corticosteroid therapy is administered. General anesthesia might be required for RA diagnosis or if other surgical/medical conditions require attention. Anesthetic protocols will vary according to the physical status of the patient.

Reactive Polyarthritis

This type of immune-mediated polyarthritis has been observed in association with chronic systemic infectious diseases, neoplasia, drug administration, or disease of the gastrointestinal tract. Therefore, arthritis is a secondary clinical manifestation of immune complexes seen in association with bacterial endocarditis, pleuritis, dirofilariasis, or drug-induced polyarthritis with the use of sulfadiazine/trimethoprim and cephalexin, among others. Thus, the complete history with a full physical examination is essential for the differential diagnosis if one considers that clinical signs (cyclic fever, stiffness, and reluctance to walk) may be similar to other syndromes. Treatment should focus on eliminating the underlying cause, which can play an important role in the anesthetic management of the case (e.g., endocarditis or dirofilariasis that may cause cardiovascular depression). The anesthetic protocol will be based on a thorough physical examination and preoperative screening of patients with systemic conditions. The use of short-acting drugs with minimal cardiorespiratory depression is advised for premedication; opioids (morphine 0.2–0.3 mg kg^{-1} or hydromorphone 0.05 mg kg^{-1} IM) with or without midazolam (0.1–0.2 mg kg^{-1} IV or IM) are recommended. Opioids produce mild sedation and bradycardia in dogs; bradycardia is typically well tolerated when clinical doses are employed but may be treated with anticholinergics (glycopyrrolate 0.01 mg kg^{-1} IV) as needed. Morphine may induce histamine release followed by short-lived hypotension after rapid IV administration. Slow and cautious administration of propofol (1–5 mg kg^{-1} IV) or alfaxalone (1–4 mg kg^{-1}) in combination with benzodiazepines (0.25–0.5 mg kg^{-1} IV) may be used for induction of anesthesia. Etomidate (1–2 mg kg^{-1} IV) with or without diazepam or midazolam (0.2 mg kg^{-1} IV) may be used for the induction of anesthesia if cardiovascular disease is observed. Pain management should be addressed accordingly.

Skin (Intradermal) Testing

Drugs including anesthetics and analgesics may affect the cutaneous allergic reaction to intradermal testing [128]. The intradermal test is used as an indirect measure of cutaneous mast cell reactivity to a selection of allergens in the presence of IgE. The American College of Veterinary Dermatology task force on canine atopic dermatitis has published information on the subject [129]. Detailed guidelines for the diagnosis and allergen identification have also been published [130] by a subgroup of the International Committee on Allergic Diseases of Animals. The procedure is usually performed under heavy sedation to increase patient compliance and to improve the quality of intradermal testing. Oxygenation and "hands-on" monitoring that may also include pulse oximetry are required during chemical restraint. Intradermal injections are painful and there is a need to adjust sedation levels accordingly during the procedure. In summary, veterinarians should be aware that antihistamines, glucocorticoids, opioid analgesics, progestational compounds, beta-adrenergic receptor agonists, phenothiazines, and tricyclic antidepressants can produce changes in skin test reactivity in different ways. However, veterinary-specific studies are lacking, and most information is extrapolated from the human literature. More specifically, veterinarians should be aware that:

- Oral hydroxyzine suppresses skin reactivity to histamine and flea antigens. Overall, antihistamines should not be administered in dogs and cats undergoing intradermal testing.
- Acepromazine has antihistaminic properties and should be avoided.
- The administration of glucocorticosteroids including topical agents may change skin reactivity depending on the dosage regimens, duration of treatment, and type of corticosteroid.
- The use of propofol for intradermal testing is controversial, as it may or may not change histamine reactions [131, 132]. It is unknown if the administration of alfaxalone has an impact on intradermal results.
- Withdrawal times for anti-inflammatory drugs before intradermal testing should be followed: antihistamines (7 days), short-acting oral glucocorticoids (14 days), long-acting injectable glucocorticoids (at least 28 days), topical glucocorticoids (14 days), cyclosporin (probably not needed), and pentoxifylline (none) [133]. The withdrawal period for other antihistamines with long half-lives can be longer.
- In general, the use of alpha-2-adrenergic receptor agonists, barbiturates, and inhalant anesthetics does not interfere with skin reactivity to intradermal testing [134].
- Dexmedetomidine alone or in combination with butorphanol administered through an IV catheter is often used to effect for profound sedation.
- Butorphanol minimally impacts intradermal testing results. However, some still avoid its use [135].
- Other opioids such as morphine and meperidine should be avoided due to the potential of histamine release, especially after IV injection. The administration of oxymorphone has also been contraindicated for intradermal testing [134, 136].
- Ketamine-based protocols may produce anti-inflammatory effects and should not be administered.

Summary

- An understanding of the pathophysiology, diagnosis, and treatment of skin and musculoskeletal disease is important for the anesthetic management of patients with these conditions.
- Some of these diseases are relatively uncommon, but they may be presented as an anesthetic challenge, a secondary complication, and/or a life-threatening scenario to the clinician.
- Emergency treatment is required with burns and MH and, potentially, with MG.
- Analgesia is normally needed as part of the anesthetic protocol if one considers that pre-existing acute or chronic pain, hyperalgesia, and/or central sensitization are commonly observed with these diseases.

- The anesthetic plan should be chosen on a case-by-case basis where the physical status of the individual and the presence of other concomitant diseases/drug therapies are considered.
- A thorough physical examination and appreciation of the pharmacology of sedatives/analgesics and anesthetics will facilitate the selection of drugs for premedication, induction, and maintenance of anesthesia.

References

1 Quist, E.M., Tanabe, M., Mansell, J.E.K.L. et al. (2012). A case series of thermal scald injuries in dogs exposed to hot water from garden hoses (garden hose scalding syndrome). *Vet. Dermatol.* 23: 162–166.

2 Steagall, P.V.M. and Monteiro-Steagall, B.P. (2013). Multimodal analgesia for perioperative pain in three cats. *J. Feline Med. Surg.* 15: 737–743.

3 Kawalilak, L.T., Fransson, B.A., and Alessio, T.L. (2017). Management of a facial partial thickness chemical burn in a dog caused by bleach. *J. Vet. Emerg. Crit. Care (San Antonio)* 27: 224–231.

4 Pavletic, M.M. and Trout, N.J. (2006). Bullet, bite, and burn wounds in dogs and cats. *Vet. Clin. North Am. Small Anim. Pract.* 36: 873–893.

5 Pope, E. (2003). Thermal, electrical, and chemical burns and cold injuries. In: *Textbook of Small Animal Surgery*, 3e (ed. D. Staller), 356–372. Philadelphia: Saunders Elsevier.

6 Sumner, J.P., Pucheu-Haston, C.M., Fowlkes, N. et al. (2016). Dorsal skin necrosis secondary to a solar-induced thermal burn in a brown-coated dachshund. *Can. Vet. J.* 57: 305–308.

7 Schwartz, S.L., Schick, A.E., Lewis, T.P. et al. (2018). Dorsal thermal necrosis in dogs: a retrospective analysis of 16 cases in the southwestern USA (2009–2016). *Vet. Dermatol.* 29: 139–e55.

8 Garzotto, C.K. (2009). Thermal burn injury. In: *Small Animal Critical Care Medicine* (eds. D.C. Silverstein and K. Hopper), 683–686. St. Louis: Saunders Elsevier.

9 Frantz, K. and Byers, C.G. (2011). Thermal injury. *Compend. Contin. Educ. Vet.* 33: E1.

10 Rong, Y., Liu, W., Wang, C. et al. (2011). Temperature distribution in the upper airway after inhalation injury. *Burns* 37: 1187–1191.

11 Neff, T.A., Doelberg, M., Jungheinrich, C. et al. (2003). Repetitive large-dose infusion of the novel hydroxyethyl starch 130/0.4 in patients with severe head injury. *Anesth. Analg.* 96: 1453–1459.

12 Capan, L.M. and Miller, S.M. (2009). Anesthesia for trauma and burn patients. In: *Clinical Anesthesia*, 6e (eds. P.G. Barash, B.F. Cullen, R.K. Stoelting, et al.), 889–926. Philadelphia: Lippincott Williams & Wilkins.

13 Taverner, T. and Prince, J. (2016). Acute neuropathic pain assessment in burn injured patients: a retrospective review. *J. Wound Ostomy Continence Nurs.* 43: 51–55.

14 Patterson, D.R., Tininenko, J., and Ptacek, J.T. (2006). Pain during burn hospitalization predicts long-term outcome. *J. Burn Care Res.* 27: 719–726.

15 Bouhassira, D., Lantéri-Minet, M., Attal, N. et al. (2008). Prevalence of chronic pain with neuropathic characteristics in the general population. *Pain* 136: 380–387.

16 Schneider, J.C., Harris, N.L., El Shami, A. et al. (2006). A descriptive review of neuropathic-like pain after burn injury. *J. Burn Care Res.* 27: 524–528.

17 Ruel, H.L.M. and Steagall, P.V. (2019). Adjuvant analgesics in acute pain management. *Vet. Clin. North Am. Small Anim. Pract.* 49: 1127–1141.

18 Weil, A.B., Ko, J., and Inoue, T. (2007). The use of lidocaine patches. *Compend. Contin. Educ. Vet.* 29: 208–210, 212, 214-6.

19 Mikawa, K., Akamatsu, H., Nishina, K. et al. (1997). Inhibitory effect of local anaesthetics on reactive oxygen species production by human neutrophils. *Acta Anaesthesiol. Scand.* 41: 524–528.

20 Nellgård, P., Jönsson, A., Bojö, L. et al. (1996). Small-bowel obstruction and the effects of lidocaine, atropine and hexamethonium on inflammation and fluid losses. *Acta Anaesthesiol. Scand.* 40: 287–292.

21 Steagall, P.V., Benito, J., and Monteiro, B.P. (2018). Analgesic effects of gabapentin and buprenorphine in cats undergoing ovariohysterectomy using two pain-scoring systems: a randomized clinical trial. *J. Feline Med. Surg.* 20: 741–748.

22 Crociolli, G.C., Cassu, R.N., Barbero, R.C. et al. Gabapentin as an adjuvant for postoperative pain management in dogs undergoing mastectomy. *J. Vet. Med. Sci.* 77: 1011–1015.

23 TerRiet, M.F., DeSouza, G.J.A., Jacobs, J.S. et al. (2000). Which is most pungent: isoflurane, sevoflurane or desflurane? *Br. J. Anaesth.* 85: 305–307.

24 Dehuisser, V., Bosmans, T., Kitshoff, A. et al. (2017). Cardiovascular effects, induction and recovery characteristics and alfaxalone dose assessment in alfaxalone versus alfaxalone-fentanyl total intravenous anaesthesia in dogs. *Vet. Anaesth. Analg.* 44: 1276–1286.

25 Cha, S.I., Kim, C.H., Lee, J.H. et al. (2007). Isolated smoke inhalation injuries: acute respiratory dysfunction, clinical outcomes, and short-term evolution of pulmonary functions with the effects of steroids. *Burns* 33: 200–208.

26 Toon, M.H., Maybauer, M.O., Greenwood, J.E. et al. (2010). Management of acute smoke inhalation injury. *Crit. Care Resusc.* 12: 53–61.

27 Tobias, K.M. (2010). Onychetomy. In: *Manual of Small Animal Soft Tissue Surgery*, 1e (ed. K.M. Tobias), 443–454. Ames: Wiley-Blackwell.

28 Ruch-Gallie, R., Hellyer, P.W., Schoenfeld-Tacher, R. et al. (2016). Survey of practices and perceptions regarding feline onychectomy among private practitioners. *J. Am. Vet. Med. Assoc.* 249: 291–298.

29 Kogan, L.R., Little, S.E., Hellyer, P.W. et al. (2016). Feline onychectomy: current practices and perceptions of veterinarians in Ontario, Canada. *Can. Vet. J.* 57: 969–975.

30 Steagall, P.V., Monteiro, B.P., Ruel, H.L.M. et al. (2017). Perceptions and opinions of Canadian pet owners about anaesthesia, pain and surgery in small animals. *J. Small Anim. Pract.* 58: 380–388.

31 Simon, B.T., Scallan, E.M., Von Pfeil, D.J.F. et al. (2018). Perceptions and opinions of pet owners in the United States about surgery, pain management, and anesthesia in dogs and cats. *Vet. Surg.* 47: 277–284.

32 Clark, K., Bailey, T., Rist, P. et al. (2014). Comparison of 3 methods of onychectomy. *Can. Vet. J. La. Rev. Vet. Can.* 55: 255–262.

33 Martell-Moran, N., Solano, M., and Townsend, H. (2018). Pain and adverse behavior in declawed cats. *J. Feline Med. Surg.* 20: 280–288.

34 Monteiro, B.P. and Steagall, P.V. (2019). Chronic pain in cats: recent advances in clinical assessment. *J. Feline Med. Surg.* 21: 601–614.

35 Tobias, K. (1994). Feline onychechtomy at a teaching institution: a retrospective study of 163 cases. *Vet. Surg.* 23: 274–280.

36 Patronek, G.J. (2001). Assessment of claims of short- and long-term complications associated with onychectomy in cats. *J. Am. Vet. Med. Assoc.* 219: 932–936.

37 Robertson, S. and Lascelles, D. (2010). Long-term pain in cats. How much do we know about this important welfare issue. *J. Feline Med. Surg.* 12: 188–199.

38 Gerard, A.F., Larson, M., Baldwin, C.J. et al. (2016). Telephone survey to investigate relationships between onychectomy or onychectomy technique and house soiling in cats. *J. Am. Vet. Med. Assoc.* 249: 638–643.

39 Wilson, D.V. and Pascoe, P.J. (2016). Pain and analgesia following onychectomy in cats: a systematic review. *Vet. Anaesth. Analg.* 43: 5–17.

40 Breitreiter, K. (2019). Late-onset osteosarcoma after onychectomy in a cat. *J. Feline Med. Surg. Open Rep.* 5: 1–6.

41 Kidney, B.A. (2008). Role of inflammation/wound healing in feline oncogenesis: a commentary. *J. Feline Med. Surg.* 10: 107–109.

42 Romans, C.W., Gordon, W.J., Robinson, D.A. et al. (2005). Effect of postoperative analgesic protocol on limb function following onychectomy in cats. *J. Am. Vet. Med. Assoc.* 227: 89–93.

43 Liehmann, L., Mosing, M., and Auer, U. (2006). A comparison of cardiorespiratory variables during isoflurane–fentanyl and propofol-fentanyl anaesthesia for surgery in injured cats. *Vet. Anaesth. Analg.* 33: 158–168.

44 Carroll, G.L., Howe, L.B., and Peterson, K.D. (2005). Analgesic efficacy of preoperative administration of meloxicam or butorphanol in onychectomized cats. *J. Am. Vet. Med. Assoc.* 226: 913–919.

45 Ingwersen, W., Fox, R., Cunningham, G. et al. (2012). Efficacy and safety of 3 versus 5 days of meloxicam as an analgesic for feline onychectomy and sterilization. *Can. Vet. J.* 53: 257–264.

46 Skarda, R.T. and Tranquilli, W.J. (2007). Local and regional anesthetic and analgesic techniques: cats. In: *Lumb & Jones Veterinary Anesthesia and Analgesia*, 4e (eds. W.J. Tranquilli, J.C. Thurmon and K.A. Grimm), 595–604. Ames: Blackwell.

47 Enomoto, M., Lascelles, B.D.X., and Gerard, M.P. (2016). Defining the local nerve blocks for feline distal thoracic limb surgery: a cadaveric study. *J. Feline Med. Surg.* 18: 838–845.

48 Elanco. Nocita. https://www.elanco.us/products-services/dogs/nocita (accessed 24 June 2021).

49 Gaynor, J.S. (2005). Chronic pain syndrome of feline onychectomy. *Clin. Br.* 3: 11–13.

50 Catbagan, D.L., Quimby, J.M., Mama, K.R. et al. (2011). Comparison of the efficacy and adverse effects of sustained-release buprenorphine hydrochloride following subcutaneous administration and buprenorphine hydrochloride following oral transmucosal administration in cats undergoing ovariohysterectomy. *Am. J. Vet. Res.* 72: 461–466.

51 Gruen, M.E., Thomson, A.E., Griffith, E.H. et al. (2016). A feline-specific anti-nerve growth factor antibody improves mobility in cats with degenerative joint disease-associated pain: a pilot proof of concept study. *J. Vet. Intern. Med.* 30: 1138–1148.

52 Enomoto, M., Mantyh, P.W., Murrell, J. et al. (2019). Antinerve growth factor monoclonal antibodies for the control of pain in dogs and cats. *Vet. Rec.* 184: 23.

53 Radlinsky, M.G. and Mason, D.E. (2004). Diseases of the ear. In: *Textbook of Veterinary Internal Medicine*, 6e (eds. S.J. Ettinger and E.C. Feldman), 1168–1186. St. Louis: Saunders Elsevier.

54 Gotthelf, L.N. (2004). Diagnosis and treatment of otitis media in dogs and cats. *Vet. Clin. North Am. Small Anim. Pract.* 34: 469–487.

55 Bischoff, M.G. and Kneller, S.K. (2004). Diagnostic imaging of the canine and feline ear. *Vet. Clin. North Am. Small Anim. Pract.* 34: 437–458.

56 Smeak, D.D. and Kerpsack, S.J. (1993). Total ear canal ablation and lateral bulla osteotomy for management of end-stage otitis. *Semin. Vet. Med. Surg.* 8: 30–41.

57 Smeak, D.D. (2011). Management of complications associated with total ear canal ablation and bulla osteotomy in dogs and cats. *Vet. Clin. North Am. Small Anim. Pract.* 41: 981–994.

58 Albarellos, G., Montoya, L., Ambros, L. et al. (2004). Multiple once-daily dose pharmacokinetics and renal safety of gentamicin in dogs. *J. Vet. Pharmacol. Ther.* 27: 21–25.

59 Murphy, M.R. and Hug, C.C. (1982). The anesthetic potency of fentanyl in terms of its reduction of enflurane MAC. *Anesthesiology* 57: 485–488.

60 Steagall, P.V.M., Aucoin, M., and Monteiro, B.P. (2015). Clinical effects of a constant rate infusion of remifentanil, alone or in combination with ketamine, in cats anesthetized with isoflurane. *J. Am. Vet. Med. Assoc.* 246: 976–981.

61 Buback, J.L., Boothe, H.W., Carroll, G.L. et al. (1996). Comparison of three methods for relief of pain after ear canal ablation in dogs. *Vet. Surg.* 25: 380–385.

62 Stathopoulou, T.R., Pinelas, R., Haar, G.T. et al. (2018). Description of a new approach for great auricular and auriculotemporal nerve blocks: a cadaveric study in foxes and dogs. *Vet. Med. Sci.* 4: 91–97.

63 Wolfe, T.M., Bateman, S.W., Cole, L.K. et al. (2006). Evaluation of a local anesthetic delivery system for the postoperative analgesic management of canine total ear canal ablation a randomized, controlled, double-blinded study. *Vet. Anaesth. Analg.* 33: 328–339.

64 Radlinsky, M.G., Mason, D.E., Roush, J.K. et al. (2005). Use of a continuous, local infusion of bupivacaine for postoperative analgesia in dogs undergoing total ear canal ablation. *J. Am. Vet. Med. Assoc.* 227: 414–419.

65 Burbidge, H.M. (1995). A review of laryngeal paralysis in dogs. *Br. Vet. J.* 151: 71–82.

66 Schachter, S. and Norris, C.R. (2000). Laryngeal paralysis in cats: 16 cases (1990–1999). *J. Am. Vet. Med. Assoc.* 216: 1100–1103.

67 Monnet, E. (2003). Laryngeal paralysis and devocalizaton. In: *Textbook of Small Animal Surgery*, 3e (ed. D. Slatter), 837–845. Philadelphia: Saunders Elsevier.

68 Stanley, B.J., Hauptman, J.G., Fritz, M.C. et al. (2010). Esophageal dysfunction in dogs with idiopathic laryngeal paralysis: a controlled cohort study. *Vet. Surg.* 39: 139–149.

69 Thieman, K.M., Krahwinkel, D.J., Sims, M.H. et al. (2010). Histopathological confirmation of polyneuropathy in 11 dogs with laryngeal paralysis. *J. Am. Anim. Hosp. Assoc.* 46: 161–167.

70 MacPhail, C.M. and Monnet, E. (2001). Outcome of and postoperative complications in dogs undergoing surgical treatment of laryngeal paralysis: 140 cases (1985–1998). *J. Am. Vet. Med. Assoc.* 218: 1949–1956.

71 Jeffery, N.D., Talbot, C.E., Smith, P.M. et al. (2006). Acquired idiopathic laryngeal paralysis as a prominent feature of generalised neuromuscular disease in 39 dogs. *Vet. Rec.* 158: 17.

72 Rangel, J.P.P., Monteiro, E.R., Bitti, F.S. et al. (2020). Hemodynamic, respiratory and sedative effects of progressively increasing doses of acepromazine in conscious dogs. *Vet. Anaesth. Analg.* 47: 447–453.

73 Radkey, D.I., Hardie, R.J., and Smith, L.J. (2018). Comparison of the effects of alfaxalone and propofol with acepromazine, butorphanol and/or doxapram on laryngeal motion and quality of examination in dogs. *Vet. Anaesth. Analg.* 45: 241–249.

74 Wilson, D.V., Evans, A.T., and Miller, R. (2005). Effects of preanesthetic administration of morphine on gastroesophageal reflux and regurgitation during anesthesia in dogs. *Am. J. Vet. Res.* 66: 386–390.

75 Wilson, D.V., Evans, A.T., and Mauer, W.A. (2007). Pre-anesthetic meperidine: associated vomiting and gastroesophageal reflux during the subsequent anesthetic in dogs. *Vet. Anaesth. Analg.* 34: 15–22.

76 Wilson, D.V., Evans, A.T., and Mauer, W.A. (2006). Influence of metoclopramide on gastroesophageal reflux in anesthetized dogs. *Am. J. Vet. Res.* 67: 26–31.

77 Ogden, J., Ovbey, D., and Saile, K. (2019). Effects of preoperative cisapride on postoperative aspiration pneumonia in dogs with laryngeal paralysis. *J. Small Anim. Pract.* 60: 183–190.

78 Johnson, R.A. (2014). Maropitant prevented vomiting but not gastroesophageal reflux in anesthetized dogs premedicated with acepromazine-hydromorphone. *Vet. Anaesth. Analg.* 41: 406–410.

79 Dyson, D.H., Doherty, T., Anderson, G.I. et al. (1990). Reversal of oxymorphone sedation by naloxone, nalmefene, and butorphanol. *Vet. Surg.* 19: 398–403.

80 Miller, C.J., McKiernan, B.C., Pace, J. et al. (2002). The effects of doxapram hydrochloride (dopram-V) on laryngeal function in healthy dogs. *J. Vet. Intern. Med.* 16: 524–528.

81 Tobias, K.M., Jackson, A.M., and Harvey, R.C. (2004). Effects of doxapram HCl on laryngeal function of normal dogs and dogs with naturally occurring laryngeal paralysis. *Vet. Anaesth. Analg.* 31: 258–263.

82 Labuscagne, S., Zeiler, G.E., and Dzikiti, B.T. (2019). Effects of chemical and mechanical stimulation on laryngeal motion during alfaxalone, thiopentone or propofol anaesthesia in healthy dogs. *Vet. Anaesth. Analg.* 46: 435–442.

83 Gross, M.E., Dodam, J.R., Pope, E.R. et al. (2002). A comparison of thiopental, propofol, and diazepam-ketamine anesthesia for evaluation of laryngeal function in dogs premedicated with butorphanol-glycopyrrolate. *J. Am. Anim. Hosp. Assoc.* 38: 503–506.

84 Jackson, A.M., Tobias, K., Long, C. et al. (2004). Effects of various anesthetic agents on laryngeal motion during laryngoscopy in normal dogs. *Vet. Surg.* 33: 102–106.

85 Ambros, B., Gaunt, M.C., Duke-Novakovski, T. et al. (2018). Effects of alfaxalone, thiopental, or propofol and diazepam on laryngeal motion in healthy dogs. *Can. Vet. J. La. Rev. Vet. Can.* 59: 791–795.

86 Norgate, D., Ter Haar, G., Kulendra, N. et al. (2018). A comparison of the effect of propofol and alfaxalone on laryngeal motion in nonbrachycephalic and brachycephalic dogs. *Vet. Anaesth. Analg.* 45: 729–736.

87 Smalle, T.M., Hartman, M.J., Bester, L. et al. (2017). Effects of thiopentone, propofol and alfaxalone on laryngeal motion during oral laryngoscopy in healthy dogs. *Vet. Anaesth. Analg.* 44: 427–434.

88 Hammel, S.P., Hottinger, H.A., and Novo, R.E. (2006). Postoperative results of unilateral arytenoid lateralization for treatment of idiopathic laryngeal paralysis in dogs: 39 cases (1996–2002). *J. Am. Vet. Med. Assoc.* 228: 1215–1220.

89 Thunberg, B. and Lantz, G.C. (2010). Evaluation of unilateral arytenoid lateralization for the treatment of laryngeal paralysis in 14 cats. *J. Am. Anim. Hosp. Assoc.* 46: 418–424.

90 Brunson, D.B. and Hogan, K.J. (2004). Malignant hyperthermia: a syndrome not a disease. *Vet. Clin. North Am. Small Anim. Pract.* 34: 1419–1433.

91 Roberts, M.C., Mickelson, J.R., Patterson, E.E. et al. (2001). Autosomal dominant canine malignant hyperthermia is caused by a mutation in the gene encoding the skeletal muscle calcium release channel (RYR1). *Anesthesiology* 95: 716–725.

92 Cosgrove, S.B., Eisele, P.H., Martucci, R.W. et al. (1992). Evaluation of greyhound susceptibility to malignant hyperthermia using halothane-succinylcholine anesthesia and caffeine-halothane muscle contractures. *Lab. Anim. Sci.* 42: 482–485.

93 Kirmayer, A.H., Klide, A.M., and Purvance, J.E. (1984). Malignant hyperthermia in a dog: case report and review of the syndrome. *J. Am. Vet. Med. Assoc.* 185: 978–982.

94 O'Brien, P.J., Cribb, P.H., White, R.J. et al. (1983). Canine malignant hyperthermia: diagnosis of susceptibility in a breeding colony. *Can. Vet. J. La. Rev. Vet. Can.* 24: 172–177.

95 Adami, C., Axiak, S., Raith, K. et al. (2012). Unusual perianesthetic malignant hyperthermia in a dog. *J. Am. Vet. Med. Assoc.* 240: 450–453.

96 Chohan, A.S. and Greene, S.A. (2011). Anesthesia case of the month. Malignant hyperthermia. *J. Am. Vet. Med. Assoc.* 239: 936–940.

97 Bellah, J.R., Robertson, S.A., Buergelt, C.D. et al. (1989). Suspected malignant hyperthermia after halothane anesthesia in a cat. *Vet. Surg.* 18: 483–488.

98 Fruen, B.R., Mickelson, J.R., and Louis, C.F. (1997). Dantrolene inhibition of sarcoplasmic reticulum Ca2x release by direct and specific action at skeletal muscle ryanodine receptors. *J. Biol. Chem.* 272: 26965–26971.

99 Schwartz, J.J. (2008). Skin and musculoskeletal diseases. In: *Stoelting's Anesthesia and Co-Existing Disease*, 5e (eds. R.L. Hines and K.E. Marschall), 437–467. Philadelphia: Saunders Elsevier.

100 Drachman, D.B. (1994). Myasthenia gravis. *N. Engl. J. Med.* 330: 1797–1810.

101 Stoelting, R.K. and Hillier, S.C. (2006). Anticholinesterase drugs and cholinergic agonists. In: *Pharmacology & Physiology in Anesthetic Practice*, 4e (eds. R.K. Stoelting and S.C. Hillier), 251–265. Philadelphia: Lippincott Williams & Wilkins.

102 Shelton, G.D., Schule, A., and Kass, P.H. (1997). Risk factors for acquired myasthenia gravis in dogs: 1,154 cases (1991–1995). *J. Am. Vet. Med. Assoc.* 211: 1428–1431.

103 Dewey, C.W., Shelton, G.D., Bailey, C.S. et al. (1995). Neuromuscular dysfunction in five dogs with acquired myasthenia gravis and presumptive hypothyroidism. *Prog. Vet. Neurol.* 6: 117–123.

104 Shelton, G.D., Ho, M., and Kass, P.H. (2000). Risk factors for acquired myasthenia gravis in cats: 105 cases (1986–1998). *J. Am. Vet. Med. Assoc.* 216: 55–57.

105 Khorzad, R., Whelan, M., Sisson, A. et al. (2011). Myasthenia gravis in dogs with an emphasis on treatment and critical care management. *J. Vet. Emerg. Crit. Care (San Antonio)* 21: 193–208.

106 Dewey, C.W., Bailey, C.S., Shelton, G.D. et al. (1997). Clinical forms of acquired myasthenia gravis in dogs: 25 cases (1988–1995). *J. Vet. Intern. Med.* 11: 50–57.

107 Shilo, Y., Pypendop, B.H., Barter, L.S. et al. (2011). Thymoma removal in a cat with acquired myasthenia gravis: a case report and literature review of anesthetic techniques. *Vet. Anaesth. Analg.* 38: 603–613.

108 Jones, R.S. and Sharp, N.J. (1985). Use of the muscle relaxant atracurium in a myasthenic dog. *Vet. Rec.* 117: 500–501.

109 Jones, R.S., Brown, A., and Watkins, P.E. (1988). Use of the muscle relaxant vecuronium in a myasthenic dog. *Vet. Rec.* 122: 611.

110 Fox, S.M. (2010). Pathophysiology of osteoarthritic pain. In: *Chronic Pain in Small Animal Medicine* (ed. S.M. Fox), 75–96. London: Manson Publishing Ltd.

111 Eitner, A., Hofmann, G.O., and Schaible, H.-G. (2017). Mechanisms of osteoarthritic pain. Studies in humans and experimental models. *Front. Mol. Neurosci.* 10: 349.

112 Mobasheri, A. and Batt, M. (2016). An update on the pathophysiology of osteoarthritis. *Ann. Phys. Rehabil. Med.* 59: 333–339.

113 Knazovicky, D., Helgeson, E.S., Case, B. et al. (2016). Widespread somatosensory sensitivity in naturally occurring canine model of osteoarthritis. *Pain* 157: 1325–1332.

114 Cimino, B.D. (2017). What can we learn from osteoarthritis pain in companion animals? *Clin. Exp. Rheumatol.* 35 (Suppl. 1): 53–58.

115 Lascelles, B.D.X. (2010). Feline degenerative joint disease. *Vet. Surg.* 39: 2–13.

116 Lascelles, B.D.X., Henry, J.B., Brown, J. et al. (2010). Cross-sectional study of the prevalence of radiographic degenerative joint disease in domesticated cats. *Vet. Surg.* 39: 535–544.

117 Lascelles, B.D.X. and Robertson, S.A. (2010). DJD-associated pain in cats. What can we do to promote patient comfort? *J. Feline Med. Surg.* 12: 200–212.

118 Marshall, W.G., Bockstahler, B.A., Hulse, D.A. et al. (2009). A review of osteoarthritis and obesity: current understanding of the relationship and benefit of obesity treatment and prevention in the dog. *Vet. Comp. Orthop. Traumatol.* 22: 339–345.

119 Sanderson, R.O., Beata, C., Flipo, R.-M. et al. (2009). Systematic review of the management of canine osteoarthritis. *Vet. Rec.* 164: 418–424.

120 Webster, R., Anderson, G.I., and Gearing, D.P. (2014). Canine brief pain inventory scores for dogs with osteoarthritis before and after administration of a monoclonal antibody against nerve growth factor. *Am. J. Vet. Res.* 75: 532–535.

121 Adrian, D., Papich, M., Baynes, R. et al. (2017). Chronic maladaptive pain in cats: a review of current and future drug treatment options. *Vet. J.* 230: 52–61.

122 Gearing, D.P., Virtue, E.R., Gearing, R.P. et al. (2013). A fully caninised anti-NGF monoclonal antibody for pain relief in dogs. *BMC Vet. Res.* 9: 226.

123 Johnson, K.C. and Mackin, A. (2012). Canine immune-mediated polyarthritis: part 2: diagnosis and treatment. *J. Am. Anim. Hosp. Assoc.* 48: 71–82.

124 Fournel, C., Chabanne, L., Caux, C. et al. (1992). Canine systemic lupus erythematosus. I: a study of 75 cases. *Lupus* 1: 133–139.

125 Stull, J.W., Evason, M., Carr, A.P. et al. (2008). Waldner C. canine immune-mediated polyarthritis: clinical and laboratory findings in 83 cases in western Canada (1991–2001). *Can. Vet. J. La. Rev. Vet. Can.* 49: 1195–1203.

126 Smee, N.M., Harkin, K.R., and Wilkerson, M.J. (2007). Measurement of serum antinuclear antibody titer in dogs with and without systemic lupus erythematosus: 120 cases (1997–2005). *J. Am. Vet. Med. Assoc.* 230: 1180–1183.

127 Ben-Menachem, E. (2010). Systemic lupus erythematosus. *Anesth. Analg.* 111: 665–676.

128 Martin, D.D. and Martin, A.L. (2006). Pain management and anesthesia in veterinary dermatology. *Vet. Clin. North Am. Small Anim. Pract.* 36: 1–14.

129 Hillier, A. and DeBoer, D.J. (2001). The ACVD task force on canine atopic dermatitis (XVII): intradermal testing. *Vet. Immunol. Immunopathol.* 81: 289–304.

130 Hensel, P., Santoro, D., Favrot, C. et al. (2015). Canine atopic dermatitis: detailed guidelines for diagnosis and allergen identification. *BMC Vet. Res.* 11: 196.

131 Graham, L.F., Torres, S.M.F., Jessen, C.R. et al. (2003). Effects of propofol-induced sedation on intradermal test reactions in dogs with atopic dermatitis. *Vet. Dermatol.* 14: 167–176.

132 Kennis, R.A., Robertson, S.A., Rosser, E.J. et al. (1998). Effects of propofol anesthesia on intradermally injected histamine phosphate in clinically normal dogs. *Am. J. Vet. Res.* 59: 7–9.

133 Olivry, T., Saridomichelakis, M., and International Committee on Atopic Diseases of Animals (ICADA) (2013). Evidence-based guidelines for anti-allergic drug withdrawal times before allergen-specific intradermal and IgE serological tests in dogs. *Vet. Dermatol.* 24: 225–e49.

134 Moriello, K.A. and Eicker, S.W. (1991). Influence of sedative and anesthetic agents on intradermal skin test reactions in dogs. *Am. J. Vet. Res.* 52: 1484–1488.

135 Milosevic, M.A., Cain, C.L., Frank, L.A. et al. (2013). Effects of butorphanol versus dexmedetomidine sedation on intradermal allergen and histamine responses in dogs with atopic dermatitis. *Vet. Dermatol.* 24: 582–586, e139-40.

136 Beale, K.M., Kunkle, G.A., Chalker, L. et al. (1990). Effects of sedation on intradermal skin testing in flea-allergic dogs. *J. Am. Vet. Med. Assoc.* 197: 861–864.

16

Infectious Disease

Bradley T. Simon[1] *and Jusmeen Sarkar*[2]

[1] *Department of Small Animal Clinical Sciences, College of Veterinary Medicine and Biomedical Science, Texas A&M University, College Station, TX, 77843, USA*
[2] *Anesthesia and Pain Management Service, Veterinary Specialty Center, Buffalo Grove, IL, 60089, USA*

Introduction

The One Health Initiative alleges "to promote, improve, and defend the health and well-being of all species" [1]. It utilizes collaborative endeavors integrating fields of science to educate and improve human and animal quality of life. Anesthetists play a vital role in this initiative. Zoonosis, iatrogenic administration of contaminated anesthetic drugs, unsafe injection practices, multidrug-resistant bacterial infections, postoperative surgical site infections (SSIs), work-area- and equipment-related infectious transmission, and active infectious diseases compromising a multitude of body systems are among some of the considerations for anesthetists. Understanding how these considerations integrate into the perioperative period allows the anesthetist to reduce risk factors predisposing animals to morbidity and mortality.

Contamination and Cleaning of Anesthetic Equipment

Breathing Circuits

Bacterial colonization of anesthetic breathing circuits is reported in human [2–7] and veterinary medicine [8], most prevalent in the breathing circuit components closest to the patient (i.e., mask or elbow adapter) [2, 8, 9]. Opinions have varied on whether breathing circuits are considered safe for extended use [3, 4, 8, 10, 11]. One veterinary teaching hospital evaluated bacterial colonization in anesthetic breathing circuits subjected to routine use over a 2-month period [8]. The presence of microorganisms of low pathogenicity was reported (*Bacillus* spp., coagulase-negative *Staphylococcus* spp., or *Micrococcus* spp.), but none likely to cause postoperative pneumonia even in immunocompromised patients [8]. Cooler temperatures of anesthetic and compressed gases, evaporation following breathing circuit disconnection from the patient, bactericidal effects of high oxygen concentrations, bacteriostatic properties of the circuit, and alkaline condensate in the carbon dioxide absorbent all reduce the risk for bacterial and viral colonization associated with reusable breathing circuits [2, 8, 12, 13]. A filter placed between the patient and breathing circuit [8] or between the breathing expiratory limb and anesthesia machine may reduce the risk for bacterial and viral colonization (figure 16.1). Buildup of moisture within anesthetic circuit breathing filters may increase airway resistance, impeding adequate ventilation [14], and filters should be

Canine and Feline Anesthesia and Co-Existing Disease, Second Edition. Edited by Rebecca A. Johnson, Lindsey B. C. Snyder and Carrie A. Schroeder.

Companion website: www.wiley.com/go/johnson/canine

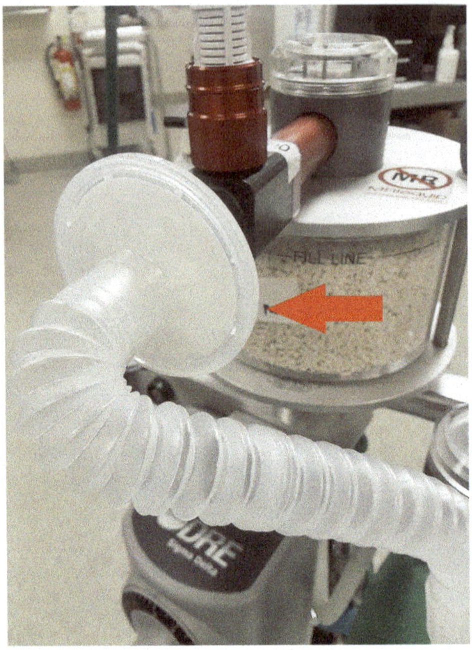

Figure 16.1 A particulate-air filter placed at the end of the expiratory limb between rebreathing circuit and the anesthesia machine (red arrow). These filters are used to protect the internal surfaces of the breathing circuit and do not allow more than 5% of particles 0.3 µm in diameter or larger to penetrate through the filter.

replaced with buildup of moisture, prolonged use, or excessive coughing.

Endotracheal Tubes

Endotracheal tubes are recommended for single use, as they come in direct contact with the patient's tracheal mucosal surfaces. Single-use endotracheal tubes may not always be practical in the veterinary setting; however, it is the anesthetist's obligation to ensure that adequate decontamination protocols are followed (Table 16.1) [15]. Disinfection of experimentally contaminated endotracheal tubes with *Streptococcus zooepidemicus* and *Bordetella bronchiseptica* was achieved with a 5-min 0.5% chlorhexidine gluconate solution soak [16]. Spraying all surfaces of the endotracheal tube with an accelerated hydrogen peroxide solution is effective to a lesser extent [16]. A cold-water soak is not effective in disinfecting endotracheal tubes and is not recommended. Intubation equipment, laryngoscope blades, and laryngoscope handles also require disinfection, as they are a potential source of contamination [17]. Decontamination with a 2% chlorhexidine/70% alcohol wipe was effective against several species of microorganisms including methicillin-resistant *Staphylococcus aureus* (MRSA) [18].

Anesthetic Equipment and Monitors

Blood contamination on anesthetic equipment and monitors is a source for infectious disease transmission. A total of 418 surfaces on anesthesia machines, anesthesia carts, and monitors frequently handled by anesthesia personnel were evaluated in one human hospital for blood contamination [19]. Prior to examination, each surface was deemed ready for use by a member of the anesthesia staff. Of the surfaces examined, 137 (33%) were positive for blood contaminants and only three had blood visible to the unaided eye [19]. The highest prevalence of blood contamination was found on anesthesia monitoring cables (82%), drawer handles (64%), and pulse oximeter probes (59%) [19]. Commercially available disinfecting wipes containing sodium hypochlorite as the active ingredient are effective in cleaning most types of microbes from anesthesia equipment [20, 21]. Wiping with 70% isopropanol does not adequately clean and disinfect reusable pulse oximetry sensors [21]. Utilizing standard operating procedures (SOPs) for routine cleaning of anesthesia equipment and monitors may improve the efficiency and quality of care, and reduce incidences of nosocomial transmission during the perianesthetic period.

Multidrug-Resistant Organisms and Surgical Site Infection

Multidrug-Resistant Organisms

The emergence of multidrug-resistant organisms (MDRO) in hospital settings is of growing concern and is an important cause of morbidity

Table 16.1 Cleaning processes, the microbiological organisms they render nonviable, and methods for implementation.

	Microorganisms rendered nonviable						
Process	**Bacteria**	**Viruses**	**Fungi**	**Bacterial spores**	**Methods**	**Required for items**	**Examples**
Sterilization	Yes	Yes	Yes	Yes	Pressurized steam, dry heat, ethylene oxide and hydrogen peroxide	Intended to contact a normally sterile body area/cavity That may inadvertently be inserted into a normally sterile body area/cavity	Surgical equipment and single-use disposables (e.g., needles, scalpels, ventilation tubing and filters, endotracheal tube, urinary catheter and drains) Esophageal stethoscope
High-level disinfection	Yes	Yes	Yes	No	Aldehydes, peracetic acid and chlorine dioxide	That contact mucous membranes, but do not penetrate the membrane or come in touch with blood	Ventilation masks, components of the laryngoscope, endoscopes, oral and nasal airways, and connectors
Intermediate-level disinfection	Yes	Most Not small viruses without envelopes	Yes	No	Alcohol, sodium, hypochlorite, phenols, and iodophors	That contact the external parts of the body (i.e., skin and hair)	Blood pressure cuffs, stethoscopes, pulse oximeter probes, head rests and straps, and ECG electrodes
Low-level disinfection	Most	Some	Some	No	Alcohol and quaternary ammonium compounds	Noncritical patient-care surfaces and equipment that contacts intact skin	Bedrails, over-the-bed table or stand, and medical devices and equipment

All contaminated equipment/devices must first be cleaned (thus decreasing their bacterial load) in order to achieve appropriate disinfection or sterilization. When items have been within the vicinity of a patient with a multidrug-resistant organism (MDRO; i.e., in the same room), disposable items should generally be discarded even if they have not been used and multiple-use items should be assumed to have been in direct contact with the patient. *Source:* Adapted with permission from Einav and Wiener-Well [15].

and mortality [22]. Currently, MRSA, extended-spectrum beta-lactamase *Enterobacteriaceae* and MDR *Enterococcus*, *Acinetobacter*, and *Pseudomonas* spp. are of most concern [22]. Factors predisposing patients to the development of MDROs include duration and type of antibiotic use, disruption of intrinsic protective barriers of the body, age extremes, presence of diabetes mellitus, and immune suppression [15]. To decrease MDRO transmission and SSIs, anesthetists should receive training in identifying patient risk factors, aseptic techniques and antibiotic regimens, and appropriate decontamination procedures. Surgical patients receiving antibiotics for their MDRO should receive an additional dose [15] 30–60 min before surgical incision [23, 24]. Locations and transport of anesthetized patients diagnosed with MDROs should be kept to a minimum. The anesthesia team should wear disposable gowns, gloves, surgical caps and masks, and avoid contact to nearby surfaces, staff, and patients. An in-line breathing circuit filter can be added to reduce the risk of cross-contamination [25]. Staff members without MDRO patient contact should assist in opening doors, cages, kennels, and elevators as required. Anesthetic equipment should be cleaned and disinfected as previously described, but, in MDRO patients, breathing circuits and endotracheal tubes should be kept to single use.

Surgical Site Infections

SSIs have tremendous clinical and financial impact in veterinary medicine [26, 27]. In humans, it is estimated that SSIs reach more than $3.5–$10 billion annually in health care expenditures [28]. The Centers for Disease Control and Prevention (CDC) Healthcare-Associated Infections guidelines have defined SSI to be an infection that occurs in the part of the body (incision or organ) where the surgery took place [28]. The rate of SSI in small-animal veterinary medicine is approximately 5.5–5.8% [29, 30]. *Staphylococcus* spp., a bacteria commonly found within the skin, is the most common cause for SSI in dogs and cats [31]. The incidences of SSI in dogs and cats for clean, clean-contaminated, contaminated, and dirty procedures are 2.5–4.9%, 4.5%, 5.8–9.1%, and 17.8–18.1%, respectively [29, 32]; with the potential of being as high as 13.3% following clean orthopedic procedures [33]. Minimally invasive surgery may be associated with a lower incidence of SSI when compared to open surgery in dogs and cats [34]. Dogs with SSIs, when compared to those without infections, have higher mean postoperative costs, longer duration from surgery to final closure of the case, and more postoperative visits [26]. Currently there is no association between SSI and long-term effects on functional outcome in dogs following orthopedic surgery [35]; however, additional studies are required. Anesthetists are an important factor in the prevalence of SSI during the perioperative period (Table 16.2) [36]. Anesthesia-specific factors associated with the development of SSI include hypoxemia, increasing American Society of Anesthesiologists (ASA) physical status, hypothermia, hyperglycemia, administration of contaminated propofol, inadequate antibiotic prophylaxis, prolonged anesthesia duration, contaminated anesthesia gurneys, and postoperative anemia [27, 31, 37–41]. Additional factors include concurrent endocrinopathy (diabetes mellitus, hyperadrenocorticism, hypothyroidism), prolonged surgery time, increasing number of people in the operating room, additional days spent in the intensive care unit (ICU), obesity, extremes in age, intact males, dirty surgical site, surgical site clipped before anesthetic induction, surgery performed during the warmer summer months, and prolonged use of antibiotics in clean wounds [29, 30, 42–45]. Inhalant-based anesthesia techniques also may increase the risk for SSI when compared to neuraxial techniques [46, 47]; however, there are conflicting reports [48]. The influence of forced-air warming blankets on the spread of nosocomial

Table 16.2 Risk factors for the development of surgical site infections.

Patient factors	Environmental factors	Treatment factors
Ascites	Contaminated medications (i.e., propofol)	Drains
Chronic inflammation	Contaminated anesthesia gurneys	Emergency procedure
Corticosteroid therapy	Inadequate disinfection/ sterilization	Hypothermia
Obesity	Inadequate skin antisepsis	Inadequate antibiotic prophylaxis
Diabetes or hyperglycemia	Inadequate ventilation	Oxygenation (controversial)
Extremes of age	Dirty surgical site	Prolonged preoperative hospitalization
Hypocholesterolemia	Surgery performed during warmer summer months	Prolonged operative time
Hypoxemia	Increased number of people in the surgical suite	Prolonged anesthesia time
Peripheral vascular disease		Prolonged use of antibiotics in clean wounds
Postoperative anemia		
Prior site irradiation		
Remote infection		
Skin carriage of *Staphylococci* spp.		
Skin disease in the area of infection		
Malnutrition		
Surgical site clipped before anesthetic induction		
Hyperadrenocorticism		
Hypothyroidism		
ASA physical status > II		

Source: Adapted with permission from Barie and Eachempati [36]. Data from: National Nosocomial Infections Surveillance System (NNIS) System Report: Data Summary from January 1992–June 2001, issued August 2001. *Am J Infect Control* 2001; 29: 404–21.

infections has been of much debate [49, 50]. Currently, there is no strong evidence to suggest that these warming devices increase the risk for SSI [49, 51]. On the contrary, forced-air warming devices may provide benefit in reducing SSI by minimizing perioperative hypothermia [50, 52]. Pharmacological and nonpharmacological factors that reduce the incidence of SSI include appropriate volume resuscitation and fluid therapy, normothermia, adequate analgesia, intraoperative and postoperative oxygen supplementation, normoglycemia, and prophylactic antibiotic therapy [53, 54]. Furthermore, lidocaine, thiopental, and diphenhydramine all possess bacteriostatic properties, and, when combined with propofol, may decrease the potential risk for bacterial contamination [55–58]. Recommendations from the CDC guidelines of SSI are represented in Table 16.3 [27, 28, 59].

Suboptimal timing, duration, and choice of perioperative antibiotics are still being practiced in veterinary medicine [33, 60]. Inappropriate use of prophylactic antibiotics may be due to failure of the veterinarian to keep up to date on current practices or failure to transition to evidence-based practices [60]. Examples of inappropriate use include the use of antibiotics for clean surgical procedures (except surgeries involving surgical implants), administration of prophylactic antimicrobials postoperatively, and the continued administration of antibiotics for longer than 24 h following surgery [61]. In contrast to the latter examples, recent evidence suggests that postoperative antibiotics may reduce the incidence of SSI following clean orthopedic implant surgery in dogs [62, 63]; however, duration of administration may be an important factor in their effectiveness [64].

Table 16.3 Recommendations from Centers for Disease Control and Prevention guidelines for the prevention of surgical site infection, 2017 [27, 28, 59].

Parenteral antimicrobial prophylaxis
- Administer antimicrobial agents only when indicated based on published guidelines
- Time administration such that bactericidal concentration is established in serum and tissues at initial incision
Glycemic control
- Implement perioperative glycemic control using blood glucose target levels <200 mg dl^{-1} in patients with and without diabetes
Normothermia
- Maintain perioperative normothermia
Oxygenation
- Administer increased fractions of inspired oxygen intraoperatively and in the immediate postoperative period following extubation for all patients with normal pulmonary function undergoing general anesthesia with endotracheal intubation
Antiseptic prophylaxis
- Instruct owners to perform full body bathing the night before surgery with either soap or an antiseptic agent. Allow complete drying of densely haired patients to avoid skin irritation
- Clipping of hair adjacent to the surgical site with clean, appropriately serviced clippers after induction of anesthesia and immediately before the surgical procedure
- Intraoperative skin preparation should be performed with an antiseptic agent containing alcohol unless contraindicated
- Nail polish, jewelry, and artificial nails should be avoided or removed in all members of the anesthesia and surgery team prior to handling of the patient during the perioperative period

In most veterinary settings, the anesthetist administers the prophylactic antibiotics to the surgical patients. Withholding prophylactic antibiotics can increase the rate of SSI. For most antibiotics, complete distribution into tissues can occur within 30–60 min following intravenous administration [61]. In a patient not previously exposed to antibiotics, an initial IV dose of cefazolin administered 10–30 min before skin incision and at the completion of the procedure is recommended. For procedures lasting longer than 2 h, additional intraoperative doses should be administered every 90 min following the initial dose [61]. For most surgical procedures, a first-generation cephalosporin such as cefazolin is effective. For surgeries in which the bowel is entered, coverage of Gram-negative organisms is important, and anaerobic coverage is appropriate if the large bowel or female genital tract is entered. Additional studies are needed to determine the recommended duration of postoperative prophylactic antibiotic administration in veterinary medicine.

Respiratory Infections

Aspiration, Bacterial, and Viral Pneumonia

Aspiration Pneumonia

Aspiration pneumonia is one of the leading causes of infectious pneumonia in human patients hospitalized in the ICU [65], with an overall mortality rate of approximately 45% [66]. Mortality rate is lower in dogs than in humans but can be as high as 25% [67, 68]. A retrospective study evaluating over 140 000 dogs anesthetized or sedated over a 10-year period reported a 0.17% incidence of postanesthetic aspiration pneumonia [69]. Several factors may predispose a patient to the development of aspiration pneumonia (Table 16.4) [69–72]. Two or more anesthesia-related events, increased anesthetic duration, regurgitation and hydromorphone administration at induction, postanesthetic vomiting and regurgitation, and procedures such as laparotomy, upper

Table 16.4 Factors associated with aspiration pneumonia in dogs and cats [69–72].

Gastrointestinal disease	**Neurologic disease**
Recent history of vomiting	Polyneuropathy
Pancreatitis	Myasthenia gravis
Intussusception	Seizure
Foreign body obstruction	Conditions leading to prolonged recumbency
Ileus	Preanesthetic tetraparesis
Chronic gastrointestinal disease	
Enteral nutrition	
Esophageal disease	**Procedures**
Megaesophagus	Laparotomy
Esophageal motility disorder	Upper airway surgery
Hiatal hernia	Neurosurgery
Esophageal stricture	Thoracotomy
Esophagitis	Endoscopy
	Magnetic resonance imaging
Pharyngeal and laryngeal disease	**Anesthesia**
Muscular dystrophy	Increased duration of anesthesia
Oropharyngeal dysphagia	Recent history of anesthesia
Laryngeal disease or trauma	Two or more anesthesia related events
	Regurgitation during anesthesia
	Administration of hydromorphone at induction
Respiratory disease	**Breed**
Upper respiratory disease	Brachycephalic (Bulldog, Pug)
Postprocedural upper airway obstruction	Golden Retriever
	Cocker Spaniel
	English Springer Spaniel
	Domestic Shorthair

Source: Adapted with permission from O'Hara et al. [59].

airway surgery, neurosurgery, thoracotomy, magnetic resonance imaging (MRI), and endoscopy were associated with the development of aspiration pneumonia [69, 70, 73, 74]. Megaesophagus, history of preexisting respiratory (i.e., laryngeal paralysis or brachycephalic syndrome) or neurologic disease, preanesthetic tetraparesis, and cervical lesions were also associated with aspiration pneumonia [69, 70, 73, 75]. There are no reported incidences of postanesthesia aspiration pneumonia in cats; however, one retrospective analysis reported an 11% mortality rate following aspiration pneumonia [72]. Risk factors in cats are likely similar to those observed in dogs.

Inhalation of sterile (aspiration pneumonitis) or septic (aspiration pneumonia) acidic orogastric contents irritates the pulmonary mucosa and fosters an environment in which bacterial colonization can occur. Damage associated with aspiration pneumonia can be categorized into two distinct phases. The first phase results from the direct chemical burn of acidic gastric contents resulting in pulmonary parenchymal inflammation. Pulmonary gas exchange is compromised, and the lungs become susceptible to bacterial colonization leading to bacterial pneumonia [76, 77]. Acidic contents stimulate alveolar macrophages and type II pneumocytes to release inflammatory cytokines, which occurs during the second phase. Inflammatory cytokines recruit neutrophils in high concentrations which release proteases and oxidants, compromising the integrity of the vascular endothelial walls in the pulmonary parenchyma [78]. This increases permeability to proteins and fluid, with associated accumulation of edema, fibrin, hemorrhage, and neutrophils. These infiltrates result in the development of atelectasis, airway collapse, and disruptions to the mucociliary action causing bacterial entrapment and infection [76, 78].

Bacterial and Viral Pneumonia

Bacterial pneumonia is one of the most common clinical diagnoses in dogs with respiratory disease and is often associated with viral infections or aspiration of gastrointestinal (GI) contents. In dogs, it is often due to canine infectious respiratory disease (CIRD) complex, a syndrome that involves a multitude of viral (canine respiratory coronavirus, influenza virus, herpesvirus, pneumovirus, parainfluenza, bocavirus, hepacivirus, picornavirus) and bacterial (*B. bronchiseptica*, *Streptococcus canis*, *Streptococcus equi subsp. zooepidemicus*, and *Mycoplasma cynos*) pathogens [71, 79]. Pathogens associated with infectious pneumonia in cats include *Pasteurella* spp., *Escherichia coli*, *Staphylococcus* spp., *Streptococcus* spp., *Pseudomonas* spp., *B. bronchiseptica*, and *Mycoplasma* spp. [71]. If the innate immune system is unable to clear the pathogens from the lower respiratory system, bronchopneumonia or bronchointerstitial pneumonia develops, damaging the type I pneumocytes and the respiratory epithelium. Progression of the disease is similar to that seen during aspiration pneumonia [71, 80].

Clinical Signs

Clinical signs are dependent on the patient's physical status and severity and chronicity of disease. In cases of aspiration pneumonia, clinical signs also depend on the volume and pH of aspirated orogastric contents. Anesthetized or neurologic patients have a less pronounced cough reflex, which makes them prone to aspiration and the development of acute respiratory distress syndrome (ARDS) [69, 81]. Fatalities in dogs and cats with ARDS following aspiration pneumonia are approximately 84% and 100%, respectively [81]. Early clinical signs include soft coughing, but as the disease worsens, productive coughing, dyspnea, exercise intolerance, lethargy, decreased appetite, syncope, cyanosis, and orthopnea may develop. Cats exhibit less pronounced clinical signs when compared to dogs. Increased respiratory effort, anorexia, vomiting, and lethargy were among the most common presenting complaints for cats diagnosed with pneumonia [72]. Other clinical signs in cats include coughing, drooling, oral bleeding, regurgitation, weight loss, and tachypnea with short, shallow breaths and nasal flaring [71, 72]. Increased work of breathing from decreased pulmonary compliance and increased pulmonary shunting contributes to the development of hypoxemia in patients with pneumonia [72, 80].

Diagnosis

A thorough history and physical examination are extremely important in the diagnosis of pneumonia. Recent history of an anesthetic event may be indicative of aspiration pneumonia. Anesthetists should pay close attention to the patient's respiratory rate and effort. Thoracic auscultation may reveal harsh lung sounds, crackles, and/or wheezes. Thoracic radiographs are an important tool in diagnosing and determining the severity of pneumonia in dogs and cats (Figure 16.2). Patients with pneumonia can develop concurrent upper airway disease (nasal congestion or discharge) and therefore upper auscultation should also be performed prior to sedation or anesthesia [71]. Fever does not always accompany pneumonia in dogs and cats and is not a reliable indicator of disease [68, 72]. In cats with pneumonia, 71%, 18%, and 11% had an alveolar pattern, unstructured interstitial pattern, and

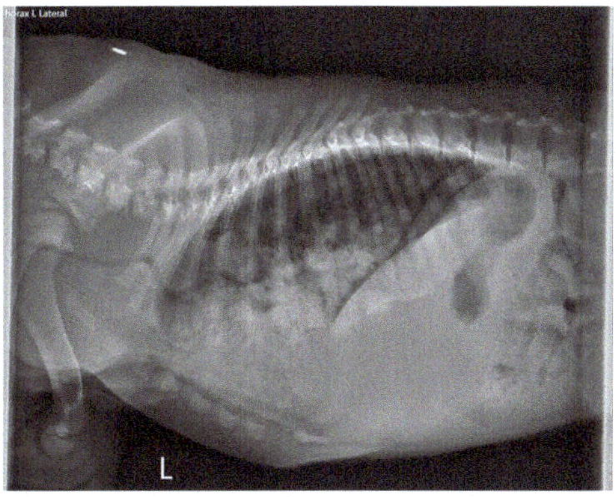

Figure 16.2 Radiographic evidence of a dog diagnosed with aspiration pneumonia. *Source:* Photo courtesy of Dr. Jessica Vallone.

mixed alveolar–interstitial pattern, respectively, with the right middle lung and left cranial lung lobes most affected [72]. Cats commonly had an inflammatory leukogram on complete blood count with occasional band neutrophils [72].

Anesthetic Management

In cases of acute pneumonia, anesthesia and surgery should be postponed until the patient is deemed stable following antimicrobial therapy, intravenous fluids to correct hydration deficits, nebulization and coupage, oxygen supplementation, and oral mucolytic agents such as *N*-acetylcysteine. Patients diagnosed with pneumonia that require emergent anesthesia should be ventilated using protective ventilation strategies. Goals for protective ventilation include optimization of patient–ventilator synchrony, reduction in iatrogenic injury, and supporting gas exchange (Figure 16.3) [82]. Tidal volume should not exceed 6–8 $ml\,kg^{-1}$ of lean body weight with a rate of 8–15 breaths min^{-1} to achieve adequate oxygenation (SpO_2>95%) and ventilation (end-tidal carbon dioxide [$EtCO_2$] between 35 and 50 mmHg) [82]. Hypercapnia is generally well tolerated when pH is maintained between 7.20 and 7.45 in nonpregnant hemodynamically stable patients with normal intracranial pressures. A fractional inspired oxygen concentration of 100% is recommended in moderate to severe cases of pneumonia. Positive end-expiratory pressure (PEEP) of 5–10 cm H_2O can be provided in hypoxemic patients (PaO_2<60 mmHg; SpO_2<90%) (Figure 16.4). To decrease the likelihood of desaturation during anesthesia induction, preoxygenation via face mask at 100 $ml\,kg^{-1}\,min^{-1}$ for a minimum of 3 min is recommended [83]. Elevating the head approximately 30° and placement of an orogastric tube can prevent the aspiration of gastric contents [84]. Endotracheal intubation with a cuffed endotracheal tube inflated to 20 cm H_2O is recommended for the prevention of aspiration pneumonia. Active suctioning should be readily available to the anesthetist to remove any buildup of secretions within the oropharynx and endotracheal tube. Prevention of aspiration is key in patients with predisposing risk factors. Reductions in pure μ-opioid receptor agonist administration, minimizing changes in position during intubation and recovery, prophylactic treatment of nausea with maropitant, metoclopramide, ondansetron, proton-pump inhibitors, or H_2-receptor antagonists, providing optimal timing for endotracheal tube cuff deflation, and aseptic handling of intubation equipment are preventative measures in reducing the development of pneumonia [74].

Prognosis

Lactate and the pneumonia severity index (PSI) have been used to determine morbidity and mortality in human patients diagnosed with pneumonia (Table 16.5) [80, 85]. For example, more intensified monitoring and diagnostic evaluations are recommended in human patients with lactate levels >1.8 $mmol\,l^{-1}$ or PSI scores >71 (Class II) [80, 85]. Mortality rate is approximately 25% in dogs [67, 68] and 11% in cats [72].

Canine Influenza A Virus

Canine influenza viruses (CIVs) are among the family Orthomyxoviridae that includes the Influenza A viruses (IAVs). The two major IAVs found in dogs include H3N2 and H3N8. Not until recently did evidence exist that dogs

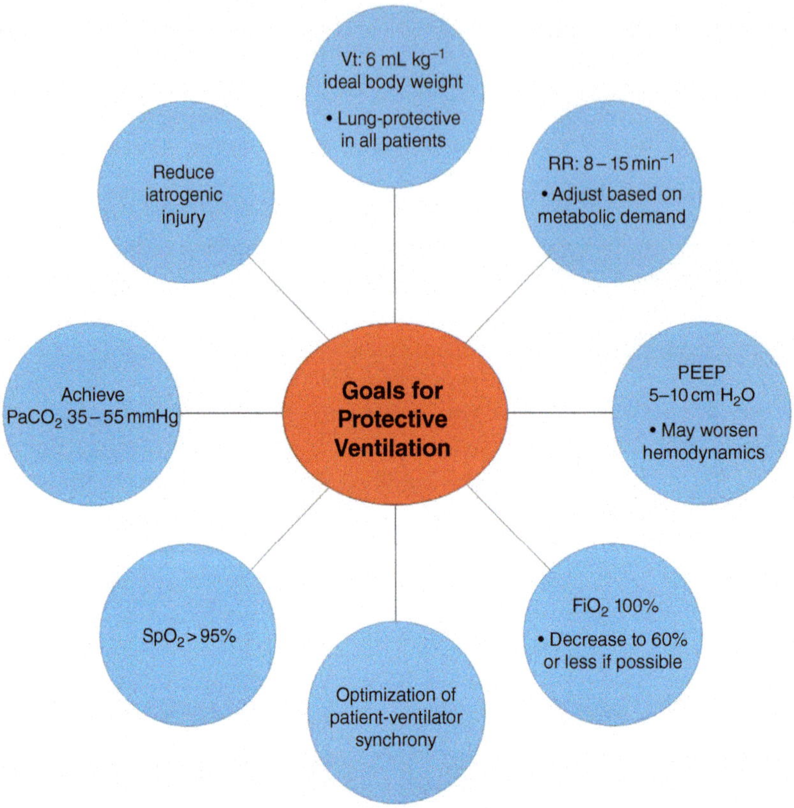

Figure 16.3 Goals for providing protective ventilation in dogs and cats with aspiration or bacterial pneumonia [82]. Vt: tidal volume; RR: respiratory rate; PEEP: positive end-expiratory pressure; FiO_2: fractional inspired oxygen; SPO_2: blood oxygen saturation; $PaCO_2$: arterial carbon dioxide pressure.

could be responsible for an epidemic spread and considered a natural host. H3N8 appears to be isolated among animal shelter dogs [86]. In 2015, another IAV, H3N2, was first introduced into the United States and is currently an ongoing widespread epidemic [87]. Transmission of H3N2 from dogs to cats has been reported in Korea and the United States but appears to be mainly found in shelter populations [88]. Humans are not susceptible to either form of IAV. Typically, these viruses are inactivated within minutes to hours in most environments; however, there is potential for them to persist longer (days) in cool, dark, damp conditions [86]. Transmission via the respiratory route usually requires direct contact and often is associated with animal shelters and boarding kennels [89]. Most commercially available disinfecting wipes and hot water will inactivate the IAV.

The H3N8 and H3N2 CIVs predominately bind to the surface of epithelial cells in the bronchus, nasal mucosa, trachea, and type II pneumocytes [90]. This results in necrosis and exfoliation of the tracheal and bronchial mucosa (tracheitis and bronchitis, respectively), promoting the infiltration of lymphocytes and serous effusion in the alveolar spaces [89, 90].

Clinical Signs

CIV infections result in rapid onset of clinical signs associated with upper respiratory tract disease (coughing, sneezing, lethargy, fever, ocular and nasal discharge, and inappetence) [91]. Initially, CIV-positive patients develop a persis-

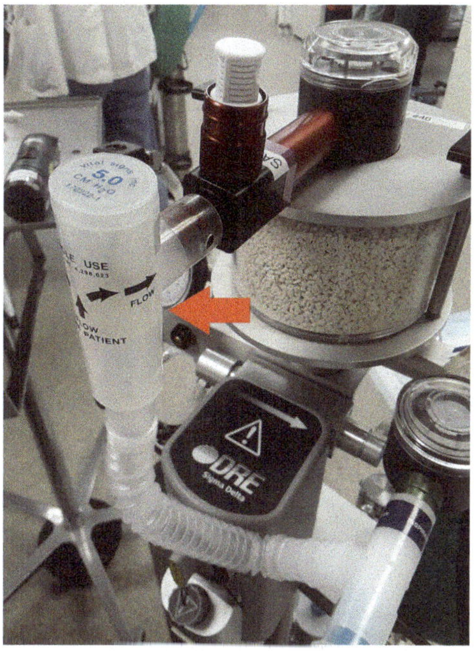

Figure 16.4 A positive end-expiratory pressure valve of 5 cm H_2O mounted vertically on the expiratory side of a circle system (red arrow).

tent, dry, and nonproductive cough which can last for several weeks. As the disease continues and lung defenses become compromised via damage to the ciliary epithelium [92], secondary pneumonia may develop [89, 92]. In some instances, vomiting, diarrhea, and respiratory distress have been reported [91]. Despite the latter signs, both forms are associated with a low fatality rate (<5%) [91].

Diagnosis

A confirmed diagnosis of CIV is usually difficult due to the short incubation (2 days) and shedding (2–4 days) periods of the virus. Using reverse transcription polymerase chain reaction (RT-PCR) on nasal swabs is the test of choice to detect CIV. Alternatively, hemagglutination inhibition titers are rapid and can detect antibody responses in dogs at 7 days post infection [89].

Anesthetic Management

CIV has the potential to spread rapidly among immunologically naïve or compromised

Table 16.5 A pneumonia severity index used to determine the prognosis in patients diagnosed with pneumonia.

Factors	Points	Score and stratification		
		Point total	**Risk class**	**Mortality**
Geriatric	Age + 10	≤70 low risk	I	0.1–0.4%
Neoplastic disease	30	71–90 low	II	0.6–0.7%
Congestive heart failure	10	91–130 moderate	III	0.9–2.8%
Cerebrovascular disease	10	>130 high	IV	8.2–12.5%
Renal disease	10		V	27.1–31.1%
Liver disease	20			
Altered mental status	20			
Tachycardia	10			
Tachypnea	20			
Systolic blood pressure <90 mmHg	20			
Temperature <35 °C or ≥40 °C	15			
Arterial pH <7.35	30			
BUN ≥30 mg dl^{-1}	20			
Sodium <130 mmol l^{-1}	20			
Glucose ≥250 mg dl^{-1}	10			
Hematocrit <30%	10			
PaO_2 60 mmHg or SpO_2 90%	10			

Adapted with permission from: Rider and Frazee [80].

animals. Patients suspected or diagnosed with CIV should be kept in isolation with limited contact to other patients. Changes from routine anesthetic management are dependent on the patient's history, physical examination, and severity of clinical signs. Dehydration should be quantified and managed with a balanced crystalloid solution prior to general anesthesia. Oxygenation and ventilation should be assessed prior to anesthesia via use of capnometry, pulse oximetry, and/or arterial blood gas analysis. Side-stream capnography can be used to acquire an estimate of the end-tidal carbon dioxide concentration prior to induction (Figure 16.5). High (>50 mmHg) $EtCO_2$ values may indicate inadequate ventilation due to upper airway disease, nasal congestion, or severe lower airway disease. Clinical signs of hyperventilation ($EtCO_2$ <25 mmHg) or increased respiratory rate may be an indicator for hypoxia. Oxygen supplementation may be required following anesthesia. Clinical signs associated with hypoxia include tachypnea, tachycardia, restlessness, and cyanosis. The anesthetist should closely monitor ventilation and oxygenation during the recovery period. Preoxygenation and protective ventilation strategies are recommended especially in patients diagnosed with a secondary pneumonia. A balanced anesthetic regimen with the use of local regional techniques would minimize the respiratory depressant and immunosuppressant effects associated with inhalant anesthetics. Opioids may be beneficial in patients feeling pain with a dry nonproductive cough due to their high analgesic efficacy and antitussive properties, respectively [93, 94]. All airway management equipment should be sterilized prior to and following use to avoid secondary bacterial pneumonia or cross-contamination, respectively.

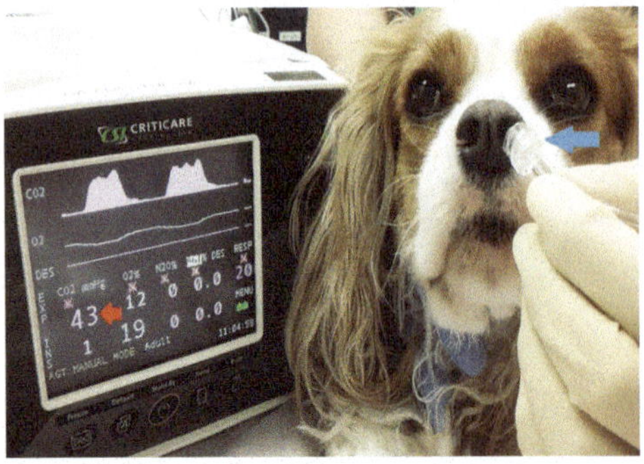

Figure 16.5 The use of side-stream capnography (blue arrow) prior to induction of anesthesia to estimate the patient's end-tidal carbon dioxide concentration (red arrow) and ability to ventilate.

Feline Respiratory Disease Complex

Feline respiratory disease complex (FRDC) or feline upper respiratory tract infection (URI) refers to an acutely contagious respiratory or ocular disease caused by one or multiple pathogens (viral, bacterial, and/or fungal) [95]. Cats housed in crowded or densely populated housing are most often affected, and it is rarely diagnosed in singly housed indoor cats [95]. Stress and poor air quality may further exacerbate the severity of the disease and increase the transmission of FRDC [96]. For example, approximately 54% of cats were reported having mild to severe clinical signs associated with FRDC in eight United States animal shelters [97]. The most common pathogens include feline calicivirus, feline herpesvirus-1 (feline rhinotracheitis), *Chlamydophila felis*, *B. bronchiseptica*, and *Mycoplasma* spp. [97]. *Cryptococcus neoformans* var. *neoformans* and *Cryptococcus gattii* have also been reported [98]. These organisms are often spread via bodily secretions (respiratory, ocular, and oral). Pending on the etiology, aerosol transmission can occur, but most often is due to contact with contaminated surfaces or direct exposure to infected cats [95].

Clinical Signs

Clinical signs are similar among etiologies and can range from mild to severe. Patients with FRDC often present with one or more of the following clinical signs: serious, mucoid, or mucopurulent nasal discharge, sneezing, conjunctivitis and ocular discharge, ulcerations of the lips, tongue, gums, or nasal planum, hypersalivation, coughing, fever, lethargy, and inappetence [95]. In severe cases, secondary bacterial pneumonia may also be present.

Diagnosis

Most often, if FRDC is suspected, the causative agent need not be determined because supportive treatment is similar among pathogens [95]. Determining the etiology in patients with lower respiratory tract disease has been previously discussed in this chapter. If a definitive diagnosis is desired, PCR testing, bacterial cultures, serologic assays, and viral isolation have been used, but false-negatives and false-positives commonly occur [95].

Anesthetic Management

Patients with FRDC may be at an increased risk of respiratory complications, particularly those with excessive ocular–nasal discharge and nasal congestion. Those with systemic signs of infection undergoing elective procedures are also at considerable risk for perioperative morbidity. Elective procedures should be delayed until clinical signs of disease have resolved. In humans, it has been suggested that anesthesia should not commence for at least 4–6 weeks following URIs to allow for adequate healing of the airways [99]. Anesthetic management should be focused around maintaining adequate hydration and reducing oronasal secretions and handling of the infected airway. Adverse events such as bronchospasm, laryngospasm, airway obstruction, and hypoxia may occur during the peri-anesthetic period [99]. Airway management is a priority; additional endotracheal tubes, airway equipment, and induction drugs should always be readily available before, during, and after the anesthetic event. Following extubation, hypoxia is alleviated with supplemental oxygen. Equipment should be disinfected as with all infectious diseases and was previously discussed.

Gastrointestinal Infections

Infectious Gastroenteritis

Infectious gastroenteritis (GE) may be of viral, bacterial, or parasitic origins. Common viral etiologies include canine parvovirus, canine coronaviral enteritis, feline parvoviral enteritis, feline immunodeficiency virus (FIV)-associated diarrhea, and feline leukemia virus (FeLV)-associated panleukopenia. *Campylobacter jejuni*, *Salmonella* spp., *Helicobacter* spp., *Clostridium perfringens*, and *Clostridium difficile* are among some causes of bacterial GE. Except for parvovirus, FIV, FeLV, and parasites, the primary pathogen is rarely confirmed; however, clinical features and management are similar among pathogens.

Clinical Signs

Vomiting and diarrhea are the two most common clinical signs associated with infectious GE. Vomiting is a result of the activation of the emetic center in the reticular formation of the medulla oblongata, the chemoreceptor trigger zone located in the fourth ventricle of the brain, and the stimulation of receptors and autonomic nervous system within the abdominal viscera [100]. Reduced intestinal absorption and/or increased intestinal secretion results in an accumulation of fecal water leading to diarrhea [100]. Infectious agents compromise the GI mucosa by blunting the absorptive properties of the villi or disrupting the ion pumps in the GI epithelium [100]. A thorough history and physical examination should be performed in patients with GE. The anesthetist should look for historical indications (chronic vomiting and diarrhea) and clinical signs associated with dehydration (Table 16.6) [100]. Skin tenting should be performed over the dorsum of the neck or lateral thorax [101]. Fever, depression, anorexia, and abdominal pain are also associated with infectious GE.

Diagnosis

Patients exhibiting mild clinical signs of GE typically do not require extensive diagnostic

Table 16.6 Subjective parameters used to assess the degree of dehydration.

Estimated degree of dehydration	Clinical signs
<5% (subclinical)	Nonapparent on physical examination
5% (mild)	Tacky or dry mucous membranes (MM)
6–8% (moderate)	Dry MM Decreased skin elasticity Tachycardia Normal pulse quality Normal arterial blood pressure
8–10% (severe)	Dry MM Further decrease in skin elasticity Small increase in capillary refill time (CRT) Weak pulses
Approximately 12% (hypovolemia)	Dry MM Increased CRT Skin tent does not return to normal Tachycardia or bradycardia Weak to absent pulses Altered mentation Hypotension Cold extremities Hypothermia

Source: Adapted with permission from: Tello and Perez-Freytes [100].

tests. In patients with moderate to severe illness, parasites can be identified using centrifugal flotation with zinc sulfate flotation solution and direct fecal examination, fecal enzyme-linked immunosorbent assay (ELISA) for canine parvovirus, and serologic analysis for FeLV and FIV. Gastric biopsy from the body, fundus, and antrum of the stomach may be helpful in diagnosing *Helicobacter* in cats; however, this requires general anesthesia.

Anesthetic Management

Dehydration from GI losses must be assessed and treated prior to general anesthesia. Appropriate fluid therapy is dependent on the patient's history, physical examination, and diagnostic tests (complete blood count, serum biochemistry, and acid–base status). General anesthetics negatively impact the cardiovascular system, and it is best to volume-resuscitate and stabilize the patient prior to anesthesia. This may require delaying anesthesia and surgery if possible. A balanced crystalloid solution (lactated Ringer's solution [LRS], Plasma-Lyte, Normosol-R, etc.) should be administered intravenously, with the dose and rate dependent upon the extent of dehydration and colloidal oncotic pressure or total protein. In severe cases, colloids can be administered at doses of 3 ml kg^{-1} and 5 ml kg^{-1} over 15 min to cats and dogs, respectively. Care should be taken to not exceed approximately 20 ml kg^{-1} day^{-1} of these solutions, as colloids have been reported to interfere with the function of platelets, von Willebrand's factor, and factor VIII in critically ill patients [102]. Vomiting is routinely associated with hyponatremia, hypochloremia, and hypokalemia. Diarrhea also contributes to hypokalemia via the loss of potassium ions in the feces. Potassium chloride (KCl) may be added to a replacement isotonic crystalloid solution to correct hypokalemia (Table 16.7) [100]. The rate of potassium administration should not exceed 0.5 mEq kg^{-1} h^{-1}. The anesthetist should be cautious when bolusing fluids containing potassium chloride. If bradycardia or electrocardiogram changes associated with hyperkalemia are observed, the bolus should be discontinued, and patient's serum potassium concentrations evaluated. Elevations in lactate, packed cell volume (PCV), and total protein may also be good laboratory indicators for dehydration. Blood pressure should be assessed prior to and during general anesthesia. Low blood pressure (mean arterial pressure <70 mmHg) may indicate hypovolemia and warrants immediate fluid therapy prior to

Table 16.7 Recommended amount of potassium chloride and rate of infusion so as not to exceed $0.5\,\text{mEq}\,\text{kg}^{-1}\,\text{h}^{-1}$.

Serum potassium concentration ($\text{mEq}\,\text{l}^{-1}$)	Potassium chloride (mEq) to add to fluid (250 ml)	Potassium (mEq) to add to fluid (1 l)	Maximal fluid infusion rate ($\text{ml}\,\text{kg}^{-1}\,\text{h}^{-1}$)
<2.0	20	80	6
2.1–2.5	15	60	8
2.6–3.0	10	40	12
3.1–3.5	7	28	18
3.6–5.0	5	20	25

Source: Adapted with permission from: Tello and Perez-Freytes [100].

induction of anesthesia. Alternatively, pulse pressure variation (PPV) and plethysmographic variability index (PVI) can be useful for identifying a patient's response to volume replacement with increases in stroke index and cardiac index [103]. Briefly, cyclic oscillations in the amplitude of the plethysmographic waveform recorded by pulse oximetry during positive pressure ventilation are a result of decreased venous return (Figure 16.6). This is often associated with hypovolemia and additional fluid therapy is recommended. A metabolic acidosis routinely accompanies patients with GI disease and dehydration. This can be corrected with a balanced crystalloid solution

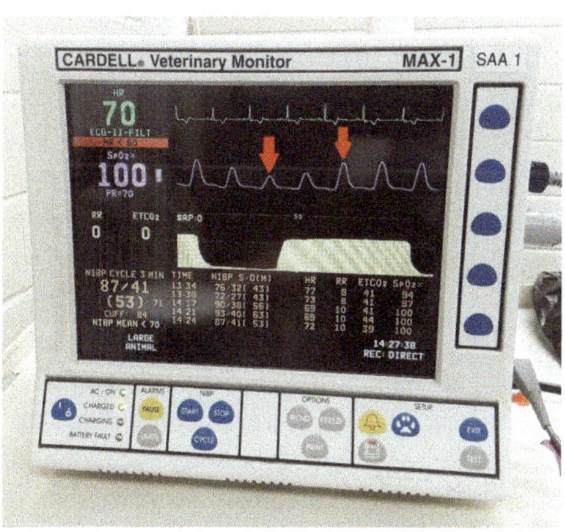

Figure 16.6 An example of plethysmographic variability. Note the cyclic oscillations in the amplitude of the plethysmographic waveform recorded by pulse oximetry during positive pressure ventilation (red arrows).

such as LRS or Plasma-Lyte. The crystalloid solution 0.9% sodium chloride is considered more acidic (pH is approximately 5.0) than other balanced solutions (LRS, pH is approximately 6.5) and is not recommended for resuscitation in patients with a metabolic acidosis.

Gurneys, operating tables, and anesthesia equipment should be thoroughly disinfected prior to next use. Particular attention should focus on equipment that could result in fecal–oral transmission (i.e., esophageal temperature probes). Contact with nonessential personnel should be kept to a minimum and it is recommended that those involved with the patient perioperatively wear disposable gloves and gowns. If possible, patients with GI infections should be scheduled for surgery toward the end of the day to allow for the operating room to undergo additional cleaning to minimize transmission between patients.

Bloodstream Infections

Catheter- and Drug-Related Infections

Bloodstream infections (BSIs) are associated with the use of central venous catheters (CVCs) and contaminated injectable anesthetics (i.e., propofol). Mortality associated with human catheter-related BSIs is as high as 10%, and is usually related to endocarditis, metastatic pulmonary infection, and septic shock [104, 105].

In veterinary medicine, jugular-catheter-associated infections were reported to be between 4% and 25%, with a mortality rate of <1% [106, 107]. CVCs are useful for the administration of fluids, blood products, parenteral nutrition and medications, repeat blood sampling, and central venous pressure measurements. However, they can be a biofilm surface and port for infections into the bloodstream. Organisms isolated from CVCs in humans tend to be multidrug-resistant Gram-positive and Gram-negative bacteria and fungi. In veterinary medicine, more than 50% of organisms isolated from positive bacterial cultured CVCs were *Klebsiella* spp. and *Enterobacter* spp. [108]. Risk factors for BSI with CVCs include hospitalization in the ICU, immunosuppression, neutropenia, parenteral nutrition, dextrose administration, multilumen catheters, jugular vein site, increased blood sampling, changing of fluid lines, inadequate skin preparation, inexperience of the placer, and catheter duration (>72 h) [108, 109]. Extraluminal colonization occurs from contaminants found on the skin around the catheter insertion site or from the hands of the individual placing the catheter. Intraluminal colonization occurs from seeding of the catheter hematogenously, infusion of a contaminated solution, or over guidewire exchange of the catheter [110]. Strict aseptic technique should be followed during placement of intravascular catheters and that proper care and maintenance are performed to reduce the risk for contamination. The use of povidone-iodine or alcohol is less effective than chlorhexidine as a sole decontamination agent [111].

Contaminated propofol also contributes to BSIs [40, 112]. The lipophilic nature of propofol supports the growth of bacterial and fungal microorganisms. The most common microorganisms associated with propofol-related iatrogenic infections include *Candida albicans*, *Staphylococcus* spp., *Enterobacter* spp., *Klebsiella pneumoniae*, *Enterococcus coli*, and *Serratia marcescens* [40, 113]. In one healthy dog requiring a routine dental scaling, *Ochrobactrum anthropi*–contaminated propofol resulted in mortality within 24 h following its administration [112]. Strict aseptic handling of propofol is strongly recommended. This includes disinfection of the surface of the vial's rubber stopper and for the anesthetist to draw up propofol just before use [41] (Figure 16.7). Propofol left unopened and unrefrigerated for >12 h should be discarded. Alfaxalone supports the growth of some microorganisms (*E. coli*), but less than that of propofol. Bacteria required a longer lag phase (>24 h) when growing in alfaxalone, suggesting it is a poorer growth medium when compared to propofol [113]. The coadministration of lidocaine or thiopental with propofol may result in bacteriostatic activity against *E. coli* or bactericidal activity against *S. aureus* and *E. coli*, respectively [56, 113].

Clinical Signs

Dogs with bacteremia exhibit some combination of lethargy, anorexia, vomiting, diarrhea, fever, lameness, and muscle pain. Infective or immune-mediated arthritis may develop. Abdominal or lumbar pain on palpation may indicate inflammation of the kidney or spleen (septic embolization, abscess, or infarction) or discospondylitis. Bacteremic or septic patients can develop organ failure and septic shock. In dogs, organ systems most affected and the order in which they are affected are as follows: GI tract, liver, kidneys, and lungs. A cardiac murmur and/or arrhythmia may indicate endocarditis. In cats with bacteremia, anorexia, fever, and shifting leg lameness are clinical signs. Heart murmurs are present with endocarditis. The lung is the shock organ in the cat, and respiratory failure can occur early in sepsis. Serum chemistry abnormalities such as an albumin of $<2.5\,\mathrm{mg\,dl^{-1}}$, a twofold or greater increase in alkaline phosphatase (ALP), and hypoglycemia ($<80\,\mathrm{mg\,dl^{-1}}$) are indicative of bacteremia. Hyperbilirubinemia, bilirubinuria, and icterus can occur [114].

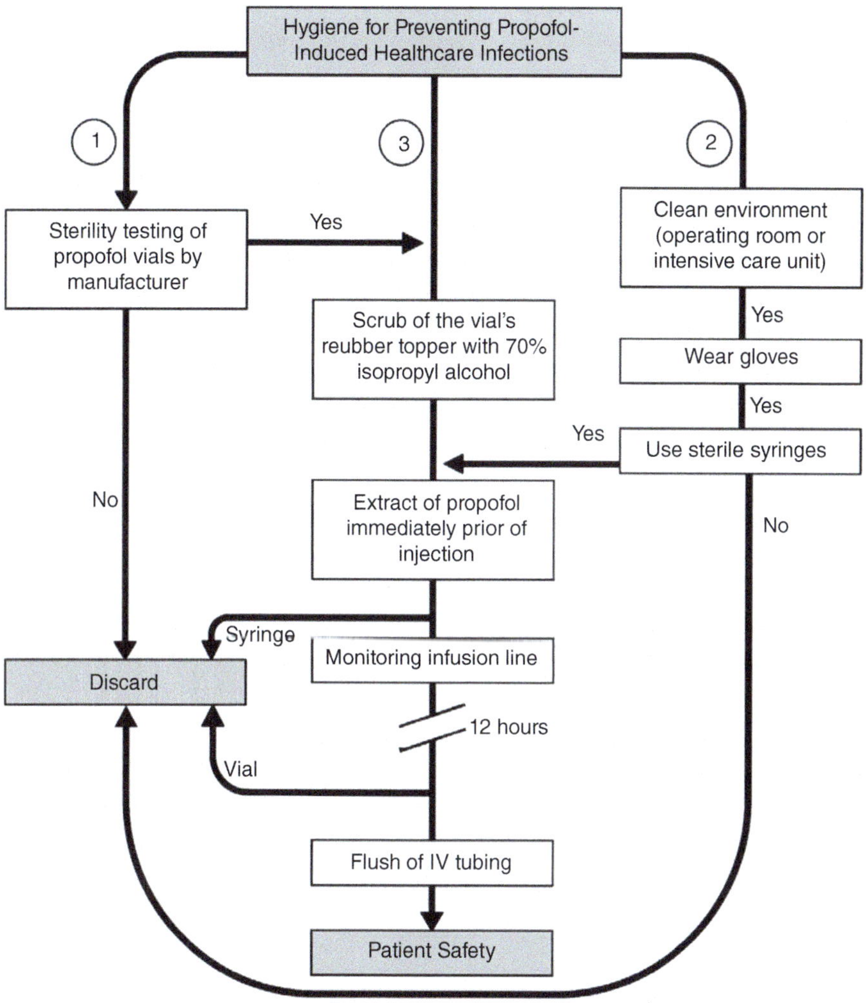

Figure 16.7 Algorithm to reduce the likelihood of infectious disease events when using propofol. To avoid intrinsic contamination, sufficient quality control during the manufacturing process is required (1). Personnel must be aware of the importance of performing healthcare procedures in a clean environment and the use of gloves and sterile syringes for anesthetic procedures. Syringes and needles must never be reused (2). Also, the aseptic technique for administration of propofol includes cleaning of the rubber bung, if present, with isopropyl alcohol, leaving it to dry. Propofol should be drawn up immediately before its use and not left standing. Intravenous (IV) infusion lines and stopcock dead spaces should be completely flushed to ensure no residual propofol remains. Vials must be discarded after opening for single use, no matter the amount of the remainder (3) [40].

Diagnosis

Catheter- and drug-related BSIs are diagnosed via clinical signs (fever, hypotension, tachycardia, depressed mentation, lethargy, hypoglycemia, and leukocytosis), no other obvious source of a BSI, and culture of the suspect organism from both peripheral blood and the CVC or contaminated drug vial. The catheter can be removed, and the tip and subcutaneous portions cultured. Diagnosis can be made without removing the catheter by obtaining positive cultures from the CVC and peripheral blood [115].

The catheter site should be inspected before removal for signs of discharge, swelling, redness, or pain at or below the site of insertion. In any patient with a persistent fever of unknown origin and negative blood cultures, the catheter should be removed, and the tip cultured. Antimicrobial therapy should be empirically instituted using the following guidelines: the patient is critically ill, the catheter was indwelling for >48 h, evidence of catheter site infection, fever (>103.5 °F), systolic blood pressure <90 mmHg, tachycardia, or leukocytosis (Table 16.8) [105, 108, 116, 117, 118].

Table 16.8 Strategies to reduce the incidence of BSI [105, 108, 116, 117, and 118].

Wash hands and use aseptic technique when placing and handling all catheters.
Prepare the skin aseptically before insertion of any catheter.
Central venous catheters should be placed by skilled individuals, using sterile technique.
The number of ports and catheter manipulations should be minimized.
Catheters should be secured in a way to reduce movement, and the site should be clean and protected from contamination.
Central venous catheters should be removed as soon as possible.

Non-catheter- or drug-related sources for BSI include infections of the GI, genitourinary and respiratory tracts, skin, wounds, abdomen, and biliary tree. In cats with bacteremia, causes include pyothorax, GI tract disease, septic peritonitis, pyelonephritis, pneumonia, pyometra, endocarditis, osteomyelitis, and bite wounds (Table 16.9) [114].

The time course of the bacteremia should be related to the infecting organism; however, this is not always possible. Several stages of bacteremia exist and are described in the following sections (Table 16.10) [114].

Anesthetic Management

In many perioperative settings, anesthesiologists are responsible for the placement of CVCs, but may not be informed of the best practices to reduce contamination. The CDC has identified six key interventions to reduce the incidences of catheter-related BSIs (Table 16.11) [118]. Due to the increased rate of BSIs in patients with medical disease or higher ASA status (≥4) [107], anesthetists should be extremely stringent regarding CDC recommendations. Immunocompromised patients should be administered a new vial of propofol for sedation or induction of anesthesia.

Table 16.9 Risk factors for bacteremia in dogs and cats [114].

Infectious diseases	Sources of infection	Causes of immunocompromise	Iatrogenic causes
Ehrlichiosis	Abscesses	Diabetes mellitus	Dental prophylaxis
FIV	Burns	Hepatic failure	Oral, abdominal, urogenital, or perianal surgery
FeLV	Colitis	Renal failure	Invasive or protracted surgery
Canine parvoviral enteritis	Gingivitis	Tumors	Endoscopic procedures
Feline panleukopenia	Stomatitis	Hematologic malignancies	IV catheterization
	Pyoderma	Glucocorticoids	Narrow-spectrum or low-dose antimicrobial therapy
	Urogenital infection	Cytotoxic drugs	Urogenital tract manipulation
	Penetrating wounds	Phagocytic defects	Immunosuppressive therapy
	Bowel injuries	Shock	
	Musculoskeletal infection	Splenectomy	
		Congenital heart defects	
		Advanced age	

FeLV: feline leukemia virus; FIV: feline immunodeficiency virus.

Table 16.10 Stages of bacteremia [114].

	Time course	Likely organism	Comments
Peracute	Several hours	Gram-positive or Gram-negative	Debilitated or immunosuppressed
Acute	12–24 h	Gram-negative or staphylococcal	
Subacute	Weeks	Gram-positive or anaerobic	
Chronic	Weeks to months	Microorganisms of low toxicity (*Staphylococcus intermedius, Brucella canis*)	Sequestration of bacteria on heart valves, in bone; abscess in liver, spleen, kidney, or muscle; partial response to antimicrobial therapy

Table 16.11 The Centers for Disease Control's six key interventions to reduce the incidence of catheter-related blood system infections [118].

1) Appropriate hand hygiene with handwashing with soap and water or an alcohol cleanser immediately prior to placement
2) Use of personal protective equipment and maximal sterile barrier precautions (surgical cap, mask, sterile gown, and sterile drape)
3) Aseptic prep of the insertion area with >0.5% chlorhexidine and alcohol
4) Conduct routine inspections of the catheter area and remove when deemed unnecessary
5) Educate healthcare personnel regarding proper procedures for insertion and maintenance, periodically assess knowledge of and adherence to guidelines, and designate only trained personal who demonstrate CVC placement and maintenance competence
6) Use of sterile gauze or sterile transparent, semipermeable dressing to cover the catheter site

Anesthetists should avoid the accidental injection of environmental air into the vial during extraction, sun exposure and high temperatures to the vial, and repeated withdrawals from the same vial [112]. Anesthetic management of patients with bacteremia is similar to those with septicemia.

Sepsis

Sepsis is as a clinical syndrome involving one or multiple organ systems caused by a bacterial, viral, protozoal, or fungal infection and the patient's systemic inflammatory response to that infection [119]. Sepsis starts out localized and becomes systemic. Sepsis can be life-threatening because of the causative organisms themselves, their toxins, and the body's own inflammatory response. Mortality rates associated with sepsis in dogs and cats are approximately 47% and 44%, respectively [120, 121]. Origins of sepsis include the peritoneal cavity (GI perforation), soft tissue (bite wounds, necrotizing fasciitis [NF]), bone (osteomyelitis), blood-borne (intravenous catheter, contaminated drugs), and the pulmonary (pneumonia), GI (bacterial translocation), reproductive (pyometra, prostatitis), urinary (pyelonephritis), and cardiovascular (endocarditis) systems. Sources for sepsis associated with Gram-negative bacteria (*Enterococcus* spp.) sources include the GI tract and genitourinary systems. Gram-positive bacteria (*Staphylococci* spp. and *Streptococci* spp.) sources include the skin, soft tissue, and intravenous catheters. The most commonly involved organisms are thought to be *Staphylococci* spp., *Streptococci* spp., and *E. coli* [114].

Cell wall components of Gram-negative (lipopolysaccharide) and Gram-positive (lipoteichoic acid and peptidoglycan) bacteria activate macrophages, neutrophils, and the production of proinflammatory factors such as tumor necrosis factor alpha (TNF-α), interleukin (IL)-1, IL-6, IL-8, and interferon γ, as well as counter-inflammatory mediators such as IL-4, IL-10, IL-13, transforming growth factor β, and glucocorticoids. Counter-inflammatory host responses turn off production of the pro-inflammatory cytokines [122]. There is normally a balance between proinflammatory and anti-inflammatory responses; however, the compensatory anti-inflammatory response makes the patient more susceptible to infection from the causative and opportunistic organisms. With sepsis, a systemic inflammatory response syndrome (SIRS) can occur, and the result is activation of the complement system and coagulation cascade. The clinical result ranges from multiple organ dysfunction syndrome (MODS) to death.

Clinical Signs

Signs are nonspecific, and the presenting complaint depends on the source of the infection. Sepsis is often associated with loss of vasomotor tone, a hypercoagulable state, increased vascular permeability, and microcirculatory derangements. Cardiovascular, pulmonary, renal, hepatic, and intestinal dysfunction, hypothermia, oliguria, respiratory failure, and lactic acidosis may also be present [114]. SIRS is a defining component of sepsis and is described by the following: fever, tachycardia, tachypnea, and an inflammatory leukogram. Definitions for SIRS in dogs and cats have been published. For dogs, SIRS is diagnosed based on the presence of two or more of the following criteria: body temperature $<38\,°C$ or $>42\,°C$, heart rate >120 beats min^{-1} in a calm dog, hyperventilation ($PaCO_2 <30$ mmHg), white blood cell count $>18\,000\,ml^{-1}$ or $<5000\,ml^{-1}$ or $>5\%$ bands [119]. For cats, SIRS is diagnosed based on the presence of two or more of the following criteria: body temperature $<38\,°C$ or $>42\,°C$, heart rate >140 beats min^{-1} in a calm cat, respiratory rate >20 breaths min^{-1} or $PaCO_2 <28$ mmHg, white blood cell count $>18\,000\,ml^{-1}$ or $<5000\,ml^{-1}$ or $>5\%$ bands [46]. Septic shock is defined by SIRS coupled with hypotension, lactic acidosis, and progressive organ dysfunction. Clinical findings of MODS and their implications are listed in the following section. Disseminated intravascular coagulation (DIC) and respiratory distress syndrome are terminal states (Table 16.12).

Diagnosis

The patient's history, physical examination findings, diagnostic findings, and isolation of the specific causative organisms can aid in the diagnosis of sepsis (Table 16.13) [119, 123]. Cultures should be submitted from blood, urine, wounds, body cavity fluid, and all suspected sources of organism growth.

Anesthetic Management

Anesthesia and surgery should be postponed until the sepsis is at least partially treated and the patient is stable. However, the source of sepsis sometimes requires urgent surgical intervention. Therapy consists of removing

Table 16.12 Multiple organ dysfunction syndrome.

Clinical findings	Implication
Cool extremities, oliguria, lactic acidosis	Tissue hypoperfusion
Oliguria	Renal failure
Hyperbilirubinemia	Liver failure
Respiratory distress syndrome	Pulmonary compromise
DIC (disseminated intravascular coagulation): prolonged PT and aPTT, low fibrinogen, increased fibrinogen degradation products	Failure of the coagulation system

Table 16.13 Diagnostic criteria for sepsis in people.

	Human parameters
General variables	
Fever	Core temperature > 38.3 °C
Hypothermia	Core temperature < 36 °C
Heart rate	> 90 beats min^{-1}
Tachypnea	
Altered mental status	
Edema or positive fluid balance	> 20 ml kg^{-1} per 24 h
Hyperglycemia	> 120 mg dl^{-1} in the absence of diabetes
Inflammatory variables	
Leukocytosis	WBC count > 12 000 μl^{-1}
Leukopenia	WBC count < 4000 μl^{-1}
Normal WBC count with > 10% immature forms	
Plasma C-reactive protein	> 2 SD above normal value
Plasma procalcitonin	> 2 SD above normal value
Tissue perfusion variables	
Hyperlactatemia	> 1 mmol l^{-1}
Decreased capillary refill or mottling	
Other variables	
$ScvO_2$	> 70%
Cardiac index	> 3.5 l min^{-1}

WBC: white blood cell count; SD: standard deviation; $ScvO_2$: central venous oxygen saturation. *Source:* Adapted with permission from: Boller and Otto [119].

the infection, aggressive and appropriate antimicrobial administration, goal-directed fluid therapy, and treatment of multisystem disturbances. Antimicrobial drugs and doses should be administered 30 min before surgical incision and repeated every 90 min during surgery. Optimization of renal function should be performed before anesthesia with appropriate fluid therapy and diuresis to maximize intravascular volume and support renal blood flow. Albumin and total protein levels should be monitored, and colloids and/or plasma should be administered to support oncotic pressure and minimize edema formation and third spacing of fluids. PCV should be monitored, and transfusion of red blood cells may be required to maintain a PCV of approximately 20–25% or greater. Patients with sepsis often are hypoglycemic, and blood glucose should be monitored, and dextrose supplementation provided to maintain normoglycemia.

Hemodynamic stabilization is best performed before anesthesia, with the goals of optimizing tissue perfusion, oxygen delivery to the tissues, and cardiac output. Fluid resuscitation should be targeted to achieve a mean arterial pressure > 65 mmHg, central venous pressure of 8–12 mmHg, a normal pH without metabolic acidosis, a mixed venous oxygen saturation > 70%, and adequate urine output [124]. Heart rate, pulse rate and quality, mucous membrane color, capillary refill time, respiratory rate, lung sounds, mentation, blood pressure, and an assessment of urine production should be documented before anesthesia and could be good indicators of resuscitative efforts. Thoracic radiographs can establish the status of the pulmonary system. Patients with respiratory signs or evidence of pulmonary disease should have blood oxygen saturation levels monitored perioperatively.

A balanced multimodal premedication, induction, and maintenance protocol should be used in patients with sepsis. Acepromazine should be avoided because of its long-lasting vasodilatory properties, hypotension, and inhibition of platelet function. The use of dexmedetomidine, an alpha-2 adrenoreceptor agonist, is controversial due to its dose-dependent negative effects on cardiac output. However, recently it has been suggested that dexmedetomidine may decrease mortality and inhibit inflammation in humans with sepsis [125]. Specifically, it has been shown to alleviate heart injury during sepsis and provide neuro-, hepatic-, renal-, pulmonary-, and splenic-protective properties when administered as a bolus or constant rate infusion (CRI) [125]. Currently, there are limited studies evaluating its efficacy in septic veterinary patients and therefore should be used with caution. If incorporated into the anesthesia regimen, doses likely should be kept to a minimum (approximately $\leq 0.5\,\mu g\,kg^{-1}\,h^{-1}$). Opioids can be used for premedication, with or without a benzodiazepine. These classes of drugs have very little impact on cardiovascular variables, and heart rate, cardiac output, and blood pressure remain stable. Pure mu-opioid receptor agonists are recommended over mixed and partial mu-opioid receptor agonists because of their superior analgesia- and inhalant-sparing properties. Caution should be used with morphine administration due to its histaminic effects. Etomidate transiently suppresses the hypothalamic–pituitary–adrenal axis. There is concern that the adrenal insufficiency may be worsened by even a single dose of etomidate in patients with sepsis [126]; however, a single dose of etomidate during induction in critical human patients diagnosed with severe sepsis and septic shock did not increase mortality, vasopressor use, or length of stay in the ICU [127]. Locoregional techniques should be incorporated when possible, except epidural analgesia which is contraindicated in patients with septicemia and bacteremia [128]. Performing an epidural in these patients may result in bacterial contamination of the spinal canal, particularly with accidental puncture of a venous plexus. If locoregional techniques cannot be administered, analgesia should be provided via a CRI of fentanyl or another opioid with a short half-life, lidocaine and/or ketamine. Lidocaine provides analgesia, inhalant-sparing effects, and possesses anti-inflammatory properties [129]. At clinical doses, it also has been reported to attenuate the hypotensive effects associated with endotoxemia in rabbits [130]. Lidocaine CRIs should be used with caution in feline patients due to its deleterious effects on cardiac output [131]. Higher lidocaine doses can further contribute to vasodilation and hypotension, and, therefore, lower clinical doses are recommended. Subanesthetic doses of ketamine ($0.5\,mg\,kg^{-1}$ IV followed by $0.12\,mg\,kg^{-1}\,h^{-1}$) administered to dogs with lipopolysaccharide-induced endotoxemia suppressed TNF-α activity [132]. Further benefits of ketamine in small-animal septic patients require additional investigation. Isoflurane, sevoflurane, or desflurane are also used for the maintenance of anesthesia but should be administered cautiously due to their dose-dependent cardiopulmonary depressant effects.

Hypotension should be treated by reducing the vaporizer concentration, administering adequate crystalloids and colloids, and incorporating positive inotropes or vasopressors (Table 16.14) [133]. The addition of a positive inotrope, such as a dobutamine, dopamine, or norepinephrine CRI, may be needed to treat myocardial depression. It is not uncommon for septic patients to require massive volumes of IV fluids during general anesthesia. Venous access is imperative, and direct arterial blood pressure monitoring, central venous pressure (CVP), PPV, and PVI monitoring can be useful for goal-directed fluid therapy. The mean arterial blood pressure should be at a minimum of 60 mmHg to support blood flow to the brain, heart, and kidneys. Ventilation should be assisted manually or mechanically, if needed, to maintain normocapnia and adequate oxygenation. Septic patients may already have pulmonary compromise and be tachypneic

Table 16.14 Dosages for commonly used positive inotropes and vasopressors [133].

Drug	Dose (IV)	Comments
Dobutamine	2–10 mcg kg^{-1} min^{-1} (dogs)	Increases contractility. Arrhythmogenic at high doses (>10 mcg kg^{-1} min^{-1})
Dopamine	3–20 mcg kg^{-1} min^{-1}	Increases contractility. Increases vascular tone at high doses (>10 mcg kg^{-1} min^{-1}). Potentially arrhythmogenic at high doses (>10 mcg kg^{-1} min^{-1})
Ephedrine	0.05–0.2 mg kg^{-1}	Increases contractility, vascular tone, and heart rate. Can be administered IV or IM
Phenylephrine	0.4–3 mcg kg^{-1} min^{-1}	May cause profound bradycardia. May reduce cardiac output and skeletal muscle blood flow
Norepinephrine	0.05–2 mcg kg^{-1} min^{-1}	Increases heart rate, systemic and pulmonary vascular resistance, coronary blood flow, and cardiac output. Results in less tachycardia than epinephrine
Epinephrine	0.005–1 mcg kg^{-1} min^{-1}	Increases heart rate, contractility, and systemic vascular resistance. Dramatic increases in vascular tone may result in tissue hypoxia. Decreases the threshold for ventricular fibrillation and increased incidence of premature ventricular contractions
Vasopressin	0.5–2 mcg kg^{-1} min^{-1}	Potent nonadrenergic vasoconstrictor via V_{1a} receptors. Vasoconstriction is dose-dependent and at low doses can cause cerebral, renal, pulmonary, and mesenteric vessel vasodilation

IV: intravenous; IM: intramuscular; V_{1a}: Vasopressin receptor 1a.

and hypoxic before anesthesia. Caution should be taken with overventilating septic patients because positive pressure ventilation decreases venous return and may impair cardiac output. In patients with normal pH and oxygenation, permissive hypercapnia ($PaCO_2$ is approximately 50–55 mmHg) is well tolerated and may be beneficial (increases heart rate and cardiac output via sympathetic nervous system stimulation) [134]. Arterial blood gas and serum biochemistry values should be monitored throughout the perioperative period. Frequency of monitoring blood work is dependent on the severity of abnormalities.

Postoperative care should continue to support cardiovascular, respiratory, and renal functions, and adequate analgesia should be provided. Multisystem monitoring is highly recommended for at least the first 48–72 h following general anesthesia and surgery. Arterial blood gas, PCV, total protein, lactate, glucose, and electrolytes should be analyzed during the recovery period. It should be ascertained that the patient is ventilating adequately on its own before extubation ($ETCO_2$ between 35 and 50 mmHg). Supplemental oxygen should be provided if the SpO_2 on room air is <93% or the PaO_2 is <80 mmHg. Continuation of blood pressure support drugs throughout the recovery period may be required.

Cutaneous Infections

Necrotizing Fasciitis

Necrotizing Fasciitis (NF) is a rapidly progressive and potentially life-threatening condition. It originates in the fascial and subcutaneous tissues with the possibility of spreading systemically resulting in septic shock [135, 136]. There are few reports of NF in dogs and cats, but beta-hemolytic *Streptococcus* is the most common bacteria cultured [137]. *S. marcescens*, *Streptococcus* spp., *E. coli*, MRSA, and *Pasteurella multocida* have also been reported in dogs and cats [138–143]. In 10% of cats, *S. canis* is present in the nasal cavity and can cause fatal NF and septic arthritis [143]. In addition, streptococci of Lancefield group G is a rare cause of NF in humans, but it appears to be the major cause in dogs [144, 145].

Most often, the bacteria are commensal organisms in dogs and cats, and infection of fascial tissues may occur when the normal skin barrier is damaged; for example, following dog or cat bites, cat scratch, history of surgery or radiation therapy, minor trauma, and skin infection [136, 141, 142]. In most cases, there is a history of mild injury to the skin several days before the onset of clinical signs. One canine patient developed NF at a site in which it received radiation therapy 33 months prior [142]. In some cases, there was no previous history of trauma [138]. People with diabetes mellitus, peripheral vascular disease, or other immunosuppressive conditions may have an increased risk of developing NF [135, 146]. It is not known whether the same is true for small animals.

After the invasion of the subcutaneous space, local tissue destruction is secondary to bacterial production of exotoxins and proteinases. Necrotic tissue provides a medium for bacterial growth and further tissue destruction. The damage initially spreads horizontally within the subcutaneous tissues and superficial fascia. With progression, the underlying muscle and overlying skin may develop ischemic necrosis from bacterial toxin-induced vasoconstriction or thrombosis of vessels [137].

Clinical Signs

Initial clinical signs include localized edema, erythema, and pain at the affected site with tachycardia and fever. In people, most cases involve an extremity, but the perineum and trunk are also common sites. In the cases of canine NF, 77% of the dogs had limb involvement. The other reported sites were the neck and ventral thorax [145, 147]. Systemic signs of shock including fever, tachycardia, lethargy, tachypnea, mental depression, anorexia, and poor peripheral perfusion are common. Patients may even show signs of lameness if isolated to the extremities. Streptococcal toxic shock syndrome (STSS) is the term used to describe the rapidly progressive, hypotensive shock and multiple organ failure that occur with severe streptococcal infection. The syndrome can occur secondary to NF or because of streptococcal infections of other organs. The pathogenesis of STSS involves bacterial exotoxin production, secondary cytokine release in large amounts, and subsequent shock and organ failure. Mortality increases in dogs with NF and STSS [144].

Diagnosis

Diagnosis is based on clinical signs, surgical findings, histopathologic results, and a positive culture (Figure 16.8). However, because the disease progresses so rapidly, successful management depends on starting therapy before culture and histopathology results are available. People exhibit extreme pain that does not match the

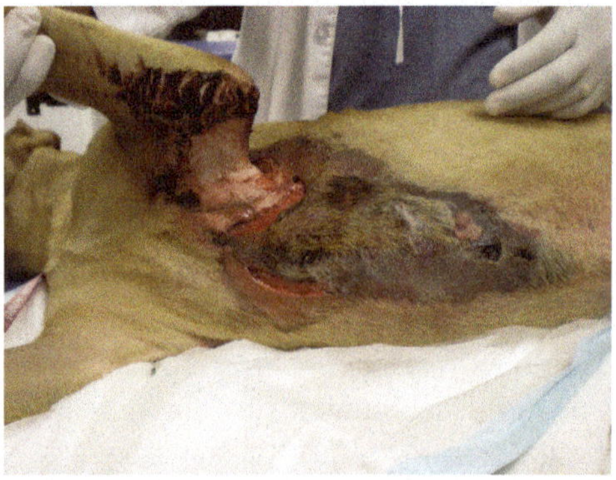

Figure 16.8 A patient diagnosed with necrotizing fasciitis along the right axillary and ventral thoracic regions. *Source:* Photo courtesy of Dr. Kelley Thieman.

appearance of the affected area. In humans, computed tomography (CT) and MRI have been used to document fascial involvement and delineate the extent of tissue damage. In one reported case in a dog, a fistulogram was used to show extension of contrast material along the fascial planes [147]. The absence of such findings on diagnostic imaging should not exclude the diagnosis of NF. Results of blood tests are often nonspecific and reflect systemic inflammation, sepsis, vasculitis, or organ dysfunction. There may be a leukocytosis, thrombocytopenia, coagulopathy, electrolyte abnormalities, hyperglycemia, and acidosis [122]. The hallmark surgical finding in people and dogs is the ease of separation of fascia from other tissues by blunt dissection. Large amount of exudative fluid in the subcutaneous spaces of the affected area is another common finding. To get a definitive diagnosis, tissue for culture should be obtained from the leading edge of the affected area. Samples from the center of the wound are more likely to contain secondary invading organisms [147]. Gram staining of fine-needle aspirates or impression smears may reveal chains of Gram-positive cocci.

Treatment

Successful treatment of NF depends on early and complete surgical debridement of necrotic tissues, and multiple surgeries are often required. Surgery performed within the first 24 h of diagnosis leads to survival rates as high as 70%; however, if postponed to ≥24 h, it can be as low as 35% [147]. In people, surgical exploration is performed every 24–48 h, until the infection is completely removed. Amputation of a limb is sometimes needed to completely remove infected tissues. Other essential components of therapy are hemodynamic support, wound care, appropriate antibiotics, analgesia, and nutritional support. Initial broad-spectrum antimicrobial therapy is recommended while waiting for culture results. In humans, the combination of penicillin, an aminoglycoside, and metronidazole or clindamycin is the most frequently suggested regime for NF [135, 148]. One retrospective study in humans showed a trend toward increased survival if the therapy included clindamycin [149]. The efficacy of enrofloxacin in dogs with NF has been questioned. The theory is that the use of enrofloxacin in dogs with *S. canis* infections may contribute to the emergence of NF and STSS. Bacterial virulence may be increased because fluoroquinolones may induce bacteriophages that encode superantigen genes [150]. A broad-spectrum antibiotic regimen that includes clindamycin is recommended.

Anesthetic Management

Anesthetic management for cases of NF is similar to cases with sepsis. The extent of the necrosis and severity of the infection may not be clear. The patient should be managed analogous to a case with septic shock and should be fluid-resuscitated before anesthesia. However, surgical debridement should not be postponed. Reliable venous access is essential, and blood should be crossmatched and available because of the risk of bleeding [122]. Postoperatively, these patients are at risk for developing multiple organ failure, and they should be managed in the ICU with continued hemodynamic support, antimicrobial therapy, analgesia, oxygen supplementation, and nutritional support.

Additional Common Infectious Diseases

Lyme Disease

Lyme disease is caused by the spirochete *Borrelia burgdorferi*. While cats can be infected, clinical disease from natural infection has not been reported in this species. The primary mode of transmission is from the three-host tick *Ixodes scapularis* in northeastern, mid-Atlantic, and adjacent areas of Canada; *Ixodes pacificus* in the Pacific states and Canada; and *Ixodes ricinus* in Europe [151]. Wild animal reservoirs for adult ticks are deer, birds, and small and large mammals. Domestic hosts are humans, dogs, and cats.

Clinical Signs

Most *B. burgdorferi*-seropositive dogs show no clinical signs. However, the two most common clinical manifestations include Lyme arthritis and Lyme nephritis [151]. On the rare occasion, a genetic breed disposition for fatal myocarditis has been reported in Boxer puppies [152]. It is currently unknown if infected cats will develop clinical illness. Clinical signs of systemic infection in dogs include fever, anorexia, joint swelling, lymphadenomegaly, and lethargy. These signs are usually responsive to antimicrobials. Polyarthritis marked by shifting leg lameness is a common clinical sign. The arthritis is transient, but the pathologic joint changes are progressive.

Dogs with Lyme nephropathy present with renal failure and anorexia, vomiting, lethargy, dehydration, polyuria, polydipsia, and muscle wasting. Protein-losing glomerulopathy has been described in naturally infected dogs. There can also be clinical signs attributable to vasculitis, thromboembolism, hypertension, uremia, and hypoproteinemia [151].

Diagnosis

Serology is the only recommended modality to evaluate for exposure to *B. burgdorferi* in dogs [151]. Validated serologic tests in North America include the SNAP 4Dx and SNAP 4Dx Plus, Quant C6, VETSCAN Rapid, and AccuPlex 4.

Anesthetic Management

Anesthetic management of dogs with Lyme disease should include a complete evaluation of renal function and diagnostics to document the level of hypoproteinemia and any associated clinical signs such as edema, ascites, pleural effusion, etc. Beta-lactams and tetracyclines are effective in reducing the clinical signs associated with Lyme arthritis in dogs. Doxycycline is recommended as the first choice of therapy because of its efficacy against coinfections (*Ehrlichia* spp., *Leptospira* spp.) and has anti-arthritic and anti-inflammatory properties [151]. Patients with moderate to severe arthritis may require analgesics effective against neuropathic and "wind-up" pain such as ketamine, gabapentin, and/or amantadine. In cases of Lyme nephropathy, blood pressure should be measured, and hypertension should be noted and treated accordingly. Dogs should be as stable as possible regarding renal function before anesthesia and should be treated as a patient with renal dysfunction (see Chapter 6). Anesthetic protocols should support renal function, and treatment of hypoproteinemia should be instituted if clinically indicated. Hypoproteinemia, especially hypoalbuminemia, decreases colloid oncotic pressure, resulting in peripheral edema, hypovolemia, and hypotension. It also prolongs the duration of action of anesthetic drugs that routinely require protein binding for inactivation. Further information on management of hypoproteinemia can be found elsewhere. Patients with concurrent nausea and vomiting may also benefit from antiemetics.

Ehrlichiosis

The genus Ehrlichia is made up of Gram-negative intracellular bacteria that are transmitted both trans- and intra-stadially by the brown dog tick (*Rhipicephalus sanguineus*) and infect monocytes, macrophages, and granulocytes. Canine monocytotropic ehrlichiosis (CME) is caused by *Ehrlichia canis*, an obligate intracellular coccoid bacterium. *Ehrlichia chaffeensis* is the cause of human monocytotropic ehrlichiosis. *E. canis* is a known cause of morbidity and mortality in dogs in Asia, Europe, Africa, and the United States. Members of the family Canidae are hosts, and reservoir hosts are the domestic dog, fox, coyote, and jackal [153].

After a 1–3-week incubation period following blood transfusion or tick attachment, there are three phases of infection: (i) acute (duration of 14–28 days), (ii) subclinical (months to years), and (iii) chronic phases. Most dogs in the acute phase will recover with adequate treatment, whereas dogs that are not treated or those treated inappropriately may enter the subclinical phase. Dogs in this phase may have subnormal platelet counts, and they may be clinically healthy carriers of *E. canis* for months to years [153]. Persistently infected dogs may spontaneously recover or develop chronic disease. Chronic disease is associated with bone marrow aplasia and peripheral blood pancytopenia. Significantly lower platelets, leukocytes, and hematocrit are linked with a high mortality risk. Severe leukopenia and anemia, prolonged activated partial thromboplastin time (aPTT), and hypokalemia are all reliable predictors of mortality with 100% probability [154]. The most common hematologic abnormality of dogs infected with *E. canis* is thrombocytopenia, and this occurs in all phases of the disease. The pathogenesis of thrombocytopenia is multifactorial. Increased platelet consumption and decreased half-life are likely secondary to immune-mediated destruction and splenic sequestration. Dogs with *E. canis* infections have circulating antiplatelet antibodies and platelet migration-inhibition factor (PMIF), a serum cytokine produced by lymphocytes when they are exposed to infected monocytes [153]. Thrombocytopenia is accompanied by platelet dysfunction, and this combination contributes to bleeding seen with infection.

Clinical Signs

Dogs with acute disease are likely to be infested with ticks. Clinical signs of CME are multisystemic and include depression, lethargy, weight loss, anorexia, and bleeding. Abnormal hemostasis can manifest as epistaxis, hematuria, melena, prolonged bleeding following venipuncture, mucosal pallor, and petechiae and/or ecchymoses. Lymphadenomegaly and splenomegaly may be present in 20% and 25% of patients, respectively [155]. Ocular changes can include anterior uveitis and retinal changes. Dogs may develop changes in eye color or appearance or blindness secondary to paraproteinemia, systemic hypertension, hyphema, subretinal hemorrhage, and retinal detachment [156]. Meningitis or meningeal hemorrhage can result in seizures, stupor, acute central or peripheral vestibular dysfunction, cerebellar dysfunction, anisocoria, ataxia, intentional tremors, cervical pain, or hyperesthesia. Myelosuppression may develop during the acute or subclinical phases [157]. Concurrent infection with other tick-borne diseases or secondary bacterial, fungal, or protozoal infections are possible in dogs with ehrlichiosis. Patients with unresolved chronic disease may also develop ulcerative stomatitis and necrotic glossitis, and hind limb and/or scrotal edema [158]. Septicemia with the chronic illness is associated with a high mortality rate.

Diagnosis

Diagnosis is based on travel history, living in an endemic area, tick infestation, clinical signs, hematologic abnormalities, and diagnostic tests such as serology and polymerase chain reaction. The typical hematologic abnormalities are a moderate to severe thrombocytopenia, mild anemia, and leukopenia.

Treatment

Treatment of *E. canis* consists of antimicrobial agents and supportive care. Therapy should begin as early as possible, as chronically infected dogs are generally unresponsive to treatment because of multisystemic infection and myelosuppression [153]. Efficacious drugs include tetracycline and chloramphenicol. Doxycycline $10\,\mathrm{mg\,kg^{-1}}$ by mouth once a day for 21–28 days is recommended by the 2002 American College of Veterinary Internal Medicine's ehrlichial consensus statement [159]. Clinical improvement can be seen within 24 h of starting therapy in dogs in the acute or mild chronic phase. The platelet count is usually within the reference range by 10–14 days after starting treatment. Dogs can become reinfected after treatment. Supportive treatment with intravenous fluids and blood transfusions may be indicated.

Anesthetic Management

Anesthesia should be postponed if possible until platelet numbers and function are improving. Supportive treatment with fluids and blood transfusions or blood products may be indicated. Patients should be blood-typed and crossmatched prior to anesthesia and surgery. Platelet-rich plasma or platelet concentrate may be required in an emergency in patients with continued blood loss and thrombocytopenia. If neither is available, fresh whole blood may be considered in a life-threatening situation. Fresh whole blood administered to a 20-kg dog at appropriate doses may increase platelet count by approximately 20 000–30 000 per microliter [160]. Desmopressin acetate (DDAVP) may be administered to treat platelet dysfunction at 1 $\mu g\,kg^{-1}$ subcutaneously 20–30 min before surgery and then every 24 h for a total of three treatments [161]. Acepromazine should be avoided because it may inhibit platelet function and results in the sequestration of red blood cells. Clinical signs such as tachypnea, tachycardia, and hypotension associated with blood loss and decreased oxygen delivery to tissues should be monitored closely. Aspirin should not be administered in the perioperative period because this drug irreversibly inhibits platelet function. Treatment with low immunosuppressive doses of glucocorticoids (e.g., 1–2 $mg\,kg^{-1}$ of prednisolone by mouth) for 2–7 days may be of benefit early on when the thrombocytopenia is severe [153]. Monitoring the response to treatment of ehrlichiosis is important because infection can persist for months to years. Platelet counts should be rechecked at least 1–3 months after treatment has been stopped. Further information on anesthesia of thrombocytopenic and anemic patients can be found in Chapter 14.

Leptospirosis

Leptospirosis, a zoonotic disease with worldwide distribution, is caused by the bacterial spirochete *Leptospira* species. Disease in dogs is caused mainly by *Leptospira interrogans* and *Leptospira kirschneri*. Cats do seroconvert after exposure to leptospires, but clinical disease is rarely reported. Infection occurs via direct or indirect transmission. Direct transmission is by contact with infected urine, placental and venereal transfer, bite wounds, or ingestion of infected tissue. Indirect transmission, which is more common, occurs by exposure of intact mucous membranes or broken skin to urine-contaminated water, soil, bedding, or food. Leptospires do not replicate outside of the host, but they can remain viable for months in soil that has been saturated with urine. A wide range of wild and domestic animals can host leptospires, including, but not limited to, rodents, raccoons, foxes, skunks, pigs, horses, sheep, goats, dogs, cats, cows, and deer [162]. Leptospires penetrate intact mucous membranes of the mouth, nose, or eyes, or abrasions of the skin, leading to a bacteremic phase, which can last up to 10 days [163]. Bacteria then replicate and invade the kidney, spleen, liver, central nervous system, genital tract, and eyes. The host immune response is activated, and once serum antibody levels increase, the host can clear the leptospires from most organs. Organisms can remain in the kidneys and be shed in the urine for weeks to months. Damage can occur to renal, hepatic, pulmonary, vascular, cardiac, and coagulation systems. Interstitial nephritis and tubular dysfunction are thought to result from kidney swelling, decreased renal blood flow, and decreased glomerular filtration. Acute tubular necrosis can occur. Vasculitis may also contribute to renal parenchymal damage. Hepatic dysfunction can occur without major histologic changes, and the degree of icterus usually correlates with the extent of hepatic necrosis. Chronic active hepatitis has been reported in dogs with leptospirosis. It is thought that hepatocellular injury and leptospires in the liver result in altered blood flow, fibrosis, and immune stimulation that perpetuate the chronic inflammatory response [162]. Acute pulmonary damage occurs secondary to the toxins from the organisms. Vasculitis can cause fluid exudation within the lungs. Rarely, severe acute pulmonary hemorrhage may occur.

Clinical Signs

Clinical signs include fever, anorexia, vomiting, muscle tenderness, myositis, reluctance to move, dehydration, cardiovascular collapse, petechiae, ecchymoses, melena, epistaxis, oliguria or anuria, icterus, hematemesis, hematochezia, conjunctivitis, or uveitis [162, 163]. Hematologic abnormalities are neutrophilia, lymphopenia, thrombocytopenia, prolonged coagulation times, and a mild nonregenerative anemia. Biochemistry abnormalities are azotemia, hypoalbuminemia, hyperbilirubinemia, hyperphosphatemia, hyperglycemia, hyponatremia, hypochloremia, hypokalemia, or hyperkalemia, and increases in ALP, alanine aminotransferase, aspartate aminotransferase, amylase, creatine kinase, and lipase. Normal serum potassium concentrations have been reported in patients with oliguria due to inhibition of Na^{+}-K^{+}-ATPase by bacterial endotoxins [164]. Abnormalities on the urinalysis include specific gravity ≤1.029, proteinuria, glucosuria, bilirubinuria, hematuria, increased granular casts, white blood cells, or an increased urine protein to creatinine ratio [162]. Thoracic radiographs may reveal a mild to moderate interstitial pattern [163]. Rarely, severe nodular interstitial to alveolar pattern is observed in cases with concurrent pulmonary hemorrhage [165]. Abdominal ultrasound may show renomegaly, intestinal wall thickening, increased echogenicity of the renal cortices, mild pyelectasia, medullary rim sign, and perirenal fluid [166]. Hepatomegaly, evidence of biliary sludge, and hypoechoic parenchyma have also been reported [166].

Diagnosis

The use of multiple diagnostic tests has been suggested due to the uncertainty of the timing of infection and the limitations of the tests themselves. Recommendations for the diagnosis of leptospirosis in dogs presenting with clinical signs include PCR of both blood and urine prior to antibiotic therapy along with paired microscopic agglutination test titers [167].

Treatment

Treatment consists of supportive care with intravenous fluids, centrally acting antiemetics, colloid administration to support vascular oncotic pressure, and antibiotics. Urine production should be monitored, and treatment of oliguria ($<2\,ml\,kg^{-1}\,h^{-1}$) may require the administration of mannitol, furosemide, and dopamine to promote diuresis. Persistent oliguria warrants consideration of peritoneal dialysis, hemodialysis, or continuous renal replacement therapy because acute renal dysfunction may be reversible [168]. Antibiotics should be administered as soon as leptospirosis is suspected because early treatment increases the chance for reversing tissue damage. Penicillin or ampicillin can be administered in the vomiting dog. Once oral medication can be tolerated, doxycycline $5\,mg\,kg^{-1}$ should be administered by mouth, every 12 h for 14 days. Concurrent administration of fluoroquinolones is not recommended because it contributes to antibiotic resistance, and efficacy has not been demonstrated [167]. Successful treatment results in gradual correction of azotemia within 10–14 days; damaged renal tissue may continue to regenerate for 4 weeks after treatment. Platelet counts usually improve within 1 week of starting treatment. Dogs treated late in the course of the disease may have permanent kidney damage.

Zoonotic Potential

Leptospirosis is a zoonotic disease, and precautions should be taken to avoid exposure to other animals and people caring for the patient. Gloves and a disposable gown should be worn when handling the patient to prevent contact with urine or blood. If aerosolization of urine is possible, such as when handling urinary catheters or collection systems or when cleaning, protective eyewear and a face mask should be worn [166]. An indwelling urinary catheter and collection system should be placed to reduce urine contamination of the environment. Leptospires are inactivated with routine disinfectants.

Anesthetic Management

Anesthetic management consists of optimizing renal function and hemodynamic stability. Anesthesia should be postponed until some improvement in renal function has been demonstrated. The degree of organ dysfunction should be noted, and hypovolemia, dehydration, electrolyte derangements, and acid–base disturbances should be corrected before anesthesia. Acepromazine should be avoided because of the associated vasodilation and hypotension. Opioids should be used to reduce induction drug requirements, reduce inhalant requirements, and provide analgesia. Drugs that are reversible or have a short duration of action should be used in patients with hepatic dysfunction. Remifentanil, a pure mu-opioid receptor agonist, is metabolized by nonspecific tissue and plasma cholinesterases, making it a good CRI option in patients with hepatic disease. Adequate intravenous fluids should be administered to support cardiovascular function and renal blood flow. Colloids may be required in cases with hypoalbuminemia. Close monitoring of the pulmonary system and serial arterial blood gas analysis are recommended in patients with pulmonary disease. Guidelines for anesthetic management of renal and hepatic dysfunction can be found in Chapters 4 and 6.

Feline Immunodeficiency Virus and Feline Leukemia Virus

FIV and FeLV belong to the retroviral family and are classified as a lentivirus and γ-retrovirus, respectively. FIV has many properties in common with other lentiviruses such as human immunodeficiency virus (HIV). FIV and FeLV are common around the world and are considered some of the most common infectious diseases among cats. Approximately 2% of healthy and 30% of high-risk or sick cats are infected in the United States [169]. FIV and FeLV are transmitted by inoculation of virus in saliva or blood, through biting or fighting wounds. Risk factors for FIV include male gender, adulthood, and outdoor access [170]. Kittens are more likely to develop severe clinical signs with FeLV [171]. Infection can be subclinical or clinical. Both infections result in immunologic dysregulation, affecting neutrophils, lymphocytes, cytokine production, immunoglobulin production, and other immune functions. Infected cats are at an increased risk for opportunistic infections, neurologic diseases, and neoplasia. Clinical stages of infection include an acute phase, a clinically asymptomatic phase, and a terminal phase. Progression is variable with a mortality of approximately 18% within the first five years after time of infection [170]. Unlike HIV-infected humans, cats that are in the feline acquired immunodeficiency syndrome (AIDS) phase may recover and become asymptomatic again. The asymptomatic phase can last weeks to years.

Clinical Signs

Cats infected with FeLV generally develop more severe clinical syndromes when compared to FIV-infected cats. The most common findings in cats with FeLV include various coinfections (FIV, feline infectious peritonitis, upper respiratory infection, hemotropic mycoplasmosis, and stomatitis), anemia, lymphoma, leukopenia or thrombocytopenia, and leukemia or myeloproliferative disease [170]. FeLV cats may also develop immune-mediated diseases such as autoimmune hemolytic anemia, glomerulonephritis, uveitis, and polyarthritis. A reduction in lymphocyte proliferation and function is also common.

During symptomatic FIV phases, clinical signs reflect secondary infections, myelosuppression, neoplasia (lymphoma and cutaneous squamous cell carcinoma), and neurologic disease. Reductions in $CD4^+$ cells in the peripheral blood and primary lymphoid tissue impair the body's humoral- and cell-mediated immune response. FIV-infected cats may have respiratory disease secondary to bacterial, fungal, protozoal, or parasitic infections. Chronic ulceroproliferative stomatitis is a common condition in FIV-infected cats and is thought to be from immune dysregulation or an immune response to chronic antigenic stimulation. Compared to noninfected cats, experimentally infected FIV cats have a higher prevalence of odontoclastic resorptive lesions [172]. Neurologic signs in FIV-infected cats can include behavioral changes, loss of bladder and rectal control, compulsive roaming, twitching of the face and tongue, seizures, weakness, and motor abnormalities. FIV-infected cats can have ocular inflammation (uveitis and chorioretinitis), renal insufficiency, lower urinary tract disease, and endocrinopathies such as hyperthyroidism and diabetes mellitus. Cats with FIV are also five times more likely to develop FeLV than noninfected cats [1]. Blood work abnormalities in FIV-infected cats may include a nonregenerative anemia, leukopenia, neutropenia, thrombocytopenia, and hyperglobulinemia. Cats that are FIV-positive should have an annual physical examination, complete blood count, biochemistry panel, and a urinalysis. Intensive diagnostics should be performed earlier in FIV-infected cats that are sick, so that a prompt diagnosis of secondary illness can be made; this enables timely therapeutic action and a successful treatment outcome [1].

Anesthetic Management

In humans, general anesthesia causes immunosuppression that occurs within 15 min of induction and that may last for 3–11 days [122]. Although this immunosuppression may not have a clinical impact in healthy patients, HIV-infected patients may be more susceptible to postoperative infections. Likewise, FIV- and FeLV-positive cats may be more susceptible to complications from the immunosuppression of anesthesia. The anesthetic period should be as short as possible, and anesthetic management and practice should minimize stress and optimize analgesia. Locoregional techniques should be used whenever possible to provide preemptive analgesia and to minimize inhalant requirements. Inhalants have been reported to further suppress the immune system and therefore total intravenous anesthesia may provide a better alternative [173]. The specific anesthetic plan would depend on the systems involved. Specific anesthetic management of these system abnormalities can be found elsewhere in this book.

References

1. Sellon, R.K. and Hartmann, K. (2012). Feline immunodeficiency virus infection. In: *Infectious Diseases of the Dog and Cat*, 4e (ed. C. Greene), 136–149. Philadelphia: WB Saunders Elsevier.
2. Richard, V.S., Mathai, E., and Cherian, T. (2001). Role of anaesthetic equipment in transmitting nosocomial infection. *J. Assoc. Phys. India* 49: 454–458.
3. Dubler, S., Zimmermann, S., Fischer, M. et al. (2016). Bacterial and viral contamination of breathing circuits after extended use - an aspect of patient safety? *Acta Anaesthesiol. Scand.* 60: 1251–1260.
4. Carter, J.A. (2006). The reuse of breathing systems in anesthesia. *Respir. Care Clin. North Am.* 12: 275–286.
5. Hogarth, I. (1996). Anaesthetic machine and breathing system contamination and the efficacy of bacterial/viral filters. *Anaesth. Int. Care* 24: 154–163.
6. Dugani, S., Kumar, A., and Wilkes, A.R. (2010). Influence of patient factors on the efficacy of breathing system filters at preventing contamination of breathing systems. *Anaesthesia* 65: 468–472.
7. Magath, T.B. (1938). Method for preventing cross-infection with gas machines. *Anesth. Analg.* 17: 215–217.

8 Pelligand, L., Hammond, R., and Rycroft, A. (2007). An investigation of the bacterial contamination of small animal breathing systems during routine use. *Vet. Anaesth. Analg.* 34: 190–199.

9 Leijten, D.T., Rejger, V.S., and Mouton, R.P. (1992). Bacterial contamination and the effect of filters in anaesthetic circuits in a simulated patient model. *J. Hosp. Infect.* 21: 51–60.

10 Hartmann, D., Jung, M., Neubert, T.R. et al. (2008). Microbiological risk of anaesthetic breathing circuits after extended use. *Acta Anaesthesiol. Scand.* 52: 432–436.

11 McGain, F., Algie, C.M., O'Toole, J. et al. (2014). The microbiological and sustainability effects of washing anaesthesia breathing circuits less frequently. *Anaesthesia* 69: 337–342.

12 Das, I. and Fraise, A.P. (1997). How useful are microbial filters in respiratory apparatus? *J. Hosp. Infect.* 37: 263–272.

13 du Moulin, G.C. and Hedley-Whyte, J. (1982). Bacterial interactions between anesthesiologists, their patients, and equipment. *Anesthesiology* 57: 37–41.

14 Buckley, P.M. (1984). Increase in resistance of in-line breathing filters in humidified air. *Br. J. Anaesth.* 56: 637–643.

15 Einav, S. and Wiener-Well, Y. (2017). Anesthesia in patients with infectious disease caused by multi-drug resistant bacteria. *Curr. Opin. Anaesthesiol.* 30: 426–434.

16 Crawford, S. and Weese, J.S. (2015). Efficacy of endotracheal tube disinfection strategies for elimination of *Streptococcus zooepidemicus* and *Bordetella bronchiseptica*. *J. Am. Vet. Med. Assoc.* 247: 1033–1036.

17 Negri de Sousa, A.C., Levy, C.E., and Freitas, M.I. (2013). Laryngoscope blades and handles as sources of cross-infection: an integrative review. *J. Hosp. Infect.* 83: 269–275.

18 Howell, V., Thoppil, A., Young, H. et al. (2013). Chlorhexidine to maintain cleanliness of laryngoscope handles: an audit and laboratory study. *Eur. J. Anaesthesiol.* 30: 216–221.

19 Hall, J.R. (1994). Blood contamination of anesthesia equipment and monitoring equipment. *Anesth. Analg.* 78: 1136–1139.

20 Gonzalez, E.A., Nandy, P., Lucas, A.D. et al. (2015). Ability of cleaning-disinfecting wipes to remove bacteria from medical device surfaces. *Am. J. Infect. Control* 43: 1331–1335.

21 Nandy, P., Lucas, A.D., Gonzalez, E.A. et al. (2016). Efficacy of commercially available wipes for disinfection of pulse oximeter sensors. *Am. J. Infect. Control* 44: 304–310.

22 Weese, J.S. (2008). A review of multidrug resistant surgical site infections. *Vet. Comp. Orthop. Traumatol.* 21: 1–7.

23 Albarellos, G.A., Montoya, L., Passini, S.M. et al. (2017). Cefazolin pharmacokinetics in cats under surgical conditions. *J. Feline Med. Surg.* 19: 992–997.

24 Gonzalez, O.J., Renberg, W.C., Roush, J.K. et al. (2017). Pharmacokinetics of cefazolin for prophylactic administration to dogs. *Am. J. Vet. Res.* 78: 695–701.

25 Sehulster, L. and Chinn, R.Y. (2003). Guidelines for environmental infection control in health-care facilities. Recommendations of CDC and the Healthcare Infection Control Practices Advisory Committee (HICPAC). *MMWR Recomm. Rep.* 52: 1–42.

26 Nicoll, C., Singh, A., and Weese, J.S. (2014). Economic impact of tibial plateau leveling osteotomy surgical site infection in dogs. *Vet. Surg.* 43: 899–902.

27 Nelson, L.L. (2011). Surgical site infections in small animal surgery. *Vet. Clin. North Am. Small Anim. Pract.* 41: 1041–1056.

28 Berrios-Torres, S.I., Umscheid, C.A., Bratzler, D.W. et al. (2017). Centers for Disease Control and prevention guideline for the prevention of surgical site infection, 2017. *JAMA Surg.* 152: 784–791.

29 Eugster, S., Schawalder, P., Gaschen, F. et al. (2004). A prospective study of postoperative surgical site infections in dogs and cats. *Vet. Surg.* 33: 542–550.

30 Brown, D.C., Conzemius, M.G., Shofer, F. et al. (1997). Epidemiologic evaluation of postoperative wound infections in dogs and cats. *J. Am. Vet. Med. Assoc.* 210: 1302–1306.

31 Andrade, N., Schmiedt, C.W., Cornell, K. et al. (2016). Survey of intraoperative bacterial contamination in dogs undergoing elective orthopedic surgery. *Vet. Surg.* 45: 214–222.

32 Vasseur, P.B., Levy, J., Dowd, E. et al. (1988). Surgical wound infection rates in dogs and cats. Data from a teaching hospital. *Vet. Surg.* 17: 60–64.

33 Nazarali, A., Singh, A., and Weese, J.S. (2014). Perioperative administration of antimicrobials during tibial plateau leveling osteotomy. *Vet. Surg.* 43: 966–971.

34 Mayhew, P.D., Freeman, L., Kwan, T. et al. (2012). Comparison of surgical site infection rates in clean and clean-contaminated wounds in dogs and cats after minimally invasive versus open surgery: 179 cases (2007–2008). *J. Am. Vet. Med. Assoc.* 240: 193–198.

35 Brown, G., Maddox, T., and Baglietto Siles, M.M. (2016). Client-assessed long-term outcome in dogs with surgical site infection following tibial plateau levelling osteotomy. *Vet. Rec.* 179: 409.

36 Barie, P.S. and Eachempati, S.R. (2005). Surgical site infections. *Surg. Clin. North Am.* 85: 1115–1135.

37 Beal, M.W., Brown, D.C., and Shofer, F.S. (2000). The effects of perioperative hypothermia and the duration of anesthesia on postoperative wound infection rate in clean wounds: a retrospective study. *Vet. Surg.* 29: 123–127.

38 Gachabayov, M., Senagore, A.J., Abbas, S.K. et al. (2018). Perioperative hyperglycemia: an unmet need within a surgical site infection bundle. *Tech. Coloproctol.* 22: 201–207.

39 Heldmann, E., Brown, D.C., and Shofer, F. (1999). The association of propofol usage with postoperative wound infection rate in clean wounds: a retrospective study. *Vet. Surg.* 28: 256–259.

40 Zorrilla-Vaca, A., Arevalo, J.J., Escandon-Vargas, K. et al. (2016). Infectious disease risk associated with contaminated propofol anesthesia, 1989-2014(1). *Emerg. Infect. Dis.* 22: 981–992.

41 Bennett, S.N., McNeil, M.M., Bland, L.A. et al. (1995). Postoperative infections traced to contamination of an intravenous anesthetic, propofol. *New. Engl. J. Med.* 333: 147–154.

42 Ireifej, S., Marino, D.J., Loughin, C.A. et al. (2012). Risk factors and clinical relevance of positive intraoperative bacterial cultures in dogs with total hip replacement. *Vet. Surg.* 41: 63–68.

43 Nicholson, M., Beal, M., Shofer, F. et al. (2002). Epidemiologic evaluation of postoperative wound infection in clean-contaminated wounds: a retrospective study of 239 dogs and cats. *Vet. Surg.* 31: 577–581.

44 Martin, E.T., Kaye, K.S., Knott, C. et al. (2016). Diabetes and risk of surgical site infection: a systematic review and meta-analysis. *Infect. Control Hosp. Epidemiol.* 37: 88–99.

45 Durkin, M.J., Dicks, K.V., Baker, A.W. et al. (2015). Postoperative infection in spine surgery: does the month matter? *J. Neurosurg. Spine* 23: 128–134.

46 Zorrilla-Vaca, A., Grant, M.C., Mathur, V. et al. (2016). The impact of neuraxial versus general anesthesia on the incidence of postoperative surgical site infections following knee or hip arthroplasty: a meta-analysis. *Reg. Anesth. Pain Med.* 41: 555–563.

47 Wilson, J.M., Farley, K.X., Erens, G.A. et al. (2019). General vs spinal anesthesia for revision total knee arthroplasty: do complication rates differ? *J. Arthroplasty* 34: 1417–1422.

48 Kopp, S.L., Berbari, E.F., Osmon, D.R. et al. (2015). The impact of anesthetic management on surgical site infections in patients undergoing total knee or total hip arthroplasty. *Anesth. Analg.* 121: 1215–1221.

49 Ackermann, W., Fan, Q., Parekh, A.J. et al. (2018). Forced-air warming and resistive heating devices. Updated perspectives on safety and surgical site infections. *Front Surg* 5: 64.

50 Memarzadeh, F. (2010). Active warming systems to maintain perioperative normothermia in hip replacement surgery. *J. Hosp. Infect.* 75: 332–333.

51 Shirozu, K., Kai, T., Setoguchi, H. et al. (2018). Effects of forced air warming on airflow around the operating table. *Anesthesiology* 128: 79–84.

52 Huang, J.K., Shah, E.F., Vinodkumar, N. et al. (2003). The Bair Hugger patient warming system in prolonged vascular surgery: an infection risk? *Crit. Care* 7: R13–R16.

53 Sessler, D.I. (2006). Non-pharmacologic prevention of surgical wound infection. *Anesthesiol. Clin.* 24: 279–297.

54 Ueno, C., Hunt, T.K., and Hopf, H.W. (2006). Using physiology to improve surgical wound outcomes. *Plast. Reconst. Surg.* 117: 59s–71s.

55 Sakuragi, T., Yanagisawa, K., Shirai, Y. et al. (1999). Growth of *Escherichia coli* in propofol, lidocaine, and mixtures of propofol and lidocaine. *Acta Anaesthesiol. Scand.* 43: 476–479.

56 Wachowski, I., Jolly, D.T., Hrazdil, J. et al. (1999). The growth of microorganisms in propofol and mixtures of propofol and lidocaine. *Anesth. Analg.* 88: 209–212.

57 Guzelant, A., Apiliogullari, S., Kara, I. et al. (2008). The preventive effect of diphenhydramine on bacterial growth in propofol: a laboratory study. *Eur. J. Anaesthesiol.* 25: 737–740.

58 Crowther, J., Hrazdil, J., Jolly, D.T. et al. (1996). Growth of microorganisms in propofol, thiopental, and a 1:1 mixture of propofol and thiopental. *Anesth. Analg.* 82: 475–478.

59 O'Hara, L.M., Thom, K.A., and Preas, M.A. (2018). Update to the Centers for Disease Control and Prevention and the Healthcare Infection Control Practices Advisory Committee Guideline for the Prevention of Surgical Site Infection (2017): a summary, review, and strategies for implementation. *Am. J. Infect. Control* 46: 602–609.

60 Knights, C.B., Mateus, A., and Baines, S.J. (2012). Current British veterinary attitudes to the use of perioperative antimicrobials in small animal surgery. *Vet. Rec.* 170: 646.

61 Boothe, D.M. and Boothe, H.W. Jr. (2015). Antimicrobial considerations in the perioperative patient. *Vet. Clin. North Am. Small Anim. Pract.* 45: 585–608.

62 Pratesi, A., Moores, A.P., Downes, C. et al. (2015). Efficacy of postoperative antimicrobial use for clean orthopedic implant surgery in dogs: a prospective randomized study in 100 consecutive cases. *Vet. Surg.* 44: 653–660.

63 Nazarali, A., Singh, A., Moens, N.M. et al. (2015). Association between methicillin-resistant *Staphylococcus pseudintermedius* carriage and the development of surgical site infections following tibial plateau leveling osteotomy in dogs. *J. Am. Vet. Med. Assoc.* 247: 909–916.

64 Aiken, M.J., Hughes, T.K., Abercromby, R.H. et al. (2015). Prospective, randomized comparison of the effect of two antimicrobial regimes on surgical site infection rate in dogs undergoing orthopedic implant surgery. *Vet. Surg.* 44: 661–667.

65 Leroy, O., Vandenbussche, C., Coffinier, C. et al. (1997). Community-acquired aspiration pneumonia in intensive care units. Epidemiological and prognosis data. *Am. J. Respir. Crit. Care Med.* 156: 1922–1929.

66 Wei, C., Cheng, Z., Zhang, L. et al. (2013). Microbiology and prognostic factors of hospital- and community-acquired aspiration pneumonia in respiratory intensive care unit. *Am. J. Infect. Control* 41: 880–884.

67 Tart, K.M., Babski, D.M., and Lee, J.A. (2010). Potential risks, prognostic indicators, and diagnostic and treatment modalities affecting survival in dogs with presumptive aspiration pneumonia: 125 cases (2005–

2008). *J. Vet. Emerg. Crit. Care (San Antonio)* 20: 319–329.

68 Kogan, D.A., Johnson, L.R., Sturges, B.K. et al. (2008). Etiology and clinical outcome in dogs with aspiration pneumonia: 88 cases (2004–2006). *J. Am. Vet. Med. Assoc.* 233: 1748–1755.

69 Ovbey, D.H., Wilson, D.V., Bednarski, R.M. et al. (2014). Prevalence and risk factors for canine post-anesthetic aspiration pneumonia (1999–2009): a multicenter study. *Vet. Anaesth. Analg.* 41: 127–136.

70 Java, M.A., Drobatz, K.J., Gilley, R.S. et al. (2009). Incidence of and risk factors for postoperative pneumonia in dogs anesthetized for diagnosis or treatment of intervertebral disk disease. *J. Am. Vet. Med. Assoc.* 235: 281–287.

71 Dear, J.D. (2014). Bacterial pneumonia in dogs and cats. *Vet. Clin. North Am. Small Anim. Pract.* 44: 143–159.

72 Levy, N., Ballegeer, E., and Koenigshof, A. (2019). Clinical and radiographic findings in cats with aspiration pneumonia: retrospective evaluation of 28 cases. *J. Small Anim. Pract.* 60: 356–360.

73 Mercurio, A. (2011). Complications of upper airway surgery in companion animals. *Vet. Clin. North Am. Small Anim. Pract.* 41: 969–980.

74 Baetge, C., Cummings, K.J., and Deveau, M. (2019). Reduced risk of pneumonia after changes in anesthetic procedures for dogs receiving repeated anesthesia for radiation treatment. *Vet. Radiol. Ultrasound* 60: 241–245.

75 Wilson, D. and Monnet, E. (2016). Risk factors for the development of aspiration pneumonia after unilateral arytenoid lateralization in dogs with laryngeal paralysis: 232 cases (1987–2012). *J. Am. Vet. Med. Assoc.* 248: 188–194.

76 Sherman, R. and Karagiannis, M. (2017). Aspiration pneumonia in the dog: a review. *Top Companion Anim. Med.* 32: 1–7.

77 Mitsushima, H., Oishi, K., Nagao, T. et al. (2002). Acid aspiration induces bacterial pneumonia by enhanced bacterial adherence in mice. *Microbial. Pathogenesis* 33: 203–210.

78 Fry, D.E. (1993). Postoperative pneumonia in the intensive care unit. *Surg. Gynecol. Obstet.* 177 (Suppl): 41–49; discussion 65–70.

79 Maboni, G., Seguel, M., Lorton, A. et al. (2019). Canine infectious respiratory disease: new insights into the etiology and epidemiology of associated pathogens. *PLoS One* 14: e0215817.

80 Rider, A.C. and Frazee, B.W. (2018). Community-acquired pneumonia. *Emerg. Med. Clin. North Am.* 36: 665–683.

81 Boiron, L., Hopper, K., and Borchers, A. (2019). Risk factors, characteristics, and outcomes of acute respiratory distress syndrome in dogs and cats: 54 cases. *J. Vet. Emerg. Crit. Care (San Antonio)* 29: 173–179.

82 Mosier, J.M. and Hypes, C.D. (2019). Mechanical ventilation strategies for the patient with severe obstructive lung disease. *Emerg. Med. Clin. North Am.* 37: 445–458.

83 McNally, E.M., Robertson, S.A., and Pablo, L.S. (2009). Comparison of time to desaturation between preoxygenated and nonpreoxygenated dogs following sedation with acepromazine maleate and morphine and induction of anesthesia with propofol. *Am. J. Vet. Res.* 70: 1333–1338.

84 Klompas, M., Branson, R., Eichenwald, E.C. et al. (2014). Strategies to prevent ventilator-associated pneumonia in acute care hospitals: 2014 update. *Infect. Control Hosp. Epidemiol.* 35 (Suppl 2): S133–S154.

85 Frenzen, F.S., Kutschan, U., Meiswinkel, N. et al. (2018). Admission lactate predicts poor prognosis independently of the CRB/CURB-65 scores in community-acquired pneumonia. *Clin. Microbiol. Infect.* 24: e301–e306, 306.

86 Parrish, C.R. and Voorhees, I.E.H. (2019). H3N8 and H3N2 canine influenza viruses: understanding these new viruses in dogs. *Vet. Clin. North Am. Small Anim.* 49: 643–649.

87 Voorhees, I.E.H., Glaser, A.L., Toohey-Kurth, K. et al. (2017). Spread of canine influenza

A(H3N2) virus, United States. *Emerg. Infect. Dis.* 23: 1950–1957.

88 Jeoung, H.Y., Lim, S.I., Shin, B.H. et al. (2013). A novel canine influenza H3N2 virus isolated from cats in an animal shelter. *Vet. Microbiol.* 165: 281–286.

89 Dubovi, E.J. (2010). Canine influenza. *Vet. Clin. North Am. Small Anim. Pract.* 40: 1063–1071.

90 Xie, X., Ma, K., and Liu, Y. (2016). Influenza A virus infection in dogs: epizootiology, evolution and prevention - a review. *Acta Vet. Hung.* 64: 125–139.

91 Dunn, D., Creevy, K.E., and Krimer, P.M. (2018). Outcomes of and risk factors for presumed canine H3N2 influenza virus infection in a metropolitan outbreak. *J. Am. Vet. Med. Assoc.* 252: 959–965.

92 Priestnall, S.L., Mitchell, J.A., Walker, C.A. et al. (2014). New and emerging pathogens in canine infectious respiratory disease. *Vet. Pathol.* 51: 492–504.

93 Simon, B.T. and Steagall, P.V. (2017). The present and future of opioid analgesics in small animal practice. *J. Vet. Pharmacol. Ther.* 40: 315–326.

94 Morice, A.H. and Shanks, G. (2017). Pharmacology of cough in palliative care. *Curr. Opin. Support. Palliat. Care* 11: 147–151.

95 Cohn, L.A. (2011). Feline respiratory disease complex. *Vet. Clin. North Am. Small Anim. Pract.* 41: 1273–1289.

96 Helps, C.R., Lait, P., Damhuis, A. et al. (2005). Factors associated with upper respiratory tract disease caused by feline herpesvirus, feline calicivirus, *Chlamydophila felis* and *Bordetella bronchiseptica* in cats: experience from 218 European catteries. *Vet. Rec.* 156: 669–673.

97 Bannasch, M.J. and Foley, J.E. (2005). Epidemiologic evaluation of multiple respiratory pathogens in cats in animal shelters. *J. Feline Med. Surg.* 7: 109–119.

98 Scherk, M. (2010). Snots and snuffles: rational approach to chronic feline upper respiratory syndromes. *J. Feline Med. Surg.* 12: 548–557.

99 Al-Ruzzeh SK, Kurup V. 2012. Respiratory diseases. In: Hines RL, editor. *Stoelting's Anesthesia and Co-Existing Disease*. 6. pp. 181–217. Philadelphia: Elsevier.

100 Tello, L. and Perez-Freytes, R. (2017). Fluid and electrolyte therapy during vomiting and diarrhea. *Vet. Clin. North Am. Small Anim. Pract.* 47: 505–519.

101 Johnson, S.E., Sherding, R.G., and Bright, R.M. (2006). Diseases of the stomach. In: *Saunders Manual of Small Animal Practice*, 3e (eds. S.J. Birchard and R.G. Sherding), 664–690. St. Louis: WB Saunders.

102 Liu, D.T. and Silverstein, D.C. (2015). Crystalloids, colloids, and hemoglobin-based oxygen-carrying solutions. In: *Small Animal Critical Care Medicine*, 2e (eds. D.C. Silverstein and K. Hopper), 311–316. St. Louis: WB Saunders.

103 Klein, A.V., Teixeira-Neto, F.J., Garofalo, N.A. et al. (2016). Changes in pulse pressure variation and plethysmographic variability index caused by hypotension-inducing hemorrhage followed by volume replacement in isoflurane-anesthetized dogs. *Am. J. Vet. Res.* 77: 280–287.

104 Wenzel, R.P. and Edmond, M.B. (2001). The impact of hospital-acquired bloodstream infections. *Emerg. Infect. Dis.* 7: 174–177.

105 Sitges-Serra, A. and Girvent, M. (1999). Catheter-related bloodstream infections. *World J. Surg.* 23: 589–595.

106 Marsh-Ng, M.L., Burney, D.P., and Garcia, J. (2007). Surveillance of infections associated with intravenous catheters in dogs and cats in an intensive care unit. *J. Am. Anim. Hosp. Assoc.* 43: 13–20.

107 Adamantos, S., Brodbelt, D., and Moores, A.L. (2010). Prospective evaluation of complications associated with jugular venous catheter use in a veterinary hospital. *J. Small Anim. Pract.* 51: 254–257.

108 Johnson, J.A. (2002). Nosocomial infections. *Vet. Clin. North Am. Small Anim. Pract.* 32: 1101–1126.

109 Ogeer-Gyles, J.S., Mathews, K.A., and Boerlin, P. (2006). Nosocomial infections

and antimicrobial resistance in critical care medicine. *J. Vet. Emerg. Crit. Care* 16: 1–18.

110 Elliott, T. (2000). Intravascular catheter-related sepsis--novel methods of prevention. *Int. Care Med.* 26 (Suppl 1): S45–S50.

111 Maki, D.G., Ringer, M., and Alvarado, C.J. (1991). Prospective randomised trial of povidone-iodine, alcohol, and chlorhexidine for prevention of infection associated with central venous and arterial catheters. *Lancet* 338: 339–343.

112 Franci, P., Dotto, G., Cattai, A. et al. (2015). Lethal septic shock after dental scaling in a healthy dog due to *Ochrobactrum anthropi*-contaminated propofol. *J. Small Anim. Pract.* 56: 345–347.

113 Strachan, F.A., Mansel, J.C., and Clutton, R.E. (2008). A comparison of microbial growth in alfaxalone, propofol and thiopental. *J. Small Anim. Pract.* 49: 186–190.

114 Calvert, C.A. and Thomason, J.D. (2011). Cardiovascular infections. In: *Infectious Diseases of the Dog and Cat*, 4e (ed. C. Greene), 912–936. Philadelphia: WB Saunders Elsevier.

115 Raad, I. and Hanna, H. (1999). Nosocomial infections related to use of intravascular devices inserted for long-term vascular access. In: *Hospital Epidemiology and Infection Control*, 2e (ed. C. Mayhall), 165–172. Philadelphia: Lippincott Williams and Wilkins.

116 Lane, R.K. and Matthay, M.A. (2002). Central line infections. *Curr. Opin. Crit. Care* 8: 441–448.

117 Mathews, K.A., Brooks, M.J., and Valliant, A.E. (1996). A prospective study of intravenous catheter contamination. *J. Vet. Emerg. Crit. Care* 6: 33–43.

118 O'Grady, N.P., Alexander, M., Burns, L.A. et al. (2011). Guidelines for the prevention of intravascular catheter-related infections. *Am. J. Infect. Control* 39: S1–S34.

119 Boller, E.M. and Otto, C.M. (2015). Sepsis and septic shock. In: *Small Animal Critical Care Medicine*, 2e (eds. D.C. Silverstein and K. Hopper), 472–480. St. Louis: WB Saunders.

120 Parsons, K.J., Owen, L.J., Lee, K. et al. (2009). A retrospective study of surgically treated cases of septic peritonitis in the cat (2000–2007). *J. Small Anim. Pract.* 50: 518–524.

121 Culp, W.T., Zeldis, T.E., Reese, M.S. et al. (2009). Primary bacterial peritonitis in dogs and cats: 24 cases (1990–2006). *J. Am. Vet. Med. Assoc.* 234: 906–993.

122 Hernandez, C.A. (2018). Infectious diseases. In: *Stoelting's Anesthesia and Co-Existing Disease*, 7e (ed. R.L. Hines), 539–566. Philadelphia: Elsevier.

123 Levy, M.M., Fink, M.P., Marshall, J.C. et al. (2003). 2001 SCCM/ESICM/ACCP/ATS/SIS International sepsis definitions conference. *Crit. Care Med.* 31: 1250–1256.

124 Rivers, E., Nguyen, B., Havstad, S. et al. (2001). Early goal-directed therapy in the treatment of severe sepsis and septic shock. *New. Engl. J. Med.* 345: 1368–1377.

125 Dardalas, I., Stamoula, E., Rigopoulos, P. et al. (2019). Dexmedetomidine effects in different experimental sepsis in vivo models. *Eur. J. Pharmacol.* 856: 172401.

126 Jackson, W.L. Jr. (2005). Should we use etomidate as an induction agent for endotracheal intubation in patients with septic shock?: a critical appraisal. *Chest* 127: 1031–1038.

127 Dmello, D., Taylor, S., O'Brien, J. et al. (2010). Outcomes of etomidate in severe sepsis and septic shock. *Chest* 138: 1327–1332.

128 Steagall, P.V.M., Simon, B.T., Teixeira Neto, F.J. et al. (2017). An update on drugs used for lumbosacral epidural anesthesia and analgesia in dogs. *Front. Vet. Sci.* 4: 68.

129 Taniguchi, T., Shibata, K., Yamamoto, K. et al. (2000). Effects of lidocaine administration on hemodynamics and cytokine responses to endotoxemia in rabbits. *Crit. Care Med.* 28: 755–759.

130 Taniguchi, T., Shibata, K., Yamamoto, K. et al. (1996). Lidocaine attenuates the hypotensive and inflammatory responses to endotoxemia in rabbits. *Crit. Care Med.* 24: 642–646.

131 Pypendop, B.H., Barter, L.S., Stanley, S.D. et al. (2011). Hemodynamic effects of dexmedetomidine in isoflurane-anesthetized cats. *Vet. Anaesth. Analg.* 38: 555–567.

132 DeClue, A.E., Cohn, L.A., Lechner, E.S. et al. (2008). Effects of subanesthetic doses of ketamine on hemodynamic and immunologic variables in dogs with experimentally induced endotoxemia. *Am. J. Vet. Res.* 69: 228–232.

133 Murrell, J. (2015). Ardrenergic agents. In: *Veterinary Anesthesia and Analgesia*, 5e (eds. K. Grimm, L. Lamont, W.J. Tranquilli, et al.), 183–195. Ames: Wiley Blackwell.

134 Rogovik, A. and Goldman, R. (2008). Permissive hypercapnia. *Emerg. Med. Clin. North Am.* 26: 941–952.

135 Childers, B.J., Potyondy, L.D., Nachreiner, R. et al. (2002). Necrotizing fasciitis: a fourteen-year retrospective study of 163 consecutive patients. *Am. Surg.* 68: 109–116.

136 Sura, R., Hinckley, L.S., Risatti, G.R. et al. (2008). Fatal necrotising fasciitis and myositis in a cat associated with *Streptococcus canis*. *Vet. Rec.* 162: 450–453.

137 Naidoo, S.L., Campbell, D.L., Miller, L.M. et al. (2005). Necrotizing fasciitis: a review. *J. Am. Anim. Hosp. Assoc.* 41: 104–109.

138 Csiszer, A.B., Towle, H.A., and Daly, C.M. (2010). Successful treatment of necrotizing fasciitis in the hind limb of a great dane. *J. Am. Anim. Hosp. Assoc.* 46: 433–438.

139 Kulendra, E. and Corr, S. (2008). Necrotising fasciitis with sub-periosteal *Streptococcus canis* infection in two puppies. *Vet. Comp. Orthop. Traumatol.* 21: 474–477.

140 Worth, A.J., Marshall, N., and Thompson, K.G. (2005). Necrotising fasciitis associated with *Escherichia coli* in a dog. *N. Z. Vet. J.* 53: 257–260.

141 Banovic, F., Linder, K., Boone, A. et al. (2013). Cat scratch-induced *Pasteurella multocida* necrotizing cellulitis in a dog. *Vet. Dermatol.* 24 (463–5): e107–e468.

142 Mayer, M.N. and Rubin, J.E. (2012). Necrotizing fasciitis caused by methicillin-resistant *Staphylococcus pseudintermedius* at a previously irradiated site in a dog. *Can. Vet. J.* 53: 1207–1210.

143 Costa, R.S., Costa, F.B., and Barros, R.R. (2018). Antimicrobial treatment of necrotizing fasciitis and septic polyarthritis in a cat associated with *Streptococcus canis* infection. *Vet. Dermatol.* 29: 90–91.

144 Prescott, J.F., Miller, C.W., Mathews, K.A. et al. (1997). Update on canine streptococcal toxic shock syndrome and necrotizing fasciitis. *Can. Vet. J.* 38: 241–242.

145 Prescott, J.F. and DeWinter, L. (1997). Canine streptococcal toxic shock syndrome and necrotising fasciitis. *Vet. Rec.* 140: 263.

146 Elliott, D.C., Kufera, J.A., and Myers, R.A. (1996). Necrotizing soft tissue infections. Risk factors for mortality and strategies for management. *Ann. Surg.* 224: 672–683.

147 Jenkins, C.M., Winkler, K., Rudloff, E. et al. (2001). Necrotizing fasciitis in a dog. *J. Vet. Emerg. Crit. Care* 11: 299–305.

148 Cunningham, J.D., Silver, L., and Rudikoff, D. (2001). Necrotizing fasciitis: a plea for early diagnosis and treatment. *Mt. Sinai J. Med.* 68: 253–261.

149 Kaul, R., McGeer, A., Low, D.E. et al. (1997). Population-based surveillance for group. A streptococcal necrotizing fasciitis: clinical features, prognostic indicators, and microbiologic analysis of seventy-seven cases. Ontario Group A Streptococcal Study. *Am. J. Med.* 103: 18–24.

150 Ingrey, K.T., Ren, J., and Prescott, J.F. (2003). A fluoroquinolone induces a novel mitogen-encoding bacteriophage in *Streptococcus canis*. *Infect. Immun.* 71: 3028–3033.

151 Littman, M.P., Gerber, B., Goldstein, R.E. et al. (2018). ACVIM consensus update on *Lyme borreliosis* in dogs and cats. *J. Vet. Intern. Med.* 32: 887–903.

152 Detmer, S.E., Bouljihad, M., Hayden, D.W. et al. (2016). Fatal pyogranulomatous myocarditis in 10 Boxer puppies. *J. Vet. Diagn. Invest.* 28: 144–149.

153 Harrus, S., Waner, T., and Neer, T.M. (2012). Ehrlichia and anaplasma infections. In: *Infectious Diseases of the Dog and Cat*, 4e (ed. C. Greene), 227–238. Philadelphia: WB Saunders Elsevier.

154 Shipov, A., Klement, E., Reuveni-Tager, L. et al. (2008). Prognostic indicators for canine monocytic ehrlichiosis. *Vet. Parasitol.* 153: 131–138.

155 Woody, B.J. and Hoskins, J.D. (1991). Ehrlichial diseases of dogs. *Vet. Clin. North Am. Small Anim. Pract.* 21: 75–98.

156 Leiva, M., Naranjo, C., and Pena, M.T. (2005). Ocular signs of canine monocytic ehrlichiosis: a retrospective study in dogs from Barcelona, Spain. *Vet. Ophthalmol.* 8: 387–393.

157 Mylonakis, M.E., Koutinas, A.F., Breitschwerdt, E.B. et al. (2004). Chronic canine ehrlichiosis (*Ehrlichia canis*): a retrospective study of 19 natural cases. *J. Am. Anim. Hosp. Assoc.* 40: 174–184.

158 Mylonakis, M.E., Harrus, S., and Breitschwerdt, E.B. (2019). An update on the treatment of canine monocytic ehrlichiosis (*Ehrlichia canis*). *Vet. J.* 246: 45–53.

159 Neer, T.M., Breitschwerdt, E.B., Greene, R.T. et al. (2002). Consensus statement on ehrlichial disease of small animals from the infectious disease study group of the ACVIM. *J. Vet. Intern. Med.* 16: 309–315.

160 Hackner, S.G. and Rousseau, A. (2015). Bleeding disorders. In: *Small Animal Critical Care Medicine*, 2e (eds. D.C. Silverstein and K. Hopper), 554–567. St. Louis: WB Saunders.

161 Giudice, E., Giannetto, C., and Gianesella, M. (2010). Effect of desmopressin on immune-mediated haemorrhagic disorders due to canine monocytic ehrlichiosis: a preliminary study. *J. Vet. Pharmacol. Ther.* 33: 610–614.

162 Greene, C., Sykes, J., and Moore, G. (2012). Leptospirosis. In: *Infectious Diseases of the Dog and Cat*, 4e (ed. C. Greene), 431–446. Philadelphia: WB Saunders Elsevier.

163 Reagan, K.L. and Sykes, J.E. (2019). Diagnosis of canine leptospirosis. *Vet. Clin. North Am. Small Anim. Pract.* 49: 719–731.

164 Lacroix-Lamande, S., d'Andon, M.F., Michel, E. et al. (2012). Downregulation of the Na/K-ATPase pump by leptospiral glycolipoprotein activates the NLRP3 inflammasome. *J. Immunol.* 188: 2805–2814.

165 Kohn, B., Steinicke, K., Arndt, G. et al. (2010). Pulmonary abnormalities in dogs with leptospirosis. *J. Vet. Intern. Med.* 24: 1277–1282.

166 Sonet, J., Barthelemy, A., Goy-Thollot, I. et al. (2018). Prospective evaluation of abdominal ultrasonographic findings in 35 dogs with leptospirosis. *Vet. Radiol. Ultrasound* 59: 98–106.

167 Sykes, J.E., Hartmann, K., Lunn, K.F. et al. (2011). 2010 ACVIM small animal consensus statement on leptospirosis: diagnosis, epidemiology, treatment, and prevention. *J. Vet. Intern. Med.* 25: 1–13.

168 Adin, C.A. and Cowgill, L.D. (2000). Treatment and outcome of dogs with leptospirosis: 36 cases (1990–1998). *J. Am. Vet. Med. Assoc.* 216: 371–375.

169 Levy, J.K., Scott, H.M., Lachtara, J.L. et al. (2006). Seroprevalence of feline leukemia virus and feline immunodeficiency virus infection among cats in North America and risk factors for seropositivity. *J. Am. Vet. Med. Assoc.* 228: 371–376.

170 Hartmann, K. (2011). Clinical aspects of feline immunodeficiency and feline leukemia virus infection. *Vet. Immunol. Immunopathol.* 143: 190–201.

171 Hoover, E.A., Olsen, R.G., Hardy, W.D. Jr. et al. (1976). Feline leukemia virus infection: age-related variation in response of cats to experimental infection. *J. Natl. Cancer Inst.* 57: 365–369.

172 Hofmann-Lehmann, R., Berger, M., Sigrist, B. et al. (1998). Feline immunodeficiency virus (FIV) infection leads to increased incidence of feline odontoclastic resorptive lesions (FORL). *Vet. Immunol. Immunopathol.* 65: 299–308.

173 Cho, J.S., Lee, M.H., Kim, S.I. et al. (2017). The effects of perioperative anesthesia and analgesia on immune function in patients undergoing breast cancer resection: a prospective randomized study. *Int. J. Med. Sci.* 14: 970–976.

17

Neoplastic Disease

Verónica Salazar

School of Veterinary Medicine, Universidad Alfonso X El Sabio, Madrid, 28691, Spain

Introduction

Cancer is a major disease in animals of all ages and is the leading cause of death in older pet animals [1]. However, a precise estimate of cancer morbidity and mortality is difficult to obtain due to several limitations that differentiate animal from human populations. Comprehensive state-based cancer registries are available in human medicine, while only a few, very limited attempts have been made in veterinary medicine to create them [1–7]. At the time of registry publication, the cancer incidence rates were 0.4–2% in dogs and 0.1–0.4% in cats, while cancer prevalence in a set population of veterinary patients was approximately 4% [2–5, 7]. Additionally, mortality rates for veterinary cancer patients are 20–56% depending on age and breed [1, 6]. However, it is entirely possible that these figures may continue to improve as more sophisticated and advanced oncologic diagnostic and therapeutic procedures become widely available. Despite the lack of accurate epidemiological veterinary cancer data, the prevalence of cancer in pets continues to rise for several reasons, but is, at least in part, related to animals living to increasingly older ages. The greater life span is the result of better preventive and therapeutic medical practices (including better nutrition and vaccination policies) and possibly the development of a stronger human–animal bond within the last 30 years [1, 8]. As such, veterinary care for oncological pets is currently demanded by society and veterinary professionals are expected to provide expertise and proficiency in the clinical management of the cancer patient. A cornerstone of their medical care is the anesthetic/analgesic management during different stages of their clinical management that ranges from diagnostic to therapeutic or palliative procedures.

Pathophysiologic Considerations

Unfortunately, cancer patients present with many pathophysiologic derangements that derive not only from the neoplasia and/or its metastases, but also from the coexisting paraneoplastic syndromes (PNS) and the secondary effects of their therapeutic management (e.g., secondary effects of chemotherapy or radiation therapy, aggressive and invasive surgical procedures, etc.). In order to perform a safe and adequate anesthetic/analgesic management of the oncologic patient, a thorough

Canine and Feline Anesthesia and Co-Existing Disease, Second Edition. Edited by Rebecca A. Johnson, Lindsey B. C. Snyder and Carrie A. Schroeder.

Companion website: www.wiley.com/go/johnson/canine

understanding of the underlying pathophysiology is warranted.

Paraneoplastic Syndromes

PNS include neoplasm-associated systemic alterations that occur distant to the tumor but can be directly linked to the neoplastic disease [9]. Tumors can produce and release several biologically active substances such as cytokines, hormones, and growth factors that lead to clinical conditions that may occasionally present a higher morbidity than the original tumor itself. PNS can be classified according to the systemic organ they target (Table 17.1).

General Manifestations

Cancer Anorexia–Cachexia Syndrome

Cancer anorexia–cachexia syndrome (CACS) represents the most common paraneoplastic disorder in both human and veterinary patients. The incidence among veterinary patients is yet to be determined by appropriate clinical studies. However, the incidence has been estimated at only 4% [10], which may be significantly lower than the real figure [9]. Oncologic patients frequently show weight loss and metabolic alterations associated with both adequate nutritional intake (cancer cachexia) and/or poor nutritional intake (cancer anorexia). This PNS results in alterations in carbohydrate, lipid, and protein metabolism that, if left untreated, decrease the patients' quality of life, their survival time, and sometimes their chances of being suitable candidates for a more appropriate therapy [11]. Clinically, CACS is characterized by nausea, anorexia, and weight loss that ultimately leads to severe wasting due to massive body fat depletion and a dramatic decrease in muscle protein mass (Figure 17.1) [12].

Patients may also have alterations in food perception (i.e., smell and taste), which decreases the palatability of the food they are offered [12]. The metabolic disorders associated with the CACS may occur even before weight loss is first detected and they may often persist after the patient is successfully treated for the neoplastic disorder, making weight gain challenging. The underlying CACS pathophysiologic

Table 17.1 Classification of common paraneoplastic syndromes in oncologic patients.

Organic system	Manifestations	
General manifestations	Cancer anorexia–cachexia syndrome (CACS)	Fever
Hematologic manifestations	Anemia	Erythrocytosis
	Leukocytosis	Thrombocytopenia
	Thrombocyte Hyperaggregability	Coagulation disorders
	Pancytopenia	Hyperproteinemia
Endocrine manifestations	Hypercalcemia	Hypoglycemia
	Syndrome of inappropriate antidiuretic hormone secretion (SIADH)	
Gastrointestinal manifestations	Gastroduodenal ulceration	
Cutaneous manifestations	Alopecia	Cutaneous flushing
	Nodular dermatofibrosis	
Neuromuscular manifestations	Myasthenia gravis	Peripheral neuropathy
Renal manifestations	Glomerulonephritis	
Miscellaneous manifestations	Hypertrophic osteopathy	

mechanism is mediated by the production and release of serotonin and cytokines that lead to alterations in the resting energy expenditure as well as in physiologic protein, fat, and carbohydrate metabolism (Table 17.2) [12].

Oncologic patients that suffer from CACS require aggressive nutritional support to limit the adverse effects of CACS and to enhance immune system function as well as the efficacy and tolerance of different therapeutic interventions (i.e., diets rich in omega-3 fatty acids) [13]. Nasoesophageal, esophagostomy, or gastrostomy tubes are also recommended in those patients that are persistently anorexic.

As a result of the aforementioned changes associated with PNS, a low fat-to-body mass ratio and a low muscle-to-body mass ratio are commonly found in these patients. Due to the decreased availability of drug protein binding, higher circulating levels of free-fraction or active drugs (e.g., barbiturates) administered in the perianesthetic period may be present. To avoid overdose and prolonged and/or rough anesthetic recoveries, careful pharmacological choices and dosing regimens need to be applied. Additionally, due to their very low fat-to-body mass ratio, these patients may be more prone to hypothermia during the perianesthetic period. Active efforts to decrease as much as possible heat loss is warranted (i.e., insulation from cold surfaces, careful wrapping, use of heat and moisture exchange filters, warm water blankets, etc.).

Fever

Fever as a PNS is associated with a wide variety of neoplastic disorders and, although it is very common in human patients, its incidence

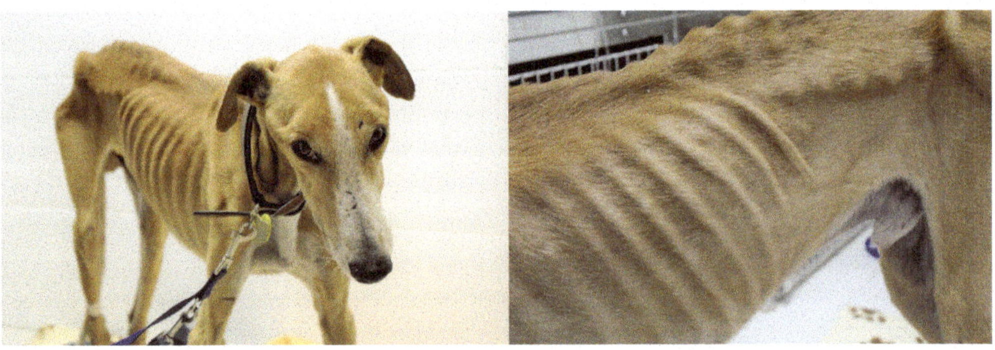

Figure 17.1 Severe wasting in a dog due to CACS. *Source:* Photo courtesy of Dr. Ana Cloquell.

Table 17.2 Cancer anorexia–cachexia syndrome (CACS): major clinical signs and pathophysiologic mechanisms.

Affected system	Pathophysiologic mechanism	Clinical signs
Protein metabolism	Decreased protein anabolism Increased protein catabolism	Muscle atrophy Poor body condition score
Carbohydrate metabolism	Altered insulin receptors Anaerobic glucose metabolism	Hyperlactatemia
Lipid metabolism	Increased lipolysis Increased lipid mobilization Decreased fatty acid extraction	Body fat loss Poor body condition score
Resting energy expenditure (REE)	Abnormal glucose metabolism	Increased REE

in veterinary medicine is unknown [14]. The pathogenesis of paraneoplastic fever is mostly due to the production and release of pyrogenic cytokines by the host immune system and/or tumor itself [15]. A thorough preanesthetic evaluation is warranted to rule out the presence of an infectious process prior to formulating an anesthetic plan. Severe elevations in body temperature are associated with an increased metabolic state and degree of oxygen consumption that may even exceed oxygen delivery to tissues. This situation may eventually lead to the development of a series of multiorgan dysfunctions (i.e., acute renal failure, myocardial arrhythmias, and disseminated intravascular coagulation [DIC]). In addition, hyperthermia is related to an increase in inhalant minimum alveolar concentrations (MAC) [20]. Anesthetic maintenance with inhalant agents may necessitate higher end-tidal inhalant concentrations. If infection is ruled out and the fever is severe or life-threatening, nonsteroidal anti-inflammatory drugs (NSAIDs) should be used to inhibit the chemical mediators responsible for fever production while still allowing for normal thermoregulation [16]. Although NSAIDs are relatively safe, they should be avoided in patients with renal disease, gastrointestinal ulceration, or bleeding disorders. Dipyrone is also an injectable NSAID with antipyretic properties via cyclooxygenase (COX-3) inhibition [17, 18] not associated with the usual NSAID contraindications. At this time, dipyrone is not used widely in small animals in the United States; however, it was recently approved by the Food and Drug Administration (FDA) for use in horses. Dipyrone may induce blood dyscrasias in human patients; however, this has not been shown in animals [19].

Hematologic Manifestations

Anemia

Tumors and their metastases can alter hematopoietic cell lines after infiltration of the bone marrow, and anemia is one of the most common PNS in veterinary patients with an incidence from 30% to 69% [21]. The most common causes are anemia of chronic disease (ACD), immune-mediated hemolytic anemia (IMHA) usually associated with hematopoietic tumors, blood loss anemia associated with paraneoplastic gastroduodenal ulceration, and microangiopathic hemolytic anemia (MAHA) most associated with microvascular tumors or any type of tumor that could lead to the development of DIC.

In the case of acute or severe anemia, stabilization is desirable before general anesthesia is considered. In ACD, blood loss anemia, and MAHA, only the tumor removal can improve the condition; however, when IMHA is present, treatment with corticosteroids with or without immunosuppressive agents such as azathioprine or cyclophosphamide may significantly improve the condition before general anesthesia is undertaken [22–26]. In addition, supportive treatment with whole blood or packed red blood cell transfusion may be necessary where hypoperfusion and hypoxia are a concern. Administration of hemoglobin-based oxygen-carrying solutions (HBOCs) may be also considered if available. In addition, measures should be taken to optimize oxygen delivery to the tissues in the anesthetized patient such as preoxygenation before induction of general anesthesia, maintaining the inspired oxygen level (FIO_2) of 1.0 throughout the procedure, and striving for optimal perfusion at all times.

Erythrocytosis

Polycythemia or erythrocytosis is uncommon in veterinary oncologic patients, and it is mainly associated with renal tumors in which an increased level of erythropoietin may be present [27, 28]. Patients present with clinical signs of tissue hypoxia, polyuria, bleeding, or thrombosis that result from hyperviscosity of the blood as well as decreased perfusion of small vessels. Stabilization via phlebotomy can be a useful temporary adjunct therapy. Serial phlebotomies of 10–20 $ml\,kg^{-1}$ of blood may be carried out until clinical symptoms have resolved or the target hematocrit is reached (usually below 50% for cats and below 55% in dogs). However, repeated phlebotomies may result in thrombotic complications or iron deficits, as well as the need for concomitant aggressive fluid therapy and potential administration of plasma [29]. Consequently, if phlebotomies are required more frequently than every 6–8 weeks, myelosuppressive therapy is advised, and hydroxyurea may be used [30]. Definitive treatment of PNS erythrocytosis implies the removal of the erythropoietin-producing tumor.

Thrombocytopenia

The incidence of thrombocytopenia in veterinary cancer patients is high, occurring in up to 58% of dogs and 20% of cats [31–33]. Clinical signs are usually not evident until the platelet count decreases below 30 000 μl^{-1}. Definitive treatment requires removal of the stimulating tumor.

Anesthetic management of PNS thrombocytopenia includes a thorough physical exam and hematological evaluation; platelet-rich plasma or plasma transfusions may be indicated. Fresh frozen plasma (FFP) transfusions of 10 and 15–18 ml kg^{-1} have been reported with favorable results [34, 35]. Transfusion reactions are rare and range from mild signs (i.e., pruritus, facial swelling, and rash) to more severe (i.e., anaphylactic reactions or even death). Patients being transfused should always be closely monitored. Corticosteroids (>2 mg kg^{-1} PO daily) and immunosuppressive drugs such as azathioprine (2 mg kg^{-1} PO daily then 0.5–1 mg kg^{-1} every other day) may be used in the case of immune-mediated disease [36]. Additionally, the use of lyophilized platelets in thrombocytopenic dogs has recently been reported with favorable results [37].

Thrombocyte Hyperaggregability

Veterinary oncologic patients may present with hyperaggregability and thromboembolism. Pulmonary thromboemboli (PTE) usually present with unexplained sudden hypotension, tachycardia, tachypnea, hypoxemia, or bronchospasm. Arterial blood gas analysis may reveal hypoxemia, hypocapnia, and an increased alveolar–arterial oxygen gradient. A decrease in end-tidal CO_2 levels is also suggestive of pulmonary embolism, although it is not specific. Definitive diagnosis of intraoperative PTE may require selective pulmonary angiography or computed tomography with contrast angiography. However, these techniques are highly sophisticated and may not be readily available. Oxygen therapy should be instituted in a timely manner and definitive therapy may include thrombolytic therapy (streptokinase, 90 000 U as an IV infusion over 20–30 min, followed by 45 000 U as an IV infusion over 3–7 h) [38] as well as anticoagulation with heparin and warfarin therapy (low-molecular-weight heparin at 75–100 U kg^{-1} SC every 8 h followed by warfarin at 0.1 mg kg^{-1} every 24 h) [39]. Prophylactically, the selection of short-acting or reversible anesthetic agents is warranted in patients prone to suffering PTE, as these protocols may allow early postoperative ambulation, therefore decreasing the incidence of additional thromboembolic episodes. Additionally, in animals considered at risk for PTE, prophylactic anticoagulant therapy may be instituted (low-molecular-weight heparin at 75–100 U kg^{-1} SC every 8 h) [39].

Coagulation Disorders

PNS coagulopathies may be present, especially if alterations in platelet number and functionality are also present and DIC is the most frequent clinical abnormality [40]. Thrombocytopenia, prolongation of activated partial thromboplastin time (APTT), increased levels of fibrin degradation products (FDPs and D-dimers), hypofibrinogenemia, and decreased antithrombin III (AT III) levels may be clear indicators of the presence of DIC (Table 17.3) [41]. Appropriate stabilization of any coagulation disorders is warranted prior to undertaking of general anesthesia.

Table 17.3 Disseminated intravascular coagulation (DIC).

Stage	Controlled non-overt DIC	Controlled overt DIC	Noncontrolled overt DIC
Pathophysiologic mechanism	Activated but compensated coagulation Thrombin generation contained or balanced by inhibitors Platelet activation	Activated and uncompensated coagulation Thrombin-inhibitors overwhelmed Inflammation–hemostasis feedback loop	Platelets and coagulation factors are consumed
Clinical signs	Microvascular thrombosis	Macrovascular thrombosis Organ dysfunction	Hemorrhage
Diagnosis	Predisposing disease Altered trend in PT Altered trend in fibrinolytic products (FDP and D-dimers)	Increased PT, PTT Increased FDP and D-dimers Low fibrinogen	Increased PT, PTT Increased FDP and D-dimers Low fibrinogen Severe thrombocytopenia

The DIC continuum as defined by the scientific subcommittee of the International Society on Thrombosis and Haemostasis (ISTH) on DIC [41] and modification for DIC in dogs [410].

Hyperproteinemia

Hyperproteinemia occurs in animals with multiple myeloma, where monoclonal immunoglobulins are secreted in large quantities producing paraproteinemia [42, 43]. Clinical signs associated with hyperproteinemia are associated with bleeding disorders (as a result of poor platelet aggregation and interference with coagulation factors) [44] and by blood hyperviscosity (due to the protein–protein interactions of large, long molecules with high intrinsic viscosity) [43]. Clinical signs of hyperviscosity result from tissue hypoxia due to the sludging of blood and include ocular disturbances, severe central nervous system (CNS) deficits, and cardiac disease or failure [43, 45]. Stabilization prior to general anesthesia through plasmapheresis may be necessary to reduce protein concentrations [46].

Endocrine Manifestations

Hypercalcemia

Approximately two-thirds of dogs and one-third of cats that present with hypercalcemia are diagnosed with neoplasia [47, 48]. The most common neoplasia associated with hypercalcemia of malignancy (HM) is lymphoma, but it may also be seen with mammary gland (adeno)carcinoma, parathyroid gland neoplasia, thyroid carcinoma, bone neoplasia, anal sac apocrine gland carcinoma, multiple myeloma, thymoma, squamous cell carcinoma, melanoma, and primary lung neoplasia [49–54]. Hypercalcemia occurs via bone resorption by osteoclasts and subsequent release of circulating calcium [55]. However, additional differentials include acute renal failure, hypoadrenocorticism, granulomatous disease, hypervitaminosis D, or a laboratory artifact (due to hemolysis or lipemia) [56]. Additionally, in the case of acidemia, an increase in the free ionized fraction of calcium can occur [9]. Similarly, the relationship between calcium and serum albumin should be evaluated, and the following correction formula could be used:

$$\text{Adjusted calcium}\left(\text{mg dl}^{-1}\right) = \left[\text{calcium}\left(\text{mg dl}^{-1}\right) - \text{albumin}\left(\text{g dl}^{-1}\right)\right] + 3.5.$$

Total calcium levels $>18\,\text{mg dl}^{-1}$ should be approached as a medical emergency [57].

Systemic signs include twitching, shaking, weakness, hypertension, bradycardia, depression, stupor, or even coma. Deposition of calcium salts in the renal parenchyma leads to pre-renal and renal azotemia, while severe vasoconstriction causes a decrease in renal blood flow and glomerular filtration rate [58]. Decreased responsiveness to the antidiuretic hormone (ADH) at the distal tubule is responsible for the inability to concentrate urine. The urinary epithelium may then undergo degeneration and, eventually, necrosis [57]. Vomiting, polydipsia, and polyuria may develop and lead to progressive deterioration and dehydration of the patient. Since some of the symptomatic therapies to treat hypercalcemia could impair the ability to reach a final diagnosis or a final resolution of the etiology (e.g., glucocorticoids), the primary goal when managing a patient with HM should always be to elucidate and treat the underlying cause (for this reason, the use of corticosteroids in cases of hypercalcemia with undiagnosed neoplasia is strongly discouraged) [9, 59, 60].

General anesthesia should be performed with caution when calcium levels are significantly above the normal range (total calcium $>12\,\text{mg dl}^{-1}$ or ionized calcium $>1.5\,\text{mmol l}^{-1}$ in dogs and $1.4\,\text{mmol l}^{-1}$ in cats) due to hemodynamic and renal consequences (i.e., bradyarrhythmias, asystole and cardiac arrest, hypertension, azotemia, polyuria, polydipsia). Complete normalization of calcium levels may not be achieved prior to anesthesia, as excision of the tumor will likely be the only definitive treatment in many cases. Nevertheless, treatment should be directed at promoting external loss of calcium, increasing renal excretion of calcium, and inhibiting bone reabsorption [9]. For example, in the case of mild hypercalcemia ($12\text{–}15\,\text{mg dl}^{-1}$) and no clinical signs, rehydration with 0.9% saline could result in normocalcemia. With moderate hypercalcemia ($15\text{–}18\,\text{mg dl}^{-1}$), rehydration and consequent diuresis with 0.9% saline and furosemide ($1\text{–}4\,\text{mg kg}^{-1}$ every 8–24 h IV, in dogs; $1\text{–}2\,\text{mg kg}^{-1}$ every 8–24 h IV, in cats) should be initiated to inhibit calcium reabsorption by the ascending loop of Henle. If the final diagnosis has been reached and lymphoma has been ruled out, prednisone ($1\,\text{mg kg}^{-1}$ every 12 h PO, both dogs and cats) could be administered. In cases of refractory hypercalcemia, administration of salmon calcitonin (4–10 MRC units kg^{-1} every 24 h SC) and bisphosphonates such as zoledronate ($0.25\,\text{mg kg}^{-1}$ IV, every 4–5 weeks) or pamidronate ($1\text{–}1.5\,\text{mg kg}^{-1}$ IV in dogs and $1.5\text{–}2\,\text{mg kg}^{-1}$ IV in cats, every 2–4 weeks) should be considered [61–63].

Hypoglycemia

Hypoglycemia is mainly associated with insulin-producing islet cell pancreatic tumors [64]. However, it has been described in patients suffering from leiomyoma, leiomyosarcoma, hepatoma, hepatocellular carcinoma, and hemangiosarcoma [65]. Pathophysiologic mechanisms include increased tumor utilization of glucose, decreased hepatic gluconeogenesis, secretion of insulin-like growth factors I and II, or upregulation of insulin receptors [66], and the most common clinical signs include weakness, disorientation, seizures, and coma. With severe hypoglycemia, IV bolus of 50% dextrose ($1\,\text{ml kg}^{-1}$ diluted 1:2–1:4 over 5 min) and an IV infusion of 2–2.5% dextrose or glucagon should be initiated [67]. However, care must be taken when treating hypoglycemia in patients with suspected insulinoma or other tumors secreting insulin-like analogs, since IV dextrose may stimulate the release of even larger amounts of insulin from the tumor, further aggravating the hypoglycemic state. Dextrose infusions should be formulated by adding the appropriate amount of 50% dextrose to an isotonic crystalloid fluid (such as Lactated Ringers, 0.9% NaCl, or Plasma-Lyte) and then administered at fluid therapy maintenance rate ($40\,\text{ml kg}^{-1}\,\text{d}^{-1}$). Care must be taken to not administer 5% dextrose in water, since the solution is hypotonic and devoid of electrolytes. Glucagon can also be administered. It should be reconstituted and diluted in 0.9% saline, resulting in a $1000\,\text{ng ml}^{-1}$ solution. It may be first administered as a 50 ng kg^{-1} bolus followed by a 5–40 ng kg^{-1} min^{-1} constant rate infusion. Some oncologic patients may be already receiving various treatments aimed at fighting hypoglycemia such as diazoxide (10–60 mg kg^{-1} every 12 h PO, in dogs), as it increases glucose levels by enhancing epinephrine-induced glycogenolysis and by inhibiting insulin release and uptake by cells [68]. Others may be receiving hydrochlorothiazide (2–4 mg every 12 h PO, in dogs and cats) to potentiate the effects of diazoxide, or somatostatin (5–20 g every 8–12 h PO or SC) [9, 68, 69].

Gastrointestinal Manifestations

Gastroduodenal ulceration is associated with mast cell tumors (MCTs) or gastrinomas (gastrin-secreting non-islet cell pancreatic tumor) [70]. Mast cell granules contain several biologically active substances such as histamine, heparin, and proteolytic enzymes and are associated with gastric mucosal damage and ulceration due to increased gastric acid secretion [70–72]. Oncologic patients diagnosed with MCT or gastrinoma should be treated with a histamine-2 receptor antagonist such as famotidine (0.5–1 mg kg^{-1} slow IV or PO every 12 h, dogs and cats) or ranitidine (2 mg kg^{-1} slow IV, every 12 h, dogs and cats) to prevent gastrointestinal complications [70]. The use of NSAIDs or corticosteroids should be avoided whenever possible due to the adverse effects on gastrointestinal mucosa.

Cutaneous Manifestations

PNS alopecia is usually bilaterally symmetrical and nonscarring and has been associated with pancreatic carcinomas with metastasis to the liver [73–75]. Patients that suffer from PNS alopecia are clinically anorexic, lose weight, are lethargic, and have difficulties standing or walking [73–75]. During the preanesthetic evaluation, several differential diagnoses should be ruled out such as hyperadrenocorticism, self-induced alopecia, or symmetrical alopecia.

Renal Manifestations

Oncologic patients may suffer glomerulonephritis due to precipitation of tumor-related immune complexes on the glomeruli as well as hypercalcemic nephropathy in those patients that suffer hypercalcemia [9, 70]. Careful renal function evaluation during the preanesthetic evaluation is warranted to stabilize an oncologic patient that may need general anesthesia for different diagnostic and therapeutic procedures.

Neuromuscular Manifestations

Myasthenia Gravis

Acquired myasthenia gravis (MG) can occur in oncologic patients diagnosed with thymoma, osteosarcoma, lymphoma, and bile duct carcinoma [76–80]. Antibodies to nicotinic acetylcholine receptors are produced because of the tumor, and, as a consequence, failure of transmission across the neuromuscular junction occurs. Clinical signs include exercise intolerance, episodic muscular weakness, dysphagia, megaesophagus, and secondary aspiration pneumonia. Improvement of this tumor-associated disorder may be observed after surgical removal of the tumor itself. However, the occurrence of megaesophagus is a negative prognostic factor [76]. The administration of immunosuppressive doses of prednisone (over 2 mg kg^{-1} every 24 h PO, dogs and cats) may be attempted if surgical therapy is not an option. Since these patients frequently present with skeletal muscle weakness, perianesthetic concerns may include diaphragm insufficiency requiring ventilator support and/or megaesophagus (see Chapter 15). Patients may show resistance to depolarizing neuromuscular blockers (i.e., succinylcholine) [81]. On the other hand, acute sensitivity to the effects of nondepolarizing blockers (i.e., vecuronium, rocuronium, or atracurium) may also occur [82]. Consequently, approximately one-tenth of the initial dose is advised in these patients. Assessment of the neuromuscular block using a nerve stimulator with or without acceleromyography or electromyography should always be established in patients requiring neuromuscular blockade.

Peripheral Neuropathy

Peripheral neuropathy affects both human and veterinary oncologic patients with lymphoma, multiple myeloma, primary lung neoplasia, mammary neoplasia, hemangiosarcoma, and MCTs [83–86]. The underlying pathophysiologic mechanism is due to autoantibodies targeting antigens expressed both on the tumor and the peripheral nerves [70]. Clinical signs range from weakness and progressive paraparesis to tetraparesis with lower motor neuron symptoms with or without polyneuropathy. Pain management is particularly important with these patients. Administration of gabapentin or pregabalin as adjuvant analgesics in addition to the standard pain management plan may be extremely beneficial in treating the neuropathic component of pain [87–93]. The most used dose of gabapentin in dogs is 10 mg kg^{-1} PO every 8 h, while in cats the dose is of 10 mg kg^{-1} PO every 12 h [94, 95]. Pregabalin dosages recommended by pharmacokinetic studies in both canine and feline patients are 4 mg kg^{-1} PO every 12 h [96, 97].

Osseous Manifestations

Hypertrophic osteopathy (HO) is characterized by progressive periosteal proliferation of new bone along the shafts of long bones of the appendicular skeleton and is commonly associated with primary lung tumors, although HO has also been described in tumors that metastasize to the lungs (Figure 17.2) [98–102].

The precise pathophysiologic mechanism is unknown; however, it is partly related to afferent neurologic stimulation through irritation of the vagal and/or intercostal nerves which subsequently enhances blood flow to the limbs [103]. Clinical signs include shifting leg lameness and reluctance to move when several limbs are affected. The extremities are usually warm, swollen and manipulation is painful. Diagnosis is usually achieved by radiography of the affected limb, and thorough screening for the tumor responsible for the development of this PNS should be initiated in a timely manner. Management of pain associated with HO relies on the administration of NSAIDs, opioids (e.g., fentanyl transdermal patches), tramadol (not as a sole agent due to questionable efficacy following PO administration), and bisphosphonates [104, 105]. Other treatments include vagotomy or intercostal nerve

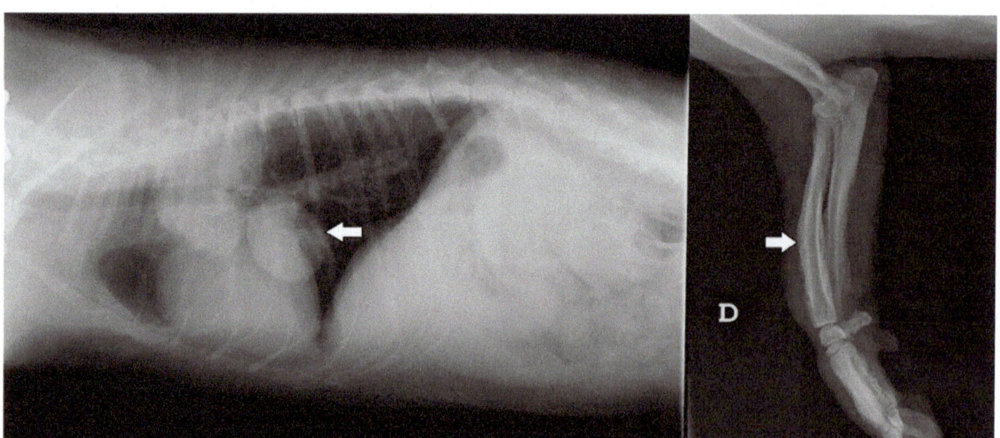

Figure 17.2 Primary lung tumor (white arrow in left picture) in a patient suffering hypertrophic osteopathy with periosteal proliferation in the same patient (white arrow in right picture). *Source:* Photo courtesy of Dr. Sergio Monteagudo.

resection to disrupt the neurologic afferent input that causes blood flow to increase [106]. However, these therapeutic options have not been extensively studied in veterinary patients.

Treatment

Chemotherapy

The increased incidence and prevalence of cancer in the small-animal population has led to an expansion in knowledge and availability of sophisticated treatment options for cancer patients. Currently, most of these therapeutic options depend on complex chemotherapeutic interventions that are associated with several complications. Since most chemotherapy drugs exert their effects in the active phases of the cellular cycle [107], their toxic effects take place most commonly in tissues with a constant cellular turnover. As some normal tissues present a growth rate that resembles that of tumoral tissue (i.e., mucosa, gametes, epidermis, or hematopoietic cells) [108], chemotherapeutic agents will therefore affect not only tumoral tissues, but some normal tissues as well. Additionally, most chemotherapeutic drugs present a very narrow therapeutic margin, as their desired effect is cellular toxicity. These effects can alter the way anesthetic plans are formulated, since many patient systems, including the bone marrow, gastrointestinal, dermatologic, neurologic, and urologic systems, are affected; hypersensitivity reactions and acute tumor lysis syndrome (TLS) can also occur.

Myelosuppression is commonly associated with the cytotoxic effects of chemotherapeutic agents. Anemia is rarely seen secondary to chemotherapy, as the life span of red cells is longer than other cells. However, certain drugs such as doxorubicin can cause recurrent bone marrow suppression and consequent exhaustion after longer periods of chemotherapy. Thrombocytopenia resulting from chemotherapeutic toxicity is rare, although rebound thrombocytosis can be observed. Neutropenia is often present after the administration of cytotoxic chemotherapeutic agents 7–21 days post-treatment, especially at the nadir of the treatment [107]. Frequently, treatment is not necessary, as patients are asymptomatic and cell counts return to normal limits within a few days, but prophylactic antibiotic therapy may be used when neutrophil counts drop below 1000 cells μl^{-1}. Anorexia, vomiting, and cachexia are the most common side effects of chemotherapy on the gastrointestinal tract due to its cytotoxic effects. Depending on the severity of the symptoms, fluid therapy, antibiotics, and hospitalization for close observation are recommended. Hydration and volume status should be optimized prior to general anesthesia.

Extravasation of the chemotherapeutic agents is a viable concern. Severe local tissue reactions may lead to necrosis of the area; doxorubicin is the agent that most commonly causes the most severe reactions due to large extravasated volumes. Clinical signs may include moist dermatitis, erythema, pruritus, pain, and eventually necrosis of the area within 7–10 days after extravasation; veins should be evaluated prior to administration for catheterization viability (Figure 17.3).

Local tissue reactions should be treated symptomatically by applying topical antibiotic or steroid preparations. Within 3 h of doxorubicin extravasation, dexrazoxane should be administered IV at a dose 10 times the extravasated dose and then daily for 3 days. If a vinca alkaloid is acutely extravasated, the area should be infiltrated with sterile saline ± 8.4% sodium bicarbonate and dexamethasone SP. Peripheral neuropathies are the main signs of neurotoxicity after administration of chemotherapeutic agents. These include partial paralysis, hind limb weakness, and even ileus that could lead to abdominal pain and constipation, especially if vinca alkaloids are being administered. Platinum products have been reported to cause cortical blindness. Nephrotoxicity and renal failure have also been reported secondary to cisplatin and doxorubicin administration, respectively, and stabilization of the patient

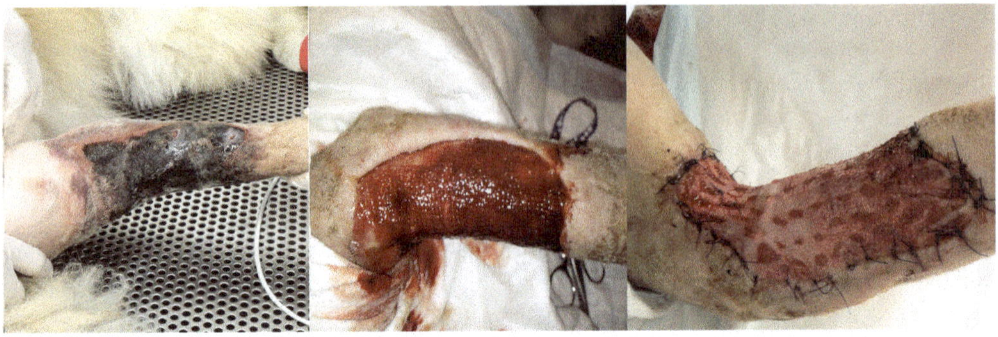

Figure 17.3 Forelimb necrosis in a canine patient after doxorubicin treatment (left) and surgical repair in the same patient (center and right). *Source:* Photo courtesy of Dr. Cavadonga Sanchez-Mellado.

may be necessary if azotemia or electrolyte derangements are present.

Acute, type I hypersensitivity reactions have been reported secondary to administration of certain chemotherapy agents such as L-asparaginase or etoposide, while other agents such as doxorubicin have been associated with anaphylactoid reactions due to direct stimulation of mast cell degranulation [107]. Emergency treatment should include epinephrine administration if severe vasodilation and bronchoconstriction are present, as well as fluid therapy, histamine-2 receptor antagonists (i.e., diphenhydramine), and steroids (i.e., dexamethasone), if necessary. TLS may also occur secondary to chemotherapy and is associated with rapid tumor cell destruction leading to release of intracellular ions and metabolic byproducts into the extracellular environment and intravascular space [109]. The most common metabolic derangements of TLS include hyperkalemia, metabolic acidosis, azotemia, and hyperphosphatemia that could secondarily induce hypocalcemia. Clinical signs of TLS include vomiting, diarrhea, lethargy, bradyarrhythmias (secondary to hypocalcemia), and pale mucous membranes (secondary to decreased cardiac output). Initial treatment should include restoration of tissue perfusion with aggressive fluid therapy and hemodynamic stabilization, correction of electrolyte and acid–base disturbances, and renal stabilization [109].

Radiation Therapy

Current radiation therapy is based on the use of ionizing radiation for local and regional eradication of malignant and, occasionally, benign tumors while preserving normal healthy tissue structure and function. The biological effect of ionizing radiation is based on its ability to cause ionization and excitation of atoms and molecules in cells that lead to the synthesis of a number of short-lived ions and unstable free radicals capable of causing molecular damage [110]. This molecular damage compromises cell survival by interaction of free radicals with cellular DNA, causing tumoral cells to enter mitosis with unrepaired DNA damage. This type of cell death is particularly relevant for tumors, as tumoral cells possess a characteristic ability to divide indefinitely. The side effects of radiation therapy on normal tissues are usually restricted to the treatment site, and they are classified chronologically into acute (during or immediately after treatment) and late effects (months to years after completion of treatment). Acute effects occur primarily from radiation-induced stem cell depletion that exceeds cell production in rapidly proliferating parenchymal tissues and usually affect mucous membranes and skin. These lesions are commonly self-limiting and resolve naturally after treatment; however, they may be temporarily painful and require supportive treatment. Late effects are considered true complications of radiation therapy and are mainly due to lesions of the vasculoconnective stroma in slowly proliferating parenchymal tissues of organs such as lungs, heart, bone, cartilage, spinal cord, or kidneys. These lesions are not self-limited and tend to irreversibly progress to severe fibrosis, necrosis, loss of function, or even death. They are usually treated conservatively, although occasionally extremely severe complications may require surgical treatment.

Mucositis usually presents in the oral cavity, pharynx, and/or esophagus when tumors of the neck and head are irradiated; colitis may be present when caudal portions of the gastrointestinal system receive radiation therapy. Clinical signs include tender mouth and thickened saliva that lead to dysphagia and eventually anorexia, dehydration and malnutrition with mucositis, and severe large intestine diarrhea with colitis. Symptoms usually develop 1–2 weeks after the beginning of therapy and reach maximum development by the end of therapy, although oral mucositis should resolve 2–3 weeks after the end of therapy. Owner compliance is essential during these weeks and interventions such as hand-feeding low-salt diets and detailed instruction on caloric and fluid requirements of the animal may be helpful. Placement of an esophagostomy/gastrostomy tube (Figure 17.4) or administration of subcutaneous fluids may be necessary in some instances to preserve the patient's hydration and nutritional status.

The preanesthetic evaluation should assess hydration and electrolyte status, body condition score (BCS), and the degree of oral mucositis. Oral lesions should be evaluated carefully, and special care should be taken when endotracheal intubation is performed by thoroughly lubricating the endotracheal tube (ETT), handling the laryngoscope with care, and securing the ETT in a gentle way, avoiding lesion areas.

Dermatological early side effects are usually restricted to the radiation field and their severity is dose related. They include several lesions such as erythema, subcutaneous fibrosis, pigmentation abnormalities, epilation, moist desquamation, and even self-mutilation of the lesion areas if care is not taken. Pain management strategies should focus on pain relief for these lesions and every effort should be made to provide padded and careful positioning to avoid the development of decubitus ulcers. Special care should be taken to avoid burning lesions by the warming devices in those sensitive areas that have radiation side effects.

Ophthalmological consequences are dose-related and vary in severity depending on the proximity of the eyes to the radiation field. Every effort is usually made to keep the eyes out of the radiation field; however, depending on the location of the tumor, it is not always possible. Acute effects include blepharitis, blepharospasm, conjunctivitis, keratoconjunctivitis sicca (KCS), and ulceration. Care must be taken to provide

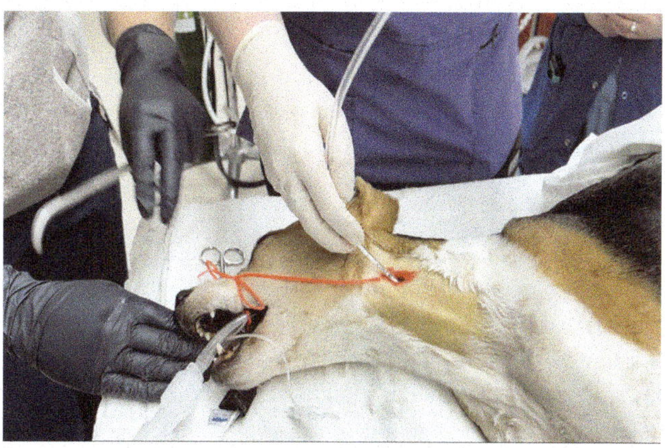

Figure 17.4 Esophagostomy tube placement in a dog.

excellent lubrication of the eyes during the anesthetic period in those patients that suffer from KCS.

Cancer Pain

Pain is not just a sensation, but rather an "experience" that includes both sensory-discriminative and motivational-affective components [111]. Cancer-related pain results from one or more of the following: (i) tumor-related pain from direct invasion of different organs, bones, and nerves, (ii) treatment-related pain following surgical intervention, chemotherapy, or radiation therapy, (iii) indirect etiologies including metabolic imbalances due to PNS, vascular obstruction, and by secondary infection, and/or (iv) unrelated factors associated with inactivity and deconditioning [112–115]. Combinations of these different etiologies result in complex pain patterns that are difficult to accurately diagnose in the veterinary cancer patient. In addition, processes related to chronification of pain such as hyperalgesia, central sensitization, synaptic remodeling, novel gene expression, and behavioral adjustment develop rapidly after persistent tissue injury, making pain management complex and challenging [116, 117].

Pain Pathophysiology

Neoplastic-associated pain can be either neuropathic, nociceptive, or a combination of the two. Neuropathic pain is related to central or peripheral neural tissue lesions and is characterized by aberrant somatosensory processing [113]. Nociceptive pain is associated with unhealed injury to either visceral or somatic tissues and can be dull and diffuse (visceral or deep somatic) or sharp, pricking, and well-localized (superficial somatic). Neuropathic pain in cancer patients is very complex, as tumor involvement of the peripheral nervous system presents many different clinical manifestations that may range from local invasion or compression of nerves to direct infiltration or perineural spread. Some of these lesions may also be associated with inflammatory changes that may lead to additional pain. The pathophysiologic mechanism underlying nerve infiltration or compression includes reparative and reactive biochemical changes that affect dendrites, soma, and axons of the entire primary afferent neuron so that it will eventually lose its neuropeptides and atrophy, and degenerate [118, 119]. In addition, tumors contain endothelin and inflammatory substances that may sensitize or directly or indirectly (through tissue acidosis) excite the nociceptors of primary afferent neurons [120].

Following repeated stimulation at both peripheral and central levels, sensitization can occur, and manifest as an enhanced response to noxious stimulation or a newly acquired responsiveness to a wider range of stimuli that includes non-noxious stimuli. Peripheral sensitization occurs when nociceptors are sensitized. Central sensitization occurs when activated N-methyl-D-aspartate (NMDA) receptors increase excitability of secondary afferent neurons in the dorsal horn. This phenomenon is also known as "central wind-up" and has two main consequences: (1) pain is more difficult to manage; larger doses and multiple drugs need to be administered, and (2) patients perceive heightened levels of pain due to the altered interpretation of stimuli (see Chapter 22).

Pain Evaluation

One of the most challenging aspects in management of the veterinary oncologic patient is related to the identification, evaluation, and quantification of pain, since, unlike humans, self-report is not an option in veterinary patients. Additionally, the tolerance of pain varies greatly from one individual to another, and the innate ability of animals to mask significant disease and pain on certain occasions complicates things further. Therefore, in veterinary medicine, the recognition of pain relies heavily on the interpretation of the animal's behavior by an observer as well as the physiological responses. Although behavioral changes vary between species, a number of changes have been identified and are used in a vigorously validated animal pain scoring system for hospitalized patients called the Glasgow Composite Measure Pain Scale (CMPS), for dogs, and the Glasgow Feline Composite Measure Pain Scale (CMPS-Feline), for cats (Figures 17.5 and 17.6) [121, 122]. They include the assessment of spontaneous and evoked behaviors, interactions with the animal, and clinical observations. These two scales were developed to assess acute pain in canine and feline patients, respectively, and should only take a few minutes to perform. The behaviors and interactions listed in the CMPS will obviously vary with animal nature and temperament, but these assessments are relevant in most patients.

Analgesia should never be withheld due to the difficulty recognizing pain in an animal. Both clinicians and technicians must be proactive in looking for signs of pain in patients, and, if in doubt, the administration of analgesia with subsequent assessment of response to treatment is recommended. Moreover, if a type of tumor and/or its location is painful in humans, it is appropriate to assume that it is so in animals as well. Since pain is not a static process, a pain assessment should be performed prior to a procedure and frequent post-procedure assessments are necessary, including home assessments.

During the past decades, many efforts have been devoted to the assessment of quality of life in human patients, and several methods have been developed and validated in clinical trials. However, validated, and standardized criteria for measuring quality of life in animals are rare. Any assessment of the quality of life of an animal must come indirectly from a proxy informant, most commonly, the owner. In 2005, Yazbek and Fantoni validated a health-related quality-of-life scale for dogs with signs of pain secondary to cancer which can be used to evaluate the cancer management plan (Table 17.4) [123].

Specific Pain Characteristics

Tumor pain characteristics differ according to the type and stage of tumor development. Osseous tumor infiltration is the most common cause of pain in oncologic patients (Figure 17.7) [113].

The pathophysiologic pain mechanisms elicited by infiltrative bone or bone marrow tumors are associated with lesions causing periosteal elevation, release of chemical mediators that sensitize nociceptors, increased intraosseous pressure, or loss of stability. Nociceptive pain originates from nociceptors located in the bone itself, but also in the bone marrow and in the periosteum.

Tumors of encapsulated organs such as kidneys, spleen, liver, or brain can enlarge the organ to several times the organ's normal size (Figure 17.8). As the organ capsule grows less rapidly than the tumor, pain ensues from

Figure 17.5 Guidance for use of the CMPS-SF. The short form composite measure pain score (CMPS-SF) can be applied quickly and reliably in a clinical setting and has been designed as a clinical decision-making tool which was developed for dogs in acute pain. It includes 30 descriptor options within 6 behavioral categories, including mobility. Within each category, the descriptors are ranked numerically according to their associated pain severity and the person carrying out the assessment chooses the descriptor within each category which best fits the dog's behavior/condition. It is important to carry out the assessment procedure as described on the questionnaire, following the protocol closely. The pain score is the sum of the rank scores. The maximum score for the 6 categories is 24, or 20 if mobility is impossible to assess. The total CMPS-SF score has been shown to be a useful indicator of analgesic requirement and the recommended analgesic intervention level is 6/24 or 5/20. *Source:* Adapted with permission.

SHORT FORM OF THE GLASGOW COMPOSITE MEASURE PAIN SCALE

Dog's name_ **Date** / / **Time**

Hospital Number __________

Procedure or Condition____

____

In thes ections below please circle the appropriate score in each list and sum these to give the total score

A. Look at dog in Kennel

Is the dog

(i)

Quiet	0
Crying or whimpering	1
Groaning	2
Screaming	3

(ii)

Ignoring any wound or painful area	0
Looking at wound or painful area	1
Licking wound or painful area	2
Rubbing wound or painful area	3
Chewing wound or painful area	4

In the case of spinal, pelvic, or multiple limb fractures, or where assistance is required to aid locomotion, do not carry out section **B** and proceed to **C**
Please tick if this is the case ☐ then proceed to C

B. Put lead ondog and lead out of the kennel

When the dog rises/walks is it?

(iii)

Normal	0
Lame	1
Slow or reluctant	2
Stiff	3
It refuses to move	4

C. If it has a wound or painful area including abdomen, apply gentle pressure 2 inches round the site

Does it?

(iv)

Do nothing	0
Look round	1
Flinch	2
Growl or guard area	3
Snap	4
Cry	5

D. Overall

Is the dog?

(v)

Happy and content or happy and bouncy	0
Quiet	1
Indifferent or non-responsive to surroundings	2
Nervous or anxious or fearful	3
Depressed or non-responsive to stimulation	4

Is the dog?

(vi)

Comfortable	0
Unsettled	1
Restless	2
Hunched or tense	3
Rigid	4

Total Score (i+ii+iii+iv+v+vi) = ________

Glasgow Feline Composite Measure Pain Scale: CMPS - Feline

Choose the most appropriate expression from each section and total the scores to calculate the pain score for the cat. If more than one expression applies choose the higher score

LOOK AT THE CAT IN ITS CAGE:

Is it?

Question 1

Slient / puming / meowing	0
Crying/growling / groaning	1

Question 2

Relaxed	0
Licking lips	1
Restless/cowering at back of cage	2
Tense/crouched	3
Rigid/hunched	4

Question 3

Ignoring any wound or painful area	0
Attention to wound	1

Question 4

a) Look at the following caricatures. Circle the drawing which depicts the cat's ear position?

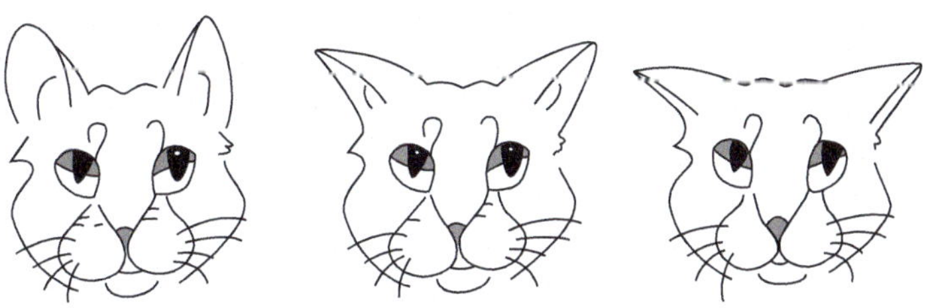

0 | 1 | 2

b) Look at the shape of the muzzle in the following caricatures. Circle the drawing which appears most like that of the car?

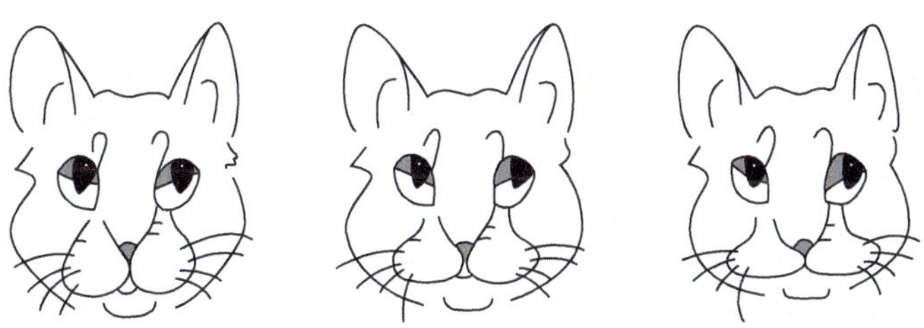

0 | 1 | 2

Figure 17.6 Guidance for use of the Glasgow Feline Composite Measure Pain Scale (CMPS-Feline), which can be applied quickly and reliably in a clinical setting, has been designed as a clinical decision-making tool for use in cats in acute pain. It includes 28 descriptor options within 7 behavioral categories. Within each category, the descriptors are ranked numerically according to their associated pain severity and the person carrying out the assessment chooses the descriptor within each category which best fits the cat's behavior/condition. It is important to carry out the assessment procedure as described on the questionnaire, following the protocol closely. The pain score is the sum of the rank scores. The maximum score for the 7 categories is 20. The total CMPS-Feline score has been shown to be a useful indicator of analgesic requirement and the recommended analgesic intervention level is 5/20. *Source:* Adapted with permission.

APPROACH THE CAGE, CALL THE CAT BY NAME & STROKE ALONG ITS BACK From HEAD TO TAIL

Question 5

Does it?	
Respond to stroking	0
Is it?	
Unresponsive	1
Aggressive	2

IF IT HAS A WOUND OR PAINFUL AREA, APPLY GENTLE PRESSURE 5 CM AROUND THE SITE. THE ABSENCE OF ANY PAINFUL AREA APPLY SIMILAR PRESSURE AROUND THE HIND LEG ABOVE THE KNEE

Question 6

Does it?	
Do nothing	0
Swish tail/flatten ears	1
Cry/hiss	2
Growl	3
Bite/lash out	4

Question 7

General impression

Is the cat?	
Happy and content	0
Disinterested/quiet	1
Anxious/fearful	2
Dull	3
Depressed/grumpy	4

Pain Score ... /20

Figure 17.6 (Continued)

increased intracapsular pressure, direct capsule infiltration, or from traction or pressure on the tissue suspending the organ.

Tumors and metastases in digestive and urogenital hollow organs are frequently painful (Figure 17.9). Pain results from intestinal dilation, motility disorders, ulcerations, and blood flow impairment. Pain in urogenital organs may be caused by arteritis, perineural tumor infiltration, or perineural inflammatory reactions.

Solid organs such as the pancreas suffer specific pain symptoms subsequent to tumor-induced necrosis that results in autodigestive pancreatitis. The autodigestion most likely results from tumorous destruction of the parenchyma as well as from tumor infiltration and stenosis of the excretory ducts.

Tumor infiltration of soft tissues elicits pain by compressing individual nerves and plexus, as well as by affecting organs that are responsible of the patient's movement, such as tendons or muscles (Figure 17.10). Infiltration of the interstitium and destruction of lymphatic vessels, nerves, and blood vessels prevent these organs from normal function.

Tumor infiltration and inflammation of serosa and mucosa also cause pain. Although pleural carcinomas do not usually cause pain (most likely due to the development of pleural effusion that prevents the pleurae from rubbing against each other), peritoneal carcinosis does. Pain results from either direct contact of the metastases with peripheral nerves or from the inflammatory reaction resulting from tumor-induced perforation or penetration of an abdominal hollow organ.

Peripheral nerve pain usually arises due to entrapment of individual nerves and plexus by tumor growth. However, pain can also result as tumor infiltration causes the neural cleft to

Table 17.4 Questionnaire for evaluating health-related quality of life in dogs with signs of pain secondary to cancer.

Questionnaire
How much do you think that the disease is disturbing your dog's quality of life?
Very much (0)
Much (1)
A little (2)
Not at all (3)
Does your dog still do what it likes (e.g., play or go for a walk)?
No (0)
Rarely (1)
Frequently (2)
In a normal way (3)
How is your dog's mood?
Totally altered (0)
Some episodes of alteration (1)
Changed a little bit (2)
Normal (3)
Does your dog keep its hygienic habits (i.e., clean itself)?
No (0)
Rarely (1)
Less than before (2)
Yes (3)
How often do you think that your dog feels pain?
All the time (0)
Frequently (1)
Rarely (2)
Never (3)
Does your dog have an appetite?
No (0)
Only eats when forced; will eat more of what it likes (1)
Little (2)
Normal (3)
Does your dog get tired easily?
Yes, always (0)
Frequently (1)
Rarely (2)
No (3)
How is your dog sleeping?
Very badly; not sleeping at all (0)
Badly (1)
Almost normally (2)
Normally (3)

(*continued*)

Table 17.4 (Continued)

Questionnaire
How often does your dog vomit?
Always (0)
Frequently (1)
Rarely (2)
Never (3)
How are the intestines of your dog functioning?
Very badly (0)
Badly (1)
Almost normally (2)
Normally (3)
Is your dog able to position itself to defecate and urinate?
Never (0)
Rarely (1)
Sometimes (2)
Urinates and defecates normally (3)
How much attention is your dog giving to the family?
Indifferent (0)
Little attention (1)
Increased attention; the dog is needy (2)
Has not changed (3)

Scores (values in parentheses) for all 12 questions were summed to determine the health-related quality-of-life score. Possible scores ranged from 0 to 36 [123]. *Source:* Adapted with permission.

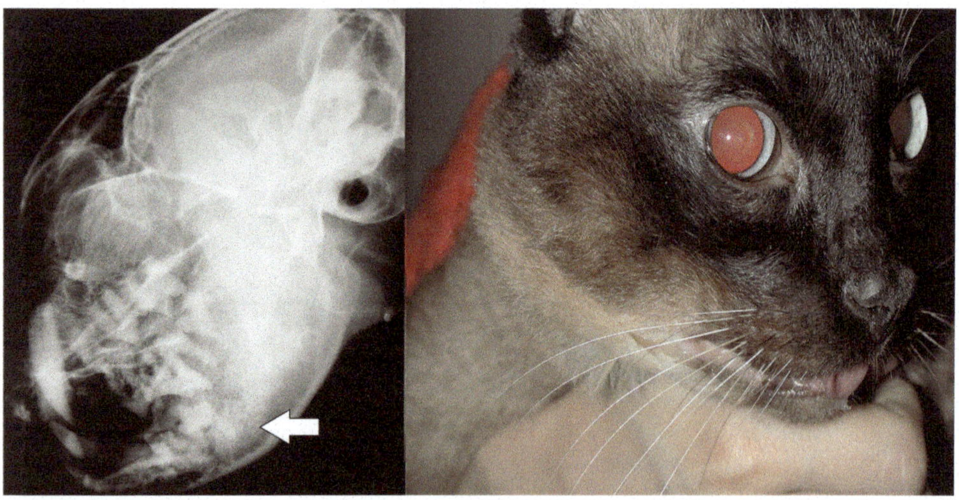

Figure 17.7 Osteosarcoma in the mandible of a feline patient (white arrow on radiograph). *Source:* Photo courtesy of Dr. Ana Ríos.

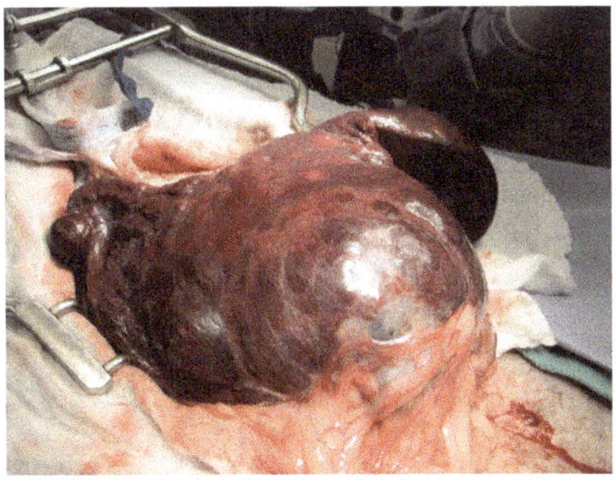

Figure 17.8 Splenic hemangiosarcoma in a canine patient. *Source:* Photo courtesy of Dr. Sara Colopy.

widen, and infiltration of the tumor into the nerve itself takes place.

Blood and lymphatic vessels are invaded as malignant neoplasia begins to metastasize. Although small vessel infiltration and obstruction are rarely painful, when large veins are affected, edema and pain in the affected area of venous drainage are often present (Figure 17.11).

Cancer Pain Management

Treatment of acute pain should be a priority not only for obvious ethical reasons, but also to minimize

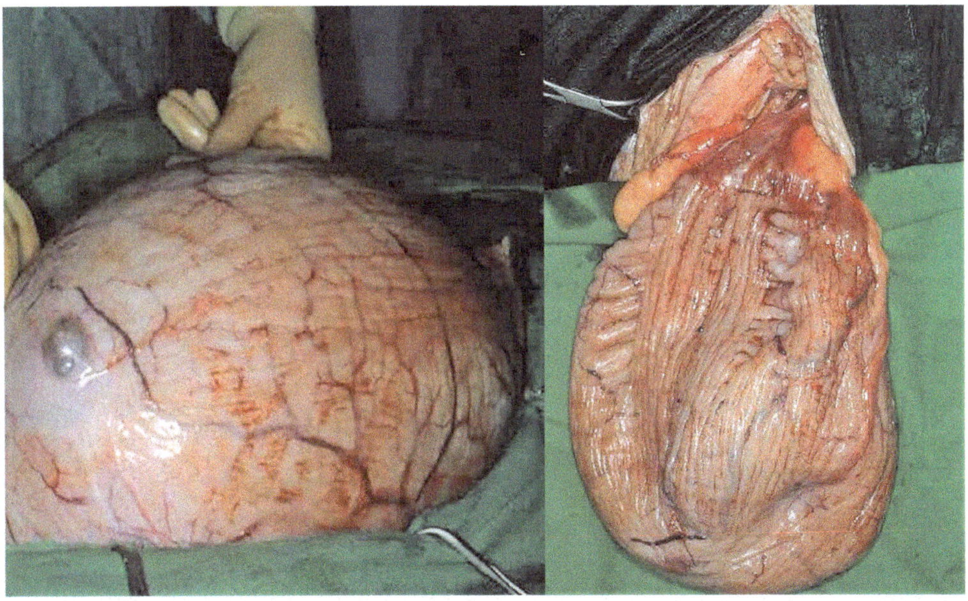

Figure 17.9 Transitional cell carcinoma invading the entire bladder of a canine patient. *Source:* Photo courtesy of Dr. Hilde de Rooster and Dr. Alejandro Rubio.

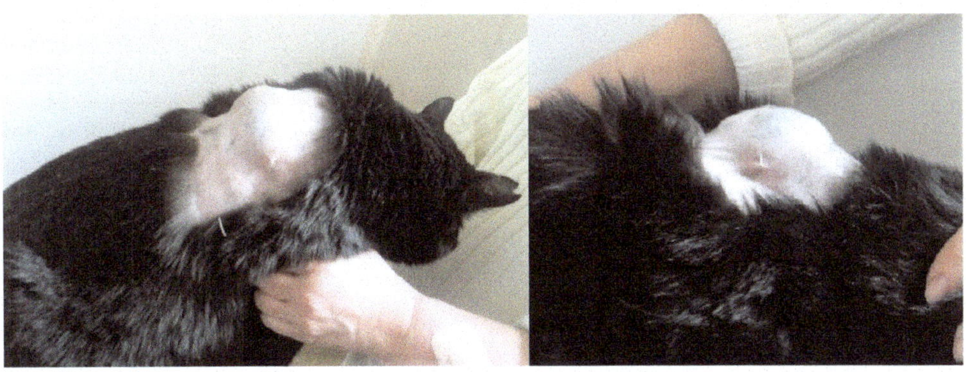

Figure 17.10 Fibrosarcoma in the interscapular region of a feline patient.

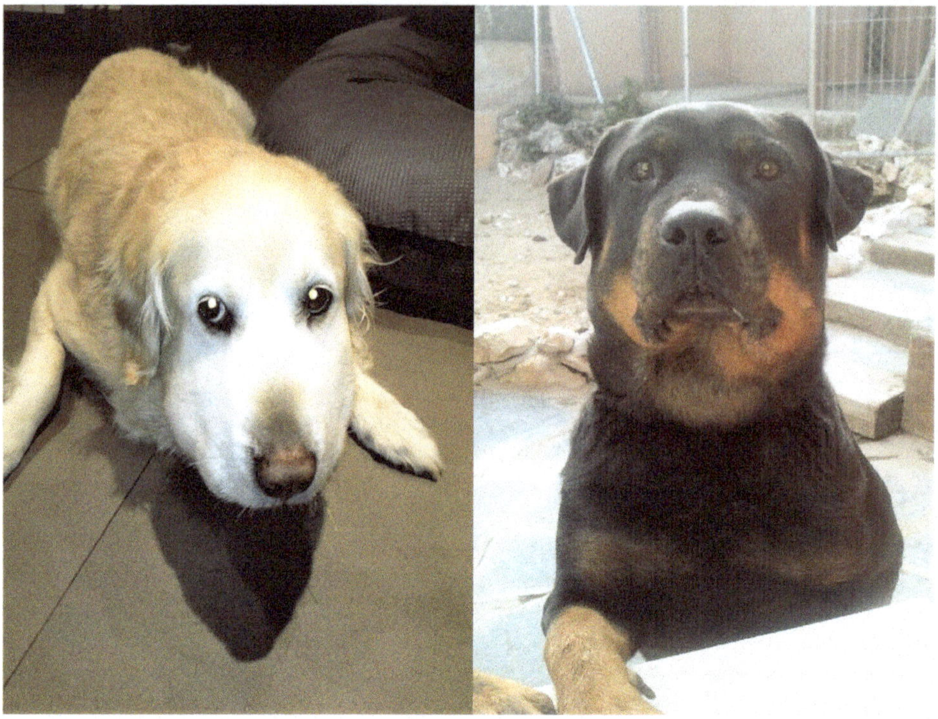

Figure 17.11 Facial edema as part of superior vena cava syndrome in two canine patients. *Source:* Photos courtesy of Dr. Noemi del Castillo and Dr. Sonia Fernandez.

its negative influence on postoperative morbidity and mortality (such as decreased rate of healing, hypertension, tachycardia, or ileus). Treating perioperative pain significantly reduces the tumor-promoting effects of surgery, as surgery itself suppresses natural killer (NK) cell activity which may enhance metastasis [124, 125]. Although drugs are the mainstay of cancer pain management, nonpharmacologic interventions are becoming increasingly popular. Overall, cancer pain management therapeutic interventions may be divided into two categories: pharmacologic and nonpharmacologic.

Pharmacologic Interventions

Multimodal analgesia should be used to alter more than one point along the nociceptive pathway including nociceptive transduction, transmission to the CNS, modulation within the CNS, or perception at the cortex (see Chapter 22). This analgesic approach reduces individual drug doses, thereby reducing the potential for adverse effects. The use of preemptive analgesia should also be used to reduce central hypersensitivity or wind-up pain. Additionally, providing effective multimodal and preemptive analgesia will not only reduce postoperative pain, but will also form part of a balanced anesthesia plan that may allow significant reductions in anesthetic agent requirements. All these interventions may ultimately lead to a smoother plane of anesthesia and optimal recovery characteristics.

The first line of analgesia should be the use of "traditional" analgesics such as opioids, NSAIDs, and local anesthetic techniques. Recently, other "adjunctive" analgesics such as NMDA receptor antagonists (i.e., ketamine, amantadine), alpha-2-adrenergic receptor agonists, bisphosphonates, and anticonvulsant (i.e., gabapentin) drugs have gained popularity. The World Health Organization

(WHO) has outlined a ladder or general approach to cancer pain management in humans based on these drug groups: nonopioids, opioids for mild-to-moderate pain, opioids for moderate to severe pain, and adjuvant drugs [126]. However, "WHO is discontinuing these guidelines considering new scientific evidence that has emerged since the time of their publication in 2019. And although WHO remains fully committed to ensuring that people suffering severe pain have access to effective pain relief medication, including opioids, it also recognizes that the need for access to pain relief must be balanced with concerns about the harm arising from the misuse of medications prescribed for the management of pain, including opioids. Scientific evidence indicates there are risks associated with the use of these medications, such as the development of dependence, overdose, and accidental death. Recent research in the fields of palliative care and pain management has identified many strategies for managing pain, beyond drug treatment alone" [127]. In fact, at the end of 2019, a task force for the reevaluation of pain management guidelines was appointed by WHO [128]. Regardless of all the recent reevaluation of this therapeutic management in human medicine, there are two potential problems with the use of the WHO analgesic ladder in veterinary medicine. First, there is a lack of information on which drugs are most effective on which type of cancer pain in veterinary patients. Second, this approach may not be appropriate for many veterinary cancer patients, as they often present at an already advanced stage of disease and may already be in a moderate to severe state of pain. Once pain has been allowed to become chronic, central sensitization and hyperalgesia are already taking place. To manage this very complex type of pain, an analgesic reverse pyramid approach may be required, which relies on the use of multiple different classes of drugs until the intensity of pain decreases, at which point the amounts and types of drugs may be minimized.

Opioids

Opioids such as morphine, hydromorphone, methadone, fentanyl, buprenorphine, and butorphanol exert their analgesic effects and their side effects through actions on the different opioid receptors (μ, δ, and κ). The most frequent side effects of opioids include dose- and drug-dependent cardiovascular depression due to a reduction in sympathetic tone. This often results in varying degrees of bradycardia, while no direct effects on systemic blood pressure or myocardial contractility are commonly seen [19]. Vasodilation from histamine release can also be observed, mainly after IV administration of morphine and meperidine [129]. Dose- and drug-dependent respiratory depression may be described after opioid administration and may be especially noticeable when given in conjunction with anesthetic induction agents and volatile anesthetics. Ileus decreases gastric emptying time and constipation may be observed as well as short-term urinary retention. Dysphoria may occur after opioid administration; however, it is infrequent if administered to animals in pain or in combination with sedatives or tranquilizers. Finally, alterations in thermoregulation, such as hypothermia and/or panting, are usually observed, while cats may exhibit hyperthermia after opioid administration.

All the previously mentioned parenteral opioids may be administered by an intermittent IV or IM route [19]. However, with intermittent dosing, patients often feel pain before their subsequent dose and may become sedated after dose administration. Alternatively, continuous rate infusions (CRI) of a shorter-acting, potent opioid analgesic agent can be used (e.g., fentanyl, alfentanil, remifentanil). Fentanyl administered as a CRI provides constant and reliable plasma levels that provide excellent analgesia and allow sparing of inhalant agent; therefore, reducing its systemic adverse effects [130–134]. Fentanyl may also provide postoperative analgesia; due to potential respiratory depression, patients should be under constant and vigilant observation.

Intramuscular, slow IV bolus, or CRI administration of morphine is efficacious, although histamine release may limit its use in MCTs [129]. Fentanyl transdermal patches provide another route of opioid administration and analgesia can be provided for several days [135–137]. However, the degree of analgesia can be unpredictable, especially in cats, probably due to failure of patch application or inappropriate dosing, and frequent patient monitoring is essential [138, 139]. Since plasma levels do not reach peak values until 12–24 h post placement, additional analgesia should be provided in the immediate postoperative period. Fentanyl patches are a suitable option for patients that may need prolonged opioid administration and for those that do not tolerate oral medication. Fentanyl patches should not be prescribed when young children are in the household, since potential removal and ingestion are of concern [140, 141]. Finally, opioids such as morphine and fentanyl have been administered epidurally to prolong perioperative analgesia [142–145]. With placement of an epidural catheter, epidural opioids can be administered for days to weeks in patients suffering from peritoneal or pancreatic pain, as well as following amputations.

Nonsteroidal Anti-Inflammatory Drugs

NSAIDs such as meloxicam or carprofen are used widely to treat mild-to-moderate pain associated with inflammation and to reduce opioid consumption. However, they possess a much lower therapeutic index than opioids and are not reversible. NSAIDs inhibit COX enzymes, thereby preventing the production of prostaglandins (PG), thromboxanes, and prostacyclin from membrane phospholipids. However, the isoenzyme COX-2 is also related to the pathogenesis and progression of certain types of tumors. The synthesis of PGE_2 by COX-2 has been associated with the promotion of tumorigenesis, and COX-2 overexpression inhibits apoptosis, facilitates the adhesion and invasiveness of tumor cells, increases cell growth, suppresses the immune system, and enhances angiogenesis [146, 147]. Overexpression of COX-2 has been implicated in a number of canine carcinomas, such as those affecting the bladder, kidneys, mammary tissues, and intestines, squamous cell carcinoma, and some sarcomas such as osteosarcoma [148–152]. As a result, the use of selective COX-2 inhibitors is widespread not only for their analgesic effects in patients with these types of tumors, but also for their beneficial effects on the tumor therapy [153–165].

The most common side effects of NSAIDs include impairment of gastrointestinal protection, inhibition of platelet aggregation and vasoconstriction, and impairment of renal perfusion [166]. Oncologic patients are at greater risk of toxic effects due to their potential for pre-existing renal disease or the concurrent administration of nephrotoxic oncologic therapies. The use of NSAIDs is not recommended in patients, regardless of their tumor, that present with gastrointestinal disorders, coagulopathies, impaired renal and hepatic function, patients that are dehydrated or hypovolemic, and those that are already receiving other NSAIDs or corticosteroids. Additionally, it should be remembered that cats have longer and inconsistent rates of metabolism and excretion of NSAIDs compared to other species (particularly through glucuronidation), and chronic dosing (longer than 5 days) is likely to be associated with greater risks in cats than other species and therefore should be used cautiously [167]. Renal monitoring of the patient that is receiving NSAID-based therapy is warranted. The owner should be informed of the potential for toxicity as well as instructed for monitoring of adverse events (depression, lethargy, vomiting, melena, and polyuria). Baseline blood work and urinalysis should also be performed at the beginning of therapy and repeated every 2–4 weeks and up to 1–4 months depending on the individual patient and evolution of the case.

Local Anesthetics

Local anesthesia is the only effective way of providing complete analgesia, as the main mechanism of action is via blockage of sodium channels. Perineural administration completely blocks transmission of nociception, thereby minimizing central sensitization for the duration of block. Local anesthetics (LAs) can be used by topical application, local infiltration, IV administration, interpleural administration, body cavity instillation, through wound-soaker catheters, by transdermal patches, and through epidural catheters. Neurological side effects are biphasic, first shown as excitatory signs (tremors, visual disturbances, and eventually seizures) and then signs of neurological depression (coma and apnea). Cardiovascular side effects include direct myocardial depression from blockade of cardiac sodium channels.

The use of topical LAs as a eutectic mixture of 2.5% lidocaine and 2.5% prilocaine (EMLA) cream has been suggested to minimize pain and discomfort during venipuncture or intravenous catheterization [168, 169]. LAs may be deposited directly over selected nerves prior to transection during surgical procedures. Ring blocks around the distal end of affected limbs or around a mass that needs to be excised may also be performed through infiltration of tissues. Ideally, the infiltration should be performed prior to surgery, paying attention to a gentle and cautious application if dealing with aggressive tumors (i.e., sarcoma); however, infiltrative blocks can also be employed during closure of surgical wounds, applying the traditional or liposome-encapsulated local anesthetic at various levels during wound closure. Finally, administration of the local anesthetic adjacent to the wound during closure has been shown to reduce pain postoperatively and reduce opioid requirements following laparotomy [170].

Wound diffusion catheters (also known as wound-soaker catheters) may be used to provide analgesia to large surgical wounds (e.g., amputations, tumor resection, mastectomies; Figure 17.12). They are usually well-tolerated and, if correctly placed, may not only improve patient comfort but significantly decrease opioid requirements. The incidence of wound infections or breakdown appears to be the same as in dogs where wound-soaker catheters are not placed [171]. Occasionally, catheters may fail to provide analgesia for the full extent of the surgical site; this may be due to uneven distribution of local anesthetic, incorrect placement, or catheter blockage. LAs may be administered every 6–8 h (1–2 $mg\,kg^{-1}$ ropivacaine or bupivacaine) [171]. The catheters can be removed 48 h after placement or remain in place for longer, if required.

LAs may be administered interpleurally to provide analgesia post thoracotomy and to manage pain in a variety of pleural conditions.

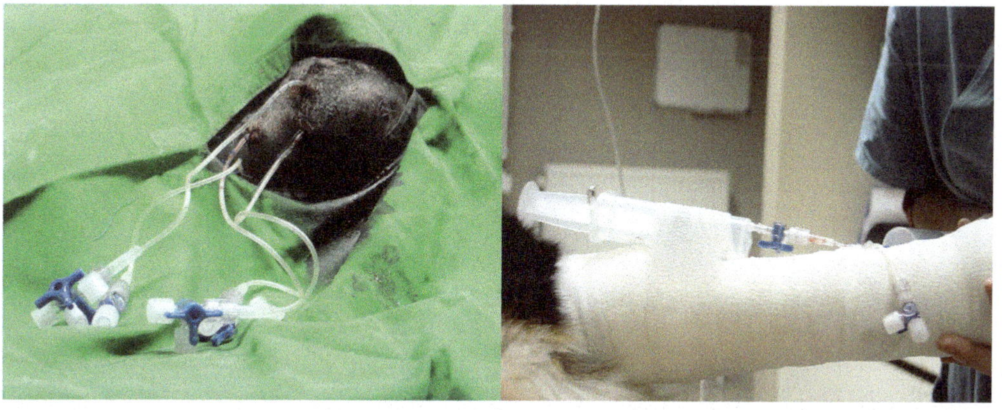

Figure 17.12 Surgical placement of wound-soaker catheter (left) with drainage and analgesic administration through the same soaker catheter (right). *Source:* Photo courtesy of Dr. Hilde de Rooster and Dr. Alejandro Rubio.

After drainage of the chest is performed, a 0.25% solution of bupivacaine ($1.5\,mg\,kg^{-1}$) may be slowly administered through the drain (Figure 17.13). This technique will usually provide up to 6 h of analgesia, while the pleural cavity may still be drained every hour if necessary, without affecting the efficacy of analgesia [172–176].

LAs may also be administered intraperitoneally. It has been found that the combination of intraperitoneal bupivacaine administered preoperatively with subcutaneous wound infiltration with bupivacaine postoperatively provided improved analgesia in dogs [170]. Similarly, sprayed, and injected intraperitoneal bupivacaine relieves postoperative pain behavior and biochemical stress responses after surgery in dogs [177, 178].

Newer techniques such as IV lidocaine infusions are efficacious and safe in dogs while decreasing isoflurane MAC [179]. In addition, longer-term epidural analgesia may be preferable for pain management of certain procedures and conditions (e.g., pancreatic pain, extensive hind limb surgery, amputations) and an epidural catheter may be placed to allow repeated administration of LAs (Figure 17.14). Drugs may be epidurally administered intermittently as a bolus or as an infusion using a syringe pump. Preservative-free morphine ($0.1\,mg\,kg^{-1}$) may be administered every 12–24 h, while bupivacaine ($0.06–0.12\,mg\,kg^{-1}$) can be administered intermittently as required. Alternatively, a CRI into the epidural catheter of morphine ($0.0125 mgkg^{-1}\,h^{-1}$) and bupivacaine ($0.03\,mg\,kg^{-1}\,h^{-1}$) has been reported [180].

Lidocaine 5% patches may be applied alongside wounds that present allodynia. Studies in both dogs and cats suggest that local skin lidocaine concentrations are high while plasma levels are low, suggesting that the analgesia seen following placement is most likely due to the local effect rather than to a systemic effect [181–184].

NMDA Antagonists

The use of subanesthetic doses of NMDA antagonists such as ketamine and amantadine may reduce the chances of central sensitization developing postoperatively and may also be particularly helpful for the management of pain derived from nerve damage. Side effects of this drug class include dose-dependent cardiovascular stimulation via sympathetic activation, increased salivation and respiratory tract secretions, cerebral vasodilation, and elevated systemic blood pressure that may lead to significant increases in cerebral blood flow and intracranial pressure. However, at the doses used for analgesia, these effects are minimized.

Bolus administration of ketamine and low-dose ketamine infusions for adjunctive analgesia have become common practices in the perioperative setting (e.g., hemilaminectomies, amputations). Several studies have proven the MAC-sparing properties of ketamine; however, only few studies evaluate the analgesic effects of ketamine which suggest that ketamine decreases postoperative

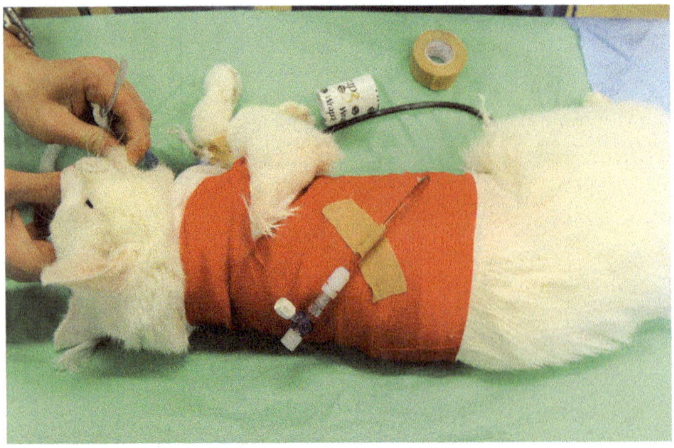

Figure 17.13 Chest drain and interpleural administration of local anesthetic in a cat. *Source:* Photo courtesy of Dr. Hilde de Rooster and Dr. Alejandro Rubio.

wound hyperalgesia and pain scores and rescues analgesic requirements [185–187].

Amantadine is an antiviral drug that was originally approved to treat influenza A in people. It is also used clinically to reduce symptoms of Parkinson's disease and other drug-induced extrapyramidal syndromes. Similar to ketamine, it is an NMDA receptor antagonist. However, it differs from ketamine, as it does not block the flow of current through open channels, but it stabilizes channels in the closed state. Numerous laboratory animal studies suggest that amantadine's NMDA antagonist activities may make it a useful adjunctive analgesic agent [188–190], but there are a limited number of controlled trials documenting its safety and efficacy in dogs and cats. It has been included in a multimodal analgesic regimen for the alleviation of refractory canine osteoarthritis pain and dogs had activity and lameness scores [191]. Amantadine may come to play a key role in managing chronic pain in dogs in the future and it may be an interesting therapeutic option for oncology patients.

Alpha-2-Adrenergic Receptor Agonists

Alpha-2-adrenergic receptor agonists such as dexmedetomidine are commonly used as adjunctive analgesics, although they are not considered first-line analgesics. Alpha-2-adrenergic receptors and opioid receptors appear to interact and coadministration of these two classes of drugs may achieve synergistic analgesic effects. However, the alpha-2 receptor-mediated analgesic effect is of shorter duration than the sedative effects [192, 193]. They are particularly useful in cardiovascular stable patients that require anxiolysis in addition to analgesia. Side effects include vasoconstriction, decreased cardiac contractility, reflex bradycardia and atrioventricular blocks, nausea and vomiting, polyuria, hyperglycemia, and increased myometrial contractility.

Dexmedetomidine CRIs may help manage both intraoperative and postoperative pain and have been found to be equally effective as morphine CRIs at providing postoperative analgesia, with no significant adverse clinical effects [194]. In addition, the incorporation of low-dose medetomidine or dexmedetomidine into an epidural protocol may achieve additive or synergistic analgesic effects when combined with standard doses of opioids or LAs due to actions at spinal alpha-2-adrenergic receptors [195–198]. In addition to the epidural route, alpha-2-adrenergic receptor agonists may be administered intraarticular and perineural, where they contribute to analgesia by inhibition of norepinephrine release and by enhancing peripheral nerve block intensity.

Tramadol

Tramadol is a synthetic codeine analog that exerts weak agonist properties at all opioid

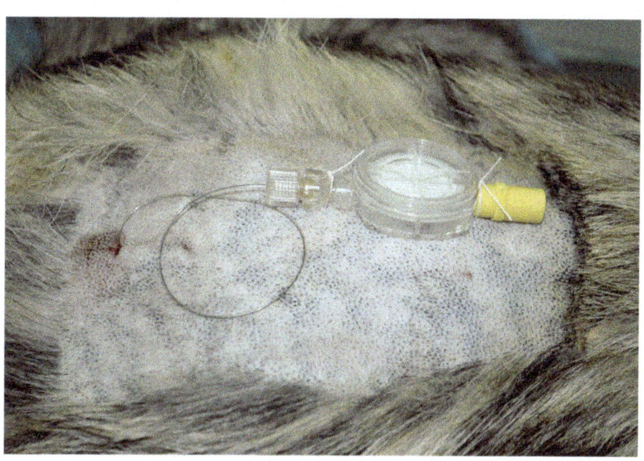

Figure 17.14 Epidural catheter placement in a cat. *Source:* Photo courtesy of Dr. Veronica Vieitez.

receptors (particularly at μ-opioid receptors). In addition, it stimulates presynaptic serotonin release and inhibits the reuptake of serotonin and noradrenaline [199]. Its analgesic potency is one-tenth that of morphine; however, recent studies comparing the effects of IV tramadol and morphine administered before ovariohysterectomy concluded that IV tramadol was comparable to morphine in its analgesic efficacy for this type of surgical pain [200, 201]. On the other side, oral administration of tramadol has shown to provide an unreliable degree of absorption as well as low concentrations of the pharmacologically active metabolite (O-desmethyltramadol, ODM) [202]. In fact, pharmacokinetic studies in dogs have shown that dogs do not produce ODM as a substantial metabolite after tramadol administration; therefore, dogs are not expected to have substantial opioid effects after tramadol administration [203, 204]. However, pharmacokinetics in cats are different, since they produce high concentrations of ODM after tramadol administration and, as a result, can show significant opioid effects. Common side effects include sedation and dysphoria (especially in cats), while constipation and respiratory depression seem to be generally milder than those caused by opioids. Its administration is contraindicated in patients with hepatic insufficiency and in those that are seizure-prone, as it decreases the seizure threshold in humans. Because of its inhibitory effect on serotonin uptake, tramadol should not be administered to patients that may have received monoamine oxidase inhibitors, such as selegiline.

Anticonvulsants

Neuromodulating drugs, such as anticonvulsants, have become the mainstay of neuropathic pain treatment in human patients in the past decades. Both pregabalin and gabapentin share a similar mechanism of action by binding to the $\alpha_2\delta$ subunit of the voltage-gated calcium channels and inhibiting the release excitatory neurotransmitters involved in pain transmission. Side effects are minimal, and they are limited to mild ataxia and sedation.

Although gabapentin is widely used in the treatment of human patients [205–207], only a few investigations have documented its effectiveness to treat chronic neuropathic pain, chronic cancer pain, chronic osteoarthritis pain, and perioperative pain in veterinary medicine [87–89, 92, 94, 208–211]. Dosing guidelines in veterinary medicine have been largely based on human recommendations despite some key species differences in pharmacokinetics. In dogs, it undergoes significant hepatic metabolism to N-methyl-gabapentin before renal elimination [94]. Gabapentin disposition has also been studied in cats [95]. The most used dose of gabapentin in dogs is $10\,\text{mg}\,\text{kg}^{-1}$ PO every 8 h, while in cats the dose is $10\,\text{mg}\,\text{kg}^{-1}$ PO every 12 h [94, 95].

Pregabalin was designed as the developmental successor of gabapentin to present a higher potency and a linear pharmacokinetic profile [96, 212, 213]. In human medicine, the analgesic efficacy of pregabalin has been extensively studied [214–229], and several large clinical trials substantiate its safety and efficacy [214–231]. Analgesic effects of pregabalin have been investigated in veterinary species with promising results [90, 91, 93, 232]. Pharmacokinetic studies in both dogs and cats suggest oral administration of pregabalin at $4\,\text{mg}\,\text{kg}^{-1}$ every 12 h as an appropriate dosing regimen [96, 97].

Tricyclic Antidepressants

Tricyclic antidepressants such as amitriptyline, clomipramine, and imipramine block the reuptake of norepinephrine and serotonin in the CNS. Their use in human medicine has been described for the treatment of neuropathic and chronic pain at doses considerably lower than those used to treat depression. Although there are no studies in the veterinary field that can support their use to this extent, clinical experience by many veterinarians substantiates their analgesic use in small animals.

Bisphosphonates

Bisphosphonates such as pamidronate and zoledronate accumulate on bone surfaces and inhibit osteoclast-induced resorption, favoring bone formation. They decrease pain and potentially increase survival rates in dogs with osteosarcoma [233] and may aid in the treatment of malignant hypercalcemia and inhibition of bone metastasis [61, 234–236]. They are safe and efficacious in dogs [237–241]. Currently, the recommended pamidronate protocol for dogs is 1–2 $mg\,kg^{-1}$ administered IV over 2 h in 250 ml of 0.9% saline administered every 21–28 days. Several studies investigating clinical effects of zoledronate have demonstrated significant inhibition of homeostatic osteolytic activity associated with single-dose IV administration (0.25 $mg\,kg^{-1}$) [242–248]. Although zoledronate may possess similar bone analgesic properties as pamidronate, its use in veterinary oncology is limited because of the substantial cost associated with the drug. Based on these initial studies, it seems that further investigation into the efficacy of IV bisphosphonates in canine oncologic patients is clearly warranted.

Transdermal Applications

Formulation of transdermal liposomal absorptive gels, creams, and sprays containing a wide range of agents such as morphine, methadone, lidocaine, ketamine or gabapentin, and capsaicin may help to desensitize the innervation of painful areas or may allow the oral absorption of substances that may otherwise not be orally bioavailable [249, 250]. Evidence supporting or denying efficacy of these treatments is lacking; however, reports of anecdotal successful use encourage their use.

Nonpharmacologic Interventions

Analgesic Radiation Therapy

Fractionated radiation therapy is used to palliate pain, particularly in those patients with bone metastases [251]. Traditionally, the analgesic effects of radiation therapy were believed to derive from elimination of tumoral cells and reduction of tumor size. However, effects such as inhibition of prostaglandin-secreting cells, moderate bone healing, and activation and induction of transforming growth factor-beta isoforms may all account for the analgesic effects observed [252].

Neurolysis

Physical destruction of nerve roots or major nerve trunks to alleviate pain in limited areas of the body may be attempted. Neurolysis may be achieved by perineural, intrathecal, or epidural administration of chemical neurolytic agents, cryoneurolysis, or radiofrequency (RF) blockade. These last two techniques are the most used in the United States for human patients [253]. Cryoneurolysis consists in destruction of the nerve by the application of extreme cold, whereas radiofrequency blockade requires the insertion of a small, insulated electrode with a noninsulated tip near a nerve that innervates the painful area to treat. Both techniques may require a test block to guarantee motor function is not being altered. They both provide months of analgesia to an area; however, they are not devoid of adverse effects such as neuroma formation, neuritis of adjacent nerves, or regrowth of nerves [254]. In veterinary medicine, the fact that patients cannot verbally indicate the exact location of the painful area may lead to significant difficulties to correctly identify motor and sympathetic from sensory function. Caution should be exercised with this technique and only practitioners well-versed in the application and adverse effects of these techniques should perform them.

Surgical Analgesic Techniques

Several different surgical techniques are currently being used in human medicine in an effort to alleviate pain in certain patients suffering from specific types of tumors, particularly those involving osseous tumors and metastases affecting vertebrae. Kyphoplasty and percutaneous vertebroplasty are performed in human medicine to stabilize fractures [255].

More extreme surgical options include neuroablative techniques that can be both peripheral (neurectomy, dorsal rhizotomy, or sympathectomy) and central (myelotomy, cordotomy, or even hypophysectomy and thalamotomy) [256]. Finally, technologically sophisticated surgical therapies such as gamma knife and stereotactic radiofrequency surgery will hopefully become available in veterinary medicine in the future.

Nursing Care of Hospitalized Patients

Pain is a complex phenomenon that not only has a physical dimension, but also includes many psychological components. It is well known that anxiety and fear may exacerbate pain and vice versa; therefore, taking care of an animal's perceived emotional needs and comfort may reduce stress and, consequently, pain levels. Patients with special needs, such as deaf and blind animals, may suffer bigger degrees of stress due to their disabilities. Special measures are warranted to minimize extra stress. Additionally, animals' perception of pain may be affected by environmental factors; therefore, rendering their surrounding more familiar by the presence of a favorite toy or blanket may help decrease stress. In the feline patient, being hospitalized in an exclusively feline ward may be extremely helpful in reducing anxiety and fear. While some animals are likely to recover better in a quiet environment, others may be better when distracted by exposure to a more active area of the hospital. Owner visits may also be planned carefully, as some animals may benefit hugely from the time spent with their families, while it may be a source of anxiety and distress for others. Simple changes in the daily plan of nursing care and interventions may play a fundamental role in a comprehensive pain management plan. Venipuncture and injections are painful; therefore, planning and coordination of treatments and laboratory tests should be performed to minimize the total number of painful events. The establishment of patient-protective policies such a "two-stick rule" (venipuncture and/or IV catheter placement should only be attempted a maximum of two times by any individual) may be an easy and effective measure. Likewise, grouping treatments to allow for longer periods of undisturbed rest and sleep should be kept in mind. Dimming the lights during the night period will allow for better rest and sleep. Additionally, every effort should be made so that patients do not associate human contact with unpleasant and stressful experiences. Therefore a "three-one rule" policy may be instituted where each patient that is exposed to one uncomfortable situation or invasive procedure is subsequently immediately exposed to three positive experiences such as feeding, petting, or grooming. Other simple nursing care steps may also allow the animal to feel more comfortable. For example, the bladder should be emptied at the end of surgery if possible and, if recumbency is predicted, an indwelling urinary catheter should be placed at the time of surgery. Finally, cage preparation and maintenance are key factors in contributing to patient comfort. Apart from obvious measures such as keeping the cage clean and dry, a cage should be of appropriate size and padding, with careful animal positioning to reduce pressure on painful areas that may be due to neoplasia or comorbidities such as arthritis. Ideally, the patient's cage should be designated as a safe zone, and all procedures considered noxious should be performed in a different area (whenever safe movement and transport are possible) so that the animal feels comfortable and safe when in the cage.

Considerations for General Anesthesia

Cancer is a major cause of morbidity and mortality in animals of all ages in present-day society and veterinarians are expected to provide advanced and compassionate clinical management of oncologic patients daily. A fundamental component of this clinical care relies on their anesthetic/analgesic management, since it is often required to perform a wide range of diagnostic, therapeutic, and palliative procedures.

Preanesthetic evaluation of these patients should be thorough to rule out major complications that should be corrected or stabilized in the preanesthetic period. Hematological evaluations as well as comprehensive coagulation tests are important, since alterations such as neutropenia, anemia, erythrocytosis, thrombocytopenia, thrombocyte hyperaggregability, and coagulation disorders could be present in some oncologic patients. Likewise, dangerous derangements in fundamental biochemical parameters such as calcium, glucose, total protein, and indicators of kidney and liver damage and function could also be present. For this reason, a meticulous evaluation of a comprehensive biochemical analysis is warranted. The preanesthetic evaluation should also include a detailed physical exam to assess BCS, hydration status, and the existence of oral mucositis or KCS if the patient is receiving radiation therapy. A comprehensive evaluation of three-view thoracic radiographs, abdominal ultrasound, and echocardiogram is also recommended. Preanesthetic stabilization of any identified derangements is one of the most critical steps in the anesthetic/analgesic management of these patients. Once stabilization of life-threatening tumor- or treatment-related derangements has been achieved, any underlying pathophysiologic changes need to be individually considered, and, as a result, there is no single anesthetic protocol that can be recommended for all oncologic patients.

When choosing a premedication combination and dosages, it is important to note that low fat-to-body mass ratio and low muscle-to-body mass ratio are commonly found in patients that suffer CACS; these patients may have higher circulating levels of unbound or active drugs that could result in overdose and/or prolonged recoveries. Premedication should include the combination of an opioid with short-acting or reversible sedatives such as alpha-2-adrenergic agonists or gamma aminobutyric acid (GABA) receptor agonists such as midazolam. Although midazolam is not a very reliable sedative in dogs and cats when administered on its own, it has proven useful in older animals when combined with opioids or other sedatives. It also provides excellent muscle relaxation, and the very favorable cardiovascular profile makes it an excellent choice to obtain sedation in older or critically ill animals. Additionally, many cancer patients require general anesthesia for short procedures on daily basis for a period of time (such as radiation therapy sessions) and short-acting or reversible drugs are warranted. Acepromazine is frequently avoided in these patients due to the lack of drug antagonist and its relatively long duration of action. Furthermore, caution should be exercised in patients that present with thrombocytopenia or coagulation disorders, as it may impair platelet aggregation [257]. Opioid choice is based on the patient's analgesic needs, but agents such as methadone or butorphanol may be acceptable options, as they are devoid of severe hemodynamic or gastrointestinal side effects when administered at clinically relevant doses, while they still provide mild-to-moderate sedation and analgesia. The use of butorphanol is probably not a good option for the treatment of severely painful conditions, as it is an agonist/antagonist opioid and provides minimal analgesia. However, the sedation obtained after butorphanol administration may be more intense compared to pure μ agonist opioids, while the intensity of its cardiovascular and gastrointestinal side effects is significantly milder.

Propofol is an excellent choice for anesthetic induction since it is short-acting and has at least some extrahepatic metabolism with very little accumulation when moderate induction doses are used (2–8 $mg\,kg^{-1}$ IV) [258]. However, repeated use of propofol should be avoided in those cats that may need repeated episodes of general anesthesia, as its use has been associated with oxidative hematological lesions (characterized by increased production of Heinz bodies) as well as increased recovery times from anesthesia and anorexia [259]. Ketamine, alfaxalone, and etomidate are also suitable options for anesthetic induction if there are no specific contraindications.

Any of the currently used inhalant agents (isoflurane, sevoflurane, and desflurane) may be used for anesthetic maintenance and there are no clear advantages of one over the others. In addition, total intravenous administration (TIVA) of injectable agents such as propofol (0.3–0.7 $mg\,kg^{-1}\,min^{-1}$ IV) or alfaxalone (0.1–0.15 $mg\,kg^{-1}\,min^{-1}$ IV, in dogs, 0.11–0.18 $mg\,kg^{-1}\,min^{-1}$, in cats) can also be used, depending on the disease pathophysiology and the therapeutic or diagnostic procedure to be performed. It is important to titrate the dosages of agents used in TIVA to effect to provide necessary anesthesia while minimizing cardiovascular and respiratory adverse effects. Intensive and continuous anesthetic monitoring of patients during anesthesia is necessary. As such, continuous electrocardiography (ECG), pulse oximetry (SpO_2), capnography ($ETCO_2$), and temperature and direct or indirect blood pressure monitoring should always be implemented. In certain patients, blood gas analysis may also be necessary to monitor partial pressures of O_2 and CO_2 in arterial blood. Cachectic patients may be more prone to hypothermia during the perianesthetic period; active efforts to decrease heat loss are warranted (i.e., insulation from cold surfaces, careful wrapping, use of heat and moisture exchange filters, warm water blankets, etc.).

Effects of Perioperative Management on Postoperative Oncologic Outcomes

Surgery is one of the main treatment modalities for most of the solid organ tumors and is potentially curative; over 80% of human patients with cancer will undergo at least one surgical procedure during their treatment period [260]. Unfortunately, tumor recurrence following oncologic surgery of curative intent does happen, and usually results in refractory disease and patient death. Postoperative recurrence is responsible for high morbidity and mortality rate in oncologic patients and metastatic disease is typically refractory to treatment; many human cancer-related deaths are due to metastasis [261].

Tumor recurrence after surgical resection varies significantly and is influenced by many factors, including tumor grade, stage, and primary organ affected. Surgical technique obviously affects recurrence risk; as such, there are two obvious goals in surgical oncology: to minimize tumor handling to prevent the spread of tumor cells and to achieve clear sample margins. What is less clear is whether anesthetic, analgesic, or other perioperative interventions (e.g., the use of steroids, beta-adrenergic receptor antagonists, or systemic lidocaine) may also have an influence on cancer recurrence [262].

Much of the available evidence on these clinical interventions comes from experimental *in vitro* and *in vivo* models, with clinical evidence largely limited to retrospective observational studies or post-hoc analysis of randomized clinical trials (RCTs) originally designed to evaluate noncancer outcomes. Therefore, proving a causal link requires data from prospective RCTs with oncological outcomes as primary endpoints. Until those studies are performed, there is insufficient evidence to recommend any particular anesthetic or analgesic technique for patients undergoing tumor resection surgery on the basis that it might alter the risk of recurrence or appearance of metastasis.

Surgery

Surgery and other perioperative interventions can induce a biological state that promotes not only the survival of residual cancer cells released from the primary tumor intraoperatively, but also their growth. The mechanisms underlying postsurgical cancer recurrence are complex, and the likelihood that individual cancer cells will "seed" in tissues and progress to a clinically significant metastatic disease is influenced by pathophysiological changes induced by surgery. Cancer cells exist in a complex tumor microenvironment that involves the interplay of surrounding noncancerous stromal cells, extracellular matrix, immune system cells, chemokines, and cytokines [263]. This delicate microenvironment is easily disrupted by tissue trauma, and the surgical intervention may inadvertently create conditions that promote not only survival but also progression, proliferation, and spread of residual cancer cells. Such surgery-induced physiological changes are numerous and include inflammation, tissue hypoxia that may promote the occurrence of angiogenesis, and surgical stress response and pain, both of which may directly lead to immunosuppression [264]. In summary, all these pathophysiologic events may eventually lead to metastatic growth of the circulating tumor cells (CTCs) that are released intraoperatively during tumor excision.

Anesthetic Drugs

There is limited and contradictory evidence as to whether anesthetic technique affects long-term outcome or recurrence of the tumor after oncologic surgery. However, most evidence suggests that the anesthetic and analgesic interventions performed during surgical excision of tumors could have a direct effect over many of the previously mentioned pathophysiological processes, influencing risk of cancer recurrence in either a beneficial or detrimental way.

Inhalant Agents

Halogenated agents are probably the most used drugs for the maintenance of general anesthesia worldwide and volatile anesthetic agents affect the immune system and the inflammatory response [265, 266]. However, conflicting evidence exists as to whether volatile anesthetic agents activate or inhibit these pathways and it remains unclear whether clinical outcomes are influenced.

In vitro studies suggest the ability of volatile agents to modulate the immune response via several cellular targets, including acetylcholine, serotonin, GABA, and glycine receptors present on immune cells, such as NK cells, macrophages, and neutrophils [267]. Additionally, inhalants can potentially exert direct effects on cancer cells themselves. Inhalants may stimulate *in vitro* ovarian cancer cell migration and other prometastatic processes, while sevoflurane increases *in vitro* breast cancer cell proliferation and migration [268, 269]. Conversely, other studies suggest that inhalational agents may directly inhibit cellular mechanisms that drive metastasis, and that any overall effect on recurrence may be related to cancer type [270]. Finally, volatile anesthetic agents may be protective against ischemia–reperfusion injury in different organs and clinical settings by inducing HIF1A expression, an angiogenesis-regulating factor [271]. However, this usually protective mechanism may be related to malignant recurrence in oncologic surgery [272].

Clinical studies comparing inhalants to propofol-based techniques suggest that inhalants can either decrease the overall survival, increase the risk of cancer recurrence, or have the same outcomes as propofol-based techniques [273–276]. However, the clinical relevance of these findings is questionable, as none of those studies are RCT specifically designed to measure these specific oncologic clinical outcomes.

In an *in vitro* prospective veterinary study, sevoflurane effects on canine mammary tumor cell proliferation and on the expression of neuroepithelial transforming gene 1 (NET1) were studied [277]. Both primary (CIPp) and metastatic (CIPm) canine tubular adenocarcinoma cell lines were seeded and incubated with different concentrations of sevoflurane which modified the cell proliferation rate in both cell lines, causing a decrease or increase when applied to CIPm or CIPp, respectively. Expression of the NET1 gene also increased after treatment with the higher sevoflurane concentration in CIPm, suggesting that the role of sevoflurane on cancer recurrence still needs to be further investigated before clear clinical recommendations can be made.

Propofol

Propofol is one of the most used IV anesthetic agents for induction and maintenance of anesthesia. Propofol may possess anti-inflammatory properties as well as stimulatory effects on immune function, potentially resulting in beneficial effects on cancer recurrence, although definitive clinical evidence of this remains unclear [278]. However, other retrospective studies examining a variety of cancer surgeries reported no difference in either survival or recurrence between TIVA and volatile-based groups [276, 279, 280]. Thus, although retrospective studies suggest that propofol may have beneficial effects in resisting metastasis and improving survival, definitive evaluation in prospective, randomized controlled clinical trials is still necessary. Several large RCTs examining cancer recurrence comparing propofol and volatile anesthetics for oncologic surgery are currently underway; however, none of these trials have been completed at the time of publication [281].

Alpha-2-Adrenergic Receptor Agonists

Although alpha-2-adrenergic receptor agonists (i.e., dexmedetomidine) are used routinely as sedative and analgesic agents, the effects of these drugs on cancer recurrence and survival after oncologic surgery have rarely been studied. It has been hypothesized that similarly to catecholamines, drugs that activate adrenoceptors such as this class may potentially exert cancer-promoting effects.

Laboratory studies in both animal and human cancer cells point to a detrimental effect of alpha-2-adrenergic receptor agonists in oncologic surgery, since protumoral effects and detrimental effects on innate immune system cells were observed [282–284]. However, one small RCT suggested a potentially beneficial antitumor effect since a reduction in the levels of proinflammatory cytokines and catecholamines was observed [285]. Although most of the laboratory evidence points toward a detrimental effect, it must be also remembered that the administration of these agents may allow for reduced volatile anesthetics and opioids requirements, both of which may have a role in cancer recurrence and reduced survival. To that end, the role that alpha-2-adrenergic receptor agonists play in cancer recurrence and survival after oncologic surgery is still unknown; laboratory results are conflicting and clinical studies are scarce and retrospective. Additionally, it may be difficult to completely differentiate the origin of the clinical outcomes observed, as they could be due to either a direct effect or secondary to the reduced requirements of other drugs.

Analgesic Agents and Analgesic Techniques

Opioids

Opioids are potent analgesics that are essential for pain management in cancer patients. Besides being widely used perioperatively for oncologic surgery, they are also the standard of care for the treatment of cancer-related pain in patients with advanced stage disease. However, basic cancer cell biology suggests that opioid analgesics may inhibit both cellular and humoral immune functions and this may facilitate tumoral cell proliferation (such as migration, invasion, and angiogenesis) [262, 279, 286]. Although opioid administration may be detrimental in oncologic patients, some laboratory studies have shown the opposite effect and suggest that opioids may exert an inhibitory effect on tumoral cells. These studies suggest that, depending on the opioid and the animal model studied, these agents may not always enhance metastatic spread and tumor recurrence [287]. Also, definitive prospective clinical data are not yet available regarding this topic.

Studies show that opioids act indirectly to release biological amines (that may inhibit NK cytotoxicity and thus attenuate innate immunity) and stimulate the hypothalamic–pituitary–adrenal (HPA) axis, triggering glucocorticoid release that may indirectly lead to immunosuppression [288, 289]. On the other hand, immune function may be directly affected through opioid receptors (such as the mu-opioid receptor, MOR), or nonopioid receptors expressed by immune cells (such as NK cells) [288, 290]. In addition, different opioids likely produce different physiological effects on immune function. For example, buprenorphine may prevent the depression of NK cell cytotoxicity and metastasis enhancement caused by surgery, opposite in fentanyl and morphine, while tramadol may possess immune-stimulating properties and enhances NK cytotoxicity in rats [289, 291]. Moreover, a small number of *in vitro* and *in vivo* studies show that morphine may exert potentially beneficial antitumoral effects, suggesting that morphine may not possess unequivocal detrimental effects on cancer biology [292–294]. Finally, mouse models have shown that opioid receptor antagonists (methylnaltrexone and naloxone) may possess antitumoral effects [295, 296].

Several retrospective clinical studies have investigated oncologic surgery outcomes related to the type and dose of opioids administered perioperatively. Taking into consideration the currently available evidence regarding the influence of opioids on postsurgical oncologic outcomes, it is extremely difficult to justify a major change in clinical practice, since the nature of the studies and experimental designs vary widely. Results are contradictory in most cases, as some show a reduction in overall survival or recurrence-free survival, others show no effect, and yet others show beneficial increases in the same parameters [297–301]. The same conclusion has been obtained by some of the most accurate and recent meta-analyses of this topic, since publications are too heterogeneous to quantify an effect of the different clinical practices [302, 303].

Despite the hypothesized cancer-promoting effects of some opioids, it must not be forgotten that there is current evidence that proves that poorly controlled pain may stimulate malignant processes and may be associated with poorer survival in certain oncologic patients [125, 304]. The underlying mechanisms are unknown, although an increase in activity of both the HPA axis and the sympathetic nervous system (SNS) may be implicated, leading to an increase in circulating glucocorticoids, catecholamines, and a certain degree of immunosuppression [305]. Thus, it is clear that pain should be treated in these patients with a multimodal technique that does not solely rely on opioids [306].

Regional Anesthesia and Local Anesthetics

LAs effectively inhibit all neurotransmission through sodium channel inhibition. In addition, they may play a role in reducing cancer recurrence via potential direct antitumor properties, attenuation of the stress response that may reduce the associated immunosuppression, preservation of the innate immune system's ability to eliminate residual cancer cells, and/or the reduction in inhalant agent and opioid requirements, potentially reducing their possible detrimental effect on cancer recurrence. However, *in vitro* study results are conflicting, although amide LAs (i.e., lidocaine, bupivacaine) compellingly inhibit tumor cells [307–310]. Proposed underlying molecular mechanisms may include DNA demethylation, inhibition of the proto-oncogene tyrosine-protein kinase Src, or even their more commonly known sodium channel inhibitory effect [311–313].

In comparison, several older retrospective clinical studies suggest that regional techniques could exert a protective role against cancer recurrence [314, 315]. More recent retrospective clinical studies show results with some suggesting a beneficial effect of regional anesthesia on overall survival, recurrence-free survival, or biochemical recurrence, while others report no difference, and a small minority even detects detrimental effects [316–318]. A recent Cochrane review of the topic concluded that evidence for a benefit of regional anesthesia on tumor recurrence or survival remains inadequate [319]. To clarify this dilemma, ongoing prospective RCTs are currently under consideration (Table 17.5).

Nonsteroidal Anti-Inflammatory Drugs

The inflammatory response to surgery likely plays an important role in metastatic spread or recurrence of cancer. As such, it has been hypothesized that inhibition of inflammation may reduce postoperative recurrence [320]. There is growing evidence to support the beneficial role of NSAIDs; however, most information comes from epidemiological studies that may not always be set in surgical context [321].

Prostaglandin reduction may play a role in decreased tumorigenesis; however, other NSAID-related mechanisms such as impaired cancer cell viability, proliferation and migration, reduced vascular endothelial growth factor (VEGF) expression, downregulation of the SOX2 oncogene, altered signaling proteins (such as epidermal growth factor receptor), or expression of transcription factors (such as NF-kB) may also be considered [322–325].

Long-term NSAID administration may provide some benefits to oncologic patients [326–328], whereas perioperative use of NSAIDs has resulted in variable outcomes [329–333]. Interestingly, prospective studies on COX-2 inhibitors and oncologic outcomes have been very limited or have even been interrupted due to the occurrence of potential cardiovascular side effects [334], and most are either too heterogeneous or of suboptimal quality to attempt a meta-analysis. Thus, a beneficial effect of perioperative NSAIDs is still lacking, although studies are underway currently (Table 17.5) [335].

Opioid-Free Anesthesia and Cancer

The concept of opioid-free anesthesia (OFA) is based on the preoperative, intraoperative, and postoperative administration of analgesics other than opioids that have shown promising evidence in the reduction of cancer recurrence. As such, NSAIDs and LA could be considered promising therapeutic alternatives for surgical cancer patients. This strategy not only targets analgesic techniques but also other perianesthetic interventions. OFA strategies may aim to include the use of propofol as an anesthetic maintenance agent, the provision of analgesia based on locoregional techniques to avoid or reduce the use of opioids, the administration of a coadjuvant CRI of lidocaine during maintenance, the use of beta-adrenergic receptor antagonists, and the perioperative administration of NSAIDs [336]. However, current evidence is still too weak to support such a radical change in the anesthetic management of surgical oncologic patients. Further prospective, randomized, controlled clinical trials that compare the administration of perioperative opioid-based analgesia for primary tumor resection surgery with alternative anesthetic–analgesic techniques are required to verify their effects on long-term oncologic outcomes such as recurrence-free survival and overall survival. Unfortunately, such studies take years to complete, since patient enrolment may be slow and follow-up is, by definition and design, intentionally long.

Other Perioperative Interventions

Blood Transfusion

Blood product transfusion is frequently required during aggressive oncologic surgery. However, this clinical intervention is not harmless, since it has proven to cause in vitro immunosuppression and inflammation, two key adverse factors in cancer recurrence [337]. Mechanisms underlying this transfusion-related immunomodulation (TRIM) may include compromised phagocytic activity of endogenous macrophages, and cytokines contained in transfused blood products multiple, contributing to inflammation [338, 339]. Interestingly, *in vivo* studies have suggested that the cancer-stimulating effects are directly proportional to the length of storage duration [340].

When studying multiple cancer types such as bladder, gastric, and prostate cancer, a

Table 17.5 Classification of common paraneoplastic syndromes in oncologic patients

Study ID	Title	Intervention	Oncologic Outcome	Experimental Design	Completion (estimated)
NCT00418457	Regional Anesthesia and Breast Cancer Recurrence	Inhalant+opioids vs propofol TIVA+RA	Cancer recurrence rate	Multicenter prospective RCT (n=1311)	March 2019
NCT03034096	General Anesthetics in Cancer Resection Surgery	Propofol TIVA vs inhalant	Overall survival; recurrence-free survival	Multicenter prospective RCT (n=2000)	December 2020
NCT02786329	Influence of Anesthesia on Postoperative Outcome and Complications in Colorectal Cancer Patients	2x2: Propofol vs inhalant; lidocaine vs placebo	Overall survival and recurrence rate	Single center prospective 2x2 factorial RCT (n=450)	December 2021
NCT02840227	Effect of Combined GA/RA on Cancer Recurrence on Patients Having Lung Cancer Resections	GA+epidural vs GA+opioids	Cancer-free survival	Multicenter prospective RCT (n=2000)	December 2021
NCT03172988	Dexamethasone, Flurbiprofen Axetil and Long-Term Survival After Lung Cancer Surgery	2x2: Flurbiprofen, dexamethasone, saline, and lipid microspheres	Overall survival at 3 years; recurrence-free survival	Multicentre prospective 2x2 factorial RCT (n=844)	August 2023
NCT03109990	Impact of Dexmedetomidine on Postoperative Tumor Recurrence in Patients with Breast Cancer	Intraoperative dexmedetomidine CRI vs placebo	Overall survival and recurrence rate	Multicenter prospective RCT (n=460)	April 2024

CRI = constan trate infusion; GA = general anesthesia; RA = regional anesthesia; RCT = randomized, controlled trial; TIVA = total intravenous anesthesia negative effect of blood transfusion on oncologic outcomes (such as recurrence-free survival, cancer-specific survival, and overall survival) has been shown [341–343]. However, proving causality between the administration of blood transfusions and cancer recurrence is problematic, as this association could be attributable to patients with more aggressive tumors presenting a larger need of blood transfusions and not to a true effect of the transfusions themselves on cancer recurrence.

Beta-Adrenergic Receptor Antagonists

Stress may be linked with the onset and progression of cancer, and beta-adrenergic receptor antagonist administration may ameliorate the effects of surgery-induced stress and SNS activation. Therefore, the administration of beta-adrenergic receptor antagonists (e.g., propranolol, esmolol) may help limit the cancer-promoting effects of catecholamines. Catecholamines are not only the major transmitters of the stress response, but they may also play a role in certain tumor pathogenesis, as beta-adrenergic receptors have been identified on breast, ovarian, and pancreatic cancer cells [344–348]. In addition, beta-adrenergic receptor stimulation increases angiogenesis, tumor invasion, and integrin-mediated cell adhesion, and beta-adrenergic receptor antagonists may have beneficial effects, including antimetastatic properties [347, 349–355]. Similar to other treatment modalities, a recent meta-analysis suggested that beta-adrenergic receptor antagonists had no evident effect on cancer recurrence, while effects on disease-free and overall survival rates were variable depending on tumor type, ranging from beneficial to harmful [356]. Therefore, the currently available evidence in human medicine is weak and limited; appropriately designed randomized controlled trials studying the effect of beta-adrenergic receptor antagonists on recurrence of different types of tumors are necessary.

Corticosteroids

The potential role of corticosteroids on cancer recurrence is based on the anti-inflammatory effects that may counterbalance the inflammation resulting from surgery. As such, corticosteroids may reduce the cancer-stimulating effects of the surgical inflammatory response. However, at higher doses, corticosteroids also induce immunosuppression, which may potentially increase the recurrence risk [357]. It is currently unknown where the balance of these two effects lies, as it has not been widely studied in relation of postsurgical oncologic outcomes such as cancer recurrence, disease-free survival, or overall survival as primary endpoints. Studies are again sparse with inconsistent results [358–361].

Perioperative Nutrition

In human medicine, adequate and patient-tailored nutrition plays a major role in the perioperative period, particularly when it is related to oncologic surgery. Not only does it help the patient to recover faster from surgical trauma, but also decreases the postoperative complications [362]. A complication-free recovery in a nutritionally optimized patient allows timely and optimal dosing administration of oncological treatments. Recently, nutritional status in the perioperative period of the oncologic patient has been related to overall disease-free survival, and patients who suffer from nutrition-related postoperative complications have worse survival rates [363].

The Enhanced Recovery After Surgery (ERAS) paradigm has been proven safe and beneficial in most surgical fields including surgical oncology, and oncologic patients should be managed within an ERAS program in which the main therapeutic goals are to maintain nutritional status, minimize surgical stress, reduce the incidence of complications, and optimize recovery rate [364–366]. Key aspects of this therapeutic strategy include minimal opiate-based pain management, early mobilization of the patient, early return of gastrointestinal function, and, if possible, minimally invasive surgery [367]. Nutritional components of ERAS include avoiding fasting, preoperative fluid and carbohydrate loading, and early reintroduction of oral diet on the first postoperative day [368].

Prehabilitation

Prehabilitation is defined as the physical activity performed before surgery with the aim of improving the functional capacity of an individual, in anticipation of a stressful event (such as a surgical procedure). The main goals are to improve the patient's postoperative outcome, to decrease the associated hospital care expenses, and to enhance quality of life during the perioperative period [369, 370]. Physical activity is known to reduce the risk for cancer development [371]. Similarly, prehabilitation consisting of inspiratory muscle training, aerobic exercise, and resistance training has proven to not only improve immune function and metabolism and reduce length of hospital stay and complications, but also reduce cancer recurrence and overall mortality from some types of tumors [372–374]. However, since there are currently no available veterinary studies and the number of available studies in human medicine is still small, this additional therapeutic strategy to reduce cancer recurrence and improve overall survival currently remains only a promising option that deserves better study in appropriately designed, randomized, controlled trials.

Palliative Care

Owners must fully understand that the word "palliation" means treatment for comfort and supportive care, not cure. Often palliation is clearly the preferred mode of care for certain oncology patients instead of curative treatment or euthanasia. If an oncologic patient is in the advanced or terminal stage of cancer at the time of diagnosis, various levels of palliative and/or hospice care can be recommended as highly effective options.

Palliative care is currently a growing medical specialty that aims to alleviate suffering resulting from both serious illness and/or its treatment. It may be provided to patients of any age at any time over the course of an illness and it consists in providing relief from the symptoms, pain, and stress of serious illness, as well as emotional support to the owners of the sick patients. While palliative care is commonly associated with hospice, these terms are not synonymous. In fact, hospice is a specialized form of palliative care that focuses on caring for patients in the end stages of an illness. It is rather a philosophy of care that considers death as a natural process, prioritizes comfort and quality of life over quantity of life as death draws near, and supports the cultural and spiritual aspects of dying [375].

While many veterinarians are already providing palliative care daily for their patients and clients (particularly oncologic patients), palliative care is still an emerging discipline within veterinary medicine. In fact, it is quite a recent phenomenon that hospice and palliative care have split in two separate disciplines and are evolving as distinct areas of veterinary practice. Moreover, a number of programs have been developed in academia and private practice settings, as well as curricular initiatives have taken place in the past few years as a consequence of the growth of this emerging field of veterinary care [376–379] and organizations such as the American Veterinary Medical Association (AVMA) and American Animal Hospital Association (AAHA) recently developed official guidelines for hospice and end-of-life care [380, 381]. For further information, a recent monographic issue edited by Katherine Goldberg on "Advances in Palliative Medicine" has been published elsewhere [375].

Hospice Care Programs

Families are now requesting pet hospice services, and veterinary teaching curriculums have created veterinary hospice programs to meet this need [376–378]. In addition, veterinary private practices have not been unaware of this emerging need. For example, Angell's Pain and Palliative Care Service was created as a small division of an independent, nonprofit, teaching institution that is the flagship hospital of the Massachusetts Society for the Prevention of Cruelty to Animals (MSPCA). The Angell's Pain and Palliative Care Service was first developed as a pain medicine service, and now incorporates palliative care as well [382].

It is a reality that some oncologic patients will not be treated due to owner reluctance, financial constraints, concurrent illness, or a logistical problem. However, care for the well-being of the patient should always remain first of our concerns. Consultation programs are available as end-of-life hospice care programs that consist of staff helping clients to provide end-of-life care at home for their ill pet. In order to objectively assess the quality of life, an itemized scale has been designed. Although not peer-reviewed or scientifically validated, the quality-of-life scale provides guidelines for the objective assessment of a patient to help with their management. The scale includes seven descriptors: hurt, hunger, hydration, hygiene, happiness, mobility, and more good days than bad (Table 17.6).

Palliative home care is founded on several interventions that start with evaluation and modification of the patient's environment (i.e., ramps, rugs to cover slippery floors), comprehensive nutrition, adaptation to new bladder/bowel habits, and setting up a routine and schedule that will likely help the mental health and well-being of the patient. Additionally, creating and following a pain diary to include notes on the quality-of-life scale as well as regular "call back" sessions will facilitate home care. Many psychological factors may decrease the pain threshold in people (i.e., insomnia, boredom, fear of worsening pain, anxiety, isolation, or frustration) and although we cannot prove that veterinary oncology patients feel or sense similar emotions, it seems reasonable to make every effort to strive for reduction of uncomfortable environments, provide a steady sleep/rest schedule, and offer diversional activities.

Table 17.6 Quality-of-life scale.

The HHHHHMM Scale
Hurt (0–10)
No pain. Adequate pain control and breathing ability are of top concern. If the pet cannot breathe, intervene. Is the pet's pain successfully managed? Is oxygen necessary?
Hunger (0–10)
No hunger. Is the pet eating enough? Does hand feeding help? Does the patient require a feeding tube?
Hydration (0–10)
Is the patient dehydrated? For patients not drinking enough, use subcutaneous fluids to supplement fluid intake.
Hygiene (0–10)
The patient should be kept brushed and cleaned, particularly after elimination. Avoid pressure sores, and keep all wounds clean.
Happiness (0–10)
Does the patient express joy and interest? Is the patient responsive to things around him (family, toys, etc.)? Is the pet depressed, anxious, bored, or afraid? Can the pet's bed be close to the family activities and not be isolated?
Mobility (0–10)
Can the patient get up without assistance? Does the pet need human or mechanical assistance? Does the pet feel like going for a walk?
More good days than bad (0–10)
When there are too many bad days in a row, quality of life is too compromised. The caretaker must be aware the end is near.

A score of 5 is acceptable in each category. A total of 35 points or greater is accountable for a good Pawspice.
Source: Adapted from Villalobos [411]. Adapted with permission.

Acupuncture for the Oncologic Patient

Acupuncture and complementary medicine may help alleviate tension and create a sense of well-being that offsets pain. Acupuncture sessions can be extremely helpful to the cancer patient and may bring comfort to the distressed owner as well. The empirical principles on which acupuncture is founded are based largely on traditional Chinese medicine (TCM). Acupuncture exerts neuromodulation by the insertion of thin, sterile needles into precise anatomic locations with very minimal side effects. A few considerations need to be considered when performing acupuncture in cancer patients, such as reducing the number of beads and semi-permanent needles in coagulopathic or neutropenic animals and avoiding inserting needles in the proximity of the neoplastic tissue. Beneficial effects in humans include reduction of malignant pain as well as phantom limb pain, appetite stimulation, decreased nausea and constipation, reduced toxic side effects of radiation and chemotherapy (such as gastrointestinal reactions or leukopenia), and reduction of lymphedema and surgical swelling [383]. For a comprehensive review of the mechanism of action of acupuncture, the reader is directed to reviews published elsewhere [384].

Alternative Analgesic Options in Palliative Care

Pain management as part of palliative and hospice care is based on the use of a wide variety of drugs and procedures, ranging from simple, oral analgesics to novel drugs and sophisticated interventional techniques. Currently used analgesic interventions (both pharmacological and nonpharmacological) have already been covered in this chapter: several very solid state-of-the-art reviews have previously been published [385–388]. Many of these procedures are tremendously promising for the pain management of conditions that are unresponsive to currently available therapies, and urgently deserve further attention and investigation.

Nonopiate IV Infusions

Intravenous infusions of lidocaine, ketamine, dexmedetomidine, or bisphosphonates are currently used in human patients to treat neuropathic and cancer pain. One of their most beneficial characteristics is that the effects of the infusions often outlast their duration by weeks to months [389], making them a very interesting therapeutic option when dealing with chronic painful conditions. Although minimal data exist to support their use for relief of chronic oncologic pain in veterinary medicine, the expenses and logistics associated to their administration are minimal, and it could be a suitable therapeutic option for the general practice setting.

Epidural Injection

Epidural steroid injections (ESI) are one of the interventional pain management procedures most performed in human medicine. They can be performed at the cervical, thoracic, lumbar, or caudal level [390, 391]. The most frequently administered steroids include dexamethasone, methylprednisolone, and triamcinolone, although other drugs such as LAs are often combined with the steroids [392].

Although some veterinarians perform this procedure in patients with confirmed lumbosacral (LS) stenosis or intervertebral disc diseases (IVDD), ESI for pain management is not well established in veterinary medicine. This is mainly due to the lack of evidence in the scientific literature to support its use. In fact, only one study has evaluated the effect of methylprednisolone acetate in dogs with confirmed LS stenosis [393]. Almost 80% of the dogs in this study showed some improvement; however, the study was retrospective, not blinded, and had no positive or negative control groups. In summary, ESI in veterinary patients deserves further study, as it may be an excellent option in oncologic patients that suffer from chronic pain that requires long-term analgesic management.

Subcutaneous Opioid Infusion and Other Opioid Delivery Routes

An alternative route of administration has become available when human patients with cancer are no longer able to take oral opioids during the final stages of their disease. Continuous subcutaneous infusion (CSCI) is an effective alternative, and opioids such as morphine, hydromorphone, methadone, or fentanyl can be administered with similar efficacy and safety to conventional routes such as transdermal, rectal, or IV [394, 395]. Most frequently, this technique consists in the insertion of a SC catheter after aseptic preparation, which exits the skin under a sterile dressing and connects to an external pump worn by the patient. In some other instances, when long-term pain management is considered, a totally implantable device can be aseptically inserted SC under light sedation and local anesthetic infiltration. Both SC options can then be connected to a pump that may run the continuous infusion.

Unfortunately, no suitable commercial device is currently available for use in small animals. This modality of pain management would be particularly interesting in oncologic patients that have very poor peripheral vasculature, those whose families may prefer to continue treatment at home at the end of their disease, or even in those patients that may need pain control in anatomical areas difficult to reach by locoregional anesthetic techniques (such as oropharyngeal neoplasia).

Joint Injections for Osteoarthritis

The use of intraarticular (IA) steroid injections is a common procedure performed in humans with osteoarthritis (OA) when conservative treatments fail, for their analgesic and anti-inflammatory effects [396]. In veterinary medicine, steroid administration in joints with OA has been extensively studied in the equine patient [397, 398]. However, this clinical intervention seems to be applied less frequently in small animals than in equine athletes or human patients, possibly due to lack of data on analgesic effects, chondrotoxicity, and systemic effects associated with systemic absorption in these species [398]. Empirical administration of IA steroid injections has shown excellent analgesia in canine patients with OA when patients with moderate to severe pain do not respond to conservative treatment [388]. However, administration of low doses can only be recommended at this point and caution needs to be exerted until more published data become available regarding their side effects.

Myofascial Injections

Myofascial pain is a chronic regional pain syndrome that has been identified not only in human patients but in veterinary patients as well; however, many veterinarians are unaware of its existence [399, 400]. Myofascial trigger points are irritable, palpable, knots, or taut bands within a muscle that are responsible for eliciting pain that radiates into specific "reference pain zones." In animals, palpation of these trigger points often elicits escape behaviors, anxiety, and/or vocalization. Some authors have empirically and successfully injected small volumes of LAs on trigger points [388].

Toxins

In human medicine, several novel drugs that come from toxins produced by animals or other organisms have recently been generated to treat chronic painful conditions. In fact, these toxins have proven to be able to selectively modulate receptors and ion channels (such as voltage-gated calcium channels, CaV; voltage-gated sodium channels, NaV; transient receptor potential channels, TRP; NMDA; G protein-coupled receptors, GPCRs; or norepinephrine transporter, NET) at different levels of the nociceptive pathway [401].

In veterinary medicine, the paucity of published studies makes the routine use of these substances still not a clinical reality. So far, preclinical studies have provided positive outcomes in dogs with naturally occurring pain from bone malignancy after the intrathecal administration of substance P-saporin (a chemical conjugate of substance P and a recombinant version of the neurotoxin saporin) [402] and resiniferatoxin (an agonist of the nonselective cation channel TRPV1 found in the plant *Euphorbia resinifera*) [403]. Toxins continue to yield some of the most exciting leads for developing novel nonopioid analgesics both in human and veterinary medicine.

Neurolysis

Long-term relief of intractable pain can be achieved by destruction of nervous tissue (neurolysis), as opposed to a locoregional block, which does not damage nervous tissue. Three methods are currently used: chemical neurolysis, cryoneurolysis, and radiofrequency therapy. Except for the first method, most of these interventions lack data that support its routine use in veterinary patients, although their potential use seems promising in palliative care patients.

Chemical neurolysis is still used in veterinary patients; however, its use has mainly been limited to treatment of pain from terminal neoplasia as in human patients. This method is based on the injection of a neurolytic agent into a given ganglion or plexus, since nociceptive primary afferent neurons pass through several sympathetic ganglia/plexuses on their way to the dorsal horn of the spinal cord, and the injections can relieve pain from specific anatomic structures [404]. Complications are uncommon.

Cryoneurolysis is based on the freezing of nerves using a special probe using N_2O or CO_2 and is capable of generating temperatures around −80 °C at its tip [405]. Wallerian degeneration occurs, but the nerve does eventually regenerate [405].

RF therapy consists of applying an alternating current at radio wave frequency through an insulated cannula that delivers the current directly to the specific nerve, to produce long-term analgesia [406, 407]. The current delivered generates an electromagnetic field that eventually generates heat resulting in Wallerian degeneration of neurons, which prevents transmission of nociceptive impulses. In humans, the procedure is typically performed under local anesthesia, and steroids are usually injected perineurally to prevent neuritis and provide analgesia [408].

Spinal Cord Stimulation

Spinal cord stimulations (SCSs) consist in the insertion of electrodes into the epidural space (percutaneously or via a small laminotomy), so that neurons can be stimulated with electricity and chronic intractable pain can be replaced with paresthesia. Its underlying mechanism is based on the gate control theory that explains how electrical energy interrupts nociceptive transmission [409]. Several companies manufacture neurostimulation devices; however, no data from veterinary patients are currently available.

References

1 Bronson, R.T. (1982). Variation in age at death of dogs of different sexes and breeds. *Am. J. Vet. Res.* 43: 2057–2059.

2 Dorn, C.R., Taylor, D.O., Schneider, R. et al. (1968). Survey of animal neoplasms in alameda and contra costa counties, California.

II. Cancer morbidity in dogs and cats from Alameda County. *J. Natl. Cancer Inst.* 40: 307–318.

3 Dorn, C.R., Taylor, D.O., Frye, F.L. et al. (1968). Survey of animal neoplasms in alameda and contra costa counties, California. I. Methodology and description of cases. *J. Natl. Cancer Inst.* 40: 295–305.

4 MacVean, D.W., Monlux, A.W., Anderson, P.S. et al. (1978). Frequency of canine and feline tumors in a defined population. *Vet. Pathol.* 15: 700–715.

5 Egenvall, A., Bonnett, B.N., Olson, P. et al. (2000). Gender, age and breed pattern of diagnoses for veterinary care in insured dogs in Sweden during 1996. *Vet. Rec.* 146: 551–557.

6 Craig, L.E. (2001). Cause of death in dogs according to breed: a necropsy survey of five breeds. *J. Am. Anim. Hosp. Assoc.* 37: 438–443.

7 Proschowsky, H.F., Rugbjerg, H., and Ersbøll, A.K. (2003). Morbidity of purebred dogs in Denmark. *Prev. Vet. Med.* 58: 53–62.

8 Lagoni, L., Butler, C., and Hetts, S. (1994). *The Human-Animal Bond and Grief.* Philadelphia: Saunders.

9 Bergman, P. (2007). Paraneoplastic syndromes. In: *Withrow & MacEwen's Small Animal Clinical Oncology*, 4e (eds. J. Withrow and D.M. Vail), 77–94. St. Louis: Saunders Elsevier.

10 Michel, K.E., Sorenmo, K., and Shofer, F.S. (2004). Evaluation of body condition and weight loss in dogs presented to a veterinary oncology service. *J. Vet. Intern. Med.* 18: 692–695.

11 Howard, J. and Senior, D.F. (1999). Cachexia and nutritional issues in animals with cancer. *J. Am. Vet. Med. Assoc.* 214: 632–637.

12 Arnold, S.M., Lowry, A.M., Patchell, R., and Foon, K. (2001). Paraneoplastic syndromes. In: *Cancer: Principles and Practice of Oncology* (eds. D.V. VD, S. Hellman and S.A. Rosenberg), 2511. Philadelphia: Lippincott, Williams and Wilkins.

13 Ogilvie, G.K., Fettman, M.J., Mallincrkrodt, C.H. et al. (2000). Effect of fish oil, arginine, and doxorubicin chemotherapy on remission and survival time for dogs with lymphoma: a double-blind, randomized placebo-controlled study. *Cancer* 88: 1916–1928.

14 John, W.J., Patchell, R.A., and Foon, K.A. (1997). Paraneoplastic syndromes. In: *Cancer: Principles and Practice of Oncology* (eds. V.D. DeVita, S. Hellman and S.A. Rosenberg). Philadelphia: Lippincott-Raven.

15 Saper, C.B. and Breder, C.D. (1994). The neurologic basis of fever. *N. Engl. J. Med.* 330: 1880–1886.

16 Miller, J.B. (2009). Hyperthermia and fever. In: *Small Animal Critical Care Medicine* (eds. D.C. Silverstein and K. Hopper), 21–26. Philadelphia: Saunders-Elsevier.

17 Levy, M., Zylber-Katz, E., and Rosenkranz, B. (1995). Clinical pharmacokinetics of dipyrone and its metabolites. *Clin. Pharmacokinet.* 28: 216–234.

18 Chandrasekharan, N.V., Dai, H., Roos, K.L.T. et al. (2002). COX-3, a cyclooxygenase-1 variant inhibited by acetaminophen and other analgesic/antipyretic drugs: cloning, structure, and expression. *Proc. Natl Acad. Sci. USA* 99: 13926–13931.

19 Lamont, L.A. and Mathews, K.A. (2007). Opioids, nonsteroidal anti-inflammatories, and analgesic adjuvants. In: *Lumb & Jones Veterinary Anesthesia and Analgesia*, 4e (eds. W.J. Tranquilli, J.C. Thurmon and K.A. Grimm), 241–271. Ames: Blackwell Publishing.

20 Quasha, A.L., Eger, E.I., and Tinker, J.H. (1980). Determination and applications of MAC. *Anesthesiology* 53: 315–334.

21 Madewell, B.R. and Feldman, B.F. (1980). Characterization of anemias associated with neoplasia in small animals. *J. Am. Vet. Med. Assoc.* 176: 419–425.

22 Ogilvie, G.K., Felsburg, P.J., and Harris, C.W. (1988). Short-term effect of cyclophosphamide and azathioprine on selected aspects of the canine blastogenic response. *Vet. Immunol. Immunopathol.* 18: 119–127.

23 Burgess, K., Moore, A., Rand, W. et al. (2000). Treatment of immune-mediated hemolytic anemia in dogs with cyclophosphamide. *J. Vet. Intern. Med.* 14: 456–462.

24 Mason, N., Duval, D., Shofer, F.S. et al. (2003). Cyclophosphamide exerts no beneficial effect over prednisone alone in the initial treatment of acute immune-mediated hemolytic anemia in dogs: a randomized controlled clinical trial. *J. Vet. Intern. Med.* 17: 206–212.

25 Balch, A. and Mackin, A. (2007). Canine immune-mediated hemolytic anemia: treatment and prognosis. *Compend. Contin. Educ. Vet.* 29: 230–238; quiz 239.

26 Piek, C.J., van Spil, W.E., Junius, G. et al. (2011). Lack of evidence of a beneficial effect of azathioprine in dogs treated with prednisolone for idiopathic immune-mediated hemolytic anemia: a retrospective cohort study. *BMC Vet. Res.* 7: 15.

27 Sato, K., Hikasa, Y., Morita, T. et al. (2002). Secondary erythrocytosis associated with high plasma erythropoietin concentrations in a dog with cecal leiomyosarcoma. *J. Am. Vet. Med. Assoc.* 220: 486–490, 464.

28 Wiesener, M.S., Seyfarth, M., Warnecke, C. et al. (2002). Paraneoplastic erythrocytosis associated with an inactivating point mutation of the von Hippel-Lindau gene in a renal cell carcinoma. *Blood* 99: 3562–3565.

29 Benjamin, D., Yeshurun, D., Charnilas, J. et al. (1978). Hyperlipidemia and myocardial infarction among 118 patients with polycythemia vera. *Am J Med Sci* 276: 23–26.

30 Campbell, K.L. (1990). Diagnosis and management of polycythemia in dogs. *Compend.. Contin. Educ. Pract. Vet. Small Anim. Pract.* 12: 543–550.

31 Jordan, H.L., Grindem, C.B., and Breitschwerdt, E.B. (1993). Thrombocytopenia in cats: a retrospective study of 41 cases. *J. Vet. Intern. Med.* 7: 261–265.

32 Ruslander, D. and Page, R. (1995). Perioperative management of paraneoplastic syndromes. *Vet. Clin. North Am. Small Anim. Pract.* 25: 47–62.

33 Childress, M.O. (2012). Hematologic abnormalities in the small animal cancer patient. *Vet. Clin. North Am. Small Anim. Pract.* 42: 123–155.

34 Logan, J.C., Callan, M.B., Drew, K. et al. (2001). Clinical indications for use of fresh frozen plasma in dogs: 74 dogs (October through December 1999). *J. Am. Vet. Med. Assoc.* 218: 1449–1455.

35 Snow, S.J., Ari Jutkowitz, L., and Brown, A.J. (2010). Trends in plasma transfusion at a veterinary teaching hospital: 308 patients (1996–1998 and 2006–2008). *J. Vet. Emerg. Crit. Care (San Antonio)* 20: 441–445.

36 O'Marra, S.K., Delaforcade, A.M., and Shaw, S.P. (2011). Treatment and predictors of outcome in dogs with immune-mediated thrombocytopenia. *J. Am. Vet. Med. Assoc* 238: 346–352.

37 Davidow, E.B., Brainard, B., Martin, L.G. et al. (2012). Use of fresh platelet concentrate or lyophilized platelets in thrombocytopenic dogs with clinical signs of hemorrhage: a preliminary trial in 37 dogs. *J. Vet. Emerg. Crit. Care (San Antonio)* 22: 116–125.

38 Ramsey, C.C., Burney, D.P., Macintire, D.K. et al. (1996). Use of streptokinase in four dogs with thrombosis. *J. Am. Vet. Med. Assoc.* 209: 780–785.

39 Johnson, L. (2009). Pulmonary thromboembolism. In: *Small Animal Critical Care Medicine* (eds. D.C. Silverstein and K. Hopper), 114–117. St. Louis: Saunders-Elsevier.

40 Maruyama, H., Miura, T., Sakai, M. et al. (2004). The incidence of disseminated intravascular coagulation in dogs with malignant tumor. *J. Vet. Med. Sci.* 66: 573–575.

41 Taylor, F.B., Toh, C.H., Hoots, W.K. et al. (2001). Towards definition, clinical and laboratory criteria, and a scoring system for disseminated intravascular coagulation. *Thromb. Haemost.* 86: 1327–1330.

42 MacEwen, E.G. and Hurvitz, A.I. (1977). Diagnosis and management of monoclonal gammopathies. *Vet. Clin. North Am.* 7: 119–132.

43 Somer, T. and Meiselman, H.J. (1993). Disorders of blood viscosity. *Ann. Med.* 25: 31–39.

44 O'Keefe, D.A. and Couto, C.G. (1988). Coagulation abnormalities associated with neoplasia. *Vet. Clin. North Am. Small Anim. Pract.* 18: 157–168.

45 McGrath, M.A. and Penny, R. (1976). Paraproteinemia: blood hyperviscosity and clinical manifestations. *J. Clin. Invest.* 58: 1155–1162.

46 Matus, R.E., Leifer, C.E., Gordon, B.R. et al. (1983). Plasmapheresis and chemotherapy of hyperviscosity syndrome associated with monoclonal gammopathy in the dog. *J. Am. Vet. Med. Assoc.* 183: 215–218.

47 Uehlinger, P., Glaus, T., Hauser, B. et al. (1998). Differential diagnosis of hypercalcemia--a retrospective study of 46 dogs. *Schweiz. Arch. Tierheilkd.* 140: 188–197.

48 Savary, K.C., Price, G.S., and Vaden, S.L. (2000). Hypercalcemia in cats: a retrospective study of 71 cases (1991–1997). *J. Vet. Intern. Med.* 14: 184–189.

49 Elliott, J., Dobson, J.M., Dunn, J.K. et al. (1991). Hypercalcaemia in the dog: a study of 40 cases. *J. Small Anim. Pract.* 32: 564–571.

50 Sheafor, S.E., Gamblin, R.M., and Couto, C.G. (1996). Hypercalcemia in two cats with multiple myeloma. *J. Am. Anim. Hosp. Assoc.* 32: 503–508.

51 Pressler, B.M., Rotstein, D.S., Law, J.M. et al. (2002). Hypercalcemia and high parathyroid hormone-related protein concentration associated with malignant melanoma in a dog. *J. Am. Vet. Med. Assoc.* 221: 263–265, 240.

52 Anderson, T.E., Legendre, A.M., and McEntee, M.M. (2000). Probable hypercalcemia of malignancy in a cat with bronchogenic adenocarcinoma. *J. Am. Anim. Hosp. Assoc.* 36: 52–55.

53 Klausner, J.S., Bell, F.W., Hayden, D.W. et al. (1990). Hypercalcemia in two cats with squamous cell carcinomas. *J. Am. Vet. Med. Assoc.* 196: 103–105.

54 Meuten, D.J., Cooper, B.J., Capen, C.C. et al. (1981). Hypercalcemia associated with an adenocarcinoma derived from the apocrine glands of the anal sac. *Vet. Pathol.* 18: 454–471.

55 Rosol, T.J. and Capen, C.C. (1996). Pathophysiology of calcium, phosphorus, and magnesium metabolism in animals. *Vet. Clin. North Am. Small Anim. Pract.* 26: 1155–1184.

56 Schenck, P.A., Chew, D.J., Nagode, L.A. et al. (2012). Disorders of calcium: hypercalcemia and hypocalcemia. In: *Fluid, Electrolyte, and Acid-Base Disorders in Small Animal Practice*, 4e (ed. S.P. DiBartola), 120–194. St. Louis: Saunders Elsevier.

57 Bergman, P.J. (2012). Paraneoplastic hypercalcemia. *Top. Companion Anim. Med.* 27: 156–158.

58 Kruger, J.M., Osborne, C.A., Nachreiner, R.F. et al. (1996). Hypercalcemia and renal failure. Etiology, pathophysiology, diagnosis, and treatment. *Vet. Clin. North Am. Small Anim. Pract.* 26: 1417–1445.

59 Price, G.S., Page, R.L., Fischer, B.M. et al. (1991). Efficacy and toxicity of doxorubicin/cyclophosphamide maintenance therapy in dogs with multicentric lymphosarcoma. *J. Vet. Intern. Med.* 5: 259–262.

60 Green, T. and Chew, D.J. (2009). Calcium disorders. In: *Small Animal Critical Care Medicine* (eds. D.C. Silverstein and K. Hopper), 233–239. St. Louis: Elsevier.

61 Hostutler, R.A., Chew, D.J., Jaeger, J.Q. et al. (2005). Uses and effectiveness of pamidronate disodium for treatment of dogs and cats with hypercalcemia. *J. Vet. Intern. Med.* 19: 29–33.

62 Milner, R.J., Farese, J., Henry, C.J. et al. (2004). Bisphosphonates and cancer. *J. Vet. Intern. Med.* 18: 597–604.

63 Martin, C.K., Welbeck, J.L., Thudi, N.K. et al. (2010). Zoledronic acid reduces bone loss and tumor growth in an orthotopic xenograft model of osteolytic oral squamous cell carcinoma. *Cancer Res.* 70: 8607–8616.

64 Caywood, D.D., Klausner, J.S., and O'Leary, T.P. (1988). Pancreatic insulin-secreting neoplasms: clinical, diagnostic, and prognostic features in 73 dogs. *J. Am. Anim. Hosp. Assoc.* 24: 577–584.

65 Beaudry, D., Knapp, D.W., Montgomery, T. et al. (1995). Hypoglycemia in four dogs with smooth muscle tumors. *J. Vet. Intern. Med.* 9: 415–418.

66 Zapf, J. (1993). Role of insulin-like growth factor (IGF) II and IGF binding proteins in extrapancreatic tumour hypoglycaemia. *J. Intern. Med.* 234: 543–552.

67 Koenig, A. (2009). Hypoglycemia. In: *Small Animal Critical Care Medicine* (eds. D.C. Silverstein and K. Hopper), 295–298. St. Louis: Saunders-Elsevier.

68 Meleo, K. (1990). Management of insuloma patients with refractory hypoglycemia. *Probl. Vet. Med.* 2: 602–609.

69 Leifer, C.E. and Peterson, M.E. (1984). Hypoglycemia. *Vet. Clin. North Am. Small Anim. Pract.* 14: 873–889.

70 Gaschen, F. (2005). Paraneoplastic syndrome. In: *Textbook of Veterinary Internal Medicine*, 6e (eds. S.J. Ettinger and E. Feldman), 789–795. St. Louis: Elsevier Saunders.

71 Ishiguro, T., Kadosawa, T., Takagi, S. et al. (2003). Relationship of disease progression and plasma histamine concentrations in 11 dogs with mast cell tumors. *J. Vet. Intern. Med.* 17: 194–198.

72 Fox, L.E., Rosenthal, R.C., Twedt, D.C. et al. (1990). Plasma histamine and gastrin concentrations in 17 dogs with mast cell tumors. *J. Vet. Intern. Med.* 4: 242–246.

73 Godfrey, D.R. (1998). A case of feline paraneoplastic alopecia with secondary Malassezia-associated dermatitis. *J. Small Anim. Pract.* 39: 394–396.

74 Barrs, V.R., Martin, P., France, M. et al. (1999). What is your diagnosis? Feline paraneoplastic alopecia associated with pancreatic and bile duct carcinomas. *J. Small Anim. Pract.* 40 (559): 595–596.

75 Tasker, S., Griffon, D.J., Nuttall, T.J. et al. (1999). Resolution of paraneoplastic alopecia following surgi, cal removal of a pancreatic carcinoma in a cat. *J. Small Anim. Pract.* 40: 16–19.

76 Atwater, S.W., Powers, B., Park, R. et al. (1994). Thymoma in dogs: 23 cases (1980–1991). *J. Am. Vet. Med. Assoc.* 205: 1007–1013.

77 Krotje, L.J., Fix, A.S., and Potthoff, A.D. (1990). Acquired myasthenia gravis and cholangiocellular carcinoma in a dog. *J. Am. Vet. Med. Assoc.* 197: 488–490.

78 Lainesse, M.F., Taylor, S.M., Myers, S.L. et al. (1996). Focal myasthenia gravis as a paraneoplastic syndrome of canine thymoma: improvement following thymectomy. *J. Am. Anim. Hosp. Assoc.* 32: 111–117.

79 Moore, A.S., Madewell, B.R., Cardinet, G.H. et al. (1990). Osteogenic sarcoma and myasthenia gravis in a dog. *J. Am. Vet. Med. Assoc.* 197: 226–227.

80 Joseph, R.J., Carrillo, J.M., and Lennon, V.A. (1988). Myasthenia gravis in the cat. *J. Vet. Intern. Med.* 2: 75–79.

81 Eisenkraft, J.B., Book, W.J., Mann, S.M. et al. (1988). Resistance to succinylcholine in myasthenia gravis: a dose-response study. *Anesthesiology* 69: 760–763.

82 Martyn, J.A., White, D.A., Gronert, G.A. et al. (1992). Up-and-down regulation of skeletal muscle acetylcholine receptors. Effects on neuromuscular blockers. *Anesthesiology* 76: 822–843.

83 Braund, K.G., Steiss, J.E., Amling, K.A. et al. (1987). Insulinoma and subclinical peripheral neuropathy in two dogs. *J. Vet. Intern. Med.* 1: 86–90.

84 Braund, K.G. (1990). Remote effects of cancer on the nervous system. *Semin. Vet. Med. Surg.* 5: 262–270.

85 Villiers, E. and Dobson, J. (1998). Multiple myeloma with associated polyneuropathy in a German shepherd dog. *J. Small Anim. Pract.* 39: 249–251.

86 Mariani, C.L., Shelton, S.B., and Alsup, J.C. (1999). Paraneoplastic polyneuropathy and subsequent recovery following tumor removal in a dog. *J. Am. Anim. Hosp. Assoc.* 35: 302–305.

87 Ruel, H.L.M., Watanabe, R., Evangelista, M.C. et al. (2020). Pain burden, sensory profile and inflammatory cytokines of dogs with naturally-occurring neuropathic pain treated with gabapentin alone or with meloxicam. *PLoS One* 15: e0237121.

88 Plessas, I.N., Volk, H.A., Rusbridge, C. et al. (2015). Comparison of gabapentin versus topiramate on clinically affected dogs with Chiari-like malformation and syringomyelia. *Vet. Rec.* 177: 288.

89 Crociolli, G.C., Cassu, R.N., Barbero, R.C. et al. (2015). Gabapentin as an adjuvant for postoperative pain management in dogs undergoing mastectomy. *J. Vet. Med. Sci.* 77: 1011–1015.

90 Thoefner, M.S., Skovgaard, L.T., McEvoy, F.J. et al. (2020). Pregabalin alleviates clinical signs of syringomyelia-related central neuropathic pain in Cavalier King Charles Spaniel dogs: a randomized controlled trial. *Vet. Anaesth. Analg.* 47: 238–248.

91 Sanchis-Mora, S., Chang, Y.M., Abeyesinghe, S.M. et al. (2019). Pregabalin for the treatment of syringomyelia-associated neuropathic pain in dogs: a randomised, placebo-controlled, double-masked clinical trial. *Vet. J.* 250: 55–62.

92 Goich, M., Bascuñán, A., Faúndez, P. et al. (2019). Multimodal analgesia for treatment of allodynia and hyperalgesia after major trauma in a cat. *J. Feline Med. Surg. Open Reports* 5:1–8.

93 Schmierer, P.A., Tunsmeyer, J., Tipold, A. et al. (2020). Randomized controlled trial of pregabalin for analgesia after surgical treatment of intervertebral disc disease in dogs. *Vet. Surg.* 49: 905–913.

94 Kukanich, B. and Cohen, R.L. (2011). Pharmacokinetics of oral gabapentin in greyhound dogs. *Vet. J.* 187: 133–135.

95 Siao, K.T., Pypendop, B.H., and Ilkiw, J.E. (2010). Pharmacokinetics of gabapentin in cats. *Am. J. Vet. Res.* 71: 817–821.

96 Salazar, V., Dewey, C.W., Schwark, W. et al. (2009). Pharmacokinetics of single-dose oral pregabalin administration in normal dogs. *Vet. Anaesth. Analg.* 36: 574–580.

97 Esteban, M.A., Dewey, C.W., Schwark, W.S. et al. (2018). Pharmacokinetics of single-dose oral pregabalin administration in normal cats. *Front. Vet. Sci.* 5: 136.

98 Seaman, R.L. and Patton, C.S. (2003). Treatment of renal nephroblastoma in an adult dog. *J. Am. Anim. Hosp. Assoc.* 39: 76–79.

99 Barrand, K.R. and Scudamore, C.L. (2001). Canine hypertrophic osteoarthropathy associated with a malignant Sertoli cell tumour. *J. Small Anim. Pract.* 42: 143–145.

100 Becker, T.J., Perry, R.L., and Watson, G.L. (1999). Regression of hypertrophic osteopathy in a cat after surgical excision of an adrenocortical carcinoma. *J. Am. Anim. Hosp. Assoc.* 35: 499–505.

101 Randolph, J.F., Center, S.A., Flanders, J.A. et al. (1984). Hypertrophic osteopathy associated with adenocarcinoma of the esophageal glands in a dog. *J. Am. Vet. Med. Assoc.* 184: 98–99.

102 Halliwell, W.H. and Ackerman, N. (1974). Botryoid rhabdomyosarcoma of the urinary bladder and hypertrophic osteoarthropathy in a young dog. *J. Am. Vet. Med. Assoc.* 165: 911–913.

103 Hara, Y., Tagawa, M., Ejima, H. et al. (1995). Regression of hypertrophic osteopathy following removal of intrathoracic neoplasia derived from vagus nerve in a dog. *J. Vet. Med. Sci.* 57: 133–135.

104 Nguyen, S. and Hojjati, M. (2011). Review of current therapies for secondary hypertrophic pulmonary osteoarthropathy. *Clin. Rheumatol.* 30: 7–13.

105 King, M.M. and Nelson, D.A. (2008). Hypertrophic osteoarthropathy effectively treated with zoledronic acid. *Clin. Lung Cancer* 9: 179–182.

106 Brodey, R.S. (1980). Hypertrophic osteoarthropathy. In: *Spontaneous Animal Models of Human Disease* (eds. E.J.

Andrews, B.C. Ward and N.H. Altman), 241–246. Waltham: Academic Press.

107 Frimberger, A. (2005). Principles of chemotherapy. In: *Textbook of Veterinary Internal Medicine*, 6e (eds. D.S. Ettinger and E. Feldman), 708–712. St. Louis: Elsevier Saunders.

108 Chun, R., Garrett, L.D., and Vail, D. (2007). Cancer chemotherapy. In: *Withrow & MacEwen's Small Animal Clinical Oncology*, 4e (eds. S.J. Withrow, D. Vail and E.G. MacEwen), 163–192. St. Louis: Elsevier Saunders.

109 Bergman, P. (2009). Tumor lysis syndrome. In: *Small Animal Critical Care Medicine* (eds. D. Sliverstein and K. Hopper), 737–738. St. Louis: Saunders-Elsevier.

110 Fornace, A. (2001). Molecular basis of cancer therapy: radiation therapy. In: *The Molecular Basis of Cancer* (ed. J. Mendelson), 423–465. Philadelphia: WB Saunders.

111 Molony, V. and Kent, J.E. (1997). Assessment of acute pain in farm animals using behavioral and physiological measurements. *J. Anim. Sci.* 75: 266–272.

112 Vainio, A. and Auvinen, A. (1996). Prevalence of symptoms among patients with advanced cancer: an international collaborative study. Symptom Prevalence Group. *J. Pain Symptom Manag.* 12: 3–10.

113 Fitzgibbon, D. and Loeser, J. (2010). Characteristics of cancer pain. In: *Cancer Pain: Assesment, Diagnosis and Management* (eds. D. Fitzgibbon and J. Loeser), 32–41. Philadelphia: Lippincott, Williams and Wilkins.

114 Talamo, G., Angtuaco, E., Walker, R.C. et al. (2005). Avascular necrosis of femoral and/or humeral heads in multiple myeloma: results of a prospective study of patients treated with dexamethasone-based regimens and high-dose chemotherapy. *J. Clin. Oncol.* 23: 5217–5223.

115 Fitzgibbon, D. and Loeser, J. (2010). The process of pain in the cancer patient. In: *Cancer Pain: Assesment, Diagnosis and Management* (eds. D. Fitzgibbon and J. Loeser), 17–23. Philadelphia: Lippincott, Williams and Wilkins.

116 Mitchell, B.S., Schumacher, U., and Kaiserling, E. (1994). Are tumours innervated? Immunohistological investigations using antibodies against the neuronal marker protein gene product 9.5 (PGP 9.5) in benign, malignant and experimental tumours. *Tumour Biol.* 15: 269–274.

117 Besson, J.M. (1999). The neurobiology of pain. *Lancet* 353: 1610–1615.

118 Jessell, T., Tsunoo, A., Kanazawa, I. et al. (1979). Substance P: depletion in the dorsal horn of rat spinal cord after section of the peripheral processes of primary sensory neurons. *Brain Res.* 168: 247–259.

119 Vega, F., Davila, L., Mazarin, P. et al. (1993). Experimental carcinomatous plexopathy. *J. Neurol.* 240: 54–58.

120 Asham, E.H., Loizidou, M., and Taylor, I. (1998). Endothelin-1 and tumour development. *Eur. J. Surg. Oncol.* 24: 57–60.

121 Reid, J., Scott, E.M., Calvo, G. et al. (2017). Definitive Glasgow acute pain scale for cats: validation and intervention level. *Vet. Rec.* 180: 449.

122 Calvo, G., Holden, E., Reid, J. et al. (2014). Development of a behaviour-based measurement tool with defined intervention level for assessing acute pain in cats. *J. Small Anim. Pract.* 55: 622–629.

123 Yazbek, K.V.B. and Fantoni, D.T. (2005). Validity of a health-related quality-of-life scale for dogs with signs of pain secondary to cancer. *J. Am. Vet. Med. Assoc.* 226: 1354–1358.

124 Bar-Yosef, S., Melamed, R., Page, G.G. et al. (2001). Attenuation of the tumor-promoting effect of surgery by spinal blockade in rats. *Anesthesiology* 94: 1066–1073.

125 Page, G.G., Blakely, W.P., and Ben-Eliyahu, S. (2001). Evidence that postoperative pain is a mediator of the tumor-promoting effects of surgery in rats. *Pain* 90: 191–199.

126 World Health Organization. 2018. WHO guidelines for the pharmacological and radiotherapeutic management of cancer pain in adults and adolescents. Available at: https://www.who.int/publications/i/item/who-guidelines-for-the-pharmacological-and-radiotherapeutic-management-of-cancer-pain-in-adults-and-adolescents (accessed February 2021).

127 World Health Organization (2020). Retraction of WHO guidance on opioid use. *Bull. World Health Organ.* 98: 3.

128 World Health Organization. 2021. Revision of pain management guidelines. Available at: https://www.who.int/news/item/27-08-2019-who-revision-of-pain-management-guidelines (accessed February 2021)

129 Baldo, B.A. and Pham, N.H. (2012). Histamine-releasing and allergenic properties of opioid analgesic drugs: resolving the two. *Anaesth. Intensive Care* 40: 216–235.

130 Reilly, S., Seddighi, R., Egger, C.M. et al. (2013). The effect of fentanyl on the end-tidal sevoflurane concentration needed to prevent motor movement in dogs. *Vet. Anaesth. Analg.* 40: 290–296.

131 Aguado, D., Benito, J., and Gómez de Segura, I.A. (2011). Reduction of the minimum alveolar concentration of isoflurane in dogs using a constant rate of infusion of lidocaine-ketamine in combination with either morphine or fentanyl. *Vet. J.* 189: 63–66.

132 Ueyama, Y., Lerche, P., Eppler, C.M. et al. (2009). Effects of intravenous administration of perzinfotel, fentanyl, and a combination of both drugs on the minimum alveolar concentration of isoflurane in dogs. *Am. J. Vet. Res.* 70: 1459–1464.

133 Andreoni, V. and Hughes, J.M.L. (2009). Propofol and fentanyl infusions in dogs of various breeds undergoing surgery. *Vet. Anaesth. Analg.* 36: 523–531.

134 Lemmens, S., Stienen, P.J., Jaramillo, L.G. et al. (2008). The cardiorespiratory effects of a fentanyl infusion following acepromazine and glycopyrrolate in dogs. *Tijdschr. Diergeneeskd.* 133: 888–895.

135 Gilbert, D.B., Motzel, S.L., and Das, S.R. (2003). Postoperative pain management using fentanyl patches in dogs. *Contemp. Top. Lab. Anim. Sci.* 42: 21–26.

136 Wilson, D., Pettifer, G.R., and Hosgood, G. (2006). Effect of transdermally administered fentanyl on minimum alveolar concentration of isoflurane in normothermic and hypothermic dogs. *J. Am. Vet. Med. Assoc.* 228: 1042–1046.

137 Bellei, E., Roncada, P., Pisoni, L. et al. (2011). The use of fentanyl-patch in dogs undergoing spinal surgery: plasma concentration and analgesic efficacy. *J. Vet. Pharmacol. Ther.* 34: 437–441.

138 Egger, C.M., Glerum, L.E., Allen, S.W. et al. (2003). Plasma fentanyl concentrations in awake cats and cats undergoing anesthesia and ovariohysterectomy using transdermal administration. *Vet. Anaesth. Analg.* 30: 229–236.

139 Egger, C.M., Glerum, L., Haag, K.M. et al. (2007). Efficacy and cost-effectiveness of transdermal fentanyl patches for the relief of post-operative pain in dogs after anterior cruciate ligament and pelvic limb repair. *Vet. Anaesth. Analg.* 34: 200–208.

140 Reed, F., Burrow, R., Poels, K.L.C. et al. (2011). Evaluation of transdermal fentanyl patch attachment in dogs and analysis of residual fentanyl content following removal. *Vet. Anaesth. Analg.* 38: 407–412.

141 Schmiedt, C.W. and Bjorling, D.E. (2007). Accidental prehension and suspected transmucosal or oral absorption of fentanyl from a transdermal patch in a dog. *Vet. Anaesth. Analg.* 34: 70–73.

142 Sabbe, M.B., Grafe, M.R., Mjanger, E. et al. (1994). Spinal delivery of sufentanil, alfentanil, and morphine in dogs. Physiologic and toxicologic investigations. *Anesthesiology* 81: 899–920.

143 Naganobu, K., Maeda, N., Miyamoto, T. et al. (2004). Cardiorespiratory effects of epidural administration of morphine and fentanyl in dogs anesthetized with sevoflurane. *J. Am. Vet. Med. Assoc.* 224: 67–70.

144 Almeida, T.F., Fantoni, D.T., Mastrocinque, S. et al. (2007). Epidural anesthesia with bupivacaine, bupivacaine and fentanyl, or bupivacaine and sufentanil during intravenous administration of propofol for ovariohysterectomy in dogs. *J. Am. Vet. Med. Assoc.* 230: 45–51.

145 Novello, L. and Corletto, F. (2006). Combined spinal-epidural anesthesia in a dog. *Vet. Surg.* 35: 191–197.

146 Zweifel, B.S., Davis, T.W., Ornberg, R.L. et al. (2002). Direct evidence for a role of cyclooxygenase 2-derived prostaglandin E2 in human head and neck xenograft tumors. *Cancer Res.* 62: 6706–6711.

147 Rüegg, C. and Dormond, O. (2001). Suppression of tumor angiogenesis by nonsteroidal anti-inflammatory drugs: a new function for old drugs. *Sci. World J.* 1: 808–811.

148 Koki, A., Khan, N.K., Woerner, B.M. et al. (2002). Cyclooxygenase-2 in human pathological disease. *Adv. Exp. Med. Biol.* 507: 177–184.

149 Kulkarni, S., Rader, J.S., Zhang, F. et al. (2001). Cyclooxygenase-2 is overexpressed in human cervical cancer. *Clin. Cancer Res.* 7: 429–434.

150 Soslow, R.A., Dannenberg, A.J., Rush, D. et al. (2000). COX-2 is expressed in human pulmonary, colonic, and mammary tumors. *Cancer* 89: 2637–2645.

151 Buckman, S.Y., Gresham, A., Hale, P. et al. (1998). COX-2 expression is induced by UVB exposure in human skin: implications for the development of skin cancer. *Carcinogenesis* 19: 723–729.

152 Chan, G., Boyle, J.O., Yang, E.K. et al. (1999). Cyclooxygenase-2 expression is up-regulated in squamous cell carcinoma of the head and neck. *Cancer Res.* 59: 991–994.

153 Howe, L.R., Subbaramaiha, K., Patel, J. et al. (2002). Celecoxib, a selective cyclooxygenase 2 inhibitor, protects against human epidermal growth factor receptor 2 (HER-2)/neu-induced breast cancer. *Cancer Res.* 62: 5405–5407.

154 Koki, A.T. and Masferrer, J.L. (2002). Celecoxib: a specific COX-2 inhibitor with anticancer properties. *Cancer Control* 9: 28–35.

155 Knottenbelt, C.M., Simpson, J.W., Tasker, S. et al. (2000). Preliminary clinical observations on the use of piroxicam in the management of rectal tubulopapillary polyps. *J. Small Anim. Pract.* 41: 393–397.

156 Schmidt, B.R., Glickman, N.W., DeNicola, D.B. et al. (2001). Evaluation of piroxicam for the treatment of oral squamous cell carcinoma in dogs. *J. Am. Vet. Med. Assoc.* 218: 1783–1786.

157 Knapp, D.W., Richardson, R.C., Bottoms, G.D. et al. (1992). Phase I trial of piroxicam in 62 dogs bearing naturally occurring tumors. *Cancer Chemother. Pharmacol.* 29: 214–218.

158 Knapp, D.W., Richardson, R.C., Chan, T. et al. (1994). Piroxicam therapy in 34 dogs with transitional cell carcinoma of the urinary bladder. *J. Vet. Intern. Med.* 8: 273–278.

159 Knapp, D.W., Chan, T.C., Kuczek, T. et al. (1995). Evaluation of in vitro cytotoxicity of nonsteroidal anti-inflammatory drugs against canine tumor cells. *Am. J. Vet. Res.* 56: 801–805.

160 Knapp, D.W., Glickman, N.W., Widmer, W.R. et al. (2000). Cisplatin versus cisplatin combined with piroxicam in a canine model of human invasive urinary bladder cancer. *Cancer Chemother. Pharmacol.* 46: 221–226.

161 Mohammed, S.I., Bennett, P.F., Craig, B.A. et al. (2002). Effects of the cyclooxygenase inhibitor, piroxicam, on tumor response, apoptosis, and angiogenesis in a canine model of human invasive urinary bladder cancer. *Cancer Res.* 62: 356–358.

162 Lavalle, G.E., De Campos, C.B., Bertagnolli, A.C. et al. (2012). Canine malignant mammary gland neoplasms with advanced clinical staging treated with carboplatin and cyclooxygenase inhibitors. *in vivo* 26: 375–379.

163 Royals, S.R., Farese, J.P., Milner, R.J. et al. (2005). Investigation of the effects of deracoxib and piroxicam on the in vitro viability of osteosarcoma cells from dogs. *Am. J. Vet. Res.* 66: 1961–1967.

164 Sonzogni-Desautels, K., Knapp, D.W., Sartin, E. et al. (2011). Effect of cyclooxygenase inhibitors in a xenograft model of canine mammary tumours. *Vet. Comp. Oncol.* 9: 161–171.

165 McMillan, S.K., Boria, P., Moore, G.E. et al. (2011). Antitumor effects of deracoxib treatment in 26 dogs with transitional cell carcinoma of the urinary bladder. *J. Am. Vet. Med. Assoc.* 239: 1084–1089.

166 Papich, M.G. (2008). An update on nonsteroidal anti-inflammatory drugs (NSAIDs) in small animals. *Vet. Clin. North Am. Small Anim. Pract.* 38: 1243–1266, vi.

167 Court, M.H. (2013). Feline drug metabolism and disposition: pharmacokinetic evidence for species differences and molecular mechanisms. *Vet. Clin. North Am. Small Anim. Pract.* 43: 1039–1054.

168 van Oostrom, H. and Knowles, T.G. (2018). The clinical efficacy of EMLA cream for intravenous catheter placement in client-owned dogs. *Vet. Anaesth. Analg.* 45: 604–608.

169 Crisi, P.E., DeSantis, F., Giordano, M.V. et al. (2020). Evaluation of eutectic lidocaine/prilocaine cream for jugular blood sampling in cats. *J. Feline Med. Surg.* 23: 185–189.

170 Carpenter, R.E., Wilson, D.V., and Evans, A.T. (2004). Evaluation of intraperitoneal and incisional lidocaine or bupivacaine for analgesia following ovariohysterectomy in the dog. *Vet. Anaesth. Analg.* 31: 46–52.

171 Abelson, A.L., McCobb, E.C., Shaw, S. et al. (2009). Use of wound soaker catheters for the administration of local anesthetic for post-operative analgesia: 56 cases. *Vet. Anaesth. Analg.* 36: 597–602.

172 Thompson, S.E. and Johnson, J.M. (1991). Analgesia in dogs after intercostal thoracotomy. A comparison of morphine, selective intercostal nerve block, and interpleural regional analgesia with bupivacaine. *Vet. Surg.* 20: 73–77.

173 Conzemius, M.G., Brockman, D.J., King, L.G. et al. (1995). Analgesia in dogs after intercostal thoracotomy: a clinical trial comparing intravenous buprenorphine and interpleural bupivacaine. *Vet. Surg.* 23: 291–298.

174 Stobie, D., Caywood, D.D., Rozanski, E.A. et al. (1995). Evaluation of pulmonary function and analgesia in dogs after intercostal thoracotomy and use of morphine administered intramuscularly or intrapleurally and bupivacaine administered intrapleurally. *Am. J. Vet. Res.* 56: 1098–1109.

175 Dhokarikar, P., Caywood, D.D., Stobie, D. et al. (1996). Effects of intramuscular or interpleural administration of morphine and interpleural administration of bupivacaine on pulmonary function in dogs that have undergone median sternotomy. *Am. J. Vet. Res.* 57: 375–380.

176 Vadeboncouer, T.R., Riegler, F.X., and Pelligrino, D.A. (1990). The effects of two different volumes of 0.5% bupivacaine in a canine model of interpleural analgesia. *Reg. Anesth.* 15: 67–72.

177 Kim, Y.K., Lee, S.S., Suh, E.H. et al. (2012). Sprayed intraperitoneal bupivacaine reduces early postoperative pain behavior and biochemical stress response after laparoscopic ovariohysterectomy in dogs. *Vet. J.* 191: 188–192.

178 Campagnol, D., Teixeira-Neto, F.J., Monteiro, E.R. et al. (2012). Effect of intraperitoneal or incisional bupivacaine on pain and the analgesic requirement after ovariohysterectomy in dogs. *Vet. Anaesth. Analg.* 39: 426–430.

179 Valverde, A., Doherty, T.J., Hernández, J. et al. (2004). Effect of lidocaine on the minimum alveolar concentration of isoflurane in dogs. *Vet. Anaesth. Analg.* 31: 264–271.

180 Hansen, B.D. (2001). Epidural catheter analgesia in dogs and cats: technique and review of 182 cases (1991–1999). *J. Vet. Emerg. Crit. Care* 11: 95–103.

181 Ko, J., Weil, A., Maxwell, L. et al. (2007). Plasma concentrations of lidocaine in dogs following lidocaine patch application. *J. Am. Anim. Hosp. Assoc.* 43: 280–283.

182 Ko, J.C.H., Maxwell, L.K., Abbo, L.A. et al. (2008). Pharmacokinetics of lidocaine following the application of 5% lidocaine patches to cats. *J. Vet. Pharmacol. Ther.* 31: 359–367.

183 Weiland, L., Croubels, S., Baert, K. et al. (2006). Pharmacokinetics of a lidocaine patch 5% in dogs. *J. Vet. Med. Series A* 53: 34–39.

184 Weil, A.B., Ko, J., and Inoue, T. (2007). The use of lidocaine patches. *Compend. Contin. Educ. Vet.* 29: 208–210, 212, 214-6.

185 Bergadano, A., Andersen, O.K., Arendt-Nielsen, L. et al. (2009). Plasma levels of a low-dose constant-rate-infusion of ketamine and its effect on single and repeated nociceptive stimuli in conscious dogs. *Vet. J.* 182: 252–260.

186 Sarrau, S., Jourdan, J., Dupuis-Soyris, F. et al. (2007). Effects of postoperative ketamine infusion on pain control and feeding behaviour in bitches undergoing mastectomy. *J. Small Anim. Pract.* 48: 670–676.

187 Lee, S.-E., Seo, J.-M., Liu, J. et al. (2006). The comparison on changes of the body heats in electroacupuncture analgesia and anesthesia by ketamine hydrochloride in dogs. *Am. J. Chin. Med.* 34: 69–76.

188 Snijdelaar, D.G., van Rijn, C.M., Vinken, P. et al. (2005). Effects of pre-treatment with amantadine on morphine induced antinociception during second phase formalin responses in rats. *Pain* 119: 159–167.

189 Kleinböhl, D., Görtelmeyer, R., Bender, H.-J. et al. (2006). Amantadine sulfate reduces experimental sensitization and pain in chronic back pain patients. *Anesth. Analg.* 102: 840–847.

190 Chen, S.-R., Samoriski, G., and Pan, H.-L. (2009). Antinociceptive effects of chronic administration of uncompetitive NMDA receptor antagonists in a rat model of diabetic neuropathic pain. *Neuropharmacology* 57: 121–126.

191 Lascelles, B.D.X., Gaynor, J.S., Smith, E.S. et al. (2008). Amantadine in a multimodal analgesic regimen for alleviation of refractory osteoarthritis pain in dogs. *J. Vet. Intern. Med.* 22: 53–59.

192 Kuusela, E., Raekallio, M., Anttila, M. et al. (2000). Clinical effects and pharmacokinetics of medetomidine and its enantiomers in dogs. *J. Vet. Pharmacol. Ther.* 23: 15–20.

193 Slingsby, L.S. and Taylor, P.M. (2008). Thermal antinociception after dexmedetomidine administration in cats: a dose-finding study. *J. Vet. Pharmacol. Ther.* 31: 135–142.

194 Valtolina, C., Robben, J.H., Uilenreef, J. et al. (2009). Clinical evaluation of the efficacy and safety of a constant rate infusion of dexmedetomidine for postoperative pain management in dogs. *Vet. Anaesth. Analg.* 36: 369–383.

195 Sullivan, A.F., Dashwood, M.R., and Dickenson, A.H. (1987). Alpha 2-adrenoceptor modulation of nociception in rat spinal cord: location, effects and interactions with morphine. *Eur. J. Pharmacol.* 138: 169–177.

196 Sullivan, A.F., Kalso, E.A., McQuay, H.J. et al. (1992). The antinociceptive actions of dexmedetomidine on dorsal horn neuronal responses in the anaesthetized rat. *Eur. J. Pharmacol.* 215: 127–133.

197 Campagnol, D., Teixeira Neto, F.J., Giordano, T. et al. (2007). Effects of epidural administration of dexmedetomidine on the minimum alveolar concentration of isoflurane in dogs. *Am. J. Vet. Res.* 68: 1308–1318.

198 Pohl, V.H., Carregaro, A.B., Lopes, C. et al. (2012). Epidural anesthesia and postoperatory analgesia with alpha-2 adrenergic agonists and lidocaine for ovariohysterectomy in bitches. *Can. J. Vet. Res.* 76: 215–220.

199 Stoelting, R. (2006). Opioid agonists and antagonists. In: *Pharmacology and Physiology in Anesthetic Practice*, 4e (eds. R. Stoelting and S. Hillier), 87–126. Philadelphia: Lippincott, Williams and Wilkins.

200 Kongara, K., Chambers, J.P., and Johnson, C.B. (2012). Effects of tramadol, morphine or their combination in dogs undergoing ovariohysterectomy on peri-operative electroencephalographic responses and post-operative pain. *N. Z. Vet. J.* 60: 129–135.

201 Mastrocinque, S. and Fantoni, D.T. (2003). A comparison of preoperative tramadol and morphine for the control of early postoperative pain in canine ovariohysterectomy. *Vet. Anaesth. Analg.* 30: 220–228.

202 Benitez, M.E., Roush, J.K., Kukanich, B. et al. (2015). Pharmacokinetics of hydrocodone and tramadol administered for control of postoperative pain in dogs following tibial plateau leveling osteotomy. *Am. J. Vet. Res.* 76: 763–770.

203 Pypendop, B.H., Siao, K.T., and Ilkiw, J.E. (2009). Effects of tramadol hydrochloride on the thermal threshold in cats. *Am. J. Vet. Res.* 70: 1465–1470.

204 Kukanich, B. and Papich, M.G. (2011). Pharmacokinetics and antinociceptive effects of oral tramadol hydrochloride administration in greyhounds. *Am. J. Vet. Res.* 72: 256–262.

205 Cheng, J.-K. and Chiou, L.-C. (2006). Mechanisms of the antinociceptive action of gabapentin. *J. Pharmacol. Sci.* 100: 471–486.

206 Mathiesen, O., Møiniche, S., and Dahl, J.B. (2007). Gabapentin and postoperative pain: a qualitative and quantitative systematic review, with focus on procedure. *BMC Anesthesiol.* 7: 6.

207 Menda, F., Koner, O., Sayin, M. et al. (2010). Effects of single-dose gabapentin on postoperative pain and morphine consumption after cardiac surgery. *J. Cardiothorac. Vasc. Anesth.* 24: 808–813.

208 Aghighi, S.A., Tipold, A., Piechotta, M. et al. (2012). Assessment of the effects of adjunctive gabapentin on postoperative pain after intervertebral disc surgery in dogs. *Vet. Anaesth. Analg.* 39: 636–646.

209 Wagner, A.E., Mich, P.M., Uhrig, S.R. et al. (2010). Clinical evaluation of perioperative administration of gabapentin as an adjunct for postoperative analgesia in dogs undergoing amputation of a forelimb. *J. Am. Vet. Med. Assoc.* 236: 751–756.

210 Wolfe, K.C. and Poma, R. (2010). Syringomyelia in the Cavalier King Charles spaniel (CKCS) dog. *Can. Vet. J.* 51: 95–102.

211 Cashmore, R.G., Harcourt-Brown, T.R., Freeman, P.M. et al. (2009). Clinical diagnosis and treatment of suspected neuropathic pain in three dogs. *Aust. Vet. J.* 87: 45–50.

212 Guay, D.R.P. (2005). Pregabalin in neuropathic pain: a more 'pharmaceutically elegant' gabapentin? *Am. J. Geriatr. Pharmacother.* 3: 274–287.

213 Bockbrader, H.N., Wesche, D., Miller, R. et al. (2010). A comparison of the pharmacokinetics and pharmacodynamics of pregabalin and gabapentin. *Clin. Pharmacokinet.* 49: 661–669.

214 Dworkin, R.H., Corbin, A.E., Young, J.P. Jr. et al. Pregabalin for the treatment of postherpetic neuralgia: a randomized, placebo-controlled trial. *Neurology* 60: 1274–1283.

215 Lesser, H., Sharma, U., LaMoreaux, L. et al. (2004). Pregabalin relieves symptoms of painful diabetic neuropathy: a randomized controlled trial. *Neurology* 63: 2104–2110.

216 Aboumarzouk, O.M. and Nelson, R.L. (2012). Pregabalin for chronic prostatitis. *Cochrane Database Syst. Rev.* 8: CD009063.

217 Matsutani, N. and Kawamura, M. (2012). Significant improvement of chronic pain by pregabalin after thoracotomy: report of four cases. *Surg. Today* 43: 915–917.

218 Gray, P., Kirby, J., Smith, M.T. et al. (2011). Pregabalin in severe burn injury pain: a double-blind, randomised placebo-controlled trial. *Pain* 152: 1279–1288.

219 Kim, S.Y., Song, J.W., Park, B. et al. (2011). Pregabalin reduces post-operative pain after mastectomy: a double-blind, randomized, placebo-controlled study. *Acta Anaesthesiol. Scand.* 55: 290–296.

220 Durkin, B., Page, C., and Glass, P. (2010). Pregabalin for the treatment of postsurgical pain. *Expert. Opin. Pharmacother.* 11: 2751–2758.

221 Cabrera Schulmeyer, M.C., de la Maza, J., Ovalle, C. et al. (2010). Analgesic effects of a single preoperative dose of pregabalin after laparoscopic sleeve gastrectomy. *Obes. Surg.* 20: 1678–1681.

222 Richter, R.W., Portenoy, R., Sharma, U. et al. (2005). Relief of painful diabetic peripheral neuropathy with pregabalin: a randomized, placebo-controlled trial. *J. Pain* 6: 253–260.

223 Freynhagen, R., Strojek, K., Griesing, T. et al. (2005). Efficacy of pregabalin in neuropathic pain evaluated in a 12-week, randomised, double-blind, multicentre, placebo-controlled trial of flexible- and fixed-dose regimens. *Pain* 115: 254–263.

224 van Seventer, R., Feister, H.A., Young, J.P. Jr. et al. (2006). Efficacy and tolerability of twice-daily pregabalin for treating pain and related sleep interference in postherpetic neuralgia: a 13-week, randomized trial. *Curr. Med. Res. Opin.* 22: 375–384.

225 Stacey, B.R., Dworkin, R.H., Murphy, K. et al. (2008). Pregabalin in the treatment of refractory neuropathic pain: results of a 15-month open-label trial. *Pain Med.* 9: 1202–1208.

226 Satoh, J., Yagihashi, S., Baba, M. et al. (2011). Efficacy and safety of pregabalin for treating neuropathic pain associated with diabetic peripheral neuropathy: a 14 week, randomized, double-blind, placebo-controlled trial. *Diabet. Med.* 28: 109–116.

227 Gilron, I., Wajsbrot, D., Therrien, F. et al. (2011). Pregabalin for peripheral neuropathic pain: a multicenter, enriched enrollment randomized withdrawal placebo-controlled trial. *Clin. J. Pain* 27: 185–193.

228 Ghai, A., Gupta, M., Hooda, S. et al. (2011). A randomized controlled trial to compare pregabalin with gabapentin for postoperative pain in abdominal hysterectomy. *Saudi J Anaesth* 5: 252–257.

229 Baron, R., Brunnmüller, U., Brasser, M. et al. (2008). A. Efficacy and safety of pregabalin in patients with diabetic peripheral neuropathy or postherpetic neuralgia: open-label, non-comparative, flexible-dose study. *Eur. J. Pain* 12: 850–858.

230 Toth, C. (2012). Drug safety evaluation of pregabalin. *Expert Opin. Drug Saf.* 11: 487–502.

231 Ogawa, S., Satoh, J., Arakawa, A. et al. (2012). Pregabalin treatment for peripheral neuropathic pain: a review of safety data from randomized controlled trials conducted in Japan and in the West. *Drug Saf.* 35: 793–806.

232 Mishra, S., Bhatnagar, S., Goyal, G.N. et al. (2012). A comparative efficacy of amitriptyline, gabapentin, and pregabalin in neuropathic cancer pain: a prospective randomized double-blind placebo-controlled study. *Am. J. Hosp. Palliat. Care* 29: 177–182.

233 Fan, T.M., de Lorimier, L.-P., O'Dell-Anderson, K. et al. (2007). Single-agent pamidronate for palliative therapy of canine appendicular osteosarcoma bone pain. *J. Vet. Intern. Med.* 21: 431–439.

234 Kadar, E., Rush, J.E., Wetmore, L. et al. (2004). Electrolyte disturbances and cardiac arrhythmias in a dog following pamidronate,

calcitonin, and furosemide administration for hypercalcemia of malignancy. *J. Am. Anim. Hosp. Assoc.* 40: 75–81.

235 Rumbeiha, W.K., Fitzgerald, S.D., Kruger, J.M. et al. (2000). Use of pamidronate disodium to reduce cholecalciferol-induced toxicosis in dogs. *Am. J. Vet. Res.* 61: 9–13.

236 Shibutani, T., Inuduka, A., Horiki, I. et al. (2011). Bisphosphonate inhibits alveolar bone resorption in experimentally-induced peri-implantitis in dogs. *Clin. Oral Implants Res.* 12: 109–114.

237 Fan, T.M., de Lorimier, L.-P., Charney, S.C. et al. (2005). Evaluation of intravenous pamidronate administration in 33 cancer-bearing dogs with primary or secondary bone involvement. *J. Vet. Intern. Med.* 19: 74–80.

238 Ashton, J.A., Farese, J.P., Milner, R.J. et al. (2005). Investigation of the effect of pamidronate disodium on the in vitro viability of osteosarcoma cells from dogs. *Am. J. Vet. Res.* 66: 885–891.

239 Fan, T.M., Charney, S.C., de Lorimier, L.P. et al. (2009). Double-blind placebo-controlled trial of adjuvant pamidronate with palliative radiotherapy and intravenous doxorubicin for canine appendicular osteosarcoma bone pain. *J. Vet. Intern. Med.* 23: 152–160.

240 Oblak, M.L., Boston, S.E., Higginson, G. et al. (2012). The impact of pamidronate and chemotherapy on survival times in dogs with appendicular primary bone tumors treated with palliative radiation therapy. *Vet. Surg.* 41: 430–435.

241 Tomlin, J.L., Sturgeon, C., Pead, M.J. et al. (2000). Use of the bisphosphonate drug alendronate for palliative management of osteosarcoma in two dogs. *Vet. Rec.* 147: 129–132.

242 de Lorimier, L.-P. and Fan, T.M. (2005). Bone metabolic effects of single-dose zoledronate in healthy dogs. *J. Vet. Intern. Med.* 19: 924–927.

243 Martín-Jiménez, T., De Lorimier, L.-P., Fan, T.M. et al. (2007). Pharmacokinetics and pharmacodynamics of a single dose of zoledronate in healthy dogs. *J. Vet. Pharmacol. Ther.* 30: 492–495.

244 Fan, T.M., de Lorimier, L.-P., Garrett, L.D. et al. (2008). The bone biologic effects of zoledronate in healthy dogs and dogs with malignant osteolysis. *J. Vet. Intern. Med.* 22: 380–387.

245 Spugnini, E.P., Vincenzi, B., Caruso, G. et al. (2009). Zoledronic acid for the treatment of appendicular osteosarcoma in a dog. *J. Small Anim. Pract.* 50: 44–46.

246 Allen, M.R., Kubek, D.J., and Burr, D.B. (2010). Cancer treatment dosing regimens of zoledronic acid result in near-complete suppression of mandible intracortical bone remodeling in beagle dogs. *J. Bone Miner. Res.* 25: 98–105.

247 Helm, N.B., Padala, S., Beck, F.M. et al. (2010). Short-term zoledronic acid reduces trabecular bone remodeling in dogs. *Eur. J. Oral Sci.* 118: 460–465.

248 Huja, S.S., Mason, A., Fenell, C.E. et al. (2011). Effects of short-term zoledronic acid treatment on bone remodeling and healing at surgical sites in the maxilla and mandible of aged dogs. *J. Oral Maxillofac. Surg.* 69: 418–427.

249 Fransson, B.A., Peck, K.E., Smith, J.K. et al. (2002). Transdermal absorption of a liposome-encapsulated formulation of lidocaine following topical administration in cats. *Am. J. Vet. Res.* 63: 1309–1312.

250 Willis-Goulet, H.S., Schmidt, B.A., Nicklin, C.F. et al. (2003). Comparison of serum dexamethasone concentrations in cats after oral or transdermal administration using pluronic lecithin organogel (PLO): a pilot study. *Vet. Dermatol.* 14: 83–89.

251 Tong, D., Gillick, L., and Hendrickson, F.R. (1982). The palliation of symptomatic osseous metastases: final results of the study by the radiation therapy oncology group. *Cancer* 50: 893–899.

252 Arcangeli, G., Micheli, A., Arcangeli, G. et al. (1989). The responsiveness of bone metastases to radiotherapy: the effect of site, histology and radiation dose on pain relief. *Radiother. Oncol.* 14: 95–101.

253 Saberski, L., Fitzgerald, J., and Ahmad, M. (2000). Cryoneurolysis and radiofrequency lesioning. In: *Practical Management of Pain* (ed. P.P. Raj), 759. Maryland Heights: Mosby.

254 Janjan, N. (2001). Bone metastases: approaches to management. *Semin. Oncol.* 28: 28–34.

255 Fourney, D.R., Schomer, D.F., Nader, R. et al. (2003). Percutaneous vertebroplasty and kyphoplasty for painful vertebral body fractures in cancer patients. *J. Neurosurg.* 98: 21–30.

256 Fenstermaker, R. (2006). Neurosurgical procedures for cancer pain management. In: *Cancer Pain: Pharmacological, Interventional and Palliative Care Approaches* (ed. D. Leon-Casasola), 453–458. Philadelphia: Saunders.

257 Barr, S.C., Ludders, J.W., Looney, A.L. et al. (1992). Platelet aggregation in dogs after sedation with acepromazine and atropine and during subsequent general anesthesia and surgery. *Am. J. Vet. Res.* 53: 2067–2070.

258 Nolan, A. and Reid, J. (1993). Pharmacokinetics of propofol administered by infusion in dogs undergoing surgery. *Br. J. Anaesth.* 70: 546–551.

259 Andress, J.L., Day, T.K., Day, D.G. et al. (1995). The effects of consecutive day propofol anesthesia on feline red blood cells. *Vet. Surg.* 24: 277–282.

260 Sullivan, R., Alatise, O.I., Anderson, B.O. et al. (2015). Global cancer surgery: delivering safe, affordable, and timely cancer surgery. *Lancet Oncol.* 16: 1193–1224.

261 Mehlen, P. and Puisieux, A. (2006). Metastasis: a question of life or death. *Nat. Rev. Cancer* 6: 449–458.

262 Byrne, K., Levins, K.J., and Buggy, D.J. (2016). Can anesthetic-analgesic technique during primary cancer surgery affect recurrence or metastasis? *Can. J. Anesth.* 63: 184–192.

263 Casey, S.C., Amedei, A., Aquilano, K. et al. (2015). Cancer prevention and therapy through the modulation of the tumor microenvironment. *Semin. Cancer Biol.* 35: S199–S223.

264 Hiller, J.G., Perry, N.J., Poulogiannis, G. et al. (2017). Perioperative events influence cancer recurrence risk after surgery. *Nat. Rev. Clin. Oncol.* 15: 205–218.

265 Stollings, L.M., Jia, L.-J., Tang, P. et al. (2016). Immune modulation by volatile anesthetics. *Anesthesiology* 125: 399–411.

266 Lee, Y.M., Song, B.C., and Yeum, K.J. (2015). Impact of volatile anesthetics on oxidative stress and inflammation. *Biomed. Res. Int.* 2015: 242709. (epub).

267 Yuki, K. and Eckenhoff, R.G. (2016). Mechanisms of the immunological effects of volatile anesthetics: a review. *Anesth. Analg.* 123: 326–335.

268 Luo, X., Zhao, H., Hennah, L. et al. (2015). Impact of isoflurane on malignant capability of ovarian cancer in vitro. *Br. J. Anaesth.* 114: 831–839.

269 Ecimovic, P., McHugh, B., Murray, D. et al. (2010). Direct effect of sevoflurane on breast cancer cell function in vitro. *Eur. J. Anaesthesiol.* 27: 1.

270 Ciechanowicz, S., Zhao, H., Chen, Q. et al. (2018). Differential effects of sevoflurane on the metastatic potential and chemosensitivity of non-small-cell lung adenocarcinoma and renal cell carcinoma in vitro. *Br. J. Anaesth.* 120: 368–375.

271 Wu, L., Zhao, H., Wang, T. et al. (2014). Cellular signaling pathways and molecular mechanisms involving inhalational anesthetics-induced organoprotection. *J. Anesth.* 28: 740–758.

272 Ma, D., Lim, T., Xu, J. et al. (2009). Xenon preconditioning protects against renal ischemic-reperfusion injury via HIF-1α activation. *J. Am. Soc. Nephrol.* 20: 713–720.

273 Jun, I.-J., Jo, J.-Y., Kim, J.-I. et al. (2017). Impact of anesthetic agents on overall and recurrence-free survival in patients undergoing esophageal cancer surgery: a retrospective observational study. *Sci. Rep.* 7: 14020.

274 Lee, J.H., Kang, S.H., Kim, Y. et al. (2016). Effects of propofol-based total intravenous anesthesia on recurrence and overall survival in patients after modified radical mastectomy: a retrospective study. *Korean J. Anesthesiol.* 69: 126–132.

275 Wu, Z.-F., Lee, M.-S., Wong, C.-S. et al. (2018). Propofol-based total intravenous anesthesia is associated with better survival than desflurane anesthesia in colon cancer surgery. *Anesthesiology* 129: 932–941.

276 Enlund, M., Berglund, A., Andreasson, K. et al. (2014). The choice of anaesthetic-sevoflurane or propofol-and outcome from cancer surgery: a retrospective analysis. *Ups. J. Med. Sci.* 119: 251–261.

277 Argano, M., De Maria, R., Vogl, C. et al. (2019). Canine mammary tumour cells exposure to sevoflurane: effects on cell proliferation and neuroepithelial transforming gene 1 expression. *Vet. Anaesth. Analg.* 46: 369–374.

278 Jiang, S., Liu, Y., Huang, L. et al. (2018). Effects of propofol on cancer development and chemotherapy: potential mechanisms. *Eur. J. Pharmacol.* 831: 46–51.

279 Oh, T.K., Kim, K., Jheon, S. et al. (2018). Long-term oncologic outcomes for patients undergoing volatile versus intravenous anesthesia for non-small cell lung cancer surgery: a retrospective propensity matching analysis. *Cancer Control* 25:1–7.

280 Kim, M.H., Kim, D.W., Kim, J.H. et al. (2017). Does the type of anesthesia really affect the recurrence-free survival after breast cancer surgery? *Oncotarget* 8: 90477–90487.

281 Wall, T., Sherwin, A., Ma, D. et al. (2019). Influence of perioperative anaesthetic and analgesic interventions on oncological outcomes: a narrative review. *Br. J. Anaesth.* 123: 135–150.

282 Szpunar, M.J., Burke, K.A., Dawes, R.P. et al. (2013). The antidepressant desipramine and α2-adrenergic receptor activation promote breast tumor progression in association with altered collagen structure. *Cancer Prev. Res.* 6: 1262–1272.

283 Wang, C., Datoo, T., Zhao, H. et al. (2018). Midazolam and dexmedetomidine affect neuroglioma and lung carcinoma cell biology in vitro and in vivo. *Anesthesiology* 129: 1000–1014.

284 Chen, G., Le, Y., Zhoe, L. et al. (2016). Dexmedetomidine inhibits maturation and function of human cord blood-derived dendritic cells by interfering with synthesis and secretion of IL-12 and IL-23. *PLoS One* 11: e0153288.

285 Wang, Y., Xu, X., Liu, H. et al. (2015). Effects of dexmedetomidine on patients undergoing radical gastrectomy. *J. Surg. Res.* 194: 147–153.

286 Connolly, C. and Buggy, D.J. (2016). Opioids and tumour metastasis: does the choice of the anesthetic-analgesic technique influence outcome after cancer surgery? *Curr. Opin. Anaesthesiol.* 29: 468–474.

287 Afsharimani, B., Doornebal, C.W., Cabot, P.J. et al. (2015). Comparison and analysis of the animal models used to study the effect of morphine on tumour growth and metastasis. *Br. J. Pharmacol.* 172: 251–259.

288 Boland, J.W. and Pockley, A.G. (2018). Influence of opioids on immune function in patients with cancer pain: from bench to bedside. *Br. J. Pharmacol.* 175: 2726–2736.

289 Franchi, S., Panerai, A.E., and Sacerdote, P. (2007). Buprenorphine ameliorates the effect of surgery on hypothalamus-pituitary-adrenal axis, natural killer cell activity and metastatic colonization in rats in comparison with morphine or fentanyl treatment. *Brain Behav. Immun.* 21: 767–774.

290 Xie, N., Gomes, F.P., Deora, V. et al. (2017). Activation of μ-opioid receptor and toll-like receptor 4 by plasma from morphine-treated mice. *Brain Behav. Immun.* 61: 244–258.

291 Gaspani, L., Bianchi, M., Limiroli, E. et al. (2002). The analgesic drug tramadol prevents the effect of surgery on natural killer cell activity and metastatic colonization in rats. *J. Neuroimmunol.* 129: 18–24.

292 Koodie, L., Yuan, H., Pumper, J.A. et al. (2014). Morphine inhibits migration of tumor-infiltrating leukocytes and suppresses angiogenesis associated with tumor growth in mice. *Am. J. Pathol.* 184: 1073–1084.

293 Afsharimani, B., Baran, J., Watanabe, S. et al. (2014). Morphine and breast tumor metastasis: the role of matrix-degrading enzymes. *Clin. Exp. Metastasis* 31: 149–158.

294 Khabbazi, S., Nassar, Z.D., Goumon, Y. et al. (2016). Morphine decreases the pro-angiogenic interaction between breast cancer cells and macrophages in vitro. *Sci. Rep.* 6: 31572.

295 Mathew, B., Lennon, F.E., Siegler, J. et al. (2011). The novel role of the mu opioid receptor in lung cancer progression: a laboratory investigation. *Anesth. Analg.* 112: 558–567.

296 Bimonte, S., Barbieri, A., Cascella, M. et al. (2018). The effects of naloxone on human breast cancer progression: in vitro and in vivo studies on MDA.MB231 cells. *Onco. Targets. Ther.* 11: 185–191.

297 Cata, J.P., Keerty, V., Keerty, D. et al. (2014). A retrospective analysis of the effect of intraoperative opioid dose on cancer recurrence after non-small cell lung cancer resection. *Cancer Med.* 3: 900–908.

298 Maher, D.P., Wong, W., White, P.F. et al. (2014). Association of increased postoperative opioid administration with non-small-cell lung cancer recurrence: a retrospective analysis. *Br. J. Anaesth.* 113: i88–i94.

299 Oh, T.K., Jeon, J.H., Lee, J.M. et al. (2017). Investigation of opioid use and long-term oncologic outcomes for non-small cell lung cancer patients treated with surgery. *PLoS One* 12: e0181672.

300 Tai, Y.-H., Wu, H.-L., Chang, W.-K. et al. (2017). Intraoperative fentanyl consumption does not impact cancer recurrence or overall survival after curative colorectal cancer resection. *Sci. Rep.* 7: 10816.

301 Du, K.N., Feng, L., Newhouse, A. et al. (2018). Effects of intraoperative opioid use on recurrence-free and overall survival in patients with esophageal adenocarcinoma and squamous cell carcinoma. *Anesth. Analg.* 127: 210–216.

302 Hooijmans, C.R., Geessink, F.J., Ritskes-Hoitinga, M. et al. (2015). A systematic review and meta-analysis of the ability of analgesic drugs to reduce metastasis in experimental cancer models. *Pain* 156: 1835–1844.

303 Diaz-Cambronero, O., Mazzinari, G., and Cata, J.P. (2018). Perioperative opioids and colorectal cancer recurrence: a systematic review of the literature. *Pain Manag.*. 8: 353–361.

304 Zylla, D., Kuskowski, M.A., Gupta, K. et al. (2014). Association of opioid requirement and cancer pain with survival in advanced non-small cell lung cancer. *Br. J. Anaesth.* 113: i109–i116.

305 Cole, S.W., Nagaraja, A.S., Lutgendorf, S.K. et al. (2015). Sympathetic nervous system regulation of the tumour microenvironment. *Nat. Rev. Cancer* 15: 563–572.

306 Barr, C. and Gianotti, G. (2019). Alternatives to opioid analgesia in small animal anesthesia. *Vet. Clin. North Am. Small Anim. Pract.* 49: 1013–1027.

307 Fant, F., Tina, E., Sandblom, D. et al. (2013). Thoracic epidural analgesia inhibits the neuro-hormonal but not the acute inflammatory stress response after radical retropubic prostatectomy. *Br. J. Anaesth.* 110: 747–757.

308 Siekmann, W., Eintrei, C., Magnuson, A. et al. (2017). Surgical and not analgesic technique affects postoperative inflammation following colorectal cancer

surgery: a prospective, randomized study. *Color. Dis.* 19: O186–O195.

309 Li, R., Xiao, C., Liu, H. et al. (2018). Effects of local anesthetics on breast cancer cell viability and migration. *BMC Cancer* 18: 666.

310 Xuan, W., Zhao, H., Hankin, J. et al. (2016). Local anesthetic bupivacaine induced ovarian and prostate cancer apoptotic cell death and underlying mechanisms in vitro. *Sci. Rep.* 6: 26277.

311 Dan, J., Gong, X., Li, D. et al. (2018). Inhibition of gastric cancer by local anesthetic bupivacaine through multiple mechanisms independent of sodium channel blockade. *Biomed. Pharmacother.* 103: 823–828.

312 Chamaraux-Tran, T.N. and Piegeler, T. (2017). The amide local anesthetic lidocaine in cancer surgery-potential antimetastatic effects and preservation of immune cell function? A narrative review. *Front. Med.* 4: 235.

313 Lirk, P., Hollmann, M.W., Fleischer, M. et al. (2014). Lidocaine and ropivacaine, but not bupivacaine, demethylate deoxyribonucleic acid in breast cancer cells in vitro. *Br. J. Anaesth.* 113: i32–i38.

314 Exadaktylos, A.K., Buggy, D.J., Moriarty, D.C. et al. (2006). Can anesthetic technique for primary breast cancer surgery affect recurrence or metastasis? *Anesthesiology* 105: 660–664.

315 Biki, B., Mascha, E., Moriarty, D.C. et al. (2008). Anesthetic technique for radical prostatectomy surgery affects cancer recurrence: a retrospective analysis. *Anesthesiology* 109: 180–187.

316 Grandhi, R.K., Lee, S., and Abd-Elsayed, A. (2017). The relationship between regional anesthesia and cancer: a metaanalysis. *Ochsner J.* 17: 345–361.

317 Weng, M., Chen, W., Hou, W. et al. (2016). The effect of neuraxial anesthesia on cancer recurrence and survival after cancer surgery: an updated meta-analysis. *Oncotarget* 7: 15262–15273.

318 Lee, B.M., Ghotra, V.S., Karam, J.A. et al. (2015). Regional anesthesia/analgesia and the risk of cancer recurrence and mortality after prostatectomy: a meta-analysis. *Pain Manag.*. 5: 387–395.

319 Cakmakkaya, O.S., Kolodzie, K., Apfel, C.C. et al. (2014). Anaesthetic techniques for risk of malignant tumour recurrence. *Cochrane Database Syst. Rev.* 11: CD008877.

320 Wang, D. and Dubois, R.N. (2010). Eicosanoids and cancer. *Nat. Rev. Cancer* 10: 181–193.

321 Basha, R., Baker, C.H., Sankpal, U.T. et al. (2010). Therapeutic applications of NSAIDS in cancer special emphasis on tolfenamic acid. *Front. Biosci.* S3: 797–805.

322 Kashfi, K., Rayyan, Y., Qiao, L.L. et al. (2002). Nitric oxide-donating nonsteroidal anti-inflammatory drugs inhibit the growth of various cultured human cancer cells: evidence of a tissue type-independent effect. *J. Pharmacol. Exp. Ther.* 303: 1273–1282.

323 Liggett, J.L., Zhang, X., Eling, T.E. et al. (2014). Anti-tumor activity of non-steroidal anti-inflammatory drugs: cyclooxygenase-independent targets. *Cancer Lett.* 346: 217–224.

324 Čeponytė, U., Paškevičiūtė, M., and Petrikaitė, V. (2018). Comparison of NSAIDs activity in COX-2 expressing and non-expressing 2D and 3D pancreatic cancer cell cultures. *Cancer Manag. Res.* 10: 1543–1551.

325 Thyagarajan, A., Saylae, J., and Sahu, R.P. (2017). Acetylsalicylic acid inhibits the growth of melanoma tumors via SOX2-dependent-PAF-R-independent signaling pathway. *Oncotarget* 8: 49959–49972.

326 Rigas, B. and Tsioulias, G.J. (2015). The evolving role of nonsteroidal anti-inflammatory drugs in colon cancer prevention: a cause for optimism. *J. Pharmacol. Exp. Ther.* 353: 2–8.

327 Ng, K., Meyerhardt, J.A., Chan, A.T. et al. (2015). Aspirin and COX-2 inhibitor use in patients with stage III colon cancer. *J. Natl. Cancer Inst.* 107: 345.

328 Huang, X., Gao, P., Sun, J.-X. et al. (2015). Aspirin and nonsteroidal anti-inflammatory drugs after but not before diagnosis are associated with improved breast cancer survival: a meta-analysis. *Cancer Causes Control* 26: 589–600.

329 Forget, P., Vandenhende, J., Berliere, M. et al. (2010). Do intraoperative analgesics influence breast cancer recurrence after mastectomy? A retrospective analysis. *Anesth. Analg.* 110: 1630–1635.

330 Forget, P., Bentin, C., Machiels, J.P. et al. (2014). Intraoperative use of ketorolac or diclofenac is associated with improved disease-free survival and overall survival in conservative breast cancer surgery. *Br. J. Anaesth.* 113: 82–87.

331 Choi, J.E., Villarreal, J., Lasala, J. et al. (2015). Perioperative neutrophil: lymphocyte ratio and postoperative NSAID use as predictors of survival after lung cancer surgery: a retrospective study. *Cancer Med.* 4: 825–833.

332 Lee, B.M., Rodriguez, A., Mena, G. et al. (2016). Platelet-to-lymphocyte ratio and use of NSAIDs during the perioperative period as prognostic indicators in patients with NSCLC undergoing surgery. *Cancer Control* 23: 284–294.

333 Huang, W.-W., Zhu, W.-Z., Mu, D.-L. et al. (2018). Perioperative management may improve long-term survival in patients after lung cancer surgery: a retrospective cohort study. *Anesth. Analg.* 126: 1666–1674.

334 Midgley, R.S., McConkey, C.C., Johnstone, E.C. et al. (2010). Phase III randomized trial assessing rofecoxib in the adjuvant setting of colorectal cancer: final results of the VICTOR trial. *J. Clin. Oncol.* 28: 4575–4580.

335 Cata, J.P., Guerra, C.E., Chang, G.J. et al. (2017). Non-steroidal anti-inflammatory drugs in the oncological surgical population: beneficial or harmful? A systematic review of the literature. *Br. J. Anaesth.* 119: 750–764.

336 Kim, R. (2018). Effects of surgery and anesthetic choice on immunosuppression and cancer recurrence. *J. Transl. Med.* 16: 8.

337 Cata, J.P., Wang, H., Gottumukkala, V. et al. (2013). Inflammatory response, immunosuppression, and cancer recurrence after perioperative blood transfusions. *Br. J. Anaesth.* 110: 690–701.

338 Youssef, L.A. and Spitalnik, S.L. (2017). Transfusion-related immunomodulation: a reappraisal. *Curr. Opin. Hematol.* 24: 551–557.

339 Hod, E.A., Zhang, N., Sokol, S.A. et al. (2010). Transfusion of red blood cells after prolonged storage produces harmful effects that are mediated by iron and inflammation. *Blood* 115: 4284–4292.

340 Atzil, S., Arad, M., Glasner, A. et al. (2008). Blood transfusion promotes cancer progression: a critical role for aged erythrocytes. *Anesthesiology* 109: 989–997.

341 Cata, J.P., Lasala, J., Pratt, G. et al. (2016). Association between perioperative blood transfusions and clinical outcomes in patients undergoing bladder cancer surgery: a systematic review and meta-analysis study. *J. Blood Transfus.* 2016: 9876394.

342 Agnes, A., Lirosi, M.C., Panunzi, S. et al. (2018). The prognostic role of perioperative allogeneic blood transfusions in gastric cancer patients undergoing curative resection: a systematic review and meta-analysis of non-randomized, adjusted studies. *Eur. J. Surg. Oncol.* 44: 404–419.

343 Li, S.L., Ye, Y., and Yuan, X.H. (2017). Association between allogeneic or autologous blood transfusion and survival in patients after radical prostatectomy: a systematic review and meta-analysis. *PLoS One* 12: e0171081.

344 Justice, A. (1985). Review of the effects of stress on cancer in laboratory animals. Importance of time of stress application and type of tumor. *Psychol. Bull.* 98: 108–138.

345 Antoni, M.H., Lutgendorf, S.K., Cole, S.W. et al. (2006). The influence of bio-behavioural factors on tumour biology: pathways and mechanisms. *Nat. Rev. Cancer* 6: 240–248.

346 Vandewalle, B., Revillion, F., and Lefebvre, J. (1990). Functional β-adrenergic receptors in breast cancer cells. *J. Cancer Res. Clin. Oncol.* 116: 303–306.

347 Thaker, P.H., Han, L.Y., Kamat, A.A. et al. (2006). Chronic stress promotes tumor growth and angiogenesis in a mouse model of ovarian carcinoma. *Nat. Med.* 12: 939–944.

348 Weddle, D.L. (2001). Beta-adrenergic growth regulation of human cancer cell lines derived from pancreatic ductal carcinomas. *Carcinogenesis* 22: 473–479.

349 Rangarajan, S., Enserink, J.M., Kuiperij, H.B. et al. (2003). Cyclic AMP induces integrin-mediated cell adhesion through Epac and Rap1 upon stimulation of the β2-adrenergic receptor. *J. Cell Biol.* 160: 487–493.

350 Wang, F., Liu, H., Wang, F. et al. (2018). Propranolol suppresses the proliferation and induces the apoptosis of liver cancer cells. *Mol. Med. Rep.* 17: 5213–5221.

351 Glasner, A., Avraham, R., Rosenne, E. et al. (2010). Improving survival rates in two models of spontaneous postoperative metastasis in mice by combined administration of a β-adrenergic antagonist and a cyclooxygenase-2 inhibitor. *J. Immunol.* 184: 2449–2457.

352 Zhou, L., Li, Y., Li, X. et al. (2016). Propranolol attenuates surgical stress–induced elevation of the regulatory T cell response in patients undergoing radical mastectomy. *J. Immunol.* 196: 3460–3469.

353 Haldar, R., Shaashua, L., Lavon, H. et al. (2018). Perioperative inhibition of β-adrenergic and COX2 signaling in a clinical trial in breast cancer patients improves tumor Ki-67 expression, serum cytokine levels, and PBMCs transcriptome. *Brain Behav. Immun.* 73: 294–309.

354 Zhong, S., Yu, D., Zhang, X. et al. (2016). β-blocker use and mortality in cancer patients: systematic review and meta-analysis of observational studies. *Eur. J. Cancer Prev.* 25: 440–448.

355 Choi, C.H., Song, T., Kim, T.H. et al. (2014). Meta-analysis of the effects of beta blocker on survival time in cancer patients. *J. Cancer Res. Clin. Oncol.* 140: 1179–1188.

356 Yap, A., Lopez-Olivo, M.A., Dubowitz, J. et al. (2018). Effect of beta-blockers on cancer recurrence and survival: a meta-analysis of epidemiological and perioperative studies. *Br. J. Anaesth.* 121: 45–57.

357 Kunicka, J.E., Talle, M.A., Denhardt, G.H. et al. (1993). Immunosuppression by glucocorticoids: inhibition of production of multiple lymphokines by in vivo administration of dexamethasone. *Cell. Immunol.* 149: 39–49.

358 Merk, B.A., Havrilesky, L.J., Ehrisman, J.A. et al. (2016). Impact of postoperative nausea and vomiting prophylaxis with dexamethasone on the risk of recurrence of endometrial cancer. *Curr. Med. Res. Opin.* 32: 453–458.

359 Sandini, M., Ruscic, K.J., Ferrone, C.R. et al. (2018). Intraoperative dexamethasone decreases infectious complications after pancreaticoduodenectomy and is associated with long-term survival in pancreatic cancer. *Ann. Surg. Oncol.* 25: 4020–4026.

360 Yu, H.C., You, Y.X., Peng, H. et al. (2015). Avoiding perioperative dexamethasone may improve the outcome of patients with rectal cancer. *Eur. J. Surg. Oncol.* 41: 667–673.

361 Singh, P.P., Lemanu, D.P., Taylor, M.H.G. et al. (2014). Association between preoperative glucocorticoids and long-term survival and cancer recurrence after colectomy: follow-up analysis of a previous randomized controlled trial. *Br. J. Anaesth.* 113: i68–i73.

362 Forget, P., Berliere, M., van Maanen, A. et al. (2013). Perioperative ketorolac in high risk breast cancer patients. Rationale, feasibility and methodology of a prospective randomized placebo-controlled trial. *Med. Hypotheses* 81: 707–712.

363 Arends, J., Bachmann, P., Baracos, V. et al. (2017). ESPEN guidelines on nutrition in cancer patients. *Clin. Nutr.* 36: 11–48.

364 Gustafsson, U.O., Scott, M.J., Schwenk, W. et al. (2012). Guidelines for perioperative care in elective colonic surgery: enhanced recovery after surgery (ERAS®) society recommendations. *Clin. Nutr.* 31: 783–800.

365 Nowakowski, M., Pisarska, M., Rubinkiewicz, M. et al. (2018). Postoperative complications are associated with worse survival after laparoscopic surgery for non-metastatic colorectal cancer – interim analysis of 3-year overall survival. *Wideochir. Inne. Tech. Maloinwazyjne* 13: 326–332.

366 Kabata, P., Jastrzebski, T., Kakol, M. et al. (2015). Preoperative nutritional support in cancer patients with no clinical signs of malnutrition—prospective randomized controlled trial. *Support Care Cancer* 23: 365–370.

367 Fearon, K.C.H., Ljungqvist, O., Von Meyenfeldt, M. et al. (2005). Enhanced recovery after surgery: a consensus review of clinical care for patients undergoing colonic resection. *Clin. Nutr.* 24: 466–477.

368 Gustafsson, U.O. and Ljungqvist, O. (2011). Perioperative nutritional management in digestive tract surgery. *Curr. Opin. Clin. Nutr. Metab. Care* 14: 504–509.

369 Chen, C.-H., Chang, H., Huang, Y.-Z. et al. (2011). Hand-grip strength is a simple and effective outcome predictor in esophageal cancer following esophagectomy with reconstruction: a prospective study. *J. Cardiothorac. Surg.* 6: 98.

370 Moran, J., Wilson, F., Guinan, E. et al. (2016). Role of cardiopulmonary exercise testing as a risk-assessment method in patients undergoing intra-abdominal surgery: a systematic review. *Br. J. Anaesth.* 116: 177–191.

371 Caprara, G. (2021). Mediterranean-type dietary pattern and physical activity: the winning combination to counteract the rising burden of non-communicable diseases (NCDs). *Nutrients* 13: 1–37.

372 Moran, J., Guinan, E., McCormick, P. et al. (2016). The ability of prehabilitation to influence postoperative outcome after intra-abdominal operation: a systematic review and meta-analysis. *Surgery (United States)* 160: 1189–1201.

373 Findlay, J.M., Gillies, R.S., Millo, J. et al. (2014). Enhanced recovery for esophagectomy: a systematic review and evidence-based guidelines. *Ann. Surg.* 259: 413–431.

374 Lemanne, D., Cassileth, B., and Gubili, J. (2013). The role of physical activity in cancer prevention, treatment, recovery, and survivorship. *Oncology (Williston Park)* 27: 580–585.

375 Goldberg, K.J. (2019). Advances in palliative medicine. *Vet. Clin. North Am. Small Anim. Pract.* 49 (A1–6): 325–586.

376 Bishop, G.A., Long, C.C., Carlsten, K.S. et al. (2008). The Colorado State University Pet Hospices Program: end-of-life care for pets and their families. *J. Vet. Med. Educ.* 35: 525–531.

377 Gore, M., Lana, S.E., and Bishop, G.A. (2019). Colorado State University, Pet Hospice Program. *Vet. Clin. North Am. Small Anim. Pract.* 49: 339–349.

378 Yaxley, P.E. (2019). Michigan State University veterinary hospice care: an academic hospice practice 2011 to 2014. *Vet. Clin. North Am. Small Anim. Pract.* 49: 351–362.

379 Goldberg, K.J. (2019). Current topics in serious illness and palliative medicine: a curricular initiative in a US veterinary teaching institution. *Vet. Clin. North Am. Small Anim. Pract.* 49: 373–386.

380 American Veterinary Medical Association (AVMA). 2007. Guidelines for Veterinary Hospice Care. Available at: http://landofpuregold.com/cancer/the-pdfs/hospiceguidelines.pdf (accessed 2 February 2021).

381 Bishop, G., Cooney, K., Cox, S. et al. (2016). AAHA/IAAHPC end-of-life care guidelines. *J. Am. Anim. Hosp. Assoc.* 52: 341–356.

382 Moses, L. (2019). Pain and palliative care service, Massachusetts society for the prevention of cruelty to animals-Angell animal medical Center. *Vet. Clin. North Am. Small Anim. Pract.* 49: 363–371.

383 Yang, J., Wahner-Roedler, D.L., Zhou, X. et al. (2021). Acupuncture for palliative cancer pain management: systematic review. *BMJ Support. Palliat. Care* Jan 13: online ahead of print.

384 Wright, B.D. (2019). Acupuncture for the treatment of animal pain. *Vet. Clin. North Am. Small Anim. Pract.* 49: 1029–1039.

385 Millis, D.L. and Ciuperca, I.A. (2015). Evidence for canine rehabilitation and physical therapy. *Vet. Clin. North Am. Small Anim. Pract.* 45: 1–27.

386 Bradbrook, C. and Clark, L. (2018). State of the art analgesia—recent developments pharmacological approaches to acute pain management in dogs and cats. Part 2. *Vet. J.* 236: 62–67.

387 Bradbrook, C.A. and Clark, L. (2018). State of the art analgesia- recent developments in pharmacological approaches to acute pain management in dogs and cats. Part 1. *Vet. J.* 238: 76–82.

388 Boesch, J.M. (2019). Advances in pain management: palliative care applications. *Vet. Clin. North Am. Small Anim. Pract.* 49: 445–461.

389 Kosharskyy, B., Almonte, W., Shaparin, N. et al. (2013). Intravenous infusions in chronic pain management. *Pain Physician* 16: 231–249.

390 Kaye, A.D., Manchikanti, L., Abdi, S. et al. (2015). Efficacy of epidural injections in managing chronic spinal pain: a best evidence synthesis. *Pain Physician* 18: E939–E1004.

391 Waldman, S. (2014). *Atlas of Interventional Pain Management E-Book*, 4e. Kansas City: Elsevier.

392 Cohen, S.P., Bicket, M.C., Jamison, D. et al. (2013). Epidural steroids: a comprehensive, evidence-based review. *Reg. Anesth. Pain Med.* 38: 175–200.

393 Janssens, L., Beosier, Y., and Daems, R. (2009). Lumbosacral degenerative stenosis in the dog. The results of epidural infiltration with methylprednisolone acetate: a retrospective study. *Vet. Comp. Orthop. Traumatol.* 22: 486–491.

394 Radbruch, L., Trottenberg, P., Elsner, F. et al. (2011). Systematic review of the role of alternative application routes for opioid treatment for moderate to severe cancer pain: an EPCRC opioid guidelines project. *Palliat. Med.* 25: 578–596.

395 Herndon, C.M. and Fike, D.S. (2001). Continuous subcutaneous infusion practices of United States hospices. *J. Pain Symptom Manag.* 22: 1027–1034.

396 McAlindon, T.E., Bannuru, R.R., Sullivan, M.C. et al. (2014). OARSI guidelines for the non-surgical management of knee osteoarthritis. *Osteoarthr. Cartil.* 22: 363–388.

397 Frisbie, D.D., Kawkac, C.E., Trotter, G.W. et al. (1997). Effects of triamcinolone acetonide on an in vivo equine osteochondral fragment exercise model. *Equine Vet. J.* 29: 349–359.

398 Vandeweerd, J.-M., Zhao, Y., Nisolle, J.-F. et al. (2015). Effect of corticosteroids on articular cartilage: have animal studies said everything? *Fundam. Clin. Pharmacol.* 29: 427–438.

399 Wall, R. (2014). Introduction to myofascial trigger points in dogs. *Top. Companion Anim. Med.* 29: 43–48.

400 Janssens, L.A. (1991). Trigger points in 48 dogs with myofascial pain syndromes. *Vet. Surg.* 20: 274–278.

401 Cardoso, F.C., Hasan, M., Zhao, T. et al. (2018). Toxins in pain. *Curr. Opin. Support. Palliat. Care* 12: 132–141.

402 Brown, D.C. and Agnello, K. (2013). Intrathecal substance P-saporin in the dog: efficacy in bone cancer pain. *Anesthesiology* 119: 1178–1185.

403 Brown, D.C., Agnello, K., and Iadarola, M.J. (2015). Intrathecal resiniferatoxin in a dog model: efficacy in bone cancer pain. *Pain* 156: 1018–1024.

404 Choi, E.J., Choi, Y.M., Jang, E.J. et al. (2016). Neural ablation and regeneration in pain practice. *Korean J. Pain* 29: 3–11.

405 Ilfeld, B.M., Preciado, J., and Trescot, A.M. (2016). Novel cryoneurolysis device for the treatment of sensory and motor peripheral nerves. *Expert Rev. Med. Devices* 13: 713–725.

406 Cosman, E.R. and Cosman, E.R. (2005). Electric and thermal field effects in tissue around radiofrequency electrodes. *Pain Med.* 6: 405–424.

407 Ball, R.D. (2014). The science of conventional and water-cooled monopolar lumbar radiofrequency rhizotomy: an electrical engineering point of view. *Pain Physician* 17: E175–E211.

408 Govind, J., King, W., Bailey, B. et al. (2003). Radiofrequency neurotomy for the treatment of third occipital headache. *J. Neurol. Neurosurg. Psychiatry* 74: 88–93.

409 Melzack, R. and Wall, P.D. (1994). Pain mechanisms: a new theory. *Pain Clin.* 7: 57–72.

410 Wiinger, B. (2006). Prospective pilot study on performance and prognostic value of a new human, ISTH based scoring system for identifying non-overt disseminated intravascular coagulation in dogs. *ACVIM Abstract 203. J Vet Intern Med* 20: 697–802.

411 Villalobos, A. (2007). Canine and feline and geriatric oncology. In: *Honoring the Human-Animal Bond* (eds. A. Villalobos and L. Kaplan). Ames: Blackwell Publishing.

18

Cesarean Section and Pregnancy

Turi K. Aarnes[1] *and Melissa A. Murdock*[2]

[1] *Department of Veterinary Clinical Sciences, College of Veterinary Medicine, The Ohio State University, Columbus, OH, 43210, USA*
[2] *BluePearl Specialty and Emergency Pet Hospital, Levittown, PA, 19056, USA*

Introduction

Anesthetic drug selection, delivery, and monitoring techniques for pregnant dogs and cats are similar to those used for the nonpregnant animal. It is, however, critically important to account for changes in maternal physiology and concerns for fetal viability, which often influences drug selection, delivery, and anesthetic monitoring. When planning for cesarean-section anesthesia, provisions should be made for neonatal resuscitation and postdelivery care. The emergent nature of many cesarean sections often results in limited availability of trained and knowledgeable staff. Puppy mortality is approximately two-thirds greater during emergent than during planned cesarean sections [1]. Maternal mortality is also significantly greater in emergent versus planned cesareans [2]. For this reason, anesthesia and delivery must be well planned before anesthetic induction. Oxygen, clean absorbent towels, a suction apparatus, and resuscitation and antagonist drugs should be available and organized before surgery.

Maternal Physiology

Pregnancy creates major maternal physiologic and anatomic adaptations associated with the increased metabolic demand imposed by the growing fetal and uterine mass [3]. Many or most of these adaptations impact periparturient anesthetic management, particularly those management aspects related to cardiorespiratory, gastrointestinal (GI), and hematological systems (Table 18.1).

Cardiorespiratory System

During pregnancy, oxygen consumption increases to meet the increased metabolic demand associated with the growing fetus(es). Changes to account for this increased demand begin to occur early during pregnancy and peak during the last trimester. Cardiovascular function returns to prepartum values within 4–12 weeks postpartum in women [4]. Cardiac output increases 30–40% and gravid uterine blood flow is 20–40 times greater than nonpregnant flow [3]. Blood flow to the mammary glands and skin also increases. The increased

Canine and Feline Anesthesia and Co-Existing Disease, Second Edition. Edited by Rebecca A. Johnson, Lindsey B. C. Snyder and Carrie A. Schroeder.

Companion website: www.wiley.com/go/johnson/canine

Table 18.1 Maternal physiology changes associated with pregnancy (see text for details).

Cardiovascular changes
Increased oxygen consumption
Increased cardiac output
Decreased vascular tone
Decreased arterial blood pressure
Increased stroke volume
Increased heart rate
Increased blood volume
Increased red blood cell mass
Decreased packed cell volume
Respiratory changes
Increased tidal volume
Increased respiratory rate
Increased minute ventilation
Decreased functional residual capacity
Gastrointestinal changes
Increased intragastric pressure
Decreased lower esophageal sphincter pressure
Decreased GI motility
Increased gastrin production
Central nervous system changes
Increased endorphins

cardiac output is associated with a decrease in vascular tone and arterial blood pressure (approximately 10%) and an increased heart rate (approximately 55%) and stroke volume [3]. Blood volume increases up to 35% in women [3] and 23% in dogs [5]. Accompanying this increased blood volume is an increase in red cell mass. However, plasma volume increases relatively more than red cell mass, resulting in a pregnancy-associated anemia. The magnitude of this anemia correlates with increasing fetal numbers [6]. Blood loss during normal parturition is buffered by this increased blood volume and red cell mass. Pregnancy-associated anemia will influence the use of packed cell volume as an index of dehydration.

Uterine and placental blood flow is not autoregulated (maintained constant over a wide range of perfusion pressure); therefore, anything that inhibits uterine arterial flow will result in decreased fetal oxygen and nutrient delivery. This includes anesthetic drug- and hemorrhage-induced hypotension. Anything causing vasoconstriction can also result in decreased uterine perfusion, including vasoactive drugs (i.e., alpha-2-adrenergic receptor agonists, norepinephrine, etc.), excitement-induced or iatrogenic hyperventilation leading to respiratory alkalosis, and sympathetic stimulation such as pain.

In supine women, uterine blood flow is compromised because of accompanying aortocaval compression. This can lead to a decrease in venous return and cardiac output with a potential for reduced fetal oxygenation. This condition may be treated with a lateral tilt position, placing a wedge or towels under the right hip to alleviate aortocaval compression by the gravid uterus. Canine studies indicate that dorsal recumbency is not associated with a decrease in systemic blood pressure or altered arterial blood gas values [7]. These studies did not, however, investigate changes in uterine blood flow. In pentobarbital-thiamylal-anesthetized pregnant dogs, ligation of the inferior vena cava caudal to the renal veins did not result in diminished venous return with radiographic evidence of ample collateral venous return [8]. Thus, dorsal recumbency during anesthesia does not result in hypotension in the hemodynamically normal pregnant dog. While research suggests that pregnant dogs do not experience significant hemodynamic effects of uterine aortocaval compression, it is important to closely monitor the cardiovascular status of the pregnant patient and note any changes or indicators of hemodynamic instability when placed in dorsal recumbency.

Vasopressor and chronotropic drugs are less effective in the parturient, possibly related to a downregulation of alpha- and beta-adrenergic receptors and possibly increased vasodilatory prostaglandins [3]. For this reason, parturients with dehydration or cardiovascular compromise should receive appropriate fluid therapy before anesthetic induction because anesthetic drugs are typically associated with varying degrees of cardiovascular depression. Blood pressure should be monitored, and hypotension treated with crystalloids or colloids. Hemorrhage decreases arterial blood pressure in pregnant dogs relatively more than in nonpregnant dogs [5]. Therefore, hemorrhage and dehydration should be aggressively treated before anesthesia. Ephedrine improves blood pressure in pregnant ewes without decreasing uterine blood flow, while dopamine and dobutamine effectively improve maternal blood pressure but decrease uterine blood flow in nonanesthetized pregnant ewes [9]. The decrease in uterine blood flow is dose-dependent and relatively greater for dopamine than dobutamine. Consequently, ephedrine is commonly used in parturient hypotensive women. Ephedrine can be used in dogs and cats as a bolus of 0.03–0.1 mg kg^{-1} intravenous (IV) and dobutamine at 2–4 μg kg^{-1} min^{-1} IV.

Tidal volume, respiratory rate, and minute ventilation increase by approximately 70% in women at term [3], despite the enlarged abdomen and anterior movement of the diaphragm. However, functional residual capacity (FRC) decreases, leading to decreased oxygen reserve within the lung. The decreased FRC and the increased oxygen consumption associated with pregnancy mean that long periods of apnea can more readily result in hypoxemia and hemoglobin desaturation. Because of this, preoxygenation before anesthetic induction is advisable, and apnea should be aggressively avoided during anesthesia. Progesterone-induced maternal hyperventilation results in mild respiratory alkalosis [10] and an accompanying mild increase in PaO_2.

Gastrointestinal System

The enlarged uterus increases intragastric pressure. Increased circulating progesterone decreases lower esophageal sphincter pressure and GI motility. The increased intragastric pressure and the decreased GI motility result in a greater risk for regurgitation and aspiration during anesthesia. Concentrations of the peptide hormone gastrin, which stimulates production of stomach acid, increase in pregnant dogs during anesthesia [11]. The decreased gastric pH and regurgitation can result in a greater incidence of aspiration pneumonia and possibly esophageal inflammation. Rapid intubation with a cuffed endotracheal tube will help prevent aspiration of stomach contents. It is currently not known if a preoperative proton-pump inhibitor or histamine H2-receptor antagonists will lessen these risks.

Central Nervous System (CNS)

Serum progesterone increases during pregnancy. This and possibly a pregnancy-associated endorphin increase are thought to be responsible for a 16–40% decrease in minimum alveolar concentration (MAC) of inhalants [12]. This decreased requirement may not be noticed during cesarean-section anesthesia, as preanesthetic tranquilizers and sedatives that reduce MAC are often limited or not used. Inhalational anesthetics depress fetal blood pressure and minute ventilation. Therefore, high inhalant concentrations should be avoided, and local anesthetic techniques and epidurals should be considered to reduce inhalant anesthetic requirement and fetal cardiopulmonary depression.

Placental Drug Transfer

Little is known regarding the extent of drug passage across the placenta of dogs and cats. Most information is extrapolated from laboratory animal studies [13]. Because of species differences in placentation, extrapolation of placental drug transfer in dogs and cats from other species can be misleading. The placenta has some ability to metabolize drugs and also some carrier proteins on the maternal and fetal sides of the placenta are capable of transferring drugs across the placenta. The extent of such placental metabolism and transport is unknown for dogs and cats. The safest approach is to assume that most drugs cross the placenta and affect the developing fetus(es). The developing fetus(es) are most vulnerable to teratogenic drug effects during the first trimester—the first 20 days of gestation in dogs and cats. Therefore, elective surgical or medical procedures requiring anesthesia should be avoided during these first 20 days of gestation.

A fundamental principle of cesarean-section anesthesia is to minimize fetal concentrations of anesthetic drugs with respiratory, cardiovascular, and CNS depressant properties. In addition, drugs that can be antagonized, such as opioids, are advantageous because their effects can be reversed using naloxone in puppies or kittens after delivery. Little is known concerning placental transfer of anesthetic drugs in dogs and cats and the respective maternal/fetal plasma concentration ratios. Studies on sheep confirm that medetomidine, propofol, ketamine, and etomidate rapidly cross the placenta to develop high fetal concentrations. Conversely, the placental barrier may be effective in decreasing fetal exposure to dexmedetomidine administered to the dam during elective cesarean sections [14]. No detectable dexmedetomidine was present in the amniotic fluid, while a detectable amount was found in the placentas. A majority of puppies were considered vigorous at birth, and no puppy required antagonism of the dexmedetomidine at birth or at hospital discharge [14].

Anesthetic drugs cross the placenta by simple diffusion according to Fick's equation of diffusion (Eq. 18.1): [15]

$$\frac{\Delta q}{\Delta t}=\frac{KA\left(C_2-C_1\right)}{d} \qquad (18.1)$$

where $\Delta q/\Delta t$ represents the rate of drug transfer, and K is a diffusion constant that relates to drug molecular weight, pK_a, lipid solubility, degree of ionization, and protein binding. A is the surface area for diffusion, $C_2 - C_1$ is the drug concentration difference across the placenta, and d is the membrane thickness. Properties favoring rapid placental drug transfer include drugs with a molecular weight <600 Da which are nonionized, highly lipid-soluble, and minimally protein-bound. Most anesthetic drugs have molecular weights <300 Da and are relatively lipid soluble. This, coupled with the relatively large placental surface area, means that most anesthetic drugs readily cross the placenta. Exceptions are glycopyrrolate, a relatively large polar molecule, and neuromuscular blocking drugs.

The relatively more acidic fetal blood favors ionic trapping within the fetus of weakly basic drugs when drug pK_a is close to plasma pH (local anesthetics, ketamine, and opioids), possibly prolonging their action in the fetus. Acidic drugs whose pK_a is close to plasma pH (thiobarbiturates) more readily transfer from fetal to maternal plasma.

The ultrashort-acting drugs propofol and etomidate are extremely lipid-soluble and almost completely nonionized at plasma pH. Propofol, a weak acid with pK_a = 11, rapidly and readily crosses the placenta in women achieving an umbilical vein/maternal vein ratio of 0.7–0.85 at fetal delivery [16]. The transfer of propofol in sheep is not as complete, and the fetal elimination half-life is longer than the maternal half-life in this species. This might relate to the thicker barrier for diffusion of the ovine placenta compared to that in women [17]. Regardless, propofol's relatively rapid clearance from maternal and fetal plasma makes it a suitable anesthetic induction drug. Etomidate, a weak base with a pK_a = 4.2, achieves an umbilical vein/maternal vein plasma ratio of between 1:2 and 1:24 (0.5 and 0.04, respectively) in women [18]. In sheep, the transfer is not as complete, but relatively high fetal concentrations do occur [19].

The effect of dexmedetomidine and propofol for induction on puppy survival, Apgar scores, maternal plasma drug concentrations, as well as placental and amniotic fluid drug concentrations has been evaluated. Both 2.0 $\mu g\, kg^{-1}$ of dexmedetomidine and 2.5 $mg\, kg^{-1}$ of propofol were found to have higher concentrations in the placenta than the dam's blood, and neither drug was detectable in the amniotic fluid. Placental drug concentrations were not correlated to placental weights. The birth weight of puppies increased with increasing placental weights, which also correlated to better Apgar scores. Dexmedetomidine may be an acceptable option in healthy bitches undergoing elective cesarean section that require additional premedication/sedation. None of the puppies in this study required reversal of the dexmedetomidine with atipamezole [14].

Fetal hemodynamic changes associated with alfaxalone administration were evaluated in pregnant ewes and were compared to propofol and etomidate. Propofol induction had no effect on fetal heart rate; use of alfaxalone increased fetal heart rate, while etomidate lowered it. No difference was found between baseline values and after administration of clinically acceptable induction drug doses in blood flow, velocities, and volumes to the umbilical arteries [20].

Inhalation anesthetics are highly lipid-soluble and readily cross the placenta. Despite achieving concentrations associated with anesthesia in the fetus(es), isoflurane, sevoflurane, and desflurane have relatively low blood:gas partition coefficients and are rapidly cleared by the newly delivered neonate if they are breathing at delivery. Excessive inhalant concentrations should be avoided to prevent neonatal apnea. Women undergoing cesarean section demonstrate no difference in neonatal viability between isoflurane, sevoflurane, and desflurane, and no difference was detected in neonatal viability in women receiving sevoflurane compared to those receiving a spinal anesthetic [21, 22]. In these studies, nitrous oxide was administered to minimize the inhalant anesthetic concentrations. Methoxyflurane was the only inhalant anesthetic associated with increased canine neonatal death in a survey of anesthesia for canine cesarean section and should be avoided for cesarean section [1]. Isoflurane was associated positively with puppy survival at 7 days after delivery. However, neonatal mortality was no different in puppies delivered during propofol/isoflurane anesthesia or epidural [23]. Sevoflurane or desflurane, because of relatively low blood: gas solubilities, are useful for cesarean-section anesthesia [21, 22, 24].

Opioid and Nonsteroidal Anti-Inflammatory Drug Effects on Maternal and Fetal Physiology

Opioids

Opioids include a variety of natural and synthetic products that produce analgesic effects because of their combination with distinct opioid receptors. The most potent opioid analgesics activate mu-opioid receptors and include morphine, hydromorphone, oxymorphone, fentanyl, methadone, and meperidine. Buprenorphine is classified as a partial mu-opioid receptor agonist. Butorphanol is a kappa-opioid receptor agonist and mu-opioid receptor antagonist.

Maternal opioid administration will result in placental transfer of these drugs to the fetus according to the previously discussed Fick's equation of diffusion (Equation 18.1). The extent of this transfer differs among opioids [25]. Placental transfer of buprenorphine tends to be low (<10% of placental buprenorphine reaches the fetus), while that of the highly lipid-soluble fentanyl is quite high, and fentanyl persists in the fetus long after clearing the maternal circulation [25–27].

Significant differences in the sensitivity to opioid-induced analgesia are observed in animals during maturation compared to adults. The source of these differences is unknown. CNS maturity and the blood–brain barrier, end-organ sensitivity to opioids, and solubility of different opioids have been postulated as the causes of the differences between age-related effects of mu-opioid receptor agonists [28]. Studies have also indicated differences in side effects from adult patients, although these differences are seemingly related to those in drug metabolism and physiology between animals of different ages. The most notable example of these differences is the development of respiratory depression. Respiratory depression, although a concern in adults, is a much more important issue in neonates because even a small change in tidal volume or respiratory rate in a neonate can result in life-threatening hypoxia. While in utero, the fetal lungs are mostly nonfunctional, and the fetus is dependent on maternal circulation for normoxia and normocarbia. However, after cesarean section, the newborn becomes dependent on its own respiratory system for gas exchange and exhaling the inhalant anesthetic; opioid-induced respiratory depression may lead to increased neonatal mortality [29].

Nonsteroidal Anti-Inflammatory Drugs (NSAIDs)

Nonsteroidal anti-inflammatory drugs inhibit inflammation and produce analgesia by decreasing prostaglandin synthesis through inhibition of cyclooxygenase (COX) and, in some cases, 5-lipoxygenase (LOX) enzymes [30]. Prostaglandins cause vasodilation, increase vascular permeability, and sensitize pain receptors to noxious stimuli. In addition, they are responsible for regulating renal blood flow, protecting GI mucosa, and aiding platelet aggregation. COX has two clinically relevant isoforms: COX-1 and COX-2. Both are constitutively expressed in select tissues, although COX-2 is upregulated in the inflammatory cascade. Differences between NSAID effects, efficacy, and toxicity are related to COX enzymes and the inhibitory effects on preexisting COX activities in the patient. LOX products (leukotriene B, leukotriene C, and leukotriene D) are responsible for recruitment of immune mediators and alteration of vascular permeability [30].

NSAIDs have minimal effects on normal cardiovascular and respiratory systems. Side effects are typically the result of COX-1 inhibition, are dose-related, and typically include GI ulceration, renal papillary necrosis, and inhibition of platelet aggregation [30].

NSAIDs should be used with caution in pregnant and young animals because of their reduced clearance and immaturity of biotransformation pathways. Fetal exposure to NSAIDs could result in significantly prolonged clearance, and prolonged and adverse effects. These drugs could impact the development of organ maturation or cause significant damage to young organs [31].

Cimicoxib, a COX-2 selective NSAID, remained below the detectable limit in plasma of most suckling puppies sampled after the dams had received one oral dose. This low level of transfer to the puppies occurred despite high concentrations of the cimicoxib detected in the milk [32]. The low level of transfer of cimicoxib in milk makes it a viable option for postoperative analgesia in the dam once the puppies have been surgically removed.

Patient Management for Cesarean Section

Preoperative Considerations

Preanesthetic evaluation should include a thorough physical examination and blood work evaluation (packed cell volume and total protein in healthy animals). A complete blood cell count and biochemistry panel may be helpful to evaluate overall health and determine calcium and blood glucose levels in animals that have been in active labor [33]. In addition, animals undergoing sedation and/or general anesthesia should be held off food for planned cesarean sections. Pregnant animals have an increased risk of regurgitation and aspiration due to decreased lower esophageal sphincter tone and prolonged gastric-emptying time [34, 35]. An IV catheter should be placed to provide IV access for the administration of anesthetic agents, access in the case of emergency, and for IV fluid administration.

Pregnant animals should be preoxygenated when possible (Figure 18.1) [36]. Preoxygenation for 3 min increases the time to desaturation in healthy dogs in which propofol was administered for anesthetic induction [37]. Placental oxygen delivery is an important factor influencing fetal mortality [35]. Some animals may be resistant to the placement of a face mask; therefore, preoxygenation may not be possible. In either case, it is important to intubate pregnant animals as soon as possible after anesthetic induction.

Most cesarean sections in dogs and cats are performed on unpremedicated animals because all commonly used anesthetic drugs will cross the placenta [38]. Sedatives and tranquilizers have cardiovascular and respiratory side effects for the dam and fetus that can result in increased fetal mortality. For quiet and relatively calm parturient dogs and cats, preanesthetic sedation can be avoided to minimize cardiorespiratory depression in the newborn. If it is possible to place an IV catheter without sedation, it would be preferable to do so. However, excitable and nervous animals

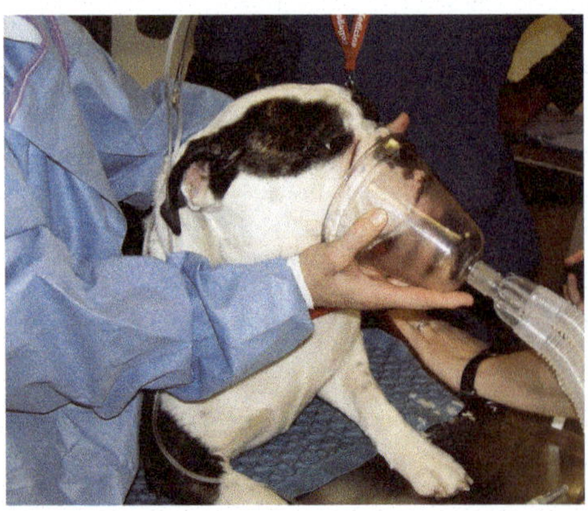

Figure 18.1 Preoxygenation of pregnant animals prior to anesthetic induction when possible may decrease the risk of hemoglobin desaturation if apnea is experienced.

will benefit from preanesthetic sedation. This may provide a smoother anesthetic induction and a decreased need for induction agent and inhalant anesthetic concentrations. Fetal exposure to relatively high inhalant anesthetic concentrations results in excessive neonate respiratory depression immediately after delivery. If a preanesthetic sedative or tranquilizer is required, it is important to carefully consider the effects on the mother and the fetus(es). Xylazine administration is associated with fetal death, but this may have been impacted by the concurrent administration of ketamine. Ketamine, xylazine, and the combination of ketamine and xylazine should be administered with caution or avoided when possible [1]. Acepromazine is highly protein-bound, and its molecular weight is relatively high compared to other sedatives. For this reason, it crosses the placenta more slowly than other anesthetic drugs. Acepromazine is not associated with increased maternal or neonatal mortality [2]. However, because it causes vasodilation, it should not be used in dehydrated parturients or those in shock. Chlorpromazine, an agent similar to acepromazine, premedication before various anesthetic combinations has an overall puppy mortality of <4% [39]. This is less than that reported in a study of overall puppy mortality [1]. The use of a low dose of dexmedetomidine before propofol for elective cesarean sections resulted in undetectable levels of the dexmedetomidine in amniotic fluid [14]. No puppy born during the study required reversal of alpha-2 agonist with atipamezole, and 77.8% of the puppies were “vigorous” at birth [14].

Opioids may be given with caution for cesarean sections. While intraoperative respiratory depression in the mother can be monitored and controlled, respiratory depression in the fetus(es) induced by opioid administration may be significant. Morphine is relatively poorly lipid-soluble and only 20–30% unionized at plasma pH. Therefore, it crosses the placenta less rapidly than the more lipid-soluble opioids such as fentanyl. Hydromorphone's lipid solubility is between that of morphine and fentanyl. Opioid respiratory depression in recently delivered neonates can be reversed using a drop of the opioid receptor antagonist naloxone sublingually.

Anesthetic Induction and Intraoperative Management

Local and regional anesthetic techniques such as subarachnoid (spinal) and epidural injections of opioids and local anesthetics as a sole anesthetic technique are commonly used for cesarean section in humans; their use is much less common in small animal veterinary practice. A textbook on regional anesthesia and analgesia is a good source to review anatomic landmarks, drug doses, and procedural steps of performing an epidural [40]. A smaller volume of local anesthetic is required for epidural administration during pregnancy due to the increased size of the epidural veins [33]. Lidocaine, for instance, may be administered at 2–3 mg kg^{-1} epidurally with no greater than 6 ml total volume in any dog [33]. Lidocaine is most often used for epidurals for cesarean section due to its short onset and short duration. Local anesthetic administration in the epidural space can result in systemic hypotension due to vasodilation [33], and sensory and motor blockade may also spread cranially, resulting in respiratory and cardiovascular depression. In cats, local anesthetic administration may result in increased severity of the previously listed effects due to cats' inherently lowered tolerance and the increased toxic effects of this drug in felines [41].

The advantage of epidural and spinal techniques is that there is minimal fetal effect. The respiratory rate of newborn puppies was significantly higher after epidural anesthesia in the dam compared to dams that were induced with midazolam/ketamine or propofol and maintained on enflurane [39]. Puppies from bitches that had received local anesthetic epidurals required less resuscitation than the puppies from bitches without epidurals. Without epidurals, bitches received higher inhalant doses, more rescue fentanyl doses, and more propofol boluses, all possibly contributing to neonatal depression [24]. While systemic local anesthetics can cross the blood–placental barrier and become ionized and trapped within the fetus, lidocaine epidurals have local effects. Systemic absorption occurs over time and should not reach the placenta before fetus removal. Local anesthetic techniques require the anesthetist to be comfortable with the technique. Patients who have received an epidural are usually conscious during the surgical procedure; if the technique was faulty or there was uneven spread of local anesthetic within the epidural space, the patient may feel the surgical stimulation. In addition, while the patient's caudal portion experiences motor and sensory blockade, the cranial portion does not, and the patient may move or vocalize during the procedure. The airway is also not protected, and the patient is in dorsal recumbency. Finally, the effects of the local anesthetic require time to wear off [23]. Dams that had received an epidural with lidocaine took 15–20 min longer to stand after recovery compared to those without an epidural [24]. Hospital-acquired infection of the newborns is possible, and, in most cases, it is preferable to send patients home as quickly as possible. Animals that have received spinals or epidurals should be monitored until motor function has returned, so their postoperative time in the hospital tend to be longer than with cesarean sections performed under general anesthesia.

Intravenous induction agents are preferable to inhalant anesthetic inductions. A relatively rapid induction with IV induction agent administration allows for a more controlled induction with less struggling and greater control of the patient's airway. Propofol is the drug of choice for anesthetic induction in cesarean section. Propofol has a short half-life, rapid hepatic and extrahepatic metabolism, and manageable respiratory and cardiovascular side effects [23]. Fetal mortality has been demonstrated to be equivalent with propofol as with mask induction using isoflurane and without the rough induction characteristics associated with inhalant anesthetic inductions [1, 42]. In addition, the concentration of inhalant in dams that have experienced a mask induction is significantly higher than that of dams that were anesthetized using propofol for anesthetic induction. Anesthetic induction using ketamine decreases puppy vigor, and thiobarbiturates increase the risk of no spontaneous puppy movement at birth [23, 42].

Alfaxalone is a neuroactive steroid IV anesthetic induction agent classified as a hypnotic. The clinical effects of alfaxalone are similar to those of propofol, and include a smooth induction, rapid redistribution and recovery, and dose-dependent respiratory and cardiovascular depression [43]. At doses of $2\,mg\,kg^{-1}$ IV, the changes in blood pressure and heart rate are well-tolerated in healthy nonparturient patients [43]. A $2\,mg\,kg^{-1}$ IV bolus results in a plasma half-life of 24 ± 1.9 min [44], but pharmacokinetics may be altered in pregnant patients due to the cardiovascular changes described in Table 18.1.

In nonparturient dogs, there was no clinically relevant difference between propofol and alfaxalone for general anesthesia induction [45]; cats reported similar findings. Cats receiving either propofol or alfaxalone experienced similar decreases in respiratory rate and diastolic blood pressure that were well-tolerated and there was no significant difference in recovery quality between propofol or alfaxalone [46]. Unfavorable recovery characteristics with alfaxalone such as paddling, vocalization, and hypersensitivity are reported [44, 45].

Puppy survival (up to 3 months) was similar between propofol and alfaxalone when administered for anesthetic induction for elective cesarean section, though Apgar scores within the first 60 min after birth were slightly better in puppies from bitches that received alfaxalone at induction. Maternal recovery time and quality were similar [47]. Alfaxalone is a suitable induction agent in pregnant bitches for cesarean section, with >95% of puppies that were born alive still alive at 24 h [48].

In addition to being an effective and safe option for IV anesthetic induction, intramuscular (IM) alfaxalone administration is well documented in nonparturient cats and dogs [49–51]. This administration route could be a good option for aggressive dams where IV access is not possible before induction. Careful monitoring is required after IM sedation with alfaxalone, as the airway is unprotected, thus increasing the risk of aspiration prior to intubation. Sedative and opioid combinations will lengthen sedation time and improve sedation quality [52], keeping in mind placental transfer of drugs that may affect overall survival and mortality. The use of IM alfaxalone has not been described in pregnant dogs or cats and the effect on neonatal health and recovery when used IM is unknown. As previously discussed, alfaxalone administered IV for anesthetic induction in cesarean section resulted in similar or slightly better Apgar scores in the first 60 min, compared to propofol [47].

Before intubation, care should be taken to position animals in sternal recumbency with their head above their abdomen. All pregnant animals undergoing general anesthesia should be intubated to protect their airway. If regurgitation occurs, the poll of the head should be positioned as the highest point to protect the airway and encourage drainage out of the mouth. In the event of regurgitation, suction may be used to remove gastric contents from the back of the mouth.

Anesthetic maintenance with isoflurane has been associated with increased puppy survival compared to methoxyflurane [1]. The primary elimination route of modern inhalant anesthetics is through ventilation; it is important to note that inhalant anesthetics cause a dose-dependent respiratory depression. It is recommended to maintain as light a plane of anesthesia as possible to minimize inhalant delivery across the placenta and encourage neonatal ventilation [42, 53].

Propofol and alfaxalone can be used for anesthetic maintenance during cesarean sections [24, 54]. Propofol constant rate infusion (CRI) caused higher mortality and lower Apgar scores due to prolonged sedation and recovery in both the dam and puppies [55]. Propofol administered as multiple boluses rather than a CRI, with and without a lidocaine epidural, was compared to sevoflurane for maintenance [24]. While neonatal mortality at birth, 12 and 24 h, was not different between groups, puppies in the epidural group required less resuscitation at birth. Also, the dam required less "rescue analgesia," fewer propofol boluses, and had lower inhalant requirements after the puppies were removed [24]. Isoflurane administration resulted in lower arterial blood pressures, but higher Apgar scores in puppies compared with alfaxalone. Overall, survival and mortality were similar between isoflurane and alfaxalone for anesthetic maintenance [54].

Local anesthetic infiltration along the incision line may be helpful to reduce inhalant concentrations and minimize systemic effects of inhalants (Figure 18.2) [33]. Bupivacaine or ropivacaine, long-acting local anesthetic drugs, can be used for this purpose. Some patients will even allow the anesthetist to perform this line block before general anesthesia induction. However, the efficacy of line blocks for analgesia in nonpregnant dogs has been questioned. There was no difference in postoperative pain using three different pain scales or pain thresholds using algometry compared between a line block with lidocaine and bupivacaine and the negative control, which received saline in the line block instead of local anesthetic [56]. Failure to find significant differences in this study may have been due to study design, difficulty in assessing pain in animals, or assessment methods not sensitive or specific enough to detect small differences. However, if a line block is the only opportunity to provide incisional analgesia, there is minimal risk and potential benefit to the patient.

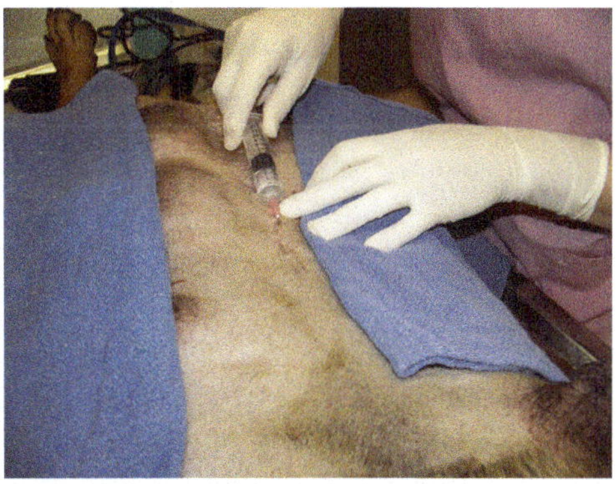

Figure 18.2 Example of a line block preoperatively with a local anesthetic to provide analgesia to the surgical incision site. It is important to aspirate with every repositioning of the needle to avoid intravascular injection of local anesthetic.

Another local anesthetic option is to use fascial plane blocks, such as the transversus abdominis plane (TAP) block. Guided by ultrasound, local anesthetic deposition within the fascial plane between the internal abdominal oblique and transversus abdominis muscles should desensitize abdominal muscles, subcutaneous tissues, mammary glands, skin, and the parietal peritoneum [57]. Anatomical dissection of the nerves contained in this fascial plane in the dog showed consistent involvement of nerves from T10–T12 spinal nerves, and variable presence of nerves from T7–T9. Blockade of lumbar nerves (L1–L3) has been reported in the TAP block as well. Based on the variable coverage of nerves by the TAP block, the efficacy of this block may vary greatly between patients [57]. Fascial plane blocks such as the TAP block in dogs could reduce systemic analgesics such as NSAIDs and opioids and should be considered for abdominal pain and incisional pain [58].

Utilizing the traditional approach for the TAP block, the patient is placed in lateral recumbency and a linear ultrasound probe placed transversely halfway from caudal to the last rib to the iliac crest, approximately 5 cm lateral from ventral midline [59]. Using ultrasound guidance, a spinal or Tuohy needle is used to pierce the external and internal oblique muscles until the fascial plane overlying the transversus abdominis muscle is reached. A successful test injection of saline or local anesthetic will show separation of the internal oblique muscle and transversus abdominis muscle, confirming the correct placement between layers, rather than within the muscle [59]. In some dogs, additional fascial sheets may make results of this block variable [57]. Introduction of the spinal needle can be from the lateral flank pointing toward midline, or from the medial aspect [60]. Keeping in mind the developed mammary tissue, the lateral flank approach is probably the most appropriate for cesarean sections. A newly described approach to blocking the abdominal wall is the rectus sheath block [61], which may avoid the developed mammary tissue. This cadaveric anatomical study was performed in nonparturient dogs and application of the rectus sheath block as well as the TAP block should be tailored to each patient.

Cardiovascular and respiratory parameters of the dam should be monitored during general anesthesia, consisting of heart rate, blood pressure, and hemoglobin saturation [38]. These parameters are important as indirect uteroplacental perfusion indices. Uterine and placental perfusion is pressure-dependent, relying on the arterial–venous uterine blood pressure difference and is inversely proportional to uterine vascular resistance. It is also important to note that there is no fetal autoregulation of blood pressure. Fetal blood flow is entirely dependent on maternal cardiac output. Ventilation should be monitored using capnometry to ensure appropriate ventilation. Hyperventilation and hypoventilation, easily measured by end-tidal CO_2, can directly and indirectly result in vasoconstriction which may decrease blood flow to the uterus [62]. This decreased uterine blood flow decreases fetal oxygen delivery, potentially resulting in fetal hypoxia and increased fetal mortality [63]. Performing a physiologic sigh (a controlled breath given by squeezing the rebreathing bag to a pressure of 15–20 cm H_2O) may enhance surfactant flow, which results in decreased atelectasis and increased blood oxygenation [36].

Animal positioning during cesarean section requires dorsal recumbency. The canine and feline uterine anatomy is such that aortocaval compression syndrome is less of an issue in dogs and cats than in humans; fetuses generally lie lateral to the caudal vena cava and abdominal aorta. Smaller dogs, between 9 and 25 kg, are not likely to develop aortocaval compression syndrome. However, in large-breed dogs, this may become a source of decreased blood flow to the uterus and hindlimbs [7, 64].

Fluid administration may be helpful to reduce dehydration in patients who have been in labor and held off food before planned cesarean section or to replace fluids lost during surgery due to evaporation or blood loss. In addition, fluid administration may help to maintain a patent IV catheter and can be used to flush in systemic drugs during an emergency. However, only approximately 53% of patients undergoing cesarean section received fluids in a study of perioperative management and mortality rates [2].

Postoperative Pain Management

Patient pain management undergoing cesarean section is controversial. Pain tolerance in pregnant patients is increased and there is a decreased anesthetic requirement in pregnant patients. Increased pain tolerance causes include increased pregnanolone (which has sedative effects) or increased endogenous endorphins [35]. Typical pain signs in these patients include lack of appetite, not allowing nursing, immobility, difficulty rising, and vocalization during activity. Local anesthetic infiltrative line blocks can be helpful in the immediate postoperative period, but the duration of action of ropivacaine is only around 4 h. Many veterinarians administer a dose of opioids to these patients IV or IM once the puppies have been surgically removed. Buprenorphine is often used for this purpose because it has a long duration of action and has minimal cardiovascular and respiratory side effects in the dam. However, milk transfer has not been evaluated for any of the opioids in lactating bitches or queens. NSAIDs are also controversial. The use of NSAIDs in pregnant dogs and cats has not been evaluated, and most available NSAIDs have not been evaluated in puppies younger than 4–6 weeks of age [31]. Milk transfer of these drugs is also possible, although unlikely [25].

Neonatal Resuscitation

Drugs and supplies for neonatal resuscitation should be available and organized before surgical delivery (Table 18.2). Excessive anesthetic concentrations can result in weak and unresponsive neonates with hypoxemia and hypercarbia. In addition, severe congenital anomalies that may be initially unidentifiable or progressing hypothermia can result in neonatal unresponsiveness.

Neonatal resuscitation involves the following: (i) supplying appropriate tactile stimulation, (ii) improving or maintaining ventilation and oxygenation, and (iii) maintaining neonatal body temperature or increasing it if hypothermic. Normally, as the fetus is expelled from the birth canal, the increased pressure on the neonate assists in stimulating the first breath and expelling fluid from the respiratory tract. This stimulation is minimized during surgical delivery. Therefore, immediately after surgical delivery and as soon as the fetal membranes are removed and the umbilicus severed, the neonate should be stimulated by vigorously drying it with an absorbent towel. Emphasis is on stimulating the perineal and abdominal areas. During this time, a suction bulb is used to clear the oral cavity of fluid. Alternatively, a variable suction source on the lowest setting may be used (Figure 18.3). Stronger suction is not useful and can damage delicate neonatal mucosa. Although it is a common practice, there is no evidence to suggest that "swinging" newborns in an arc facilitates resuscitation. It is not necessary or recommended, as it increases the likelihood that a neonate could be dropped, thrown, or otherwise traumatized [65]. The "accordion squeeze" method is another effective way to stimulate the neonate to breathe and clear excess secretions and fluids from the lungs. This is achieved by laying the puppy on its back, with the head and shoulders in one hand, and the pelvis in the other hand. The puppy is

Table 18.2 Physical and pharmacological neonatal resuscitation.

Physical resuscitation			
Vigorously dry neonates			
Clear the oral cavity of fluid using gentle suction			
Administer supplemental oxygen via face mask			
Monitor heart rate via precordial palpation			
Monitor respiratory rate, intubate if necessary			
Keep neonates warm			
Useful drugs for resuscitation[a]			
Drug	Dose	Route	Indication
Epinephrine	$10\,\mu g\,kg^{-1}$	Sublingual or via umbilical vein	Bradycardia
Naloxone	1 drop	Sublingual or via umbilical vein	Opioid reversal

[a] Drugs are typically administered only after physical resuscitation techniques have been unsuccessfully performed.

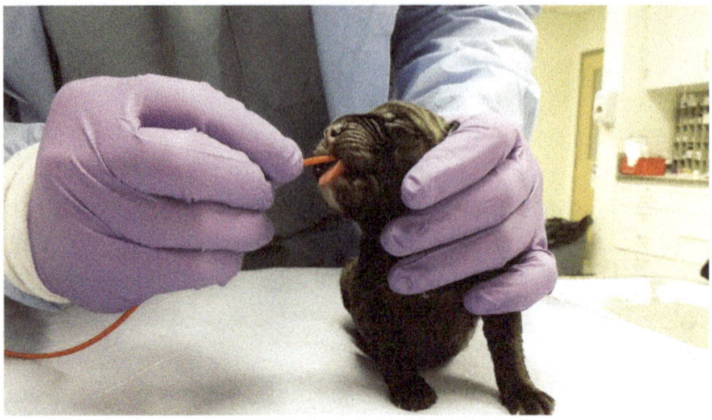

Figure 18.3 While stimulating and drying the neonate immediately after delivery, the oral cavity and nose should be suctioned of secretions. This may be required multiple times during the resuscitation process. Note if using vacuum-powered suction, use on the lowest setting to avoid damaging fragile mucosa of oral cavity and airways of the neonate.

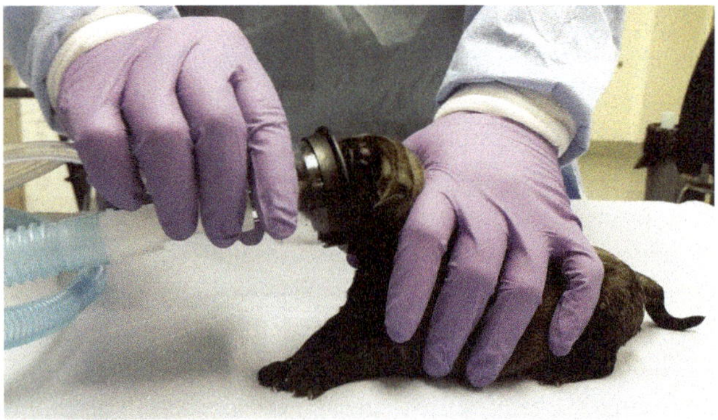

Figure 18.4 Face mask connected to a nonrebreathing anesthetic circuit used to deliver 100% oxygen.

then gently folded nose to toes and then extended. This will encourage air to move into the lungs, stimulate the heart, and push the stomach against the diaphragm to help drain fluids to the nose and mouth, where they can be adequately suctioned [66].

Spontaneous breathing should be identified by observing chest wall movement and by listening for vocalization. Bradycardia signifies developing hypoxemia. If spontaneous breathing is not obvious, vigorous rubbing should be continued and manual breaths with supplemental oxygen should be administered via an endotracheal tube. Unfortunately, the neonate's small size makes endotracheal intubation difficult. The neonate's head should be extended to facilitate endotracheal intubation. A short-bladed laryngoscope is helpful to depress the tongue and identify the tiny glottis. A flexible 14-gauge or 16-gauge IV catheter can be modified into an endotracheal tube. The oral mucosa has high water content and is thus very fragile and easily traumatized, so intubation must be performed carefully. Alternatively, delivery of a manual breath can be attempted by applying a tight-fitting face mask over the muzzle while extending the neonate's head and neck (Figure 18.4). Unfortunately, this often results in gas

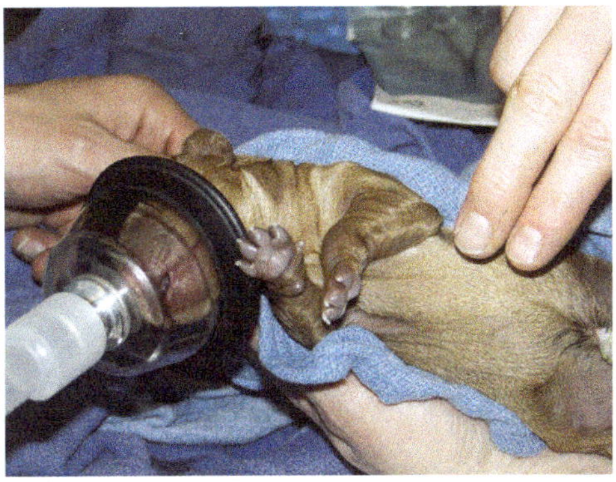

Figure 18.5 Close up of a face mask connected to a nonrebreathing anesthetic circuit used to deliver 100% oxygen. Note that multiple anesthetic circuits with available face masks may be required if the litter is large. Also note where to palpate precordial pulse.

preferentially entering the stomach rather than the lungs.

The neonate's heart rate is most easily counted by palpating a precordial pulse, with thumb and fingers lightly compressing the thoracic wall (Figure 18.5). Normal newborn heart rate should be approximately 220 beats min^{-1} [67]. Bradycardia indicates hypoxemia and should be treated by stimulation of breathing as described, supplemental oxygen, warming, and mechanical stimulation. Atropine administration to increase heart rate is ineffective because the bradycardia is not parasympathetically mediated, but rather due to anoxia of the cardiac pacemaker/conduction system [68]. If opioids were administered as part of the anesthetic regimen, the associated respiratory depression can be treated with naloxone, a complete mu-opioid receptor antagonist. It is administered sublingually (one drop) to the neonate or through the umbilical vein. The umbilical vein is the single thin-walled structure within the umbilical stump, and the umbilical arteries are paired and thicker walled. If given through the umbilical vein, drugs should be diluted in a 0.5-ml volume to facilitate injection and absorption. Often, residual inhalant anesthetics continue to suppress neonatal ventilation. No evidence demonstrates that doxapram will successfully stimulate ventilation in the newborn. However, there is also no good evidence to indicate that it is ineffective. Doxapram can be administered as described for naloxone (one drop sublingually or via the umbilical vein). Indiscriminate use of doxapram is not recommended due to increased oxygen consumption associated with its administration that may not be matched by oxygen delivery in the neonate. This agent should not be used as a first-line treatment. Cardiac massage can be accomplished by side-to-side compression of the thorax using the thumb and fingers. Epinephrine ($10\,\mu g\,kg^{-1}$) can be administered as described in Table 18.2.

Fetal Physiology

An understanding of fetal physiology is important, and the effects of many drugs on fetal physiology are unknown. Blood flow to the fetus occurs through the placenta. Maternal blood via the uterine arteries crosses the placenta to the fetal circulation [35]. Blood is carried from the placenta to the fetal circulation through the umbilical vein. Approximately 50% bypasses the liver through the ductus venosus and travels to the right atrium [69]. Some of the blood from the right atrium, returning mainly from the fetal head, travels to the right ventricle, while the majority of the right atrial volume shunts to the left atrium through the foramen ovale. Approximately 7% of the total cardiac output is pumped to the fetal lungs from the right ventricle, while approximately 60% goes through the ductus arteriosus, bypassing the lungs, and travels through the fetal circulation or to the umbilical arteries back to the placenta [69]. The blood that travels through the systemic circulation also travels to the liver. Liver metabolism in the fetus is minimal [69]. The placenta acts as a barrier similarly to the blood–brain barrier, and drugs that cross the blood–brain barrier will also cross the placenta to the fetus. The fetal environment relative to maternal is acidic, and weakly basic drugs that are relatively more ionized in a more acidic environment, such as lidocaine, can become trapped in the fetus and are inhibited from returning through the placenta to the maternal circulation for metabolism [38].

The first breath after birth is stimulated by fetal hypoxia and hypercarbia (due to separation from the placenta), a lowered body temperature, and an increase in sensory input from mechanical stimulation as the fetus passes through the birth canal. Lung inflation causes a reduction in pulmonary vascular resistance, which decreases pressure in the right atrium, right ventricle, and the pulmonary artery [69]. Systemic vascular resistance increases due to the placental circulation loss, and pressure increases in the left atrium, left ventricle, and aorta. The end result is that left atrial pressure is higher than right atrial pressure, and aortic pressure is higher than pulmonary arterial pressure. These changes reverse blood flow through the foramen ovale and ductus arteriosus, leading to their eventual closure [69]. Decreased prostaglandin concentrations are associated with ductal constriction [69].

Fetal reflex maturity varies by species. In dogs and cats, parasympathetic innervation is mature, and gag and panniculus reflexes and pain perception are present at birth. Within 4 days, the baroreceptor reflex is present and respiratory system innervation occurs in 2 weeks. Sympathetic innervation is mature at 11 days of age in cats and at 14 days in dogs. The cytochrome P450 system is at 85% of normal by 4 weeks, and full maturity occurs at 6 months of age (Figure 18.6) [31].

The fetus compared to an adult has a relatively higher hemoglobin concentration, and, due to a leftward shift of the oxyhemoglobin dissociation curve, fetal hemoglobin remains relatively saturated with oxygen at a low PO_2. The P50 of fetal dog blood is 18 mmHg, while that of adult dogs is 31 mmHg [70]. Normal fetal umbilical vein PO_2 is only 35 mmHg at which hemoglobin is 80–90% saturated [71].

Pregnant Patient Management for Noncesarean-Section Surgery

Anesthetic concerns for pregnant patients for noncesarean-section surgery are similar to those for cesarean-section patients. Surgery in pregnant patients should be avoided unless necessary due to the stress response associated with anesthesia, surgery, and hospitalization. If surgery is necessary due to traumatic injury, it is possible that the trauma itself may result in fetal loss.

Anesthetic protocols in pregnant patients for noncesarean-section surgery should incorporate the recommendations and cautions made for cesarean-section patients. Perioperative management should focus on optimizing hemodynamics and oxygen delivery to avoid decreased oxygen delivery to the fetus(es). There is little information on pharmacological treatments in veterinary medicine and the risk of such treatments to a developing fetus. In general, the fetus is at greater risk for teratogenic effects of pharmacological treatments during organogenesis (the first 20 days of pregnancy in dogs and cats) [13]. Elective procedures should not be performed in this period, if possible, to minimize stress and the effects of all drugs on the developing fetus.

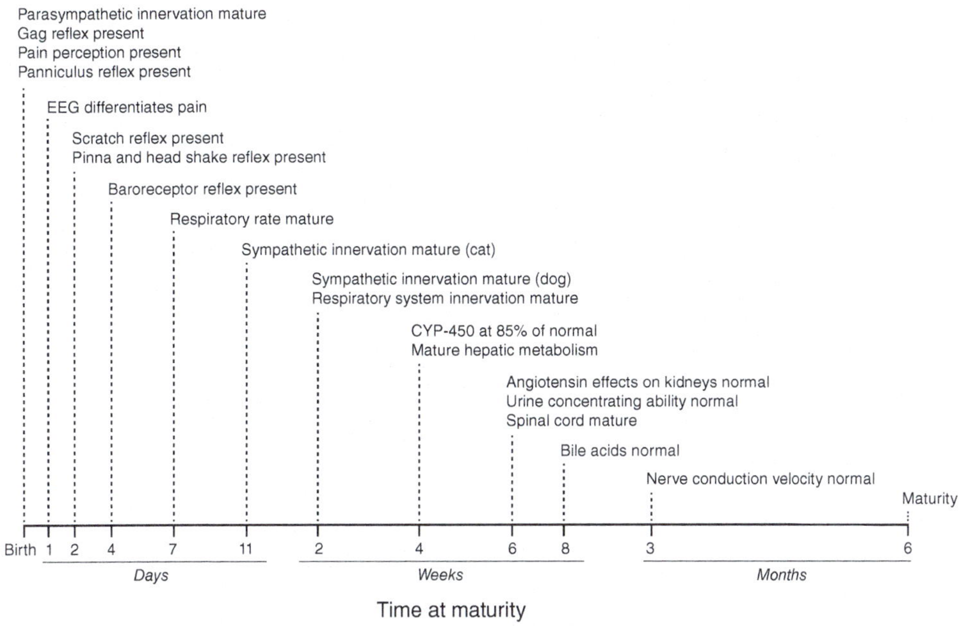

Figure 18.6 Maturation of various body systems in the dog and cat.

References

1 Moon, P.F., Erb, H.N., Ludders, J.W. et al. (2000). Perioperative risk factors for puppies delivered by cesarean section in the United States and Canada. *J. Am. Anim. Hosp. Assoc.* 36: 359–368.

2 Moon, P.F., Erb, H.N., Ludders, J.W. et al. (1998). Perioperative management and mortality rates of dogs undergoing cesarean section in the United States and Canada. *J. Am. Vet. Med. Assoc.* 213: 365–369.

3 Camann, W. and Ostheimer, G. (1990). Physiological adaptations during pregnancy. *Int. Anesthesiol. Clin.* 28: 2–10.

4 Chang, J. and Streitman, D. (2012). Physiologic adaptations to pregnancy. *Neurol. Clin.* 30: 781–789.

5 Brooks, V. and Keil, L. (1994). Hemorrhage decreases arterial pressure sooner in pregnant compared with nonpregnant dogs: role of baroreflex. *Am. J. Phys.* 266: H1610–H1619.

6 Kaneko, M., Nakayama, H., Igarashi, N. et al. (1993). Relationship between the number of fetus(es) and the blood constituents of beagles in late pregnancy. *J. Vet. Med. Sci.* 5: 681–682.

7 Probst, C.W. and Webb, A.I. (1983). Postural influence on systemic blood pressure, gas exchange, and acid/base status in the term pregnant bitch during general anesthesia. *Am. J. Vet. Res.* 44: 1963–1965.

8 Abitbol, M. (1978). Inferior vena cava compression in the pregnant dog. *Am. J. Obstet. Gynecol.* 130: 194–198.

9 Fishburne, J., Meis, P., Urban, R. et al. (1980). Vascular and uterine responses to dobutamine and dopamine in the gravid ewe. *Am. J. Obstet. Gyencol.* 137: 944–952.

10 Hollinshead, F., Hanlon, D., Gilbert, R. et al. (2010). Calcium, parathyroid hormone, oxytocin, and pH profiles in the whelping bitch. *Theriogenology* 73: 1276–1283.

11 Linden, A., Erikson, M., Carlquist, M. et al. (1987). Plasma levels of gastrin, somatostatin, and cholecystokinin immunoreactivity during pregnancy and lactation in dogs. *Gastroenterology* 92: 578–584.

12 Gin, T. and Chan, M. (1994). Decreased minimum alveolar concentration of isoflurane in pregnant humans. *Anesthesiology* 81: 829–832.

13 Rebuelto, M. and Loza, M.E. (2010). Antibiotic treatment of dogs and cats during pregnancy. *Vet. Med. Int.* 2010: 385640.

14 Groppetti, D., Di Cesare, F., Pecile, A. et al. (2019). Maternal and neonatal wellbeing during elective C-section induced with a combination of propofol and dexmedetomidine: how effective is the placental barrier in dogs? *Theriogenology* 129: 90–98.

15 Ostrea, E., Mantaring, J., and Silvestre, M. (2004). Drugs that affect the fetus and newborn infant via the placenta or breast milk. *Pediatr. Clin. North Am.* 51: 539–579.

16 Valtonen, M., Kanto, J., and Rosemberg, P. (1989). Comparison of propofol and thiopentone for induction of anaesthesia for elective caesarean section. *Anaesthesia* 44: 758–762.

17 Andaluz, A., Tusell, J., Trasserres, O. et al. (2003). Transplacental transfer of propofol in pregnant ewes. *Vet. J.* 166: 198–204.

18 Esener, Z., Sarihasan, B., Güven, H. et al. (1992). Thiopentone and etomidate concentrations in maternal and umbilical plasma, and in colostrum. *Br. J. Anaesth.* 69: 586–588.

19 Fresno, L., Andaluz, A., Moll, X. et al. (2008). Placental transfer of etomidate in pregnant ewes after an intravenous bolus dose and continuous infusion. *Vet. J.* 175: 395–402.

20 Domínguez, E., Rivera del Álamo, M.M., Novellas, R. et al. (2013). Doppler evaluation of the effects of propofol, etomidate and alphaxalone on fetoplacental circulation hemodynamics in the pregnant ewe. *Placenta* 34: 738–744.

21 Gambling, D., Sharma, S., White, P. et al. (1995). Use of sevoflurane during elective cesarean birth: a comparison with isoflurane and spinal anesthesia. *Anesth. Analg.* 81: 90–95.

22 Karaman, S., Akercan, F., Aldemir, O. et al. (2006). The maternal and neonatal effects of the volatile anaesthetic agents desflurane and sevoflurane in caesarean section: a prospective, randomized clinical study. *J. Int. Med. Res.* 34: 183–192.

23 Funkquist, P.M.E., Nyman, G.C., Lofgren, A.J. et al. (1997). Use of propofol-isoflurane as an anesthetic regimen for cesarean section in dogs. *J. Am. Vet. Med. Assoc.* 211: 313–317.

24 Vilar, J.M., Batista, M., Pérez, R. et al. (2018). Comparison of 3 anesthetic protocols for the elective cesarean-section in the dog: effects on the bitch and the newborn puppies. *Anim. Reprod. Sci.* 190: 53–62.

25 Matthews, K.A. (2008). Pain management for the pregnant, lactating, and neonatal to pediatric cat and dog. *Vet. Clin. North Am. Small Anim. Pract.* 38: 1291–1308.

26 Nanovskaya, T., Deshmukh, S., Brooms, M. et al. (2002). Transplacental transfer and metabolism of buprenorphine. *J. Pharmacol. Exp. Ther.* 300: 26–33.

27 Cooper, J., Jauniaux, E., Gulbis, B. et al. (1999). Placental transfer of fentanyl in early human pregnancy and its detection in fetal brain. *Br. J. Anaesth.* 82: 929–931.

28 Bragg, P., Zwass, M.S., Lau, M. et al. (1995). Opioid pharmacodynamics in neonatal dogs: differences between morphine and fentanyl. *J. Appl. Phys.* 79: 1519–1524.

29 Brice, J.E.H., Moreland, T.A., and Walker, C.H.M. (1979). Effects of pethidine and its antagonists on the newborn. *Arch. Dis. Child.* 54: 356–361.

30 Lamont, L.A. and Matthews, K.A. (2007). Opioids, nonsteroidal anti-inflammatories, and analgesic adjuvants. In: *Lumb and Jones' Veterinary Anesthesia and Analgesia*, 4e (eds. W.J. Tranquilli, J.C. Thurmon and K.A. Grimm), 241–271. Ames: Blackwell Publishing.

31 Aarnes, T.K. and Muir, W.W. (2011). Pain assessment and management. In: *Small Animal Pediatrics: The First 12 Months of Life* (eds. M.E. Peterson and M.A. Kutzler), 220–232. St. Louis: Elsevier Saunders.

32 Schneider, M., Kuchta, A., and Woehrlé, F. (2015). Disposition of cimicoxib in plasma and milk of whelping bitches and in their puppies. *BMC Vet. Res.* 11: 178.

33 Pascoe, P.J. and Moon, P.F. (2001). Periparturient and neonatal anesthesia. *Vet. Clin. North Am. Small Anim. Pract.* 31: 315–341.

34 Mhuireachtaigh, R.N. and O'Gorman, D.A. (2006). Anesthesia in pregnant patients for nonobstetric surgery. *J. Clin. Anesth.* 18: 60–66.

35 Shnider, S.M. and Levinson, G. (1994). Anesthesia for obstetrics. In: *Miller's Anesthesia*, 4e (ed. R.D. Miller), 2031–2076. Philadelphia: Elsevier.

36 Robertson SA. 2009. Physiology of pregnancy and anesthesia for cesarean section in dogs. Proceedings Southern European Veterinary Conference 2009. Available at: http://www.ivis.org/proceedings/sevc/2009/eng/robertson1.pdf.

37 McNally, E.M., Robertson, S.A., and Pablo, L.S. (2009). Comparison of time to desaturation between preoxygenated and non-preoxygenated dogs following sedation with acepromazine maleate and morphine and induction of anesthesia with propofol. *Am. J. Vet. Res.* 70 (133): 3–8.

38 Raffe, M.R. and Carpenter, R.E. (2007). Anesthetic management of cesarean section patients. In: *Lumb and Jones' Veterinary Anesthesia and Analgesia*, 4e (eds. W.J. Tranquilli, J.C. Thurmon and K.A. Grimm), 955–967. Ames: Blackwell Publishing.

39 Luna, S.P.L., Cassu, R.D., Castro, G.B. et al. (2004). Effects of four anaesthetic protocols on the neurological and cardiorespiratory variables of puppies born by caesarean section. *Vet. Rec.* 154: 387–389.

40 Otero, P.E. and Campoy, L. (2013). Epidural and spinal anesthesia. In: *Small Animal Regional Anesthesia and Analgesia* (eds. L. Campoy and M.R. Read), 227–259. Ames: Blackwell Publishing.

41 Robertson, S.A., Gogolski, S.M., and Pascoe, P. (2018). AAFP feline anesthesia guidelines. *J. Feline Med. Surg.* 20: 602–634.

42 Moon-Massat, P.F. and Erb, H.N. (2002). Perioperative factors associated with puppy vigor after delivery by cesarean section. *J. Am. Anim. Hosp. Assoc.* 38: 90–96.

43 Muir, W., Lerche, P., Wiese, A. et al. (2008). Cardiorespiratory and anesthetic effect of clinical and supraclinical doses of alfaxalone in dogs. *Vet. Anaesth. Analg.* 35: 451–462.

44 Ferré, P.J., Pasloske, K., Whittem, T. et al. (2006). Plasma pharmacokinetics of alfaxalone in dogs after an intravenous bolus of Alfaxan-CD RTU. *Vet. Anaesth. Analg.* 33: 229–236.

45 Maney, J.K., Shepard, M.K., Braun, C. et al. (2013). A comparison of cardiopulmonary and anesthetic effects of an induction dose of alfaxalone or propfol in dogs. *Vet. Anaesth. Analg.* 40: 237–244.

46 Martinez Taboada, F. and Murison, P.J. (2010). Induction of anaesthesia with alfaxalone or propofol before isoflurane maintenance in cats. *Vet. Rec.* 167: 85–89.

47 Doebeli, A., Michel, E., Bettschart, R. et al. (2013). Apgar score after induction of anesthesia for canine cesarean section with alfaxalone versus propofol. *Theriogenology* 80: 850–854.

48 Metcalfe, S., Hulands-Nave, A., Bell, M. et al. (2014). Multicentre, randomized clinical trial evaluating the efficacy and safety of alfaxalone administered to bitches for induction of anaesthesia prior to caesarean section. *Aust. Vet. J.* 92: 333–338.

49 Tamura, J., Ishizuka, T., Fukui, S. et al. (2015). The pharmacological effects of the anesthetic alfaxalone after intramuscular administration to dogs. *J. Vet. Med. Sci.* 77: 289–296.

50 Tamura, J., Ishizuka, T., Fukui, S. et al. (2015). Sedative effects of intramuscular alfaxalone administered to cats. *J. Vet. Med. Sci.* 77: 897–904.

51 Maney, J.K. (2017). Sedative and physiologic effects of low-dose intramuscular alfaxalone in dogs. *Vet. Anaesth. Analg.* 44: 1184–1188.

52 Tamura, J., Hatakeyama, N., Ishizuka, T. et al. (2016). The pharmacological effects of intramuscular administration of alfaxalone

combined with medetomidine and butorphanol in dogs. *J. Vet. Med. Sci.* 78: 929–936.

53 Dodman, N.H. (1979). Anaesthesia for caesarean section in the dog and cat: a review. *J. Small Anim. Pract.* 20: 449–460.

54 Conde Ruiz, C., Del Carro, A.P., Rosset, E. et al. (2016). Alfaxalone for total intravenous anesthesia in bitches undergoing elective caesarean section and its effects on puppies: a randomized clinical trial. *Vet. Anaesth. Analg.* 43: 281–290.

55 Conde Ruiz, C. (2017). Letter to the editor: poor Apgar score and high mortality in puppies born by caesarean section from bitches anesthetized with a propofol constant rate infusion. *Vet. Anaesth. Analg.* 44: 692–693.

56 McKune, C.M., Pascoe, P.J., Duncan, B. et al. (2018). The challenge of evaluating pain and a pre-incisional local anesthetic block. *Peer J.* 2: e34. https://doi.org/10.7717/peerj.341.

57 Casteñeda-Herrera, F.E., Buriticá-Gaviria, E.F., and Echeverry-Bonilla, D.F. (2017). Anatomical evaluation of the thoracolumbar nerves related to the transversus abdominis plane block technique in dogs. *Anat. Hist. Embyol.* 46: 373–377.

58 Freitag, F.A.V., Bozak, V.L., do MPW, C. et al. (2018). Letter to the editor: continuous transversus abdominis plane black for analgesia in three dogs with abdominal pain. *Vet. Anaesth. Analg.* 45: 581–583.

59 Schroeder, C.A., Snyder, L.B.C., Tearney, C. et al. (2011). Ultrasound-guided transversus abdominis plane block in dogs: an anatomical evaluation. *Vet. Anaesth. Analg.* 38: 267–271.

60 Drożdżyńska, M., Monticelli, P., Neilson, D. et al. (2017). Ultrasound-guided subcostal oblique transversus abdominis plane block in canine cadavers. *Vet. Anaesth. Analg.* 44: 183–186.

61 St James, M., Ferreira, T.H., Schroeder, C.A. et al. (2019). Ultrasound-guided rectus sheath block: an anatomic in dog cadavers. *Vet. Anaesth. Analg.* 47: 95–102.

62 Wasson, C., Kelly, A., Ninan, D. et al. (2019). Placental blood flow. In: *Absolute Obstetric Anesthesia Review* (eds. C. Wasson, A. Kelly, D. Ninan and Q. Tran), 21–23. Cham, Switzerland: Springer Nature.

63 Greene, S.A. (1995). Anesthetic considerations for surgery of the reproductive system. *Semin. Vet. Med. Surg.* 10: 2–7.

64 Probst, C.W., Broadstone, R.V., and Evans, A.T. (1987). Postural influence on systemic blood pressure in large full-term pregnant bitches during general anesthesia. *Vet. Surg.* 16: 471–473.

65 Grundy, S., Liu, S., and Davidson, A. (2009). Intracranial trauma in a dog due to being "swung" at birth. *Top. Companion Anim. Med.* 24: 100–103.

66 Greer, M.L. (2015). Managing the whelping and C-section. In: *Canine Reproduction and Neonatology* (ed. C.C. Cann), 124. Jackson: Teton NewMedia.

67 Root-Kustritz (2011). History and physical examination of the neonate. In: *Small Animal Pediatrics: The First 12 Months of Life* (eds. M.E. Peterson and M.A. Kutzler), 20–27. St. Louis: Elsevier Saunders.

68 Traas, A.M. (2008). Resuscitation of canine and feline neonates. *Theriogenology* 70: 343–348.

69 Robinson, N.E. (1997). Fetal and neonatal oxygen transport. In: *Textbook of Veterinary Physiology*, 2e (ed. J.G. Cunningham), 613–620. Philadelphia: WB Saunders Company.

70 Mueggler, P., Jones, G., Peterson, J. et al. (1980). Postnatal regulation of canine oxygen delivery: erythrocyte components affecting Hb function. *Am. J. Physiol. Heart Circ. Physiol.* 238: H73–H79.

71 Chestnutt, A. (2004). Physiology of normal pregnancy. *Crit. Care Clin.* 20: 609–615.

19

Neonatal and Pediatric Concerns

Anderson Fávaro da Cunha

Department of Specialty Medicine, College of Veterinary Medicine, Midwestern University, Glendale, AZ, 85308, USA

Introduction

The odds of anesthesia-related mortality are lower in healthy cats and dogs younger than 6 months of age in comparison to adults and older patients [1]; however, their anesthetic management is often considered a clinical challenge [2]. Further, the mortality odds increase in patients with coexisting diseases that can lead to poor functional organ capacity, such as pulmonary, central nervous system (CNS), cardiac, renal, hepatic, and endocrine diseases alone or in combination [3]. Therefore, the relationship between patient life stage and physical status needs to be considered while designing anesthetic protocols. For example, this helps the anesthetist to better understand and appreciate the possible anesthetic challenges associated with each individual and then aids in tailoring the anesthetic management protocol to meet the individual's need. Accordingly, using the American Animal Hospital Association (AAHA) guidelines, cat [4] and dog [5] life stages are classified; some terms overlap ages (Tables 19.1 and 19.2). It is important to note that defining the terms "neonatal" and "pediatric" is challenging in veterinary medicine. However, in general, the neonatal stage extends from birth to weaning, and the pediatric stage starts after weaning and ends with the beginning of the reproductive maturity [4–6] as described in Table 19.1 [5]. This chapter reviews the physiologic and pharmacologic alterations seen in neonatal and pediatric dogs and cats, as responses clearly change with age [7].

Physiological Alterations

Respiratory System

The timing for each developmental stage and the degree of lung development at birth vary significantly among species [8]. For dogs and cats, the initial development of the respiratory system happens well before birth and matures in the postnatal period [8–10]. In comparison to adults, the neonatal and pediatric rib cages are more compliant, intercostal muscles are weaker, work and pressures required to maintain tidal breathing are increased, and respiratory chemoreceptors are immature and less sensitive to increased CO_2 and/or decreased O_2 (Table 19.3) [10]. Young animals have higher resting respiratory rates and minute volume, increased tendency to develop atelectasis, higher oxygen demand, and lower functional residual capacity (FRC) [10]. Altogether, these

Canine and Feline Anesthesia and Co-Existing Disease, Second Edition. Edited by Rebecca A. Johnson, Lindsey B. C. Snyder and Carrie A. Schroeder.

Companion website: www.wiley.com/go/johnson/canine

Table 19.1 Canine life stages [5].

Stage	Definition
Neonate	Birth to weaning (approximately 4 weeks of life)
Puppy/pediatric	Weaning until reproductive maturity
Junior	Reproductively mature, yet still growing
Adult	Finished growing, fully mature

Table 19.2 Feline life stages [4].

Stage	Age
Neonate	Birth to weaning (approximately 4 weeks of life)
Kitten	Birth to 6 months of age
Junior	7 months to 2 years of age

changes are possible causes of respiratory fatigue and hypoxemia during anesthesia. Although there is minimal supportive evidence for the exact timing to reach complete adult alveolar development and lung maturity for dogs and cats, the maximum functional efficiency of the dog lungs occurs around 1 year of age [11]. By comparison, in humans, the same level of lung maturity is achieved at the age of 20 [11].

Because of the abovementioned physiologic alterations, oxygen supplementation prior to anesthesia is recommended for neonatal and pediatric patients. A minimum of 3 min of preinduction oxygenation via face mask, followed by intraoperative and postanesthetic oxygenation (including after extubation), prevents possible hypoxemia [12]. Importantly, a tight-fitting face mask should be used to efficiently increase the inspiratory fraction of oxygen [13]. For example, in dogs, high flow rates of 100% flow-by oxygen (without a mask) minimally increased the inspired concentration of oxygen from 21% to 30%, and therefore it is not considered an effective technique [13]. Further, during general anesthesia, intermittent positive pressure ventilation (IPPV) and oxygenation monitoring are recommended via pulse oximetry, capnography, and/or arterial blood gas analysis. Assisted ventilation is often recommended to maintain both normal ventilation (PCO_2 between approximately 35 and 45 mmHg) and normal oxygenation (PaO_2 higher than approximately 60 mmHg).

Cardiovascular System

The neonatal cardiovascular system undergoes dramatic changes immediately after birth to assume its own circulation and maintain homeostasis [14]. The neonatal systemic circulation is often considered a low-resistance–high-flow circuit because it is associated with low blood pressure, total blood volume, and peripheral vascular resistance [14–16].

To maintain normal tissue perfusion, the neonatal and pediatric patient must maintain a higher heart rate, cardiac output, plasma volume, and central venous pressure compared to the adult (Table 19.3) [15, 16]. Baroreceptors are not fully mature until approximately 12 weeks of age, leading to decreased vasomotor tone and vasoconstrictive properties; thus, heart rate drives normal cardiac output. To this end, anticholinergics are used frequently during anesthesia to maintain normal to higher heart rates and tissue perfusion. In the newborn, bradycardia is not vagally mediated and is often caused by hypoxemia [15].

Congenital heart defects are common in veterinary medicine. In a veterinary teaching hospital setting, approximately 17% of dogs and 5% of cats examined during a 10-year period were diagnosed with congenital heart disease. Subaortic stenosis and patent ductus arteriosus in dogs and tricuspid valve dysplasia and ventricular septal defect in cats were among the most common congenital diseases [17]. Specific details of each congenital disease can be found in Chapter 1.

Anesthetic-induced cardiovascular depression and hypotension are common cardiovascular

Table 19.3 Physiological differences observed in neonatal and pediatric dogs and cats when compared to adults.

Respiratory system	
↑	Rib cage compliance
↓	Intercostal muscle strength
↑	Inspiratory pressure
↑	Work of breathing
↑	Sensitivity to hypercarbia
↓	Sensitivity to hypoxemia
↑	Resting respiratory rate
↑	Minute volume
↑	Tendency to develop atelectasis
↑	Oxygen demand
↓	Functional residual capacity
Cardiovascular system	
↓	Blood pressure
↑	Heart rate
↑	Cardiac output
↓	Systemic vascular resistance
↓	Ability to vasoconstrict
↓	Baroreceptor maturity
↓	Central venous pressure
↑	Plasma volume
↓	Blood volume
Hepatic system	
↓	Cytochrome P-450 enzyme system maturity
↓	Albumin levels
↓	Drug metabolism
↓	Gluconeogenic ability
Central nervous system	
↓	CNS maturity
↓	Neuromuscular junction maturity
↓	Thermoregulatory center responsiveness
↑	Susceptibility to hypothermia
Renal system	
↓	Nephrogenesis
↓	Clearance rate
↓	Glomerular filtration rate
↓	Renal plasma flow
↓	Concentrating ability
↓	Filtration fraction
↓	Amino acids and phosphate reabsorption
↑	Proximal tubule natriuresis
↑	Phosphorous concentrations
↓	Creatinine concentrations
↓	Blood urea nitrogen concentrations
Pharmacokinetics	
↑	Drug elimination time
↓	Albumin–drug affinity
↓	Protein-bound
↑	Blood–brain barrier permeability
↑	Body water content
↓	Fat content
↑	Initial volume of distribution for water-soluble drugs
↓	Smaller volume of distribution for lipid-soluble drugs

↑ = Increase, ↓ = Decrease, CNS = central nervous system.

abnormalities observed during procedures; thus, adequate venous return and fluid balance must be maintained to minimize the risk of hypotension [18]. Due to decreased cardiac reserve, fluid overload can lead to congestive heart failure and pulmonary edema. Therefore, fluid rate should be chosen based on the individual need and hydration and physical status. Cardiovascular monitoring is emphasized to detect detrimental changes to the cardiovascular system of young patients that could lead to renal and hepatic insufficiency in adult life. A possible cardiovascular insult during anesthesia while the patient is young could trigger further damage to high perfusion organs that, over time, could lead to possible renal failure during their adult life [19].

Hepatic System

The cytochrome P-450 enzyme system is immature after birth but develops during postnatal life [20]. This may be associated with prolonged drug elimination times and decreased drug metabolism due to the lack of hepatic function (Table 19.3). Therefore, lower drug doses may be recommended in very young patients. Likewise, the glucose levels are frequently well maintained in normal neonatal patient; however, when stressed or fasted, they may become hypoglycemic, as glycogen stores are relatively low and gluconeogenic ability is low [21]. Monitoring intraoperative and postoperative blood glucose levels is essential during puppy and kitten anesthetic events.

Central Nervous System

The immature CNS (and neuromuscular junctions) of neonatal and pediatric patients requires less drugs to produce effective general anesthesia, local anesthesia, and neuromuscular blockage when compared to adults and doses should be adjusted (Table 19.3) [21–23]. Central thermoregulatory centers are also immature during the neonatal and pediatric stages and patients are more susceptible to anesthesia-induced hypothermia [24]. Hypothermia can be associated with bradyarrhythmias, reduced minimum alveolar concentration (MAC) of inhalants, and shivering. Further, shivering can increase oxygen consumption by up to 400% [24]. Since these patients have decreased ability to thermoregulate via shivering and cannot adequately vasoconstrict, hypothermia can be prolonged. Once again, oxygen supplementation is recommended for these patients [25] and prudent heat supplementation starting with anesthetic induction is advised.

Renal System

There is marked variation in the degree of renal maturation at birth between species [9]. In puppies, nephrogenesis is not complete until the third week of life. The canine neonatal kidney is functionally characterized by a low clearance rate, glomerular filtration, renal plasma flow, and filtration fraction (Table 19.3). It exhibits depressed amino acid and phosphate reabsorption, exaggerated proximal tubule natriuresis, and low concentrating ability [26]. In the neonate, average serum phosphorous concentrations are usually elevated (approximately 9 $mg\,dl^{-1}$), whereas serum creatinine levels (approximately 0.4 $mg\,dl^{-1}$) and blood urea nitrogen concentrations (approximately 10 $mg\,dl^{-1}$) are usually lower when compared with normal health adult animals [9].

With anesthetic induction, normal healthy patients may experience a significant reduction in renal blood flow and glomerular filtration [24] that could potentially lead to renal compromise during the patient's adult life. Cardiac disease can exacerbate the anesthetic effects on the reduction of renal blood flow and its associated side effects [24]. Therefore, for all neonatal and pediatric patients, blood pressure measurements and renal function analysis (urinalysis, blood urea nitrogen [BUN], and creatinine) are recommended. Since cardiac output is not usually monitored during veterinary anesthesia, blood pressure, mucous membrane color, urine output, and hydration status should always be monitored when possible, to predict possible decreases in cardiac output that could lead to further damage to kidneys and other vital organs.

Pharmacokinetic and Pharmacodynamic Considerations

Compared to pediatric or adult patients, neonatal patients have different drug uptake, distribution, and metabolism. For example, the neonatal patient has lower albumin levels and lower albumin–drug affinity that may lead to a decrease in protein-bound (inactive) drug. The blood–brain barrier may be more permeable, possibly potentiating CNS drug effects. Neonate and pediatric patients have higher body water content and lower fat content than adults, resulting in a higher volume of distribution for water-soluble drugs and a smaller volume of distribution for lipid-soluble drugs [21].

The alveolar rate of rise of inhaled anesthetic concentrations is faster in infants and children in comparison to adults [27]. This is likely due to the larger ratio of alveolar ventilation to FRC, greater fraction of the cardiac output to vessel-rich organs, and a greater cardiac output per kilogram. Age also can significantly affect inhalant blood–gas partition coefficients. The lower blood–gas partition coefficients in children may also explain, at least in part, the more rapid rise of alveolar anesthetic partial pressure in this age group [28]. Moreover, inhalant MAC in humans and animals varies with age, being highest in the neonate and least in the elderly; for example, the MAC of halothane in neonatal humans is 25% less than that in infants [28].

Anesthetic Management of Neonatal and Pediatric Patients

Anesthetic management of the neonatal and pediatric patient is primarily a matter of following sound anesthetic principles as they should be applied for any veterinary patient [29]. More important than drug choice is complete understanding of the individual's physical condition and directing attention to many details at once. The anesthetic protocol should start with a complete knowledge of the patient's history and a systematic physical evaluation followed by supporting laboratory data. The anesthetist should understand the relationship between anesthesia and age considering the physiological reserves of the various organ systems [29]. Patients with abnormalities should be stabilized prior to the anesthesia induction to decrease the anesthetic risks. Close monitoring of various organ systems should be performed beginning at the preinduction period and maintained until the patient regains control of vital reflexes, consciousness, body temperature, normoglycemia, and coordination [29].

Preanesthetic Evaluation

For the neonatal patient, a systematic neurological and oral exam should be performed to assess the patient's physiological health [23]. For the pediatric patient, family history of congenital disease is one of the most important factors. During the pediatric physical examination, arterial pulses, signs of cyanosis, murmurs, respiratory abnormalities, jugular venous distention, ascites, or hepatomegaly are all signs that would lead to a possible diagnosis of congenital heart defect [17]. As such, a complete physical examination to rule out those abnormalities is vital. Thoracic radiographs can be useful to evaluate cardiac size, great vessels, and pulmonary vasculature to confirm any possible congenital disease. Echocardiography is considered the cornerstone to establish the definitive diagnosis of a specific disease [18] and anesthetic plans should be tailored to each individual (see Chapter 1).

Sedation

Sedation may not be required for the neonatal cat or dog [21]. In the true neonate, mask induction may be performed without stress due to the CNS and cardiorespiratory peculiarities of an immature neonatal patient. Atropine or glycopyrrolate (anticholinergics) should be administered for any neonatal and pediatric patient before anesthetic induction to maintain a higher heart rate, which is necessary to maintain their cardiac output. Low-dose opioids and/or benzodiazepines are "not" contraindicated in neonatal patients. By contrast, the use of alpha-2-adrenergic agonists and phenothiazines (acepromazine) should be avoided in neonatal patients. Alpha-2-adrenergic agonists cause significant vasoconstriction, bradycardia, decreased cardiac output, and arrhythmias. Acepromazine administration, even in low doses, can produce hypotension [30] that could potentially lead to organ failure if severe and untreated during general anesthesia.

For the pediatric patient, mild sedation can be safely used. Like neonates, benzodiazepines in combination with opioids are often recommended and higher doses are necessary when compared to those used in neonates. Alpha-2-adrenergic agonists and acepromazine are usually not required. Due to possible drug effects on the respiratory control system (such as hypoventilation) and the potential for difficulties in airway management of small patients, a minimum of 3 min of preoxygenation with 100% oxygen via tight face mask is recommended for all neonatal and pediatric patients prior to induction of anesthesia and intubation.

Anesthetic Induction and Maintenance

Most challenges with general anesthesia of neonatal patients are related to patient size. To this end, mask induction with isoflurane or sevoflurane may be considered simple and effective in most true neonates. Inhaled anesthetic effects on blood pressure and the incidence of hypotension are similar between infants and neonates at approximately 1 MAC [31]. In addition, tracheal intubation can be difficult; the laryngeal tissues of neonatal kittens and puppies are quite fragile and great care should be taken for an atraumatic intubation [21]. Thus, the use of atraumatic (nonmetallic) stylets is highly suitable to facilitate endotracheal intubation. Application of regular monitoring equipment can be problematic; intravenous catheter placement can be difficult. Likewise, IPPV is generally needed in neonatal puppies and kittens, since neonatal patients tend to fatigue easily with increased work of breathing. Rebreathing anesthetic circuits are not recommended for patients smaller than 3 kg unless specially designed for extremely small tidal volume ventilation (i.e., Hallowell Workstation; Hallowell EMC, Pittsfield, MA). A non-rebreathing system, such as a modified Bain system, can also be used to reduce breathing resistance and to provide manual IPPV.

Young cats and dogs are frequently anesthetized for numerous procedures including ovariohysterectomy or castration with minimal complications [29]. Propofol, alfaxalone, and etomidate are usually considered safe in low doses for the pediatric population [32]. Etomidate, and possibly other injectable drugs, has higher potency in the neonatal patient and doses should be administered slowly until orotracheal intubation can be achieved. By 10 weeks of age, the etomidate dose in neonatal dogs is the same as the adult dose (1–2 $mg\,kg^{-1}$) [33]. Dissociative agents (ketamine, tiletamine) should be avoided in the first 2–3 weeks of life because they may be associated with high mortality rate [34].

Intravenous administration of warm isotonic fluids with 2.5% dextrose is often recommended [35]. Most importantly, the monitoring of core temperature and blood glucose throughout the procedure should be performed and deviations corrected as needed. For any small patient, fluid overload and heparin overdose associated with frequent intravenous catheter flushing should be avoided. Flushing with nonheparinized solutions is recommended, as 0.9% saline is less expensive and is as effective as heparinized saline to maintain patency, prevent phlebitis, and increase duration of peripheral intravenous catheters [36].

As previously mentioned, hypothermia occurs more readily in pediatric patients than in adults because of the greater body surface area, minimum amounts of subcutaneous fat, and their reduced ability to shiver. Providing a warm environment and maintaining the animal on a heat source throughout the entire procedure are essential.

Maintenance of anesthesia can be performed with inhaled or injectable anesthetics. Diligent anesthetic level monitoring is recommended, and patients should be kept in the lightest anesthetic plane required for the procedure. Isoflurane and sevoflurane are potent vasodilators and can cause significant hypotension. Continuous rate infusion of fentanyl, remifentanil, lidocaine, and ketamine alone, or in combination, is often used to decrease the MAC of inhalant anesthetics and minimize their unwanted side effects.

Age alone is not an indication for invasive monitoring; however, diligent monitoring during the entire anesthetic period and recovery is recommended. Independent of the coexisting conditions, electrocardiography, capnometry, pulse oximetry, core body temperature, and blood pressure should always be monitored, even though a caveat of hemodynamic monitoring in young patients is the paucity of studies performed regarding the accuracy of the noninvasive blood pressure monitoring in younger cats and dogs. Urinary output and blood gas analysis may also be recommended in specific circumstances.

Analgesic Techniques

Numerous lines of research demonstrate that the CNS is mature enough to transduct, transmit, modulate, and perceive pain during the last third portion of pregnancy [37] (more precisely at 29 weeks of gestation for humans) [38]. Therefore, analgesia for the neonatal and pediatric patient should always be used for any painful procedure. Surgical pain and distress can endure in the memory and result in disturbances of eating, sleeping stability, and the state of arousal in humans [39]; it is likely that the same effects happen in other species as well.

Potent opioids such as fentanyl and remifentanil can be used in neonatal and pediatric patients; however, ventilatory monitoring needs to be implemented, since they are potent respiratory depressants [40]. In addition, local anesthetic agents can be used and are very effective in all ages; dose requirements and techniques are similar in neonatal, pediatric, and adults [41]. For example, castrations are common elective surgeries in the pediatric patient; a simple intratesticular block with 2% lidocaine is very effective as an analgesic and should be performed [42, 43]. For ovariohysterectomy, the transversus abdominis plane block (TAP block; Figure 19.1) has been proposed as an effective local analgesia technique for the abdomen [44].

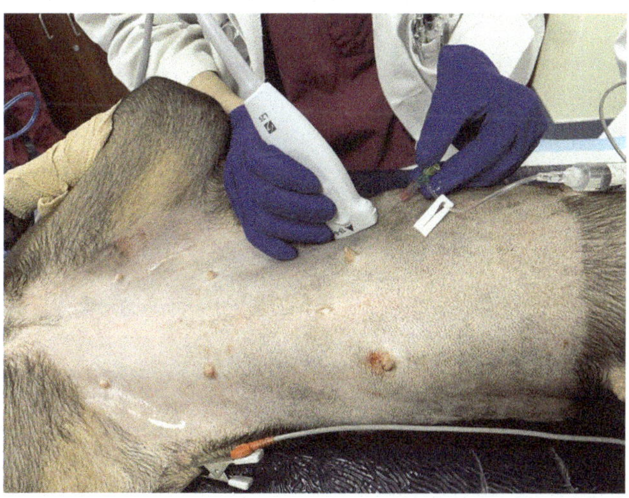

Figure 19.1 Ultrasound-guided transversus abdominis plane (TAP) block in a dog using bupivacaine before ovariohysterectomy.

Anesthetic Recovery

In the first 3 days after birth, genital or umbilical region stimulation induces reflex respiration [14] and can be attempted clinically to stimulate ventilation during anesthetic recovery. The anesthetist should be ready to provide oxygen, heat, and continuous cardiorespiratory monitoring. Maintenance of an open airway via tracheal intubation until the patient is swallowing is also important, not only to provide efficient oxygenation, but also to prevent aspiration pneumonia.

Conclusion

The anesthetist should consider age and specific coexisting diseases as a whole when designing anesthetic protocols for neonatal and pediatric patients. Age is a multifactorial, all-encompassing process; therefore, there is no one ideal anesthetic plan that would be recommended for all patients. Due to the paucity of evidence-based recommendations in veterinary medicine, many concepts described here are based on human literature. However, advances in neonatal and pediatric veterinary anesthetic procedures and investigations will become more available to fulfill the current knowledge gap.

References

1. Brodbelt, D. (2009). Perioperative mortality in small animal anaesthesia. *Vet. J.* 182: 152–161.
2. Hosgood, G. (2002 (Response 2003)). Evaluation of age and American Society of Anesthesiologists (ASA) physical status as risk factors for perianesthetic morbidity and mortality in the cat. *J. Vet. Emerg. Crit. Care* 12: 9–16; Response 13:44.
3. John, A.D. and Sieber, F.E. (2004). Age associated issues: geriatrics. *Anesthesiol. Clin. North Am.* 22: 45–58.
4. Vogt, A.H., Rodan, I., Brown, M. et al. (2010). AAFP-AAHA: feline life stage guidelines. *J. Am. Anim. Hosp. Assoc.* 46: 70–85.
5. Bartges, J.W. (2012). Chronic kidney disease in dogs and cats. *Vet. Clin. North Am. Small Anim. Pract.* 42: 669–692, vi.
6. Greer, K.A., Canterberry, S.C., and Murphy, K.E. (2007). Statistical analysis regarding the effects of height and weight on life span of the domestic dog. *Res. Vet. Sci.* 82: 208–214.
7. Kukanich, B. (2012). Geriatric veterinary pharmacology. *Vet. Clin. North Am. Small Anim. Pract.* 42: 631–642, v.
8. Thurlbeck, W.M. (1975). Postnatal growth and development of the lung. *Am. Rev. Respir. Dis.* 111: 803–844.
9. Zoetis, T. and Hurtt, M.E. (2003). Species comparison of lung development. *Birth Defects Res. B Dev. Reprod. Toxicol.* 68: 121–124.
10. Haddad, G.G. and Mellins, R.B. (1984). Hypoxia and respiratory control in early life. *Annu. Rev. Physiol.* 46: 629–643.
11. Mauderly, J.L. (1979). Effect of age on pulmonary structure and function of immature and adult animals and man. *Fed. Proc.* 38: 173–177.
12. McNally, E.M., Robertson, S.A., and Pablo, L.S. (2009). Comparison of time to desaturation between preoxygenated and nonpreoxygenated dogs following sedation with acepromazine maleate and morphine and induction of anesthesia with propofol. *Am. J. Vet. Res.* 70: 1333–1338.
13. Ambros, B., Carrozzo, M.V., and Jones, T. (2018). Desaturation times between dogs preoxygenated via face mask or flow-by technique before induction of anesthesia. *Vet. Anaesth. Analg.* 45: 452–458.
14. Grundy, S.A. (2006). Clinically relevant physiology of the neonate. *Vet. Clin. North Am. Small Anim. Pract.* 36: 443–459, v.
15. Adelman, R.D. and Wright, J. (1985). Systolic blood pressure and heart rate in the growing

beagle puppy. *Dev. Pharmacol. Ther.* 8: 396–401.

16 Magrini, F. (1978). Haemodynamic determinants of the arterial blood pressure rise during growth in conscious puppies. *Cardiovasc. Res.* 12: 422–428.

17 MacDonald, K.A. (2006). Congenital heart diseases of puppies and kittens. *Vet. Clin. North Am. Small Anim. Pract.* 36: 503–531, vi.

18 Hughes, J. (2008). Anaesthesia for the geriatric dog and cat. *Ir. Vet. J.* 61: 380–387.

19 Bartels, K., Karhausen, J., Clambey, E.T. et al. (2013). Perioperative organ injury. *Anesthesiology* 119: 1474–1489.

20 Tavoloni, N. (1985). Postnatal changes in hepatic microsomal enzyme activities in the puppy. *Biol. Neonate* 47: 305–316.

21 Pascoe, P.J. and Moon, P.F. (2001). Periparturient and neonatal anesthesia. *Vet. Clin. North Am. Small Anim. Pract.* 31: 315–340, vii.

22 Mosier, J.E. (1989). Effect of aging on body systems of the dog. *Vet. Clin. North Am. Small Anim. Pract.* 19: 1–12.

23 Lavely, J.A. (2006). Pediatric neurology of the dog and cat. *Vet. Clin. North Am. Small Anim. Pract.* 36: 475–501, v.

24 Harvey, R.C. and Paddleford, R.R. (1999). Management of geriatric patients. A common occurrence. *Vet. Clin. North Am. Small Anim. Pract.* 29: 683–699, vi.

25 Ralley, F.E., Wynands, J.E., Ramsay, J.G. et al. (1988). The effects of shivering on oxygen consumption and carbon dioxide production in patients rewarming from hypothermic cardiopulmonary bypass. *Can. J. Anaesth.* 35: 332–337.

26 Hay, D.A. and Evan, A.P. (1979). Maturation of the proximal tubule in the puppy kidney: a comparison to the adult. *Anat. Rec.* 195: 273–299.

27 Eger, E.I. 2nd, Bahlman, S.H., and Munson, E.S. (1971). The effect of age on the rate of increase of alveolar anesthetic concentration. *Anesthesiology* 35: 365–372.

28 Lerman, J., Gregory, G.A., Willis, M.M. et al. (1984). Age and solubility of volatile anesthetics in blood. *Anesthesiology* 61: 139–143.

29 Hartsfield, S.M. (1990). Anesthetic problems of the geriatric dental patient. *Probl. Vet. Med.* 2: 24–45.

30 Rangel, J.P.P., Monteiro, E.R., Bitti, F.S. et al. (2020). Hemodynamic, respiratory and sedative effects of progressively increasing doses of acepromazine in conscious dogs. *Vet. Anaesth. Analg.* 47: 447–453.

31 Lerman, J., Robinson, S., Williset, M.M. et al. (1983). Anesthetic requirements for halothane in young children 0-1 month and 1-6 months of age. *Anesthesiology* 59: 421–424.

32 Stoelting, R.K., Flood, P., Rathmett, J.P. et al. (2015). *Stoelting's Handbook of Pharmacology and Physiology in Anesthetic Practice*, 3e, 733–749. Philadelphia: Wolters Kluwer.

33 Allt-Graham, J. and Pegg, M.S. (1983). Potency changes of intravenous induction agents in the first ten weeks of life: an experiment using beagle dogs. *Vet. Res. Commun.* 7: 353–357.

34 Ikonomidou, C., Bosch, F., Miksa, M. et al. (1999). Blockade of NMDA receptors and apoptotic neurodegeneration in the developing brain. *Science* 283: 70–74.

35 Short, C.E. and Brunson, D.B. (1978). Anesthesia for small animal pediatric and geriatric patients. I. Anesthesia for small animal pediatric patients. *Cornell Vet.* 68 (Suppl 7): 9–14.

36 Goode, C.J., Titler, M., Rakel, B. et al. (1991). A meta-analysis of effects of heparin flush and saline flush: quality and cost implications. *Nurs. Res.* 40: 324–330.

37 Anand, K.J. and Hickey, P.R. (1987). Pain and its effects in the human neonate and fetus. *N. Engl. J. Med.* 317: 1321–1329.

38 Mathew, P.J. and Mathew, J.L. (2003). Assessment and management of pain in infants. *Postgrad. Med. J.* 79: 438–443.

39 Marshall, R.E., Porter, F.L., Rogers, A.G. et al. (1982). Circumcision: II. Effects upon mother-infant interaction. *Early Hum. Dev.* 7: 367–374.

40 Luks, A.M., Zwass, M.S., Brown, R.C. et al. (1998). Opioid-induced analgesia in neonatal dogs: pharmacodynamic differences between morphine and fentanyl. *J. Pharmacol. Exp. Ther.* 284: 136–141.

41 Morishima, H.O., Pedersen, H., Finster, M. et al. (1981). Toxicity of lidocaine in adult, newborn, and fetal sheep. *Anesthesiology* 55: 57–61.

42 Moldal, E.R., Eriksen, T., Kirpensteijn, J. et al. (2013). Intratesticular and subcutaneous lidocaine alters the intraoperative haemodynamic responses and heart rate variability in male cats undergoing castration. *Vet. Anaesth. Analg.* 40: 63–73.

43 Haga, H.A. and Ranheim, B. (2005). Castration of piglets: the analgesic effects of intratesticular and intrafunicular lidocaine injection. *Vet. Anaesth. Analg.* 32: 1–9.

44 Schroeder, C.A., Snyder, L.B.C., Tearney, C.C. et al. (2011). Ultrasound-guided transversus abdominis plane block in the dog: an anatomical evaluation. *Vet. Anaesth. Analg.* 38: 267–271.

20

Senior and Geriatric Concerns

Anderson Fávaro da Cunha

Department of Specialty Medicine, College of Veterinary Medicine, Midwestern University, Glendale, AZ, 85308, USA

Introduction

Age is not a disease; however, it is an important independent risk factor of morbidity and mortality [1, 2]. Age can be used as a predictor of perioperative outcome for anesthetized patients, as the odds for perioperative mortality in small-animal anesthesia are age-dependent [3, 4]. Morbidity and mortality studies suggest that a significant increase in mortality rate is observed in senior and geriatric patients, especially if they have comorbidities of the pulmonary, cardiac, renal, hepatic, and endocrine systems, alone or in combination [2, 5]. Even though age is an important variable considered during the preanesthetic evaluation, the deep understanding of the patient's physical status is even more important while formulating an anesthetic plan. This chapter critically reviews the most common physiological and pharmacological changes in the senior and geriatric dog and cat, and their differing responses to sedation and general anesthesia.

Defining the term "geriatric" is challenging in veterinary medicine. The patient's species, size, and breed are important variables used for the classification [6–8]. Accordingly, using the American Animal Hospital Association (AAHA) guidelines, the dog [6] and cat [7] senior and geriatric stages are defined in Tables 20.1 and 20.2, respectively. It is important to note that the physiological status of older patients is more relevant than their chronologic age [9, 10]. Geriatric patients can be further subclassified into different categories based on their physiological status (Table 20.3) [9].

Physiological Alterations

Respiratory System

As age progresses, respiratory function deteriorates [11–13]. The common weakening of the respiratory muscles and loss of elastic tissue observed in senior and geriatric patients, coupled with pulmonary fibrosis, lead to a decrease in chest wall compliance and elastic recoil of the lungs [14]. This is associated with a decrease in vital lung capacity, leading to a decreased functional residual capacity (FRC). These physiological changes predispose to atelectasis in senior and geriatric patients when under anesthesia or prolonged recumbency. Aged patients may also present with increased airway resistance, decreased pulmonary diffusion capacity, and decreased capillary blood

Canine and Feline Anesthesia and Co-Existing Disease, Second Edition. Edited by Rebecca A. Johnson, Lindsey B. C. Snyder and Carrie A. Schroeder.

Companion website: www.wiley.com/go/johnson/canine

Table 20.1 Definition of canine life stages [6].

Stage	Definition
Adult	Dog has reached physical maturity for breed and is no longer growing, social behavior consistent with adult of breed, lasts until dog transitions to senior
Senior	Follows adult stage and lasts until death, last 25% of dog's life span for breed
Geriatric	Time period after life expectancy has been reached

Table 20.2 Definition of feline life stages [7].

Stage	Age (years)
Young adult	3–6
Mature adult	7–10
Senior	11–14
Geriatric	>15

volume, all reducing expiratory efficiency and impairing gas exchange [13, 14]. Older patients also are increasingly susceptible to respiratory infections [14]. Altogether, these result in an increased susceptibility to perianesthetic hypoxemia, and oxygen supplementation is recommended. These patients should receive 100% oxygen for a minimum of 3 min prior to anesthetic induction via face mask (oxygen flows >150 $ml\,kg^{-1}\,min^{-1}$). Intra-anesthetic and postanesthetic oxygen support should be provided and dictated by pulse oximetry, or, in cases where hypoxemia is present or expected, arterial blood gas analysis. Oxygenation should be maintained with the goal of arterial (PaO_2) oxygen >80 mmHg or hemoglobin saturation of oxygen on the pulse oximeter (SpO_2) >95%; higher PaO_2 will be expected if 100% O_2 is delivered via endotracheal tube, as dictated by the alveolar gas equation (see Chapter 2). During anesthesia, intermittent positive pressure ventilation should be provided as necessary and dictated by capnography and blood gas analysis with the goal to maintain normal ventilation (end-tidal [$ETCO_2$] and arterial [$PaCO_2$] carbon dioxide between 35 and 45 mmHg).

Cardiovascular System

For the geriatric patient, cardiovascular diseases are a significant concern [15]. The aging process is correlated with common multifactorial

Table 20.3 Subclassification of the geriatric population [9, 11].

Classification	Definition	ASA status
1	Healthy geriatric patients—minor changes in organ function	II
2	Geriatric patients with subclinical organ dysfunction—decreased function of one or more organs such as the heart, liver, or kidneys	III
3	Geriatric patients with an obvious disease condition—severe clinical organ dysfunction (heart disease, endocrine disease, renal disease, or neoplasia)	IV, V

intrinsic physiologic changes in the cardiovascular system, including decreased baroreceptor activity and limited ability to adapt to hypotension, all leading to a reduced cardiac reserve [16]. Most of the common changes in the geriatric heart are primarily related to varying degrees of myocardial fibrosis, valvular fibrocalcification, and ventricular thickening [17]. The cardiac conduction system can also be compromised, leading to possible cardiac arrhythmias [17]. Therefore, drugs with negative inotropic or arrhythmogenic effects should be avoided or used with extreme caution.

It has been estimated that approximately 10% of dogs older than 5 years of age have mitral insufficiency and approximately 25% of dogs between 9 and 12 years of age have evidence of cardiac disease [14]. The risk increases to approximately 33% in dogs older than 13 years of age [14, 16]. The most common canine cardiovascular abnormalities are valvular heart diseases, dilated cardiomyopathy, pericardial diseases, arrhythmias, and systemic hypertension [3, 16, 18, 19]. In older cats, hypertrophic cardiomyopathy is the most common disease. These abnormalities can increase the odds of morbidity and mortality in the geriatric patient. History of exercise intolerance, arrhythmias, cyanosis, abnormal pulse quality, cardiac murmurs, and/or syncope indicates a need for a more extensive preanesthetic cardiac evaluation. Thus, in addition to a thorough history and physical exam, a complete geriatric cardiac profile includes thoracic radiography, electrocardiogram (ECG), blood work (complete blood count (CBC) and serum chemistry/electrolyte analysis), and echocardiography.

The most common cardiovascular side effect associated with sedation and general anesthesia is hypotension [20, 21]. It is essential for the anesthetist to ensure adequate blood pressure, euvolemia, venous return, and stroke volume to maintain normal tissue oxygen delivery [21]. Fluid rates should be based on individual need, hydration, and physical status. Often, older animals have compromised cardiac reserve and, therefore, fluid overload leading to congestive heart failure and/or pulmonary edema can easily occur. Total body water also decreases in the geriatric patient. Therefore, beat-to-beat cardiovascular monitoring with a dedicated anesthetist is imperative to quickly detect cardiovascular changes that could lead to anesthesia-related complications. If cardiovascular instability is expected, arterial catheterization and invasive blood pressure measurement are recommended. Treatment of possible complications such as hypotension, cardiac arrhythmias, or fluid overload should be provided as needed (see Chapter 1).

Hepatic System

With age, hepatic function deteriorates. During the geriatric phase of life, dogs and cats commonly experience decreased liver mass and hepatic blood flow secondary to reduced cardiac output, decreased microsomal enzyme activity, and generalized metabolic activity reduction [22]. Decreasing hepatic function may lead to hypoproteinemia, hypoglycemia, hypothermia, and coagulopathies. For all geriatric patients, liver function analysis and coagulation status are prudent prior to anesthesia or sedation, especially when highly metabolized drugs are to be used. Hypotension should be avoided, since it further decreases hepatic blood flow, exacerbating the possible ischemic hepatic damage that is associated with advanced age.

Central Nervous System (CNS)

The aged patient may have compromised cognitive, sensory, motor, and autonomic functions [23]. Aging may be correlated with decreasing anesthetic requirements (inhalants, benzodiazepines, opioids, barbiturates) due to a decrease in brain size, loss of neurons, increase in cerebrospinal fluid volume, depletion of neurotransmitters (dopamine, norepinephrine, tyrosine, and serotonin), [24–26] decrease in cerebral oxygen consumption, and myelin degeneration.

The geriatric thermoregulatory center is weakened and, therefore, older patients are more susceptible to anesthesia-induced hypothermia [27]. Bradyarrhythmias, hypotension, decreased minimal alveolar concentration (MAC) of volatile anesthetics, and shivering are associated with hypothermia. Moreover, shivering can increase oxygen consumption up to 400%; therefore, oxygen supplementation is important for any older patient [28].

Renal System

The incidence of renal disease has been reported to be approximately 0.5–1.5% in dogs and cats [29, 30]. The percentage increases with age; the most common renal disease occurring in elderly dogs and cats is chronic kidney disease [31]. Urinary incontinence, bladder neoplasia, and prostatic disease are also common. Decreased renal mass in senior and geriatric dogs and cats is associated with decreased tubular size and weight, decreased glomerular numbers, and filtration function [29–32]. Protein, water, and sodium reabsorption, aldosterone secretion, anionic and cationic compound secretion and reabsorption, vitamin D and renin formation, and elimination and metabolism of protein-bound compounds are all compromised in the geriatric patient [29–32]. These changes influence blood pressure regulation, acid–base status, and erythropoietin release, resulting in hyperphosphatemia, azotemia, dehydration, and hypoproteinemia.

In general terms, general anesthesia reduces cardiac output leading to an approximately 40% reduction in renal blood flow and glomerular filtration [27]. Older patients with cardiovascular diseases can have an exacerbated response. Additionally, decreases in cardiac output can worsen renal disease after general anesthesia and possibly lead to acute kidney insufficiency. Blood pressure, cardiac and urine output, hydration status, and renal function (urinalysis, blood urea nitrogen [BUN], and creatinine) monitoring is recommended. Preventing and treating any side effects as soon as possible, when necessary, and working to prevent physiologic derangements such as hypoxemia, hypervolemia, hypotension, and hypercarbia are imperative [27].

Gastrointestinal (GI) System

Patients undergoing anesthesia are at an increased risk of gastroesophageal reflux secondary to factors such as breed predisposition (Poodles, Labrador Retrievers, and German Shepherds) and positioning (Trendelenburg), among others [33]. Increased risk of gastroesophageal reflux during anesthesia, combined with possible laryngeal and pharyngeal function compromise (e.g., laryngeal paralysis or paresis), may be associated with higher risk of aspiration pneumonia in geriatric patients [34]. Proper endotracheal tube inflation and gentle esophageal suctioning before endotracheal extubation may decrease the risk of aspiration pneumonia. However, suctioning the esophagus alone does not change esophageal lumen pH, thus the risk of esophageal damage secondary to acid reflux remains. If regurgitation is observed during anesthesia or if gastric fluid is observed during esophageal suctioning prior to extubation, the following protocol may be followed to decrease the chances of esophageal damage that may lead to esophagitis and/or esophageal stricture: [35]

1) Flush the mouth well with warm saline (approximately $2\,ml\,kg^{-1}$) or until a clear solution comes out of the mouth (often five attempts are necessary).
2) Flush and suction the esophagus with warm saline (approximately $2\,ml\,kg^{-1}$) or until a clear solution comes out of suction hose (again, often five attempts are necessary).
3) Dilute sodium bicarbonate with saline to achieve a $40\,mg\,ml^{-1}$ solution.
4) Instill the bicarbonate solution into the esophagus (do not suction it out) [35].

Alternatively, the refluxate pH could be determined with pH paper. If the observed pH is higher than 4, the mouth and esophagus should be flushed well with warm saline. If the pH is less than 4, then warm bicarbonate solution (40 mg ml^{-1}) should be used for the esophageal flush as described in the preceding text. Great care must be taken to prevent the instillation of fluids into the trachea [35]. Warm tap water can be used for the oroesophageal flush using the aforementioned technique. However, if tap water is used, pulmonary aspiration of the fluid certainly must be avoided.

Gastrointestinal disorder management in the geriatric patient is similar to management in patients of any age. Management might include the addition of histamine H_2-receptor antagonists to reduce the amount of acid produced by stomach lining cells (e.g., famotidine), proton-pump inhibitors to reduce the production of acid (e.g., omeprazole), neurokinin-1 receptor antagonists used as antiemetic medications (e.g., maropitant citrate), and others. Anesthesia for gastrointestinal disorders should consider overall management of the geriatric patient and the disorder requiring anesthesia. For specifics of gastrointestinal disorders, please see Chapter 5.

Endocrine System

Hypoadrenocorticism, diabetes mellitus, and hypothyroidism are common conditions in the geriatric stage of dogs and cats. Older dogs may have decreased adrenal responsiveness to adrenocorticotropic hormone (ACTH) stimulation when compared with younger dogs [36]. Corticosteroid supplementation in the preanesthetic period may be beneficial because of the possibility of adrenal exhaustion in response to anesthetic and surgical stress [36]. Management of the geriatric patient with endocrine disorders should focus on the endocrine dysfunction itself in addition to the changes associated with aging. For specific endocrine management, please see Chapter 9.

Pharmacokinetic and Pharmacodynamic Considerations

In the elderly population, drug absorption, distribution, and elimination may be compromised. Dose adjustments are sometimes needed due to decreased drug clearance from organ dysfunction, drug–drug interactions, or greater drug sensitivity [9]. Dose adjustment or drug substitution with another of similar pharmacologic effect but different elimination route not affected by organ dysfunction or drug–drug interaction may mitigate problems [9]. For example, cats with renal dysfunction could benefit from the use of propofol, which has multiple metabolic pathways, over ketamine which is eliminated via the kidneys primarily unchanged. Choosing a drug with a wide safety margin (e.g., midazolam) is another option to minimize adverse drug effects due to decreased drug elimination in the aged patient [9]. Acepromazine can affect the geriatric patient for up to 72 h compared to the relatively short duration of midazolam in the same patient. All drug doses should be calculated on an individual basis, considering the route of metabolism and excretion [9]. The volume of distribution can also be affected by age. With a decrease in fat and muscle mass, drug dosages can typically be reduced as well.

Anesthetic Management of Senior and Geriatric Patients

Before designing an anesthetic protocol, the anesthetist should focus on understanding the possible comorbidities associated with the patient. A systematic physical evaluation followed by supporting laboratory and imaging data is always recommended [37]. Anesthetic plans should be tailored to the individual patient, but, in general, short-acting, reversible drugs are always recommended for the geriatric patient. However, the understanding of the individual physical condition is more important than drug choice, since many comorbidities can be stabilized prior to anesthetic induction, minimizing the odds of anesthesia-related complications. Close monitoring of various organ systems should start preinduction and be performed throughout the induction, maintenance, and recovery periods until the patient regains control of vital reflexes, consciousness, body temperature, normoglycemia, and coordination [36]. Monitoring should include the minimum standard of care that includes pulse oximetry, $ETCO_2$, blood pressure, and temperature. Due to anesthetic effects on the cardiovascular system, direct arterial blood pressure monitoring is recommended in the senior patient for most procedures. The ability to control ventilation is beneficial in these patients. Early detection and treatment of anesthesia-related cardiorespiratory side effects are key factors in decreasing anesthesia-related morbidity and mortality rates.

Preanesthetic Evaluation

For the senior and geriatric patient, the anesthetist must be aware of the comprehensive patient history, including current medications and their potential impact on anesthesia. This includes over-the-counter, prescription, and alternative medications and supplements [18, 37]. Special attention should be given to clinical changes and signs of pain, body weight and body condition, temperature, pulse, respirations, and cardiopulmonary auscultation. For example, a systematic physical evaluation in geriatric dogs revealed previously unrecognized (by the owners) problems in approximately 80% of one geriatric population; approximately 7.8 problems were identified per dog [37]. Pain was one important physical abnormality commonly unrecognized by the owners of that population [37]. The AAHA senior care guideline for dogs and cats suggests careful client communication before anesthesia [38].

Geriatric animals commonly have abnormalities in multiple organ systems making laboratory blood work critical to assess anesthetic-related risks, especially in patients receiving long-term medications for developing and/or chronic diseases [39]. The owner should be informed about possible procedural risks and benefits, and a written, informed consent obtained prior to anesthesia [18]. AAHA suggests that the minimum laboratory database for healthy-appearing senior dogs should include a CBC, complete urinalysis, and biochemical profile with electrolytes. For the senior and geriatric dog and cat, total T4 (cats specifically), ECG, blood pressure, cardiac auscultation, thoracic radiographs, and echocardiogram are recommended [18, 40]. However, based on initial history, examination, and laboratory results, more specific geriatric laboratory tests may be needed to assess specific organ systems [39].

Sedation

The use of reversible, short-acting drugs is typically recommended in the elderly patient. Intravenous fentanyl (2–10 $\mu g\,kg^{-1}$) or hydromorphone (0.05 $mg\,kg^{-1}$) combined with midazolam (0.1–0.2 $mg\,kg^{-1}$) causes adequate sedation in the sick patient and commonly reduces the induction agent dosage. Age itself is not a disease; however, it is often accompanied by comorbidities leading to patient compromise. In compromised patients, a fentanyl bolus in combination with midazolam may allow sufficient relaxation for endotracheal intubation without administration of induction agents. This practice is considered safe, as fentanyl and midazolam offer minimal cardiovascular side effects. The most common side effect of this drug combination is bradycardia, which is easily monitored and treated with anticholinergics. Therefore, atropine or glycopyrrolate should be readily available for the geriatric patient with cardiovascular disease associated with an intolerance to bradycardia (Chapter 1).

Alpha-2-adrenergic agonists should be used cautiously in geriatric patients, as they cause significant vasoconstriction, initial hypertension, decreased cardiac output, and bradyarrhythmias. Patient selection is essential. Acepromazine should be also avoided or used in low dosages to reduce the vasodilatory effect that can lead to hypotension.

Preoxygenation for at least 3 min with >150 ml kg^{-1} min^{-1} of 100% oxygen using a face mask prior to anesthetic induction is recommended for all patients [41]. However, this becomes increasingly important for the senior and geriatric patient (see the section titled "Respiratory System").

Anesthetic Induction and Maintenance

For the geriatric population, there is no evidence that one anesthetic drug is preferable for anesthetic induction and/or maintenance [42]. Based on the specific pharmacological properties of some drugs, they can be considered or not considered for a specific patient due to their specific coexisting disease. Drugs that heavily depend on liver metabolism and renal excretion are usually avoided or used with caution (e.g., ketamine). Alfaxalone, etomidate, and propofol are usually considered safe in the geriatric population when carefully titrated to effect, minimizing the total dose administered [43]. Alfaxalone and propofol cause dose-dependent vasodilation and decreased cardiac output [43]. Alfaxalone, etomidate, and propofol are all potent respiratory depressants; patients should be preoxygenated as described previously and immediately intubated for oxygen support. Etomidate may be recommended for the geriatric patient with an unstable cardiovascular system; however, it is associated with transient suppression of adrenocortical function and should be used cautiously in patients with adrenal disease [43].

Hypothermia and hypoglycemia are common anesthesia-related side effects in older patients. Monitoring body temperature and blood glucose throughout the procedure should be performed in any older patient and supplementation of heat and dextrose should be offered as needed [43].

Inhaled anesthetics or total intravenous anesthesia (TIVA) are often used for general anesthetic maintenance. Isoflurane and sevoflurane are potent vasodilatory agents and can cause significant hypotension when used in high concentrations. The MAC of these volatile anesthetics can be reduced by the addition of analgesic agent continuous rate infusions (CRIs); these may include fentanyl, remifentanil, lidocaine, or ketamine alone or in combination. Judicious monitoring is critical; the anesthetist must strive to maintain an ideal anesthetic plane for the procedure to minimize individual agent dosages and, therefore, adverse effects.

Fluid therapy is important in the perianesthetic period. Geriatric patients are often dehydrated, and careful fluid therapy is recommended. Geriatric patients often have limited cardiovascular reserve and a decrease in total body water and can be more prone to fluid overload. The fluid rate choice is based on the patient's hydration, cardiovascular, and electrolyte status (see Chapter 8).

Patient age (as a single parameter) is not enough justification for invasive monitoring. However, attentive monitoring during the entire anesthetic period and throughout recovery is recommended for older patients. Regardless of any coexisting conditions, ECG, $ETCO_2$, SpO_2, temperature, and blood pressure monitoring should be performed throughout anesthesia. Direct arterial blood pressure monitoring can improve the accuracy of data collected. Urinary output and arterial blood gas analysis can also be recommended. Mechanical ventilation is often recommended to provide adequate ventilation and minimize the physiological changes of age on the respiratory system.

Analgesic Techniques

Depending on CNS status of the elderly patient, the pain recognition can be challenging;

Table 20.4 Summary of the physiological differences observed in senior and geriatric dogs and cats.

Respiratory system	
↓	Rib cage compliance and elastic recoil of lungs
↓	Intercostal muscles strength
↑	Pulmonary fibrosis
↓	Vital lung capacity
↑	Airway resistance
↓	Pulmonary diffusion capacity
↓	Decreased capillary blood volume
↑	Respiratory infections
↑	Tendency to develop atelectasis
↓	Fractional residual capacity
Cardiovascular system	
↓	Blood pressure
↓	Blood volume
↓	Cardiac output
↓	Cardiac reserve
↑	Various heart diseases
↓	Baroreceptors activity
↑	Cardiac arrhythmias
Hepatic system	
↓	Hepatic blood flow
↓	Liver mass
↓	Microsomal enzyme activity
↓	Drug metabolism
↓	Gluconeogenic ability
↓	Albumin
↓	Coagulation
Central nervous system	
↓	Cognitive function
↓	Sensory function
↓	Motor and autonomic function
↓	Requirement for anesthetic drugs
↓	Cerebrospinal fluid volume
↓	Thermoregulatory center
↑	Susceptibility to hypothermia
↓	Neurotransmitters
↓	Cerebral oxygen consumption
Renal system	
↓	Renal mass
↓	Secretion of aldosterone
↓	Secretion and reabsorption of anionic and cationic compounds
↓	Formation of vitamin D and renin
↓	Elimination and metabolism of protein-bound compounds
↓	Filtration fraction
↓	Reabsorption of protein, water, and sodium
↑	Phosphatemia
↑	Creatinine
↓	Hydration status
↓	Proteinemia
Gastrointestinal system	
↑	Gastroesophageal reflux
↑	Laryngeal and pharyngeal function
↑	Risk of aspiration pneumonia
Pharmacokinetics	
↓	Drug absorption time
↓	Drug distribution time
↓	Drug elimination time
↓	Albumin–drug affinity
↓	Protein-bound

↑ = Increase, ↓ = Decrease, CNS = central nervous system.

however, common sense should be applied. For example, a painful lesion in an adult patient will very likely be painful for any other patient regardless of their age. Local anesthesia can be used and is very effective for all ages. Analgesic dose changes are often dependent on the patient's American Society of Anesthesiologist (ASA) status and/or specific disease states as opposed to patient age itself. However, geriatric patients frequently need dosage adjustments due to their aged state. Decreases in cardiac output and hepatic blood flow in the older patient can decrease or prolong metabolism and hepatic clearance of drugs [9]. Geriatric patients should always be treated for pain, but physiologic differences should be simultaneously considered.

Anesthetic Recovery

Due to age-related changes in the CNS, drug metabolism, hepatic, and renal systems, as well as a predisposition for hypotension and hypothermia, prolonged recoveries are common in elderly patients. The anesthetist should be ready to supplement oxygen and heat, and continuously monitor the cardiorespiratory system. Maintaining a controlled airway via intubation until the animal has coordinated swallowing efforts ensures less risk of aspiration pneumonia.

The same basic principles that guide pain management in the general population apply to the geriatric group [9]. Providing proper nursing care for recumbent animals, including warming, turning, human touch, and compassionate verbal encouragement, is recommended [18]. The AAHA senior care guidelines for dogs and cats also recommend that clients receive postoperative clear, concise, verbal, and written take-home instructions that include information about possible complications, drug effects, nursing care, nutritional management, home monitoring, and after-hours veterinary phone contacts [18].

Summary

Age is a multifactorial, all-encompassing process (Table 20.4). Consequently, there is not one ideal anesthetic plan that would be recommended for all geriatric patients. Individual coexisting diseases are considered more important than age itself, and, therefore, the anesthetist should understand all possible comorbidities prior to the beginning of the anesthesia process.

References

1 Brodbelt, D. (2009). Perioperative mortality in small animal anaesthesia. *Vet. J.* 182: 152–161.

2 Matthews, N.S., Mohn, T.J., Yang, M. et al. (2017). Factors associated with anesthetic-related death in dogs and cats in primary care veterinary hospitals. *J. Am. Vet. Med. Assoc.* 250: 655–665.

3 Brodbelt, D.C., Pfeiffer, D.U., Young, L.E. et al. (2008). Results of the confidential enquiry into perioperative small animal fatalities regarding risk factors for anesthetic-related death in dogs. *J. Am. Vet. Med. Assoc.* 233: 1096–1104.

4 Brodbelt, D.C., Blissitt, K.J., Hammond, R.A. et al. (2008). The risk of death: the confidential enquiry into perioperative small animal fatalities. *Vet. Anaesth. Analg.* 35: 365–373.

5 Hosgood, G. (2003). Evaluation of age and American Society of Anesthesiologists (ASA) physical status as risk factors for perianesthetic morbidity and mortality in the cat: response from 12:9, 2002. *J. Vet. Emerg. Crit. Care* 13: 44.

6 Bartges, J., Boyton, B., Vogt, A.H. et al. (2012). AAHA canine life stage guidelines. *J. Am. Anim. Hosp. Assoc.* 48: 1–11.

7 Vogt, A.H., Rodan, I., Brown, M. et al. (2010). AAFP-AAHA: feline life stage guidelines. *J. Am. Anim. Hosp. Assoc.* 46: 70–85.

8 Greer, K.A., Canterberry, S.C., and Murphy, K.E. (2007). Statistical analysis regarding the effects of height and weight on life span of the domestic dog. *Res. Vet. Sci.* 82: 208–214.

9 Kukanich, B. (2012). Geriatric veterinary pharmacology. *Vet. Clin. North Am. Small Anim. Pract.* 42: 631–642.

10 Silverstain, J.H. and Zaugg, M. (2006). Geriatrics. In: *Foundations of Anesthesia: Basic Sciences for Clinical Practice*, 2e (eds. H. HCaH and H. Philip), 835–844. Philadelphia: Mosby Elsevier.

11 Robinson, N.E. and Gillespie, J.R. (1973). Morphologic features of the lungs of aging

beagle dogs. *Am. Rev. Respir. Dis.* 108: 1192–1199.

12 Robinson, N.E. and Gillespie, J.R. (1973). Lung volumes in aging beagle dogs. *J. Appl. Phys.* 35: 317–321.

13 Robinson, N.E. and Gillespie, J.R. (1975). Pulmonary diffusing capacity and capillary blood volume in aging dogs. *J. Appl. Phys.* 38: 647–650.

14 MacDougall, D.F. and Barker, J. (1984). An approach to canine geriatrics. *Br. Vet. J.* 140: 115–123.

15 Miller, M.S., Tilley, L.P., and Smith, F.W. Jr. (1989). Cardiopulmonary disease in the geriatric dog and cat. *Vet. Clin. North Am. Small Anim. Pract.* 19: 87–102.

16 Saunders, A.B. (2012). The diagnosis and management of age-related veterinary cardiovascular disease. *Vet. Clin. North Am. Small Anim. Pract.* 42: 655–668.

17 Wei, J.Y. (1992). Age and the cardiovascular system. *N. Engl. J. Med.* 327: 1735–1739.

18 Senior Care Guidelines Task Force et al. (2005). AAHA senior care guidelines for dogs and cats. *J. Am. Anim. Hosp. Assoc.* 41: 81–91.

19 Guglielmini, C. (2003). Cardiovascular diseases in the ageing dog: diagnostic and therapeutic problems. *Vet. Res. Commun.* 27: 555–560.

20 Paddleford, R.R. (1999). Anesthetic considerations in patients with preexisting problems or concerns. In: *Manual of Small Animal Anesthesia*, 2e (ed. R.R. Paddleford), 267–317. New York: Churchill Livingstone.

21 Hughes, J. (2008). Anaesthesia for the geriatric dog and cat. *Ir. Vet. J.* 61: 380–387.

22 Mosier, J.E. (1989). Effect of aging on body systems of the dog. *Vet. Clin. North Am. Small Anim. Pract.* 19: 1–12.

23 Devaney, K.O. and Johnson, H.A. (1980). Neuron loss in the aging visual cortex of man. *J. Gerontol.* 35: 836–841.

24 Carpenter, R.E., Pettifer, G.R., and Tranquilli, W.J. (2005). Anesthesia for geriatric patients. *Vet. Clin. North Am. Small Anim. Pract.* 35: 571–580.

25 Stevens, W.C., Dolan, W.M., Gibbons, R.T. et al. (1975). Minimum alveolar concentrations (MAC) of isoflurande with and without nitrous oxide in patients of various ages. *Anesthesiology* 42: 197–200.

26 Gregory, G.A., Eger, E.I. 2nd, and Munson, E.S. (1969). The relationship between age and halothane requirement in man. *Anesthesiology* 30: 488–491.

27 Harvey, R.C. and Paddleford, R.R. (1999). Management of geriatric patients. A common occurrence. *Vet. Clin. North Am. Small Anim. Pract.* 29: 683–699.

28 Ralley, F.E., Wynands, J.E., Ramsay, J.G. et al. (1988). The effects of shivering on oxygen consumption and carbon dioxide production in patients rewarming from hypothermic cardiopulmonary bypass. *Can. J. Anaesth.* 35: 332–337.

29 Krawiec, D.R. (1989). Urologic disorders of the geriatric dog. *Vet. Clin. North Am. Small Anim. Pract.* 19: 75–85.

30 Polzin, D.J. (2011). Chronic kidney disease in small animals. *Vet. Clin. North Am. Small Anim. Pract.* 41: 15–30.

31 Bartges, J.W. (2012). Chronic kidney disease in dogs and cats. *Vet. Clin. North Am. Small Anim. Pract.* 42: 669–692.

32 Aucoin, D.P. (1989). Drug therapy in the geriatric animal: the effect of aging on drug disposition. *Vet. Clin. North Am. Small Anim. Pract.* 19: 41–47.

33 Rodriguez-Alarcon, C.A., Beristain-Ruiz, D.M., Rivera-Barreno, R. et al. (2015). Gastroesophageal reflux in anesthetized dogs: a review. *Rev. Colom. Cienc. Pecua.* 28: 144–155.

34 Pontoppidan, H. and Beecher, H.K. (1960). Progressive loss of protective reflexes in the airway with the advance of age. *J. Am. Med. Assoc.* 174: 2209–2213.

35 Wilson, D.V. and Evans, A.T. (2007). The effect of topical treatment on esophageal pH during acid reflux in dogs. *Vet. Anaesth. Analg.* 34: 339–343.

36 Hartsfield, S.M. (1990). Anesthetic problems of the geriatric dental patient. *Probl. Vet. Med.* 2: 24–45.

37 Davies, M. (2012). Geriatric screening in first opinion practice – results from 45 dogs. *J. Small Anim. Pract.* 53: 507–513.

38 Creevy, K.E., Grady, J., Little, S.E. et al. (2019). 2019 AAHA canine life stage guidelines. *J. Am. Anim. Hosp. Assoc.* 55: 267–290.

39 Edinboro, C.H., Scott-Moncrieff, J.C., and Glickman, L.T. (2010). Feline hyperthyroidism: potential relationship with iodine supplement requirements of commercial cat foods. *J. Feline Med. Surg.* 12: 672–679.

40 Metzger, F.L. and Rebar, A.H. (2012). Clinical pathology interpretation in geriatric veterinary patients. *Vet. Clin. North Am. Small Anim. Pract.* 42: 615–629.

41 Ambros, B., Carrozzo, M.V., and Jones, T. (2018). Desaturation times between dogs preoxygenated via face mask or flow-by technique before induction of anesthesia. *Vet. Anaesth. Analg.* 45: 452–458.

42 Hines, R.L. and Marschall, K.E. (2018). Diseases of aging. In: *Stoelting's Anesthesia and Co-existing Disease*, 7e (eds. K.E. Marschall and R.L. Hines), 327–343. Philadelphia: Elsevier.

43 Short, C.E. and Brunson, D.B. (1978). Anesthesia for small animal pediatric and geriatric patients. *Cornell Vet.* 68: 9–14.

21

Disorders Related to Trauma

Andre Shih[1, 2]

[1] *Department of Large Animal Clinical Sciences, University of Florida, Gainesville, FL, 32608, USA*
[2] *Capital Veterinary Specialists, Jacksonville, FL, 32609, USA*

Introduction

Anesthesia for the trauma patient can be one of the most difficult subcategories of anesthesia, since trauma is not one specific disease. In physiologic terms, trauma is a combination of severe tissue injury, hemorrhage, and inflammation, and can vary in degree of intensity, type of trauma, and injury location. Examples may include, but are not limited to, contusions, penetrating trauma, trauma of the head, thorax, or abdomen, and orthopedic injury. Each carries a subset of triage parameters.

Anesthesia for severe trauma patients is very challenging and best performed by experienced and well-trained personnel. Patients should be stabilized before anesthesia if possible. All anesthetic/analgesic agents promote some degree of cardiovascular impairment and there is no completely safe anesthetic protocol. All cases should be evaluated individually, and protocols modified according to the disease pathophysiology and clinician's physical examination of the patient. Continuous patient monitoring and reevaluation, together with a vigilant anesthetist, is probably the best solution to reduce morbidity during the perianesthetic period.

Vital sign evaluation, including level of consciousness and airway adequacy, breathing, and circulation, should be the first step in the triage of severe traumatic injury patients. Initial treatment should be rapid and center on improvement of oxygen delivery. In this chapter, we will discuss anesthetic and analgesic options to be used in patients with severe traumatic injury.

According to the veterinary literature, trauma patients represent more than 13% of all referred cases [1, 2]. Trauma is defined as transfer of energy to a living tissue, producing injury and pathology [3]. In humans, the presence of concurrent traumatic injuries affecting multiple body areas can be considered severe trauma or polytrauma [4]. The term polytrauma has been better defined in humans via an Injury Severity Score (ISS) [5]. The body regions evaluated for ISS determination are the head, face, thorax, abdomen, and extremities. The injury severity to each of the three most severely affected body regions is assigned a score on a scale from 1 to 6 (1 for minor trauma and 6 for untreatable trauma). Each score is squared, and the patient's ISS is obtained by summation of these three scores. Polytrauma is then defined as an ISS value greater than 16, a level that has been correlated with increased

Canine and Feline Anesthesia and Co-Existing Disease, Second Edition. Edited by Rebecca A. Johnson, Lindsey B. C. Snyder and Carrie A. Schroeder.

Companion website: www.wiley.com/go/johnson/canine

mortality, morbidity, and hospitalization time [4]. Unfortunately, in veterinary medicine, there is neither any unanimous consensus on the definition of severe trauma, nor on the classification of the severity of injury [6].

Initial Patient Evaluation

Severe trauma patients usually present with reduced vital organ reserve capacity, hypovolemic shock, tissue hypoxia, electrolyte disturbances, anaerobic metabolism, and a hypermetabolic state. Initial stabilization is recommended before anesthesia is attempted. In 1989, the American College of Surgeons Committee on Trauma created trauma protocols, which are also known as the "ABCDE" of trauma [3, 7]. The main objective of the initial trauma protocol is to ensure efficient reestablishment of vital organ perfusion and to maximize oxygen delivery (DO_2). Cardiac output (CO), blood hemoglobin concentration, and hemoglobin oxygen saturation are major factors in determination of global oxygen delivery [8]. Initial patient evaluation should be rapid and centered on provision of life support. Vital sign evaluation, including level of consciousness and adequacy of airway, breathing, and circulation, should be the first step of triage. Initial treatment should make sure the "airway" (A) is patent with no signs of obstruction. Head and face trauma patients are at risk of tracheal tear or maxillary fracture. Both can cause complete airway obstruction and will need immediate intubation. Following that, it is necessary to ensure the patient is "breathing" (B) with no signs of hypoxia. Most trauma patients benefit from an enriched oxygen environment (such as flow-by oxygen or via tight face mask). Preoxygenation will replace function residual capacity (FRC) nitrogen with oxygen decreasing risk of hypoxia during induction time [3, 8].

As patients are preoxygenated, monitoring equipment should simultaneously be connected. The "circulation" (C) should be assessed through heart rate, pulse quality, blood pressure monitoring, and biochemical markers such as lactate and hematocrit [3, 9, 10]. Before anesthesia, patients should receive a thorough physical examination, complemented by basic hemodynamic monitoring and relevant blood work [11].

Venous access is imperative in trauma patients for fluid, blood product, and inotrope administration. Animals should have, at a minimum, a large bore catheter preplaced before anesthetic induction. Animals with a low hematocrit (<22%) or are in severe hemorrhagic shock may benefit from red blood cell (RBC) transfusion [11]. During anesthesia, the hematocrit can drop by 3–5%, making even small blood losses significant and warranting blood transfusion [10, 11].

Finally, (D) represents "neurological disturbance" and involves assessing the patient's mental status and any neurological damage (spinal or lower neuron). It is a common mistake to miss step (D). For example, a polytrauma patient arrives with an open femur fracture; you quickly assess airway, breathing, and circulation, and start setting up a plan for surgical limb stabilization. However, it is important to ensure that the patient has an intact sciatic nerve and can feel pain in the distal limb. It is also important to ensure there is no spinal trauma. Neurological disturbance will dramatically change the prognosis and how one may proceed with surgery.

The (E) represents "external wounds." Examine the entire body to ensure that puncture or penetrating wounds are not missed. Even a small external puncture wound may represent a deep internal injury. This is particularly true in dog bites and gunshot wounds. External wounds will prompt one to rule out life-threatening internal injuries such as pneumothorax or intracavity effusion.

The implementation of point-of-care ultrasound (POCUS) has significantly impacted the emergency evaluation of trauma patients [12, 13]. Ultrasound is easy to use, noninvasive, employs no radiation, and can be moved to the patient "bed side." The abdominal-focused assessment (AFAST) and thoracic-focused assessment (TFAST) (with sonography for trauma, triage, and tracking) constitute examinations that focus on identifying the presence of fluid within the peritoneal, pleural, and pericardial spaces.

In brief, the AFAST consists of four windows: (i) the diaphragmatic–hepatic (DH), (ii) splenorenal (SR), (iii) cystocolic (CC), and (iv) hepatorenal (HR) windows [12, 13]. For the DH window, the transducer is placed in a subxiphoid location. Sufficient image depth and cranial angulation of the beam are necessary to visualize the gallbladder, hepatic parenchyma, and curvilinear diaphragm–lung interface (it is also one of the windows for TFAST). With the patient positioned in left lateral recumbency, the SR window will be located within the dependent flank behind last rib. This window is defined as the interface between the echotexture of the spleen and the kidney. To generate the CC window, the probe is placed caudally along midline, and the urinary bladder and the ventral surface of the colon are located. The HR window can be located near the last rib; the right kidney is located within the renal fossa of the caudate process of the caudate lobe of the liver. Cavitary effusions are often found adjacent to viscera and appear anechoic. Presence of effusion could indicate hemoabdomen, uroabdomen, or visceral trauma.

The TFAST examination involves assessment of both hemithorax for pleural space disease (presence of gas or effusion) and pericardial effusion. The probe position for identifying gas within the pleural space has been described as the "chest tube site": dorsolateral along the thoracic wall within the 7th–9th intercostal spaces. From this position, the interface between the pulmonary (visceral) pleural surface with the costal (parietal) pleural surface is identified. In a normal individual, the rhythmic to-and-fro motion at this interface constitutes a "glide sign." The absence of a glide sign is indicative of gas within the pleural space. If pneumothorax is identified in a dyspneic patient, therapeutic thoracocentesis is indicated. The "pericardium site" is used to evaluate pleural effusion or pericardium effusion. The probe is positioned ventrolateral along the thoracic wall, within the 5th–6th intercostal spaces. Presence of fluid within the pericardial sac can indicate cardiac tamponade [12–14].

Anesthesia in Severe Trauma Patients

As previously mentioned, aesthesia of severe trauma patients is a challenging and stressful event, since anesthetic agents have the potential to cause varying degrees of cardiovascular and respiratory depression. Furthermore, anesthetic drugs will blunt sympathetic drive and inhibit physiologic autoregulatory mechanisms that maintain adequate blood pressure and CO in trauma victims [9]. It is, therefore, common for trauma patients to suffer catastrophic cardiovascular collapse following anesthetic induction.

Before anesthetic induction, all animals should be preoxygenated for at least 3–5 min and noninvasive monitoring equipment connected. In general, essential monitoring equipment consists of an electrocardiogram (ECG) and pulse oximeter, together with noninvasive blood pressure. A capnograph should be connected once the patient is intubated and invasive blood pressure may be monitored via arterial catheterization in cardiovascular unstable patients.

Sometimes there is a need to perform emergency procedures with little "heads up" anesthesia warning time. A prewritten checklist for the anesthesia area will ensure that all equipment is working properly and that no steps have been overlooked due to haste, allowing anesthetic induction to proceed smoothly (Table 21.1) [15].

Total anesthetic time has been correlated with an increase in both morbidity and mortality [16, 17]. Longer anesthetic time increases

Table 21.1 Preoperative checklist.

( ) or N/A: oxygen source operational
( ) or N/A: anesthesia machine pressure tested
( ) or N/A: endotracheal tube and laryngoscope present
( ) or N/A: monitoring equipment operational
( ) or N/A: infusion pump/fluid setup ready
( ) or N/A: inotropes drawn and available
( ) or N/A: preoperative drugs and antibiotics present
( ) or N/A: drug cart stocked and updated
( ) or N/A: crash cart stocked and updated
( ) or N/A: patient has an IV catheter, surgical site preclipped
( ) or N/A: patient crossmatched and blood bank ready

N/A: not applicable.

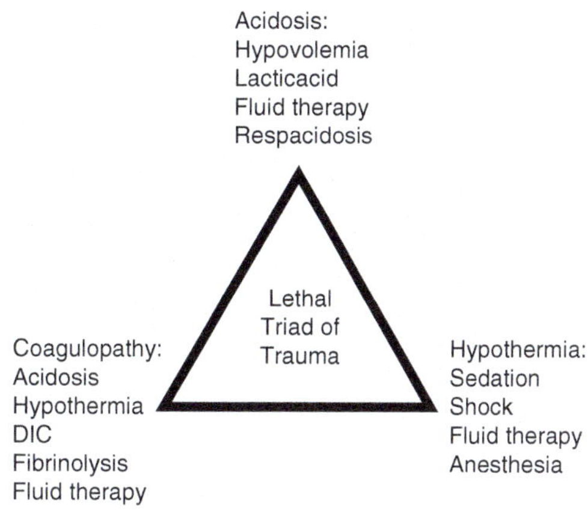

Figure 21.1 Lethal triad of trauma. These factors are interconnected and if left untreated, will increase morbidity and mortality following trauma. In animals requiring general anesthesia, the severity of one or all these factors may be compounded with increased anesthetic time.

the risk of hypothermia, acidosis, and coagulopathy. The combination of acidosis, hypothermia, and coagulopathy is known as the "lethal triad of trauma" (Figure 21.1). It is important to appreciate that those factors are interconnected, and that anesthesia may compound the triad (Figure 21.1) [18–20].

Trauma patients commonly arrive with hemorrhagic/hypovolemic shock. Low tissue oxygenation and compensatory vasoconstriction in the face of hypovolemia result in anaerobic metabolism and lactic acidosis. Acidosis can be compounded by high chloride-containing fluids such as normal (0.9% NaCl) and hypertonic (approximately 7.0–7.5% NaCl) saline. Metabolic acidosis can worsen if sedation or general anesthesia causes a superimposed respiratory acidosis (hypercapnia). Acidosis leads to denaturation of proteins, further impairing the coagulation cascade (coagulopathy), and reduces the effectiveness of many inotropes/vasopressors (i.e., epinephrine, norepinephrine, etc.) [18]. Trauma patients with altered mental status can present hypothermic. Anesthesia leads to vasodilation and decreases the shivering reflex, worsening heat loss. Hypothermia has profound implications on pharmacokinetics, glycemic control, infection risk, wound healing, dysrhythmias, and again coagulopathies.

Severe trauma can lead to excessive release of tissue factors, increases in fibrinolysis, and consumption of coagulation factors. Overzealous use of fluid therapy can also lead to dilution coagulopathy [19, 20].

Anesthetists should preserve normothermia (warm the environment/fluids, use blankets and active warmers, etc.), avoid hypoxemia/hypercarbia (secure the airway and ventilate patient if needed), and choose appropriate fluid therapy. The use of blood components and antifibrinolytic medications such as tranexamic acid or aminocaproic acid should be considered. The anesthesia, radiology, and surgery teams should actively communicate to ensure an efficient workflow with no unnecessary time under anesthesia [15]. Preclipping/cleaning of the wound(s) and having the surgical team in sterile gowns before induction can also minimize total anesthesia time. Performing an introduction of team members and verifying the patient "check list" prior to induction will also conserve anesthesia time (Table 21.1).

Anesthesia should be achieved with short-acting, reversible drugs that have minimal cardiovascular effects. Due to the wide range of trauma severity and significant homeostatic changes in traumatized patients, there is no set dosage for any given anesthetic or analgesic drug. Generally, severe trauma patients require less anesthetic agent for equivalent effect. It is recommended to start at a fraction of the published dose (Table 21.2) and then titrate based on patient response. Endotracheal intubation should always be performed in anesthetized trauma patients. Anesthetic maintenance can be obtained using inhalant anesthetics (Table 21.3), intravenous anesthetic infusion, or a combination of both [21]. One should aim for the minimum anesthetic dose necessary to keep patient relaxed. Use of analgesic infusions will greatly reduce the dose of inhalant anesthetic necessary. Appropriate use of locoregional anesthesia may also decrease the systemic anesthetic and analgesic requirements.

Essential monitoring includes ECG, blood pressure (invasive or noninvasive), capnography, and pulse oximetry. A dedicated, trained person should be constantly evaluating physiologic parameters as well as depth of anesthesia, reviewed elsewhere [22]. During recovery, the patient may still require cardiopulmonary support, and hemodynamic monitoring should be continued into the postoperative period in the intensive or critical care unit. Exercise caution when transporting patients from the surgical suite or procedure area to site of postanesthetic monitoring. Trauma patients may be hemodynamically unstable and continuous monitoring should be provided during the transport process.

Trauma patients present with a vast array of physiological derangements that require specific care. Specific trauma cases (head, thoracic/abdominal, orthopedic) are discussed in the following text.

Head Trauma

Cerebral perfusion pressure (CPP) is dictated by the difference between the mean arterial blood pressure (MAP) and the intracranial pressure (ICP). Patients with head trauma may have a reduced CPP due to a low MAP and increased ICP [23, 24]. To avoid cerebral hypoperfusion (decreased CPP), it is important to avoid (or treat) hypotension. Excessive hypertension can, however, elevate ICP and be detrimental to the CPP [10, 25]. Initial fluid therapy of choice is hypertonic saline followed by conservative dosing of isotonic crystalloid [25–27]. Early use of inotropes is also beneficial to avoid catastrophic hypotension. Patients that have been adequately fluid-resuscitated may need vasopressors to maintain MAP and CPP when inotropes are not being effective; maintaining adequate MAP is crucial in head trauma patients.

Anesthesia is often necessary in head trauma cases to allow diagnostic and curative procedures. General anesthesia can, however, have therapeutic value and may be helpful for patients with severe head trauma. Many anesthetics reduce metabolic rate and oxygen consumption and lower the cerebral oxygen requirement; general anesthesia may allow for permissive hypothermia and aggressive ventilator support to be instituted. Anesthetic drugs reduce excitatory neurotransmitters such as glutamate, which will reduce further cell damage [21, 28].

On the other hand, improper anesthesia can cause a decrease in CPP [21]. Under normal circumstances, the central nervous system (CNS) is equipped with an autoregulatory system that maintains constant blood flow and ICP despite changes in MAP. This protective mechanism maintains constant CPP and ICP despite significant fluctuation in systemic blood pressure (MAP from approximately 50 to 150 mmHg) [21, 24, 25]. In other words, autoregulation protects the brain against day-to-day fluctuations in blood pressure. Some anesthetic drugs, particularly the volatile anesthetics, will blunt the brain's autoregulation of blood flow and promote a linear shift of ICP with changes in MAP (see Chapter 3). Inhalant anesthetic drugs will also promote a dose-dependent vasodilation and increase in ICP [15, 21].

Table 21.2 Analgesic and sedative drug classes and comments.

Drug class	Effect and side effects	Use in trauma
Alpha-2 agonists (e.g., dexmedetomidine)	Reliable muscle relaxation, analgesia, and sedation. Allows for dose titration and can be reversed. Side effects include vasoconstriction, drop in cardiac output, and bradycardia.	Not recommended in patients who are hypovolemic, dehydrated, or in shock.
Nonsteroid anti-inflammatory drugs (NSAIDs)	Good analgesic and anti-inflammatory properties. Side effects include inhibition of renal protective mechanisms and gastrointestinal bleeding.	Not recommended in patients who are hypovolemic, dehydrated, or in shock.
Corticosteroids	Good analgesic and anti-inflammatory properties. Side effects include inhibition of renal protective mechanisms, gastrointestinal bleeding, immunosuppression, and hypernatremia. May compound NSAID side effects.	Not recommended in patients who are hypovolemic, dehydrated, or in shock.
Phenothiazines (e.g., acepromazine)	Reliable muscle relaxation and sedation. No analgesic properties. Side effects include vasodilation and hypotension.	Not recommended in patients who are hypovolemic, dehydrated, or in shock.
Opioids	Excellent analgesia and good sedation. Act on opioid receptors and allow for dose titration. Side effects are reversible with use of antagonists (e.g., naloxone).	Excellent for polytrauma patients. Titrate drug to effect.
Local anesthetics	Block nerve action potentials and pain recognition. Trivial systemic side effects at recommended doses.	Regional anesthesia is an excellent alternative to provide analgesia in trauma.
Systemic lidocaine	Decreases spontaneous action potential firing. Side effects include sedation, seizures, vasoconstriction, and decreases in cardiac output (worse in cats).	Not recommended for use in cats.
Benzodiazepines (e.g., midazolam)	Good muscle relaxation and sedation when combined with opioids. No analgesic properties. Minimal cardiovascular side effects.	Good adjunctive sedative drug in polytrauma patients.
NMDA receptor antagonists (e.g., ketamine)	Reduce central sensitization and "wind-up pain." Good choice for chronic pain. Decrease excitatory neurotransmitters in brain.	To be used in an intravenous infusion.
Tramadol	Good analgesic in some species in combination with NSAIDs. Acts on opioid, serotoninergic, and adrenergic receptors.	A good analgesic option in some species; however, it requires oral administration.
Trazodone	Mild sedative with little cardiovascular effects. No analgesic properties.	Must be administered orally.

Head trauma patients usually have reduced neuronal activity, making them more sensitive to anesthetic drugs. Comatose patients can be easily intubated with the use of only mild sedatives (e.g., benzodiazepines). Once the initial neurologic examination and stabilization have occurred, patients can be sedated with a combination of a benzodiazepine and an opioid.

Table 21.3 Anesthetic drug classes and comments.

Drug class	Effect and side effects	Use in trauma
Propofol	Good induction drug with rapid onset and rapid recovery. Reduces intracranial pressure. Can cause respiratory depression and hypotension.	Titrate to effect. Use with care in patients who are hypovolemic or in shock. Good option for total intravenous anesthesia (TIVA).
Alfaxalone	Good induction drug with rapid onset and rapid recovery. Patients maintain gag reflex.	Titrate to effect. Good option for trauma patients.
Etomidate	Patients maintain good cardiovascular status and gag reflex. Suppresses adrenocortical function.	Adrenal suppression is not a desired effect in trauma. Not recommended in patients who are in shock.
Benzodiazepines (e.g., midazolam)	Good muscle relaxation and sedation when combined with opioids. Used in combination with propofol or ketamine for induction.	Good adjunctive anesthetic drug in polytrauma patients.
NMDA receptor antagonists (e.g., ketamine, tiletamine)	Good induction with mild analgesic properties. Patients maintain gag reflex. Decrease CNS excitatory neurotransmitters.	Good adjunctive anesthetic/analgesic drug in polytrauma patients.
Inhalant anesthetics (isoflurane, sevoflurane)	Good maintenance drugs. Cause dose-dependent cardiovascular depression, vasodilation, and respiratory depression.	Consider addition of sedative or analgesic infusions to reduce inhalant concentration.

Vomiting, retching, and gagging can cause severe elevation of ICP; therefore, preference should be given to opioids that have a low incidence of vomiting (e.g., methadone, fentanyl, buprenorphine, or butorphanol). Preemptive use of antiemetics such as maropitant or ondansetron may also be indicated. Use of intravenous lidocaine to decrease the cough response at induction (with its possible effects on ICP) may also be useful [29].

Anesthetic induction can be achieved with propofol, which is excellent for decreasing the cerebral oxygen requirement and reducing ICP [24, 25]. Another advantage of this agent is that cerebral autoregulation remains intact [21, 24, 25]. Classically, induction with ketamine as a sole agent has been contraindicated because it can cause systemic hypertension and increased cerebral oxygen consumption. However, there is evidence that low dosages of ketamine can have a neuroprotective effect following head trauma, probably due to its N-methyl-D-aspartate (NMDA) receptor antagonist effect (Table 21.3).

Inhalant anesthetics can cause dose-dependent intracranial vasodilation, hypoventilation, and elevation of ICP. If administered at or above minimum alveolar concentration (MAC), inhalants can also promote loss of cerebral autoregulation [25]. When this occurs, fluctuations in blood pressure generate detrimental fluctuations in CPP and ICP. Inhalant anesthetic should be kept under MAC if ever used. Anesthetic maintenance for head trauma victims can be achieved with partial or total intravenous anesthesia (TIVA). This can be accomplished through propofol infusions in combination with a short-acting opioid such as remifentanil or fentanyl. Infusions in the postanesthetic period can be temporarily discontinued to conduct neurological assessment and then recommenced [30, 31].

All anesthetic drugs have the potential to cause varying degrees of hypoventilation and transient increases in carbon dioxide, which can impact cerebral vasodilation and increase ICP. Following anesthetic induction, patients should be immediately intubated and intermittent positive pressure ventilation (IPPV) commenced. During anesthesia, it is preferable to maintain normocapnia ($PaCO_2$ is approximately 30–35 mmHg) and normoxia (PaO_2>90 mmHg) to avoid increases in ICP [24, 25]. Hypothermia will lower the cerebral metabolic rate of oxygen (CMRO2); patients with head trauma may benefit from mild hypothermia (approximately 96–98 °F) throughout the procedure [30–32].

Head trauma patients release catecholamines, cytokines, and cortisol which will increase gluconeogenesis and cause hyperglycemia. Persistent hyperglycemia has a negative prognosis in head trauma patients. It will stimulate glutamate, release free radicals, and cause cerebral edema. One should monitor glucose levels every hour throughout the anesthetic period including recovery and administer (regular) insulin intraoperatively if needed [32, 33].

Other electrolyte derangements that can occur during anesthesia are hypernatremia and hyponatremia. Head injuries can lead to inappropriate release of vasopressin (antidiuretic hormone [ADH]) and excessive reabsorption of free water with a subsequent decrease in sodium levels. On the other hand, pituitary damage associated with head trauma may lead to diabetes insipidus (lack of ADH) and hypernatremia may also occur. Both high and low sodium levels are detrimental to patients and should be corrected [30–33].

A sudden reduction in heart rate accompanied by severe hypertension (Cushing reflex) may be a sign of severely elevated ICP. Intracranial hypertension can be treated with mannitol (0.5–1.0 $g\,kg^{-1}$) and hypertonic saline (2–4 $ml\,kg^{-1}$) boluses; steroid use has not been effective in reducing ICP [32]. The use of long-acting steroids has also been reported to increase morbidity in head trauma patients and is no longer indicated [32].

During anesthetic recovery, it is important to make sure that the patient can properly ventilate ($PaCO_2 < 45$ mmHg) and has a gag reflex prior to extubation. Patients that are unable to maintain normocapnia or cannot effectively maintain protective airway reflexes should remain sedated, intubated, and ventilated, as necessary. Postoperative analgesia may be achieved as necessary with the use of opioids and/or low-dose ketamine (3–5 $\mu g\,kg^{-1}\,min^{-1}$). Nonsteroidal anti-inflammatory drugs (NSAIDs) should be avoided in hypovolemic patients or patients with questionable renal function.

Thoracic and Abdominal Trauma

Most thoracic and abdominal trauma is due to blunt force or penetrating injury [10]. These patients are prone to pneumothorax, diaphragmatic hernia, pulmonary contusions, and pericardial, thoracic, and/or abdominal effusion. Following initial stabilization and physical examination, diagnostics should include chest radiographs and abdominal ultrasound (AFAST and TFAST) together with assessment of blood pressure, hematocrit, blood gases, and serum biochemical profile. Severe trauma patients can have a sudden decrease in circulating blood volume due to hemorrhage, leading to a reduction in venous return and resulting hypovolemic shock. Hypovolemic shock is characterized by a decrease in CO with an increase in systemic vascular resistance (SVR) [9, 34]. If the hypovolemia is not corrected, factors maintaining the high SVR (vasoconstriction) will no longer be able to compensate, and the patient will progress to a hypodynamic stage [35]. Hypodynamic shock is characterized by a decrease in CO accompanied by a decrease in SVR (vasodilation) and resistance to inotropes [35, 36].

Initial therapy for hypovolemic shock consists of appropriate fluid therapy and use of inotropes and/or vasopressors to ensure adequate arterial blood pressure [34–37]. As mentioned before, excessive fluid therapy can lead to hemodilution worsening of coagulopathy and increase in blood loss (Figure 21.1). Overly aggressive fluid resuscitation and aiming for supraphysiologic blood pressure values may cause blood clots to be dislodged and further increase bleeding. The combination of hypertonic saline with the minimum crystalloid dose necessary to maintain MAP at approximately 60 mmHg is an appropriate fluid therapy choice to treat moderate uncontrolled hemorrhage [35, 36]. If there are signs of severe hemorrhage or anemia (signs of low DO_2) [35], early use of blood products (fresh blood or packed RBCs) is indicated. Catastrophic uncontrolled hemorrhage requires immediate and aggressive fluid therapy to maintain CO until surgical hemostasis can be performed.

Unfortunately, an accurate assessment of the patient's volume status and the ability to predict the effects of fluid therapy are often difficult [38, 39]. Traditional variables used as indicators of preload to guide fluid resuscitation, such as central venous pressure (CVP), MAP, and blood lactate concentration, are unable to consistently predict the hemodynamic response to a fluid challenge [39–42]. A better method is therefore needed to guide fluid therapy during anesthesia [43]. Assessment of preload through monitoring of pulse pressure variation (PPV) on arterial waveforms, total end-diastolic volume from repeated cardiac echocardiograms, and/or direct CO measurements can serve as better guides to fluid therapy [43–45]. When an arterial line is not available for PPV measurements, one can use the plethysmography variability index measured from the pulse oximetry waveform.

In most severe thoracic and abdominal trauma patients, sedation can be achieved with the use of an opioid and benzodiazepine administered intravenously to effect. General anesthesia may be induced in severely affected animals with the careful titration of these agents without the need for additional induction agent. Short-acting, rapid-onset opioids (such as fentanyl or remifentanil) are preferable (Table 21.2) [21]. If necessary, administration of low-dose ketamine ($0.5–1.0\,mg\,kg^{-1}$) or careful titration of very low dosages of induction agents such as alfaxalone or propofol will allow for endotracheal intubation (Table 21.3) [21]. Anesthetic maintenance can be achieved with an inhalant anesthetic. Since all inhalant anesthetics produce dose-dependent hypotension, myocardial depression, and decreased CO, it is important to use the minimum amount necessary. Ketamine, lidocaine, and/or an opioid infusion can reduce the total amount of inhalant anesthetic necessary [46]. When appropriate, local or regional anesthetic blocks are an excellent option to reduce inhalant anesthetic use even further.

The patient should be closely monitored in the postoperative period. The first three hours after general anesthesia is the most likely period in which anesthesia-related fatalities occur [47]. Severe trauma patients may have injuries and comorbidities that make them prone to chronic (pathologic) pain syndrome (see Chapter 22). Adequate analgesia is paramount to ensure smooth recovery and decrease morbidity. In general, NSAIDs should not be administered in the perioperative period, as these patients are often hypovolemic or may have underlying organ compromise from the recent trauma.

Orthopedic Trauma

Orthopedic trauma correction is often not necessary as an emergent procedure and anesthesia can therefore be postponed until the patient is stabilized and other concomitant morbidities such as diaphragmatic hernia or abdominal/thoracic effusion are ruled out. Some fractures can lead to significant blood loss (e.g., pelvic or femur fracture) and the patient can be hypovolemic upon presentation. Along with initial patient stabilization, care should be taken to temporarily immobilize the fractured limb(s). This procedure provides significant pain relief due to reduction of movement and dislocation of bone fragments. If spinal trauma is suspected, it is necessary to restrain and immobilize the patient with a rigid backboard to avoid any further nerve damage. Use of a radiolucent backboard will facilitate diagnosis, as all diagnostic imaging procedures may be performed with the patient still immobilized. If dealing with an open fracture, a sterile wound dressing cover will prevent further contamination and nosocomial infection.

Once the patient is adequately stabilized and internal organ damage has been ruled out, anesthesia can be induced in a routine fashion. The main concern during premedication is to decrease stress and provide adequate analgesia. In patients that are adequately stabilized and are otherwise healthy, standard preanesthetic sedation considerations apply. For example, opioids, in association with a low-dose alpha-2-adrenergic agonist or acepromazine (Table 21.2), are good choices for premedication. Opioids provide adequate sedation, muscle relaxation, and analgesia in most trauma patients. The use of sedatives will reduce the induction dose and inhalant anesthetic agents required. Most short-acting intravenous induction agents are suitable for this group of patients. These include propofol, alfaxalone, dissociative anesthetics (ketamine and tiletamine), and etomidate (Table 21.3).

Inhalant agents offer a good option for anesthetic maintenance. Whenever possible, local and regional anesthetic techniques should be used to provide analgesia and reduce the amount of inhalant anesthetic necessary. An epidural is a very effective way to provide analgesia and muscle relaxation in distal limbs. The most frequently used medications for epidural analgesia are local anesthetics, opioids, or combinations of these drugs [48]. Ultrasound-guided peripheral nerve blocks such as a femoral nerve block or brachial plexus block can be utilized when epidural injection may be contraindicated. The indications and techniques for these regional blocks are reviewed elsewhere [49, 50] and are briefly discussed in the following text. NSAIDs are a good option for these patients if they are normovolemic with no signs of renal or hepatic disease.

Analgesia in Severe Trauma Patients

After severe trauma, there is a significant amount of tissue damage, organ dysfunction, and activation of inflammatory pathways; all of these may elicit significant pain and activate pain pathways. Tissue damage due to neurological traumatic injury, pulmonary contusions, soft tissue destruction, bone fractures, or vascular injury is often associated with a painful experience and may have ramifications that can last a lifetime [46]. In both veterinary and human medicine, there is still inadequate attention given to the amelioration of pain. In human polytrauma patients in an intensive care unit (ICU), approximately 75% received inadequate analgesia and rated their pain intensity as moderate to severe [51]. In addition, approximately 50% of burn patients respond poorly to analgesic treatment [52, 53]. Similar to these human patients, dental pain in cats is likely underdiagnosed and treated as well; with training, veterinary professionals may be better adept at recognizing and consequently treating chronic pain states in veterinary patients [54, 55].

Inadequately treated pain has been repeatedly shown to increase the stress response, resulting in higher morbidity in trauma patients; effective and appropriate analgesia should be a priority after initial stabilization. As pain is a major component of trauma and has several deleterious systemic effects, early pain management is of utmost importance and should be considered a basic tenet of care of trauma patients [56].

The appropriate use of local and regional anesthetic techniques is particularly important in trauma patients. If performed correctly, locoregional anesthesia allows the patient to achieve excellent analgesia while allowing the surgical procedure to be performed with minimal amounts of systemic analgesics. If a catheter is placed close to the desired nerve, repeat administration of local anesthetic can be performed throughout the hospitalization of the patient. Bandage changes, wound debridement, and splint replacements may be performed with the appropriate use of locoregional anesthesia along with sedation.

Pain Effects in Polytrauma Patients

Cardiovascular Effects

In the severe trauma patient, a cardiovascular response is present shortly after the initial insult and is characterized by an increase in sympathetic tone leading to an increase in SVR (vasoconstriction) and MAP [57]. Blood loss results in stimulation of baroreceptors causing further increases in heart rate and SVR [36]. Acute pain exacerbates the cardiovascular response to trauma through an immediate and massive catecholamine release [58]. This can lead to severe hypertension and undesirable tachyarrhythmias. Interestingly, persistent untreated pain has been shown to reduce arterial baroreceptor sensitivity and blunt the normal physiological tachycardic response to hypotension, further worsening patient hemodynamics [59].

Neuroendocrine Effects

Perhaps surprisingly, tissue damage releases both proinflammatory and anti-inflammatory cytokines [60, 61]. Massive tissue trauma leads to an excessive inflammatory response. Cytokines and other inflammatory mediators increase nociceptor sensitivity in injured tissues. Severe injury and subsequent extensive inflammation result in the release of metabolically active chemicals [23, 62]. For example, trauma causes activation of nearly all components of the immune system. It activates the neuroendocrine system and local tissue destruction, and results in lactic acid accumulation. Hormones such as adrenocorticotropic hormone (ACTH), corticosteroids, and catecholamines play important roles in the initiation and persistence of the proinflammatory response after severe injury [62]. An overwhelming proinflammatory response leads to the clinical manifestation of systemic inflammatory response syndrome (SIRS), which seems to be responsible for organ dysfunction and multiple organ failure (MOF) [63].

Pain caused by trauma is conducted to the spinal cord and then transmitted to the hypothalamus. The consequent hypothalamic activation induces corticotropin-releasing hormone secretion [62, 64]. Corticotropin-releasing hormone stimulates the secretion of ACTH and enhances adrenocortical hormone production [65]. Pain leads to an exacerbated stress response and increases corticosteroid secretion. Endogenous cortisol secretion leads to an anti-inflammatory response and immunosuppression. This overwhelming anti-inflammatory response is called compensatory anti-inflammatory response syndrome (CARS), which leads to the immunosuppression that puts traumatized patients at high risk for septic complications [66].

Long-lasting nociceptive pain also triggers NMDA receptor activation and induces acute hyperalgesia. Activation of these receptors and sensitization of peripheral nociceptors lead to the shift from adaptive (protective) to maladaptive (pathologic) inflammatory pain [67]. Maladaptive pain is the expression of abnormal sensory processing and persists long after the tissue has healed. In summary, untreated pain makes trauma patients more prone to SIRS, immunosuppression, sepsis, and long-lasting maladaptive pain, underscoring the need for effective and appropriate analgesia in trauma patients.

Effects on Wound Healing

There is a significant relationship between pain and wound healing after routine surgery; postsurgical pain is associated with delayed healing of the surgical wound via multiple mechanisms [68]. Pain increases serum cortisol levels, negatively affecting wound healing [69, 70]. Both the phagocytic and killing functions of leukocytes can be altered by repeated exposure to painful stimulation, impairing bacterial clearance and resulting in a significant increase in the incidence of opportunistic infection [71, 72]. Pain-induced catecholamine production directly impairs keratinocyte motility and wound re-epithelialization; keratinocytes express beta-2-adrenergic receptors and activation of these has been shown to delay healing of acute surgical wounds [73, 74]. Therefore, trauma patients appear to be highly predisposed to developing delayed and impaired wound healing if appropriate pain management is not initiated.

Therapeutic Analgesia Options for Trauma Patients

Pain control should be an integral part of the overall treatment plan for the trauma patient. When a patient has experienced severe trauma, the clinician should assume that the condition is extremely painful and provide appropriate treatment. Analgesic treatment in trauma represents a multistage approach involving pain assessment, intervention, and repeated reevaluation.

Some clinicians continue to work under the misconception that analgesia masks physiologic indicators of patient deterioration and delays recognition of clinical complications [75]. A meta-analysis of prospective studies performed in human polytrauma patients demonstrated the absence of adverse effects associated with the early treatment of pain, and better outcomes in patients that received early analgesic intervention [76]. Observations also exist in veterinary medicine suggesting that analgesics do not mask the signs of patient deterioration and should not be withheld for this reason [77].

Other important elements that influence pain in polytrauma are psychological factors such as stress, fear, and anxiety and the significant role of stress in the enhancement of nociceptive responses is clear [78–80]. Use of anxiety-reducing drugs and techniques for individuals experiencing pain reduces the perceived severity and intensity of the pain [81]. Therefore, anxiolysis could represent an effective, adjunctive component of the analgesic approach to traumatized veterinary patients. If the patient is still anxious despite adequate steps have been taken to ensure appropriate analgesia, sedative or anxiolytic medications may be indicated. Drugs such as trazodone (up to 5–10 mg kg^{-1} orally) and gabapentin (20–25 mg kg^{-1} orally) have little hemodynamic negative effects and can provide anxiolysis to trauma patients. Low doses of intravenous dexmedetomidine (Table 21.4) may also be an alternative if patient is not hypovolemic or dehydrated.

It is also critical to consider iatrogenic pain secondary to procedures performed during daily patient care of the polytrauma patient [82]. Traumatized human patients often report excruciating pain during even trivial and common procedures such as changes of body position and phlebotomy; this experience may be extrapolated to veterinary patients that present with varying degrees of stoicism [83].

Injuries sustained to the abdomen, pelvis, and hind limbs may benefit from epidural analgesia, reviewed elsewhere [48]. Agents may be injected into the epidural space via a single-dose technique or through an epidural catheter. Successful epidural analgesia administration leads to a reduction in systemic analgesic requirements and side effects such as sedation or nausea compared with intravenous administration. Local anesthetic agents such as bupivacaine or ropivacaine in combination

Table 21.4 Suggested constant rate infusion doses.

Drug class	Loading dose (IV)	Infusion dose	Comments
Dexmedetomidine	$1\,\mu g\,kg^{-1}$	$0.1–2.0\,\mu g\,kg^{-1}\,h^{-1}$	Excellent sedation. Not recommended in dehydrated or hypovolemic patients. May accumulate with prolonged infusion time.
Morphine	$0.1–0.3\,mg\,kg^{-1}$ SLOWLY	$0.05–0.2\,mg\,kg^{-1}\,h^{-1}$	May cause histamine release. May cause nausea and gastrointestinal (GI) stasis.
Hydromorphone	$0.02–0.05\,mg\,kg^{-1}$	$0.01–0.05\,mg\,kg^{-1}\,h^{-1}$	Excellent for polytrauma. May cause nausea and GI stasis.
Fentanyl	$2–5\,\mu g\,kg^{-1}$	$0.5–5.0\,\mu g\,kg^{-1}\,h^{-1}$	Excellent for polytrauma patients. Titrate drug to effect.
Lidocaine	$1–2\,mg\,kg^{-1}$	$20–50\,\mu g\,kg^{-1}\,min^{-1}$ ($1.2–3.0\,mg\,kg^{-1}\,h^{-1}$)	Great adjunct analgesic used with opioids. May cause nausea with prolonged infusion. Not used in cats.
Ketamine	$0.5–2.0\,mg\,kg^{-1}$	$2.0–10\,\mu g\,kg^{-1}\,min^{-1}$ ($0.12–0.6\,mg\,kg^{-1}\,h^{-1}$)	Great adjunct analgesic used with opioids.
Propofol	$1–5\,mg\,kg^{-1}$	$5–100\,\mu g\,kg^{-1}\,min^{-1}$	Excellent sedation. Respiratory depression. Can accumulate with time.

with morphine are commonly administered epidurally. Appropriate volume dosing of epidurally administered local anesthetics is important to avoid excessive cranial spread and blockade of the motor and sympathetic output to affected segments. Sympathetic blockade by local anesthetics in the epidural space leads to blockade of vasomotor tone, potentially resulting in vasodilation, hypotension, and hypothermia. Caution must also be exercised in trauma patients; epidural injection is contraindicated in patients with coagulation disorders, spinal injuries, or skin infections [48].

Ultrasound-guided peripheral nerve or fascial plane blocks are possible alternatives to epidural analgesia and can be useful in the management of patients with orthopedic, abdominal, or thoracic trauma. Sedation or general anesthesia may be required to perform ultrasound-guided or epidural injections; anesthetic risk must be considered when choosing these analgesic options. Practitioners electing to perform these advanced analgesic techniques must have sufficient training prior to performing injections. Indications, techniques, and descriptions of various locoregional techniques are beyond the scope of this chapter, but are described elsewhere [49, 50].

Trauma-associated pain is a complex and multifactorial symptom that requires a thoughtful approach using a variety of treatment modalities to obtain an optimal outcome. Multimodal (or balanced) analgesia represents an approach to pain management using a combination of several drugs with different mechanisms of action to minimize the dose of each single agent [84, 85].

Multimodal analgesics allow reductions in single-drug dosages, as many analgesics will have a synergistic effect on one another; however, it is therefore important to stress that the clinician should use the minimum number of drugs necessary to achieve optimal control of pain. Opioids have the advantages of being effective, titratable, reversible analgesics with minimal cardiovascular side effects. For these reasons, they constitute first-line analgesics for trauma patients. A possible initial approach to multimodal analgesia in trauma patients may, therefore, include an opioid combined with a regional block or a ketamine infusion (Table 21.4).

Summary

Trauma can activate several different pain pathways and should be aggressively treated. Untreated pain can cause an accentuation of the stress response leading to the development of chronic disabling pain and is associated with delayed wound healing. Multimodal analgesia and continuous patient reassessment constitute the cornerstones of pain management. Polytrauma cases will test your skills as a veterinary care provider. With knowledge of physiology, pharmacology, analgesic options, and locoregional anesthesia, one can achieve success.

References

1. Kolata, R.J. (1980). Trauma in dogs and cats: an overview. *Vet. Clin. North Am. Small Anim. Pract.* 10: 515–522.
2. Hall, K., Boller, M., and Sharp, C. (2018). ACVECC – veterinary committee on trauma report: 2013-2017. *J. Vet. Emerg. Crit. Care* 28: 497–502.
3. Futema, F. and Ferrigno, C.R. (2002). Anestesia no trauma. In: *Anestesia em caes e gatos* (eds. D.T. Fantoni and S.R. Cortopassi), 251–259. Sao Paulo: Rocca.
4. Brenneman, F.D., Boulanger, B.R., McLellan, B.A. et al. (1998). Measuring injury severity: time for a change? *J. Trauma* 44: 580–582.
5. Baker, S.P. and O'Neill, B. (1974). The injury severity score: a method for describing patients with multiple injuries and evaluating emergency care. *J. Trauma* 14: 187–196.
6. Wingfield, W.E. and Raffe, M.R. (2002). *Section X: Trauma. The Veterinary ICU Book*, 1e, 905–1004. Jackson: Teton NewMedia.
7. Chaplew, W., Al Khatib, J., and Zarour, R. (2013). Advanced trauma life support (ATLS): the ninth edition. *J. Trauma Acute Care Surg.* 74: 1363–1366.
8. Ambros, B., Valentina, M., and Jones, T. (2018). Desaturation times between dog preoxygenated via face mask or flow by technique before induction of anesthesia. *Vet. Anaesth. Analg.* 45: 452–458.
9. Mellema, M. (2009). Cardiac output monitoring. In: *Small Animal Critical Care Medicine* (eds. D. Silverstein and K. Hopper), 894–898. St Louis: Saunders Elsevier.
10. Carroll, G.L. and Martin, D. (2007). Trauma and critical patients. In: *Lumb and Jones; Veterinary Anesthesia and Analgesia*, 4e (eds. W.J. Tranquilli, J.C. Thurmon and K.A. Grimm), 969–984. Ames: Blackwell Publishing.
11. Quandt, J. (2009). Anesthesia of the critically ill patient. In: *Small Animal Critical Care Medicine* (eds. D. Silverstein and K. Hopper), 705–709. St Louis: Saunders Elsevier.
12. Stengel, D., Rademacher, G., and Mutze, S. (2015). Emergency ultrasound based algorithms for diagnosing blunt abdominal trauma. *Cochrane Database Syst. Rev.* 9: CD004446.
13. Lisciandro, G. (2011). Abdominal and thoracic focused assessment with

sonography for trauma triage and monitoring in small animals. *J. Vet. Emerg. Crit. Care* 21: 104–122.

14 Boysen, S. and Lisciandro, G.A. (2013). Use of ultrasound for dogs and ats in the emergency room. *Vet. Clin. North Am. Small Anim. Pract.* 43: 773–797.

15 Davenport, R.A., Tai, N., and West, A. (2010). A major trauma centre is a specialty hospital not a hospital of specialties. *Br. J. Surg.* 97: 109–117.

16 Phan, B., Kim, J., and Cho, S. (2017). Anesthesia duration as an independent risk factor for early postoperative complication in adults undergoing elective surgery. *Global Spine J.* 7: 727–734.

17 Laurenza, C., Ansart, L., and Portier, K. (2020). Risk factors of anesthesia-related mortality and morbidity in one equine hospital: a retrospective study on 1,161 cases undergoing elective or emergency surgeries. *J. Front. Vet. Sci.* 6: 514.

18 Palmer, L. and Martin, L. (2014). Traumatic coagulopathy – part II. Resuscitative strategies. *J. Vet. Emerg. Crit. Care* 24: 75–92.

19 Giannoudi, M. and Harwood, P. (2016). Damage control resuscitation: lessons learned. *Eur. J. Trauma Emerg. Surg.* 43: 273–282.

20 Palmer, L. (2017). Fluid management in patients with trauma: restrictive versus liberal approach. *Vet. Clin. North Am. Small Anim. Pract.* 47: 397–410.

21 Haskins, S.C. (2006). Comparative cardiovascular and pulmonary effects of sedatives and anesthetic agents and anesthetic drugs selection for the trauma patient. *J. Vet. Emerg. Crit. Care* 16: 300–328.

22 Haskins, S.C. (2015). Monitoring the anesthetized patient. In: *Veterinary Anesthesia and Analgesia: The Fifth Edition of Lumb and Jones* (eds. K.A. Grimm, L.A. Lamont, W.J. Tranquilli, et al.), 86–113. Ames: John Wiley & Sons.

23 Keel, M. and Trentz, O. (2005). Pathophysiology of polytrauma. *Injury* 36: 691–709.

24 Paulson, O., Strandgard, S., and Edvinson, L. (1990). Cerebral autoregulation. *Brain Metab. Rev.* 2: 161–192.

25 Slupe, M. and Kirsch, J. (2018). Effect of anesthesia on cerebral blood flow metabolism and neuroprotection. *J. Cereb. Blood Flow Metab.* 38: 2192–2208.

26 DiBartola, S.P. (1992). *Fluid Therapy in Small Animal Practice*. Philadelphia: Saunders.

27 Faraci, F., Mayhan, G., and Heistad, D. (1987). Segmental vascular response to acute hypertension in cerebrum and brain stem. *J. Am. Physiol.* 252: H738–H742.

28 Buggy, D., Nicol, B., and Rowbothan, D. (2000). Effect of intravenous anesthesia on glutamate release: a role of GABA receptor mediated inhibition. *Anesthesiology* 92: 1067–1073.

29 Thompson, K.R. and Rioja, E. (2016). Effects of intravenous and topical laryngeal lidocaine on heart rate, mean arterial pressure and cough response to endotracheal intubation in dogs. *Vet. Anaesth. Analg.* 43: 371–378.

30 Mrozek, S., Vardon, F., and Geeraerts, T. (2012). Brain temperature physiology and pathophysiology after brain injury. *J. Anesth. Res. Pract.* 12: 989–987.

31 Dearden, N. (1998). Mechanism and prevention of secondary brain damage during intensive care. *J. Clin. Neuropathol.* 17: 221–228.

32 DiFazio, J. and Fletcher, D. (2013). Updates in the management of small animal patients with neurologic trauma. *Vet. Clin. North Am. Small Anim. Pract.* 43: 915–940.

33 Kolmodin, L., Sekhon, M., and Griesdale, D. (2013). Hypernatremia in patients with severe traumatic brain injury: a systematic review. *J. Ann. Intensive Care* 3: 35.

34 Belonche, F., Meziani, F., and Asfar, P. (2013). Does vasopressor therapy have an indication in shock? *J. Ann. Intensive Care* 22: 11–13.

35 Rudloff, E. and Kirby, R. (2008). Fluid resuscitation and the trauma patient. *Vet. Clin. North Am. Small Anim. Pract.* 38: 645–652.

36 Heckbert, S.R., Vedder, N.B., Hoffman, W. et al. (1998). Outcome after hemorrhagic shock in trauma patients. *J. Trauma* 45: 545–549.

37 Corley, K.T. (2002). Monitoring and treating haemodynamic disturbances in critically ill neonatal foals. Part I Haemodynamic monitoring. *Equine Vet. Educ.* 4: 345–358.

38 Geeraedts, L.M. Jr., Kaasjager, H.A., van Vugt, A.B. et al. (2009). Exsanguination in trauma: a review of diagnostics and treatment options. *Injury* 40: 11–20.

39 Shippy, C.R., Appel, P.L., and Shoemaker, W.C. (1984). Reliability of clinical monitoring to assess blood volume in critically ill patients. *Crit. Care Med.* 12: 107–112.

40 Godje, O., Peyerl, M., Seebauer, T. et al. (1998). Central venous pressure, pulmonary capillary wedge pressure and intrathoracic blood volumes as preload indicators in cardiac surgery patients. *Eur. J. Cardiothorac. Surg.* 13: 533–539; discussion 539–40.

41 Kumar, A., Anel, R., Bunnell, E. et al. (2004). Pulmonary artery occlusion pressure and central venous pressure fail to predict ventricular filling volume, cardiac performance, or the response to volume infusion in normal subjects. *Crit. Care Med.* 32: 691–699.

42 Renner, J., Meybohm, P., Hanss, R. et al. (2009). Effects of norepinephrine on dynamic variables of fluid responsiveness during hemorrhage and after resuscitation in a pediatric porcine model. *Paediatr. Anaesth.* 19: 688–694.

43 Vigani, A., Shih, A., Queiroz, P. et al. (2012). Quantitative response of volumetric variables measured by a new ultrasound dilution method in a juvenile model of hemorrhagic shock and resuscitation. *Resuscitation* 83: 1031–1037.

44 Renner, J., Cavus, E., Meybohm, P. et al. (2007). Stroke volume variation during hemorrhage and after fluid loading: impact of different tidal volumes. *Acta Anaesthesiol. Scand.* 51: 538–544.

45 Shih, A., Giguere, S., Vigani, A. et al. (2011). Determination of cardiac output by ultrasound velocity dilution in normovolemia and hypovolemia in dogs. *Vet. Anaesth. Analg.* 38: 279–285.

46 Perkowski, S. (2009). Pain and sedation assessment. In: *Small Animal Critical Care Medicine* (eds. D. Silverstein and K. Hopper), 697–699. St. Louis: Saunders Elsevier.

47 Brodbelt, D.C., Blissitt, K.J., Hammond, R.A. et al. (2008). The risk of death: the confidential enquiry into perioperative small animal fatalities. *Vet. Anaesth. Analg.* 35 (5): 365–373.

48 Valverde, A. (2008). Epidural analgesia and anesthesia in dogs and cats. *Vet. Clin. North Am. Small Anim. Pract.* 38: 1205–1230.

49 Portela, D.A., Verdier, N., and Otero, P.E. (2018). Regional anesthetic techniques for the pelvic limb and abdominal wall in small animals: a review of the literature and technique description. *Vet. J.* 238: 27–40.

50 Portela, D.A., Romano, M., and Otero, P.E. (2019). Locoregional anesthesia of the thoracic limb and thorax in small animals. *Vet. Clin. North Am. Small Anim. Pract.* 49: 1063–1083.

51 Whipple, J.K., Lewis, K.S., Quebbeman, E.J. et al. (1995). Analysis of pain management in critically ill patients. *Pharmacotherapy* 15: 592–599.

52 Hedderich, R. and Ness, T.J. (1999). Analgesia for trauma and burns. *Crit. Care Clin.* 15: 167–184.

53 Payen, J.F., Chanques, G., Mantz, J. et al. (2007). Current practices in sedation and analgesia for mechanically ventilated critically ill patients: a prospective multicenter patient-based study. *Anesthesiology* 106: 687–695.

54 Steagall, P. and Monteiro, B. (2019). Acute pain in cats: recent advances in clinical assessments. *J. Feline Med. Surg.* 21: 25–34.

55 Mich, P.M., Hellyer, P.W., Kogan, L. et al. (2010). Effects of a pilot training program on veterinary students' pain knowledge, attitude, and assessment skills. *J. Vet. Med. Educ.* 37: 358–368.

56 Dobscha, S.K., Clark, M.E., Morasco, B.J. et al. (2009). Systematic review of the literature on pain in patients with polytrauma including traumatic brain injury. *Pain Med.* 10: 1200–1217.

57 Anderson, I.D., Little, R.A., Pyman, J.A. et al. (1990). Changes in cardiovascular homeostasis after injury are mediated by tissue damage and not haemorrhage. *Br. J. Surg.* 77: 1338–1341.

58 Little, R.A., Marshall, H.W., and Kirkman, E. (1989). Attenuation of the acute cardiovascular responses to haemorrhage by tissue injury in the conscious rat. *Q. J. Exp. Physiol.* 74: 825–833.

59 Quest, J.A. and Gebber, G.L. (1972). Modulation of baroreceptor reflexes by somatic afferent nerve stimulation. *Am. J. Phys.* 222: 1251–1259.

60 Smith, C., Kruger, M.J., Smith, R.M. et al. (2008). The inflammatory response to skeletal muscle injury: illuminating complexities. *Sports Med.* 38: 947–969.

61 Giannoudis, P.V. (2003). Current concepts of the inflammatory response after major trauma: an update. *Injury* 34: 397–404.

62 Lenz, A., Frankin, G., and Gheadle, W. (2007). Systemic inflammation after trauma. *J. Injury* 38: 1336–1345.

63 Douglas, R.G. and Shaw, J.H. (1989). Metabolic response to sepsis and trauma. *Br. J. Surg.* 76: 115–122.

64 Hotta, H., Sato, A., and Sumitomo, T. (1992). Hypothalamic corticotropin-releasing hormone (CRH) secretion into hypophysial portal blood is regulated by cutaneous sensory stimulation in anesthetized rats. *Jpn. J. Physiol.* 42: 515–524.

65 Egdahl, R.H. (1959). Pituitary-adrenal response following trauma to the isolated leg. *Surgery* 46: 9–21.

66 Bone, R.C. (1996). Sir Isaac Newton, sepsis, SIRS, and CARS. *Crit. Care Med.* 24: 1125–1128.

67 Kidd, B.L. and Urban, L.A. (2001). Mechanisms of inflammatory pain. *Br. J. Anaesth.* 87: 3–11.

68 McGuire, L., Heffner, K., Glaser, R. et al. (2006). Pain and wound healing in surgical patients. *Ann. Behav. Med.* 31: 165–172.

69 Padgett, D.A., Marucha, P.T., and Sheridan, J.F. (1998). Restraint stress slows cutaneous wound healing in mice. *Brain Behav. Immun.* 12: 64–73.

70 Hubner, G., Brauchle, M., Smola, H. et al. (1996). Differential regulation of pro-inflammatory cytokines during wound healing in normal and glucocorticoid-treated mice. *Cytokine* 8: 548–556.

71 Rojas, I.G., Padgett, D.A., Sheridan, J.F. et al. (2002). Stress-induced susceptibility to bacterial infection during cutaneous wound healing. *Brain Behav. Immun.* 16: 74–84.

72 Shurin, M.R., Kusnecov, A., Hamill, E. et al. (1994). Stress-induced alteration of polymorphonuclear leukocyte function in rats. *Brain Behav. Immun.* 8: 163–169.

73 Chen, J., Hoffman, B.B., and Isseroff, R.R. (2002). Beta-adrenergic receptor activation inhibits keratinocyte migration via a cyclic adenosine monophosphate-independent mechanism. *J. Invest. Dermatol.* 119: 1261–1268.

74 Pullar, C.E., Grahn, J.C., Liu, W. et al. (2006). Beta2-adrenergic receptor activation delays wound healing. *FASEB J.* 20: 76–86.

75 Whitesides, T.E. Jr. (2001). Pain: friend or foe? *J. Bone Joint Surg. Am.* 83-A: 1424–1425.

76 McHale, P.M. and LoVecchio, F. (2001). Narcotic analgesia in the acute abdomen – a review of prospective trials. *Eur. J. Emerg. Med.* 8: 131–136.

77 Brock, N. (1995). Treating moderate and severe pain in small animals. *Can. Vet. J.* 36: 658–660.

78 Chapman, C.R., Tuckett, R.P., and Song, C.W. (2008). Pain and stress in a systems perspective: reciprocal neural, endocrine, and immune interactions. *J. Pain* 9: 122–145.

79 Rivat, C., Laboureyras, E., Laulin, J.P. et al. (2007). Non-nociceptive environmental stress induces hyperalgesia, not analgesia, in pain and opioid-experienced rats. *Neuropsychopharmacology* 32: 2217–2228.

80 Imbe, H., Iwai-Liao, Y., and Senba, E. (2006). Stress-induced hyperalgesia: animal models and putative mechanisms. *Front. Biosci.* 11: 2179–2192.

81 Tang, J. and Gibson, S.J. (2005). A psychophysical evaluation of the relationship between trait anxiety, pain perception, and induced state anxiety. *J. Pain* 6: 612–619.

82 Puntillo, K.A. (1994). Dimensions of procedural pain and its analgesic management in critically ill surgical patients. *Am. J. Crit. Care* 3: 116–122.

83 Pasero, C. (2003). Pain in the critically ill patient. *J. Perianesth. Nurs.* 18: 422–425.

84 Lemke, K.A. (2008). Paravertebral blockade of the brachial plexus in dogs. *Vet. Clin. North Am. Small Anim. Pract.* 38: 1231–1241.

85 White, P.F. (2008). Multimodal analgesia: its role in preventing postoperative pain. *Curr. Opin. Investig. Drugs* 9: 76–82.

22

Nociceptive Disorders

Andrew Claude

Department of Small Animal Clinical Sciences, College of Veterinary Medicine, Michigan State University, East Lansing, MI, 48824, USA

Introduction

According to the International Association for the Study of Pain, "Pain has been defined as an unpleasant sensory and emotional experience associated with actual or potential tissue damage or described in terms of such damage" [1]. Whereas nociception is the physiological, afferent, sensory mechanism involving both the peripheral and central nervous systems (CNS), pain is the conscious product originating within the brain. Nociception and its final product, pain, are protective and essential for a living organism to survive. Pain consists of three components: a sensory-discriminatory component (physiological, temporal, spatial, thermal/mechanical), an affective component (subjective, emotional, autonomic), and an evaluative component (magnitude, severity) [2]. Although most pain descriptors are based on human experiences, controversy exists as to whether animal pain experiences are similar. The physiology of nociception (see the section titled "The Nociceptive Process") is nearly identical between humans and animals. The only process of nociception in animals that has not been well described is the supraspinal modulation or perception phase. Like all organic systems and processes within the body, nociception can also undergo pathological changes with potentially debilitating conditions. Most disorders of nociception have been recognized in humans; however, some have similar counterparts in other species.

Definitions

- *Acute pain* varies in severity from mild to severe. It is immediate and can last 3–6 months. Acute pain is typically associated with an injury or surgery and subsides as the tissues heal. Acute pain is one component of a protective mechanism by which an individual secures survival.
- *Allodynia* is pain associated with stimuli that are not considered noxious. Allodynia is a common result of central sensitization and/or wind-up, and diseases such as neuralgias and neuropathies. There are multiple forms of allodynia recognized: mechanical, which includes static and dynamic touch, thermal, and movement.
- *Analgesia* is the complete or partial loss of sensitivity to noxious stimuli.
- *Anesthesia* is the complete or partial loss of all afferent, sensory input.

Canine and Feline Anesthesia and Co-Existing Disease, Second Edition. Edited by Rebecca A. Johnson, Lindsey B. C. Snyder and Carrie A. Schroeder.

Companion website: www.wiley.com/go/johnson/canine

- *Central sensitization* (centralized pain) is an amplified response to intense and/or sustained afferent, nociceptive input at the dorsal horn of the spinal cord resulting in the activation of N-methyl-D-aspartate acid (NMDA) receptors among others. Central sensitization is most often associated with peripheral sensitization; however, it can also be caused by direct injury to central neurological structures.
- *Chronic pain* lasts greater than what would be expected considering the injury and persists beyond the expected healing time. Chronic pain is considered a pathological condition by itself and serves no purpose for survival. It is difficult to diagnose with veterinary patients, is challenging to manage, and often requires extensive periods of pain medications and other pain management modalities. Chronic pain is not defined by a specific origin; instead, it can result from injury, surgery, or disease.
- *Neuropathic pain* is a debilitating type of pain due to direct injury of neurological tissues (i.e., peripheral and/or central nervous systems). Neuropathic pain can quickly advance to a state of hyperalgesia (enhanced sensitivity to painful stimuli) and wind-up. Neuropathic pain can possibly be associated with loss of other somatosensory afferent input, motor, and autonomic functions.
- *Nociception* is the neuronal process of encoding pain and includes transduction, transmission, primary modulation, projection, and secondary modulation (perception). Nociception is the physiology (or pathophysiology) that describes the movement and processing of noxious, afferent sensory information from the periphery to the CNS.
- *Peripheral sensitization* is caused by the formation of an "inflammatory soup" due to peripheral tissue damage. Tissue injury has subsequent inflammatory components, such as adenosine triphosphatase, potassium and hydrogen ions, cytokines, chemokines, growth factors, tissue factor, and prostaglandins. These factors cause neuronal changes to occur such as quiescent nociceptor activation and neuronal sensitization that can potentiate nociception afferent input summation at the dorsal horn of the spinal cord.
- *Wind-up* is a term that describes a hypersensitization of peripheral and central nociceptive sensory structures due to a barrage of afferent noxious impulses. Wind-up is synonymous with sensitization of either peripheral (tissue injury) or central tissues and is used to describe the frequency-dependent excitability of spinal neurons [3]. Wind-up results in a high degree of stress, excessive/overreactive responses to pain, allodynia, and chronic pain conditions.

The Nociceptive Process

Nociception involves five main components (Figure 22.1), described in the following text. The peripheral nerves are extensions of the CNS and can be divided into sensory, motor, and autonomic fibers. The sensory components of the nervous system are further divided into broad categories that include tactile, proprioception, autonomic, and nociceptive afferent neuronal tissues.

Transduction

Intense thermal, mechanical, and chemical stimuli are detected by a subpopulation of peripheral nerve fibers called nociceptors. Nociceptors are excited only when stimuli reach a noxious range (i.e., low sensitivity, high threshold properties). Historically, nociceptors have been described as unmyelinated nerve endings located throughout the body tissues. Specialized cutaneous glial cells with extensive processes form a mesh-like network within the subepidermal border of the skin and are involved with conveying mechanical and thermal sensitivity [4]. There are two major classes of nociceptors; myelinated medium diameter fibers (A-delta [Aδ]-fibers) that mediate acute, localized, fast pain, and unmyelinated, small diameter fibers (C-fibers) that convey less localized, dull or slow pain.

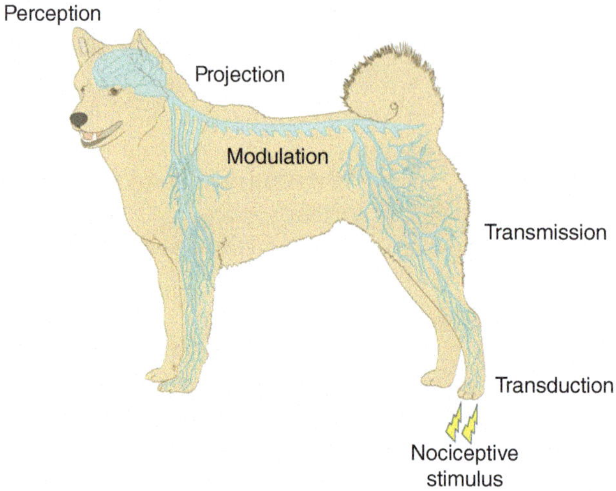

Figure 22.1 Five components of the nociceptive process. See text for details. Illustration by Jacquelyn Vargas.

Nociceptors and the specialized glial meshwork recognize environmental (thermal, mechanical, chemical) energy and transform it into electrochemical signals.

Transmission

The electrochemical signals are propagated as action potentials from the periphery to the dorsal horn of the spinal cord via afferent, sensory nerve fibers. Activation of the sensory nerve endings primarily causes the release of glutamate or substance P (SP) into the synaptic cleft. The postsynaptic effect of glutamate/SP is mediated by several inotropic receptors, chiefly α-amino-3-hydroxy-5-methyl-4-isoxazolepropionic acid (AMPA), kainite, and NMDA receptors.

Primary Modulation

The initial processing of afferent noxious stimuli occurs in the spinal cord via a complex structure of second-order neurons. The gray matter within the spinal cord is composed of cells responsible for the transmission of specific nerve fibers. Lamina I (marginal layer) contains neurons that are generally responsive to thermal input from Aδ- and C-fibers. Lamina II (substantia gelatinosa) is generally responsive to noxious stimulation from Aδ- and nonpeptidergic C-fibers. Lamina V neurons receive both innocuous A-beta (Aβ)-input (touch) and high-threshold Aδ- and C-fibers (noxious); therefore, this region is referred to as having a wide dynamic range (WDR). Although Lamina X is not physically part of the dorsal horn, it does receive nociceptive input, primarily from the visceral regions [5]. Activation of the second-order neurons produces both excitatory and inhibitory effects [6]. For example, nociceptive-specific C-fibers converge on the WDR of Lamina V which project to inhibitory interneurons. The inhibitory neurons reduce nociceptive transmission either by reducing activity in the WDR or inhibiting the release of neurotransmitters from C-fibers [4]. Although the primary projection of afferent nerve fibers is in the spinal cord segment of entry, collateral interneuron spread can send excitatory impulses to adjacent segments, resulting in multiple dermatomes being affected. In addition, neuroplasticity within intraneuronal communications and duplicated noxious sensory information across multiple spinal segments can further result in somatic-visceral and visceral-somatic reflexes (see the section titled "Central Sensitization").

Projection

Projection fibers couple both afferent and efferent neuronal activities within the spinal cord to the brain. These fibers are myelinated nerves arranged in columns within the white matter surrounding the gray matter. There are two primary ascending spinal tracts that carry nociception to the brain; the spinothalamic tract, which transmits to the thalamus and is associated with sensory-discriminative information, and the spinoreticulothalamic tract, which transmits to the brainstem and is associated with poorly localized aspects of pain. There are also spinal cord projections to the parabrachial region of the dorsolateral pons which provide a rapid connection to the amygdala and are generally considered to be associated with the aversive properties of pain.

Supraspinal Modulation (Perception)

The primary brain regions associated with the experience of pain are the cortex (perception, awareness), thalamus (integration), cingulate gyrus (behavior, emotion), periaqueductal gray zone (modulation, endorphins), locus coeruleus (arousal, vigilance), reticular formation (antinociception), hippocampus (autonomic), and the amygdala (fear, anxiety). As stated in the preceding text, the perception component of the nociception process is the least understood in animal species. However, dog and cat brains have all central regions classically associated with pain modulation; therefore, it would be logical to conclude that dogs and cats could have similar pain-related experiences as humans.

Nociception and Pain Disorders

Peripheral Sensitization (Wind-Up)

Tissue injury with subsequent inflammation can eventually elicit alterations in nociceptive afferent responses. Acceleration of ongoing (spontaneous) presynaptic afferent neurons innervating the site of tissue injury and inflammation can potentiate activation of silent nociceptors and conversion of low threshold Aβ- to behave like Aδ-fibers. There are multiple factors leading to altered peripheral afferent response characteristics. Changes in the local chemical microenvironment associated with inflammation drive the alteration and increased responsiveness in peripheral nociception within the injured tissue. Tissue damage and plasma extravasation result in an "inflammatory soup" consisting of factors including hydrogen and potassium ions, local inflammatory cells, prostaglandins, leukotrienes, histamine, serotonin, bradykinin, cytokines (tumor necrosis factor alpha [TNF-α]), and nerve growth factor. Locally released factors activate C-fibers which are perceived as slow or dull pain sensation. The degree of receptor activation is directly related to the concentrations and composition of local factors. The combination of a concentrated "inflammatory soup" coupled with the activation of silent fibers, conversion of low-threshold Aβ-fibers, and peripheral afferent axon growth (budding) relates to peripheral sensitization [7]. Peripheral sensitization and intense, monotonic afferent stimuli can result in central summation which then amplifies the degree of pain. Increased peripheral input can lead to "hyperalgesia priming" and/or wind-up and eventually to central sensitization through long-term potentiation in the CNS [8]. Changes in peripheral terminal excitability (peripheral sensitization) and the ongoing activity in the pain-activated afferent sensory nerve result in an increase response within the spinal cord (central sensitization).

Central Sensitization (Wind-Up)

Dorsal horn WDR neurons have a stimulant-dependent response to single C-fiber stimuli. The physiological result of an intense and/or persistent barrage of afferent, C-fiber stimuli within the spinal cord could result in the amplification of nociceptive messages defined as a pathophysiological pain condition called central wind-up. The combined effect of peripheral and central wind-up causes activation of adjacent spinal segments and corresponding dermatomes. The receptive field includes not only the primary area of tissue damage but also surrounding dermatomes, resulting in a debilitating condition called referred pain and/or allodynia. Another consequence of segmental recruitment due to central sensitization is the presence of somatic-visceral (or visceral-somatic) reflexes, seen clinically as chronic visceral conditions coexisting with chronic peripheral pain. When internal organs have pathological conditions, somatic zones that are innervated by the same spinal segments can exhibit increased degrees of sensitivity [9, 10]. In humans, this relationship has been seen clinically as pain-sensitive points on the abdomen and back regions in patients with gastric ulcers. The visceral-somatic Aδ- and C-fiber stimuli from peripheral afferent nociceptive neurons cause the release of a variety of neurotransmitters including glutamate and SP at the central nerve terminals. Afferent, noxious stimuli at the dorsal horn and subsequent glutamate, and SP activation of AMPA and neurokinin-1 (NK1) receptors, respectively, are considered one component of physiological nociception. However, high-intensity and/or persistent WDR C-fiber input can result in activation of NMDA and NK1 receptors, which increases the amplitude of signaling and responsiveness in the spinal cord segment(s). These neurochemical changes are examples of the neuroplastic properties of the nervous system and highlight the turning point at which the physiologic response to noxious input becomes a hypersensitized, amplified process, resulting in pathological, chronic, and debilitating conditions. Another important property of the nervous system is its memory. Once the condition of central wind-up nociception occurs, it cannot be "unlearned."

Chronic or Maladaptive Pain

Chronic or maladaptive pain is pain that lasts beyond 6 months and/or the expected time for tissue healing. Chronic pain is considered an abnormal condition or disease in and of itself. It is pain that no longer serves a protective, life-sustaining purpose. In fact, chronic pain is debilitating and tends to increase the likelihood of comorbidities and decrease life expectancy [11]. In humans, chronic pain is associated with diabetes mellitus, obesity, hypertension, heart disease, decreased exercise, depression, sleep disturbances, anxiety, and fatigue. These comorbidities reduce the quality of life and obstruct an individual from experiencing a healthy lifestyle. The term "chronic pain" was first used around the 1900s to describe painful human patients that were "often regarded as deluded or were condemned as malingers or drug abusers" [12]. Veterinary medicine still struggles with an objective means of recognizing and treating chronic pain. Unfortunately, it is still problematic for the veterinary industry to agree as to whether animal patients experience chronic pain and how to effectively treat the condition.

Animal patients have almost identical nociceptive physiology and contain all the pain-processing brain centers as human patients. It would be illogical to conclude that animals do not experience chronic pain in ways like humans. Underrecognized and undermanaged chronic pain may result in death via humane euthanasia years earlier than would otherwise be necessary [13]. Although veterinary medicine has made strides in recognizing acute pain by utilizing semi-objective pain scores (i.e., Glasgow composite pain scores for dogs and cats, Equine [and other species] Grimace Scales), we still do not have consistent, universal means to recognize chronic pain in our patients. Traditionally, veterinary practitioners have relied almost exclusively on behavior changes as indicators of chronic pain in animal patients. Examples of behaviors related to chronic pain in veterinary patients include diminished exercise or general activity, difficulty in walking, standing, eating, and taking stairs, decreased grooming, and changes in urination and/or defecation [14]. Myofascial palpation is a technique that can aid veterinarians in recognizing chronic pain in their patients. A palpatory examination of the myofascial structure may reveal clinical information that correlates to a chronic, painful condition endured by a veterinary patient. Palpatory examinations include thermal palpation, myofascial palpation, joint palpation, and structure mobility (gait). Myofascial palpatory indicators of chronic pain include trigger points, taut bands, muscle atrophy, temporal mandibular changes, areas on the body with increased and/or decreased temperature, and gait abnormalities with compensatory weight adaptations.

Neuropathic Pain

Neuropathic pain is associated with damage or disease involving the somatosensory nervous system and may or may not be associated with loss of neurological, autonomic, or motor function [15]. In humans, neuropathic pain is described as burning, shooting, stabbing, and/or electric shock sensations which can be continuous or episodic. Neuropathic pain can originate from peripheral nerve damage resulting in neuronal hyperexcitability and spontaneous pathological activity resembling peripheral sensitization described in the preceding text. Peripheral neuropathy can directly contribute to the development of central sensitization. Causes of central neuropathic pain can be related to injury or diseases involving structures associated with the spinal cord.

Central sensitization is almost always a consequence of central neuropathic pain. In fact, some believe that the two types of hypersensitized pain (central wind-up pain and central neuropathic pain) are practically synonymous. Both central, hypersensitized types of pain are associated with the activation of the NMDA postsynaptic receptors. In addition, both are related to changes in the functional properties of the afferent sensory (nociception and innocuous) and second-order neurons in the spinal cord. These changes are defined by a reduction of pain threshold and endogenous antinociceptive mechanisms and increased magnitude and duration of responses to noxious input, and innocuous sensory input is perceived as pain sensations [16]. Neuropathic pain is notoriously difficult to manage. In humans, it is estimated that between 40% and 60% of those affected by neuropathic pain achieve partial relief [17]. In addition to analgesics, treatment includes antidepressants, anticonvulsants, and topical applications.

Preventive and Multimodal Analgesia

Balanced anesthesia refers to using two or more anesthetic agents in small doses to provide a summed or greater effect. Preemptive analgesia is a form of pain control dating back to 1913 when Crile realized that postoperative pain improved if regional blocks were administered prior to surgery [18]. In 1986, Wall introduced the concept of preemptive analgesia as a protocol to reduce postoperative pain by administering analgesics preoperatively [19]. In 2011, Katz published an analgesic management protocol called "preventive analgesia" that considers three perioperative phases: preoperative, intraoperative, and postoperative [20]. Preventive analgesia is a pain management system based on the realization that some analgesic interventions or analgesic combinations influence postoperative pain by exceeding the expected drug duration of action [21]. The concept of preventive analgesia has been broadened with increasing knowledge to consider the influence of multiple factors on the generation of central sensitization, with the aim to attenuate the impact of noxious preoperative, intraoperative, and postoperative stimuli [22].

A common misunderstanding in veterinary medicine is the confusion regarding the definitions of anesthesia, analgesia, and multimodal analgesia. Anesthesia is defined as a reversible loss of all sensory input either involving a region of the body (locoregional anesthesia) or the entire body (general anesthesia). Analgesia is the complete or partial loss of the ability to feel pain and analgesics are any kind of modality that decrease the sensation of pain. Technically, analgesia should be defined as the loss of conscious nociception, and analgesic should be defined as any type of modality that decreases the physiologic process of nociception. Unfortunately, some practitioners may be unclear when employing analgesic management during surgical procedures; for example, the belief that if a patient is anesthetized and is therefore not experiencing pain, then the patient is receiving adequate analgesia. This belief is incorrect for two reasons. One, most anesthetic induction agents and inhalational agents do not provide adequate analgesia especially during the postoperative period. Second, while it is true that the anesthetized patient is unconscious, thus unable to feel pain (lack of perception), the remaining processes of nociception continue to occur. Without additional analgesic modalities, nociceptive transduction, transmission, primary modulation, and projection (Figure 22.1) continue to bombard the nervous system, which could result in peripheral and central sensitization.

Another important area of intervention is ensuring adequate analgesia for individual cases. Multimodal analgesia involves multiple analgesic modalities that impact several physiological steps during the nociceptive process (Figure 22.1). For example, one preemptive injection of an opioid will only address a limited number of anatomical areas during nociception. In addition, it is possible that one single, preemptive opioid injection may be ineffective throughout the intraoperative or postoperative phase. Based on the concept of preventive analgesia, nociception should be addressed using multimodal analgesia during all three perioperative phases (Table 22.1). Historically, there was a tendency to focus postoperative analgesia on the immediate postoperative period to several days later. A better approach would be to consider the postoperative phase to encompass the entire period that a patient requires analgesic intervention, which could be a lifetime. In human patients, both pharmaceutical and nonpharmaceutical analgesic options are commonly employed to address analgesic needs. It has only been since the mid-1990s that nonpharmaceutical analgesic modalities, such as rehabilitation, have been used in veterinary medicine. In the United States, canine rehabilitation began to show progress in the early 1990s and the start of certification programs in 1997 [23].

Practical Anesthetic and Analgesic Considerations

Common Analgesic Categories Used in Small-Animal Veterinary Medicine

There are multiple analgesic drugs that are commonly used in veterinary medicine. This section will list and discuss specific drugs, their methods of action, clinical uses, and side effects.

Opioid Receptor Agonists

Historically, opioid receptor agonists have been the backbone for analgesia in both human and veterinary medicine. Opioid drugs can be divided into mixed-opioid receptor agonists, partial mu-opioid receptor agonists, pure mu-opioid receptor agonists, mu-opioid receptor antagonist-kappa-opioid receptor agonists, and opioid receptor antagonists. The effects of opioid drugs are similar to the endogenous opioids, namely, endorphins, enkephalins, and dynorphins, which are secreted from the periaqueductal gray zone in the midbrain [24]. Although opioid receptors are found in numerous places throughout the body, the primary antinociceptive effects of opioid ligands are their interactions with mu- and kappa-opioid receptors located in the dorsal horn of the spinal cord [25]. Opioid ligands bind to mu- and kappa-opioid receptors on the

Table 22.1 Three perioperative phases with examples of analgesic considerations. Note that these should be combined to provide a multimodal analgesic approach.

Agent	Examples	Method of administration
Preemptive phase		
Opioids	Hydromorphone, morphine, methadone, buprenorphine	IM, IV
Lidocaine		IV, not to be used in cats
Locoregional blocks	Intratesticular, epidural	—
Alpha-2 agonists	Dexmedetomidine	IM, IV
NMDA antagonists	Ketamine	IM. IV
Gabapentinoids	Gabapentin, pregabalin	PO, prior to anesthesia
Intraoperative phase		
Opioids	Hydromorphone, methadone	IV, intermittent injections
Opioids	Fentanyl, morphine	IV, constant rate infusion
Lidocaine		IV, constant rate infusion
NMDA antagonists	Ketamine	IV, constant rate infusion
Alpha-2 agonists	Dexmedetomidine	IV, constant rate infusion
Postoperative phase		
Immediate postoperative		
Pharmaceutical analgesics	Opioids, NSAIDs, continued analgesic CRIs, gabapentin, amantadine, Nocita	SC, IM, IV, PO
Nonpharmaceutical	Ice, bedding, comfort, monitoring food/water intake and urination/defecation, etc.	-
Long-term postoperative		
Pharmaceutical analgesics	NSAIDs, grapiprant, gabapentinoids, amantadine	PO
Nonpharmaceutical	Physical rehabilitation, acupuncture, phototherapy, myofascial massage, chiropractic manipulation	—

presynaptic membrane of the afferent sensory neuron, resulting in a decreased release of glutamate and SP, which hinders the activation of postsynaptic AMPA and NK1 receptors, thus inhibiting the progress of noxious impulses [26]. Clinically, opioid drugs are used for their analgesic properties; however, in many species, opioids can also provide some degree of sedation and calming effects. Side effects of opioid drugs, such as dysphoria, may be related to the degree of delta-opioid receptor interaction [27]. Common adverse effects include emesis, dysphoria, bradycardia, histamine release, and decreased gastrointestinal motility, depending on the specific drug chosen. For example, the commonly used opioid morphine is considered a mixed-opioid receptor agonist because it interacts with both mu- and kappa-opioid receptors providing excellent analgesia. Morphine can also directly interact with mast cells resulting in histamine release seen clinically as a pseudoallergic reaction [28]. Hydromorphone is considered a pure mu-opioid receptor agonist with similar effects as morphine in dogs and cats, but without the histamine release. In addition to having pure mu-opioid receptor agonist properties, methadone is a commonly utilized opioid and is also an NMDA receptor antagonist, thus providing additional (multimodal) analgesia. Other commonly used opioids include buprenorphine (partial mu-opioid agonist), butorphanol (kappa receptor agonist-mu receptor antagonist), and fentanyl (mu-opioid agonist). See the section titled "Preemptive Phase" in the following text for more details.

Alpha-2-Adrenergic Receptor Agonists

Alpha-2-adrenergic receptor agonists stimulate both presynaptic and postsynaptic alpha-2 adrenoreceptors and imidazole receptors in the CNS and periphery resulting in decreased norepinephrine release and a reduction in nociceptive transmission to the spinal cord and brain [29]. The net result is decreased sympathetic tone causing a sleeplike state, central muscle relaxation, and analgesia. Alpha-2-adrenergic receptor agonists have demonstrated additive and synergistic effects when combined with opioids, thus enhancing the analgesic effects [30]. Alpha-2-adrenergic agonists can be administered intramuscularly, intravenously, via the buccal mucosa (e.g., detomidine in dogs), and as an epidural/subdural regional technique [31]. The primary adverse effects are marked increases in peripheral vascular resistance and bradycardia. Hypertension is the result of peripheral alpha-1 and alpha-2 adrenoreceptor activation, while bradycardia is due to a baroreflex and decreased CNS sympathetic outflow. Clinically, these effects can result in pale mucous membranes, sinus bradycardia, atrioventricular blocks, and hypothermia. In addition, alpha-2-adrenergic receptor agonists decrease gastrointestinal motility and can be used for gastrointestinal pain; however, this family of drugs also can induce vomiting (especially cats) and decrease insulin activity resulting in glucosuria. Although alpha-2-adrenergic agonists can decrease respiratory drive, it is usually not considered clinically significant. Patients that are highly excitable may not sedate well with alpha-2-adrenergic receptor agonists or become easily startled when sedated. Alpha-2-agonist drugs have been proven to be safe, versatile, and effective, especially when used preoperatively as a neuroleptanalgesic. The central and peripheral effects of alpha-2 receptor agonists can be antagonized by the alpha-2-adrenergic receptor antagonist atipamezole.

NMDA Receptor Antagonists

"Dissociative" anesthetic drugs include ketamine and tiletamine and produce a dose-dependent level of immobility and analgesia. Their primary mode of action includes a direct inhibition of the NMDA receptors in both the brain and spinal cord resulting a cataleptic state, increased muscle rigidity, and increased sympathetic output [32]. Clinically, this is seen as a catatonic, statue-like posture with an inability to move, increased heart rate, and analgesia. Muscle rigidity can be minimized by the coadministration of a benzodiazepine (midazolam, diazepam, zolazepam) [33]. Ketamine is the most common dissociative anesthetic used in small-animal practice and can be administered to produce analgesia, sedation, or immobility. Ketamine can also be used intraoperatively with other analgesics drugs (fentanyl, lidocaine) as a constant rate infusion to provide an isoflurane-sparing effect [34]. Tiletamine is combined with zolazepam in a 1:1 ratio and distributed as Telazol® (Zoetis, New Jersey, USA). The primary adverse effects of dissociative NMDA receptor antagonists are increased muscle tone, tachycardia, tremors, and increased cerebral blood flow (increased intracranial pressure) [35]. Cardiovascular effects include tachyarrhythmias, hypertension, and increased myocardial oxygen demand, and they should be used cautiously in patients with known cardiac disease at high doses, although analgesic dosages are considerably lower. Dissociatives, especially at high doses, are relatively contraindicated in cats with hypertrophic cardiomyopathy, as their sympathomimetic effects cause an increased myocardial contractility and heart rate [36]. Ketamine, and its metabolites, are extensively excreted via the kidneys; therefore, should be used with caution in patients with renal disease.

Nonsteroidal Anti-Inflammatory Drugs (NSAIDs)

Modern NSAIDs can be safely administered preemptively or postoperatively as part of a multimodal analgesic plan via reducing surgical inflammation through cyclooxygenase (COX) inhibitory activity [37]. Historically, NSAIDs have been classified based on their inhibitory effects on the COX enzyme of the inflammatory cascade. The most common NSAIDs used in small-animal veterinary medicine include carprofen (COX-2 preferred), ketoprofen (nonselective COX-2), meloxicam (COX-2 preferred), deracoxib (COX-2 selective), firocoxib (COX-2 selective in dogs), and robenacoxib (COX-1 and COX-2 selective) [38]. The primary adverse effects of COX-inhibitory NSAIDs are GI upset/ulceration, renal failure, platelet inhibition, liver toxicosis, and third-trimester abortions. A new family of NSAIDs, EP4-receptor antagonists, helps control inflammation via inhibition of prostaglandin E2 (PGE2). Currently, the only EP4-receptor antagonist available for dogs in veterinary medicine is grapiprant (Galliprant®, Elanco, Indiana, USA) [39]. The most common adverse effects of grapiprant are short-term vomiting and diarrhea. Grapiprant has also been used successfully in cats with little to no adverse effects [40].

Preemptive Phase

Preemptive analgesia significantly decreases the process of peripheral and central hypersensitization and wind-up. Most veterinary practitioners understand the value of preemptive analgesia and include analgesic medications in their preanesthetic protocols (Table 22.2).

Opioid receptor agonists are commonly used as preemptive analgesic due to their analgesic profile as well as the sedation that is synergistic with co-administered sedatives (neuroleptanalgesia). In veterinary medicine, butorphanol is commonly used as a preemptive opioid analgesic. Butorphanol acts as a mu-opioid receptor antagonist and a kappa-opioid receptor agonist. Unfortunately, butorphanol has limited analgesic effects and lasts less than 1.5 h in dogs with variable duration of action in cats [28]. When butorphanol is used as a preemptive analgesic, a different opioid or other analgesic should be administered during the intraoperative and postoperative phases. Other opioid options include hydromorphone and morphine (Table 22.2). A common misunderstanding is that hydromorphone should not be used in cats. While hyperthermia has been associated with its use, hydromorphone is a safe and effective opioid in cats [41]. Buprenorphine is a partial mu-opioid receptor agonist with an extended length of action in dogs and cats (4–6 h). A 24-h version (Simbadol®, Zoetis, New Jersey, USA, $0.24\,mg\,kg^{-1}$) is a highly concentrated form ($1.8\,mg\,ml^{-1}$) of buprenorphine.

Acepromazine does not have analgesic properties; however, it can act as an adjunct sedative when combined with an opioid administered preemptively [42]. Alpha-2-adrenergic receptor agonists have some analgesic properties and are a good option for preemptive pain control when combined with an opioid. Nonsteroidal anti-inflammatory agents can be safely administered preemptively in healthy veterinary patients, but caution should be taken when administering preemptively if hypotension is anticipated. Combining ketamine with a benzodiazepine (ketamine/diazepam, ketamine/midazolam) will provide a loading dose for a perioperative ketamine continuous rate infusion (CRI), which is quite useful in many painful situations. In addition, any mu-opioid receptor agonist opioid will provide a loading dose for a fentanyl or sufentanil CRI, which are short-acting mu-opioid agonists.

Local and regional anesthetic procedures are an important analgesic tool in small-animal veterinary medicine. Although the practice of regional anesthesia is beyond the scope of this chapter, local techniques should always be incorporated into anesthetic protocols. An excellent textbook reference for locoregional

Table 22.2 Examples of analgesic medications used in the perioperative phase.

Intermittent injections			
Drug family	**Representatives**	**Dosage**	**Notes**
Opioids	Morphine	0.1–0.5 mg kg^{-1} IV as needed, every 2–4 h	
	Hydromorphone	0.07–0.2 mg kg^{-1} IV as needed, every 2–4 h	
	Methadone	0.25–0.35 mg kg^{-1} IV as needed, every 2–4 h	
	Fentanyl	2.5–10 μg kg^{-1} IV as needed	Short-acting opioid, can accumulate in thin patients, cats
	Sufentanil	0.5–5 μg kg^{-1} IV as needed	Short-acting opioid, effects last 20–30 min
Local anesthetics	Lidocaine	1–3 mg kg^{-1} IV every 1–2 h (also used as a loading dose for a CRI)	Do not use IV in cats
Alpha-2 agonists	Dexmedetomidine	0.5–3 μg kg^{-1} IV	
NMDA antagonists	Ketamine	0.5–3 mg kg^{-1} IV (also used as loading dose for a CRI)	Avoid in cats with hypertrophic cardiomyopathy
Constant rate infusions			
Drugs	Dosage	Notes	
Lidocaine	1.5–6 mg kg^{-1} h^{-1}	Lidocaine alone or combined with ketamine (LK)	Do not use IV in cats
Ketamine	0.6–1.2 mg kg^{-1} h^{-1}	Ketamine alone or LK	
Morphine	0.1 mg kg^{-1} h^{-1}	Morphine alone or + LK	
Hydromorphone	0.02 mg kg^{-1} h^{-1}	Hydromorphone alone or + LK	
Fentanyl	5–15 μg kg^{-1} h^{-1}	Fentanyl alone or + LK	
Sufentanil	0.5–3 μg kg^{-1} h^{-1}	Sufentanil alone or + LK	
Dexmedetomidine	0.5–2 μg kg^{-1} h^{-1}	Dexmedetomidine alone or + LK	
Dexmedetomidine + morphine	0.5 μg dexmedetomidine + 0.2 mg kg^{-1} h^{-1} morphine	Can be combined with LK infusion	

techniques is *Small Animal Regional Anesthesia and Analgesia*, edited by Luis Campoy and Matt Read. Multiple local anesthetic agents can be chosen based on patient need and agent onset and duration of action. For example, lidocaine is a versatile local anesthetic, as it can be used as a short duration locoregional drug and/or administered systemically as an intravenous analgesic/anesthetic adjunct in dogs (Table 22.2). However, due to negative myocardial effects, lidocaine should not be used as an intravenous analgesic agent in cats [43].

Gabapentin is gaining popularity as both a preemptive and postoperative analgesic drug. Gabapentin is a structural analog to gamma-aminobutyric acid (GABA), but does not interact with the GABA receptors, is not a GABA agonist, and nor does it regulate the GABA neurotransmitter. Although the method of action is not completely understood, gabapentin appears to inhibit calcium channels on neurons [44]. Studies have shown that gabapentin may have good analgesic properties for wind-up and/or neuropathic pain in dogs [45]. However, its use in acute, surgical pain states is lacking. Ketamine can be used as an analgesic, sedative, and/or induction agent depending on the dose administered. As an NMDA receptor antagonist, ketamine is another option to help control wind-up and/or neuropathic pain. High-dose ketamine and tiletamine should be used cautiously with cats that have hypertrophic cardiomyopathy. Maropitant is a popular antiemetic in dogs and cats. Maropitant's NK1 antagonistic properties at both the spinal cord and brain provide a minimum alveolar concentration (MAC)-sparing effect during abdominal surgery in dogs and cats [46, 47]; however, definitive proof of the analgesic properties of maropitant is lacking and the administration of additional analgesics is advised.

Intraoperative Phase

Protocol choices and limitation of intraoperative analgesics are often based on a practitioner's level of comfort and/or understanding, availability of drugs, and postoperative monitoring capabilities. It is discouraged to discharge or leave a patient unattended overnight if the patient is still demonstrating sedative or central and peripheral neurotropic effects of narcotics and/or other analgesic/anesthetic drugs. Therefore, intraoperative protocols involving intravenous lidocaine (only in dogs) and subanesthetic dosages of ketamine, alone or mixed, as constant rate infusions are excellent options to help control surgical nociception with a potential for decreased postoperative sedation when discontinued appropriately. Intermittent injections can be used if CRI options are unavailable; however, most CRI cocktails can be mixed and administered via an intravenous fluid drip set or graduated-burette infusion devices. Syringe drivers/syringe pumps are more accurate and easier to use; however, they are not necessarily required for intraoperative CRIs. Opioids and/or dexmedetomidine (1-2 $\mu g\ kg^{-1}\ hr^{-1}$) are commonly used in combination with lidocaine and ketamine for CRIs. Cats do not tolerate intravenous lidocaine; therefore, combinations of ketamine, dexmedetomidine, and/or an opioid can be used. Any of the drugs listed in Table 22.2 can be used alone or in combination, depending on the need. Any single drug or combination can be tailored to desired effects.

Postoperative Phase

Immediate Postoperative Care

Monitoring for levels of pain in small-animal veterinary patients can be accomplished utilizing pain scores such as the canine and feline Glasgow composite pain scales (https://www.newmetrica.com/wp-content/uploads/2016/09/Reid-et-al-2007.pdf). Pharmaceutical options for postoperative analgesia are commonly a continuation of the preoperative and/or intraoperative protocols. Depending on the surgery, and the patient's general medical state, postoperative analgesia should be tailored according to the clinical situation. In addition, NSAIDs should not be relied upon as the primary/only analgesic choice. Although NSAIDs are a common and safe drug choice, they should be used according to the patient's needs and in conjunction with other postoperative analgesic modalities. Due to the opioid crisis and an ever-increasing availability of alternative drugs, narcotic prescriptions for veterinary patients have become less popular. To reduce hyperalgesic states, other options include gabapentin and amantadine. Amantadine is an NMDA receptor antagonist that has been shown to reduce surgical neuropathic pain in human cancer patients [48]. Amantadine has also been used to treat chronic neuropathic pain in dogs [49]. Nocita® (Elanco, Indiana, USA) is a liposome-encapsulated form of bupivacaine that provides local anesthesia at the injection site for up to 72 h. Nocita is gaining popularity as a local, postoperative, surgical site infusion, performed during surgical closure (Figure 22.2). However, Nocita is also FDA approved as a peripheral nerve block to provide preemptive regional anesthesia in cats undergoing onychectomies. For detailed instructions on its clinical use and administration guidelines, the reader is directed to the manufacturer's prescribing information and package insert (https://www.elanco.us/products-services/dogs/nocita, https://www.elanco.us/products-services/cats/nocita).

Nonpharmaceutical options for analgesia and patient welfare include icing surgical sites, cold laser, appropriate bedding, patient body temperature control, feed and water intake, urination and defecation, etc. The postoperative period is a time when anesthesia-related complications commonly occur in veterinary medicine. In addition, companion veterinary patients are accustomed to human contact, especially during stress. Therefore, postoperative veterinary patients should be monitored until they are able to swallow, maintain themselves in sternal recumbency, and/or stand and walk.

Pain scoring should be performed preoperatively (baseline score) and immediately postoperative when the patient is fully recovered. Guidelines for analgesia intervention based on pain scoring are suggested at a score

(a)

(b)

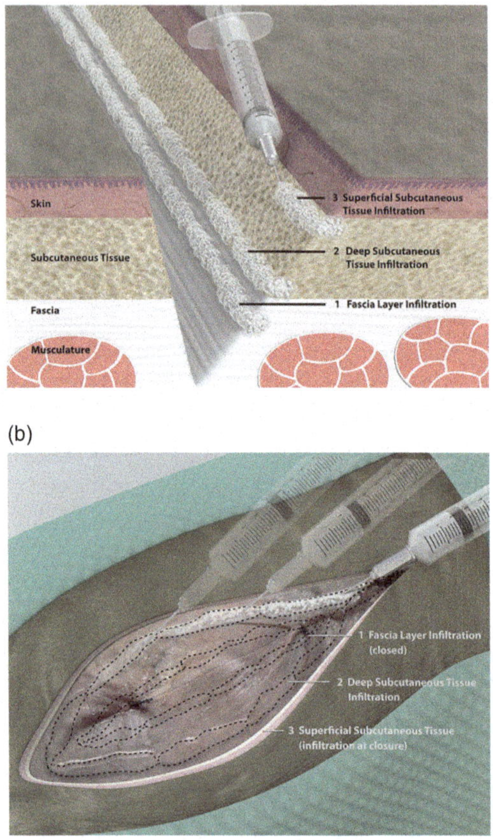

Figure 22.2 (a) Cross-sectional illustration of correct administration of the liposomal bupivacaine solution, Nocita. Infiltration should be performed at all layers of closure, including the levels of the muscle and surrounding fascia, deep subcutaneous, and superficial tissues. (b) Illustration of the moving needle technique to infiltrate incisional layers. Nocita should be infiltrated as the needle withdraws slowly along a plane of coverage. Aspiration to verify absence of blood should always be performed prior to injection of local anesthetic solutions. Source: Images courtesy of Elanco Animal Health, with permission.

of 6/24 or greater on the Glasgow Composite Pain Scale for dogs able to ambulate, or 5/20 or greater for patients unable to ambulate. For feline patients, a score of 5/20 or greater should receive additional analgesics. Pain scoring should continue at least every 30–60 min for patients receiving rescue analgesia to determine efficacy. For patients that have well-managed postoperative pain, scoring should be repeated an hour after the first score that indicates that the patient no longer needs additional analgesia, within 3 h after the first score, and then again 12 h later.

Long-Term Postoperative Care

Until recently, long-term analgesia and long-term patient recovery have been mostly ignored in veterinary medicine. With the successful applications of physical therapy in human medicine, veterinary medicine has gradually followed suit. Extended analgesia and patient recovery options include rehabilitation, acupuncture, electro-acupuncture, low-level laser therapy, therapeutic massage, and chiropractic modalities. The monitoring of patient progress, including pain control, should occur frequently depending on the patient's overall needs. Myofascial palpation should be an important aspect of long-term patient recovery. Myofascial palpation is a documented method of assessing myofascial changes related to weight transfer, tension, and chronic, progressive pathology [50]. In addition to myofascial changes, behavioral changes are also important ways to assess long-term pain management. Common behavioral signs of chronic pain with veterinary patients include gait and posture changes, reluctance to move, preferential recumbency (i.e., avoids one side of the hip when lying down), changes regarding interaction with humans (aggression, submission), changes with eating, urination, or defecation, and changes with grooming or hair coat. Other options to aid in evaluating chronic pain include the Helsinki Chronic Pain Index and the Canine Brief Pain Index [51].

The most important aspect of successful pain management with veterinary patients is practicing good client communication. Veterinary practitioners must take the role in educating their clients on what to expect immediately postoperative and in long term. Owners should receive pain management information and have questions answered before the procedure. The source of pain, potential effects related to pain, and several options to manage pain should be part of the preoperative discussion. Caregivers and the veterinarians should communicate openly about the patient's pain management.

References

1 Muir, W.W. (2015). Pain and stress: stress-induced hyperalgesia and hypoalgesia. In: *Handbook of Veterinary Pain Management*, 3e (eds. J.S. Gaynor and W.W. Muir), 42–60. St. Louis: Elsevier Mosby.

2 Farina, S., Tinazzi, M., Le Pera, D. et al. (2003). Pain-related modulation of the human motor cortex. *Neurol. Res.* 25: 130–142.

3 Arnoff, G.M. (2016). What we know about the pathophysiology of chronic pain? Implications for treatment considerations. *Med. Clin. North Am.* 100 (1): 31–42.

4 Adbo, H., Calvo-Enrique, L., Lopez, J.M. et al. (2019). Specialized cutaneous Schwann cells initiate pain sensation. *Science* 365: 695–699.

5 Wiese, A.J. and Yaksh, T.L. (2015). Nociception and pain mechanisms. In: *Handbook of Veterinary Pain Management*, 3e (eds. J.S. Gaynor and W.W. Muir), 10–41. St. Louis: Elsevier Mosby.

6 Phillips, W.J. and Currier, B.L. (2004). Analgesic pharmacology: I. Neurophysiology. *J. Am. Acad. Orthop. Surg.* 12 (4): 213–220.

7 Latremoliere, A. and Wolff, C.J. (2009). Central sensitization: a generator of pain hypersensitivity by central neural plasticity. *J. Pain* 10: 895–926.

8 Eller-Smith, O.C., Nicol, A.L., and Christianson, J.A. (2018). Potential mechanisms underlying centralized pain and emerging therapeutic interventions. *Front. Cell. Neurosci.* 13: 12–35.

9 Rong, P.J., Li, S., Ben, H. et al. (2013). Peripheral and spinal mechanisms of acupoint sensitization phenomenon. *Evid. Based Compliment Altern. Med.* 2013: 742195.

10 Cheng, B., Shi, H., Ji, C.F. et al. (2010). Distribution of the activated acupoints after acute gastric mucosal injury in the rat. *Acutpunct. Res.* 35: 193–197.

11 Romano, T. (2007). Chronic persistent pain can kill. *Pract. Pain Manag.* 7: 7.

12 Collier, R. (2018). A short history of pain management. *Can. Med. Assoc. J.* 190: E26–E27.

13 Epstein, M. (2013). Managing chronic pain in cats & dogs part 1: the two most important tools in the treatment of osteoarthritis. *TVP*. November/December:: 20–23.

14 Epstein, M., Rodan, I., Griffenhagen, G. et al. (2015). Pain management guidelines for dogs and cats. *J. Am. Anim. Hosp. Assoc.* 51: 67–84.

15 Murnion, B.P. (2018). Neuropathic pain: current definition and review of drug treatment. *Aust. Prescr.* 41: 60–63.

16 Latremoliere, A. and Woolf, C.J. (2009). Central sensitization: a generator of pain hypersensitivity by neural plasticity. *J. Pain* 10: 895–926.

17 Dworkin, R.H., O'Connor, A.B., Backonja, M. et al. (2007). Pharmacologic management of neuropathic pain: evidence-based recommendations. *Pain* 132: 237–251.

18 Crile, G.W. (1913). The kinetic theory of shock and its prevention through anoci-association (shockless operation). *Lancet* 185: 7–16.

19 Woolf, C.J. and Wall, P.D. (1986). Morphine-sensitive and morphine insensitive action of C-fiber input on the rat spinal cord. *Neurosci. Lett.* 64: 221–225.

20 Katz, J., Clarke, H., and Seltzer, Z. (2011). Preventive analgesia: quo vadiumus? *Anesth. Analg.* 113: 1242–1253.

21 Clark, L. (2014). Pre-emptive or preventive analgesia – lessons from the human literature? *Vet. Anaesth. Analg.* 41: 109–112.

22 Gurney, M.A. (2012). Pharmacological options for intra- operative and early postoperative analgesia: an update. *J. Small Anim. Pract.* 53: 377–386.

23 Van Dyke, J.B. (2012). Introduction to veterinary rehabilitation. In: *WSAVA/FECAVA/BSAVA World Congress*. Canine Rehabilitation Institute, FL.

24 Corder, G., Castro, D.C., Bruchas, M.R. et al. (2018). Endogenous and exogenous opioids in pain. *Annu. Rev. Neurosci.* 8: 453–473.

25 Epstein, M. (2015). Opioids. In: *Handbook of Veterinary Pain Management*, 3e (eds. J.S. Gaynor and W.W. Muir), 161–195. St. Louis: Elsevier Mosby.

26 Lamont, L.A. and Mathews, K.A. (2007). Opioids, non-steroidal anti-inflammatories, and analgesic adjuvants. In: *Lumb and Jones Veterinary Anesthesia and Analgesia*, 4e (eds. W.J. Tranquilli, J.C. Thurmon and K.A. Grimm), 241–271. Ames: Blackwell Publishing.

27 Trescot, A.M., Datta, S., Lee, M. et al. (2008). Opioid pharmacology. *Pain Physician* 11 (2 Suppl): S133–S153.

28 Kukanich, B. and Papich, M.G. (2009). Opioid analgesic drugs. In: *Veterinary Pharmacology & Therapeutics*, 9e (eds. J.E. Riviere and M.G. Papich), 301–335. Ames: Blackwell Publishing.

29 Posner, L.A. and Burns, P. (2009). Sedative agents: tranquilizers, alpha-2 agonists, and related agents. In: *Veterinary Pharmacology & Therapeutics*, 9e (eds. J.E. Riviere and M.G. Papich), 337–380. Ames: Blackwell Publishing.

30 Pypendop, B. (2015). α2-agonists. nociception and pain mechanisms. In: *Handbook of Veterinary Pain Management*, 3e (eds. J.S. Gaynor and W.W. Muir), 196–215. St. Louis: Elsevier Mosby.

31 Muir, W.W., Hubbell, A.E., Bednarski, R.M., and Lerche, P. (eds.) (2013). Preanesthetic and perioperative medications. In: *Handbook of Veterinary Anesthesia*, 5e, 22–57. St. Louis: Elsevier.

32 Posner, L.A. and Burns, P. (2009). Injectable anesthetic agents. In: *Veterinary Pharmacology & Therapeutics*, 9e (eds. J.E. Riviere and M.G. Papich), 265–299. Ames: Blackwell Publishing.

33 Muir, W.W., Hubbell, A.E., Bednarski, R.M. et al. (2013). Injectable anesthetic drugs. In: *Handbook of Veterinary Anesthesia*, 5e (eds. W.W. Muir, A.E. Hubbell, R.M. Bednarski and P. Lerche), 139–162. St. Louis: Elsevier.

34 Gutierrez-Blanco, E., Victoria-Mora, J.M., Ibancovichi-Camarillo, J.A. et al. (2013). Evaluation of the isoflurane-sparing effects of fentanyl, lidocaine, ketamine, dexmedetomidine, or the combination lidocaine-ketamine-dexmedetomidine during ovariohysterectomy in dogs. *Vet. Anaesth. Analg.* 40: 599–609.

35 Branson, K. (2001). Injectable anesthetics. In: *Veterinary Pharmacology and Therapeutics*, 8e (ed. H.R. Adams), 213–267. Ames: Blackwell Publishing Professional.

36 Robinson, R. and Borgeat, K. (2016). Cardiovascular disease. In: *BSAVA Manual of Canine and Feline Anaesthesia and Analgesia*, 3e (eds. T. Duke-Novakovski, M. de Vries and C. Seymour), 283–313. Gloucester: British Small Animal Veterinary Association.

37 Monteiro-Steagall, B.P., Steagall, P.V.M., and Lascelles, B.D.X. (2013). Systemic review of nonsteroidal anti-inflammatory drug-induced adverse effects in dogs. *J. Vet. Intern. Med.* 37: 1011–1019.

38 Papich, M.G. and Messenger, K. (2015). Non-steroidal anti-inflammatory drugs. In: *Lumb and Jones Veterinary Anesthesia and Analgesia*, 5e (eds. K.A. Grimm, L.A. Lamont, W.J. Tranquilli, et al.), 227–243. Ames: Wiley.

39 Shaw, K.K., Rausch-Derra, L.C., and Rhodes, L. (2015). Grapiprant: an EP4 prostaglandin receptor antagonist and novel therapy for pain and inflammation. *Vet. Med. Sci.* 21 (2): 3–9.

40 Rausch-Derra, L.C. and Rhodes, L. (2016). Safety and toxicokinetic profiles associated with daily oral administration of grapiprant, a selective antagonist of the prostaglandin E2 EP4 receptor, to cats. *Am. J. Vet. Res.* 77: 688–692.

41 Kukanich, B. and Wiese, A.J. (2015). Opioids. In: *Lumb and Jones Veterinary Anesthesia and Analgesia*, 5e (eds. K.A. Grimm, L.A. Lamont, W.J. Tranquilli, et al.), 207–226. Ames: Wiley.

42 Muir, W.W. (2015). Drug interactions, analgesic protocols and their consequences, and analgesic drug antagonism. In: *Handbook of Veterinary Pain Management*, 3e (eds. J.S. Gaynor and W.W. Muir), 335–362. St. Louis: Elsevier Mosby.

43 Pypendop, B.H. and Ilkiw, J.E. (2005). Assessment of the hemodynamic effects of lidocaine administered IV in isoflurane-anesthetized cats. *Am. J. Vet. Res.* 66: 661–668.

44 Papich, M. (2009). Anticonvulsant drugs. In: *Veterinary Pharmacology & Therapeutics*, 9e (eds. J.E. Riviere and M.G. Papich), 493–508. Ames: Blackwell Publishing.

45 Cashmore, R.G., Harcourt-Brown, T.R., Freeman, P.M. et al. (2009). Clinical diagnosis and treatment of suspected neuropathic pain in three dogs. *Aust. Vet. J.* 87: 45–50.

46 Boscan, P., Monnet, E., Mama, K. et al. (2011). Effect of maropitant, a neurokinin 1 receptor antagonist, on anesthetic requirements during noxious visceral stimulation of the ovary in dogs. *Am. J. Vet. Res.* 72: 1576–1579.

47 Niyom, S., Boscan, P., Twedt, D.C. et al. (2013). Effect of maropitant, a neurokinin-1 receptor antagonist, on the minimum alveolar concentration of sevoflurane during stimulation of the ovarian ligament in cats. *Vet. Anaesth. Analg.* 40: 425–431.

48 Pud, D., Eisenberg, E., Spitzer, A. et al. (1998). The NMDA receptor antagonist amantadine reduces surgical neuropathic pain in cancer patients: a double blind, randomized, placebo controlled trial. *Pain* 75 (2-3): 349–354.

49 Madden, M., Gurney, M., and Bright, S. (2014). Amantadine, an N-methyl-D-aspartate antagonist, for treatment of chronic neuropathic pain in a dog. *Vet. Anaesth. Analg.* 41: 440–441.

50 Ward, R.C. (1997). Integrated neuromusculoskeletal release and myofascial release. In: *Foundations for Osteopathic Medicine* (ed. R.C. Ward). Baltimore: Williams & Wilkins.

51 Hielm-Björkman, A.K., Rita, H., and Tulamo, R.M. (2009). Psychometric testing of the Helsinki chronic pain index by completion of a questionnaire in Finnish by owners of dogs with chronic signs of pain caused by osteoarthritis. *Am. J. Vet. Res.* 70: 727–734.

23

Cardiopulmonary Resuscitation and Postcardiac Arrest Care

Thomas K. Day

VCA Veterinary Emergency Service and Specialty Center, Middleton, WI, 53562, USA

Introduction

The overall incidence of cardiopulmonary arrest (CPA) during anesthesia or sedation in veterinary medicine is reported to be 0.17% in dogs and 0.24% in cats [1]. While the overall survival rate from CPA is 6–7% [2], the survival rate for dogs and cats that have CPA while anesthetized is as high as 47% [3]. Guidelines for cardiopulmonary resuscitation (CPR) in veterinary medicine have historically been determined by guidelines from human medicine, specifically by the American Heart Association (AHA) or have been developed based on veterinary expert opinion [4]. The Reassessment Campaign on Veterinary Resuscitation (RECOVER) has developed guidelines for CPR in dogs and cats and was also designed to increase our knowledge to improve the quality of these guidelines for CPA [5–11]. This chapter is based on the RECOVER guidelines for CPA in dogs and cats and is directed to CPA in the perianesthetic period.

CPR Preparedness and Prevention

The most important element of having an efficient CPR experience is to have a premade arrest station, or crash cart, that contains all of the items necessary for CPR (Figures 23.1–23.5) [4]. The crash cart should be organized in a manner that all essential equipment can readily be obtained from the cart during a CPR event. The example provided has the biphasic (BP) veterinary defibrillator with electrocardiogram (ECG) cables, attached pulse oximeter, ECG pads, and suction unit on top of the crash cart (Figure 23.1). The first drawer contains various sized syringes with and without needles, catheter flush, and CPR drugs (Figure 23.2). The second drawer contains airway management items including a portable capnometer (Figure 23.3). The third drawer contains IV catheter items (Figure 23.4). The fourth drawer contains surgical items and the internal defibrillation paddles (Figure 23.5). The

Canine and Feline Anesthesia and Co-Existing Disease, Second Edition. Edited by Rebecca A. Johnson, Lindsey B. C. Snyder and Carrie A. Schroeder.

Companion website: www.wiley.com/go/johnson/canine

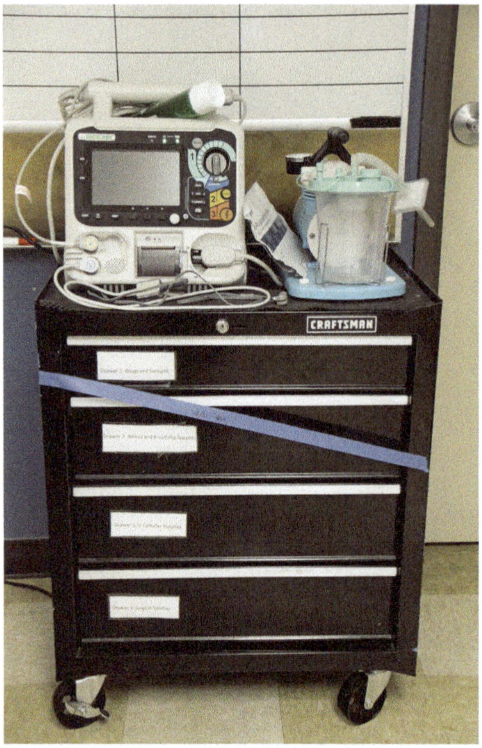

Figure 23.1 Example of a crash cart in a readily available location.

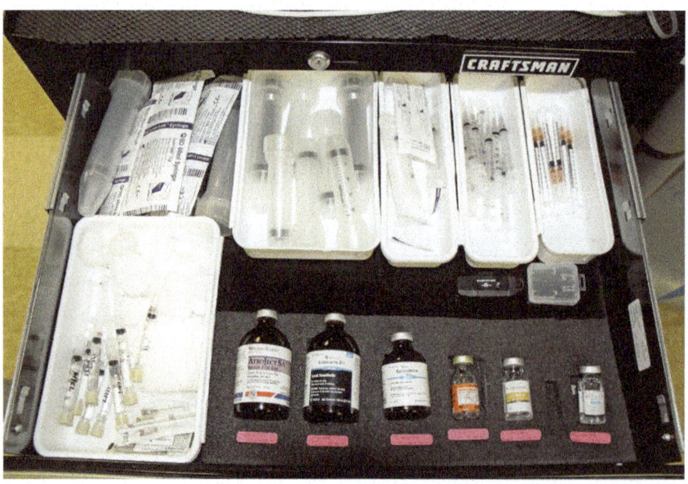

Figure 23.2 Drawer of a crash cart containing CPR drugs, needles, and syringes.

crash cart should be in an area that is readily accessible during the perianesthetic period, whether it is in the main treatment area, in an induction or surgical suite, or in the recovery area. The most common problem in human medicine involving the arrest station area is lack of returning equipment or not restocking necessary medication [12]. Therefore, some indicator such as a piece of intact tape needs to be placed on the crash cart to know that it is fully stocked, marked with date it was updated (Figure 23.1).

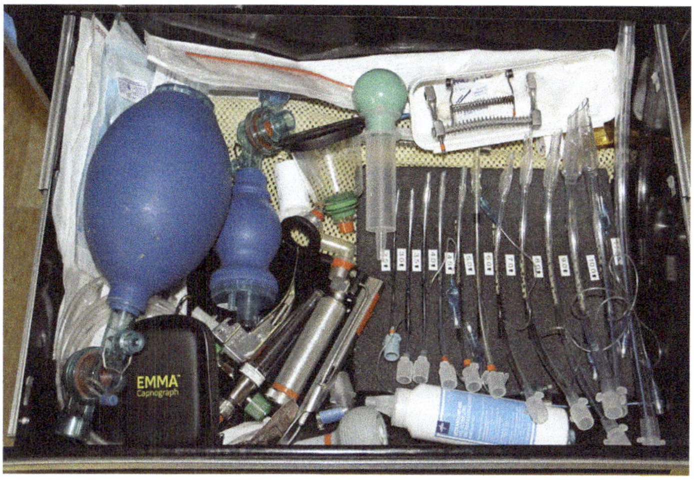

Figure 23.3 Drawer of a crash cart containing airway management items.

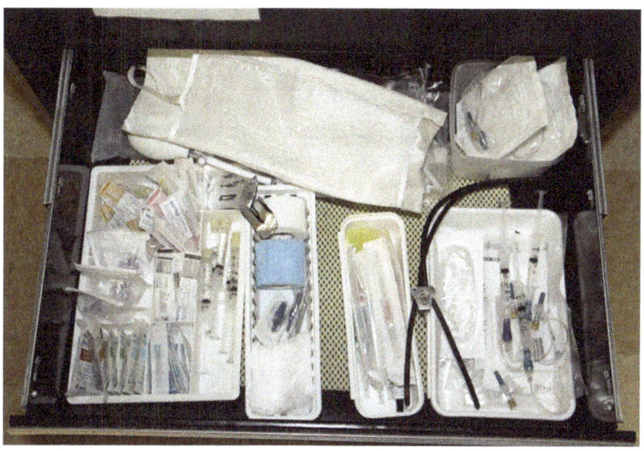

Figure 23.4 Drawer of a crash cart containing intravenous catheter items.

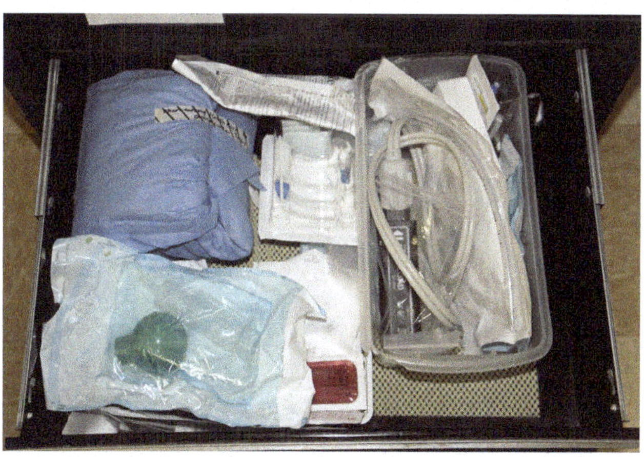

Figure 23.5 Drawer of a crash cart containing surgical items.

There is essential equipment for a crash cart (Table 23.1) including multiple sizes of needles, syringes, and IV catheters along with ready-made securing material. There should be a variety of endotracheal tubes and equipment to secure an airway, including materials to perform an emergent tracheostomy. CPR drugs are discussed later in the chapter. A defibrillator with an ECG monitor is the most expensive yet essential item in a crash cart, since no currently available drugs will effectively and reproducibly convert ventricular fibrillation (VF) to normal sinus rhythm; only electrical defibrillation can convert VF. Suction should also be readily available.

Human evidence suggests that the quality of CPR improves with continued training and the use of CPR manikins [13]. There are no current studies in veterinary medicine that investigate the effect of training, or lack of continued training, on the effectiveness of CPR. Most veterinarians and veterinary nurses learned CPR during their initial schooling and many personnel may have minimal experience with CPR unless working in an emergency environment. It is recommended that veterinary personnel review all equipment (including the defibrillator) and CPR protocols and procedures every 6 months [11]. This is especially true for anesthesia personnel considering that CPR for an anesthesia or sedation event has a higher chance of being successful [7]. Veterinarians and veterinary support staff can obtain CPR certification through the RECOVER website (www.recoverinitiative.org).

A CPA related to anesthesia or sedation has a high likelihood of being prevented. Many anesthetic drugs are cardiopulmonary depressants and are commonly used in combination, resulting in additive or synergistic decreases in cardiac and pulmonary functions (Table 23.2). Constant monitoring during anesthesia can result in recognition of early signs of CPA (see the section titled "Basic Life Support" in the following text) and early intervention. An important advantage to several anesthetic drugs is reversibility. For example, atipamezole reverses the effects of dexmedetomidine, naloxone reverses opioid effects, and flumazenil

Table 23.1 Essential crash cart items.

- Defibrillator with ECG capability—both external and internal paddles, gel for external paddles
- Intubation equipment—several sizes of endotracheal tubes, laryngoscope, several sizes of laryngoscope blades, material to tie in endotracheal tube
- Ambu bag—two sizes
- Drugs: epinephrine, atropine, lidocaine, naloxone, flumazenil, atipamezole
- Intravenous catheter material
- Surgical equipment for open chest cardiac massage
- Tracheostomy equipment

Table 23.2 Cardiac and pulmonary depressant effects of anesthetic drugs.

Drug	Heart rate	Blood pressure	Respiratory effect
Opioids (e.g., morphine, hydromorphone, methadone)	Bradycardia, AV block	No direct effect, though hypotension with bradycardia	Moderate depression
Alpha-2 agonists (e.g., dexmedetomidine)	Bradycardia, AV block	Increase or decrease	Moderate depression
Acepromazine	Tachycardia	Hypotension	No effect
Propofol	Tachycardia	Hypotension	Severe depression
Alfaxalone	Tachycardia	Hypotension	Severe depression
Benzodiazepines	Minimal effect	Minimal effect	Mild depression

AV, atrioventricular.

reverses benzodiazepine action. In addition, 100% oxygen is delivered during inhalation anesthesia and some method of oxygen delivery can be applied during sedation. It is possible that the increased survival rate for CPR in anesthetized patients could be due to higher arterial oxygen content before CPA and an increased time before tissues such as the brain and heart become hypoxic. Another possible reason for a higher success rate in anesthetized animals undergoing elective procedures is that some anesthetized patients tend to be younger in age.

Basic Life Support

Basic life support (BLS) is defined as the recognition of CPA, obtaining a patent airway, and performing ventilation and chest compressions (external or internal) [7]. Human studies suggest that the BLS quality is directly related to an increased survival rate [14, 15]. Chest compressions can be either external or internal with external chest compressions utilized far more commonly. The indications for immediate internal compressions, also termed cardiac massage, include a thoracic cage that is not intact, usually due to trauma, or if the patient is under general anesthesia during an abdominal or thoracic surgery.

With CPA during inhalation anesthesia, the most challenging aspect of BLS will be recognition of CPA, as patients are already intubated, usually have patent IV catheters with fluids being administered, and are receiving 100% oxygen. There are no studies that address the issue of recognizing CPA in anesthetized dogs and cats [7]. Identification of CPA in nonanesthetized dogs and cats involves loss of consciousness, lack of breathing efforts or agonal gasps, and/or loss of a heartbeat or pulse [7]. Other signs indicative of CPA include pale to white mucous membranes and sudden loss of blood pressure. These signs can be applied to dogs and cats that are sedated. However, identification of CPA during inhalation anesthesia can be more challenging and may be dependent on the amount of monitoring being used. Inhalation anesthetics are potent respiratory depressants, and it is expected for dogs and cats under inhalation anesthesia and breathing spontaneously to have reduced respiratory rate/tidal volume and increased arterial carbon dioxide as measured by arterial blood gas or via capnography. Cessation of all respirations (respiratory arrest) is usually followed by cardiovascular complications such as severe bradycardia and hypotension and developing sinus arrest or VF. Breath by breath decreases in end-tidal carbon dioxide (ETCO2) are a sign of impending circulatory arrest and complete, abrupt cessation of $ETCO_2$ can signify cardiac arrest [16].

Sedated dogs and cats that experience CPA should have an airway secured and ventilation begins at 10 breaths min^{-1} via an Ambu bag or anesthesia machine while chest compressions are started [7, 11]. Immediate ventilation is essential in BLS, as studies in animal models and human clinical patients show that hypoxia and hypercapnia reduce the likelihood of return of spontaneous circulation (ROSC) [17, 18]. Care should be taken to avoid hyperventilation; therefore, in addition to a rate of 10 breaths min^{-1}, an inspiratory time of 1 s should be applied, as this time equates to a tidal volume of approximately 10 ml kg^{-1} [7].

External chest compressions should begin immediately. High-quality external chest compressions can provide a maximum of 25–30% of the normal cardiac output; animal position and hand location are extremely important to achieve this goal (Figures 23.6 and 23.7) [11]. The two theories of circulation during external chest compressions are the cardiac pump theory and the thoracic pump theory. One experimental study has revealed the difference between the cardiac and thoracic pump theories of external chest compressions [19]. For example, external chest compressions over the heart result in closure of the mitral valve and direct blood flow from the heart (cardiac pump). External chest compression directed at

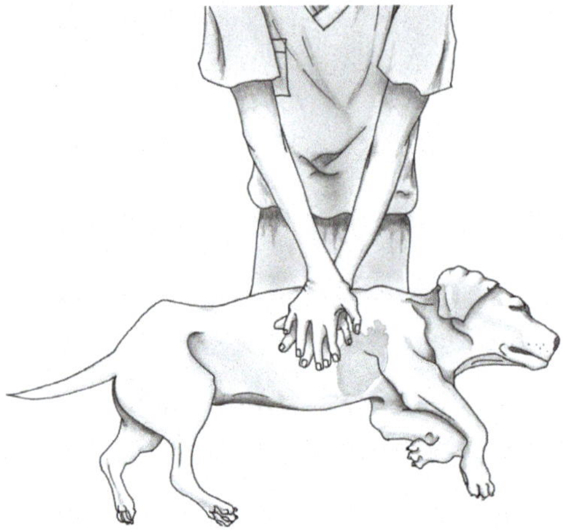

Figure 23.6 Hand position during external chest compressions in the dog. Source: Image from Fletcher et al. (2012) with permission.

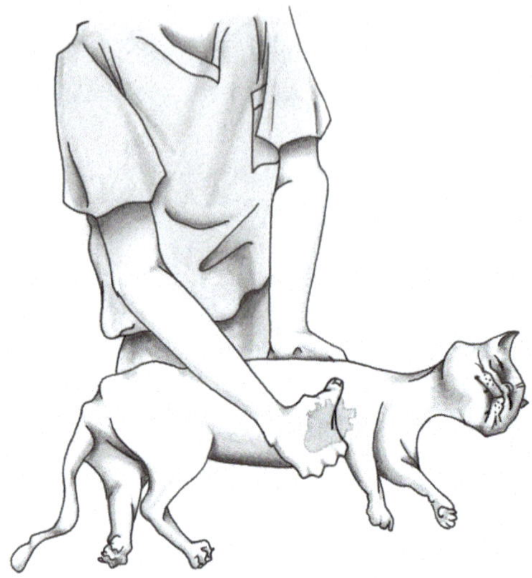

Figure 23.7 Correct hand position for external chest compressions in the cat and small dog. Source: Image from Fletcher et al. (2012) with permission.

the peak height of the thorax in lateral recumbency results in the mitral valve continuously open and blood flow circulating passively (thoracic pump). There is a difference in recommended hand placement based on the size of the dog or cat (Figures 23.6 and 23.7). A medium- to large-sized dog should have the back against the resuscitator and both hands placed at the highest part of the thorax (Figure 23.6). The thoracic pump theory is likely to prevail with this method of external chest compressions. Small dogs and cats can be placed perpendicular to the resuscitator with one hand over the thorax and one had over the sternum (Figure 23.7). Both hands compress simultaneously, as one hand will be directly over the heart and one hand will be at the highest part of the thorax. The cardiac pump theory is likely to occur during compressions using this method. Dogs with a thorax that is equally deep as wide can be in lateral or dorsal recumbency during external chest compressions, though this technique may seem uncomfortable.

The external chest compression rate in dogs and cats necessary for maximal cardiac output is between 100 and 120 beats min^{-1} [7, 11]. The ideal depth of external chest compressions has not been determined in dogs and cats. However, extrapolation from human CPR studies implies that a depth between one-third and one-half of the chest wall width is reasonable, whereas greater than one-half of the depth could damage the thoracic wall [20]. Allowing complete thoracic recoil is vital to maintain cardiac output during external chest compressions; leaning on the thorax during chest compressions in humans decreases cardiac output [21]. In addition, there should be no pause in external chest compressions when delivering breaths during CPR [7, 11]. Finally, mixed results are seen in dog and pig models concerning interposed abdominal compression with external chest compression to improve venous return and cardiac output [7]. No harm has been shown with interposed abdominal compressions, though a large benefit has not been seen; thus, while this technique may not be detrimental, it may not be advantageous and yet requires a second resuscitator to perform.

A realistic clinical factor during CPR when maintaining effective external chest compressions at 100–120 beats min^{-1} is rescuer fatigue, especially in large dogs. Human CPR studies using manikins revealed a loss of external chest compression quality over the first three minutes [22]. Recommendations for veterinary CPR are to change resuscitators every two minutes [7, 11].

The next step for CPR in a sedated dog or cat is to reverse any previously administered opioid or alpha-2-adrenergic agonist. The benzodiazepines produce minimal cardiac or pulmonary depression and may not need to be reversed, especially since seizures may occur during the postresuscitative period. Although naloxone has a very short duration of action and may be administered multiple times, atipamezole has a very long duration of action and likely will not need to be given more than once.

Decisions to either continue with advanced life support (ALS) CPR, administer electrical defibrillation, or to discontinue CPR due to ROSC should be made based on monitoring, discussed in the following text. The ECG will be an important monitor, as the electrical activity of the heart will determine how to proceed with ALS [7].

Advanced Life Support

ALS is defined as all resuscitative efforts after BLS that can include drug administration, correction of volume deficits and electrolyte abnormalities, blood product administration, and electric defibrillation [8]. The ALS domain of the RECOVER initiative determines aspects of ALS that have historically been very controversial, based on individual bias and experience, or extrapolated directly from human CPR. The most important ALS aspects directed to veterinary patients include the treatment of asystole, pulseless electrical activity (PEA), VF, vasoactive and cardioactive drug use, and supplemental treatment implementation (i.e., oxygen, fluid therapy, blood products administration, and correction of electrolyte disturbances) in an attempt to not only make species-specific recommendations but also to simplify the technique of veterinary CPR.

Primary CPR drugs intensely investigated are epinephrine and atropine. Anecdotally, many veterinarians were taught to co-administer atropine first then epinephrine second as a standard initial drug therapy during CPR. However, there is an inherent danger to this practice, as atropine lowers the VF threshold in experimental models [23]; increased vagal tone can be protective of VF [24]. No specific experimental studies address the concurrent administration of atropine followed by epinephrine as a standard first line of drug therapy for CPR. The clinical importance is that if no defibrillator is available for CPR and VF occurs, there is no drug therapy to correct VF. Also, many anesthetic drugs increase vagal tone and bradyarrhythmias. Decision-making during an arrest where a patient has received these anesthetic drugs can also be very important, as atropine takes 1–2 min to produce an effect and epinephrine takes seconds to work.

Epinephrine is a vasoactive drug with positive chronotropic and inotropic effects that provides increases in coronary perfusion, heart rate, and blood pressure. After extensive research, the recommended dose of epinephrine for veterinary patients is $0.01\,mg\,kg^{-1}$, IV [8]. Past human experimental and clinical studies investigated the "high" dose of epinephrine ($0.1\,mg\,kg^{-1}$, IV) compared to the "low" dose of epinephrine ($0.01\,mg\,kg^{-1}$, IV); children receiving "high"-dose epinephrine compared to "low"-dose epinephrine had lower survival rate [25]. There have been no studies in dogs and cats comparing "high"- and "low"-dose epinephrine [8].

A possible alternative to epinephrine is vasopressin ($0.8\,U\,kg^{-1}$, IV). Vasopressin is a vasopressor without cardiac effects, making it a possible alternative to epinephrine and lowering the chance of drug-induced VF. There is limited evidence in dogs that shows a benefit to vasopressin. Evidence in human studies shows a benefit in subsets of arrest due to hypovolemia, asystole, or prolonged CPR [8]. Vasopressin has been considered appropriate for use in veterinary CPR [8], though could be cost-prohibitive.

Atropine (0.04 mg kg^{-1}, IV) is a vagolytic drug that can be used effectively during an arrest attributed to high vagal tone [8]. Most studies suggest atropine as an additional drug for CPR and not a sole drug. Atropine should be considered in CPA associated with high vagal tone, such as animals with vomiting and ileus; however, there are no high-quality reports supporting the routine use of atropine in an arrest not related to high vagal tone [8].

A dilemma occurs in CPA where anesthetic drugs that increase vagal tone and decrease heart rate have been used. Atropine takes several minutes to take effect. Once an arrest has been identified, intubation, ventilation, and chest compressions should commence. An ECG should be placed to determine CPR drugs that should be administered. The offending drugs should have reversal agents administered as indicated. In situations where CPA is associated with anesthetic drugs, respiratory arrest is very common. If respiratory arrest has occurred and caught early, CPA could possibly be reversed with tracheal intubation and ventilation. However, if bradycardia is still present, it is reasonable to administer atropine as a first-line drug. If there is lack of circulation, a slow ventricular escape rhythm, or continued lack of spontaneous breathing, epinephrine should be administered before, and possibly instead of atropine.

Other drugs that have been historically, particularly anecdotally, used for CPR include antiarrhythmic agents, calcium, corticosteroids, and buffers. There is no evidence that supports the routine, prophylactic use of lidocaine, procainamide, bretylium, or magnesium. Amiodarone may have use in dogs with pulseless ventricular tachycardia (VT) or VF, though the drug can cause hypotension and anaphylaxis [8]. Calcium, sodium bicarbonate, and corticosteroids have no role in CPR in dogs and cats [8].

As previously mentioned, electrical defibrillation will be the only effective treatment for VF [8]. Defibrillators are classified as either monophasic (MP) or BP. Monophasic defibrillators deliver a current in one direction between electrodes, whereas BP defibrillators have a current that begins in one direction and then reverses the other direction. Biphasic defibrillators have lower delivered energy and are more effective than MP (Figure 23.8) [26, 27]. The starting energy dose for external defibrillation is 4–6 J kg^{-1} (MP) and 2–4 J kg^{-1} (BP) [8]. The energy should be increased by

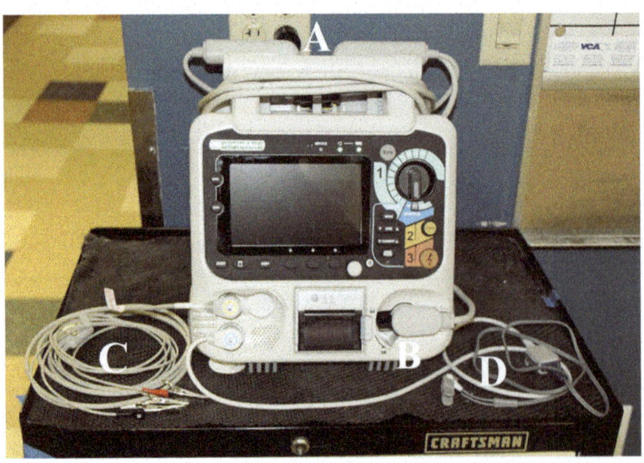

Figure 23.8 A CardioStart CS91x veterinary defibrillator (Digicare Animal Health, Digicare Biomedical, Boynton Beach, FL) with (a) external paddles that connect directly into the (b) unit, (c) ECG leads, and (d) pulse oximetry.

50% if the first delivery of energy is not successful [8]. There must be effective, solid contact with the paddles and the chest cavity with liberal use of ultrasound gel; alcohol should be avoided, as fire could be produced if electrical defibrillation is discharged on skin covered with alcohol. No personnel should be in contact with the patient or the table where the dog or cat is undergoing defibrillation.

The RECOVER guidelines recommend immediate defibrillation if VF onset is less than 4 min [8], since the ischemic heart goes through three progressive phases [28]. First is the electrical phase, in which the heart has minimal ischemic damage and can be receptive to effective defibrillation, which occurs in less than 4 min. Second is the circulatory phase in which reversible ischemic damage occurs for up to 6 min after CPA. The third and final phase is the metabolic phase, occurring after 6 min of CPA, in which potentially irreversible ischemia ensues requiring implementation of advanced CPA care procedures such as mild hypothermia and cardiopulmonary bypass to reverse the damage. It is recommended, based on the abovementioned description, that if VF has occurred for more than 4 min before defibrillation, a 2-min cycle of BLS be implemented prior to defibrillation [8].

When VF occurs during anesthesia for abdominal or thoracic surgery, the surgeon should immediately begin internal cardiac massage, either directly during a thoracotomy or by entering the thoracic cavity via incising the diaphragm during abdominal surgery. Defibrillation will need to be applied with sterile, internal paddles (Figure 23.9) placed on each side of the ventricles. The beginning energy dose is 0.5–1.0 J kg^{-1}. Note that the steps to charge the defibrillator and discharge the energy are all manual steps and care must be given to communicate each step prior to energy discharge, making certain that no personnel have contact with the patient or the surgery table. It is recommended to review the steps for external and internal defibrillation on a regular basis so that the proper communication occurs during the defibrillation process.

Monitoring During CPR

The ECG will be an important initial primary monitor used to make decisions on drug therapy or the need for defibrillation during CPR. VF is a common cause of CPA in people, though is a rare presenting rhythm in veterinary medicine [9]. Most human studies show higher survival rates with a nonshockable rhythm that then converts to pulseless VT or VF compared to when pulseless VT or VF is the initial rhythm [29, 30]. One veterinary study suggests

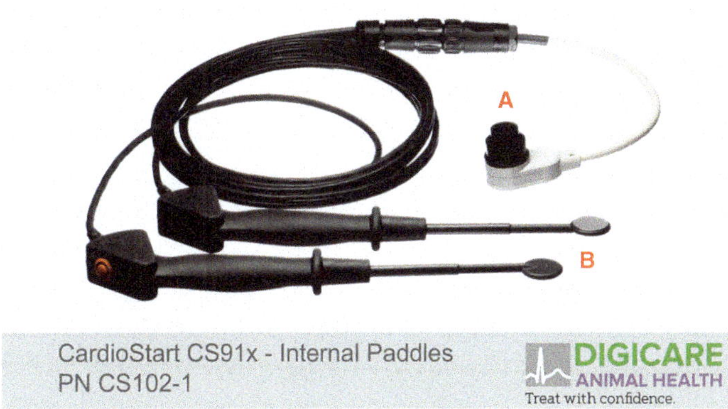

Figure 23.9 Internal defibrillation paddles. Note the connection (a) on the distal end of the paddles that will need to be connected directly to the defibrillator (Figure 23.8b). The paddles (b) will need to be placed on each side of the heart prior to discharge of the electrical energy.

that the presenting rhythm in all dogs and cats with CPA was PEA or asystole [3]. However, in sedated or anesthetized dogs and cats with CPA, the initial ECG could be related to increased vagal activity due to anesthetic drugs and concurrent hypoxemia resulting in bradyarrhythmias. Therefore, initial determination of the ECG in anesthetized patients with CPA is vital to determine the next course of CPR treatment. Experimental and clinical human studies reveal that interruptions of chest compression to assess the ECG be minimized and, if brief, do not affect overall outcome [31].

Another important reason to monitor the ECG during the initial phases of CPA is to determine whether intervention effectiveness (epinephrine administration, drug reversal, BLS commencement) is resulting in positive ECG rhythms (e.g., sinus rhythm or tachycardia). Once a more normal ECG rhythm is present, further cardiovascular monitoring such as blood pressure and perfusion parameters can commence.

Capnometry is especially useful in the immediate phases of CPR to detect ROSC and CPR effectiveness [9]. Exhalation of CO_2 requires lung perfusion and $ETCO_2$ is decreased during CPA [9]. An increase from initial $ETCO_2$ values during CPR indicates adequate perfusion during external chest compressions or ROSC. Intermittent interruptions of chest compressions will be required to observe whether or not an increased $ETCO_2$ is due to ROSC or due to external chest compressions. A steady decrease in $ETCO_2$ with constant ventilation during ALS or postcardiac arrest (PCA) care indicates impending CPA.

Postcardiac Arrest Care

Survival to discharge in veterinary patients undergoing CPA is 2–10% [32]. ROSC after application of effective ALS and BLS can occur in 35–45% of veterinary patients undergoing CPA, and, as previously discussed, survival rates of 47% have been reported in dogs and cats with CPA related to anesthesia [3]. The RECOVER initiative recognized that the discrepancy of survival rates to those that had ROSC likely occurs because of PCA syndrome, which is characterized by a combination of maladies including multiorgan failure, cardiogenic shock, anoxic brain injury, and the consequences of preexisting disease [29, 30]. Therefore, directed PCA care must be applied continuously to the specific needs of each patient. Many factors are addressed in the RECOVER initiative concerning PCA care including cardiovascular support, maintaining adequate oxygenation and ventilation, control of body temperature, neuroprotective strategies, treatment for traumatic brain injury, and advanced monitoring [10].

Cardiovascular support during PCA care is essential to a positive outcome. The approach to cardiovascular support for PCA care in human medicine is well supported; however, there is no veterinary evidence regarding the approach to cardiovascular support for PCA care. Specific optimal hemodynamic variables have not been defined in human or veterinary medicine for PCA care and have been extrapolated from recommendations in patients with sepsis [10]. Specific areas for discussion include fluid therapy and cardiovascular support with vasoactive drugs.

There are no studies that address whether fluid administration or withholding fluids after ROSC has positive or negative effects in veterinary patients with hypotension after ROSC [10]. The expectation is that patients undergoing elective sedative or anesthetic procedures will have normal blood volume and normal pulmonary function. Judicious use of fluids in a patient with normal volume is recommended, knowing that one of the cardiovascular effects of PCA is hypotension due to vasodilation [10]. Excess fluid therapy in the face of cardiovascular dysfunction could possibly result in fluid overload and pulmonary edema. The recommendation is to apply fluid therapy based on the criteria accepted by veterinary critical care specialists.

The use of cardioactive drugs or vasopressors was investigated in the RECOVER initiative, primarily on the side of human medicine, as there are no veterinary studies. Experimental CPR models investigating induction of hypertension with norepinephrine CRI (0.05–0.20 $\mu g\,kg^{-1}\,min^{-1}$) were the most promising with a target goal of mean arterial pressure (MAP) > 150 mmHg [33, 34]. Investigations showing the benefit of inotropes such as dopamine and dobutamine were lacking and do not have a place in PCA care.

An important goal immediately following ROSC in CPA is to rapidly establish normal ventilation, pH, and reoxygenation of tissues [10]. Arterial CO_2 controls cerebral vascular tone and directly regulates cerebral perfusion pressure. Hyperventilation causing hypocarbia and hypoventilation causing hypercarbia can both be potentially detrimental to cerebral perfusion and normocarbia should be maintained throughout PCA care. Alveolar oxygenation to maintain normal arterial oxygenation will help improve oxygen delivery. However, hyperoxemia can potentially be detrimental, as oxygen is a source reactive oxygen species, which could be harmful [35]. Supplementation with 100% oxygen or use of high-flow oxygen therapy (HFOT) is not routinely recommended for PCA care, though supplementation as needed to provide normal arterial oxygenation should be implemented.

Mild therapeutic hypothermia (MTH) is a common practice if a person is comatose after ROSC and results in higher survival rates [36]. Core body temperatures between 32 and 34 °C have been used in human medicine and in canine experimental studies. It is reasonable to allow mild hypothermia (33 °C) in dogs and cats for PCA care, though there is no specific method on how to induce MTH. The speed of rewarming was also investigated in several dog models to determine if slow rewarming compared to rapid warming provided any clinical benefit [37]. The RECOVER initiative recommendation is to rewarm no faster than 1 °C h^{-1} [10].

Several neuroprotective strategies used to improve outcomes during PCA care include corticosteroid administration, seizure prophylaxis, and various metabolic protectants. Corticosteroid use in PCA care showed no benefit in two large cohort studies in human medicine [38, 39]; the RECOVER initiative concludes that corticosteroids should not be administered as a part of PCA care.

Seizures have been reported to occur in 5–15% of people during the PCA care and in 40% of people who remain comatose after ROSC [37]. Seizure incidence during PCA care in dogs and cats is not known. Many antiseizure strategies have been investigated on adults and children including prophylactic thiopental, phenobarbital, phenytoin, and midazolam administration; the RECOVER initiative concluded that routine seizure prophylaxis is not warranted in dogs and cats.

Cerebral edema has been reported in people after CPA and correlates with a poor outcome [4, 40]. Treatment for cerebral edema could involve administration of mannitol or hypertonic saline (HS). Prophylactic treatment for presumed traumatic brain injury as a result of CPA with mannitol has been recommended in veterinary patients [4, 41]. One prospective, observational veterinary study reported an improved outcome when mannitol was administered during CPR, though the study was not designed to determine a causal relationship between mannitol administration and survival [3]. Mannitol and HS are reasonable treatments for cerebral edema once cerebral edema is detected by clinical parameters by advanced imaging techniques such as magnetic resonance imaging (MRI).

Several metabolic protectants have been studied with the thought of preserving cellular function after a period of hypoxia followed by reperfusion including alpha-phenyl-tert-butylnitrone (PBN), 21-aminosteroids, methylene blue, N-acetylcysteine, and superoxide dismutase. There have been no clinical veterinary studies addressing whether any of these protectants have benefits during PCA care

Table 23.3 Summary of recommendations for PCA care.

1) Judicious application of fluid therapy based on the needs of the patient, the fluid status prior to CPA, and the standards adopted by veterinary critical care
2) Maintain normoxemia and avoid hyperoxemia and hypoxemia
3) Mild hypothermia (33 °C) can be applied after prolonged CPA and rapid rewarming ($>1\,°C\,h^{-1}$) should be avoided
4) There is no evidence to support prophylactic administration of corticosteroids, mannitol, seizure prophylaxis, or metabolic protectants after CPR
5) Hypertonic saline administration could be considered in patients showing signs of cerebral edema or evidence of cerebral edema based on MRI
6) Comprehensive PCA care in a specialty center with access to more advanced monitoring, and more advanced support care may have a more positive outcome

compared to standard therapies; therefore, use is not recommended.

The final aspect of PCA care that was investigated in the RECOVER initiative was whether survival was increased in specialty centers versus nonspecialty facilities. Human studies suggest that survival is increased with centers that have more experience with PCA care and have higher caregiver-to-patient ratios [42–44]. Only one veterinary study vaguely addresses the topic of higher survival rates when there are more people involved in the resuscitation efforts [3]. It is reasonable to presume that a dog or cat that survives a CPA and attains ROSC should be transported to a 24-h facility for PCA care.

A summary of the current recommendations for PCA care outlined by the RECOVER initiative is found in Table 23.3. A 24-h facility with experience in CPA care and a board-certified or residency-trained doctor in veterinary emergency and critical care would be ideal to care for these patients. Regardless, application of the Rule of 20 (Table 23.4) for monitoring critical veterinary patients is reasonable to provide the best chance of survival to discharge.

Table 23.4 The Rule of 20 for care of critical veterinary patients.

1) Fluid balance
2) Oncotic pull and albumin level
3) Blood glucose
4) Electrolytes and acid–base balance
5) Oxygenation and ventilation
6) Neurologic status
7) Blood pressure
8) Heart rhythm, synchrony, and contractility
9) Core body temperature
10) Coagulation
11) Red blood cell parameters
12) Renal function
13) Immune status and ability to recognize infection
14) Gastrointestinal function
15) Drug dosages and metabolism
16) Nutrition
17) Analgesia
18) Nursing care
19) Wound care
20) Tender loving care

Clinical Application of the RECOVER Guidelines for Veterinary CPR

The final installation of the RECOVER initiative guidelines provides clinical application of the findings based on the five domains that were examined: (i) readiness and preparedness, (ii) BLS, (iii) ALS, (iv) monitoring, and (v) PCA care [11]. A clinical algorithm chart of BLS and ALS (Figure 23.10) has been developed and should be posted in an intensive care unit or primary treatment area. A second algorithm was developed as a guide for PCA care (Figure 23.11). A comprehensive chart of commonly used drugs with dosages and amounts to be administered based on body weight has been developed that should be posted in an appropriate area (Figure 23.12). Finally, a CPR document can be used during CPR to record events during a CPA (Figure 23.13). All charts can be purchased through the Veterinary Emergency & Critical Care Society (VECCS).

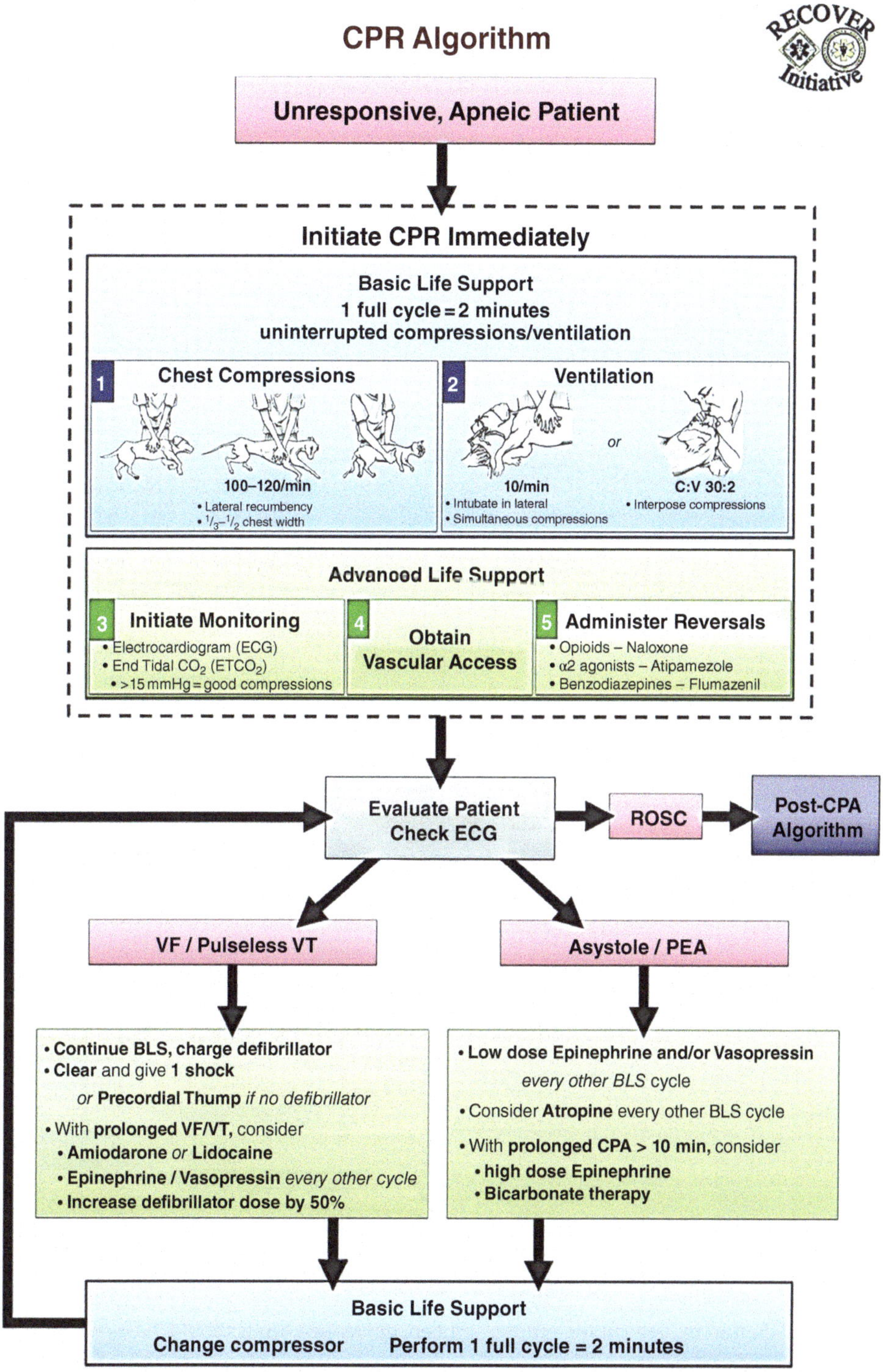

Figure 23.10 Clinical algorithm summary of BLS and ALS CPR. Source: Image from Fletcher et al. (2012) with permission.

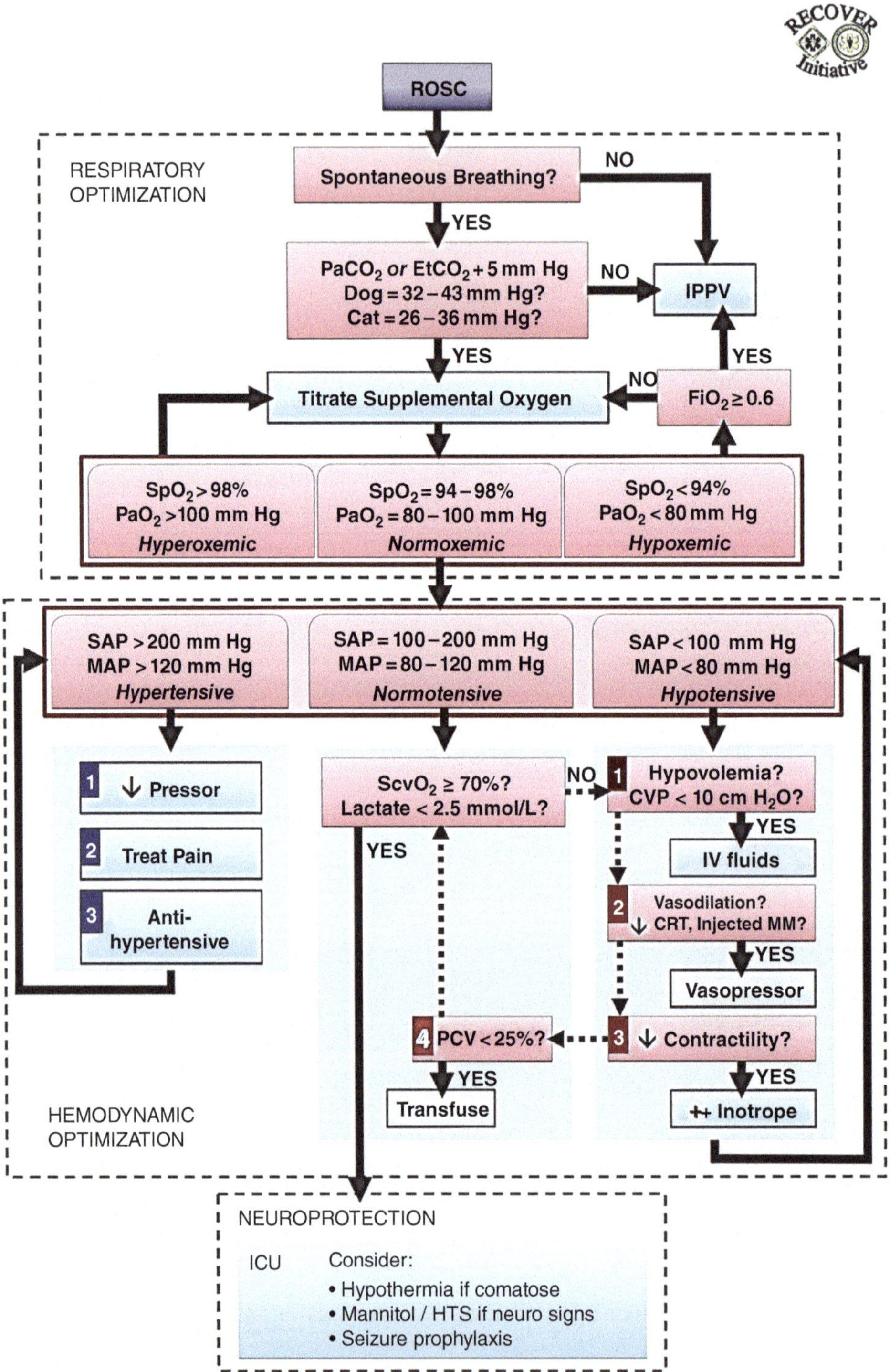

Figure 23.11 A guide for PCA care. Source: Image from Fletcher et al. (2012) with permission.

CPR Emergency Drugs and Does

RECOVER Initiative

		Weight (kg)	2.5	5	10	15	20	25	30	35	40	45	50
		Weight (lb)	5	10	20	30	40	50	60	70	80	90	100
	DRUG	DOSE	ml	ml	ml	ml	ml	ml	ml	ml	ml	ml	ml
Arrest	Epi High (1:1000; 1 mg/ml) every other BLS cycle x3	0.01 mg/kg	0.03	0.05	0.1	0.15	0.2	0.25	0.3	0.35	0.4	0.45	0.5
Arrest	Epi High (1:1000; 1 mg/ml) for prolonged CPR	0.1 mg/kg	0.25	0.5	1	1.5	2	2.5	3	3.5	4	4.5	5
Arrest	Vasopressin (20 U/ml)	0.8 U/kg	0.1	0.2	0.4	0.6	0.8	1	1.2	1.4	1.6	1.8	2
Arrest	Atropine (0.54 mg/ml)	0.04 mg/kg	0.2	0.4	0.8	1.1	1.5	1.9	2.2	2.6	3	3.3	3.7
Anti-Arrhyth	Amiodarone (50 mg/ml)	5 mg/kg	0.25	0.5	1	1.5	2	2.5	3	3.5	4	4.5	5
Anti-Arrhyth	Lidocaine (20 mg/ml)	2 mg/kg	0.25	0.5	1	1.5	2	2.5	3	3.5	4	4.5	5
Reversal	Naloxone (0.4 mg/ml)	0.04 mg/kg	0.25	0.5	1	1.5	2	2.5	3	3.5	4	4.5	5
Reversal	Flumazenil (0.1 mg/ml)	0.01 mg/kg	0.25	0.5	1	1.5	2	2.5	3	3.5	4	4.5	5
Reversal	Atipamezole (5 mg/ml)	100 Ug/kg	0.06	0.1	0.2	0.3	0.4	0.5	0.6	0.7	0.8	0.9	1
Defib Monophasic	External Defib (J)	4-6 J/kg	10	20	40	60	80	100	120	140	160	180	200
Defib Monophasic	Internal Defib (J)	0.5-1 J/kg	2	3	5	8	10	15	15	20	20	20	25

Figure 23.12 A guide for CPR drugs and defibrillation energy setting for CPR. Source: Image from Fletcher et al. (2012) with permission.

Standard Reporting of Small Animal Cardiopulmonary Resuscitation

RECOVER

Date: Time: | Patient:
Doctor: | Client Name:
Canine ☐ Feline ☐ Wt: | Sex: F ☐ M ☐ FS ☐ MN ☐
Chest Conformation: Round ☐ Keel ☐ Flat ☐ | Age: yrs mos Breed:

Time HR	MIN	
		Compressions started ☐ Not started because: DNR ☐ Futile ☐ Respiratory Arrest Only ☐
		Ventilation started ☐ ET Tube ☐ Size:_____ Breaths: Ambu bag ☐ Anesthetic circuit ☐ Mouth to Snout ☐
		Vascular Access ☐ IVC size:_____ Location:_____ Peripheral ☐ Jugular ☐ Central ☐ IO ☐
		CPR Stopped ☐ Reason: ROSC ☐ (Time:____) Unresponsive to ALS ☐ Owner Decision ☐ Clinician decision ☐

Time HR	MIN	Monitoring	mmHg	EPI mL	ATRO mL	VASO mL	mL	mL	Route IV/IT	DEFIB J	Open	Re-Arrest	Fluids Type/Rate/Dose
		PEA ☐ Asystole ☐ VF ☐ VT ☐ Brady ☐ ROSC ☐	CO2:								☐	☐	
		PEA ☐ Asystole ☐ VF ☐ VT ☐ Brady ☐ ROSC ☐	CO2:								☐	☐	
		PEA ☐ Asystole ☐ VF ☐ VT ☐ Brady ☐ ROSC ☐	CO2:								☐	☐	
		PEA ☐ Asystole ☐ VF ☐ VT ☐ Brady ☐ ROSC ☐	CO2:								☐	☐	
		PEA ☐ Asystole ☐ VF ☐ VT ☐ Brady ☐ ROSC ☐	CO2:								☐	☐	
		PEA ☐ Asystole ☐ VF ☐ VT ☐ Brady ☐ ROSC ☐	CO2:								☐	☐	
		PEA ☐ Asystole ☐ VF ☐ VT ☐ Brady ☐ ROSC ☐	CO2:								☐	☐	
		PEA ☐ Asystole ☐ VF ☐ VT ☐ Brady ☐ ROSC ☐	CO2:								☐	☐	

Time HR	MIN	Additional Notes (Drugs, lab tests, AFAST, TFAST)	Time HR	MIN	Additional Notes (Drugs, lab tests, AFAST, TFAST)

CPR Team	Drug Concentrations:	Add'l Conc.	Fluids Used:
Lead:	Epinephrine	____:	Crystalloid:
Recorder/Drugs:	Atropine	____:	Colloid:
Rotators (Airway/Vent, Compressions, Runner):	Vasopressin	____:	Blood Prod:
ROSC >20min Yes ☐ No ☐ Euthanized ☐	Dextrose	____:	____:

https://recoverinitiative.org Rev 2018.1 RECOVER Initiative ©2019

Figure 23.13 Example of a document that can be used to record events, drug administration, and defibrillation during a CPA. Source: Image from Fletcher et al. (2012) with permission.

STANDARD REPORTING OF VETERINARY SMALL ANIMAL CPR

Date of event ☐☐ ☐☐ ☐☐ (Day / Month / Year)

PERSONNEL INVOLVED

	1	2	3	4+
DVM	☐	☐	☐	☐
Technician	☐	☐	☐	☐
Students	☐	☐	☐	☐
Support Staff	☐	☐	☐	☐

Credentials (Circle one)

DACVECC/Other Specialists

LVT, CVT, RVT　VTS

VTS (ECC)

ADDITIONAL PATIENT INFORMATION

Admission Date ☐☐ ☐☐ ☐☐ (Day / Month / Year)

Disease Category at admission (all that apply)

- ☐ Medical cardiac/non-cardiac
- ☐ Surgical elective/non-elective
- ☐ Trauma
- ☐ DOA
- ☐ Unknown

Comorbid conditions (all that apply)

- ☐ Arrhythmia
- ☐ Congestive Heart Failure (prior admit)
- ☐ Congestive Heart Failure (this admit)
- ☐ Pericardial effusion/tamponade
- ☐ Hypotension/Hypoperfusion
- ☐ Respiratory insufficiency
- ☐ Pneumonia
- ☐ Renal insufficiency
- ☐ Hepatic insufficiency
- ☐ CNS disease
- ☐ SIRS
- ☐ Immune-mediated disease
- ☐ Sepsis
- ☐ Infectious disease
- ☐ Diabetes mellitus
- ☐ Metabolic/electrolyte disorder
- ☐ Malignancy
- ☐ Major trauma
- ☐ Envenomation
- ☐ Post-operative
- ☐ Coagulopathy
- ☐ Thromboembolic disease
- ☐ None
- ☐ Unknown

Location of CPA (select one)

- ☐ Out of hospital
- ☐ Emergency Room
- ☐ Intensive Care Unit
- ☐ Wards
- ☐ Anesthesia/Surgery
- ☐ Consult Room
- ☐ Diagnostic Procedures Area
- ☐ Waiting Room
- ☐ Other ________

CPR measures ALREADY in place at time of CPA (check all that apply)

Venous access	Y / N
Central Venous Catheter	Y / N
Tracheal intubation	Y / N
ECG monitoring	Y / N
Arterial catheterization	Y / N
Oxygen	Y / N
Mechanical ventilation	Y / N

ADDITIONAL ARREST INFORMATION

Suspected cause of CPA

- ☐ Life threatening arrhythmia
- ☐ Respiratory failure
- ☐ Heart failure
- ☐ Trauma
- ☐ Hemorrhage
- ☐ Hypovolemia (non-hemorrhagic/non-septic)
- ☐ Severe sepsis/Septic shock
- ☐ Brain disease
- ☐ MODS
- ☐ Metabolic/Electrolyte
- ☐ Toxicosis/Overdose
- ☐ Unknown

Mode of Death after ROSC >20 min.

- ☐ Euthanasia - decision based on → ☐ Severity of illness / ☐ Terminal illness / ☐ Economic reasons
- ☐ Re-arrest without CPR
- ☐ Re-arrest w/CPR, but w/out sustained ROSC

Previous CPA: Yes: 1 2 3 4 5+ No

Extubation: Y/N Time: ____ Date: ____

General Anesthesia at time of CPA

- ☐ Yes → ☐ Anesthetic induction / ☐ Anesthetic recovery / ☐ Procedural sedation
- ☐ No

Pre-arrest Severity of Illness　AppleFast Score ☐

Post-arrest Functional Capacity　Fletcher Score ☐

Number of hours post ☐

Hospital Discharge: Y / N Time: ____ Date: ____

In-hospital Death: Y / N Time: ____ Date: ____

Additional Outcome Information

Duration of sustained ROSC

- ☐ None
- ☐ >20 min.
- ☐ >24 hr.
- ☐ >30 days

Recorder: ____________________

Figure 23.13 (Continued)

Conclusion

The RECOVER initiative has revolutionized veterinary CPR to reveal specific needs for our veterinary patients based on an extensive review of the literature and comparison to human CPR. Adherence to these guidelines during CPR of sedated or anesthetized patients could possibly increase survival. Three examples of the application of the RECOVER initiative recommendations directly related to sedated or anesthetized patients can be found in the following text (see Appendices).

References

1 Brodbelt, D.C., Blissitt, K.J., Hammond, R.A. et al. (2008). The risk of death: the confidential enquiry into perioperative small animal fatalities. Vet. Anaesth. Analg. 35 (5): 365–373.

2 Fletcher, D.J. and Boller, M. (2013). Updates in cardiopulmonary resuscitation. *Vet. Clin. North Am. Small Anim. Pract.* 43 (4): 971–987.

3 Hofmeister, E.H., Brainard, B.M., Egger, C.M. et al. (2009). Prognostic indicators for dogs and cats with cardiopulmonary arrest treated by cardiopulmonary cerebral resuscitation at a university teaching hospital. *J. Am. Vet. Med. Assoc.* 235 (1): 50–57.

4 Cole, S.G., Otto, C.M., and Hughes, D. (2003). Cardiopulmonary cerebral resuscitation in small animals – a clinical practice review. Part II. *J. Vet. Emerg. Crit. Casre* 13: 13–23.

5 Boller, M. and Fletcher, D.J. (2012). RECOVER evidence and knowledge gap analysis on veterinary CPR. Part 1: evidence analysis and consensus process: collaborative path toward small animal CPR guidelines. *J. Vet. Emerg. Crit. Care* 22: S4–S12.

6 McMichael, M., Herring, J., Fletcher, D.J. et al. (2012). RECOVER evidence and knowledge gap analysis on veterinary CPR. Part 2: preparedness and prevention. *J. Vet. Emerg. Crit. Care (San Antonio)* 22: S13–S25.

7 Hopper, K., Epstein, S.E., Fletcher, D.J. et al. (2012). RECOVER evidence and knowledge gap analysis on veterinary CPR. Part 3: basic life support. *J. Vet. Emerg. Crit. Care* 22: S26–S43.

8 Rozanski, E.A., Rush, J.E., Buckley, G.J. et al. (2012). RECOVER evidence and knowledge gap analysis on veterinary CPR. Part 4: advanced life support. *J. Vet. Emerg. Crit. Care* 22: S44–S64.

9 Brainard, B.M., Boller, M., and Fletcher, D.J. (2012). RECOVER evidence and knowledge gap analysis on veterinary CPR. Part 5: monitoring. *J. Vet. Emerg. Crit. Care* 22: S65–S84.

10 Smarick, S.D., Haskins, S.C., Boller, M. et al. (2012). RECOVER evidence and knowledge gap analysis on veterinary CPR. Part 6: post-cardiac arrest care. *J. Vet. Emerg. Crit. Care* 22: S85–S101.

11 Fletcher, D.J., Boller, M., Brainard, B.M. et al. (2012). RECOVER evidence and knowledge gap analysis on veterinary CPR. Part 7: clinical guidelines. *J. Vet. Emerg. Crit. Care* 22: S102–S131.

12 Schade, J. (1983). An evaluation framework for code 99. *QRB Qual. Rev. Bull.* 9 (10): 306–309.

13 Andreatta, P., Saxton, E., Thompson, M. et al. (2011). Simulation-based mock codes significantly correlate with improved pediatric patient cardiopulmonary arrest survival rates. *Pediatr. Crit. Care Med.* 12 (1): 33–38.

14 Sasson, C., Rogers, M.A., Dahl, J. et al. (2010). Predictors of survival from out-of-hospital cardiac arrest: a systematic review and meta-analysis. *Circ. Cardiovasc. Qual. Outcomes* 3 (1): 63–81.

15 Rittenberger, J.C., Menegazzi, J.J., and Callaway, C.W. (2007). Association of delay

to first intervention with return of spontaneous circulation in a swine model of cardiac arrest. *Resuscitation* 73 (1): 154–160.

16 Haskins, S.C. (2015). Monitoring anesthetized patients. In: *Veterinary Anesthesia and Analgesia* The fifth edition of Lumb and Jones (eds. K.A. Grimm, L.A. Lamont, W.J. Tranquilli, et al.), 101. Ames: Wiley Blackwell.

17 Idris, A.H., Wenzel, V., Becker, L.B. et al. (1995). Does hypoxia or hypercarbia independently affect resuscitation from cardiac arrest? *Chest* 108 (2): 522–528.

18 Yeh, S.T., Cawley, R.J., Aune, S.E. et al. (2009). Oxygen requirement during cardiopulmonary resuscitation (CPR) to effect return of spontaneous circulation. *Resuscitation* 80 (8): 951–955.

19 Feneley, M.P., Maier, G.W., Gaynor, J.W. et al. (1987). Sequence of mitral valve motion and transmitral blood flow during manual cardiopulmonary resuscitation in dogs. *Circulation* 76 (2): 363–375.

20 Meyer, A., Nadkarni, V., Pollock, A. et al. (2010). Evaluation of the neonatal resuscitation program's recommended chest compression depth using computerized tomography imaging. *Resuscitation* 81 (5): 544–548.

21 Aufderheide, T.P., Pirrallo, R.G., Yannopoulos, D. et al. (2005). Incomplete chest wall decompression: a clinical evaluation of CPR performance by EMS personnel and assessment of alternative manual chest compression-decompression techniques. *Resuscitation* 64 (3): 353–362.

22 Ashton, A., McCluskey, A., Gwinnutt, C.L. et al. (2002). Effect of rescuer fatigue on performance of continuous external chest compressions over 3 min. *Resuscitation* 55 (2): 151–155.

23 Yoon, M.S., Han, J., Tse, W.W., and Rodgers, R. (1977). Effects of vagal stimulation, atropine and propranolol on fibrillation threshold of normal and ischemic ventricles. *Am. Heart J.* 93 (1): 60–65.

24 Brack, K.E., Coote, J.H., and Ng, G.A. (2011). Vagus nerve stimulation protects against ventricular fibrillation independent of muscarinic receptor activation. *Cardiovasc. Res.* 91 (3): 437–446.

25 Perondi, M.B.M., Reis, A.G., Paiva, E.F. et al. (2004). A comparison of high-dose and standard-dose epinephrine in children with cardiac arrest. *N. Engl. J. Med.* 350 (17): 1722–1730.

26 Leng, C.T., Paradis, N.A., Calkins, H. et al. (2000). Resuscitation after prolonged ventricular fibrillation with use of monophasic and biphasic waveform pulses for external defibrillation. *Circulation* 101 (25): 2968–2974.

27 Lee, S.-G., Moon, H.-S., and Hyun, C. (2008). The efficacy and safety of external biphasic defibrillation in toy breed dogs. *J. Vet. Emerg. Crit. Care* 18 (4): 362–369.

28 Weisfeldt, M.L. and Becker, L.B. (2002). Resuscitation after cardiac arrest. A 3-phase time-sensitive model. *J. Am. Med. Assoc.* 288 (23): 3035–3038.

29 Neumar, R.W., Nolan, J.P., Adrie, C. et al. (2008). Post-cardiac arrest syndrome: epidemiology, pathophysiology, treatment, and prognostication. A consensus statement from the International Liaison Committee on Resuscitation (American Heart Association, Australian and New Zealand Council on Resuscitation). *Circulation* 118 (23): 2452–2483.

30 Herlitz, J., Svensson, L., Engdahl, J. et al. (2008). Characteristics and outcome in out-of-hospital cardiac arrest when patients are found in a nonshockable rhythm. *Resuscitation* 76 (1): 31–36.

31 Steen, S., Liao, Q., Pierre, L. et al. (2003). The critical importance of minimal delay between chest compressions and subsequent defibrillation: a haemodynamic explanation. *Resuscitation* 58 (3): 249–258.

32 Kass, P.H. and Haskins, S.C. (1992). Survival following cardiopulmonary resuscitation in dogs and cats. *J. Vet. Emerg. Crit. Care* 2 (2): 57–65.

33 Sterz, F., Leonov, Y., Safar, P. et al. (1990). Hypertension with or without hemodilution after cardiac arrest in dogs. *Stroke* 21 (8): 1178–1184.

34 Safar, P., Stezoski, W., and Nemoto, E.M. (1976). Amelioration of brain damage after 12 minutes' cardiac arrest in dogs. *Arch. Neurol.* 33 (2): 91–95.

35 Neumar, R.W. (2011). Optimal oxygenation during and after cardiopulmonary resuscitation. *Curr. Opin. Crit. Care* 17 (3): 236–240.

36 The Hypothermia after Cardiac Arrest Study Group (2002). Mild therapeutic hypothermia to improve the neurologic outcome after cardiac arrest. *N. Engl. J. Med.* 346 (8): 549–556.

37 Wu, X., Drabek, T., Tisherman, S.A. et al. (2008). Emergency preservation and resuscitation with profound hypothermia, oxygen, and glucose allows reliable neurological recovery after 3 h of cardiac arrest from rapid exsanguination in dogs. *J. Cereb. Blood Flow Metab.* 28 (2): 302–311.

38 Jastremski, M., Sutton-Tyrrell, K., Vaagenes, P. et al. (1989). Glucocorticoid treatment does not improve neurological recovery following cardiac arrest. Brain Resuscitation Clinical Trial I Study Group. *J. Am. Med. Assoc.* 262 (24): 3427–3430.

39 Grafton, S.T. and Longstreth, W.T. (1988). Steroids after cardiac arrest: a retrospective study with concurrent, nonrandomized controls. *Neurology* 38 (8): 1315–1316.

40 Metter, R.B., Rittenberger, J.C., Guyette, F.X. et al. (2011). Association between a quantitative CT scan measure of brain edema and outcome after cardiac arrest. *Resuscitation* 82 (9): 1180–1185.

41 Boller, M., Kellett-Gregory, L., Shofer, F.S. et al. (2010). The clinical practice of CPCR in small animals: an internet-based survey. *J. Vet. Emerg. Crit. Care* 20 (6): 558–570.

42 Callaway, C.W., Schmicker, R., Kampmeyer, M. et al. (2010). Receiving hospital characteristics associated with survival after out-of-hospital cardiac arrest. *Resuscitation* 81 (5): 524–529.

43 Carr, B.G., Kahn, J.M., Merchant, R.M. et al. (2009). Inter-hospital variability in post-cardiac arrest mortality. *Resuscitation* 80 (1): 30–34.

44 Engdahl, J., Abrahamsson, P., Bång, A. et al. (2000). Is hospital care of major importance for outcome after out-of-hospital cardiac arrest? Experience acquired from patients with out-of-hospital cardiac arrest resuscitated by the same emergency medical service and admitted to one of two hospitals over a 16-year period in the municipality of Göteborg. *Resuscitation* 43 (3): 201–211.

CPR Recommendations in a Cat Sedated with Preanesthetic Medication Before an Elective Laceration Repair

Signalment and History

- A 2-year-old male domestic shorthair cat (7 kg) presents with a large laceration on the left rear limb.
- The cat is very fractious and a complete examination prior to sedation and anesthesia is not possible.
- Preanesthetic medication: ketamine 70 mg IM, dexmedetomidine 70 µg IM, midazolam 1.5 mg IM.
- The cat is placed in a holding cage.
- The cat is observed to be headfirst in the corner of the cage and is unresponsive.
- Initial physical examination reveals cyanotic mucous membranes, no palpable heartbeat, no efforts to breathe, and mydriatic pupils. A CPA is announced; the cat is taken to the area where the crash cart is located; and staff begins to bring monitoring equipment to the area.

CPR Efforts

- The cat is tracheally intubated with a large amount of secretions noted in the oropharynx and ventilation with an Ambu bag commences at 10 breaths min^{-1} for a 2-min cycle.
- Chest compressions begin at 120 beats min^{-1} for a 2-min cycle.
- An ECG is placed on the cat and atipamezole is administered IM.
- At the end of the 2-min BLS cycle, the ECG is noted to have a sinus bradycardia with a heart rate of 100 beats min^{-1}, the cat has pink mucous membranes and is starting to have some spontaneous breaths.
- $ETCO_2$ is 55 mmHg during spontaneous breathing and intermittent manual ventilation is continued to maintain the $ETCO_2$ between 35 and 40 mmHg.
- The atipamezole takes effect and the heart rate increases to 180 beats min^{-1}, spontaneous breathing results in a normal $ETCO_2$ and the cat recovers enough to be extubated.
- Over the next several hours of monitoring as the cat recovers from ketamine administration, he is observed to have normal behavior.

CPR Recommendations for a Dog During Anesthesia for an Elective Ovariohysterectomy

Signalment and History

- An 8-month-old female mixed-breed dog (20 kg) is presented for elective ovariohysterectomy.
- The dog is nervous, though allows a complete physical examination, which is unremarkable.
- Blood work is normal.
- Preanesthetic medication is with hydromorphone (4 mg) IM and acepromazine (0.5 mg) IM.
- Induction is with propofol with a total dose of 50 mg administered slowly IV.
- Maintenance is with isoflurane in oxygen and the dog is permitted to breathe spontaneously.
- Monitoring intraoperatively is with an ECG, Doppler blood pressure monitor, and capnometry.
- Sterile surgical preparation commences and there is a miscommunication regarding the isoflurane and oxygen setting where the oxygen flow rate remained at 3 l min^{-1} and the isoflurane setting remained at 3%.
- The only $ETCO_2$ reading that was recorded was 60 mmHg.
- The ECG shows a ventricular escape rhythm of 30 beats min^{-1}.
- The Doppler is no longer audible.
- There are no spontaneous breaths.
- A CPA is announced, and the crash cart is brought into the operating room.

CPR Efforts

- The dog is placed into lateral recumbency, as the rebreathing anesthetic tubes are removed from the endotracheal tube and ventilation commences with an Ambu bag at 10 breaths min^{-1}. The $ETCO_2$ reads at 10 mmHg with each breath.
- Chest compressions begin immediately and the $ETCO_2$ slowly begins to rise with each breath up to 20 mmHg.
- Hydromorphone is reversed by the administration of naloxone IV.
- The ECG continues to show ventricular escape complexes at a rate of 30 beats min^{-1} with no palpable pulse.
- Epinephrine (0.4 mg) is administered IV as BLS continues.
- The ECG converts to sinus tachycardia, but then progresses to VF. Chest compressions continue and the $ETCO_2$ increases to 20 mmHg.
- The defibrillator is brought into the operating room and set to 25 J of energy.
- Gel is placed on the external paddles, a paddle is placed on each side of the thorax, and

the energy is delivered. The resultant ECG is sinus tachycardia.

- A femoral pulse is palpated and the $ETCO_2$ continues to increase.
- The dog begins to breathe spontaneously and is transferred to the ICU for PCA care.

CPR Recommendations During an Abdominal Exploratory of a Dog with a Hemoperitoneum Secondary to a Ruptured Splenic Mass

History and Signalment

- A 10-year-old MN Golden Retriever (30 kg) presents on emergency for sudden collapse and abdominal distension.
- An AFAST ultrasound reveals peritoneal fluid and a splenic mass.
- Hemoperitoneum is diagnosed.
- Immediate anesthesia and surgery commences, as there is hypotension and tachycardia unresponsive to fluid therapy or administration of blood products.
- Preanesthetic medication is with midazolam (6 mg) IV and hydromorphone (3 mg) IV.
- Induction is with fentanyl (150 μg) IV.
- Anesthesia maintenance is with total intravenous anesthesia with CRI of fentanyl ($20\,\mu g\,kg^{-1}\,h^{-1}$) and CRI of midazolam ($1\,mg\,kg^{-1}\,h^{-1}$) while connected to the anesthesia machine providing 100% oxygen; ventilation is applied to maintain normal $ETCO_2$.
- Direct arterial blood pressure reveals mild hypotension with ECG monitoring revealing sinus tachycardia with occasional ventricular premature complexes (VPCs).
- Fluid therapy is with crystalloids ($5\,mL\,kg^{-1}\,h^{-1}$) and a whole blood transfusion.
- The spleen is successfully removed.
- The ECG begins to show more VPCs that progress to VT and VF.
- The $ETCO_2$ drops with each breath to 5 mmHg.
- A CPA is announced, and the crash cart is brought to the operating room (OR).

CPR Efforts

- The surgeon incises the diaphragm and begins internal cardiac massage with a result of the $ETCO_2$ increasing to 15 mmHg.
- The internal paddles are prepared and handed to the surgeon who places the paddles on each side of the heart.
- Energy is set to 25 J, appropriate communication occurs, and the defibrillator is discharged with successful conversion to VT.
- A lidocaine bolus is administered to convert VT to sinus tachycardia.
- The fentanyl and midazolam CRI are decreased, and intermittent spontaneous ventilation commences with $ETCO_2$ 55 mmHg.
- Intermittent ventilation is applied to maintain $ETCO_2$ 35–40 mmHg.
- Direct arterial pressure reveals mild hypotension.
- A CRI of norepinephrine is administered that results in mild hypertension toward the end of surgery.
- The dog is transferred to ICU for PCA care.

Index

Canine and Feline Anesthesia and Co-Existing Disease, Second Edition. Edited by Rebecca A. Johnson, Lindsey B. C. Snyder and Carrie A. Schroeder.

Companion website: www.wiley.com/go/johnson/canine

d

e

f

g

h

p

q

r